AF772857

# Atlas of Clinical Dermatology in Coloured Skin

This Atlas of Dermatology has a unique clinical orientation and lays emphasis on morphology. The disease entities are arranged according to the morphology of lesions, not etiologically. This arrangement of disease entities is more useful for both teaching and learning and serves as an important aid in making a diagnosis, as this approach is based on the way patients present themselves in out-patient departments. Key diagnostic clinical pointers too have been provided with images, which help one suspect the diagnosis and exclude clinical differentials. This Atlas would serve as a desk reference for residents and practitioners.

**Key Features**

- An atlas and text covering skin, mucosa, hair and nail diseases in skin of color
- Emphasis on key diagnostic clinical pointers
- 3000+ clinical images—multiple images of a disease to cover the clinical spectrum
- Dedicated section on Regional Dermatology and Skin changes in systemic diseases
- Clinician's desk reference for OPD practice

# Atlas of Clinical Dermatology in Coloured Skin

## A Morphological Approach

Edited by
PC Das and Piyush Kumar

CRC Press
Taylor & Francis Group
Boca Raton New York London

CRC Press is an imprint of the
Taylor & Francis Group, an **informa** business

First edition published 2023
by CRC Press
6000 Broken Sound Parkway NW, Suite 300, Boca Raton, FL 33487-2742
and by CRC Press
4 Park Square, Milton Park, Abingdon, Oxon, OX14 4RN

*CRC Press is an imprint of Taylor & Francis Group, LLC*



**Library of Congress Cataloging-in-Publication Data**

Names: Das, P. C. (Dermatologist), editor. | Kumar, Piyush, 1982- editor.
Title: Atlas of clinical dermatology in coloured skin : a morphological approach / edited by P C Das and Piyush Kumar.
Description: First edition. | Boca Raton : CRC Press, 2023. | Includes bibliographical references and index.
Identifiers: LCCN 2022033961 (print) | LCCN 2022033962 (ebook) | ISBN 9781138483682 (hardback) | ISBN 9781032399669 (paperback) | ISBN 9781351054225 (ebook)
Subjects: MESH: Skin Diseases--diagnosis | Skin Diseases--ethnicity | Skin Pigmentation | Skin Manifestations | Diagnosis, Differential | Atlas
Classification: LCC RL71 (print) | LCC RL71 (ebook) | NLM WR 17 | DDC 616.5--dc23/eng/20221128
LC record available at https://lccn.loc.gov/2022033961
LC ebook record available at https://lccn.loc.gov/2022033962

ISBN: 9781138483682 (hbk)
ISBN: 9781032399669 (pbk)
ISBN: 9781351054225 (ebk)

DOI: 10.1201/9781351054225

Typeset in Minion
by KnowledgeWorks Global Ltd.

Access the companion website: https://routledgetextbooks.com/textbooks/9781032399669/

Dedicated to my father, late Sri Surya Narayan Das, who had inherent scientific temperament, exceptional observational capacity and intent learning interest

– **PC Das**

Dedicated to my parents and teachers, who showed me the path of learning, and to my patients, who kept me walking on this path

– **Piyush Kumar**

# Contents

# Foreword by Debabrata Bandyopadhyay

During the past couple of decades, sweeping changes have occurred in all aspects of medicine. We have witnessed rapid expansion of knowledge about the molecular biology, genetics, and immunology of diseases, resulting in revolutionary transformation in the way diseases are diagnosed and managed. In this milieu of explosive change, the core competence in the specialty of dermatology has still remained largely dependent on the clinical aspects of the diseases.

It is a specialty that frequently allows the physician to make a correct diagnosis based solely on history and physical examination. The easy visibility and accessibility of the whole organ helps the clinician in this respect. This is the beauty, as well as the challenge, of the practice of this branch of medicine as there exists hundreds of named disease entities, and the clinician has to interpret a wide variety of clinical signs dependent on the morphology and distribution of the lesions to pinpoint a diagnosis.

It is with great pleasure that I welcome a new addition to dermatological literature that approaches the subject of clinical dermatology with the major emphasis on the morphologic and regional basis of differential diagnosis of the dermatoses. The coterie of mostly bright young dermatologists (many of whom I had the opportunity to teach and learn from) have done a superb job with their contributions, covering a wide spectrum of clinical topics, the arrangement of text reflecting the clinical orientation of the authors.

I have found the text to be a user-friendly, rapidly accessible source of information on dermatologic presentations and diseases. Therefore, the book will be helpful not only to dermatology residents and practicing dermatologists but also to physicians in other allied fields of medicine, particularly internal medicine, family medicine, pediatrics, and rheumatology.

**Debabrata Bandyopadhyay**
Former Professor & Head
Dept. of Dermatology, Venereology, & Leprosy
Medical College & Hospital, Kolkata

# Foreword by Eckart Haneke

Differential diagnosis in dermatology is often very challenging, sometimes not even possible without further laboratory investigations. Skin type may be a confounding factor – dark skin is difficult for practitioners used to fair-skinned patients as most skin lesions tend to be darkly pigmented or even black, whereas for those treating mainly skin of color everything appears to be strangely red. In addition, in Asia dark-complexioned people tend to live in a tropical climate and are more exposed to infections and infestations but more protected against the harmful, particularly carcinogenic action of the sun, of which they have more than plenty.

This atlas is comprised of five sections, with groups of skin signs and diseases. In fact, after a brief introduction to look at the skin to make a diagnosis, as the title promises, the atlas starts with hypo- and hyperpigmentations, which are very stigmatizing in dark skin. Even in seemingly black skin, hyperpigmentation is noted as profoundly embarrassing by the individual, and patchy hypopigmentation is extremely visible and may be a serious psychosocial burden, whereas smooth pale skin is what most people strive for.

The text continues with the classic efflorescences such as papules, nodules, plaques, tumors, blisters, pustules, and ulcers. Scaly and atrophic lesions, bleeding, erythema, telangiectasia, cysts, sinuses, and eschar complete this section.

Section 3 is devoted to regional dermatoses, ranging from the scalp to the sole of the foot. All regions that have so fundamentally different anatomical characteristics and diverse functions are covered so that each "regional specialist" will find their diagnoses well and critically discussed.

Skin, hair, and nail disorders in systemic disease follow. This will satisfy the needs of all those colleagues who are convinced that the skin is the mirror of the soul and the internal organs. Indeed, virtually no organ system or tissue of the body can be seen in isolation. It is well acknowledged that there are not only psychocutaneous but also cutaneopsychological disorders. Virtually nobody with an embarrassing or severe skin disease will not be psychologically stressed; and vice versa, psychological distress worsens or even precipitates a variety of skin diseases.

Finally, the miscellaneous chapters cover what is not yet discussed – age- and pregnancy-related dermatoses, drug reactions, physically induced skin lesions, and pediatric rashes with fever.

The 85 chapters in five sections will leave no gap. The illustrations will help to reach to the correct diagnosis, and the first three sections will facilitate the use of the atlas as they are related to signs easily recognized by any practitioner, thus allowing the practitioner to recognizing skin lesions and evaluate their importance.

I thank the editors and all authors for their tremendous work in the field of dermatology in colored skin, which represents in fact the majority of the world population.

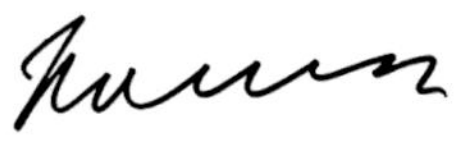

**Eckart Haneke**
Freiburg, Germany and Bern, Switzerland

# Preface

Why a new book? This was a question we too asked ourselves before starting work upon this book. The answer lies in the experience of teaching and interaction with many colleagues. Most of the textbooks and reference books follow an etiological approach (i.e., they describe viral skin conditions together), and thus, readers learn about varicella and common warts in the same chapter. This arrangement of entities does not help readers, especially the beginners, in developing their clinical acumen. Diagnostic skills depend on generating as well as excluding differentials for a given presentation based on morphology (and other details), and thus it is understandable that a book discussing dermatoses based on morphological similarities and differences will help readers improve their clinical skills. Hence, we decided to work upon an atlas of dermatology tailored to the interest and need of young clinicians and trainees.

The content of the book is divided into five sections. The first section of the atlas focuses on the basic vocabulary required to understand the language of dermatology. The different attributes of skin lesions have been elaborated with emphasis on its morphology, distribution, pattern, and arrangement. Section two is the backbone of the atlas as it incorporates the differential diagnosis of primary, secondary, and special skin lesions. As skin is not uniform all over and diseases tend to express differently over the body parts, a need for a separate section (three) on regional dermatology was felt. The subsequent fourth section is to emphasize and cover the link between skin manifestations and systemic (internal) diseases. The remaining unclassified but important topics, which could not be included in the preceding sections, have been incorporated in the concluding fifth section of miscellaneous topics (neonatal dermatoses, geriatric dermatoses, pregnancy-related dermatoses, cutaneous adverse drug reaction, and dermatoses with photosensitivity, etc.).

The introductory part of every chapter classifies various entities according to their salient clinical features (number/ color/ distribution/ presence or absence of systemic features, etc.). This clinical approach is followed by a brief description of the entities. In the description part, the entities appear as per the clinical classification referred above. This arrangement is in sync with the tone of "differential diagnosis," which is the purpose of this atlas. However, this would mean that the sequence of entities would bear relevance to morphology in priority rather than how common or rare they are. Obviously again, entities would have presence in more than one chapter, which is true to observe in this atlas. Each such repeated condition has been described in detail in one chapter, whereas at other places, it bears a brief mention only. In order to keep the atlas concise, very rare entities have been incorporated into tables and omitted from the discussion. Readers desirous of description of such entities would be advised to refer to comprehensive text books of the field.

The role of investigations and treatment protocols were not within the scope of this book, so they have been deliberately omitted. Only the salient clinical points and important differentials have been incorporated in the abridged description of disease entities.

A book covering these many aspects along with an enormous number of images would be a bulky textbook. To retain its handy shape and size, the publishers and editors converged upon a novel design of the book. The print and online versions of designated chapters in the same book have helped it achieve a suitable form and size. Of course, for convenience, the table of contents is common for online as well as print portions. Editors anticipate that this form of book will offer an advantage to its users.

Dermatology being primarily a visual science, clinching diagnosis fairly depends upon the mental image that one forms out of innumerable visual impressions absorbed during clinical training, fortified by sound theoretical learning and the knowledge of appropriate investigative methods. Adequate memory image development demands repetitive exposure to clinical cases and appreciation of minute variations in the presentation of lesions. Images in different forms such as print and digital supportive media further aid in acquiring visual skills. This atlas is enriched with numerous clinical images, depicting the spectrum of morphological changes in colored skin. We are sure the rich collection of images will appeal to every clinician dealing with dermatoses in colored skin.

This book is not intended to be an exhaustive text on dermatology but to help clinicians hone clinical skills. We hope that our book, titled *Atlas of Clinical Dermatology in the Skin of Color: A Morphological Approach*, serves its purpose and achieves popular acceptance amongst the trainees and practitioners of dermatology for whom it is intended and dedicated to.

Happy and fruitful learning!

*Education is not the learning of facts but the training of the mind to think.* – Albert Einstein

**PC Das**
**Piyush Kumar**
dermatatlas@gmail.com

# Acknowledgements


- All the patients who put trust in us and allowed us to use images for teaching purpose
- Past and present residents of Department of Dermatology, Katihar Medical College and Hospital, Katihar especially Dr. Sushil S Savant, Dr. Rizwana Barkat, Dr. Ghuncha Alam, Dr. Danish Akhtar, Dr. Talat Fatima, Dr. Priya Rajbansh, Dr. Mamta Yadav, Dr. Rashid Shahid, and Dr. Rashmi Roy
- Dr. Hiral Shah, Baroda Medical College, Vadodara for generously allowing us to borrow clinical images from her collection and for valuable inputs on various aspects of the book
- Dr. Devrashetti Srinivas, Nizamabad, India for generously allowing us to borrow clinical images from his collection
- Colleagues from "Urgent" group, where we discussed different topics for a better understanding
- Ms. Snehlata (Jha) and Mr. Harsh Narayan Jha for their invaluable help in arranging files for submission
- Ms. Shivangi, Ms. Himani, and others from CRC team for timely guidance, motivation, and cooperation throughout the project
- Many persons whose cooperation have been felt, but whom we have missed mentioning

**Editors**

- All the teachers and colleagues from the Department of Dermatology, Medical College and Hospital, Kolkata – my alma mater where I learned dermatology and where many clinical photographs used in this book were collected
- All the teachers and colleagues from the Department of Dermatology, Katihar Medical College and Hospital, Katihar where I learned and thought dermatology and where many clinical photographs used in this book were collected

**Piyush Kumar**

# Editors

**Dr. PC Das** is a senior practicing clinical dermatologist at Purnea and Katihar districts of Bihar, India. He has graduated and post-graduated from Patna Medical College, Patna University, India, in 2000. He has been practicing clinical dermatology, lasers, and dermatosurgery for over two decades. He has participated and presented papers in international, national, and regional dermatology conferences and organized some of them. His fields of special interest are newer drugs in leprosy and clinical dermatology.

**Dr. Piyush Kumar** finished his post-graduate work in dermatology from Medical College and Hospital, Kolkata in 2011 and was judged the best outgoing university medical graduate in dermatology. He received many scholarships during and after his post-graduate work to attend and present papers at national and international conferences. He has been teaching Dermatology residents for more than a decade and is currently working as Professor, Dermatology at Madhubani Medical College, Bihar, India. He has published more than 150 papers in indexed national and international journals and works as a reviewer for various national and international specialty journals. He has contributed many chapters in various books and has co-edited *Nail Disorders: A Comprehensive Approach, Clinical Cases in Disorders of Melanocytes,* and *Clinical Cases in Leprosy.* His areas of interest are clinical dermatology, dermatopathology, nail disorders, and genital dermatoses.

# Assistant editors


**Dr. Santoshdev Rathod, MD, DNB**
Professor & Head of Unit, Dermatology
SCL General Hospital, Smt. NHL Municipality Medical College
Ahmedabad, India

**Dr. Bhushan Madke, MD**
Professor & Head
Department of Dermatology, Venereology & Leprosy, Jawaharlal Nehru Medical College, Datta Meghe Institute Higher Education and Research
Wardha, India

**Dr. Shekhar Neema, MD, FEBDV**
Associate Professor
Department of Dermatology
Armed Forces Medical College
Pune, India

**Dr. Niharika Ranjan Lal, MD**
Assistant Professor
Dermatology ESIPGIMSR and ESIC Medical College
Joka, Kolkata, India

**Dr. Anup Kumar Tiwary, MD**
Consultant Dermatologist
Yashoda Hospital and Research Center
Ghaziabad, India

**Dr. Indrashis Podder, MD, DNB**
Assistant Professor
Department of Dermatology
College of Medicine and Sagore Dutta Hospital
Kolkata, India

**Dr. Dipali Rathod, DNB, DDVL, FIADVL (Dermatopathology)**
Assistant Professor, Dermatology
Seth GS Medical College and KEM Hospital
Mumbai, India

**Dr. Swetalina Pradhan, MD**
Associate Professor, Dermatology
All India Institute of Medical Sciences
Patna, India

**Dr. Somodyuti Chandra, MBBS (Hons), MD (Gold Medalist), DNB, MRCP-SCE (UK), FRGUHS**
Consultant Dermatologist
Kolkata, India

**Dr. Komal Agarwal, MBBS (Hons.) (Gold Medalist), MD (DVL), MRCP- SCE (UK)**
Senior Resident
Department of Dermatology
Calcutta National Medical College & Hospital
Kolkata, India

# Contributors

**Komal Agarwal**
Senior Resident, Dermatology
Calcutta National Medical College & Hospital
Kolkata, West Bengal, India

**Trupti Agarwal**
Consultant Dermatologist
Cloudnine Hospital
Mumbai, Maharashtra, India

**Danish Akhtar**
Senior Resident, Dermatology
Katihar Medical College and Hospital
Katihar, Bihar, India

**Amarkant Jha Amar**
Former Head of Unit, Dermatology
Patna Medical College and Hospital
Patna, Bihar, India

**Balachandar S Ankad**
Professor and Head
Department of Dermatology
S Nijalingappa Medical College
Bagalkot, Karnataka, India

**Amina Asfiya M I**
Senior Resident
Department of Dermatology
Yenepoya Medical College
Deralakatte, Mangalore, Karnataka, India

**Sasi Attili**
Consultant Dermatologist
Vizag, Andhra Pradesh, India

**Rizwana Barkat**
Senior Resident
Department of Dermatology, Venereology and Leprosy
Anugrah Narayan Magadh Medical College
Gaya, Bihar, India

**Kalgi Baxi**
Assistant Professor, Dermatology
Smt NHL Municipal Medical College
Ahmedabad, Gujrat, India

**Riti Bhatia**
Assistant Professor
Department of Dermatology and Venereology
All India Institute of Medical Sciences
Rishikesh, Uttarakhand, India

**Anirban Das**
RMO-cum-Clinical Tutor
Murshidabad Medical College & Hospital
Berhampore, West Bengal, India

**Anupam Das**
Assistant Professor, Dermatology
KPC Medical College and Hospital
Kolkata, West Bengal, India

**Nilay Kanti Das**
Professor and Head
Department of Dermatology
College of Medicine and Sagore Dutta Hospital
Kamarhati, Kolkata, India

**Gaurav Dash**
Assistant Professor
Department of Dermatology
SCB Medical College and Hospital
Cuttack, Odissa, India

**Chirag Desai**
Consultant Dermatologist
Mumbai, Maharashtra, India

**Talat Fatima**
Senior Resident, Dermatology
Nalanda Medical College and Hospital
Patna, Bihar, India

**Satyaki Ganguly**
Associate Professor, Dermatology
All India Institute of Medical Sciences
Raipur, Chhatisgarh, India

**Ramesh C Gharami**
Professor
Department of Dermatology
Medical College and Hospital
Kolkata, West Bengal, India

**Aparajita Ghosh**
Associate Professor, Dermatology
KPC Medical College and Hospital
Kolkata, West Bengal, India

**Vishal Golay**
Consultant Nephrologist
Remedy Clinic
Siliguri, West Bengal, India

**Ankan Gupta**
Associate Professor
Department of Dermatology
Christian Medical College
Vellore, Tamilnadu, India

**Sunil Kumar Gupta**
Dermatology
All India Institute of Medical Sciences
Gorakhpur, Uttar Pradesh, India

**Vishal Gupta**
Assistant Professor
Department of Dermatology and Venereology
All India Institute of Medical Sciences
New Delhi, India

**Navya Handa**
Consultant Dermatologist
New Delhi, India

**Shahid Hassan**
Professor, Dermatology
Madhubani Medical College and Hospital
Madhubani, Bihar, India

**Ravi Hiremagalore**
Consultant Dermatologist
Bangalore, Karnataka, India

**Sourabh Jain**
Assistant Professor
Dermatology
Atal Bihari Vajpayee Government Medical College
Vidisha, Madhya Pradesh, India

**Swetha Jain**
Consultant Dermatologist
Mumbai, Maharashtra, India

**Abhishek Jha**
Associate Professor, Dermatology
Patna Medical College and Hospital
Patna, Bihar, India

**Prerna**
Senior Resident
Dermatology Government Medical College and Hospital
Purnea, Bihar, India

**Bhumesh Kumar Katakam**
Assistant Professor, Dermatology
Gandhi Medical College/Hospital
Hyderabad, Telangana, India

**Manish Khandare**
Head of Department, Dermatology
Indian Naval Hospital Ship (INHS) Sanjivani
Kochi, Kerala, India

**Meenaz Khoja**
Consultant Dermatologist
Pune, Maharastra, India

**Sri Harsha Kolla**
Assistant professor, Dermatology
Mamata Academy of Medical Sciences
Bachupally, Telangana, India

**Sunil Kothiwala**
Consultant Dermatologist
Jaipur, Rajsthan, India

**Ch Venkata Krishna**
Consultant Dermatologist
Kiranya Anjana Skin and Hair Clinic
Nalgonda, Telangana, India

**Dhiraj Kumar**
Consultant Dermatologist
Patna, Bihar, India

**Ghaliyah Aziz Kutty**
Consultant Pediatrician
Mathery Medical Mission Hospital
Alappuzha, Kerala, India

**Niharika Ranjan Lal**
Assistant Professor, Dermatology
ESIPGIMSR and ESIC Medical College
Joka, Kolkata, West Bengal, India

**Rajesh Kumar Mandal**
Associate Professor, Dermatology
North Bengal Medical College and Hospital
Sushrutanagar, Siliguri, West Bengal, India

**Madhulika Mhatre**
Director, Skin Saga Centre for Dermatology
Mumbai, India

**Avijit Mondal**
Assistant Professor, Dermatology
College of Medicine and JNM Hospital
Kalyani, West Bengal, India

**Sabha Mushtaq**
Lecturer
Department of Dermatology, Venereology and Leprology
Government Medical College, Jammu
Jammu and Kashmir, India

**Shekhar Neema**
Associate Professor
Department of Dermatology
Armed Forces Medical College
Pune, Maharashtra, India

**Balakrishna Nikam**
Assistant Professor, Dermatology
Krishna Institute of Medical Sciences
Karad, Maharashtra, India

**Pooja Nupur**
Assistant Professor, Dermatology
Nalanda Medical College and Hospital
Patna, Bihar, India

**Saumya Panda**
Consultant Dermatologist
Belle Vue Clinic
Kolkata, West Bengal, India

**Col. Vikas Pathania**
Commanding Officer
180 Military Hospital
Missamari, Assam, India

**Swetalina Pradhan**
Associate Professor, Dermatology
All India Institute of Medical Sciences
Patna, Bihar, India

**Sai Prasanth Neti**
Consultant Dermatologist
G. K. Polyclinic
Hyderabad, Telangana, India

**Anuradha Priyadarshini**
Assistant Professor
Department of Dermatology
Sri Ramachandra Medical College
Chennai, Tamilnadu, India

**Priya Rajbansh**
Senior Resident, Dermatology
Katihar Medical College and Hospital
Katihar, Bihar, India

**Dipali Rathod**
Assistant Professor, Dermatology
Seth GS Medical College and KEM Hospital
Mumbai, India

**Santoshdev P Rathod**
Professor & Head of Unit, Dermatology
SCL General Hospital, Smt. NHL Municipality Medical College
Ahmedabad, Gujrat, India

**Arpita Nibedita Rout**
Assistant Professor
Department of Dermatology and Venereology
All India Institute of Medical Sciences
Bhubaneswar, Odissa, India

**Rashmi Roy**
Senior Resident, Dermatology
Lord Buddha Koshi Medical College & Hospital
Saharsa, Bihar, India

**Dilip Kumar SA**
Professor
Department of Dermatology
LSLAM Government Medical College
Raigarh, Chhattisgarh, India

**Divya Sachdev**
Consultant Dermatologist
Raipur, Chhatisgarh, India

**Abanti Saha**
Associate Professor, Dermatology
Medical College and Hospital
Kolkata, West Bengal, India

**Kananbala Sahu**
Assistant professor, Dermatology
Sri Jagannath Medical College and Hospital
Puri, Odissa, India

**(Sqn Ldr) Sunmeet Sandhu**
Assistant Professor, Dermatology
7 Air Force Hospital
Kanpur, Uttar Pradesh, India

**Satish S Savant**
Director, The Humanitarian Clinic: Skin, Hair and Laser Centre
Dr. Savant's Institute of Dermatosurgery, Cosmetology, Trichology and Laser Medicine
Mumbai, Maharashtra, India

**Sushil S. Savant**
Assistant Director, The Humanitarian Clinic: Skin, Hair and Laser Centre
Dr. Savant's Institute of Dermatosurgery, Cosmetology, Trichology and Laser Medicine
Mumbai, Maharashtra, India

**Rashid Shahid**
Senior Resident, Dermatology
All India Institute of Medical Sciences
Patna, Bihar, India

**Aseem Sharma**
Chief Dermatologist
Skin Saga Centre for Dermatology
Mumbai, India

**Preeti Sharma**
Consultant Dermatologist
Chandigarh, Punjab, India

**Rampal Sharma**
Former Head of Unit, Dermatology
LRM Government Medical College
Meerut, Uttar Pradesh, India

**Shivani Sharma**
Specialist Medical Officer, Dermatology District Hospital
Mathura, Uttar Pradesh, India

**Manjunath M. Shenoy**
Professor & Head of Unit
Department of Dermatology
Yenepoya Medical College
Deralakatte, Mangalore, Karnataka, India

**B Shiny Shulamite**
Consultant Dermatologist
Capstone Clinic
Hyderabad, Telangana, India

**Amrita Sil**
Associate Professor
Department of Pharmacology
Rampurhat Government Medical College
Rampurhat, West Bengal, India

**Gautam Kumar Singh**
Professor & Classified Specialist, Dermatology
Base Hospital
Delhi, India

**Sudhir Singh**
Associate Professor
Department of Dermatology
Datta Meghe Medical College
Nagpur, Maharashtra, India

**Anwita Sinha**
Assistant Professor, Dermatology
Base Hospital
Barrackpore, India

**Preema Sinha**
Professor & Head of Unit
Department of Dermatology
Base Hospital
Lucknow, Uttar Pradesh, India

**Chandra Sekhar Sirka**
Additional Professor
Department of Dermatology and Venereology
All India Institute of Medical Sciences
Bhubaneswar, Odissa, India

**Dependra Kumar Timshina**
Consultant Dermatologist
Remedy Clinic
Siliguri, West Bengal, India

**Anup Kumar Tiwary**
Consultant Dermatologist
Yashoda Hospital and Research Centre
Ghaziabad, Uttar Pradesh, India

**Kanya Rani Vashisht**
Consultant Dermatologist
Panchkula, Haryana, India

**Resham Vasani**
Consultant Dermatologist
Bhojani Clinic
Matunga, Mumbai, Maharashtra, India
Research Associate
B J Wadia Hospital for Children
Parel, Mumbai, Maharashtra, India

**Vignasree A**
Consultant Dermatologist
Hyderabad, Telangana, India

**Mamta Yadav**
Senior Resident, Dermatology
Maharshi Devrahawa Baba Autonomous State (MDBAS) Medical College
Deoria, Uttar Pradesh, India

# SECTION 1

# Introduction to clinical dermatology

DOI: 10.1201/9781351054225-1

E1

# Overview of skin lesions

CHANDRA SEKHAR SIRKA, SWETALINA PRADHAN, KANANBALA SAHU,
ARPITA NIBEDITA ROUT

## ABSTRACT

Description of the skin lesions is necessary to reach a clinical diagnosis. A good description of primary, secondary and foot print of the lesions can help in diagnosis. This chapter discusses various skin lesions, arrangements and distributions necessary for a good dermatological description of lesions.

The text of this chapter is available online at https://routledgetextbooks.com/textbooks/9781032399669/



DOI: 10.1201/9781351054225-2

# SECTION 2

# Approach to clinical diagnosis

PIYUSH KUMAR, PC DAS

Dermatology is a visual speciality, and diagnosing a dermatological disease is different from making a clinical diagnosis in other specialities. While some skin diseases can be diagnosed by a mere glance (such as acne vulgaris, fixed drug eruption, herpes zoster, etc.), the diagnosis of most dermatoses requires careful consideration of clues gathered from history and clinical examination. In dermatology, the diagnostic process usually involves these five steps:

1. **Brief history** – Ascertain onset, duration, symptoms, etc. Determine whether a condition is congenital or acquired, acute or chronic, symptomatic or asymptomatic, etc.
2. **Quick mucocutaneous examination** – The purpose is to document the morphology (primary, secondary, special), distribution, and arrangement of the lesions. It helps us to arrive at a provisional diagnosis or to generate a list of differential diagnosis.
3. **Detailed history** – A good history in dermatology aims at collecting positive and negative pointers for the conditions included in the list of differential diagnosis generated in the second step.
4. **Thorough examination** – This involves dermatological and systemic examination to document findings, to elicit supportive clinical signs, if any, and to assess the extent and severity of involvement of skin and other systems.
5. **Investigation and diagnosis** – A confirmatory test is done to establish the diagnosis and exclude differentials that could not be excluded clinically.

In our opinion, clinical diagnostic skills in dermatology rest on generating a list of differential diagnosis and narrowing the list clinically as far as possible. Though many dermatologists prefer to take history before clinical examination of lesions, we prefer to do a quick clinical examination first to get a list of differential diagnosis as it helps us in getting a meaningful and clinically useful history. This quick mucocutaneous examination rests on documentation and analysis of the following (acronym-**MADE**):

- **Morphology** – Identify primary and special lesions, secondary changes (if any), and the number, color, and shape of lesions.
- **Arrangement** (configuration) – The lesions in many dermatoses assume a characteristic distribution, and sometimes configuration alone is diagnostic. For example, grouped vesicles on an erythematous base, arranged in a dermatomal pattern, are diagnostic of herpes zoster and zosteriform herpes simplex.
- **Distribution** – Skin and mucosa have limited ways of expressing themselves (as primary and secondary lesions), and a variety of etiologically different conditions may present in a similar manner. The differential distribution of these etiologically different conditions allows clinical diagnosis of many conditions. For example, eczematous changes over convex parts of face and other photo-exposed areas suggest the diagnosis of photoallergic contact dermatitis, while similar changes localized to lower legs may be seen in stasis dermatitis.

DOI: 10.1201/9781351054225-3

- **Evolution** – Evolution refers to changes in the lesions over time. For example, the initial papule of lupus vulgaris expands over time to form a plaque and then further extends by central scarring. Among blistering disorders, bulla in subepidermal blistering disorders may heal with scarring and milia formation, while intraepidermal bullae heal with pigmentary changes only. Hence, it is evident that it is very important to note evolution of lesions to arrive at a diagnosis.

The main aim of this book is to help readers generate clinical differentials. The subsequent chapters will discuss some common and uncommon differential diagnosis for a given presentation.

# 1

# Hypopigmented and depigmented macules and patches: Localized

PC DAS, PRIYA RAJBANSH

## INTRODUCTION

Pigmentary changes constitute a major proportion of the patients consulting a dermatologist or general physician. In skin of color, hypo/depigmented macules and patches are more evident. Etiologically, pigmentary loss can be due to apoptosis of melanoblasts during differentiation (piebaldism), reduced melanogenesis (seen in pityriasis versicolor and steroid-induced hypopigmentation), autoimmune destruction (vitiligo), impaired dendritic transfer of melanosomes to keratinocytes (pityriasis alba), post-inflammatory (as seen in incontinentia pigmenti, lichen striatus, or annular lichenoides dermatitis of youth), or due to extreme local cutaneous vasoconstriction (nevus anemicus and Bier spots).

While approaching a patient presenting with localized hypo/depigmented disorders, one should first observe if the lesions are hypopigmented (reduced pigmentation) or depigmented (complete loss of pigmentation). There are only a few clinical differentials for localized depigmented patches, and hence this observation can be very useful in narrowing the list of differentials. Other than that, size, shape, and distribution of lesions are important clinical clues. There can be various morphologies of hypo/depigmented macules, such as guttate in idiopathic guttate hypomelanosis; confetti-like and petaloid in pityriasis versicolor; leaf-shaped in phylloid hypomelanosis; and ash-leaf macules of tuberous sclerosis – linear, large, and irregular. Additionally, a lesion can be scaly, surrounded by erythematous or hyperpigmented border, or associated with skin sclerosis or atrophy as seen in morphea. Decreased or loss of sensation in the lesion(s) favors Hansen's disease, warranting further investigation. Distribution of such hypopigmented macules is another important clue to arrive at a diagnosis or rule out differentials. Some diseases may present with only localized hypopigmentation, such as hypomelanosis of Ito, nevus depigmentosus, or piebaldism.

Therefore, detailed history regarding evolution of the lesions, careful examination of hypopigmented macules and their distribution, followed by all possible and needful investigations are always required to avoid misdiagnosis. Some clinical clues to the diagnosis of localized hypopigmented macules and patches have been summarized in **Tables 1.1** and **1.2**. Further, common dermatologic conditions have been discussed individually. [1-12]

### Pityriasis alba

- This is a common self-limiting, idiopathic condition affecting children and adolescents. It presents as ill-defined, faintly erythematous, or hypopigmented macules and patches of 1–4 cm in size with fine scaling. The number usually ranges from 4 or 5 to 20 or more.[1]
- The lesions are asymptomatic or mildly itchy.
- The face (cheeks in most cases) is the most commonly affected site (**Figure 1.1**). Upper arms, neck, or shoulders (and rarely trunk or lower extremities) may also be affected in generalized disease.
- History of atopy may be present.
- Uncommon variants are the pigmenting type (central hyperpigmented zone with hypopigmented, slightly scaly halo) and generalized type.
- Differential diagnosis (DD): Post inflammatory hypopigmentation (history of prior dermatoses), seborrheic dermatitis (affects seborrheic area), and early vitiligo (no scales).

### Nevus depigmentosus (nevus achromicus)

- It is a congenital pigmentary mosaic condition due to altered clones of melanocytes that have a decreased ability to synthesize melanin and transport it to keratinocytes.
- It usually presents at birth or in early childhood.[2]
- It presents as a solitary, asymptomatic, hypopigmented macule/patch with a well-defined serrated margin that does not cross the midline. Very often smaller macules appear around the lesion, giving it a "splashed

DOI: 10.1201/9781351054225-4

Table 1.1 Clinical clues to localized hypo/depigmented macules

| | Solitary/Few macules | Guttate macules | Variable sized macules | Linear/segmental hypopigmentation |
|---|---|---|---|---|
| Early childhood | • Nevus depigmentosus<br>• Nevus anemicus<br>• Piebaldism [D] (and Waardenburg syndrome) | • Confetti-like macules [D] in tuberous sclerosis and multiple endocrine neoplasia type 1 | • Ash-leaf macule in tuberous sclerosis<br>• Phylloid hypomelanosis | • Hypomelanosis of Ito<br>• Incontinentia pigmenti *** |
| Late childhood | • Pityriasis alba<br>• Focal vitiligo [D] | • Eruptive hypomelanosis<br>• Pityriasis lichenoides chronica<br>• Vitiligo punctata [D] | • Vitiligo vulgaris [D] | • Lichen striatus †<br>• Segmental vitiligo [D] |
| Adults | • Focal vitiligo [D]<br>• Chemical leukoderma [D]<br>• Melanoma associated leukoderma<br>• Indeterminate leprosy<br>• Tuberculoid leprosy<br>• Borderline tuberculoid leprosy<br>• Morphea<br>• Annular lichenoides dermatitis of youth (ALDY)<br>• Post-inflammatory hypopigmentation<br>• Halo nevus [D] and phenomenon<br>• Woronoff's ring | • Vitiligo punctata [D]<br>• Post-inflammatory hypopigmentation<br>• Pityriasis versicolor<br>• Idiopathic guttate hypomelanosis [D]<br>• Leukoderma punctata [D]<br>• Physiologic anemic macules (Bier spots)<br>• Lichen sclerosus et atrophicus *<br>• Tumor of follicular infundibulum ** | • Vitiligo vulgaris [D]<br>• Post-inflammatory hypopigmentation<br>• Progressive macular hypomelanosis<br>• Lepromatous leprosy<br>• Macular post kala-azar dermal leishmaniasis | • Corticosteroid-induced hypopigmentation |

*Notes:*

*It is actually an indurated plaque. It has been included here in the table for clinical similarity of vitiligo.

**The lesions in tumors of follicular infundibulum are actually tiny papules that may be misinterpreted as macules if the observer is not careful

***Atrophy is associated; hence, lesion is not macule/patch.

†The primary lesions are tiny papules. The lesions heal with post-inflammatory hypopigmentation, which may be only clinical findings observed in cases presenting late.

[D] Depigmented patches

paint" appearance (**Figure 1.2a,b**). In contrast to nevus anemicus, the lesional skin shows erythema on rubbing (**Figure 1.2c**).

- The common sites involved are trunk and proximal extremities.
- The lesion grows in size with the growth of the body and becomes stable thereafter.

Table 1.2 Approach to depigmented macules and patches

| Onset | Features | Diseases |
|---|---|---|
| Congenital/ childhood onset | Non-progressive (shows proportionate growth as child grows) | • Associated with hyperpigmented macules – piebaldism<br>• Segmental vitiligo |
| Acquired | Randomly distributed, progressive | Vitiligo and its clinical variants |
| | History of injury | Leukoderma |
| | Older population, lesion does not grow much in size | Idiopathic guttate hypomelanosis |

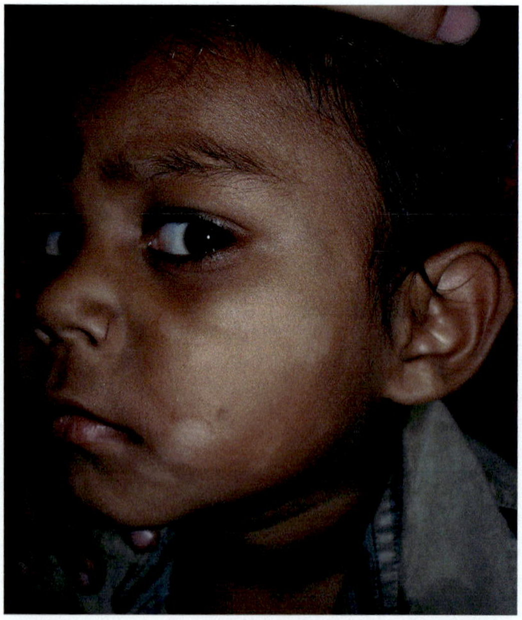

Figure 1.1 Pityriasis alba presenting as Ill-defined hypopigmented mildly scaly macules on cheeks in a child. (Courtesy: Dr. Piyush Kumar, Katihar, India.)

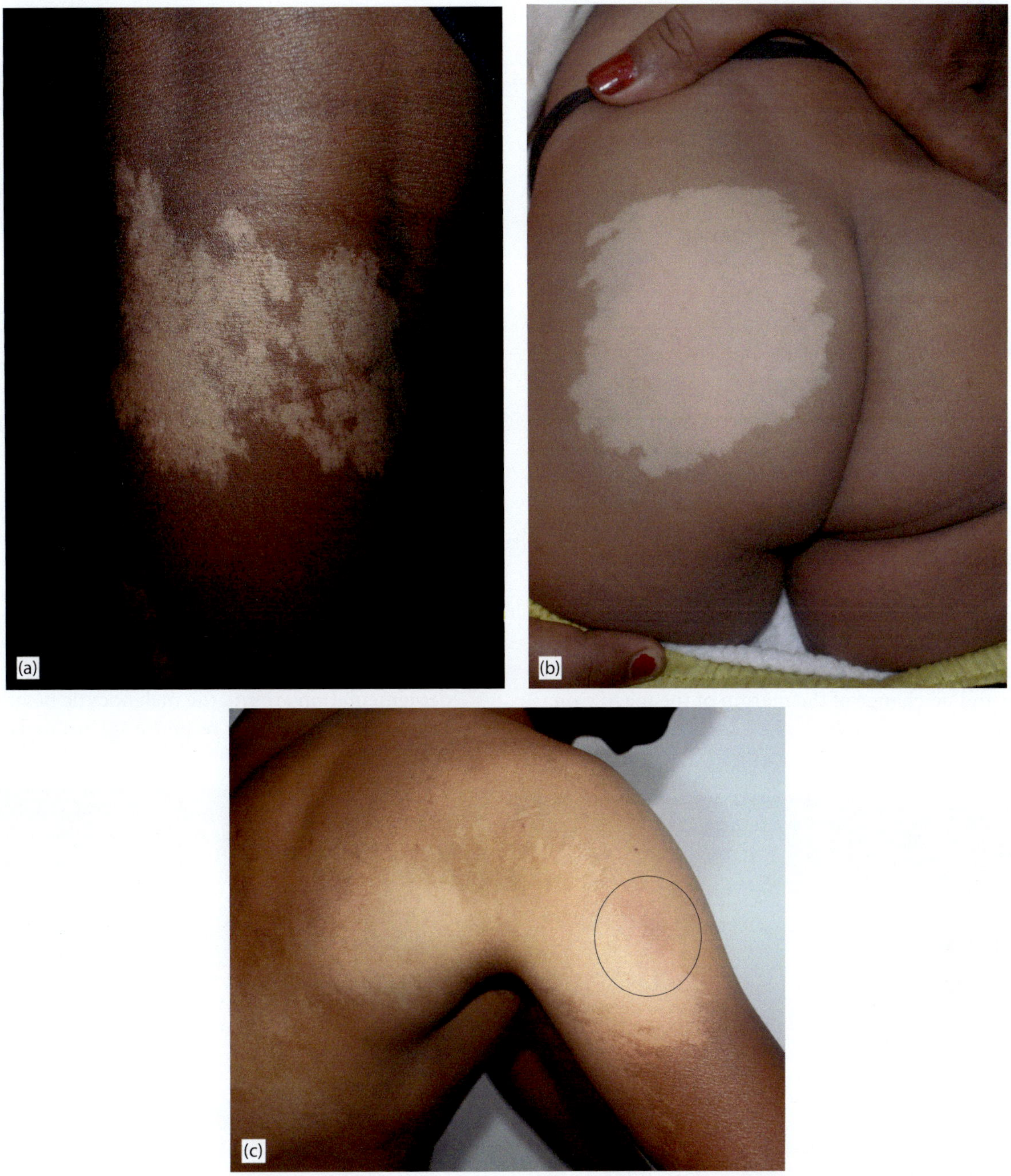


Figure 1.2 **(a)** Nevus depigmentosus with typical splash paint border on the posterior aspect of leg. **(b)** Nevus depigmentosus on the buttock. **(c)** The lesional skin (circled) as well as surrounding skin shows erythema on rubbing. (a–c – Courtesy: Dr. Piyush Kumar, Katihar, India.)

- Three clinical patterns have been observed – localized, segmental, and linear or whorled.
- The linear, or whorled, type can be extensive in distribution and associated with extra-cutaneous findings like seizures, mental retardation, hemihypertrophy, and yellow hair. It has considerable overlap with hypomelanosis of Ito, and hence its existence as a separate entity is debatable.
- Wood's lamp examination demonstrates an off-white color.
- DD: Nevus anemicus (the margin disappears on diascopy), vitiligo (chalky-white color on Wood's lamp).

## Nevus anemicus

- It is a congenital anomaly characterized by localized hypersensitivity of blood vessels to catecholamines, resulting in vasoconstriction. It may present at birth or become noticeable in early childhood and persists unchanged throughout life.
- It presents as single or a few asymptomatic, circumscribed, rounded, oval, or linear pale macules or patches with irregular margins that may be surrounded by satellite macules.[3]
- The lesion does not show erythema on rubbing, while the surrounding skin does (**Figure 1.3**).

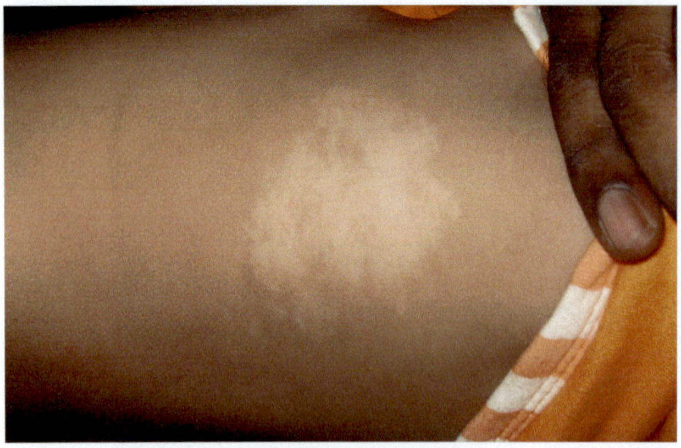

Figure 1.3 Nevus anemicus with hypopigmented patch with irregular, ill-defined margin. (Courtesy: Dr. Piyush Kumar, Katihar, India.)

- It is most commonly noted on the chest, although it can be found anywhere on the body.
- The margin becomes less prominent on diascopy.
- It is rarely associated with neurofibromatosis, tuberous sclerosis, or phakomatosis pigmentovascularis.
- DD: Nevus depigmentosus (which can be differentiated from nevus anemicus by appearance of erythema on rubbing and no change of the margin of the macule on diascopy).

## Piebaldism

- Piebaldism is an autosomal dominant disorder characterized by localized absence of melanocytes due to mutations in the c-kit proto-oncogene. The skin and hair changes are present from birth and do not progress. The characteristic feature is a midline triangular or diamond-shaped, depigmented patch with poliosis.[4]
- Hyperpigmented macules or islands of pigmentation within the patch and at its border provide an important clinical clue for diagnosis.
- The frontal area is the most commonly affected site (white forelock). The face (particularly the chin), trunk, and mid-extremities (sparing hands and feet) are other commonly affected areas (**Figure 1.4a–c**).
- It could present as an isolated anomaly or as a part of Waardenburg syndrome, along with heterochromia of the irides, lateral displacement of inner canthi, and deafness (**Figure 1.4d**).
- DD: Vitiligo.

## Halo nevus

- Synonyms are Sutton's nevus and leukoderma acquisitum centrifugum.
- It refers to melanocytic nevus with a zone of depigmentation around the melanocytic nevus due to immune-inflammatory response against melanocytes.[5]

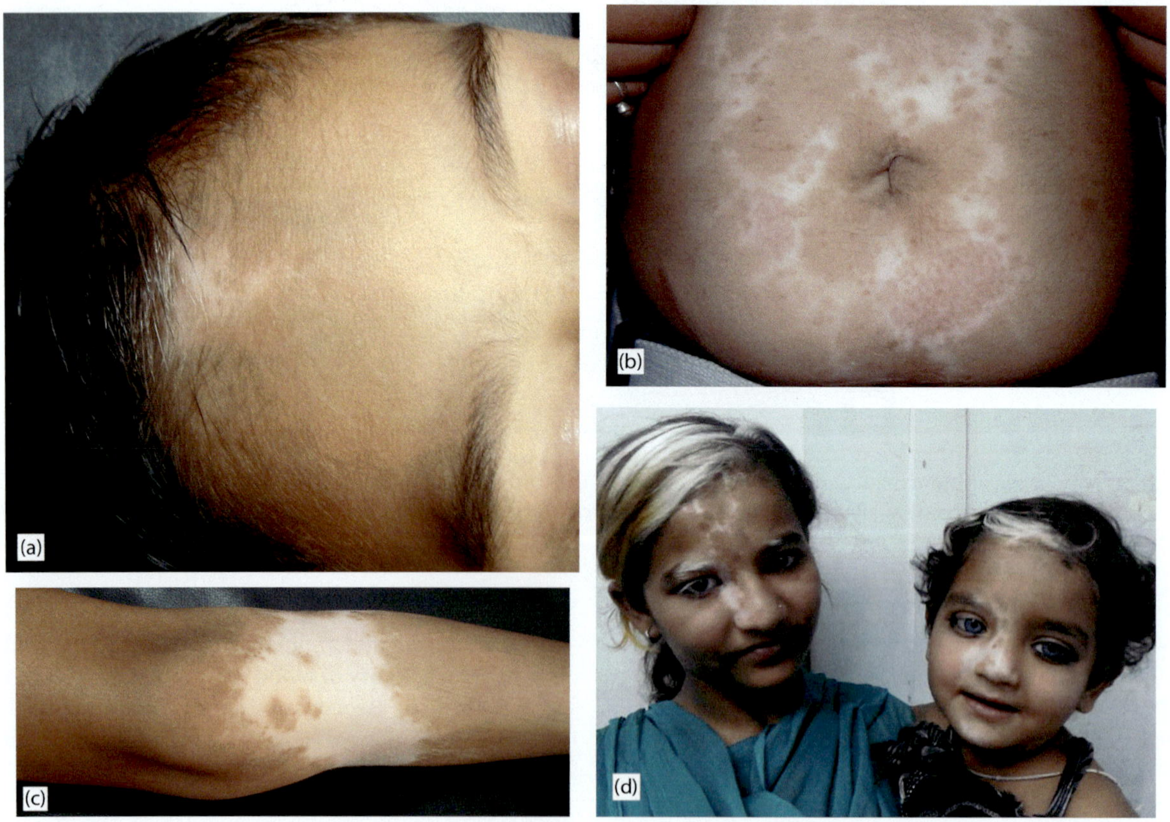


Figure 1.4 **(a)** Piebaldism affecting the forehead. Note poliosis. **(b)** Piebaldism affecting the abdomen. Note hyperpigmented macules within the depigmented patches. **(c)** Piebaldism affecting the knee. Note pigmented macules within the area of depigmentation. **(d)** Two sisters with Waardenburg syndrome. (a,c – Courtesy: Dr. Anil Patki, Pune, India; b – Courtesy: Dr. Piyush Kumar, Katihar, India; d – Courtesy: Dr. Hiral Shah, Baroda Medical College, Vadodara, India. )

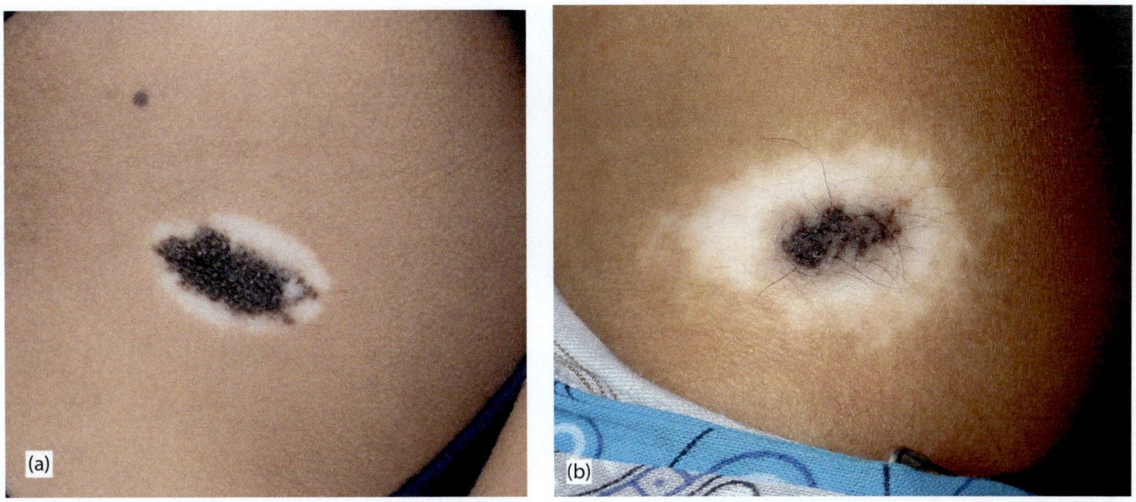

Figure 1.5 **(a)** A classical halo nevus on the hip. **(b)** Halo nevus on the shoulder region. (a,b – Courtesy: Dr. Piyush Kumar, Katihar, India.)

- Teenagers are commonly affected, and the trunk is the most common site of affliction.
- The patient develops one or multiple circular, depigmented macule(s) with a central tan or brown nevus (**Figure 1.5a,b**). Both the central nevus and zone of depigmentation may or may not involute with time.
- At times it may be associated with vitiligo.
- Over time, many other non-melanocytic and non-neoplastic conditions have been known to develop halo phenomenon.
- Conditions in which the Halo phenomenon can be seen are summarized in **Table 1.3**.
- DD: Melanoma.

## Woronoff's ring

- It is a hypopigmented halo of uniform width around a psoriatic plaque.
- This develops after phototherapy or topical treatment of psoriatic lesions (**Figure 1.6**).
- A prostaglandin E2 injection given 1cm away from the Woronoff's ring causes the hypopigmented area to develop erythema, which suggests vasoconstriction as a possible etiology.

Table 1.3 Dermatoses with halo phenomenon

| Melanocytic conditions | Non-melanocytic conditions |
|---|---|
| • Blue nevus<br>• Congenital Mongolian spots<br>• Congenital nevomelanocytic lesion<br>• Dysplastic melanocytic nevi<br>• Primary cutaneous malignant melanoma or metastasis<br>• Spitz nevus | • Basal cell epithelioma<br>• Lichen planus<br>• Molluscum contagiosum<br>• Angioma<br>• Psoriasis<br>• Seborrheic keratosis<br>• Neurofibroma<br>• Sarcoidosis<br>• Warts |

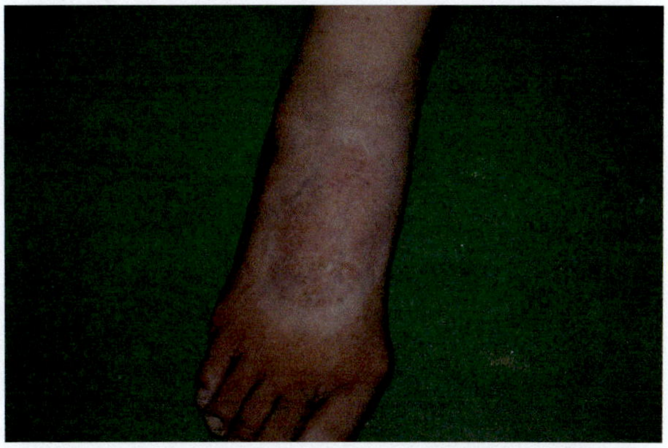

Figure 1.6 Hypopigmented Woronoff ring around the psoriasis lesion. (Courtesy: Dr. Piyush Kumar, Katihar, India.)

- DD: Halo nevus, post inflammatory hypomelanosis, pityriasis rosea.

## Vitiligo

- Vitiligo results from autoimmune destruction of melanocytes and may present as localized or generalized disease.
- Early focal vitiligo often presents with hypopigmented macules or patches with ill-defined margin with no scales.[6] With time, it becomes sharply defined and depigmented. Sometimes there may be a zone of hypopigmented skin between depigmented and normal-appearing skin (trichrome vitiligo) (**Figure 1.7a–d**).
- With treatment or spontaneously, lesions of vitiligo get repigmented frequently, and this repigmentation is either perifollicular or from the margin (**Figure 1.7e**).
- Koebnerization may be seen.
- Segmental forms of vitiligo are frequently seen and are common in children (**Figure 1.7f,g**).
- DD: Pityriasis alba (scales), lichen sclerosus (atrophy), Leprosy (sensory diminution and/or dry, anhidrotic skin), Vogt-Koyanagi-Harada syndrome, chemical leukoderma, Melanoma-associated leukoderma.

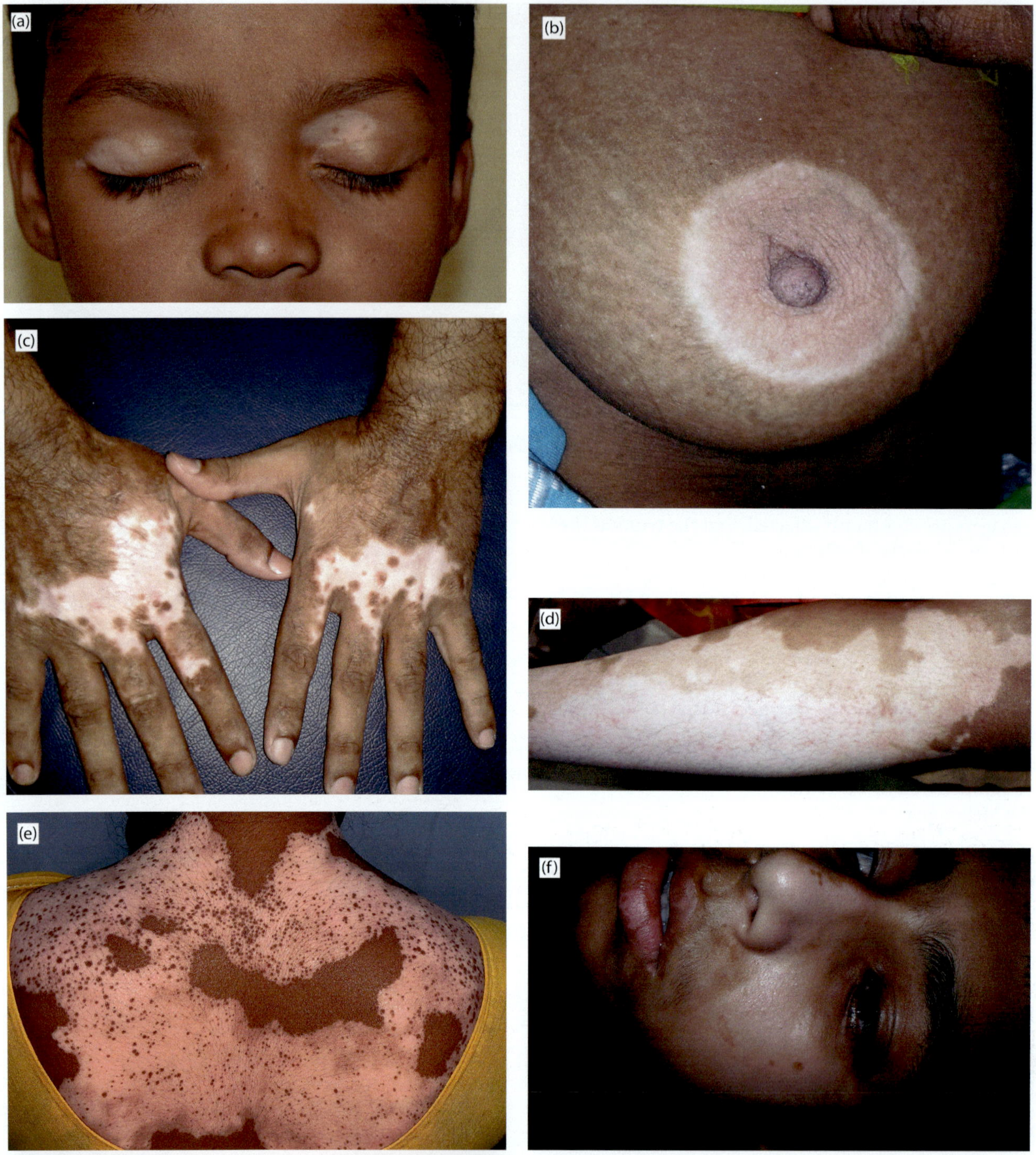


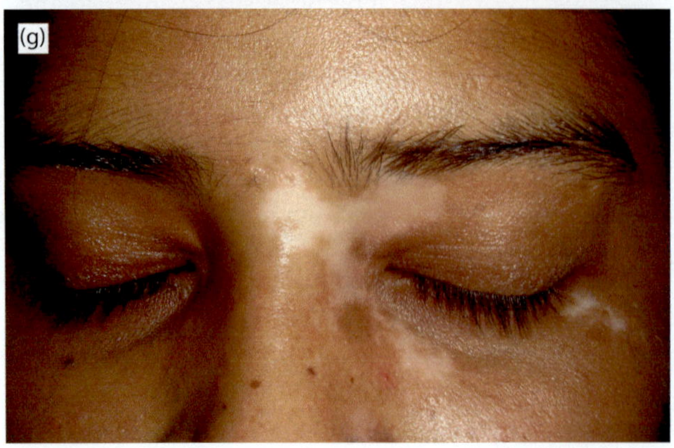


Figure 1.7 **(a)** Localized depigmented patches of vitiligo on both eyelids. **(b)** Localized vitiligo affecting areola and nipple. **(c)** Bilateral vitiligo on dorsum of hands. **(d)** Trichrome vitiligo – there is a zone of hypopigmented skin between depigmented and normal-appearing skin. **(e)** During repigmentation, perifollicular pigmented macules appear within the vitiligo lesion. **(f)** Segmental vitiligo affecting left midface. **(g)** Segmental vitiligo in the left periorbital region. (a,d,e – Courtesy: Dr. Piyush Kumar, Katihar, India.)

## Leprosy

- It is a chronic infectious disease caused by *M. leprae,* with prominent involvement of skin and peripheral nerves.
- It affects all races and age groups as well as both men and women equally.
- It has a wide spectrum of clinical findings. Leprosy is classified based on cell-mediated immunity (CMI) into polar forms, with lepromatous leprosy (LL) at one end and tuberculoid leprosy (TT) at the other end and three types of borderline leprosy in between: borderline lepromatous (BL), borderline borderline (BB) and borderline tuberculoid (BT). The term indeterminate leprosy (IL) is used to describe patients with early leprosy lesions that cannot be categorized into any pole.
- Localied hypopigmented lesions may be seen in indeterminate, tuberculoid (TT) or borderline tuberculoid (BT) leprosy (**Figure 1.8a,b**).
- Indeterminate leprosy – It is characterized by one or a few hypopigmented patches with ill-defined margins (**Figure 1.8c**). The features of nerve damage – sensory loss or loss of sweating – are not appreciable. The lesions may persist for a couple of years and then may resolve spontaneously or may develop into one of the determinate forms depending on immunity.
- TT Leprosy – Patients present with one to three hypopigmented patches with well-defined margins all around, complete or near complete sensory loss, loss of hairs, and anhidrosis.[6] Other common presentations include erythematous plaque and annular plaque.
- BT leprosy – Compared to TT leprosy, the lesions in BT are more in number and larger in size, and they demonstrate less severe features of nerve damage – sensory loss, loss of hairs, and anhidrosis. The largest diameter of BT lesions may be several centimeters, sometimes involving an extremity almost completely, and may assume annular configuration. The margin of the lesion is well defined at most places but is characteristically ill defined at others, merging with normal skin. A satellite lesion is often present and is a valuable clinical clue for the diagnosis of BT leprosy.
- DD: Early vitiligo (sensation intact, accentuation of lesions on Wood's lamp examination), morphea (indurated), lichen sclerosus (atrophy present), pityriasis alba (sensation intact, scaling), post-inflammatory hypopigmentation, hypopigmented mycosis fungoides.

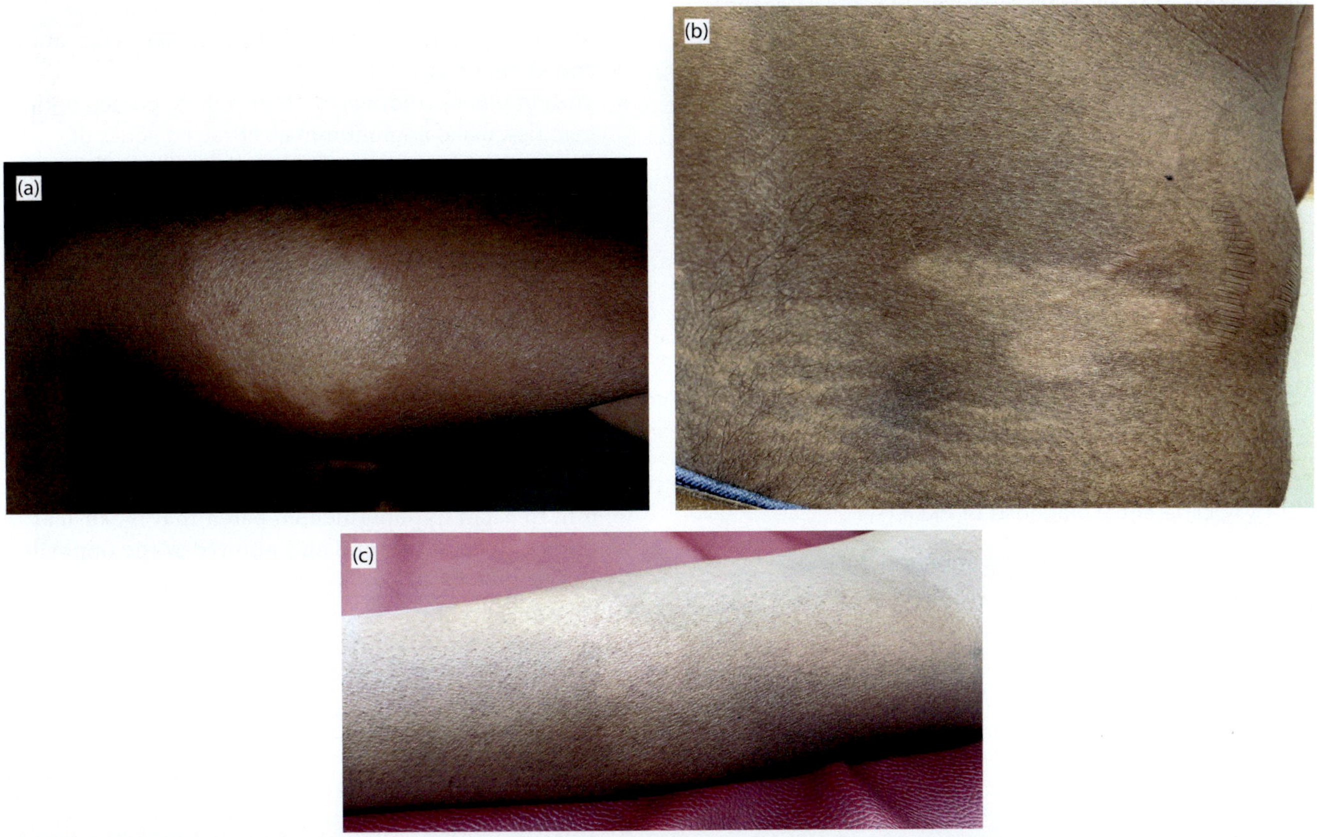


Figure 1.8 **(a)** Well defined dry, hypopigmented macule on leg in BT Hansen patient. Note epidermal atrophy appreciable as crinkles. **(b)** Hypopigmented macule on lower back along with stria distensae in BT leprosy patient. **(c)** Hypopigmented patch of indeterminate leprosy on the forearm. Note ill-defined margins. (a–c – Courtesy: Dr. Piyush Kumar, Katihar, India.)

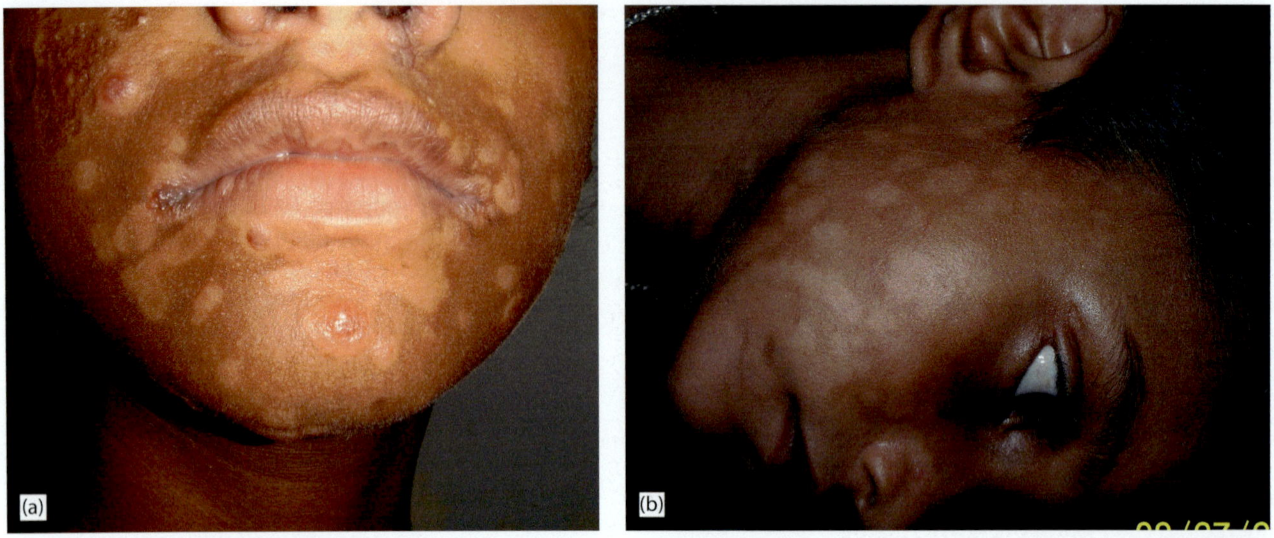


Figure 1.9 **(a)** Post kala-azar dermal leishmaniasis seen as multiple hypopigmented macules and patches predominantly seen over the muzzle area of the face. In addition, there are some erythematous juicy papules. **(b)** Hypopigmented patches in post kala-azar dermal leishmaniasis. Lesions are most prominent in perioral area. (b – Courtesy: Dr. Piyush Kumar, Katihar, India.)

## Post kala-azar dermal leishmaniasis

- It develops after partially treated or untreated visceral leishmaniasis (Kala azar). However, in some cases there is no history of prior kala azar.
- Although in advanced cases hypopigmented macules and patches are widespread, in early stages, patients present with hypopigmented macules and patches localized over the face.
- The typically affected area of the face is "muzzle area"– around the nose and mouth (**Figure 1.9a,b**).
- It characteristically presents as asymptomatic hypopigmented non scaly macules, with a tendency to coalesce to form larger patches. If left untreated, patients develop juicy erythematous papules and nodules over it.[6]
- DD: See **Table 1.4**.

Table 1.4 Differential diagnosis of PKDL

| | Differential diagnosis |
|---|---|
| Localized disease | • BT leprosy (sensory loss)<br>• Early vitiligo |
| Widespread disease (h/o kala-azar) | • Lepromatous leprosy (earlobe infiltration)<br>• Guttate vitiligo (accentuation on Wood's lamp)<br>• Pityriasis lichenoides chronica<br>• Leucoderma syphiliticum |

## Ash-leaf macules

- Ash-leaf macules (ALMs) are classically seen in tuberous sclerosis (TS) – an autosomal dominant disorder characterized by seizures, mental retardation, and skin findings.[7]
- The cutaneous findings in TS include hypomelanotic macules, facial angiofibromas, fibrous plaques of forehead, periungual and gingival fibromas, Shagreen patches, and café'-au-lait macules.
- The hypomelanotic macules in TS are usually present at birth or appear within the first few months of life and are the most common cutaneous findings.[7]
- They adopt various configurations – polygonal hypopigmented macules, ash-leaf macules, and confetti macules.
- Polygonal hypopigmented macules are the most common and can appear anywhere over the body.
- ALMs are characteristic of TS and appear as a few mm to 5-cm hypopigmented patch that is ash-leaf shaped, oval at one end and pointed at the opposite end. It is most often found on the trunk and buttocks (**Figure 1.10a,b**).
- Confetti macules are most specific and mostly seen on extremities.
- Lesional leucotrichia and poliosis have also been described.
- Subtle lesions are better visualized during Wood's lamp examination
- Three or more ALMs are a feature of tuberous sclerosis.
- DD: Nevus depigmentosus (serrated margin), nevus anemicus (margin disappears on diascopy), piebaldism (depigmented rather than hypopigmented, midline distribution), vitiligo (occasionally develops

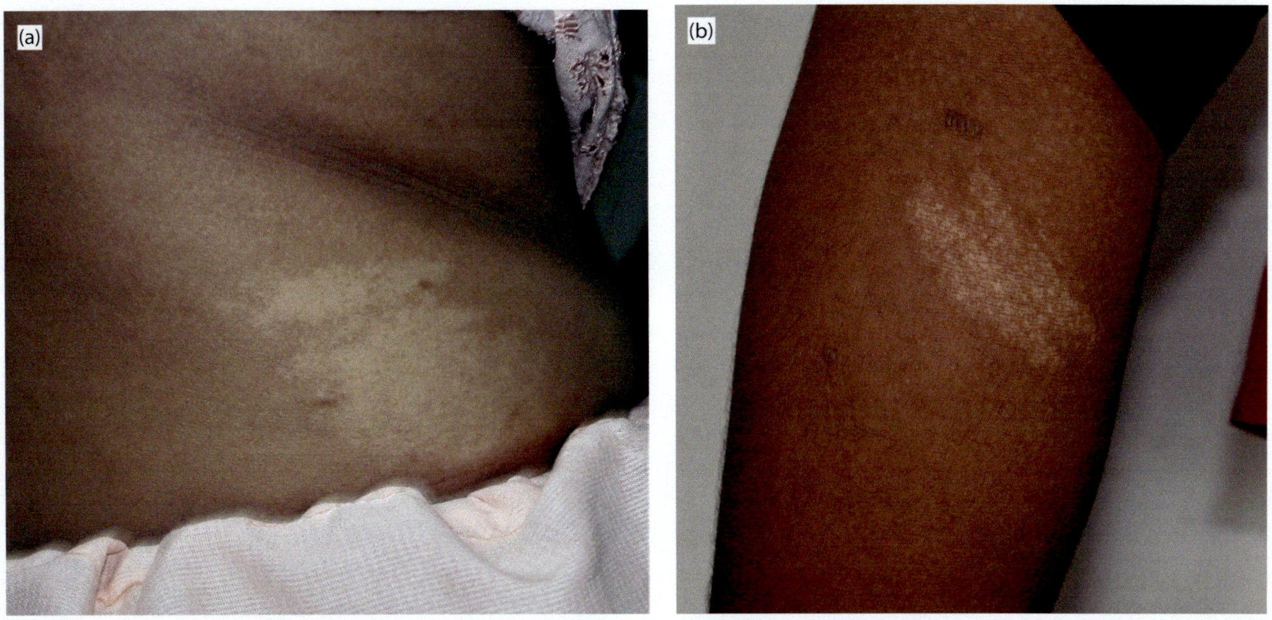


Figure 1.10 **(a)** Typical ash-leaf macule on lumbar area. **(b)** Ash-leaf macule on upper limb.

soon after birth, lesion is depigmented), multiple endocrine neoplasia type 1 (MEN 1) (multiple facial angiofibromas, collagenomas, gingival papules, confetti-like hypomelanotic macules and CALMs), post-inflammatory hypopigmentation (due to atopic or seborrheic dermatitis in infants).

## Phylloid hypomelanosis

- Phylloid hypomelanosis is a distinct pattern of hypomelanosis that occurs in patients with mosaic forms of trisomy 13.
- It is characterized by congenital hypochromic macules resembling a floral ornament with various elements such as round or oval patches, asymmetrical macules resembling begonia leaves, and pear-shaped or oblong lesions.
- Additional cutaneous features include telangiectatic macules and hypertrichosis.
- Associated extra cutaneous anomalies include cerebral defects (especially absence of corpus callosum), conductive hearing loss, choroidal and retinal colobomas, craniofacial anomalies, and digital malformations.
- DD: Post-inflammatory hypopigmentation, segmental vitiligo.

## Pityriasis versicolor (Tinea versicolor)

- It is a common, superficial cutaneous fungal infection caused by the dimorphic, lipophilic fungus of the genus *Malassezia (Malassezia furfur, M. globosa, M. sympodialis).*
- Risk factors are warm, humid environments; oil application; topical or systemic steroid use; immunosuppression; malnutrition; pregnancy; and Cushing disease.
- It is commonly seen after puberty (when activity of sebaceous glands is high) and in summer.
- Common sites are the upper trunk and upper extremities. Facial involvement is less common but may be more commonly seen in infants and immunocompromised patients.[8]
- It typically presents as asymptomatic or mildly itchy perifollicular hypopigmented to hyperpigmented macules with fine non-adherent scales and mild erythema. The lesions have a tendency to coalesce to form larger polycyclic patches, but the periphery may still show perifollicular lesions (an important clinical clue) (**Figure 1.11a–d**). The lesions become more prominent when wet (during bathing or after sweating) – another important clinical clue.
- Inverse variant – Lesions predominantly affect the flexural regions, the face, or isolated areas of the extremities. It may be more commonly noted in immunocompromised persons.
- *Pityrosporum* folliculitis – Patients develop multiple, asymptomatic, 2- to 3-mm, monomorphic, follicular, erythematous papules and pustules on trunk.
- Atrophic variant – This rare form is clinically characterized by atrophic, ivory-colored to erythematous, oval to round lesions. The surface has a wrinkled appearance, and the atrophy is limited to the areas affected by tinea versicolor.
- DD: Pityriasis alba, vitiligo (non-scaly, Wood's lamp accentuation), lepromatous leprosy (loss of sensation, non-scaly, presence of earlobe infiltration, co-existent nodular lesions, peripheral nerve thickening), seborrheic dermatitis (scalp and face involvement, more itching).

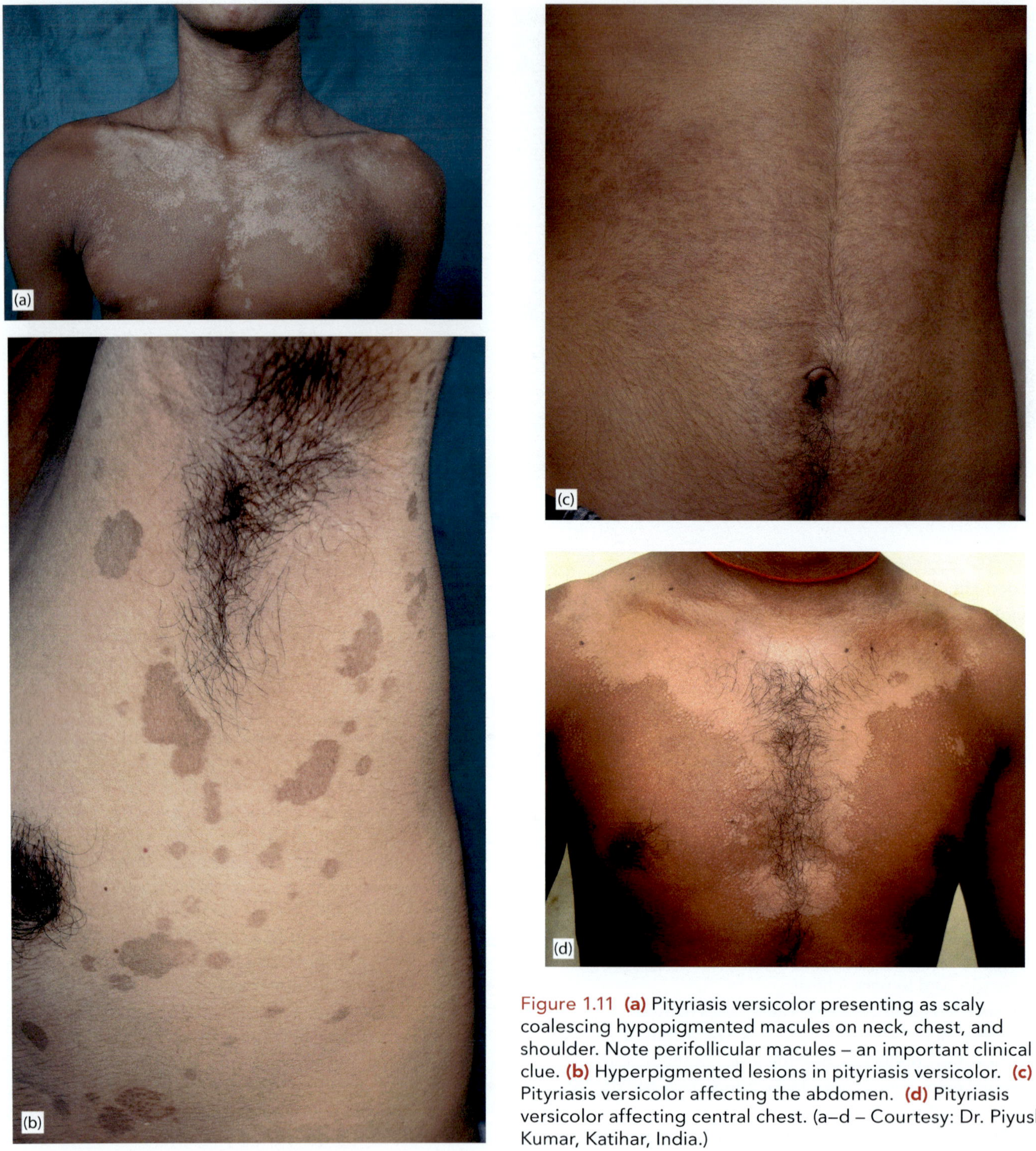


Figure 1.11 **(a)** Pityriasis versicolor presenting as scaly coalescing hypopigmented macules on neck, chest, and shoulder. Note perifollicular macules – an important clinical clue. **(b)** Hyperpigmented lesions in pityriasis versicolor. **(c)** Pityriasis versicolor affecting the abdomen. **(d)** Pityriasis versicolor affecting central chest. (a–d – Courtesy: Dr. Piyush Kumar, Katihar, India.)

## Idiopathic guttate hypomelanosis (IGH)

- It is an acquired leukoderma of unknown etiology.
- It is most commonly seen in middle-aged to older people and has no sex predilection.
- Most commonly affected sites are shins and forearms. But it may be seen anywhere on the body.
- Lesions are generally asymptomatic but can be mildly pruritic.
- IGH presents as randomly distributed, discrete, angular or circular, hypopigmented or depigmented macules of usually 1–3 mm.[6] However, lesions may be as large as 10 mm. The number of lesions increases gradually, but the size of individual lesions remains the same (**Figure 1.12a,b**).
- DD: Post inflammatory hypopigmentation, guttate vitiligo (Wood's lamp accentuation), guttate lichen sclerosus (atrophic lesion), leukoderma punctuate.

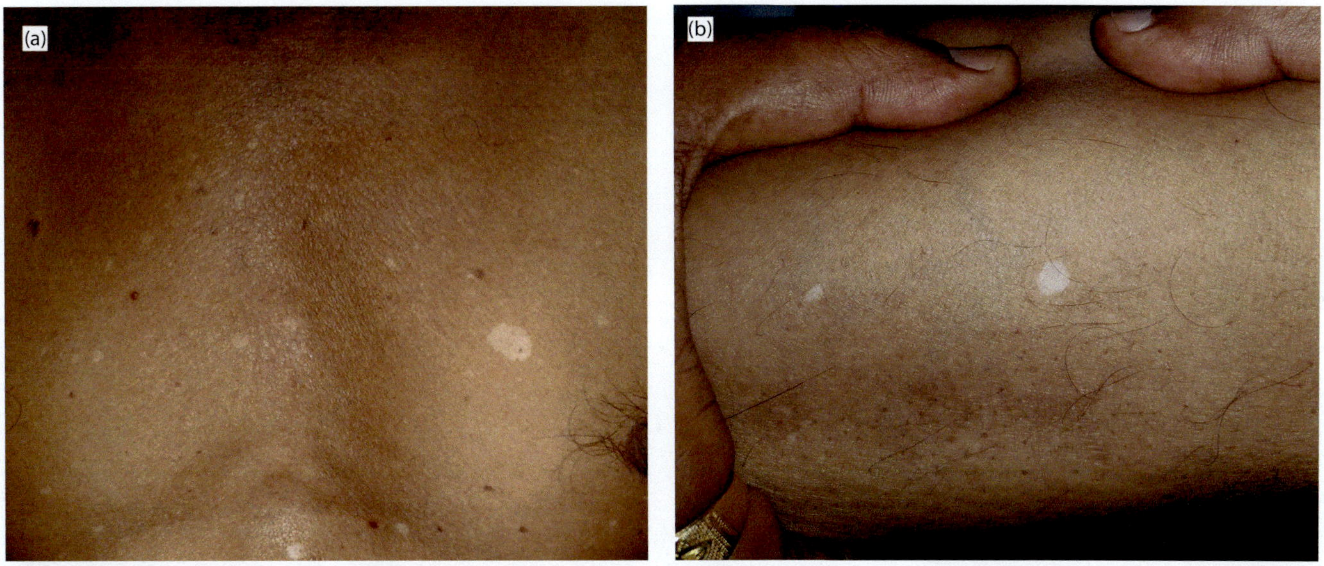

Figure 1.12 **(a)** Idiopathic guttate hypomelanosis as depigmented macule on the shin. **(b)** Idiopathic guttate hypomelanosis lesion on the chest.

## Physiologic anemic macules (Bier spots)

- Bier spots are pale macules seen on the extremities due to localized vasoconstriction.[9]
- They are seen most often in young females between 20 and 40 years of age and have no racial preponderance. However, most cases have been reported among the Chinese population.
- The lesions become more prominent when the limbs are placed in a dependent position for a long time and resolve when limbs are elevated.
- They can sometimes be seen in association with cryoglobulinemia and scleroderma renal crisis.
- Bier spots with insomnia and tachycardia are called "Marshall-White syndrome."
- DD: Punctate vitiligo, pityriasis versicolor, nevus anemicus.

## Annular lichenoides dermatitis of youth (ALDY)

- ALDY is a recently described condition of unknown etiology; most cases are from Mediterranean area. It has been documented in other parts of the world – central Europe, Japan, and Korea.
- It is predominantly seen in adolescents and has a male predilection. ALDY presents as asymptomatic, sharply demarcated annular erythematous macules and patches with central hypopigmentation. Lesions may or may not show a bilateral and symmetrical distribution. The central hypopigmentation may not be noticeable in some cases.[10]
- Most commonly affected sites are flanks and groin. Other common sites include axilla and neck.
- DD: morphea (induration present), hypopigmented mycosis fungoides.

## Tumour of follicular infundibulum

- It is a rare benign cutaneous adnexal neoplasm arising from the infundibular part of hair follicle.
- It is mostly seen in the older population, with a slight female preponderance.
- It has two variants – solitary and multiple.
- The most common form is solitary, which presents as asymptomatic papulonodular scaly lesion measuring about 1–2 cm.
- The eruptive or multiple form (infundibulomatosis) presents with a sudden onset of multiple, bilaterally symmetric, hypopigmented macules and papules over face, neck, and upper trunk. The surface may show scaling.[11]
- DD: Pityriasis versicolor, post kala-azar dermal leishmaniasis.

## Hypomelanosis of ITO (incontinentia pigmenti achromicans)

- It is a condition of pigmentary mosaicism characterized by various patterns of unilateral or bilateral hypopigmentation following the lines of Blaschko.[12] The hypopigmentation is due to presence of a clone of melanocytes with decreased ability to produce pigment.
- It usually manifests in the first year of life, with a female predominance (F:M= 2.5:1).
- Trunk and extremities are the most commonly affected sites.

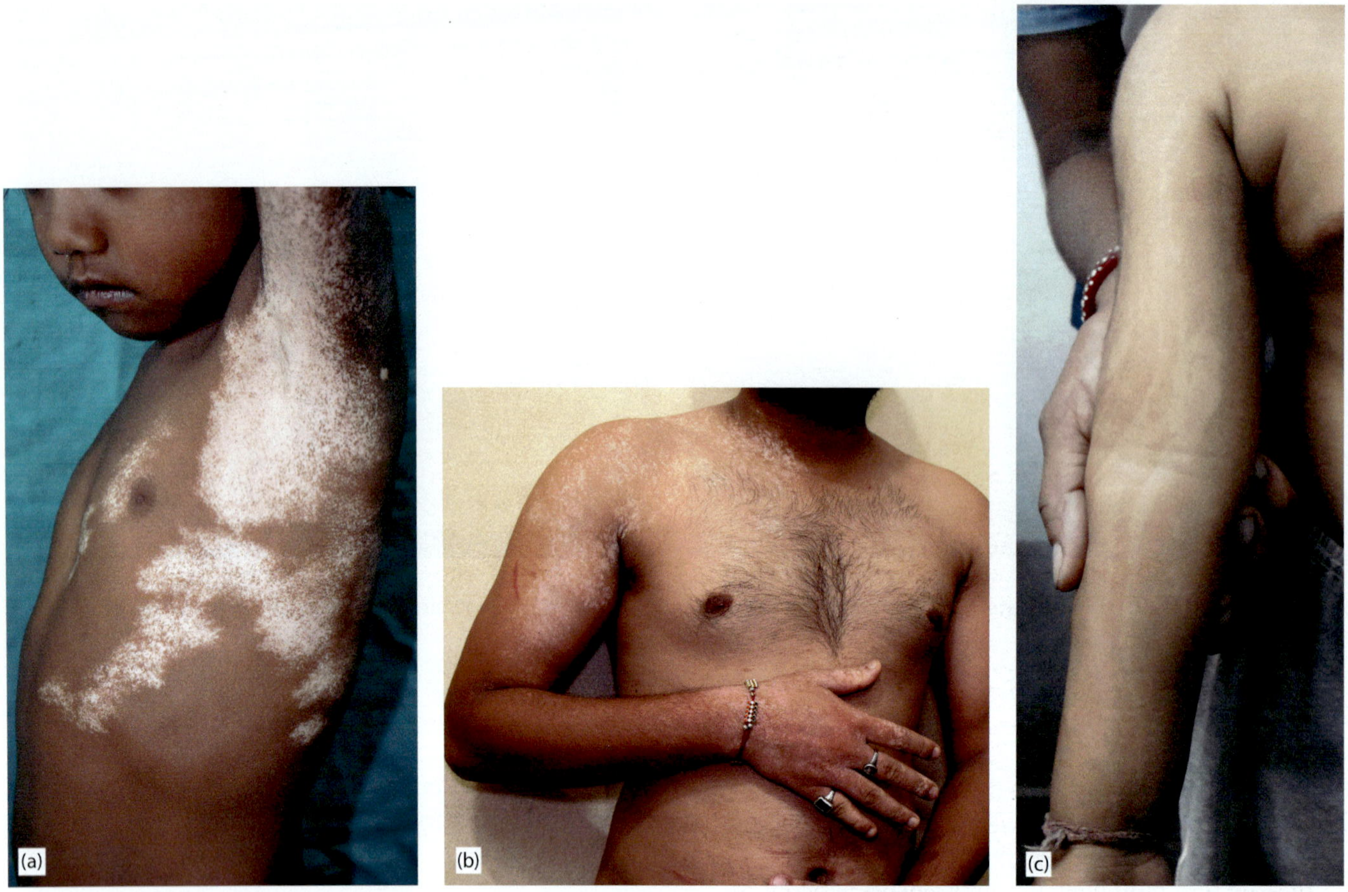


Figure 1.13 **(a)** Multi-dermatomal hypopigmented bands of hypomelanosis of Ito. **(b)** Hypomelanosis of Ito affecting the right shoulder region and right upper extremity. **(c)** Hypomelanosis of Ito in a young boy. (a,b – Courtesy: Dr. Piyush Kumar, Katihar, India; c – Courtesy: Dr Hiral Shah, Baroda Medical College, Vadodara, India.)

- It consists of asymptomatic, small hypopigmented macules coalescing to form large linear and whorl-like patches following the lines of Blaschko. It can be unilateral or bilateral. The lesion covers more than one dermatome (**Figure 1.13a–c**).
- Neurological and musculoskeletal abnormalities may be associated and should be looked for (**Table 1.5**).
- DD: Linear and whorled nevoid hypomelanosis.

## Corticosteroid induced hypopigmentation

- This occurs after topical or injectable corticosteroids used for the treatment of certain dermatosis (e.g., lichen planus, keloid) or orthopedic conditions such as tennis elbow.
- It usually develops after a few weeks of injection/topical use and may resolve spontaneously in several months.
- Asymptomatic, non-scaly, hypopigmented macules and patches with or without atrophy are present at the site of injection/application (**Figure 1.14a,b**).

Table 1.5 Neurological and musculoskeletal abnormalities in hypomelanosis of Ito

| Musculoskeletal abnormalities | Neurological abnormalities |
|---|---|
| • Cleft palate | Mental retardation |
| • Hemihypertrophy | Seizures |
| • Limb, hand, and/or foot abnormalities | Neural tumors |
| • Nail abnormalities | |
| • Hypotonia | |
| • Teeth abnormalities | |
| • Hair anomalies | |
| • Face and/or skull anomalies | |

- It may extend along the blood vessels and lymphatics, resulting in hypopigmentation in linear and branch-like fashion, tailing venous, and lymphatic drainage.
- DD: Linear vitiligo, post inflammatory hypopigmentation.

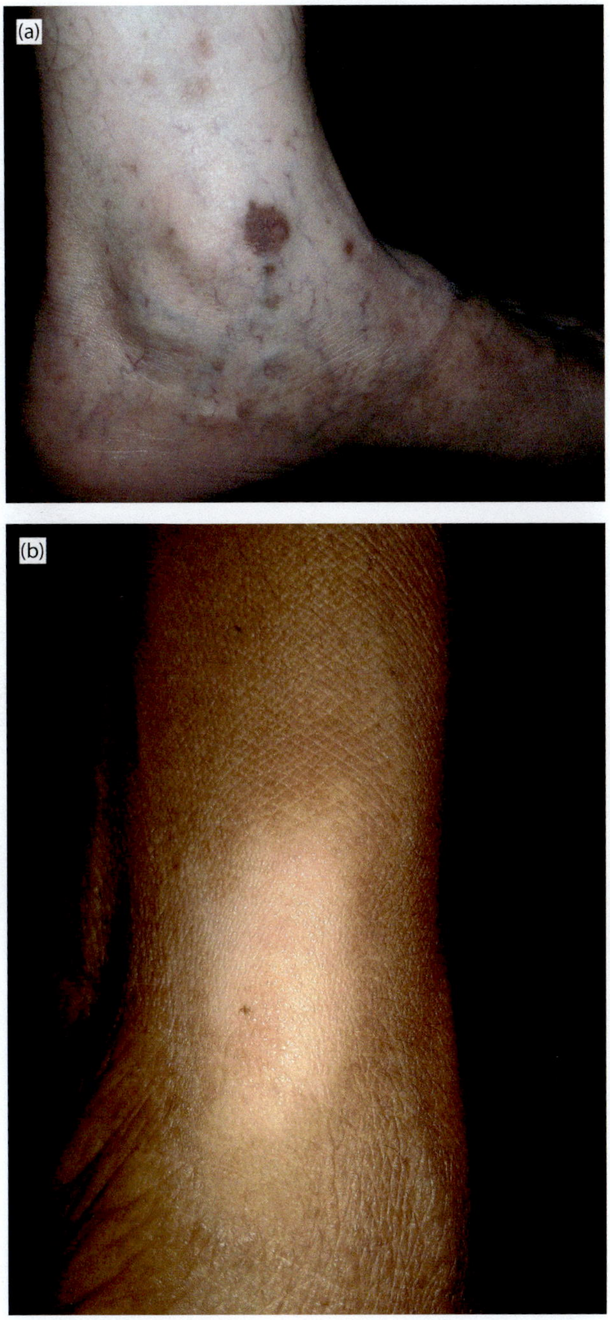

Figure 1.14 **(a)** Steroid (used for lichen planus) induced depigmentation on left ankle and lower leg. **(b)** Injectable steroid induced localized depigmented patch. (a – Courtesy: Dr. Piyush Kumar, Katihar, India.)

### Post-inflammatory hypopigmentation

- This clinically presents as hypopigmented macules or patches with or without erythema; lesions can be rough and scaly.
- History of dermatoses, infection, trauma, or burn is suggestive.
- Causes of post-inflammatory hypopigmentation are summarized in **Table 1.6**.

Table 1.6 Causes of post-inflammatory hypopigmentation

| Inflammatory skin disease | Infections |
|---|---|
| • Allergic contact dermatitis<br>• Atopic dermatitis<br>• Discoid lupus erythematosus<br>• Insect bite reactions<br>• Lichen planus<br>• Lichen striatus<br>• Pityriasis lichenoides chronica<br>• Psoriasis<br>• Sarcoidosis<br>• Scleroderma<br>• Stevens-Johnson syndrome | • Chickenpox<br>• Herpes zoster<br>• Impetigo<br>• Onchocerciasis<br>• Pinta<br>• Pityriasis versicolor<br>• Syphilis |
| **Procedure related** | **Miscellaneous** |
| • Chemical peels<br>• Cryotherapy<br>• Dermabrasion<br>• Laser | • Burns |

## REFERENCES


1. Lee D, Kang JH, Kim SH, Seo JK, Sung HS, Hwang SW. A case of extensive pityriasis alba. Ann Dermatol 2008;20(3):146–148.
2. Deb S, Sarkar R, Samanta AB. A brief review of nevus depigmentosus. Pigment Int 2014;1:56–58.
3. Sethi A, Kaur T, Puri K. Giant nevus anemicus: A rare case report. Indian J Paediatr Dermatol 2013;14:39–40.
4. Nargis T, Pinto M, Shenoy MM. Piebaldism with complete poliosis: A rare presentation. Indian J Paediatr Dermatol 2018;19:183–185.
5. Vasani R. Meyerson phenomenon. Indian J Paediatr Dermatol 2019;20:78–80.
6. Kumarasinghe P, Uprety S, Sarkar R. Hypopigmentary disorders in Asian patients. Pigment Int 2017;4:13–20.
7. Cardis MA, De Klotz CMC. Cutaneous manifestations of tuberous sclerosis complex and the paediatrician's role. Arch Dis Child 2017;102:85863.
8. Ghosh SK, Dey SK, Saha I, Barbhuiya JN, Ghosh A, Roy AK. Pityriasis versicolor: A clinicomycological and epidemiological study from a tertiary care hospital. Indian J Dermatol 2008;53:182–185.
9. Mahajan VK, Khatri G, Singh R, Chauhan PS, Mehta KS. Bier spots: An uncommon cause of mottled skin. Indian Dermatol Online J 2015;6(2):128–129.
10. Di Mercurio M, Gisondi P, Colato C, et al. Annular lichenoid dermatitis of youth: Report of six new cases with review of the literature. Dermatology 2015;231:195–200.
11. Suchonwanit P, Ruangchainikom P, Apibal Y. Eruptive Tumors of the Follicular Infundibulum: An unexpected diagnosis of hypopigmented macules. Dermatol Ther 2015;5(3):207–211.
12. Chethan C J, Ashique K T, Sukumar D, Nanda Kishore B. Hypomelanosis of ITO. Indian J Dermatol 2006;51:65–66.


## SUGGESTED READING


1. Hypopigmentation. Edited by Electra Nicolaidou, Clio Dessinioti, Andreas Katsambas. 1st edition. 2020. CRC Press.
2. The Pigmentary System: Physiology and Pathophysiology. Edited by James J. Nordlund Raymond E. Boissy Vincent J. Hearing Richard A. King William S. Oetting Jean-Paul Ortonne. 2nd edition. 2006. Blackwell Publishing Ltd.

# E2

# Hypopigmented and depigmented macules and patches: Generalized

PC DAS, MAMTA YADAV

## ABSTRACT

Hypopigmentation refers to lack of melanin pigment. Hypopigmentary disorders may be congenital or acquired, diffuse, or localized, and may occur in isolation or may be associated with a wide range of congenital or acquired disorders. This chapter reviews the common causes and salient features of hypopigmentary disorders presenting in a generalized manner.

The text of this chapter is available online at https://routledgetextbooks.com/textbooks/9781032399669/


DOI: 10.1201/9781351054225-5

# 2

# Hyperpigmented macules and patches: Localized

PC DAS, DANISH AKHTAR

## INTRODUCTION

Increased skin pigmentation results from increased number and/or activity of melanocytes. Other pathomechanisms, such as increased thickness of stratum corneum (as in acanthosis nigricans), too might be responsible. The list of clinical differentials for localized cutaneous hyperpigmentation is long and includes many congenital as well as acquired conditions. A purposeful history and physical examination offer valuable clues to the underlying cause. Some conditions are congenital (e.g., congenital melanocytic nevus), while others are acquired during childhood (freckles, Becker's nevus). A review of medications and exposure to plants and ultraviolet radiation can help determine prior drug reaction or phototoxic reaction resulting in post-inflammatory hyperpigmentation. Noting the distribution of lesions is also important. Melasma, actinic lichen planus, nevus of Ota, etc. typically occur on sun-exposed parts such as the face; Schamberg's disease is mostly seen on the lower limbs in symmetrical fashion. This chapter discusses the clinical approach to conditions presenting with localized pigmentation outlined in **Table 2.1** and their salient features are

Table 2.1 Clinical approach to localized hyperpigmented macules and patches

| Onset | Color | Diseases |
|---|---|---|
| Congenital | Blue-gray | • Face – nevus of Ota<br>• Shoulder region – nevus of Ito<br>• Lower back – Mongolian spot |
| | Brown-tan | • Uniformly pigmented – café-au-lait macule<br>• Speckled – nevus spilus |
| | Brown-black | Congenital melanocytic nevus |
| Acquired | Blue-gray | Lichen planus pigmentosus, melasma |
| | Brown-black | Macules – freckles, lentigines<br>Patches<br>• Face (*see Chapter 3*) – melasma, lichen planus pigmentosus, solar lentigo, erythema dyschromicum perstans, actinic lichen planus, post-chikungunya pigmentation (nose – chik sign), periorbital hyperpigmentation, nevus of Hori, tanning<br>• Neck – atopic dirty neck, acanthosis nigricans<br>• Trunk – pityriasis versicolor (scaly), Becker's nevus (hypertrichosis), notalgia paresthetica, progressive cribriform and zosteriform hyperpigmentation, macular amyloidosis (upper back), lifa disease (chest)<br>• Extensor extremities – macular amyloidosis<br>• Legs – Schamberg's disease, diabetic dermopathy, melanoma (acral lentiginous type)<br>• Anywhere – post-inflammatory hyperpigmentation, morphea (indurated skin), terra firma-forme dermatosis, frictional melanosis<br>Patterned – linea nigra, progressive cribriform and zosteriform hyperpigmentation, linear and whorled nevoid hypermelanosis |

DOI: 10.1201/9781351054225-6

Table 2.2 Diagnostic pitfalls

- Acanthosis nigricans – thick, velvety plaques involving flexures
- Morphea – indurated plaque, atrophy
- Atrophoderma of Pierini and Pasini – slightly depressed areas with well-defined "cliff-drop" borders and no obvious induration
- Terra firma-forme dermatosis – brown-gray, velvety, pigmented patches or plaques

discussed below. Certain diagnostic pitfalls, which need a consideration while evaluating for localized pigmentation, are enlisted in **Table 2.2**.[1–9]

## Nevus of Ota

- This is also known as oculomucodermal melanocytosis or nevus fusco-ceruleus ophthalmo-maxillaris.
- It is a hamartoma of dermal melanocytes, seen in the distribution of the ophthalmic and maxillary branches of the trigeminal nerve and thought to result from failure of migration of melanocytes from neural crest to epidermis.
- The lesion is asymptomatic, with an onset at birth or puberty and a predilection for females.
- It presents as unilateral, persistent, speckled, slate brown or bluish gray, coalescing macules and patches over the forehead, malar area, periorbital area, temple, nose, and oral mucosa (**Figure 2.1a,b**). Rarely, bilateral lesions may be seen.
- Pigmentation of the ipsilateral sclera is common and is a useful diagnostic clue (**Figure 2.1c–e**). Glaucoma may develop in the affected eye.
- The lesion remains unchanged in adulthood. Malignant transformation (malignant melanoma) is very rare and has been reported mostly with ocular lesions.
- DD: Pigmentary demarcation line (PDL), melanocytic nevus, melasma.

## Nevus of Ito

- Nevus of Ito is a dermal melanocytic hamartoma affecting the shoulder area in the distribution of the posterior supraclavicular and lateral cutaneous brachial nerves.
- This asymptomatic condition is noted at birth or soon thereafter and is seen frequently in patients with nevus of Ota.
- It presents as slate-brown or bluish-gray hyperpigmentation in the shoulder region.
- DD: PDL, melanocytic nevus, extrafacial melasma, bruise, post-inflammatory hyperpigmentation.

## Mongolian spot (congenital dermal melanocytosis)

- It is a developmental anomaly resulting from failure of migration of melanocytes from neural crest to epidermis.
- It manifests at birth or in the first few weeks of life and usually disappears in childhood; rarely, it may persist lifelong.
- The most commonly affected site is the lumbosacral area. Buttocks, flanks, and shoulders may be affected in extensive lesions.
- It presents as solitary or multiple, asymptomatic, blue-gray or dark blue, round or oval or irregularly shaped patches with ill-defined margins (**Figure 2.2a–c**). The blue color is because of the Tyndall effect, whereby the shorter wavelength light is reflected more via scattering.
- Variants include generalized (entire trunk and extremities), speckled, or persistent types.
- Extra cutaneous signs – Few cases of extensive Mongolian spots have been reported with inborn errors of metabolism (e.g., GM1 gangliosidosis, Hurler syndrome, Niemann-Pick disease, and Hunter syndrome).
- DD: bruise, blue nevus.

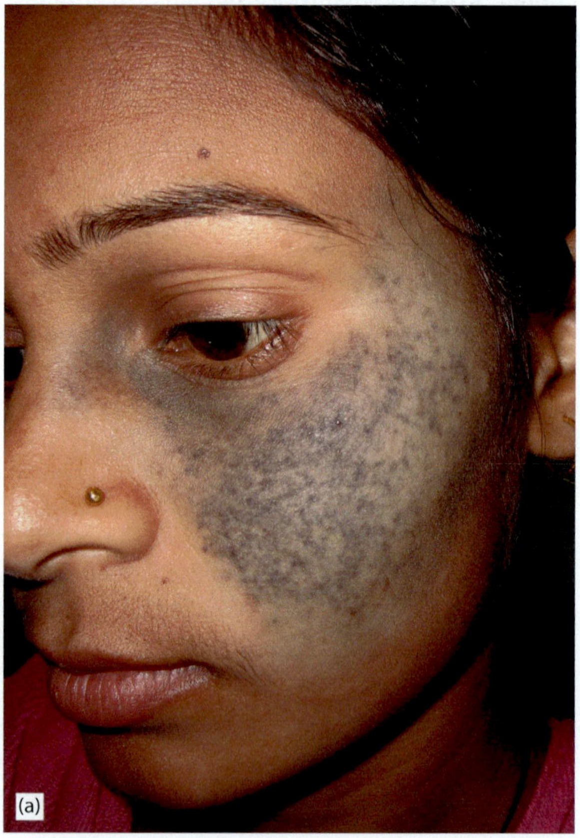


Figure 2.1 **(a)** Blue-gray speckled pigmentation on a bluish background in nevus of Ota. *(Continued)*

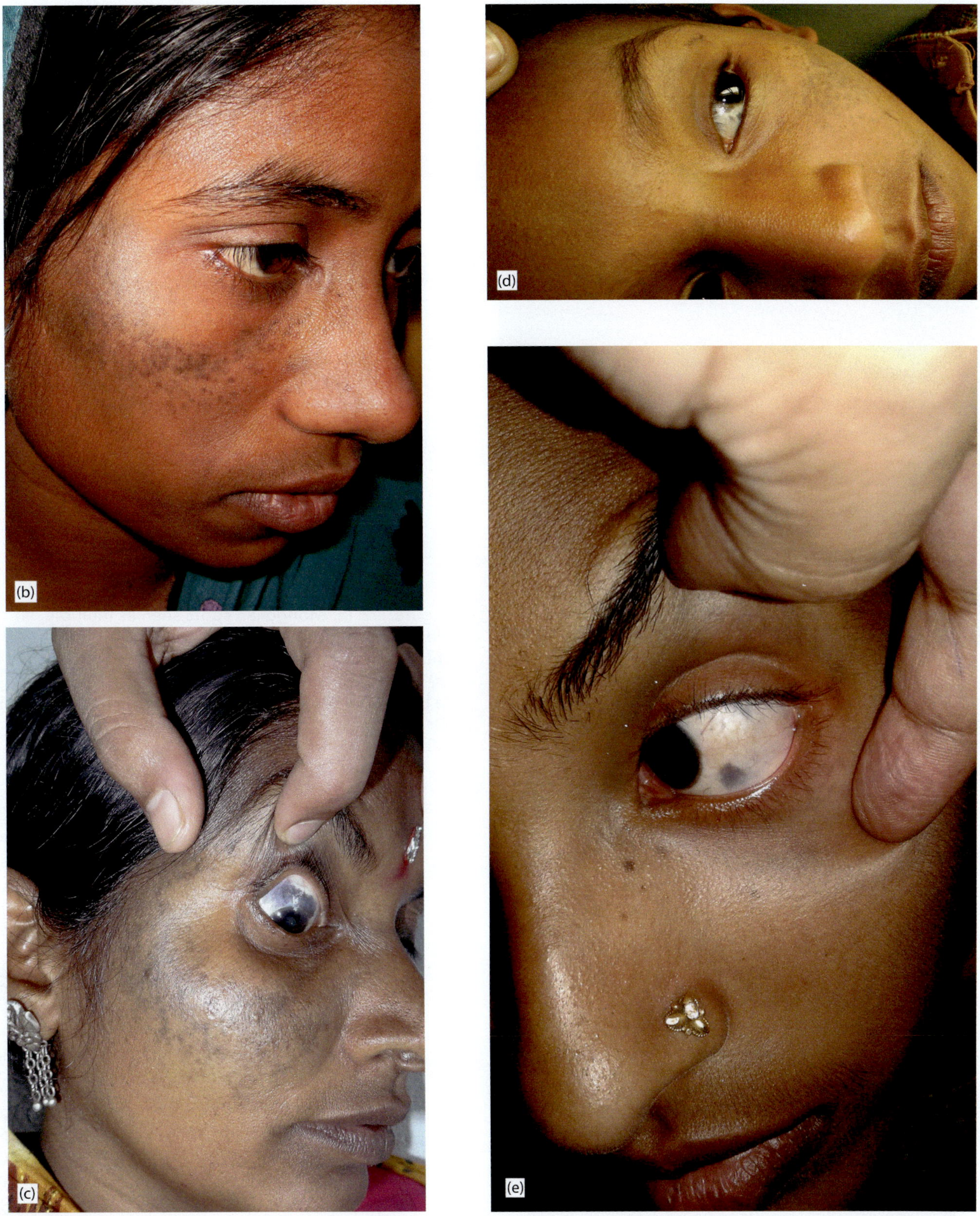


Figure 2.1 (*Continued*) **(b)** A young lady with nevus of Ota on right maxillary region. **(c)** Ocular involvement in nevus of Ota. **(d)** A young boy with ocular and cutaneous lesions of nevus of Ota. **(e)** More prominent ocular lesions. (c,d – Courtesy: Dr. Piyush Kumar, Katihar, India.)

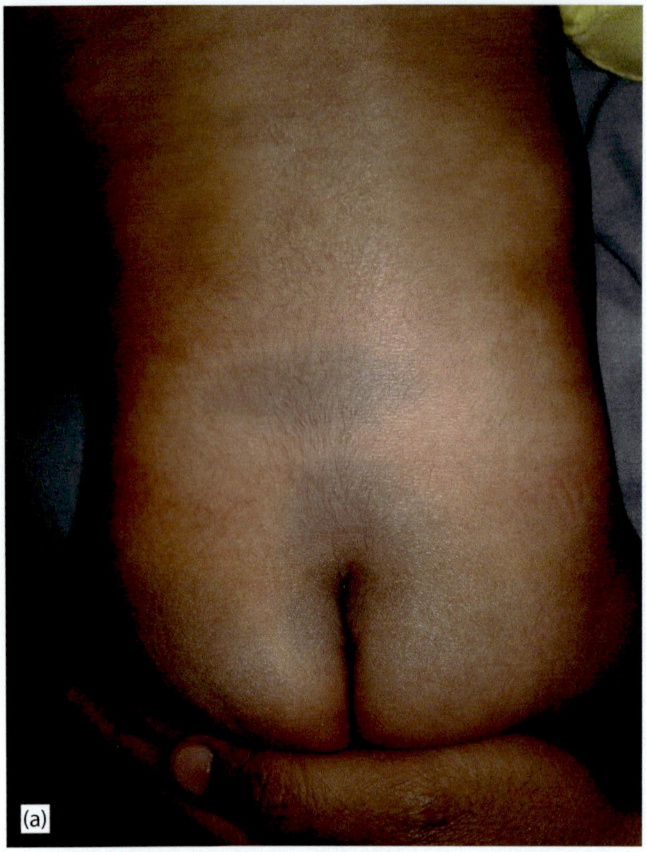

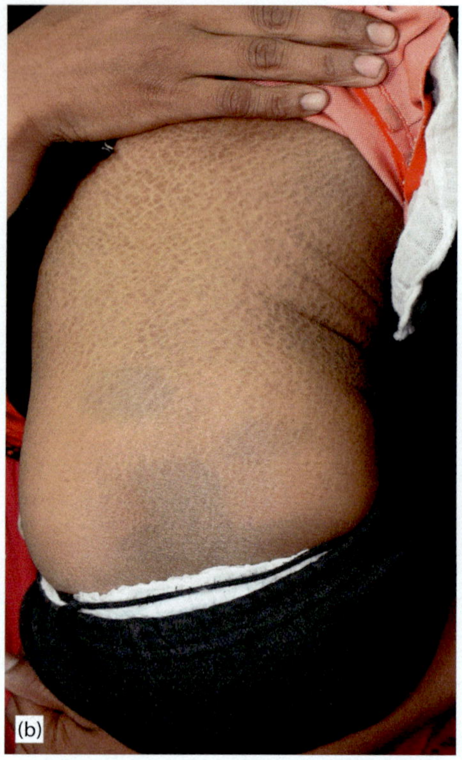

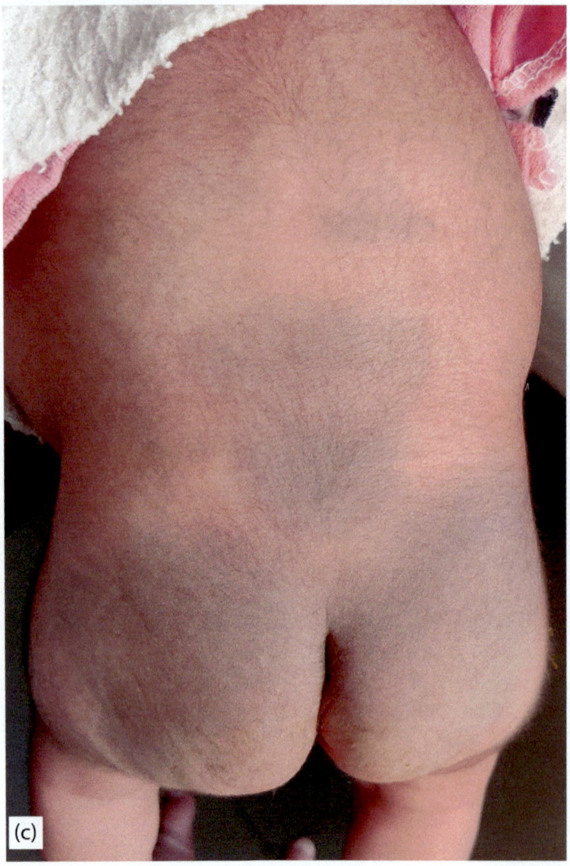

Figure 2.2 **(a)** Mongolian spots seen as multiple, ill-defined bluish patches on lumbosacral region. **(b)** An infant with ichthyosis vulgaris and Mongolian spots. **(c)** Mongolian spots seen on lumbosacral region. (a,b – Courtesy: Dr. Piyush Kumar, Katihar, India; c – Courtesy: Dr Kamlesh Kumar Agrawal, Pediatric Medicine, SMS Medical College, Jaipur, India.)

## Café-au-lait macules (CALMs)

- CALMs are light-brown to dark-brown macules and patches commonly seen in association with various genetic conditions (**Table 2.3**). Also, isolated CALM without any underlying condition may be seen.
- They may be seen at birth or during infancy and may affect any site of the body. A solitary CALM is commonly noted on buttocks.
- They may be single or multiple, well circumscribed, discrete, pale-brown to dark-brown, oval macules and patches varying in size from 0.5–20 cm (**Figure 2.3a,b**).
- Six or more CALMs of a size more than 5 mm in pre-pubertal individuals and 15 mm

Table 2.3 Conditions associated with CALMs

1. Neurofibromatosis type 1 and, less commonly, type 2
2. McCune Albright syndrome
3. Legius syndrome
4. Tuberous sclerosis
5. LEOPARD syndrome
6. Cowden disease
7. Bloom syndrome
8. Fanconi syndrome

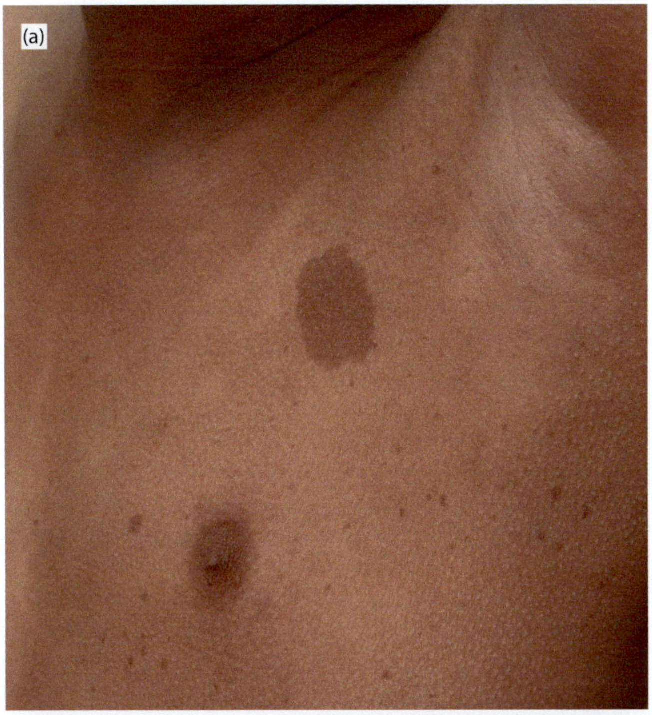

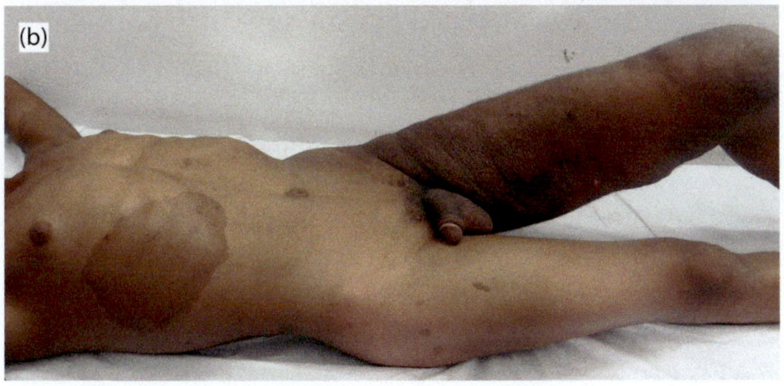

Figure 2.3 **(a)** Uniformly pigmented, tan brown patch of café-au-lait macule (CALM). Many smaller lesions of CALM are appreciable. **(b)** Giant lesion of CALM on the chest with plexiform neurofibroma involving the left thigh. (a,b – Courtesy: Dr. Piyush Kumar, Katihar, India.)

in post-pubertal individuals are suggestive of neurofibromatosis type 1 (NF1).

- Smaller CALMs affecting axilla (axillary freckling, Crowe sign) and inguinal regions (inguinal freckling) are common in NF1.
- DD: Lentigines, nevus spilus, melanocytic nevi.

## Nevus spilus (speckled lentiginous nevus)

- Nevus spilus is a localized hyperpigmented lesion arising due to focal proliferation of melanocytes along the basal layer of the epidermis.
- This asymptomatic condition presents at birth or during infancy and may appear anywhere on the body, the trunk being the most commonly affected site.
- Nevus spilus presents as a well-demarcated, light brown or tan patch, speckled with black, brown, or red-brown macules or papules of 2–3 mm (**Figure 2.4a–c**).
- The background hyperpigmentation is usually oval in shape of 3–6 cm size. But the lesion may be linear or zosteriform (**Figure 2.4d**) or may be as large as 60 cm.
- The macules and papules may be pathologically lentigines or junctional, compound, or dermal nevi. Less commonly, Spitz nevus and blue nevus may be seen.

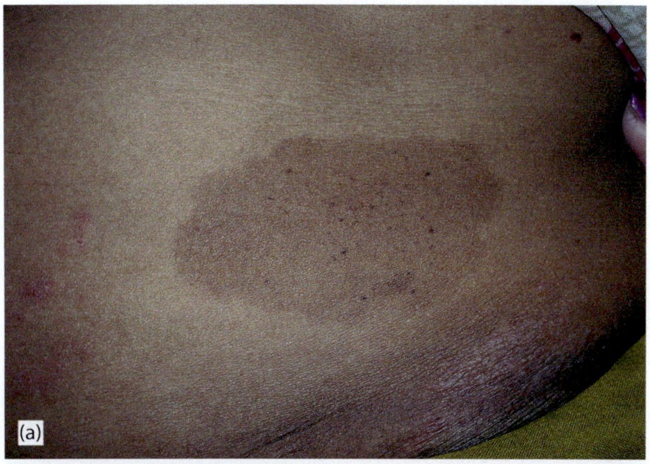

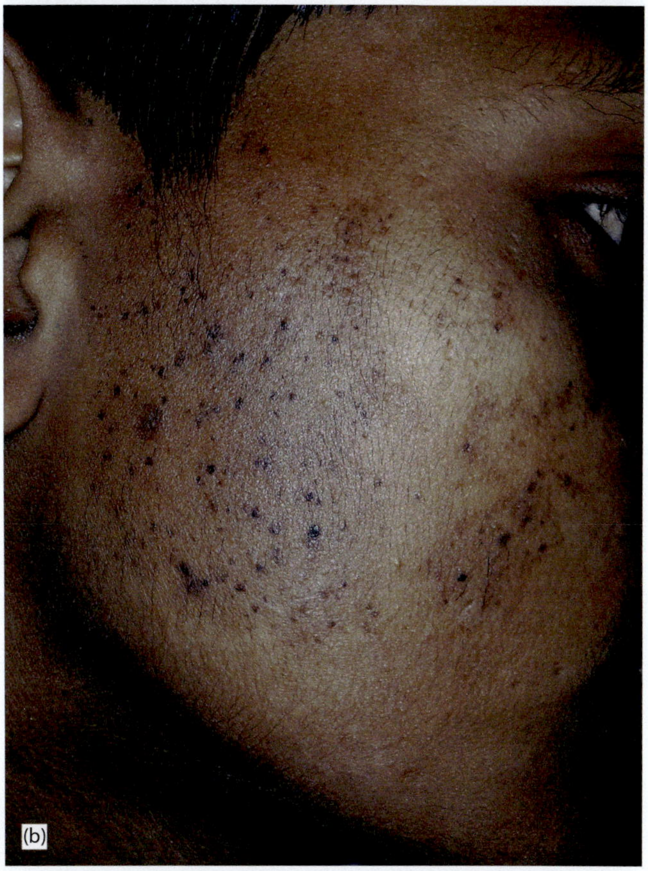

Figure 2.4 **(a)** Nevus spilus seen as well-defined tan brown patch with a few brown black macules and papules. **(b)** Nevus spilus on the face. (*Continued*)

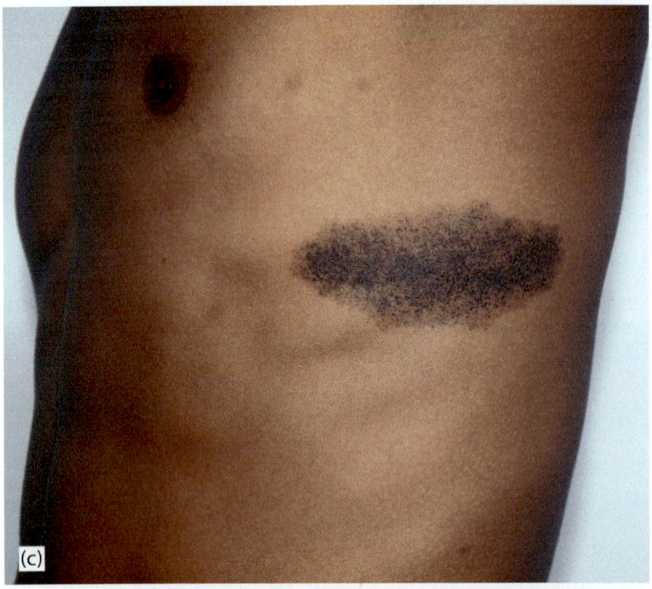

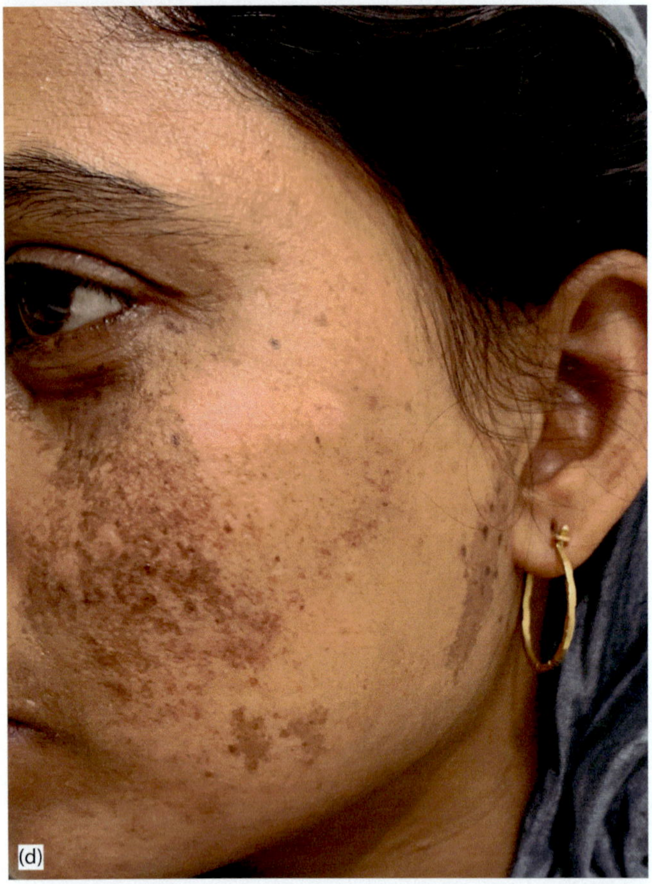

Figure 2.4 (*Continued*) **(c)** Nevus spilus on the trunk. **(d)** Zosteriform nevus spilus. (a–d – Courtesy: Dr. Piyush Kumar, Katihar, India.)

- Speckled lentiginous nevus syndrome refers to a neurocutaneous condition in which ipsilateral neurological abnormalities are noted in association with SLN.
- Extracutaneous sign – Nevus spilus may be associated with phacomatosis pigmentovascularis; phacomatosis pigmentokeratotica; and facial features, anorexia, cachexia, eye, and skin lesions (FACES) syndrome.
- DD: Partial unilateral lentiginosis, café-au-lait macules.

## Congenital melanocytic nevus (CMN)

- Congenital melanocytic nevus is a benign proliferation of melanocytes in nests (nevus cells) in epidermis and dermis.
- This asymptomatic condition usually presents at birth but may appear later on in the first two years of life (sometimes referred to as CMN tardive).
- These present as single or multiple, round or oval, well-demarcated pigmented patches and plaques. They may have increased hair growth (hypertrichosis), and the surface may be papular, rough, warty, or cerebriform with time.
- Though many more classification systems exist, they are usually classified as small (<1.5 cm in diameter), medium (1.5–19.9 cm), and large or giant nevi (20 cm or greater) (**Figure 2.5a,b**).
- The large or giant nevi is surrounded by satellite naevi.
- Over time, CMN may darken or lighten and may develop a more heterogeneous or homogeneous pigmentation. There is an increase in hair growth, and the surface becomes irregular and rough (**Figure 2.5c,d**). Usually the lesion becomes thicker and develops nodularity. Rarely the lesion may develop a halo phenomenon and may regress spontaneously.
- Giant CMN – It usually affects the trunk and extremities. It may affect more than one body segment and may be present in "bathing trunk," "stole," or "coat sleeve" distribution. Satellite lesions are frequent. When a limb is affected, the limb may have a reduced girth. Risk of developing melanoma in giant CMN is high, and such melanoma carries a poor prognosis.
- Neurocutaneous melanosis (NCM) is characterized by the presence of benign or malignant melanocytic proliferations in the leptomeninges associated with the occurrence of congenital melanocytic lesions (one giant CMN, or three or more CMNs). Central nervous system symptoms result from increased intracranial pressure and include headache, vomiting, irritability, increased head circumference, seizures, papilledema, and sometimes cranial nerve palsies.
- DD: Becker's nevus, nevus of Ota/Ito.

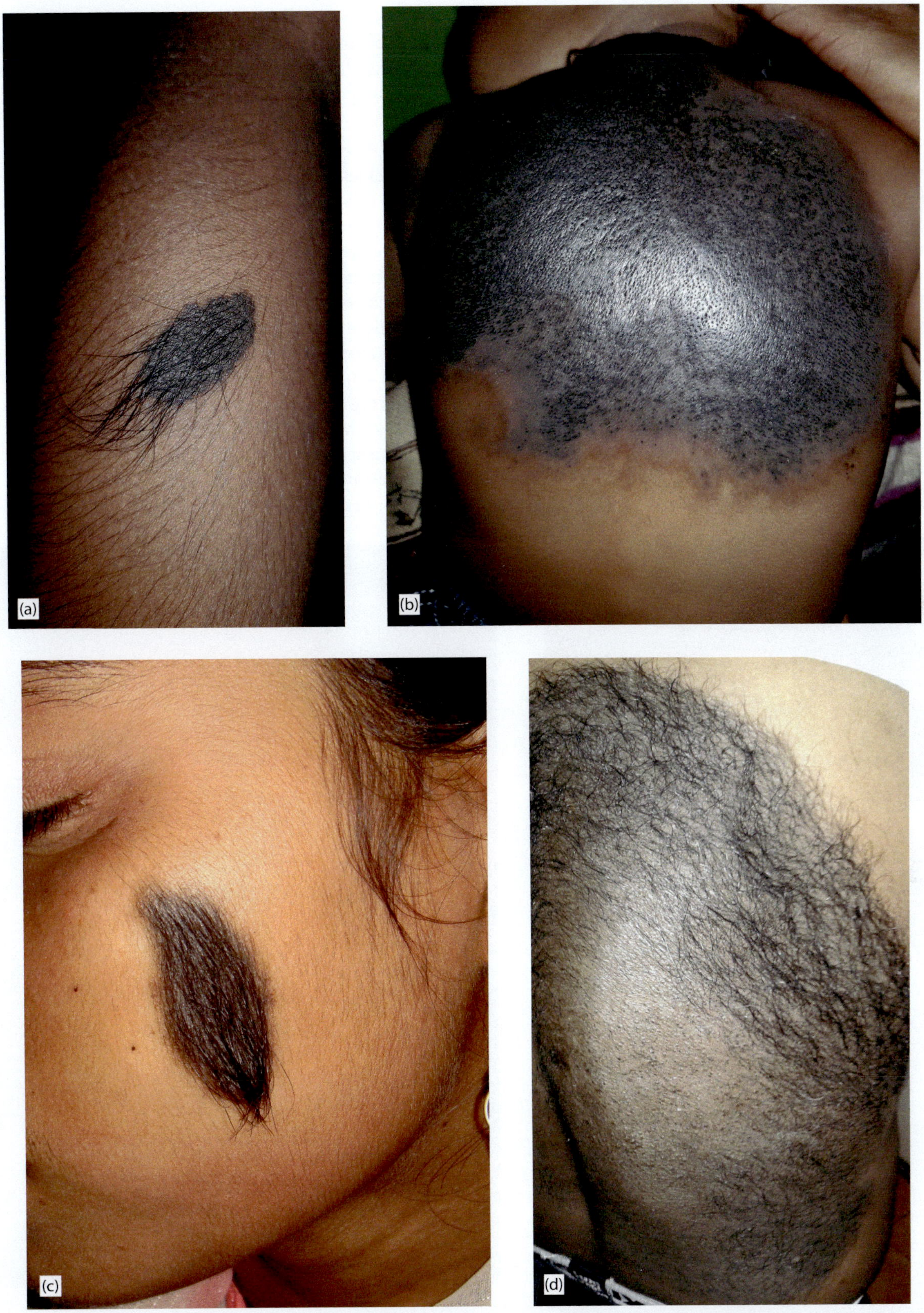


Figure 2.5 **(a)** Well-defined, black patch with lesional hypertrichosis in congenital melanocytic nevus (CMN). **(b)** Giant congenital melanocytic nevus (CMN) on the back of an infant. **(c)** Lesional hypertrichosis in CMN. **(d)** Giant CMN with hypertrichosis. (c – Courtesy: Dr. Piyush Kumar, Katihar, India.)

## Lichen planus pigmentosus (LPP)

- This is a variant of lichen planus with unknown etiology.
- It most commonly occurs in young to middle-aged adults, with an increased predilection in darker-skinned people.
- Triggering factors are sunlight, hepatitis C infection, exposure to dye, and application of mustard oil or amla oil.
- The disease usually starts on the face and neck, spreading later to the upper extremities and trunk.
- The initial lesions are small, brown, oval macules with diffuse borders. Later, they merge to form pigmented areas that are gray or brown (**Figure 2.6a–c**).
- The pigmentation may be diffuse, reticulate, blotchy, or perifollicular. The patches are usually symmetrical in distribution but may be found in a segmental, zosteriform, or Blaschkoid pattern.
- The rare sites of involvement are axilla, inframammary area, and groin; palm, soles, oral mucosa, and nails are spared.
- Lesions are asymptomatic, but mild pruritus and burning can be seen in some patients.
- DD: Erythema dyschromicum perstans (raised erythematous border and lesions in sun-protected areas), fixed drug eruption, actinic lichen planus (fine scaling over violaceous lesions).

## Freckles (ephelides)

- Freckles are an acquired pigmentary condition.
- The condition typically affects sun-exposed areas.
- Both genetic and environmental factors have role in its development.
- Both the sexes are affected.
- It may occur in any age group and race, with predominance among skin types I and II.
- It is characterized by brown macules of irregular shape and < 0.5 cm of size (**Figure 2.7**).
- It is typically seen on sun-exposed areas such as face, neck, shoulder, and dorsum of hand.
- Summer aggravation is also characteristic, with fading of lesion during winter.
- DD: Lentigines.

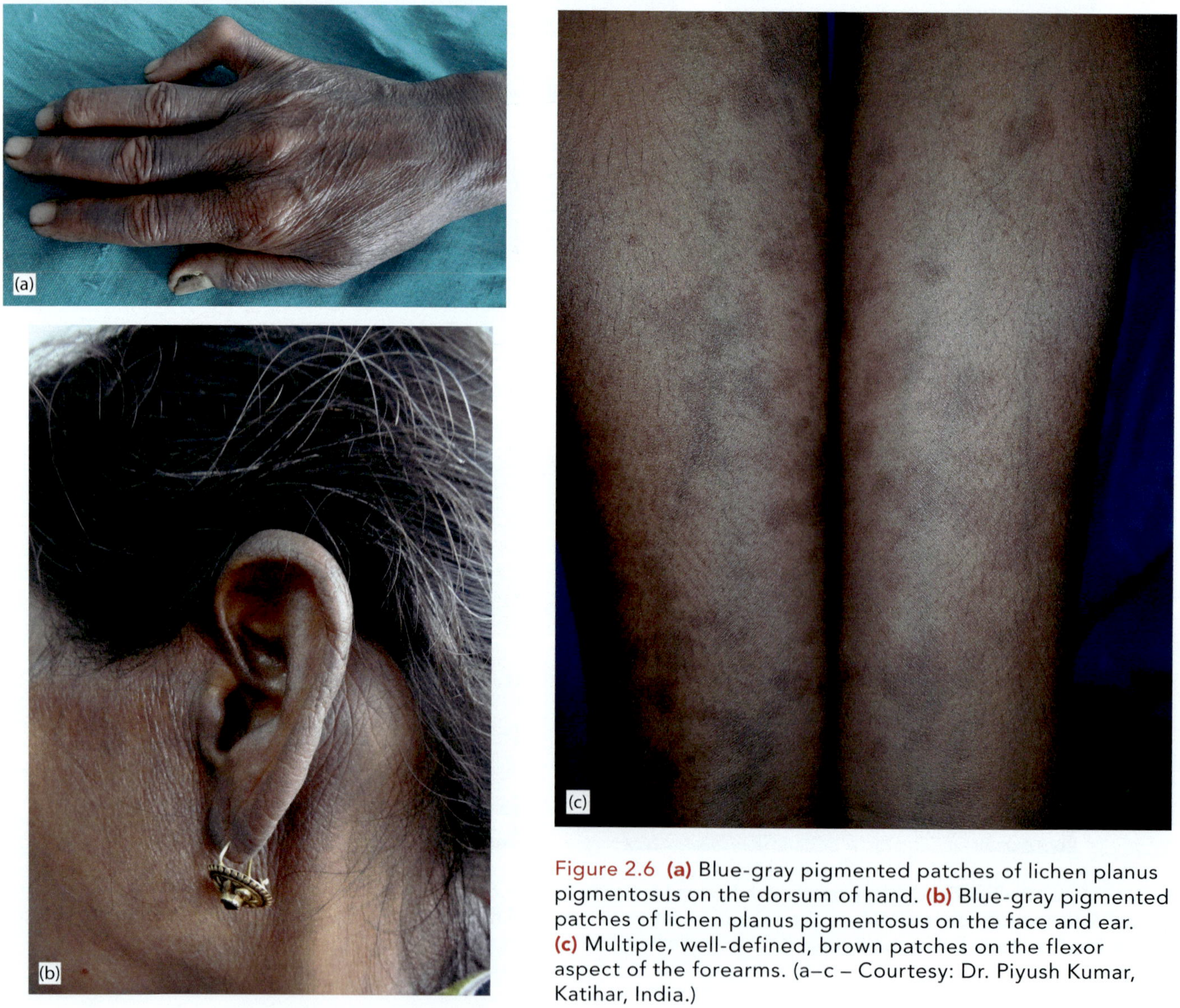


Figure 2.6 **(a)** Blue-gray pigmented patches of lichen planus pigmentosus on the dorsum of hand. **(b)** Blue-gray pigmented patches of lichen planus pigmentosus on the face and ear. **(c)** Multiple, well-defined, brown patches on the flexor aspect of the forearms. (a–c – Courtesy: Dr. Piyush Kumar, Katihar, India.)

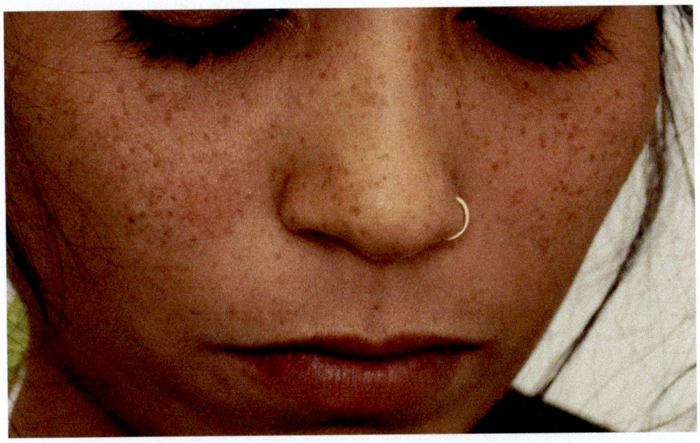

Figure 2.7 Multiple brown macules on the sun-exposed parts of the face. (Courtesy: Dr. Piyush Kumar, Katihar, India.)

## Solar lentigo

- This is an acquired benign pigmentary skin condition due to chronic sun exposure.
- Synonyms are sun spots, liver spots, or senile lentigo.
- It is most commonly seen in the 30 to 50 year old age group but can occur in any age group having chronic exposure to sun.
- It is not associated with any systemic condition.
- The condition is typically seen in fair-skinned individuals with red hair.
- It is most commonly seen on the face, shoulder, upper chest, and dorsum of the hand.
- It presents as hyperpigmented, brown to black, round to oval macules in sun-exposed areas (**Figure 2.8a,b**).
- The macules gradually increase in size and number.
- In long-standing cases, many lesions coalesce to from larger lesions.
- DD: Lichenoid keratosis, seborrhoeic keratosis, junctional melanocytic nevus.

## Lentigo simplex

- This is the most common type of lentigo.
- The exact etiology of the condition is unknown, but both environmental and genetic factors are found to have a role in its development.
- It is seen in childhood but can appear at birth also.
- It may occur in both sexes and any age group, but genetically determined lesions are common among children.
- It is not associated with sun exposure or systemic disease.
- It is characterized by asymptomatic sharply defined, round to oval, dark-brown to black (evenly distributed

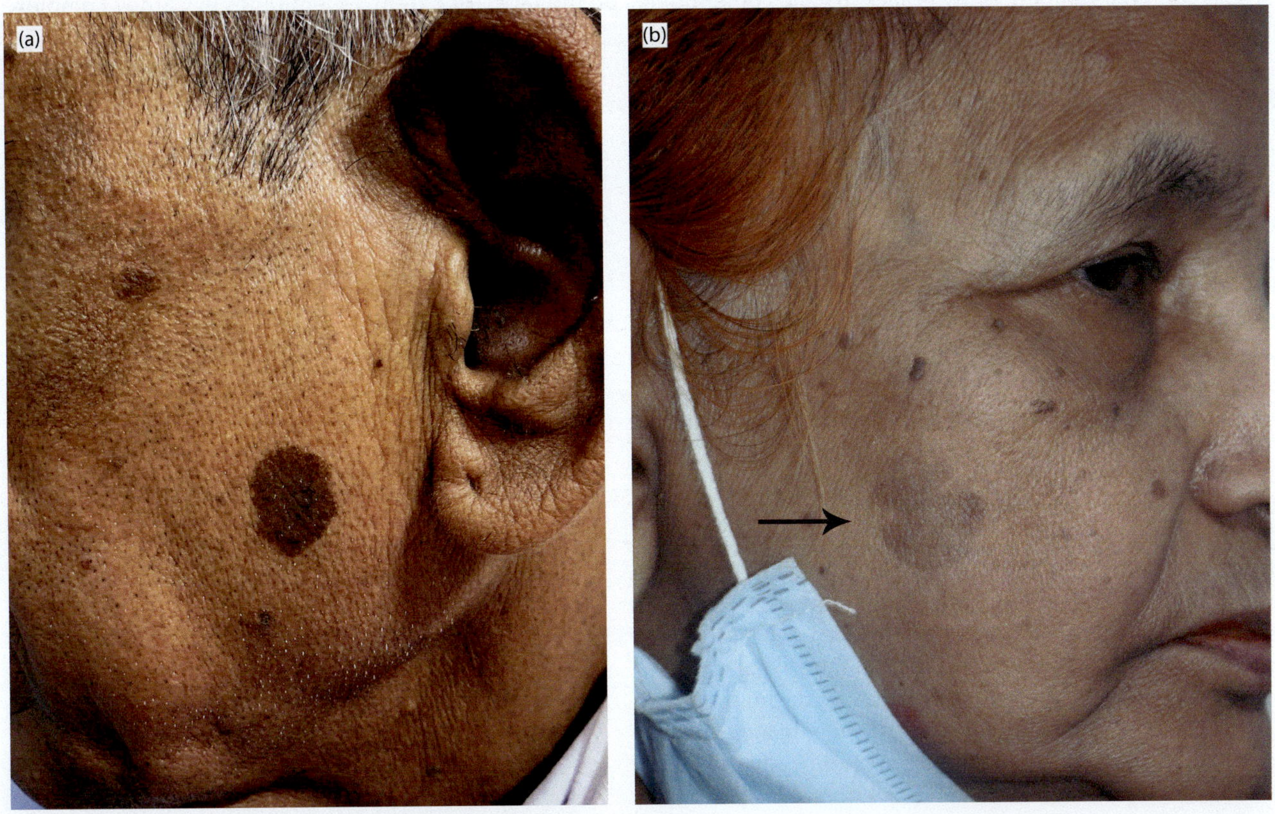


Figure 2.8 **(a)** Well-defined, brown-black, smooth-surfaced patch of solar lentigo. **(b)** Brown smooth-surfaced patch (arrow) of solar lentigo. Also, seborrheic keratosis are appreciable as pigmented papules. (a,b – Courtesy: Dr. Piyush Kumar, Katihar, India.)

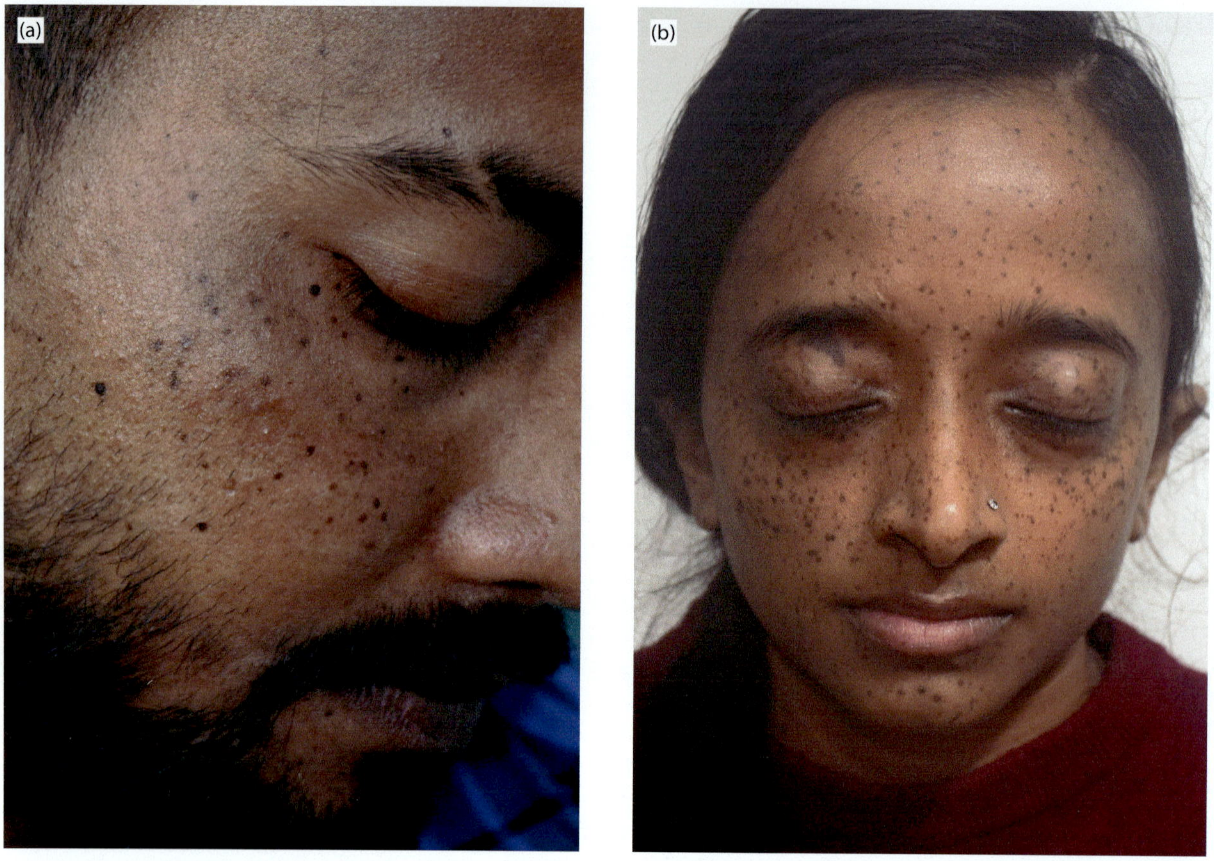

Figure 2.9 **(a)** Well-defined, brown-black macules of lentigines on the face. **(b)** Extensive lentigines in Carney complex. (Courtesy: Dr. Piyush Kumar, Katihar, India.)

pigmentation) macules that are 3–15 mm in diameter (**Figure 2.9a**).

- Lesions may occur anywhere in skin and mucosa and are not associated with sun exposure.
- Genetic syndromes associated with lentiginosis are Carney complex (**Figure 2.9b**), LEOPARD syndrome, Peutz-Jeghers syndrome, Bannayan-Riley-Ruvalcaba syndrome, progressive cribriform and zosteriform hyperpigmentation, phakomatosis pigmentovascularis, transient pustular melanosis, and multiple Mongolian spots.
- DD: Freckles, multiple lentigines syndrome.

## Segmental lentigines

- Lentigines are benign proliferation of melanocytes (without forming nests).
- Segmental lentigines have their onset in early childhood and do not aggravate on sun-exposure.
- The patient presents with numerous, grouped, brown to black lentigines within an area of normal skin, along one or more dermatomes, and the lesion respects the midline (**Figure 2.10**). The lesions may be unilateral or bilateral or present in a checkerboard pattern or in midline clusters.

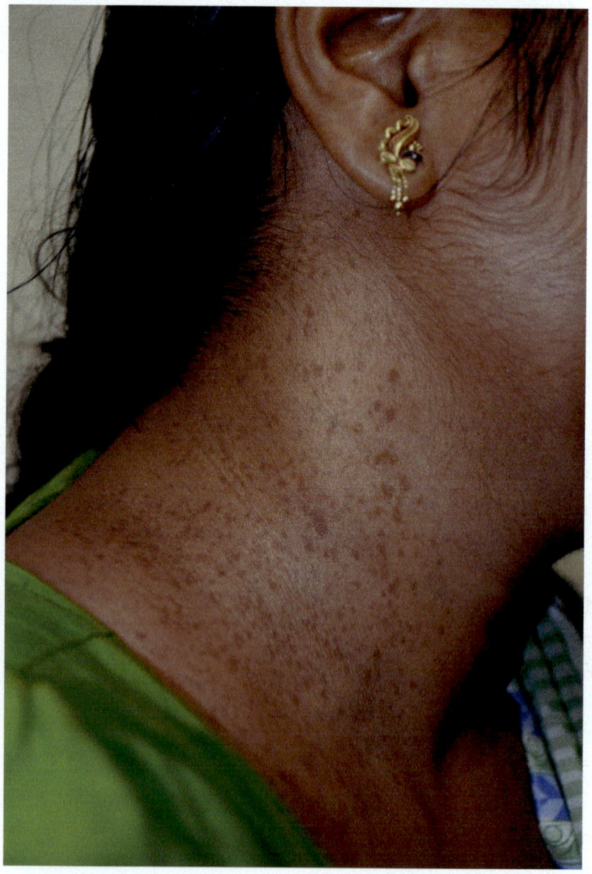

Figure 2.10 Lentigines in segmental distribution. The intervening skin between the macules appears normally pigmented. (Courtesy: Dr. Piyush Kumar, Katihar, India.)

- DD: Nevus spilus (background skin is tan to light-brown patch).

## Melasma

- It typically affects women of reproductive age with Fitzpatrick skin types IV–VI, though the condition can occur in men also.
- Genetic predisposition; ultraviolet (UV) radiation exposure; hormonal factors such as female sex hormones, thyroid disease, pregnancy, taking contraceptive pills; and drugs like phenytoin are known risk factors.
- Pigmentation usually fades after delivery or on stopping the pill, but it may persist.
- It manifests as symmetric hyperpigmented macules, and patches on the face, involving the forehead, cheeks, and moustache area and occasionally V-area of the neck. The lesions darken after sun exposure.
- According to the distribution of lesions, three clinical patterns of melasma are recognized:
    1. Centrofacial pattern is the most common pattern and involves the forehead, cheeks, upper lip, nose, and chin (**Figure 2.11a,b**).
    2. Malar pattern involving the cheeks and nose (**Figure 2.11c**).
    3. Mandibular pattern involving the ramus of the mandible.

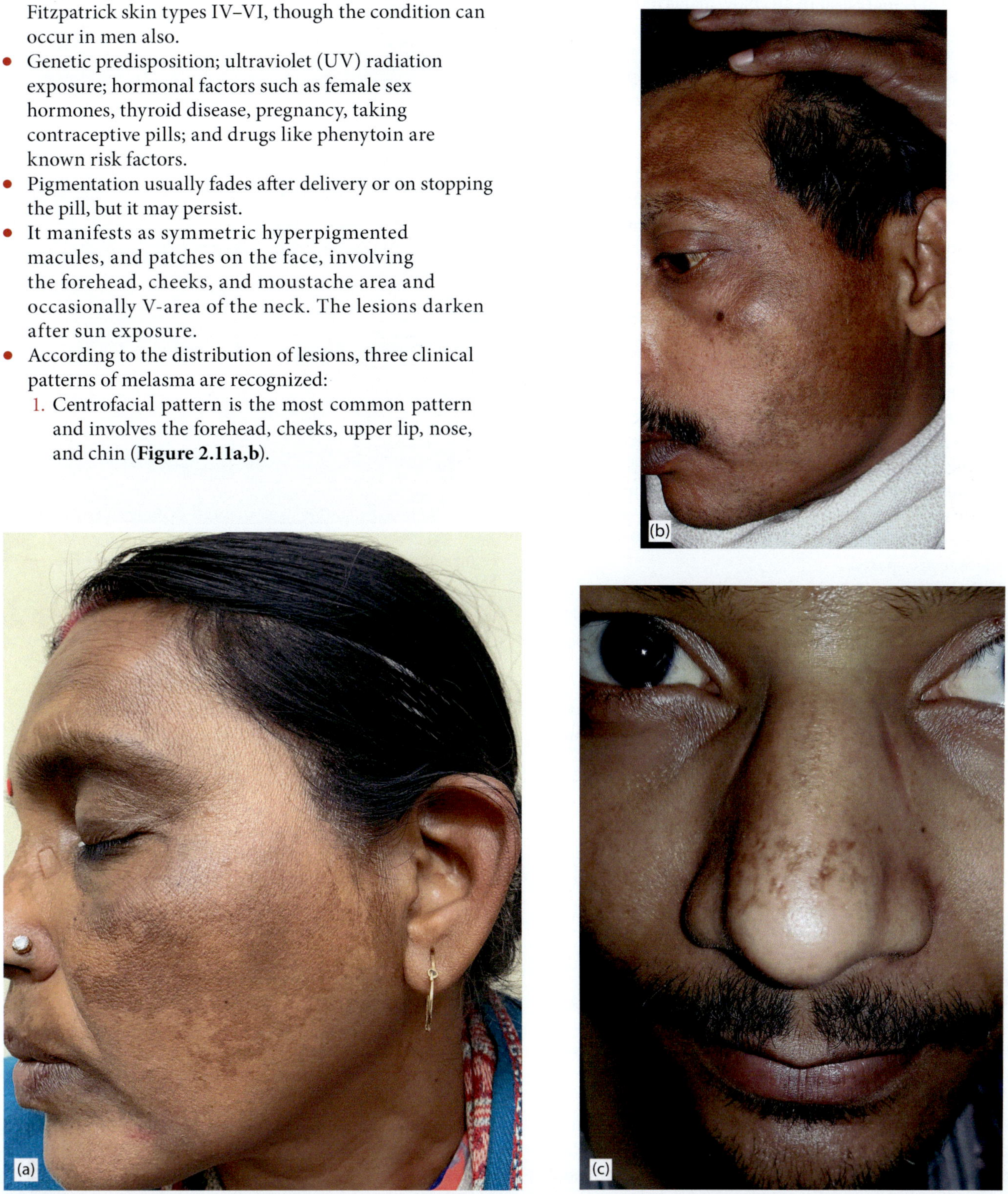


Figure 2.11 **(a)** Melasma as brown-pigmented patches on the cheek, forehead, nose, and upper lip area. **(b)** Melasma in a man. **(c)** Melasma affecting the nasal tip. (a,b – Courtesy: Dr. Piyush Kumar, Katihar, India.)

- Using the Wood's light examination, melasma can be classified into four major histological types depending upon the depth of pigment deposition:
  1. Epidermal type: Pigmentation is intensified under Wood's light and is the most common type. Melanin is increased in all epidermal layers.
  2. Dermal type: There is no accentuation of pigmentation under Wood's light.
  3. Mixed type: Pigmentation becomes more apparent in some areas, while in others there is no change.
  4. Indeterminate type: Pigment is apparent in the Wood's light in individuals with skin type VI.
- DD: Freckles, solar lentigo, Riehl's melanosis, post-inflammatory hyperpigmentation, frictional melanosis, ochronosis (endogenous and exogenous), acanthosis nigricans.

### Erythema dyschromicum perstans (EDP)

- It is present in the second to third decade of life but can occur even in younger patients.
- Individuals with skin phototypes III and IV are more frequently affected.
- It presents as symmetrical distribution of slate-gray to brown-blue asymptomatic macules and patches of variable shapes and sizes (0.5–3 cm).
- It is mostly distributed over the face, neck, trunk, and proximal upper extremities. The palms, soles, and scalp are rare sites of involvement.
- Mucosae are spared.
- Mild pruritus can be noted.
- Early lesions present with a thin, raised, erythematous border that tends to resolve over months.
- Peripheral hypopigmentation can be seen in older lesions.
- DD: Lichen planus pigmentosus (dark brown macules, sun-exposed areas), lichenoid drug eruptions (PIH and alopecia), generalized fixed drug eruptions (sharply demarcated, dusky, violaceous hue).

### Actinic lichen planus (LP)

- Actinic LP is a variant of LP seen mostly in dark-skinned people. Unlike classical LP, Koebner phenomenon is not seen in actinic LP.
- The condition is mostly noted in young adults, and onset is frequently in spring and summer.
- Actinic LP typically affects the sun-exposed areas. The lateral aspects of the forehead, the dorsa of hands, the extensor parts of upper extremities, the lower lips, the cheeks, and the neck are the most commonly involved sites. Sun-covered areas may be involved rarely (**Figure 2.12**).
- Oral mucosa and nails are spared. The most common clinical presentation is single or multiple annular plaques with thready rolled border and hyperpigmented center. The lesions are frequently surrounded by a hypopigmented halo.

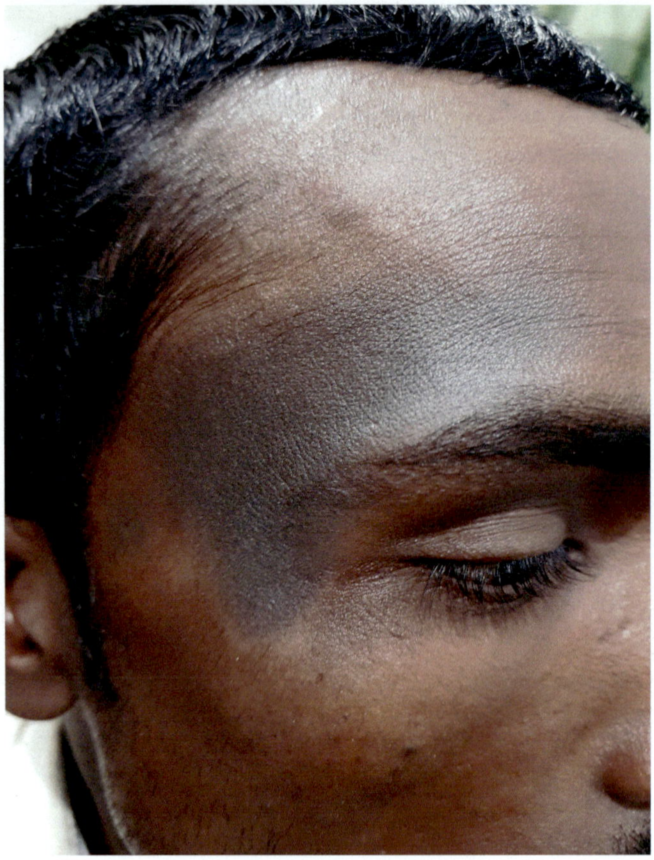

Figure 2.12 Well-defined gray-black patch of actinic lichen planus with perilesional halo.

- Lichenoid papules and plaques may occur simultaneously with annular lesions or may occur independently as a sole manifestation of actinic LP.
- DD: Fixed drug eruption, actinic prurigo, actinic keratosis, lichenoid drug eruption, granuloma annulare.

### Post-Chikungunya pigmentation (PCP)[10]

- Chikungunya fever is an acute, usually self-limiting, febrile illness caused by the Chikungunya virus.
- In the acute stage, the patient complains of fever, intense asthenia, arthralgia, myalgia, headache, sore throat, conjunctivitis, and maculopapular or other skin eruptions.
- Pigmentation develops usually two weeks after the rash, when febrile symptoms have already subsided; hence, the pigmentation is called post-Chikungunya pigmentation.
- Pigmentation manifests as hyperpigmented macules and patches over the nose (chik sign) and cheeks without any preceding erythema during the febrile illness (**Figure 2.13**). However, the pigmentation may also involve the trunk, flexures, palmar creases, and mucosa.
- Other patterns of pigmentation are discrete confetti-like macules, freckle-like, diffuse, flagellate, Addisonian

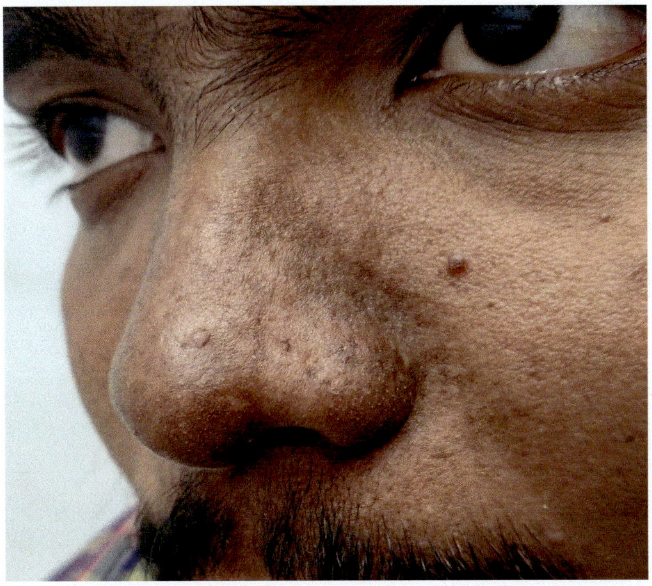

Figure 2.13 Post-chikungunya nasal tip pigmentation (chik sign). (Courtesy: Dr. Deverashetti Srinivas, Nizamabad, India.)

type of palmar pigmentation, periorbital melanosis, and pigmentation of pre-existing acne lesions.
- Patients may have persistent asthenia and joint pain in the convalescence period.
- DD: Melasma, freckles, and lentigines (PCP has an acute onset and follows febrile illness).

## Nevus of Hori[11]

- This is also known as acquired bilateral nevus of Ota-like macules (ABNOM) and nevus fuscocaeruleus zygomaticus.
- It is mostly seen in Asian women after the third decade of life.
- It presents as asymptomatic, multiple, speckled brown or slate-gray macules occurring bilaterally on malar regions without ocular or mucosal pigmentation (**Figure 2.14**).
- Forehead, upper eyelids, cheeks, and nose are less commonly affected.
- The color of lesions varies with the maturity of the lesions. Initially, these macules are usually brown and discrete and become bluish-gray and diffuse over the time.
- This may coexist with other facial pigmentary disorders like melasma, freckles, solar lentigines, and nevus of Ota.
- DD: Nevus of Ota (mucosal and conjunctival involvement), melasma, Riehl's melanosis.

## Periorbital hyperpigmentation

- Dark circles or periorbital hyperpigmentation is a common complaint affecting individuals of both genders of all ages and races.
- The condition is characterized by bilateral homogeneous hyperchromic areas in the periorbital region.
- Lesions may vary in intensity according to fatigue or lack of sleep and may worsen with aging due to sagging, thinning of skin, and loss of subcutaneous fat.

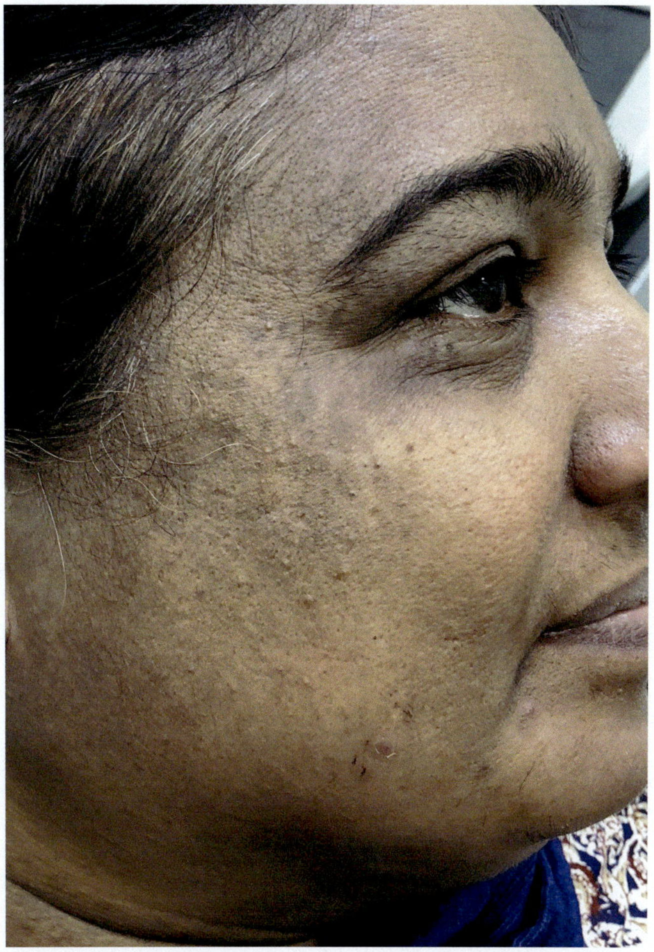

Figure 2.14 Speckled, slaty gray macules on side of the face in nevus of Hori in a woman. (Courtesy: Dr. Zubin Mandlewala, Mumbai, India.)

## Atopic dirty neck

- Atopic dirty neck is acquired hyperpigmentation, characteristically seen in patients with atopic dermatitis.
- Pigmentation has a rippled pattern; it occurs due to the combined effect of both frictional melanosis and post-inflammatory hyperpigmentation in patients with atopic dermatitis.
- It is aggravated by itching, heat and sweat.
- It usually affects the anterolateral aspect of neck, axilla, and flexures.
- DD: Acanthosis nigricans.

## Poikiloderma of Civatte

- This condition is also known as cervical idiopathic poikiloderma.
- It is characterized by irregular pigmentary alterations, with hypo- and hyperpigmentation, superficial atrophies and telangiectasias (**Figure 2.15**).
- It is usually asymptomatic; burning or pruritus may be present rarely.

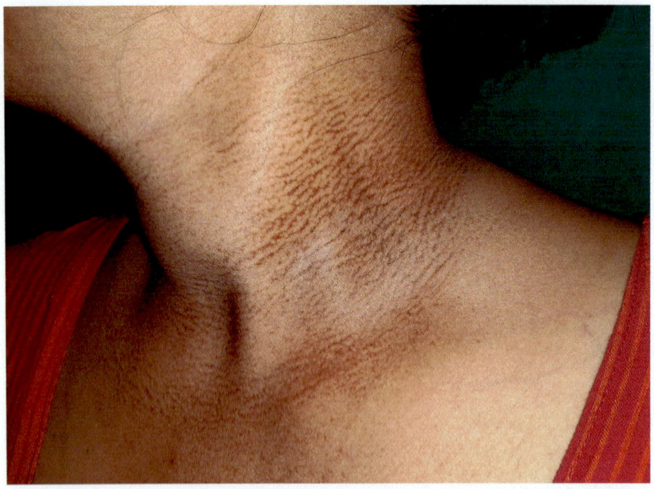

Figure 2.15 Reddish-brown, reticulate hyperpigmentation on neck in poikiloderma of Civatte. (Courtesy: Dr. Hiral Shah, Baroda Medical College, Vadodara, India.)

- Pigmentation is reticulate, reddish to brown, irregular and symmetrically distributed.
- It affects the face, neck, and upper third of chest; it spares the shaded chin area.
- DD: Acanthosis nigricans, atopic dirty neck, pigmented contact dermatitis.

## Schamberg's disease

- This is an acquired condition characterized by extravasation of erythrocytes in the skin with marked hemosiderin deposition.
- Risk factors are hypertension, diabetes mellitus, venous stasis, strenuous exercise, and occupations involving prolonged standing.
- The legs are affected in a bilateral symmetrical manner. Rarely, other sites such as the trunk and upper extremities may be involved (**Figure 2.16**).
- The initial clinical presentation is characteristic orange-brown, speckled macules and papules (cayenne pepper–like spots).
- In most cases, lesions rarely progress proximal to the knee.
- DD: Venous stasis, post-inflammatory hyperpigmentation, diabetic dermopathy.

## Diabetic dermopathy

- Diabetic dermopathy is characterized by light brown or reddish, oval or round, slightly indented scaly patches most often appearing on the shins.
- Although these lesions may appear in anyone, particularly after an injury or trauma to the area, they are one of the most common skin problems found in patients with diabetes mellitus.
- Established lesions are characterized by asymptomatic, round or elongated, brown, atrophic patches of 1 cm to 2.5 cm size.

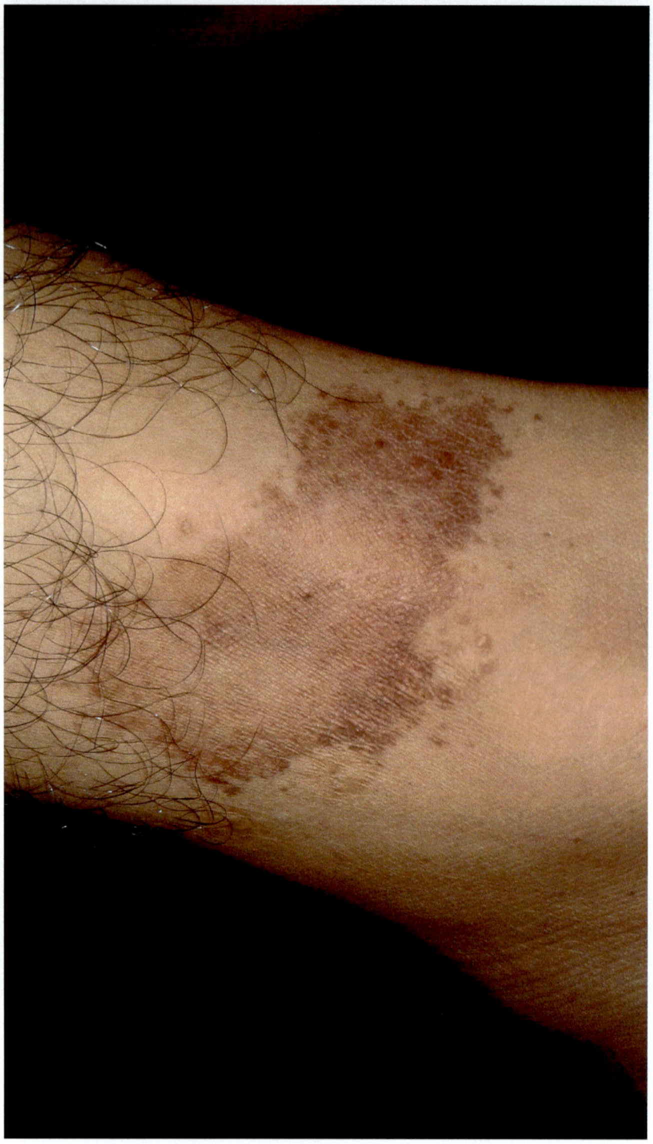

Figure 2.16 Localized brown macules and patches on the lower leg. Some erythematous macules are still appreciable.

- Individual lesions persist for months together (average 18–24 months), and then either the pigmentation fades or the lesion clears completely.
- DD: healed lesions of prurigo nodularis and lichen planus, pretibial myxedema.

## Acral lentiginous melanoma (ALM) (see Chapter E27)

- ALM presents as a slowly expanding, solitary, pigmented patch on the palm or sole. The lesion typically shows color variation (brown, blue-gray, black) and is flat and smooth-surfaced to begin with. Gradually the lesion becomes thicker and the surface shows hyperkeratosis, ulceration, and bleeding (**Figure 2.17a,b**).

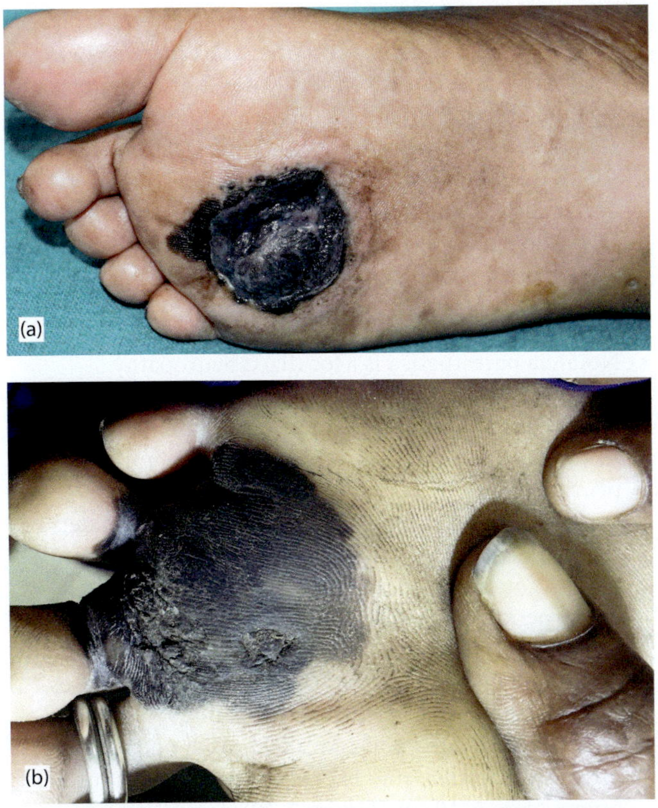


Figure 2.17 **(a)** solitary hyperpigmented patch on sole in acral lentiginous melanoma with surface ulceration and hyperkeratosis. **(b)** Acral lentiginous melanoma. (a – Courtesy: Dr. Piyush Kumar, Katihar, India; b – Courtesy: Dr. Sasi Kiran Attili, Visakha Institute of Skin and Allergy, Visakhapatnam, India.)

- Clinical pointers of ALM (ABCDE)
  - **A**symmetry of lesion
  - **B**order – irregular
  - **C**olor – variegated
  - **D**iameter – > 6 mm
  - **E**volution – increasing size and thickness; development of ulceration

## Pityriasis versicolor (tinea versicolor)

- Though hypopigmented lesions are more common, some patients may develop hyperpigmented lesions too. Sometimes, both types of lesions co-exist.
- The lesions may be asymptomatic or mildly itchy.
- A history of hyperhidrosis is often present.
- It commonly affects the trunk, neck, and arms.
- Patients present with hyperpigmented macules and patches with bran-like (furfuraceous) scales (**Figure 2.18**).
- Lesions start at perifollicular locations and coalesce to form bigger patches.
- Stretching the skin of hyperpigmented scaly macules and patches reveals fine scaling (Besnier sign).

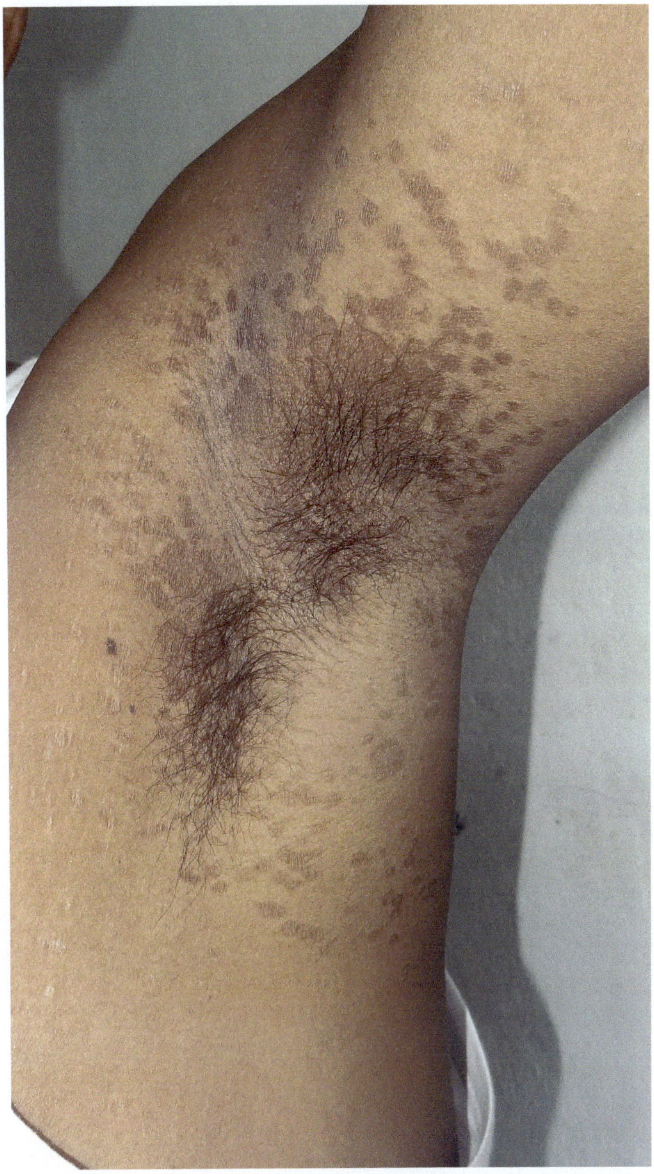

Figure 2.18 Pityriasis versicolor seen as hyperpigmented patches with fine scaling. (Courtesy: Dr. Piyush Kumar, Katihar, India.)

- Wood's lamp examination – yellow green fluorescence.
- DD: Post-inflammatory hyperpigmentation (for hyperpigmented lesions of PV).

## Acquired brachial cutaneous dyschromatosis (ABCD)[12]

- ABCD is an acquired pigmentary disorder of unknown etiology. Chronic sun-exposure is thought to play a role.
- This condition is mostly reported in older women.
- ABCD presents as asymptomatic, reticulated, gray-brown patches with an irregular geographical border, interspersed with hypopigmented macules, present bilaterally on the extensor surface of the forearms.
- DD: Extrafacial melasma, macular amyloidosis.

## Becker's nevus

- Becker's nevus is an acquired disorder of pigmentation of unknown etiology. The lesional skin shows increased androgen receptors.
- This asymptomatic condition has its onset in the peripubertal period, with a male preponderance.
- The most commonly affected areas are the shoulder region, upper chest, and back.
- Patients present with asymptomatic, unilateral, irregular tan or brown patches. New pigmented macules and patches develop at the periphery and coalesce with the larger patch (**Figure 2.19a,b**). Frequently, thick hairs develop in and around the lesions several months after appearance of pigmentation. The central area in the patch thickens over time and develops acneiform lesions. Rarely, bilateral lesions may be observed.
- Becker's nevus syndrome occurs when Becker's nevus is found in association with unilateral breast hypoplasia and muscle, skin, and/or skeletal abnormalities.
- DD: Congenital melanocytic nevus, nevus of Ito, Linear and whorled nevoid hypermelanosis.

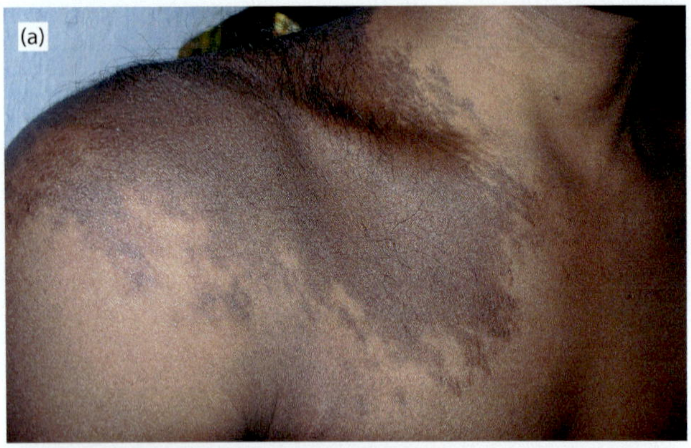


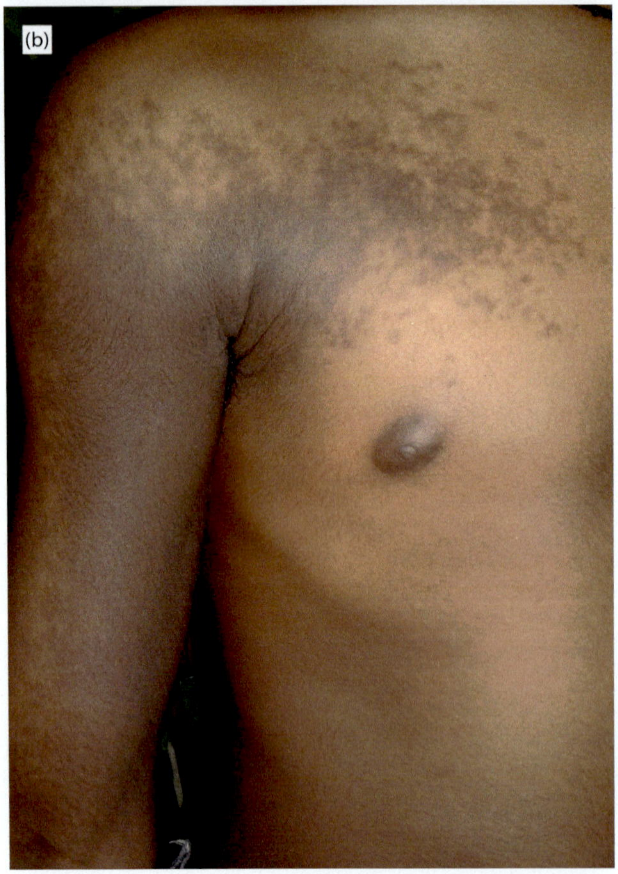


Figure 2.19 **(a)** Brownish patch with lesional hypertrichosis in Becker's nevus. **(b)** Becker's nevus involving right chest and arm. (a – Courtesy: Dr. Piyush Kumar, Katihar, India.)

## Notalgia paresthetica (NP)

- Notalgia paresthetica is a localized neuropathy and dysesthesia syndrome classically affecting the infrascapular area unilaterally. Many patients have associated cervical disease and/or brachioradial pruritus.
- The condition is primarily noted in adults and older populations and may have a female preponderance.
- Patient complains of localized burning, pain, tenderness, hyperalgesia, or dysesthesias. Infrascapular area is typically affected, but upper back, neck, scalp, and shoulder areas too may be affected in some cases.
- The skin finding is a unilateral, ill-defined, tan, or hyperpigmented non-indurated patch on the infrascapular area (mid back). The size of lesion usually ranges from 3–10 cm (**Figure 2.20**).
- Skin changes secondary to itching and chronic rubbing include excoriations, secondary infection, lichenification, lichen amyloid, eczematous changes, and xerosis.
- The disease runs a chronic course, with a natural tendency to wax and wane.
- DD: Macular amyloidosis, café-au-lait macule.

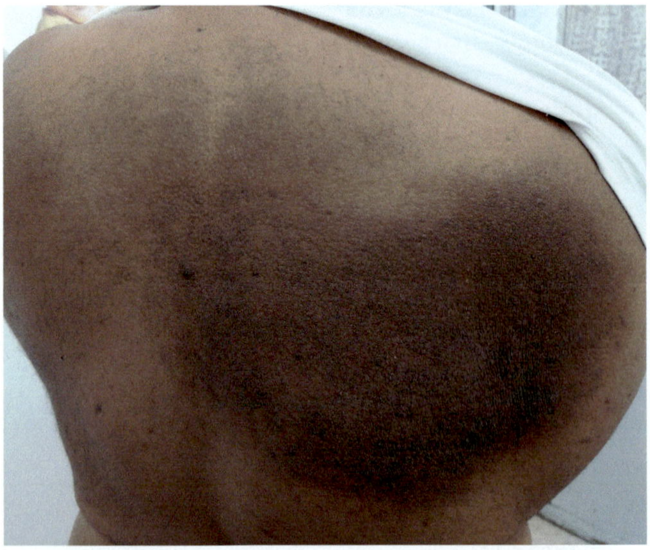

Figure 2.20 Localized pigmentation on the scapular region in notalgia paresthetica. Bottom part of lesion shows slight lichenification. (Courtesy: Dr. Deverashetti Srinivas, Nizamabad, India.)

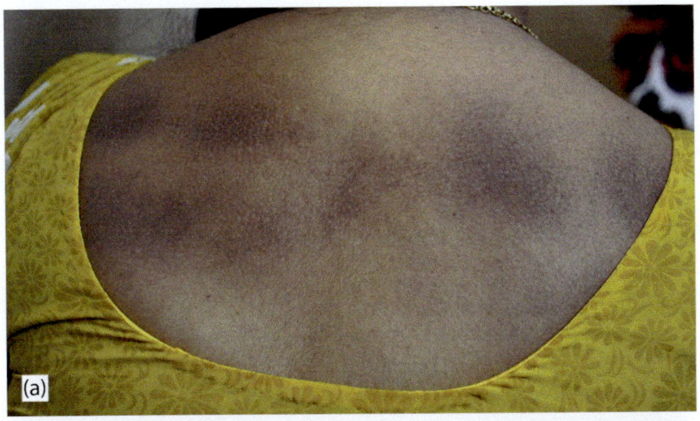

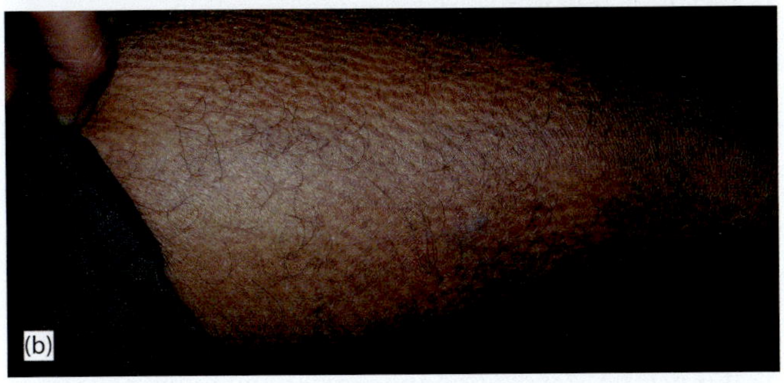

Figure 2.21 **(a)** Dirty-looking patch of pigmentation on the upper back in macular amyloidosis. **(b)** Pigmented macules in the rippled pattern in macular amyloidosis. (a,b – Courtesy: Dr. Piyush Kumar, Katihar, India.)

## Macular amyloidosis (MA)

- Macular amyloidosis (MA) is the most subtle form of cutaneous amyloidosis, characterized by brownish macules in a rippled pattern, distributed predominantly over the trunk and extremities.
- Clinically, MA presents as poorly delineated hyperpigmented patches of grayish-brown macules with a rippled pattern, associated with deposition of amyloid material in the papillary dermis (**Figure 2.21a,b**).
- The sites most commonly involved are the interscapular area and extremities (shins and forearms), although involvement of the clavicles, breast, face, neck, and axilla have also been reported.
- DD: Tinea versicolor, post-inflammatory hyperpigmentation, notalgia paresthetica.

## Lifa disease[13]

- Lifa disease (frictional dermal melanosis) is a common pigmentary disfiguring problem, especially among females, and is usually seen in the people in the Middle East and other parts of Asia.
- It most probably appears as a result of using rough washing agents during bathing, such as lifa, scrub pads, or nylon towels.
- The disease mainly affects slim subjects and is characterized by pigmentation that occurs bilaterally and symmetrically over bony prominences such as clavicular areas, upper back, upper arms, and shins (**Figure 2.22**).

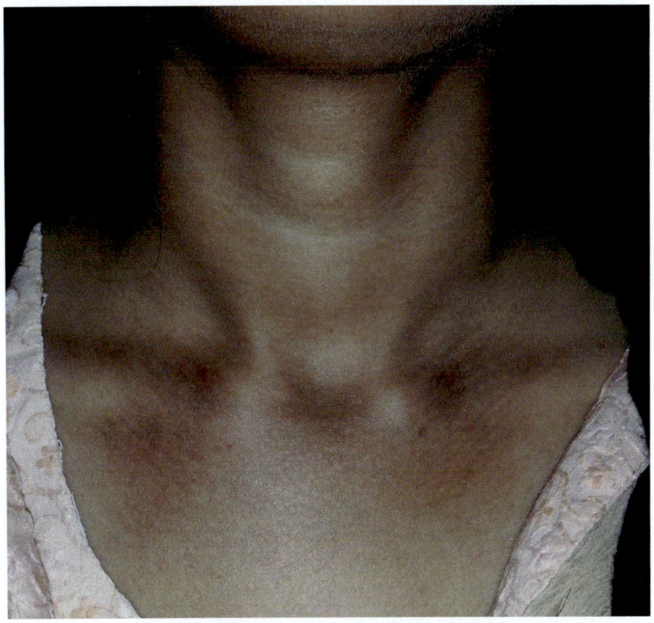

Figure 2.22 Localized pigmentation of the skin over clavicles in lifa disease. (Courtesy: Dr. Piyush Kumar, Katihar, India.)

- The epidermis, especially the basal layer, gets squeezed between the washing agent and the underlying bone, which leads to pigmentary incontinence.
- DD: macular amyloidosis, post-inflammatory hyperpigmentation.

## Post-inflammatory hyperpigmentation (PIH)[14]

- Post-inflammatory hyperpigmentation (PIH) is a common, acquired pigmentary disorder caused by various cutaneous endogenous inflammatory conditions, external injury, or cutaneous procedures (**Table 2.4**) and is common in dark-skinned individuals.

Table 2.4 Common causes of post-inflammatory hyperpigmentation

| | |
|---|---|
| Inflammatory dermatoses | Acne/acneiform eruption, eczema, psoriasis, lichen planus, dermatomyositis, lupus erythematosus, vasculitis, pemphigs vulgaris, bullous pemphigoid |
| Infections | Impetigo, viral exanthem, chickenpox, herpes zoster, dermatophytosis |
| Cutaneous adverse drug reactions | Phototoxic dermatitis, erythema multiforme, fixed drug eruption, Stevens-Johnson syndrome/toxic epidermal necrolysis |
| Dermatological procedures | Chemical peel, dermabrasion, laser treatment |
| Trauma | Mechanical trauma, friction |
| Miscellaneous | Neurotic excoriation, sunburn |

- There is a history of inflammatory dermatoses, trauma, or cutaneous procedures, and PIH lesions are preceded by erythema.
- Two clinical forms are recognized – epidermal and dermal. Some patients may have mixed patterns.
- Epidermal PIH presents as well circumscribed, light to dark brown macules and patches at the site of prior dermatoses/trauma, etc. (**Figure 2.23a,b**).
- Dermal PIH presents as blue-gray patches with ill-defined margins.
- Epidermal PIH may disappear spontaneously within months or years, whereas dermal PIH usually persists.
- PIH due to fixed drug eruption (FDE) is usually round and brown black or gray-blue black in color. The appearance of PIH is so characteristic that it allows recognition of prior FDE. History of intermittent erythema, edema, and burning on exposure to certain drug confirms the diagnosis of FDE (**Figure 2.23c**). Common offending drugs are analgesics, antibiotics, muscle relaxants, and anticonvulsants.
- Of note, pseudoephedrine, piroxicam, cotrimoxazole, sorafenib, and tadalafil may be associated with non-pigmenting FDE, and no PIH is seen.
- DD: Freckles, lentigines, melasma.

## Linea nigra

- Linea nigra is a physiological hyperpigmentation occurring during pregnancy.
- It is clinically characterized by linear hyperpigmentation that appears over the central abdomen during pregnancy; it is mainly seen in the darker-skinned population (skin types IV and V).
- It develops due to the combined effect of placental hormone, metabolic factors, and immunological factors; increased melanin production is associated with hyperestrogenic state of pregnancy.
- DD: Post-inflammatory hyperpigmentation.

## Progressive cribriform and zosteriform hyperpigmentation (PCZH)[15]

- This condition appears usually after the second decade of life.
- It presents as hyperpigmented, progressive, and asymptomatic macules and patches that are uniformly tan with zosteriform distribution with cribriform configuration.
- It is arranged in whorls and streaks and follows the lines of Blaschko.

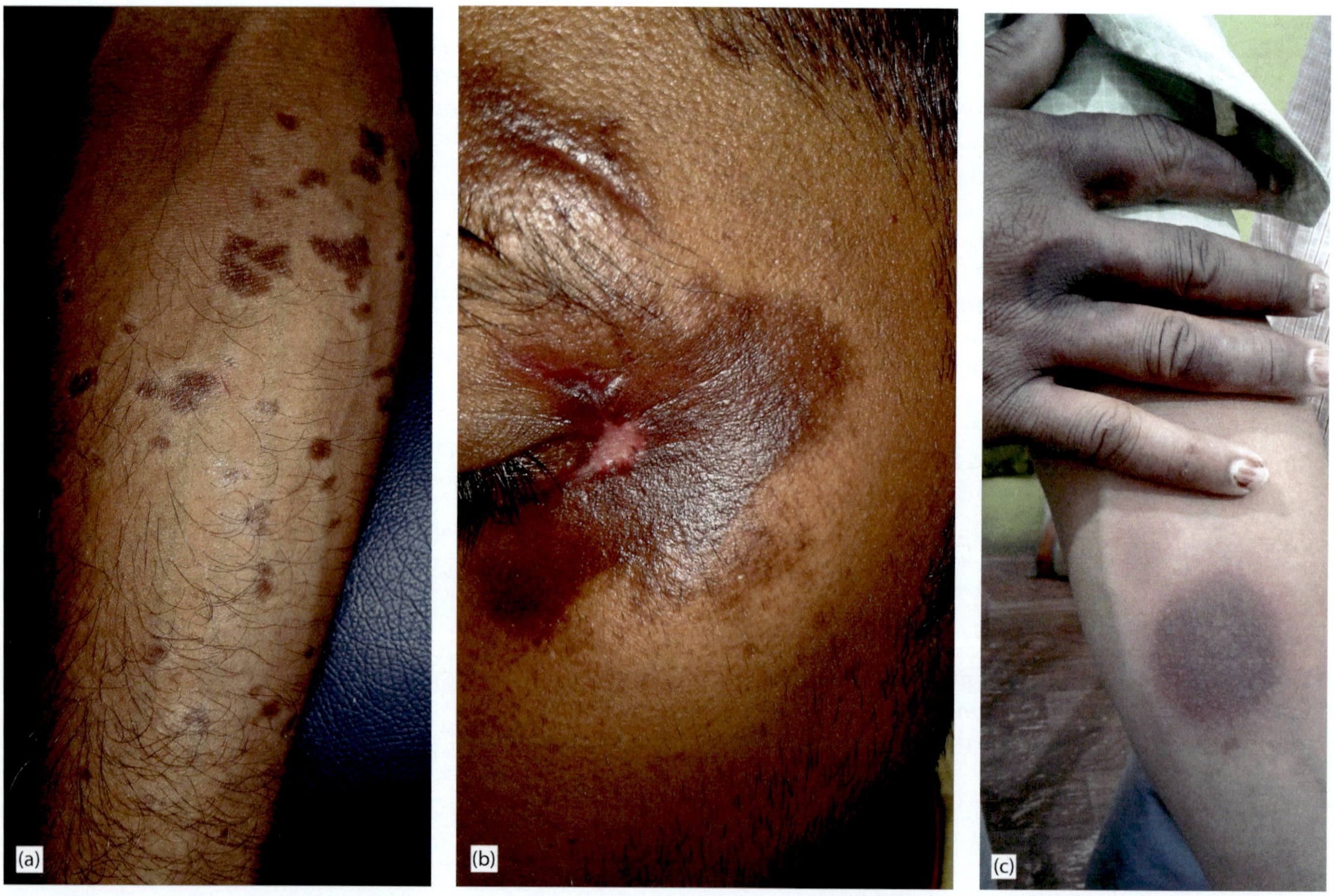


Figure 2.23 **(a)** Post-inflammatory hyperpigmentation following resolution of lichen planus. **(b)** Post-inflammatory hyperpigmentation after traumatic injury to skin. **(c)** Round-shaped, post-inflammatory hyperpigmentation following fixed drug eruption. Some erythema is appreciable as there is reactivation of lesions.

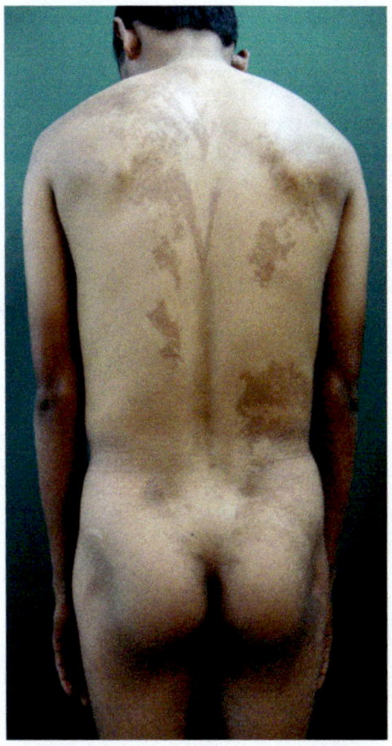

Figure 2.24 Hyperpigmented macules in a whorled pattern along Blaschko's lines in linear and whorled nevoid hypermelanosis. (Courtesy: Dr. Shekhar Neema, Armed Force Medical College, Pune, India.)

- The trunk is mainly involved, and it may extend into pubic areas.
- DD: Linear and whorled nevoid hypermelanosis (childhood), linear lichen planus (violaceous color), third stage of incontinentia pigmenti (congenital).

### Linear and whorled nevoid hypermelanosis (LWNH)[16]

- Linear and whorled nevoid hypermelanosis (LWNH) is a rare disorder of pigmentation.
- It is characterized by hyperpigmented macules in a streaky configuration along lines of Blaschko without preceding inflammation or atrophy (**Figure 2.24**).
- It is distributed mainly on the trunk and extremities, sparing palms, soles, and mucosae.
- The onset of hyperpigmentation usually occurs within the first few weeks of life and continues to progress for a year or two before stabilization.
- Various skeletal anomalies, central nervous system diseases (microcephaly, arhinencephaly and epilepsy), congenital heart diseases (ventricular septal defect and tetralogy of Fallot), psychomotor delay, deafness, and brachydactyly have been mentioned in the literature in association with LWNH.
- DD: Incontinentia pigmenti, hypomelanosis of Ito, epidermal nevus, PCZH (**Tables 2.5** and **2.6**).

Table 2.5 Difference between linear and whorled nevoid hypermelanosis and progressive cribriform and zosteriform hyperpigmentation

| LWNH | PCZH |
|---|---|
| Appear early in life, progress in first two years and then eventually stabilize | Usually appear after second decade of life |
| Diffuse lesions appearing in streaks and swirls | Localized pigmentation |
| Associated with other anomalies | No such association |

Table 2.6 Pigmentary mosaicism – the unifying concept[17,18]

- The term "pigmentary mosaicism" is proposed to encompass all pigment anomalies caused by chromosomal mosaicism. It refers to patterned hypo- or hyperpigmentation resulting from a clone of cells with altered ability to produce melanin.
- Three major clinical patterns are established:
  - Streaks and swirls following the Blaschko lines: It includes previously described entities like hypomelanosis of Ito, linear and whorled nevoid hypermelanosis, progressive cribriform and zosteriform hyperpigmentation, etc.
  - Segmental or "checkerboard" distribution: It includes segmental nevus depigmentosus, segmental pigmentation disorder, etc.
  - Phylloid (leaf-like) pattern: It includes leaf-like, pear-shaped, and oblong lesions of pigmentary alteration as seen in mosaic abnormalities of chromosome 13.
- Individuals showing pigmentary mosaicism may have multiple congenital abnormalities, developmental delays, and mental retardation.
- Sometimes both hypopigmented and hyperpigmented patches may be seen (cutis tricolor).

## REFERENCES


1. Stulberg DL, Clark N, Tovey D. Common hyperpigmentation disorders in adults: Part I. Diagnostic approach, café au lait macules, diffuse hyperpigmentation, sun exposure, and phototoxic reactions. Am Fam Physician 2003;68(10):1955–1960.
2. Stulberg DL, Clark N, Tovey D. Common hyperpigmentation disorders in adults: Part II. Melanoma, seborrheic keratoses, acanthosis nigricans, melasma, diabetic dermopathy, tinea versicolor, and post-inflammatory hyperpigmentation. Am Fam Physician 2003;68(10):1963–1968.
3. Vashi N, Kundu R. Congenital and inherited hyperpigmentation disorders. In: Stratman E, Corona R, editors. UpToDate. Available from https://www.uptodate.com/contents/congenital-and-inherited-hyperpigmentation-disorders
4. Taıeb A, Ezzedine K, Morice-Picard F. Diagnosis of some common and uncommon hyperpigmentation disorders in children. Dermatologica Sinica 2014;32:211–216.
5. Sori T, Jaisankar T J, Thappa DM, Nath AK. Hyperpigmentary disorders in children: A hospital-based study in a tertiary care center. Indian Dermatol Online J 2013;4:148–152.
6. Plensdorf S, Livieratos M, Dada N. Pigmentation disorders: Diagnosis and management. Am Fam Physician 2017;96(12):797–804.
7. Rendon MI. Hyperpigmentation disorders in Hispanic population in the United States. J Drugs Dermatol 2019;18(3):s112–s114.
8. Lipsker D, Lenormand C. Hyperpigmentations [Hyperpigmentation]. Ann Dermatol Venereol 2019;146(10):666–682.
9. Nieuweboer-Krobotova L. Hyperpigmentation: Types, diagnostics and targeted treatment options. J Eur Acad Dermatol Venereol 2013;27 Suppl 1:2–4.
10. Ghosh S, Das A, Kumar P. Chikungunya and pigmentation: A tale of two cases. Pigment Int 2018;5:59.

11. Park JM, Tsao H, Tsao S. Acquired bilateral nevus of Ota-like macules (Hori nevus): Etiologic and therapeutic considerations. J Am Acad Dermatol 2009;61(1):88–93.
12. Rongioletti F, Rebora A. Acquired brachial cutaneous dyschromatosis: A common pigmentary disorder of the arm in middle-aged women. J Am Acad Dermatol 2000;42(4):680–684.
13. Sharquie KE, Al-Dorky MK. Frictional dermal melanosis (lifa disease) over bony prominences. J Dermatol 2001;28(1):12–15.
14. Kaufman BP, Aman T, Alexis AF. Postinflammatory hyperpigmentation: Epidemiology, clinical presentation, pathogenesis and treatment. Am J Clin Dermatol 2018;19(4):489–503.
15. Das A, Bandyopadhyay D, Mishra V, Gharami RC. Progressive cribriform and zosteriform hyperpigmentation. Indian J Dermatol Venereol Leprol 2015;81:321–323.
16. Sinha P, Chatterjee M, Singh KK, Sood A. Linear and whorled nevoid hypermelanosis with depigmentation. Indian Dermatol Online J 2017;8:131–133.
17. Thapa R. Pigmentary mosaicism: An update. Indian J Dermatol 2008; 53(2):96–97.
18. Kromann AB, Ousager LB, Ali IKM, Aydemir N, Bygum A. Pigmentary mosaicism: a review of original literature and recommendations for future handling. Orphanet J Rare Dis. 2018;13(1):39.

## SUGGESTED READING

1. Dimitris Rigopoulos, Alexander C. Katoulis (Eds). Hyperpigmentation. 1st edition. 2017. CRC Press.
2. James J. Nordlund, Raymond E. Boissy, Vincent J. Hearing, Richard A. King, William S. Oetting, Jean-Paul Ortonne (Eds). The Pigmentary System: Physiology and Pathophysiology. 2nd edition. 2006. Blackwell Publishing Ltd.

# 3

# Acquired facial melanosis

PREETI SHARMA, ANUPAM DAS

## INTRODUCTION

Acquired facial melanosis is a common presentation in the dermatology out-patient department (OPD). It adversely affects the psycho-social life of the patient and creates a great diagnostic dilemma for the treating dermatologist, especially because of overlapping clinical presentations. This chapter discusses the clinical approach to common disorders causing facial melanosis, as outlined in **Figure 3.1** and **Table 3.1**.[1–5] Face may be involved in many congenital or acquired pigmentary disorders causing widespread involvement of the body; they are not discussed here.

### Melasma

- Melasma is common in darker individuals, more common in women than in men (9:1), and seen mostly in reproductive-age groups.
- Various risk factors implicated are
  1. Ultraviolet radiation
  2. Elevated levels of estrogens and progesterone(like in pregnancy)
  3. Thyroid disorders (Thyroid-stimulating hormone [TSH] and adrenocorticotropic hormone [ACTH] resemble α-melanocyte-stimulating hormone [α-MSH])
  4. Genetic factors
  5. Drugs like phenytoin, griseofulvin, NSAIDs, etc.
- Melasma presents as bilateral, symmetrical, asymptomatic, hyperpigmented macules over sun-exposed areas of the face (malar areas, nose, forehead, mandibular areas) (**Figure 3.2a–c**).
- The lesions tend to coalesce to form larger patches.
- The lesions may follow various patterns, such as blotchy, polycyclic, arcuate, and irregular.
- Facial melasma is clinically divided into the following three types:
  1. Centrofacial
  2. Malar
  3. Mandibular

Patients frequently develop more than one pattern of involvement.

- Extrafacial lesions are uncommon but may affect the neck, sternum, and forearms.
- DD: Ephelids, lentigines, acanthosis nigricans, pigmentary demarcation lines, Hori's nevus, exogenous ochronosis, Riehl's melanosis, lichen planus pigmentosus.

### Lichen planus pigmentosus (LPP)

- LPP, a variant of lichen planus, occurs more predominantly in Fitzpatrick skin types IV–VI.
- Various photosensitizers, such as cosmetic fragrances, hair dyes, and mustard oil, have also been implicated.
- Patient presents with symmetrical, diffuse or patchy, gray-brown to dark-brown macules and patches over sun-exposed areas and sun-protected flexural skin over inguinal and axillary areas (**Figure 3.3a–d**).
- Over time, lesions coalesce to form bigger patches and new lesions appear.
- The morphological variants that have been described are diffuse, reticular, blotchy, perifollicular, and annular.
- If it predominantly affects the trunk and flexural areas, it is known as LPP inversus, which is a variant of LPP. Sometimes, linear or variants overlapping with lichen planus can be present.
- DD: Erythema dyschromicum perstans (EDP), melasma, post-inflammatory hyperpigmentation, phytophotodermatitis (**Figure 3.3e**).

### Erythema dyschromicum perstans (EDP)

- EDP is also known as erythema chronicum figuratum melanodermicum, and ashy dermatosis of Ramirez.
- The exact etiology is not known; various factors, such as ammonium nitrite, cobalt, HIV, radiocontrast media, drugs (such as ethambutol, penicillin, and BZDs), and whipworm infestation, are implicated.
- EDP commonly affects the trunk and is distributed symmetrically. Face involvement may be seen.

DOI: 10.1201/9781351054225-7

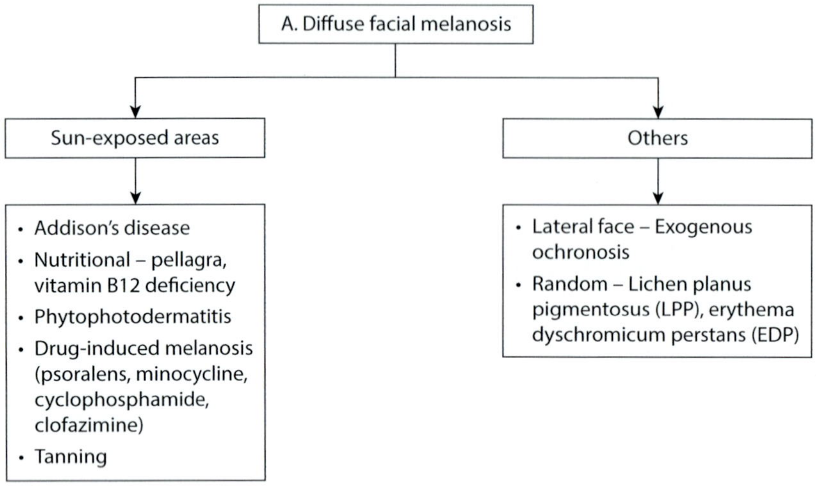


Figure 3.1 Approach to diffuse facial hyperpigmentation.

Table 3.1 Approach to acquired focal facial melanosis

| Site | Diseases |
|---|---|
| Periorbital | • Brown/brown-black – Pigmentary demarcation lines type F and G, periocular melanosis<br>• Slate-gray – Post-inflammatory hyperpigmentation due to fixed drug eruptions<br>• Blue-gray – nevus of Ota, nevus of Hori |
| Perioral | • Peribuccal pigmentation of Brocq<br>• Pigmentary demarcation line type H |
| Nose | • Nasal tip – melasma, post-Chikungunya pigmentation (chik sign)<br>• Alar groove – seborrheic melanosis<br>• Nasal salute (transverse nasal line – atopic dermatitis) |
| Malar area | • Predominantly discrete macules – freckles, lentigines<br>• Macules and patches<br>  ◦ Brown-black – melasma<br>  ◦ Blue-gray – nevus of Ota, nevus of Hori<br>• Scattered depigmented macules, caviar like papules – exogenous ochronosis |
| Cheeks/ lateral face | • Extending from infraorbital area – pigmentary demarcation lines<br>• Associated tiny papules – erythromelanosis follicularis faciei et colli<br>• Pebbly appearance, textural changes – acanthosis nigricans<br>• Others – Riehl's melanosis, maturational hyperpigmentation<br>• Lichen planus pigmentosus – face and flexures |
| Forehead | • Along hairline – Riehl's melanosis<br>• Convex areas – macular amyloidosis, frictional melanosis<br>• Concave areas – facial acanthosis nigricans<br>• Sun exposed – melasma |

- Early lesions start as erythematous macules with erythematous raised borders; they later develop brown or gray macules.
- DD: LPP (**Table 3.2**), Riehl's melanosis, Lichenoid drug reaction.

## Maturational pigmentation[6]

- This presents as darkening of sun-exposed skin in the fourth to fifth decade.

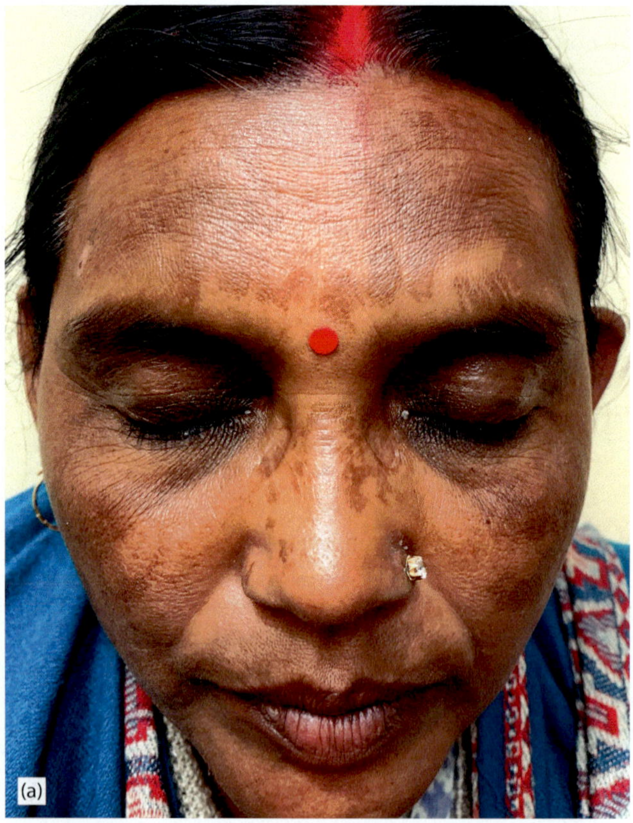


Figure 3.2 **(a)** Melasma as symmetric, brown patches on the face, mainly affecting forehead, cheeks, and nose. (*Continued*)

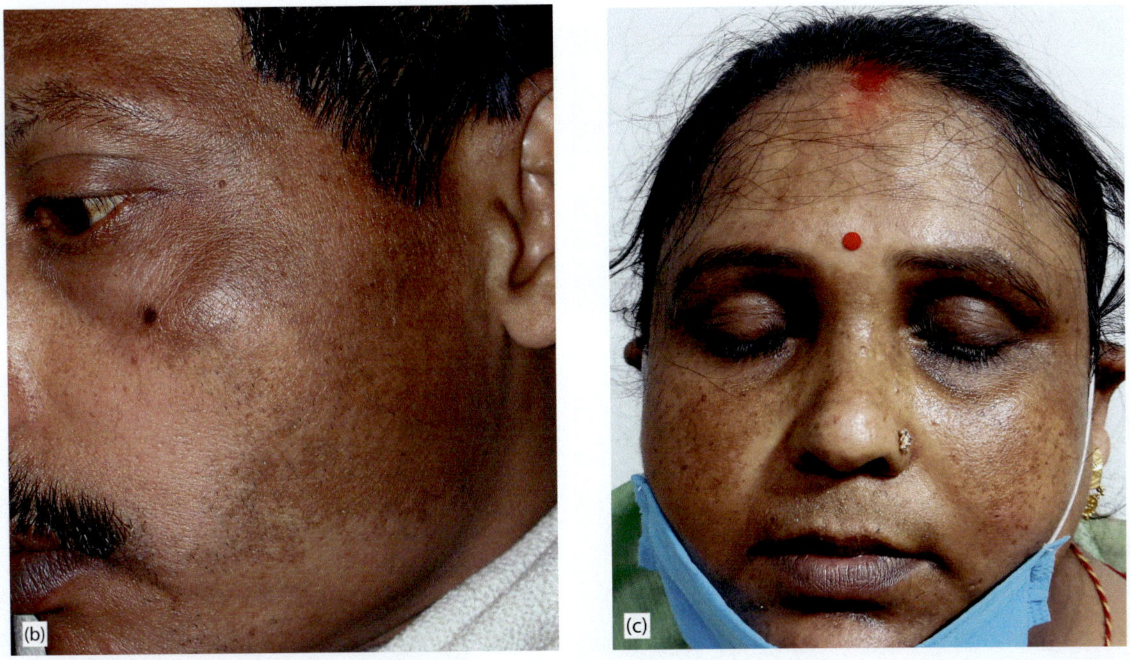

Figure 3.2 *(Continued)* **(b)** Melasma on lateral face in a middle-aged male. **(c)** Extensive melasma involving forehead, malar areas, and nose. Lentigines and freckles too are noted. (a–c – Courtesy: Dr. Piyush Kumar, Katihar, India.)

- It appears especially in skin types V and VI.
- It affects the lateral aspects of face (zygomatic areas) and merges with surrounding skin with blurred, ill-defined margins (**Figure 3.4a,b**).
- The dorsum of hands and feet may also be affected.
- The separate existence of this entity is debatable, and some authors consider it as early facial acanthosis nigricans or frictional melanosis.

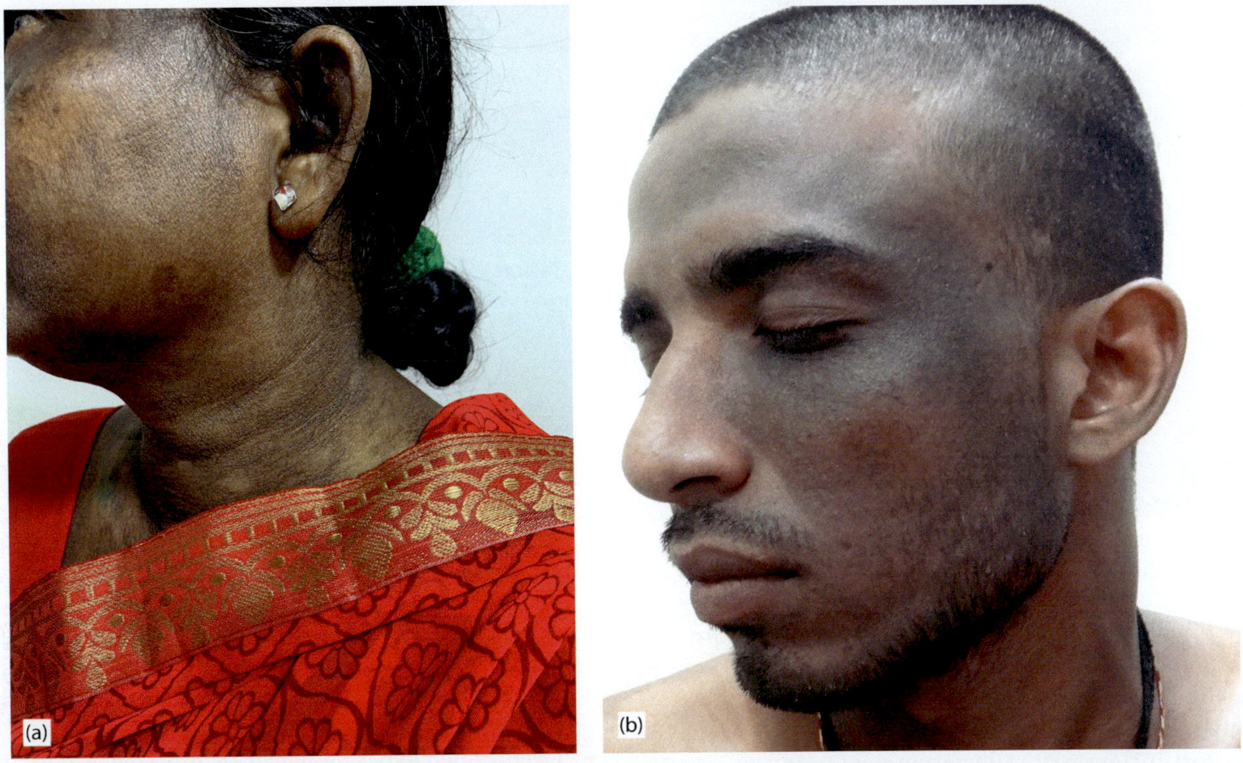

Figure 3.3 **(a)** Sometimes lichen planus pigmentosus may be extensive and may cause extensive involvement of the face and neck. **(b)** Diffuse lesions of lichen planus pigmentosus in a young male. *(Continued)*

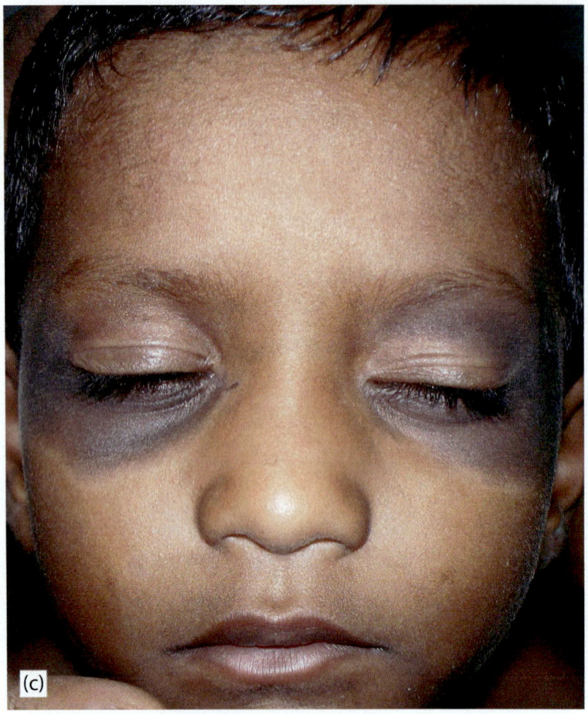

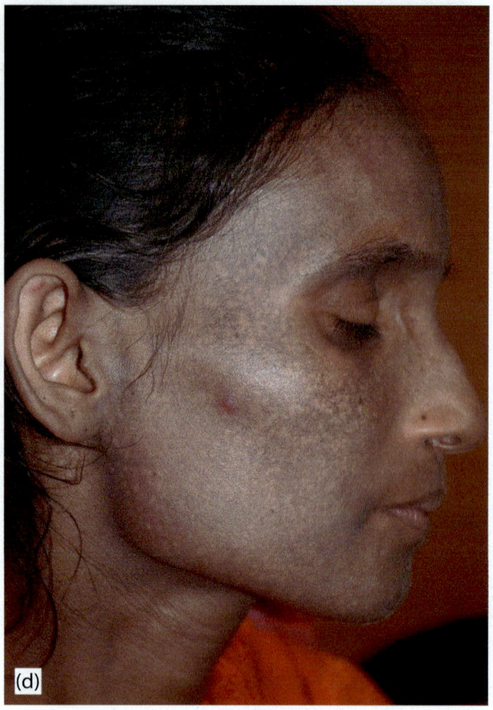

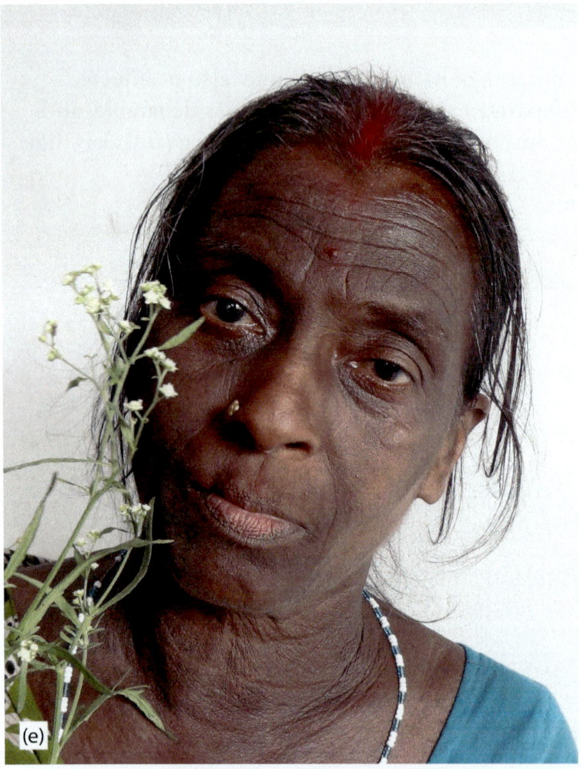

Figure 3.3 (*Continued*) **(c)** Bilateral periorbital lichen planus pigmentosus in a child. **(d)** Reticular pattern of facial pigmentation in lichen planus pigmentosus. (**e**) Diffuse facial pigmentation following resolution of airborne contact dermatitis due to parthenium. (a–e – Courtesy: Dr. Piyush Kumar, Katihar, India.)

Table 3.2 Differences between lichen planus pigmentosus (LPP) and erythema dyschromicum perstans (EDP)

| | LPP | EDP |
|---|---|---|
| Sex | More common in females | Equal in both males and females |
| Color of lesion | Slate-gray to brownish-black | Ash-colored |
| Site | Mainly on sun-exposed areas | Mainly involving the trunk |
| Borders | Discrete macules with diffuse/ill-defined borders | Polycyclic macules with elevated, erythematous border like a piece of string |

## Periorbital melanosis[7]

- This is also known as idiopathic cutaneous hyperchromia of the orbital region or dark circles.
- Periorbital melanosis is not an entity but rather a presentation of different etiologies including
  - Post-inflammatory hyperpigmentation secondary to atopic dermatitis, seborrheic dermatitis
  - Increased melanogenesis
  - Genetics
  - Loose subcutaneous tissue
  - Increased vascularity
  - Prominent tear-trough
- Deep-brown hyperpigmentation is present around periorbital skin and sometimes extends over to the upper nose and glabella (**Figure 3.5a,b**).

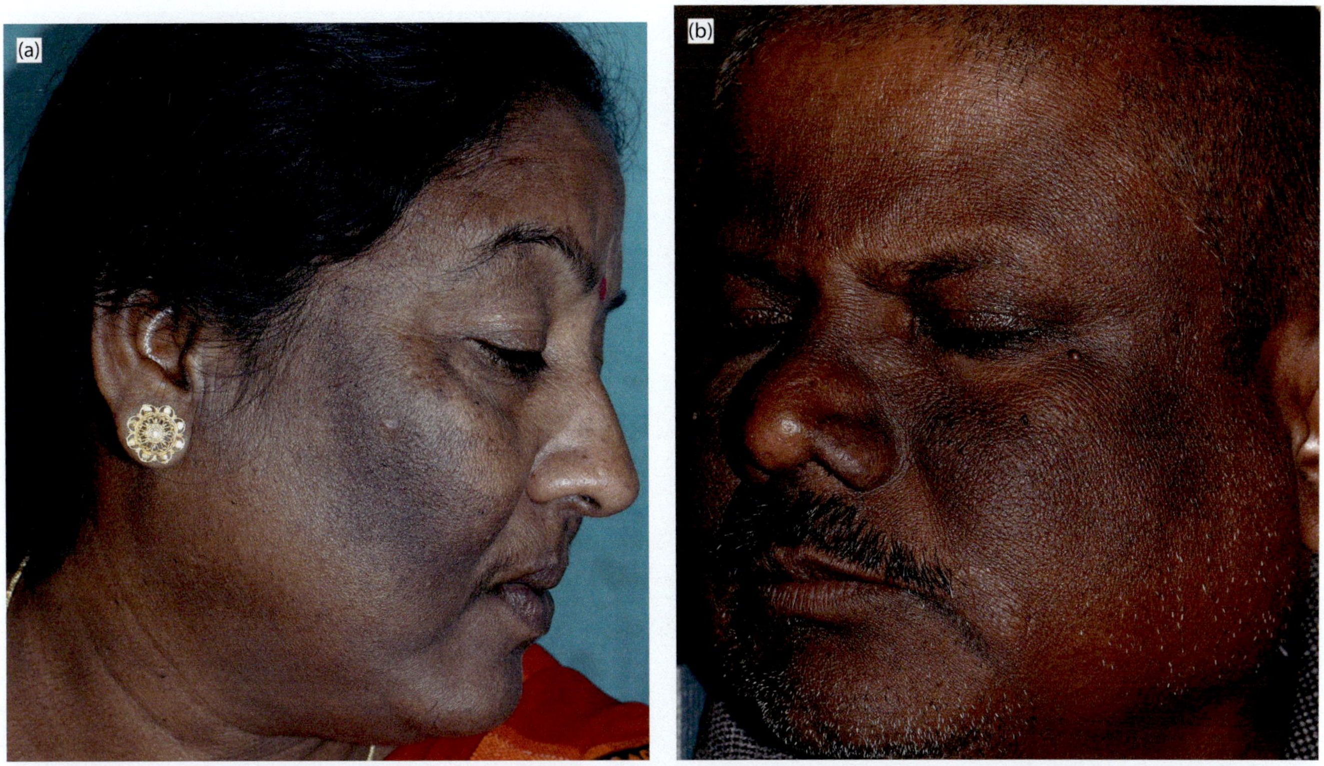


Figure 3.4 **(a)** A middle aged lady with maturational pigmentation – central face is involved and skin appears thickened. **(b)** Maturational pigmentation in a middle-aged obese man. (a,b – Courtesy: Dr. Piyush Kumar, Katihar, India.)

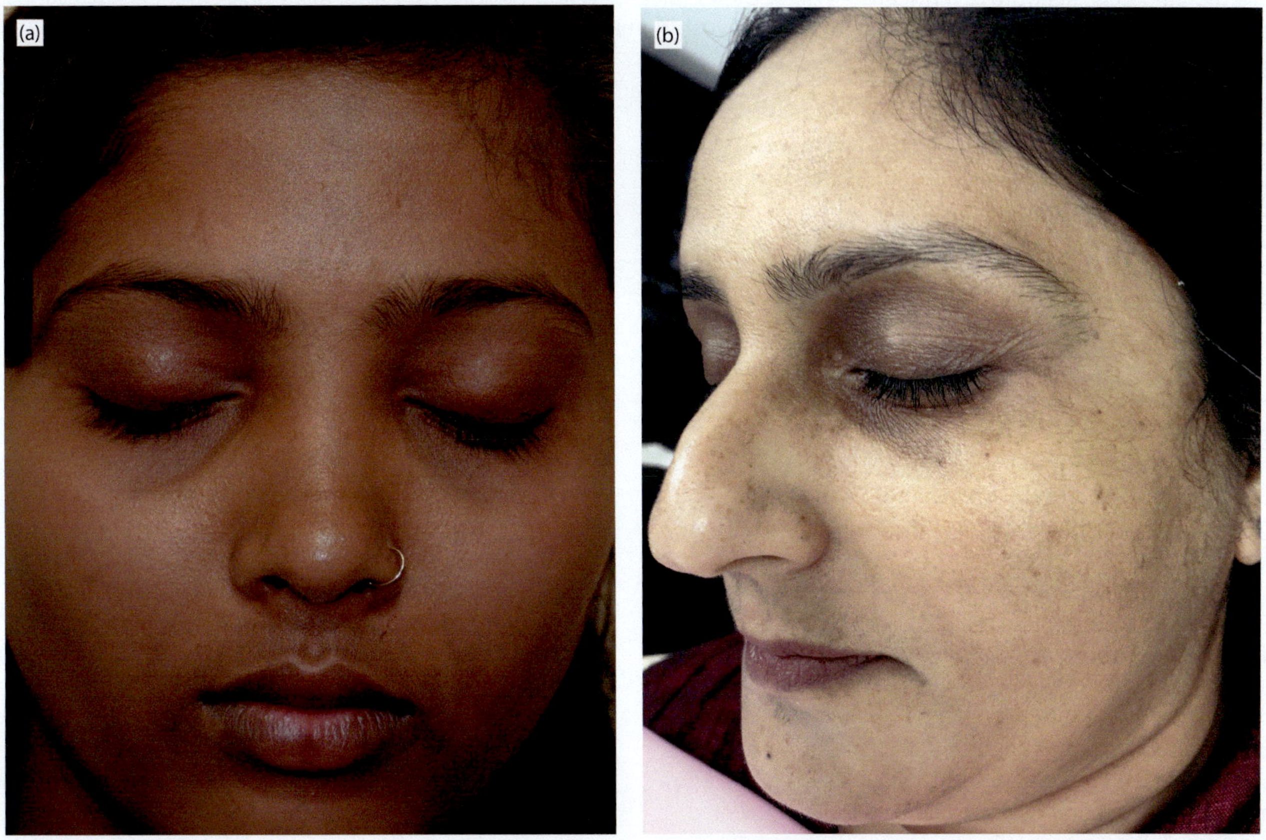


Figure 3.5 **(a)** Periorbital melanosis in a young female. **(b)** Periorbital melanosis in a lady. (a – Courtesy: Dr. Piyush Kumar, Katihar, India; b – Courtesy: Dr. Vishwas Patel, Viksha skin clinic, Ahmedabad, India.)

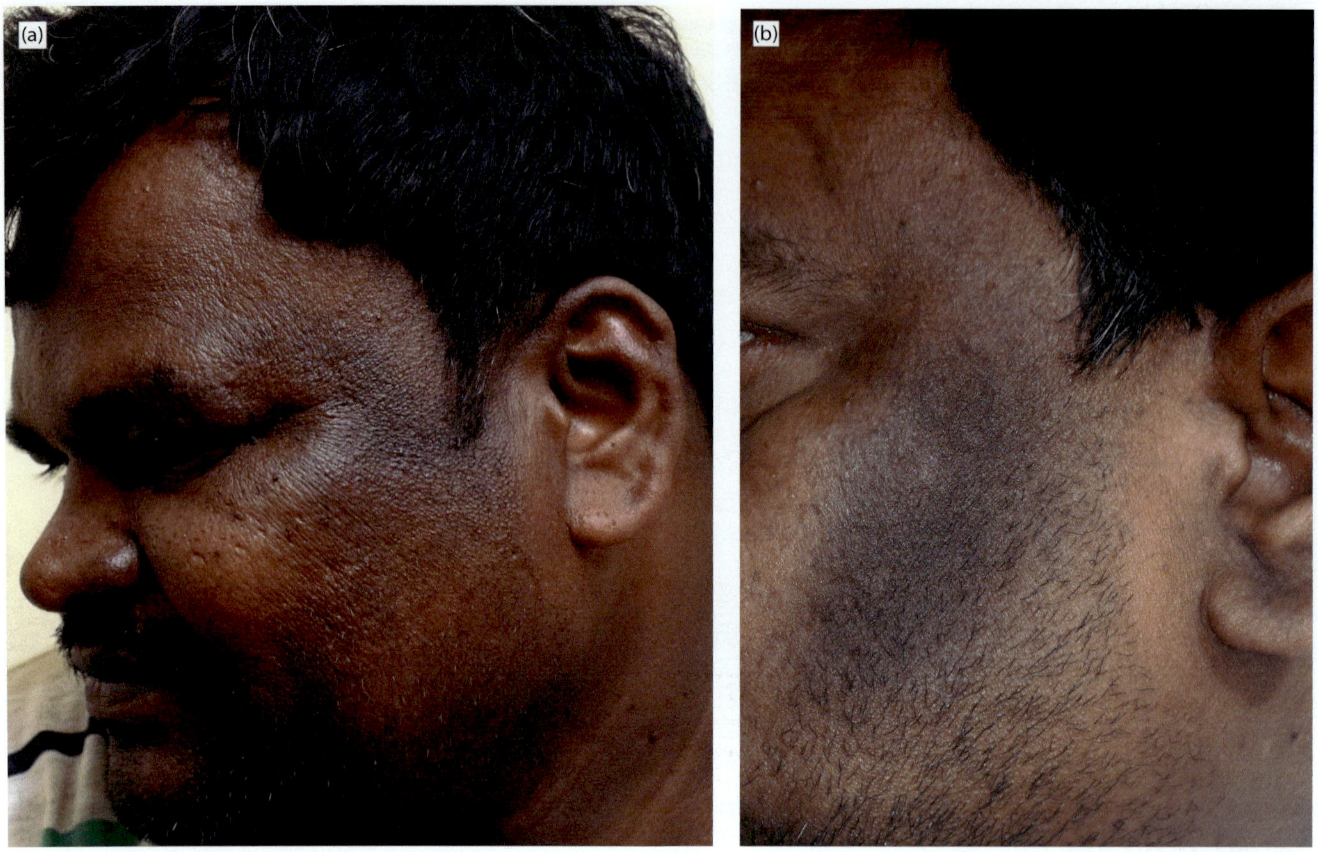

Figure 3.6 **(a)** Facial acanthosis nigricans – skin appears thickened and pebbly. **(b)** Facial acanthosis nigricans with thickened, pigmented, pebbly skin. (a,b – Courtesy: Dr. Piyush Kumar, Katihar, India.)

- On stretching the skin, if pigmentation decreases it is because of the vascular component; if it remains the same it is because of increased melanogenesis. In many cases, both components are present.

## Acanthosis nigricans

- Facial acanthosis nigricans (AN) mainly involves the forehead, temporal region, zygomatic region, and sometimes periocular and perioral regions (**Figure 3.6a,b**).
- Facial AN is associated with AN of other parts of the body, especially neck and axilla, and is a good pointer toward diagnosis.
- Facial AN is associated with metabolic syndrome involving higher BMI, hyperinsulinemia, hypertension, and dyslipidemia.

## Exogenous ochronosis (EO)

- The etiology is homogentisic acid accumulation due to prolonged use of hydroquinone, resorcinol, phenol, picric acid, oral antimalarials, and/or mercury.
- EO presents as asymptomatic, bilaterally symmetrical, speckled blue-black macules with caviar-like papules. The affected area is remarkable for interspersed depigmented macules. Telangiectasias may be present (**Figure 3.7a**).
- Three clinical stages are described by
  - Stage I: erythema and mild hyperpigmentation
  - Stage II: progressive hyperpigmentation, pigmented colloid milium (caviar-like lesions), and atrophy **(Figure 3.7b)**
  - Stage III: papulonodular (sarcoid-like) lesions

## Riehl's melanosis

- It is also known as pigmented contact dermatitis.
- It is a non-eczematous variant of contact dermatitis that is clinically characterized by hyperpigmentation with little or no signs of dermatitis. It is a type four hypersensitivity reaction to low concentration of allergens, not enough to cause spongiosis but can cause basement membrane damage and melanin incontinence.
- Common chemicals implicated in pigmented contact dermatitis include:
  - Fragrances – benzyl salicylate, sandalwood oil, eugenol, cinnamic acid derivatives, and balsam of Peru
  - Pigments – aniline dyes and kumkum (a red powder commonly used by Hindu women)
  - Optical whiteners used in washing powder containing Tinopal or CH3566
  - Coal tar derivatives, which increase photosensitivity
  - Bactericidals – carbanilides such as trichlorocarbanilide and Irgasan CF3

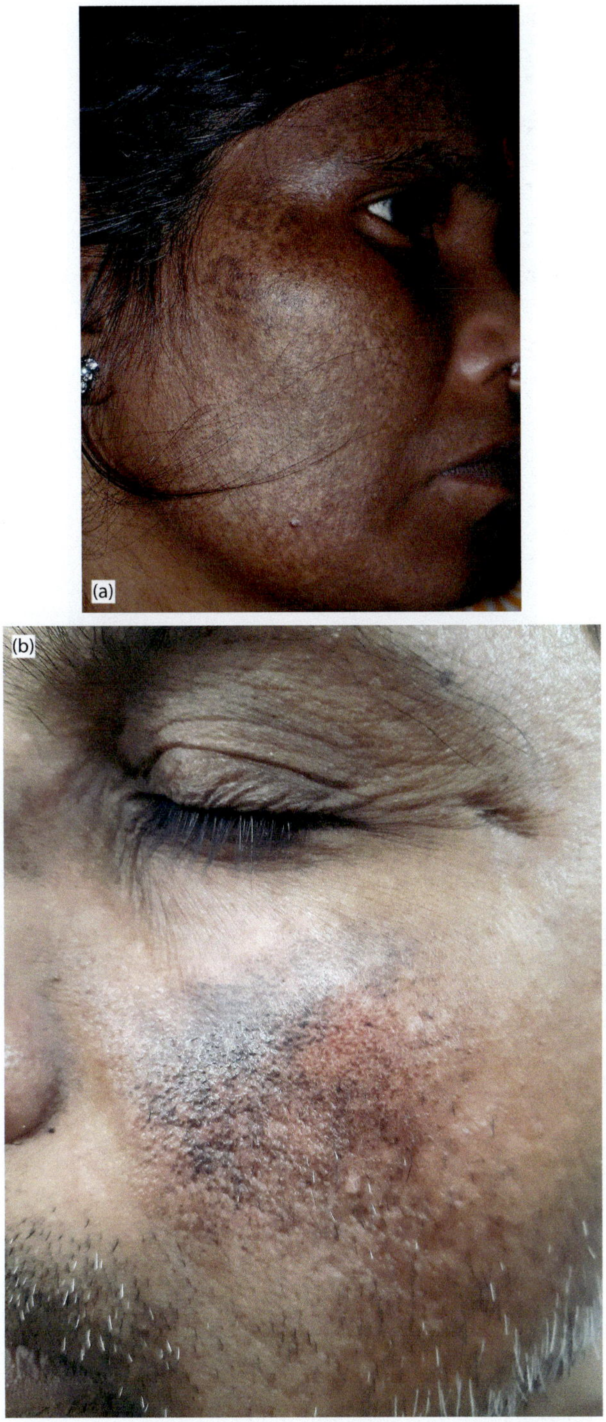


Figure 3.7 **(a)** Exogenous ochronosis with scattered hypopigmented macules in a background of diffuse pigmentation. **(b)** Exogenous ochronosis with hyperpigmentation and caviar like papules. (a – Courtesy: Dr. Piyush Kumar, Katihar, India; b– Courtesy: Dr. Hiral Shah, Baroda Medical College, Vadodara, India.)

- It presents as reddish-brown to slate-gray pigmentation in a reticulate pattern (**Figure 3.8a,b**).
- There is no active or preceding clinical dermatitis or pruritus, thus making the clinical diagnosis difficult in many cases.

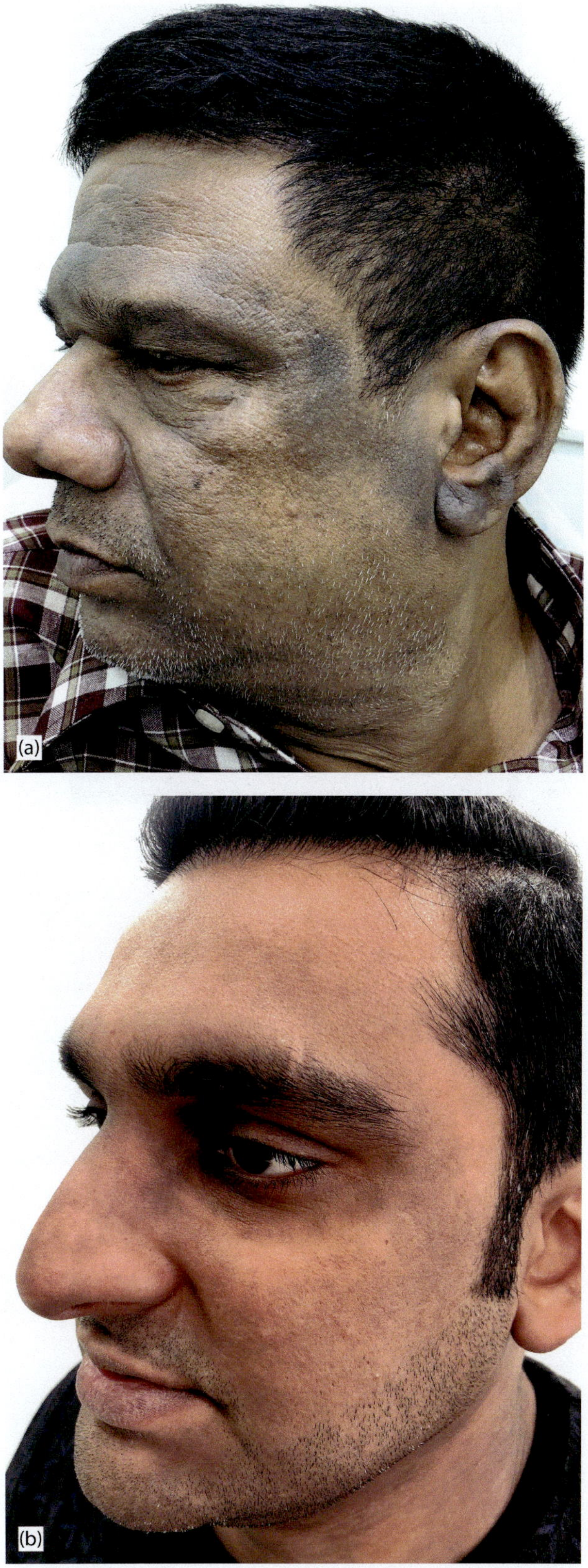


Figure 3.8 **(a)** Riehl's melanosis due to hair dye, presenting as pigmented macules and patches on the upper face and ears. **(b)** Cosmetic-induced Riehl's melanosis. (a – Courtesy: Dr. Zubin Mandlewala, Mumbai, India; b – Courtesy: Dr. Vishwas Patel, Viksha skin clinic, Ahmedabad, India.)

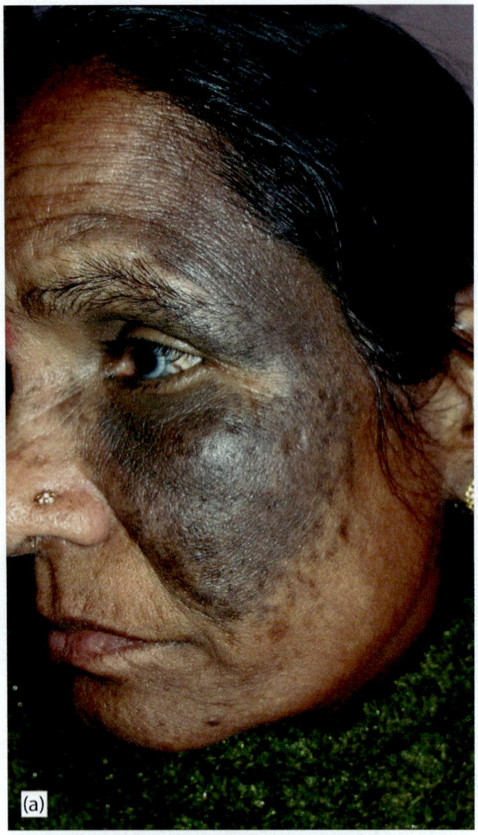


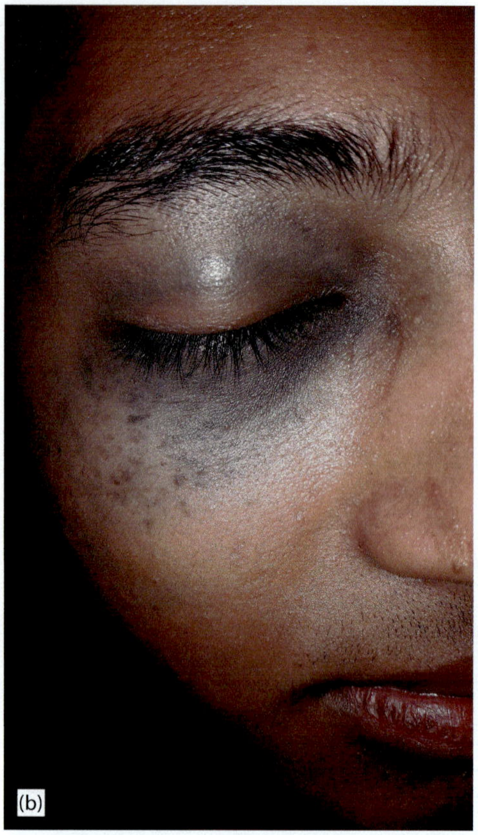


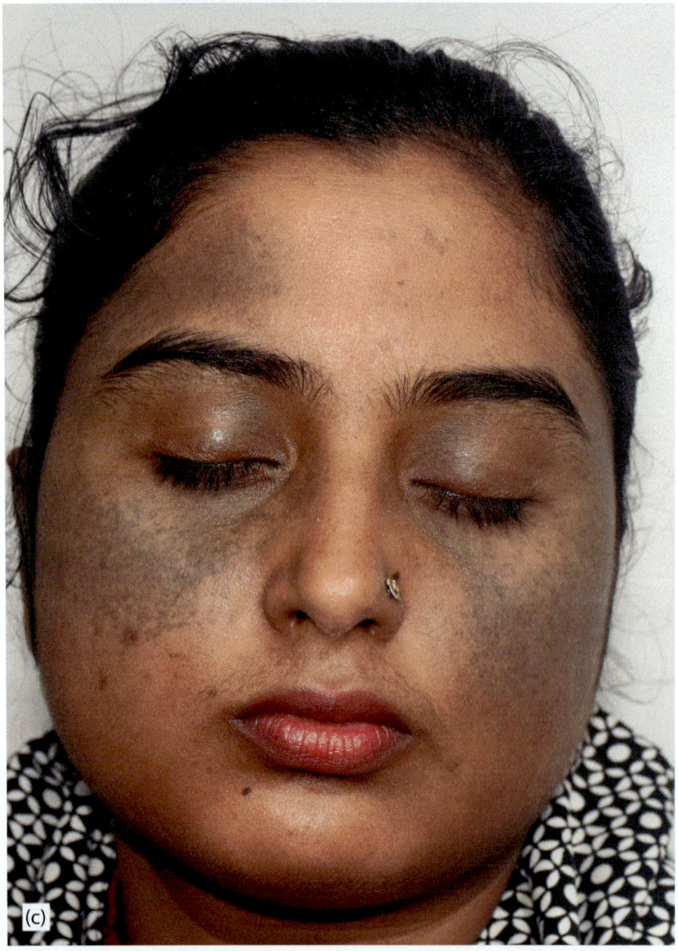


Figure 3.9 **(a)** Nevus of Ota as unilateral bluish-pigmented macules and patches on the mid face. Note involvement of ipsilateral sclera. **(b)** Localized nevus of Ota affecting the right orbital area and eyelids. **(c)** Bilateral nevus of Ota. (a – Courtesy: Dr. Hiral Shah, Baroda Medical College, Vadodara, India; b – Courtesy: Dr. Dependra Kumar Timshina, Remedy Clinics, Siliguri, India; c – Courtesy: Dr. Piyush Kumar, Katihar, India.)

- The face is the most common site affected; however, lips, axillary borders, and thighs may be affected due to lipstick color, shirt dye, and trouser dyes respectively.

## Nevus of OTA (nevus fusco caeruleus ophthalmo-maxillaris)

- Nevus of Ota is nine times more common in women than in men and presents more commonly around the perinatal period (50%) and puberty (30%).
- It is characterized by speckled blue-gray pigmentation of the area supplied by ophthalmic and maxillary divisions of trigeminal nerve, which may also involve oral mucosa and conjunctiva, sclera, retrobulbar fat, and cornea and retina in the eye. In the eye, conjunctiva is stained brown and the sclera is stained blue (**Figure 3.9a,b**).
- It is unilateral in 90% of cases but may be bilateral too (**Figure 3.9c**).
- Based on the extent, it is classified into
  - Type I (mild):
    - IA: Mild orbital type: on upper and lower eyelids, periocular and temple region

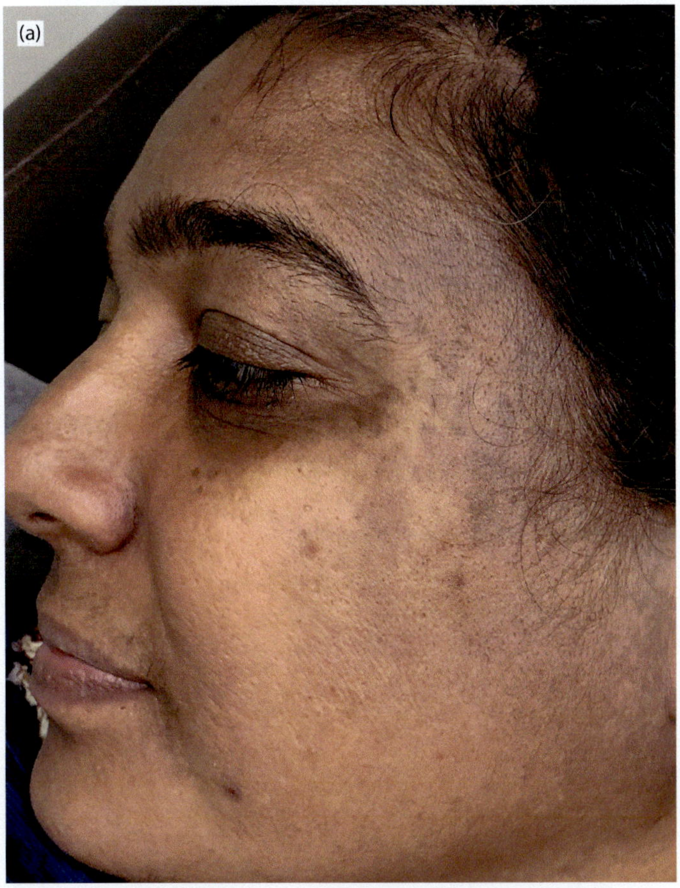


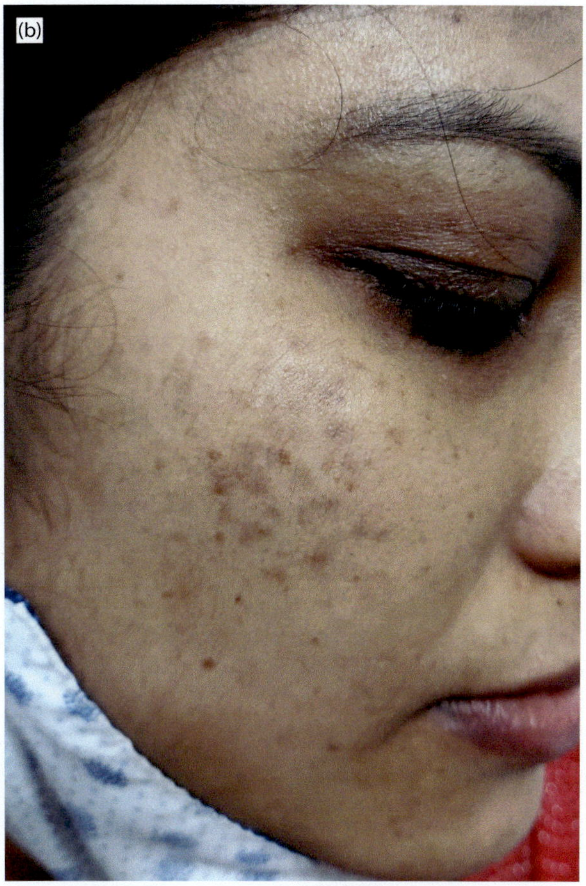


Figure 3.10 **(a)** Hori nevus as bilateral brown-blue macules and patches near the lateral canthus and on adjacent skin of temple region. **(b)** Hori nevus seen as brown-blue macules and patches. (a – Courtesy: Dr. Zubin Mandlewala, Mumbai, India; b – Courtesy: Dr. Piyush Kumar, Katihar, India.)

  - IB: Mild zygomatic type: on the infra palpebral fold, nasolabial fold and zygomatic region
  - IC: Mild forehead type: on forehead only
  - ID: on ala nasi only
- Type II (moderate): on upper and lower eyelids, periocular, zygomatic, cheek, and temple regions
- Type III (severe): on scalp, forehead, eyebrow, and nose
- Type IV (bilateral type): Bilateral

### Hori nevus/acquired bilateral nevus of Ota-like macules (ABNOM)

- It is an acquired variant.
- It is characterized by bilaterally symmetrical speckled or confluent brownish-blue pigmentation over malar region, temples, root of nose, ala nasi, eyelids, and forehead (**Figure 3.10a,b**).
- It spares the mucosa and presents in late adulthood.

### Freckles (ephelides) and lentigines

- Freckles and lentigines present as pigmented macules **(Table 3.3) (Figure 3.11a,b)**.

### Pigmentary demarcation lines (PDLs)[8]

- PDLs, also known as Futcher's or Voight's lines, are physiological, abrupt transitions from deeper pigmented skin to lighter pigmented skin. It becomes more prominent after puberty, and that is the reason most patients with PDL presents after puberty. There is a familial tendency for the development of PDL.
- PDLs, labeled A-H, have been described. Briefly, they appear as follows:
  - PDL type A – On the lateral aspect of the upper arm extending over the pectoral area
  - PDL type B – On the posteromedial portion of the lower limb
  - PDL type C – On the medio-sternal line, a vertical hypopigmented line in the pre and parasternal area
  - PDL type D – On the posteromedial area of the spine
  - PDL type E – As bilateral hypopigmented streaks, bands, or lanceolate areas over the chest in the zone between the mid third of the clavicle and the periareolar skin
  - PDL type F – As V-shaped hyperpigmented lines between the malar prominence and the temple (**Figure 3.12a,b**)

Table 3.3 Freckles and lentigines

| Differentiating features | Freckles | Lentigines |
|---|---|---|
| Color | Light brown | Dark-brown to black |
| Borders | Less defined, Irregular | Well-defined, regular |
| Genetic | MC1R gene mutation | Not familial* |
| Syndrome association | Not present | Centrofacial lentiginosis, Carvajal syndrome, and Naxos syndrome are associated |
| Sites | Present over sun-exposed areas | Present over sun-exposed as well as sun-protected areas. |
| Mucosa | Usually not affected | Frequently affected |
| Sun exposure | Increases with sun exposure and disappears when sun exposure is removed | Increases with sun exposure but doesn't disappear when there is no sun exposure. |
| Seasonal variation | Increases in summer season | No seasonal variation |
| Histopathology | Increase in melanosome concentration, melanocyte number remains the same. | Linear increase in melanocyte number present. |

* There are syndromes (e.g., LEOPARD syndrome) associated with lentigines, which may be familial.

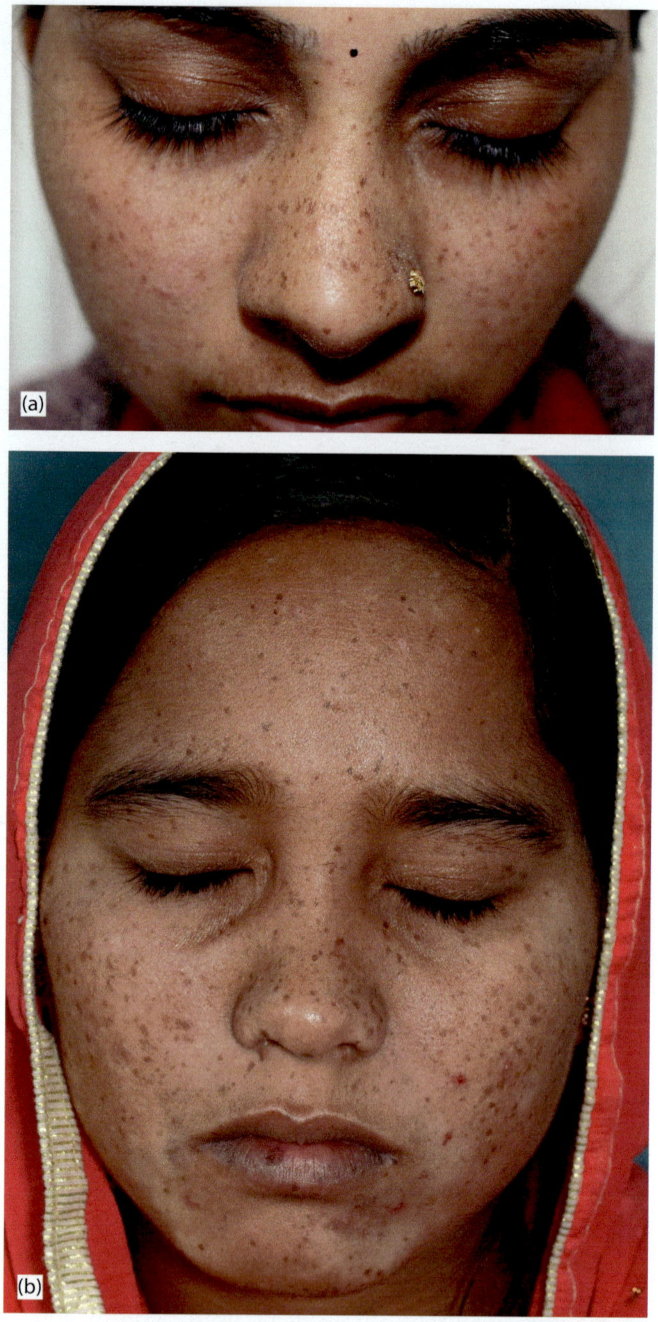

Figure 3.11 **(a)** Light-brown, ill-defined macules of freckles. **(b)** Dark-brown to black, well-demarcated macules in lentigines. Note involvement of lip. (a – Courtesy: Dr. Divya Sachdev, Raipur, India; b – Courtesy: Dr. Piyush Kumar, Katihar, India.)

- PDL type G – As W-shaped hyperpigmented lines between the malar prominence and the temple
- PDL type H –As linear bands of hyperpigmentation from the angle of the mouth to the lateral aspects of the chin (**Figure 3.12c**)

## Erythromelanosis follicularis faciei *et* colli (EFF)

- EFF is seen in young/middle-aged men.
- It is an unusual condition characterized by the triad of hyperpigmentation, follicular plugging, and well-defined erythema of the face and neck (**Figure 3.13**).
- It has been considered as a variant of keratosis pilaris – in view of the follicular papules, blotchy erythema, and associated keratosis pilaris, although EFF is distinguished by the extension onto the neck and the presence of pigmentation.

## Erythrose péribuccale pigmentaire de Brocq (peribuccal pigmentation of Brocq)

- This predominantly affects middle-aged women. It is a type of pigmented contact dermatitis affecting the perioral area.

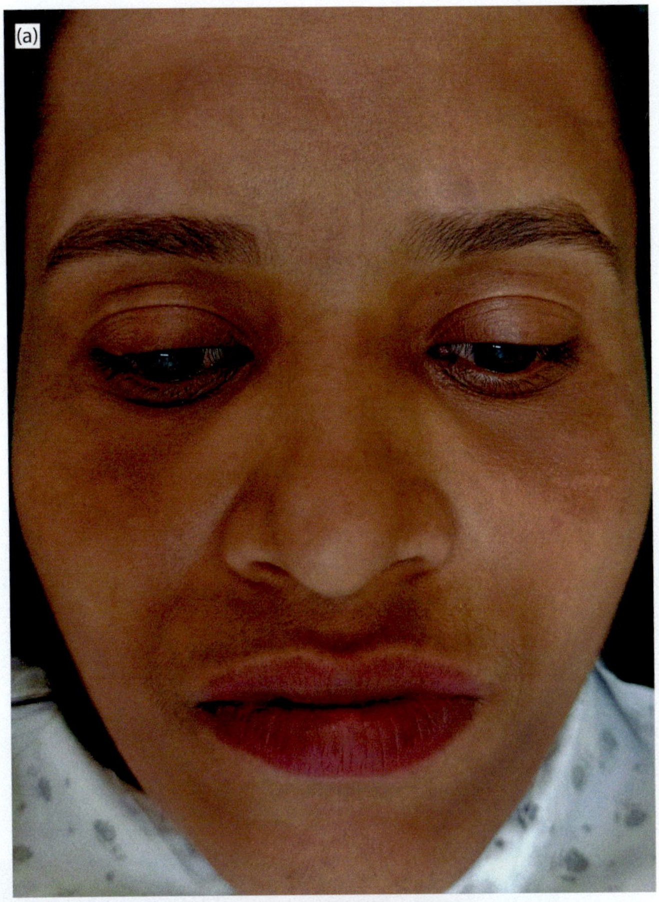

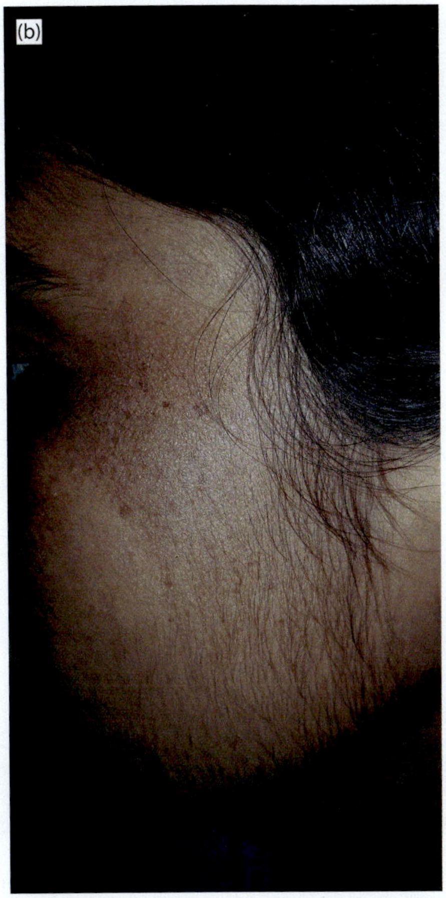

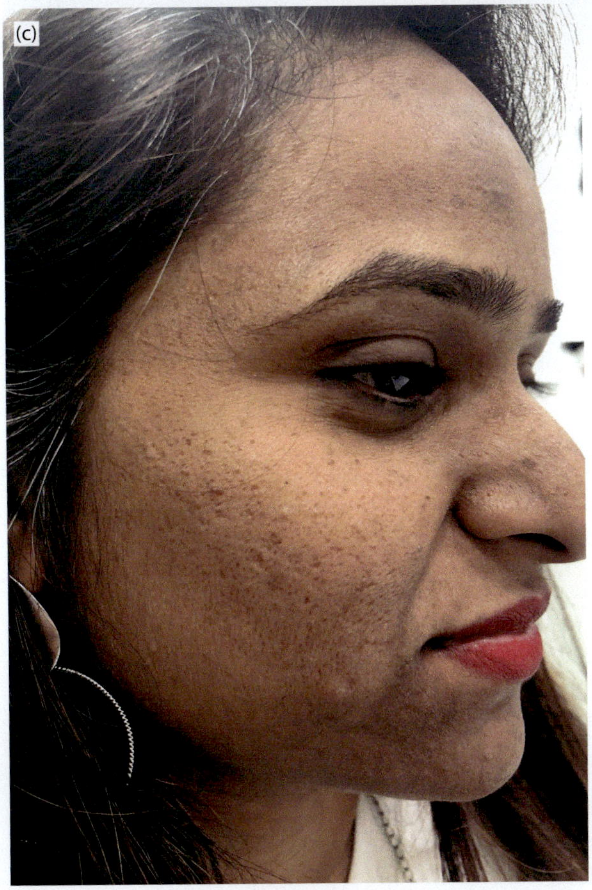

Figure 3.12 **(a)** Bilateral pigmentary demarcation line type F on the face. **(b)** Well-demarcated, brownish, V-shaped patch of pigmentary demarcation line type F. **(c)** Pigmentary demarcation line type H. (a – Courtesy: Dr. Pooja Manwar, Mahatma Gandhi Institute of Medical Sciences, Sevagram, India; b – Courtesy: Dr. PC Das, Katihar, India; c – Courtesy: Dr. Vishwas Patel, Viksha skin clinic, Ahmedabad, India.)

- The etiology is that it is due to photodynamic substance in cosmetics.
- Diffuse brownish-red pigmentation with erythema develops symmetrically around the mouth (**Figure 3.14a**).
- It spares a narrow perioral rim.
- DD: Post-inflammatory hyperpigmentation due to lip licking dermatitis (**Figure 3.14b**).

## Seborrheic melanosis[9]

- This term is commonly used among Indian dermatologists for a particular pattern of pigmentation affecting certain seborrheic areas of the face – the alar grooves, angles of the mouth and labio-mental crease.
- Such a pattern of pigmentation is known among darker people from Asia and Africa and in Hispanic populations.

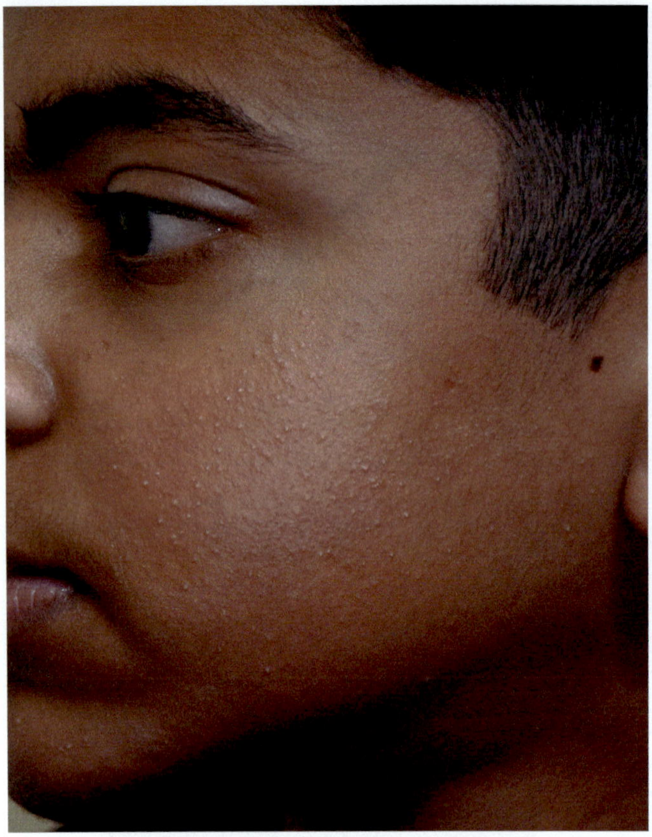

Figure 3.13 Erythromelanosis follicularis faciei presenting as erythema, pigmentation, and tiny papules on the lateral face. (Courtesy: Dr. Piyush Kumar, Katihar, India.)

- Patients may have a prior history of erythema, which frequently goes unnoticed in skin of color. Patients usually present with hyperpigmentation of the alar grooves, angles of the mouth, and labio-mental crease. It may be accompanied by scaling and seborrhea (**Figure 3.15a–c**).
- The nosology of this entity is debatable and many authors have stated that acanthosis nigricans and post-inflammatory hyperpigmentation are responsible for the clinical presentation.

## Poikiloderma of Civatte

- Long-term exposure to UV light, genetic predisposition, certain cosmetic ingredients, hormonal influences, and age contribute to its causation.
- Reddish-brown reticulate pigmentation with atrophy and telangiectasia are present in symmetrical fashion over the sides of cheeks and neck (**Figure 3.16**).
- Submental and submandibular areas that are sun protected are characteristically spared.

## Post-Chikungunya pigmentation

- This is seen in patients with Chikungunya infection from *Aedes* mosquitoes.

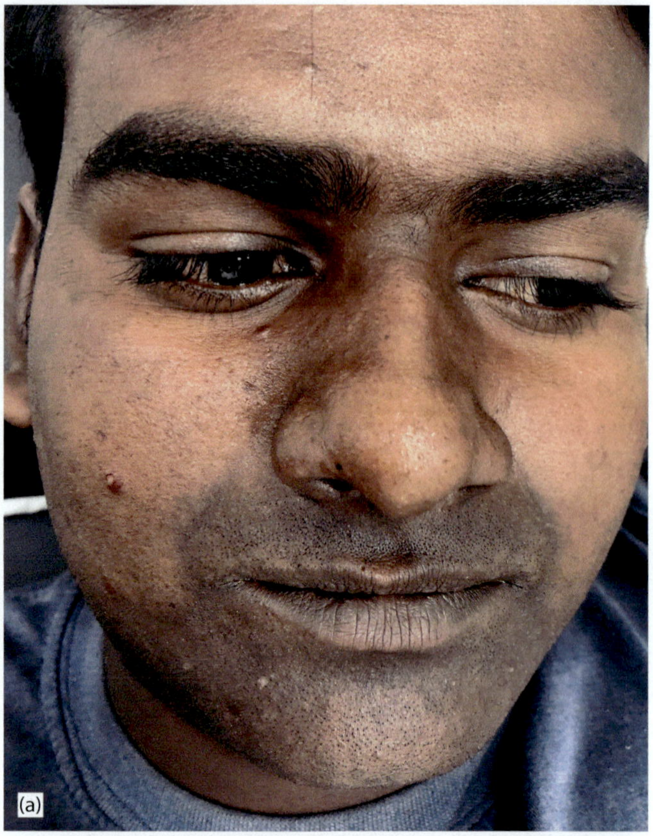

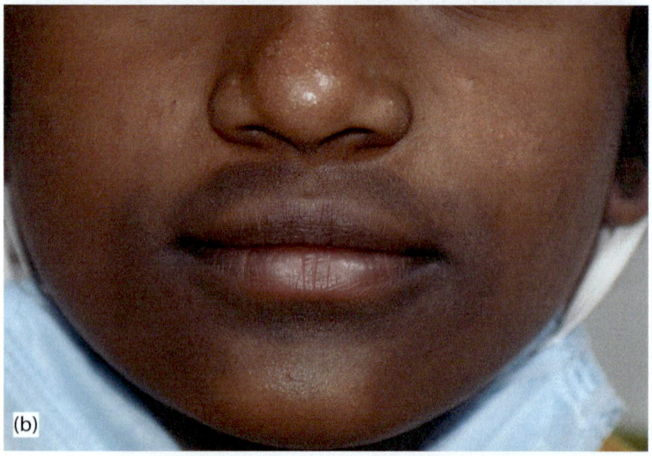

Figure 3.14 **(a)** Peribuccal pigmentation of Brocq. **(b)** Perioral pigmentation due to lip licking dermatitis. (a – Courtesy: Dr. Vishwas Patel, Viksha skin clinic, Ahmedabad, India; b – Courtesy: Dr. Piyush Kumar, Katihar, India.)

- Patients present with hyperpigmented macules mainly on the nose (chik sign). It can also appear similar to melasma or periorbital melanosis or with flagellate patterns on the trunk, extremities, abdomen, and palms (**Figure 3.17**).

## Addison's disease

- Tuberculosis is the predominant cause of Addison's disease in developing countries; however, nowadays autoimmune pathology is gaining attention.

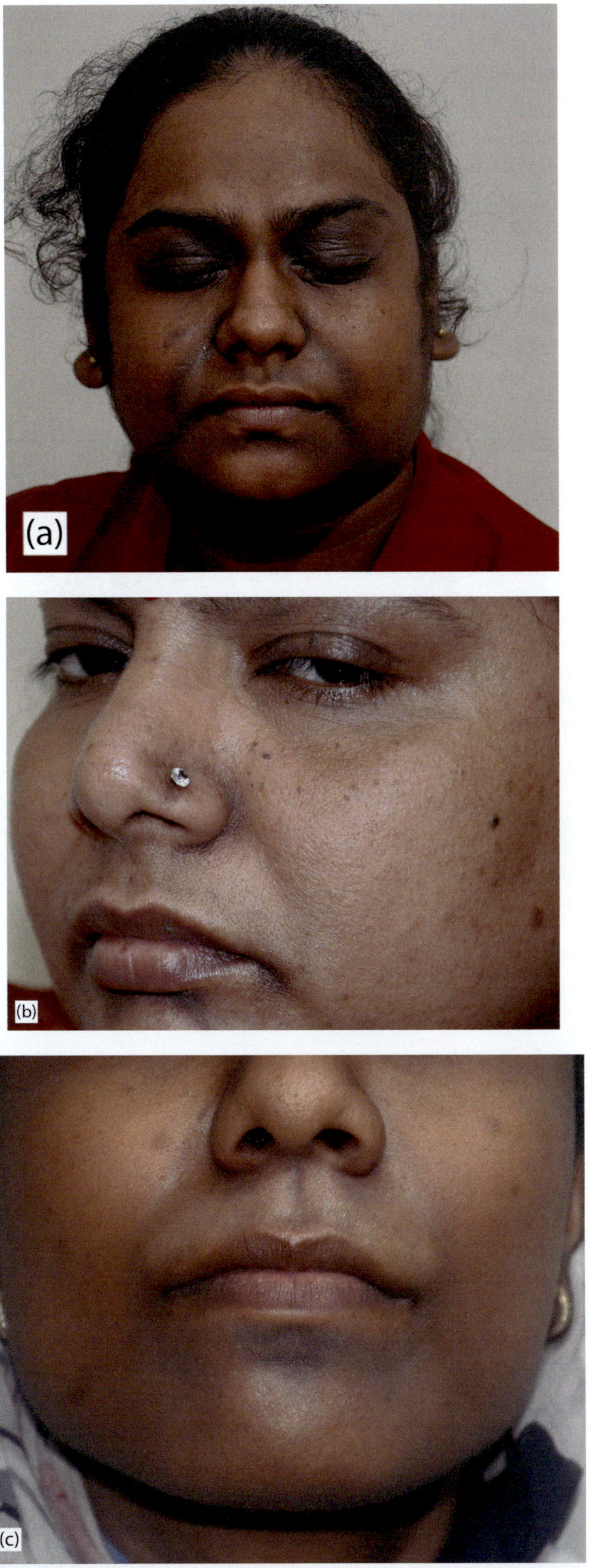


Figure 3.15 **(a, b)** Hyperpigmentation in alar groove and angle of mouth in seborrheic melanosis. **(c)** Seborrheic melanosis in a young lady. (a–c – Courtesy: Dr. Piyush Kumar, Katihar, India.)

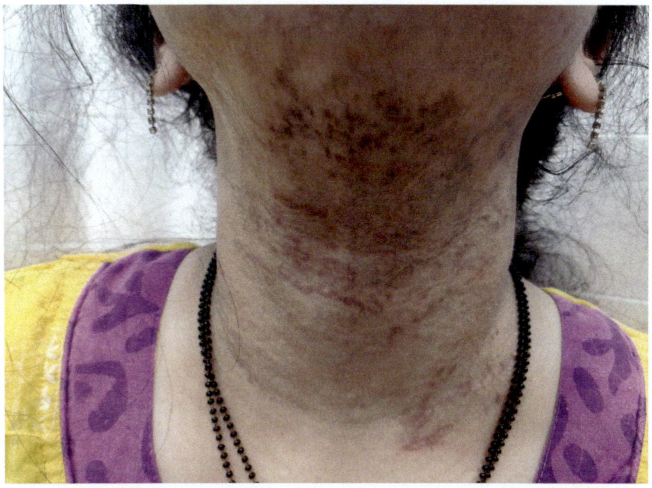

Figure 3.16 Poikiloderma of Civatte affecting the neck in a middle-aged lady. (Courtesy: Dr. Ganesh Avhad, Mumbai, India.)

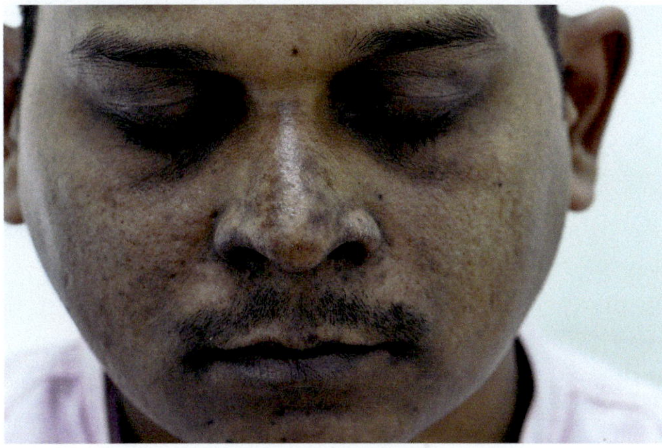

Figure 3.17 Grayish macular pigmentation of the nose and cheeks following Chikungunya. (Courtesy: Dr. Sushil S Savant, Consultant Dermatologist, Mumbai, India.)

- Increased ACTH or B-lipotropin simulates MSH, which results in melanocyte production.
- Cutaneous features of Addison's disease appear before other clinical features appear.
- There is generalized hyperpigmentation of sun-exposed and trauma-prone areas, along with oral mucosal pigmentation (**Figure 3.18a,b**).
- There is hyperpigmentation of palmar creases, genitals, nipples, and existing scars.
- There is development of new pigmented nevi, and older nevi darken.
- Other clinical features are fatigue, abdominal pain, hypotension, nausea, vomiting, diarrhea, and craving for salt.

### Vitamin $B_{12}$ deficiency[10]

- The pigmentation in vitamin $B_{12}$ deficiency mimics that of Addison's disease.
- Inadequate intake, low consumption of animal-source foods and pernicious anemia due to deficient intrinsic factor are major causes in younger adults.

Malabsorption, in part due to gastric atrophy, is a major contributing factor in elderly persons.

- Mucocutaneous features include diffuse and patchy hyperpigmentation, graying of hairs, and mucosal changes (mucosal pigmentation, atrophic glossitis and angular stomatitis).
- Hyper pigmentation of friction- and pressure-prone areas, such as the dorsum of the hands and feet, with accentuation over the interphalangeal joints and terminal phalanges is a classical feature of vitamin B12 deficiency (**Figure 3.19a,b**).
- Systemic features include fatigue, weight loss, and anorexia.

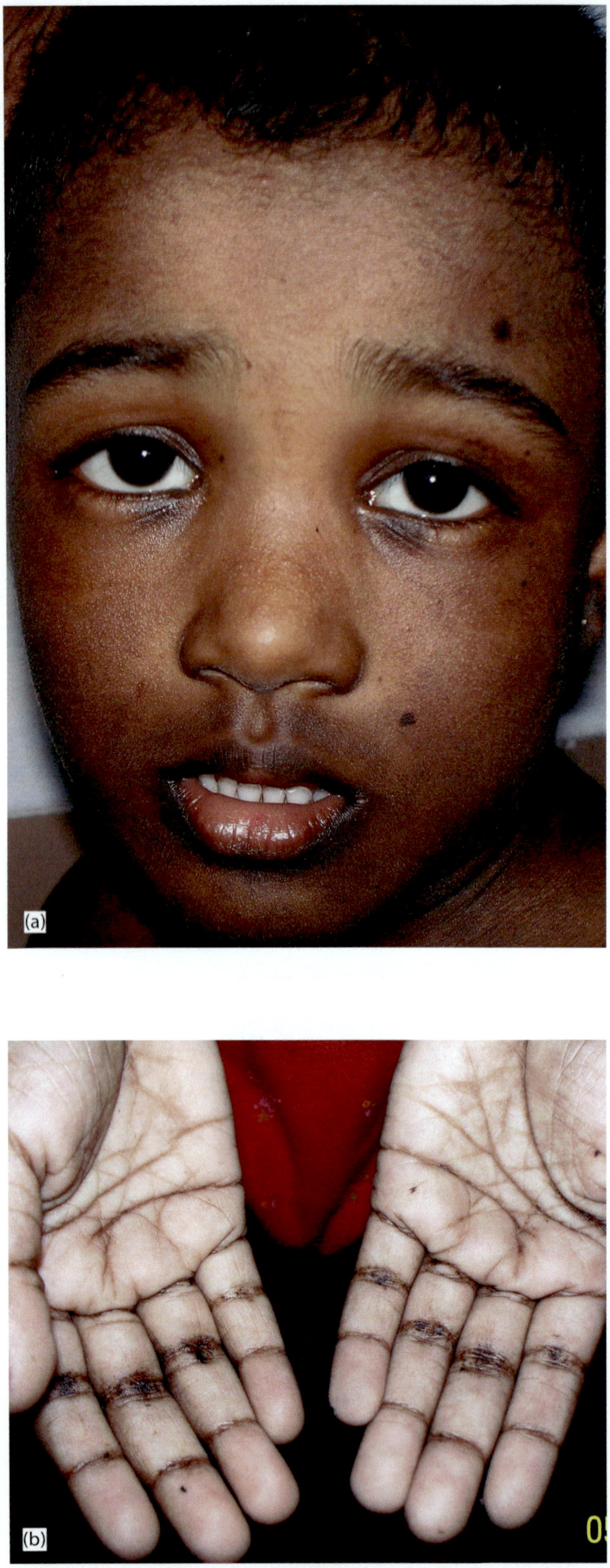


Figure 3.18 **(a)** Diffuse brownish pigmentation of the face in Addison's disease. **(b)** Same patient with pigmented palmar creases. (a,b – Courtesy: Dr. Piyush Kumar, Katihar, India.)

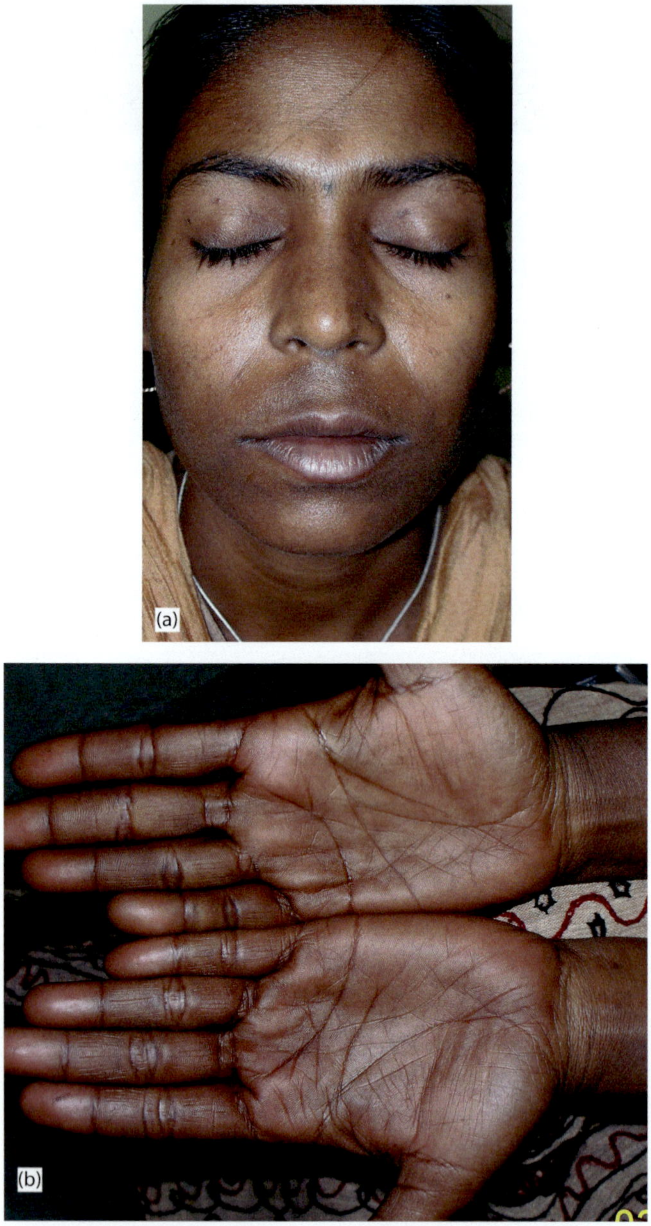


Figure 3.19 **(a)** Facial pigmentation in vitamin $B_{12}$ deficiency. **(b)** Same patient with pigmentation of both palms. (a,b – Courtesy: Dr. Piyush Kumar, Katihar, India.)

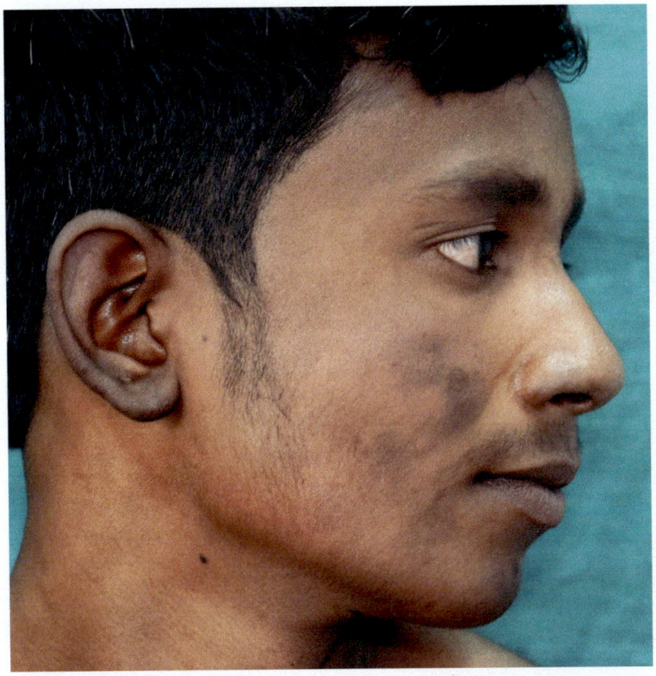

Figure 3.20 Clofazimine induced patchy pigmentation of the face and ear. (Courtesy: Dr. Piyush Kumar, Katihar, India.)

### Drug induced pigmentation

- Various patho-mechanisms involved are accumulation of melanin, accumulation of the drug itself, nonspecific inflammation, deposits of iron following trauma to vessels, aggravation by sun exposure, formation of complexes between melanin and causative drug, and drug particles engulfed by dermal macrophage.
- Drugs implicated are nonsteroidal anti-inflammatory drugs, antimalarials, amiodarone, tetracyclines, psychotropic drugs, clofazimine (**Figure 3.20**), heavy metals, etc.
- Drug-induced pigmentation can be over photo-exposed areas, mucosae, nails, or even Addisonian-like.

### Macular amyloidosis[11]

- It commonly affects the upper back and interscapular area but may occasionally affect the forehead.
- It presents as small dusky-brown to gray pigmented macules associated with pruritus. It may be associated with severe itching. These macules may later coalesce into patches.
- DD: frictional melanosis, post-inflammatory hyperpigmentation, lichen planus pigmentosus.

### Frictional melanosis

- In a tropical country like India, people sweat a lot and use handkerchiefs or other material to wipe away the sweat. The repeated acts of friction result in pigmentation of the face.

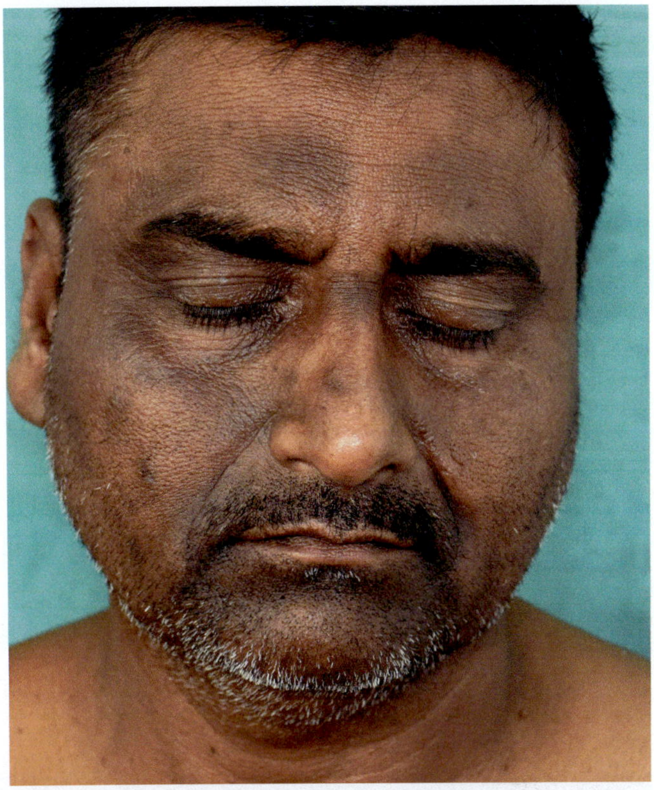

Figure 3.21 Dark-brown pigmentation over the forehead in frictional melanosis. Also note seborrheic melanosis in the alar groove and mento labial crease. (Courtesy: Dr. Piyush Kumar, Katihar, India.)

- The pigmentation typically affects the skin over bony prominences, sparing the mid forehead and nose (**Figure 3.21**).
- The pigmentation is usually symmetric, uniform, deep dark brown. The affected skin usually does not show textural changes, but that may be present in longstanding cases.
- Stopping the acts of friction may hasten the resolution of the condition.
- DD: melasma, facial macular amyloidosis, facial acanthosis nigricans, lichen planus pigmentosus, pigmented contact dermatitis, post-inflammatory hyperpigmentation.

### Post-inflammatory hyperpigmentation (PIH)

- It is a common sequelae of inflammatory dermatosis (such as acne vulgaris, impetigo and atopic dermatitis). It may be epidermal, dermal, or mixed, depending on the trauma or insult to skin. When inflammation causes damage to the basement membrane, it results in melanin incontinence and PIH, which is dermal.
- It tends to affect Fitzpatrick skin types IV–VI.
- It presents as tan, brown, or dark-brown macules on any part of the face along with a history of a preceding dermatosis in the same region (**Figure 3.22a–c**).

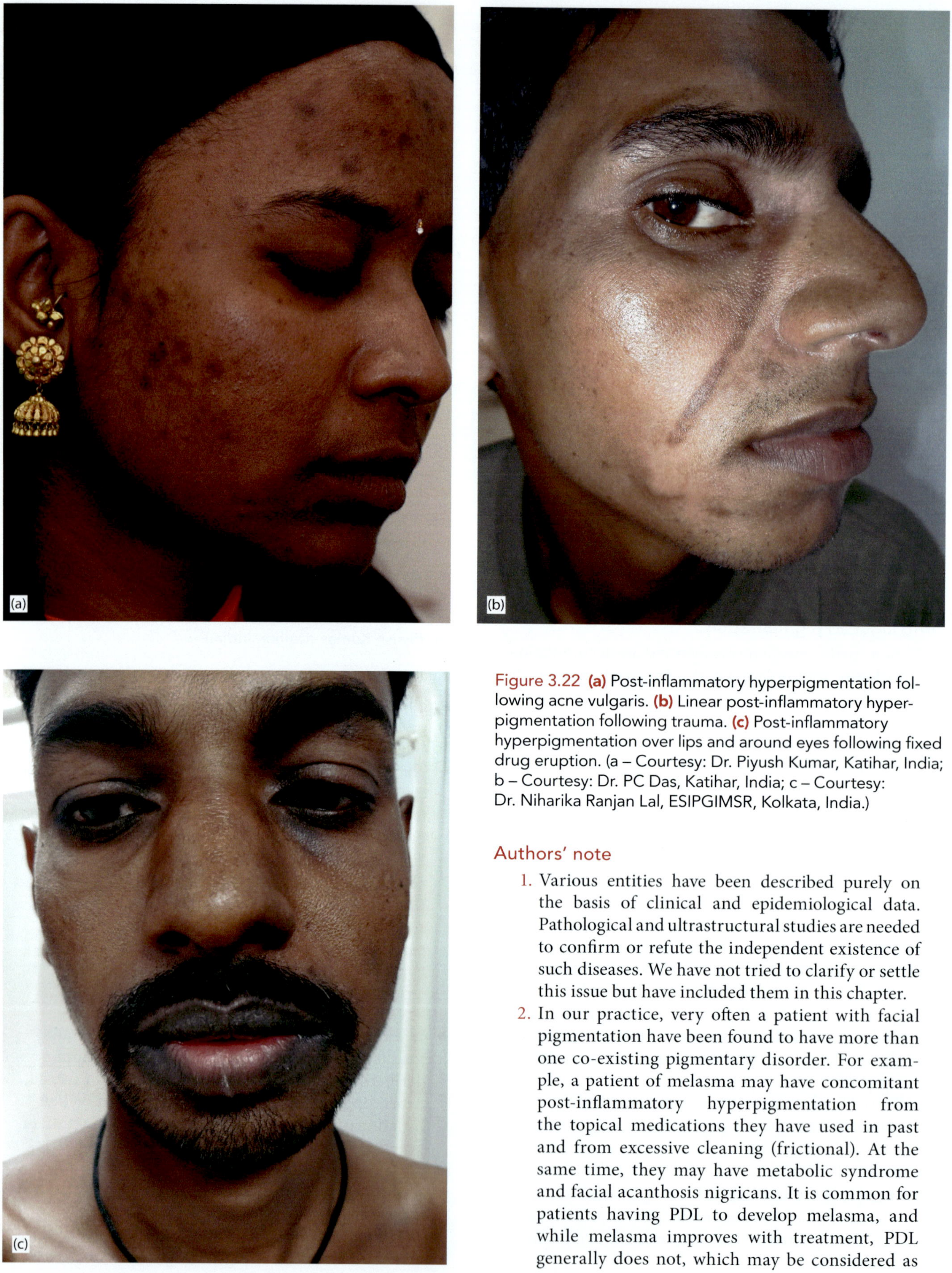

Figure 3.22 **(a)** Post-inflammatory hyperpigmentation following acne vulgaris. **(b)** Linear post-inflammatory hyperpigmentation following trauma. **(c)** Post-inflammatory hyperpigmentation over lips and around eyes following fixed drug eruption. (a – Courtesy: Dr. Piyush Kumar, Katihar, India; b – Courtesy: Dr. PC Das, Katihar, India; c – Courtesy: Dr. Niharika Ranjan Lal, ESIPGIMSR, Kolkata, India.)

## Authors' note

1. Various entities have been described purely on the basis of clinical and epidemiological data. Pathological and ultrastructural studies are needed to confirm or refute the independent existence of such diseases. We have not tried to clarify or settle this issue but have included them in this chapter.
2. In our practice, very often a patient with facial pigmentation have been found to have more than one co-existing pigmentary disorder. For example, a patient of melasma may have concomitant post-inflammatory hyperpigmentation from the topical medications they have used in past and from excessive cleaning (frictional). At the same time, they may have metabolic syndrome and facial acanthosis nigricans. It is common for patients having PDL to develop melasma, and while melasma improves with treatment, PDL generally does not, which may be considered as

treatment failure. Hence, we encourage our readers to examine the complete face thoroughly and make multiple diagnoses, if needed, as one diagnosis does not exclude the possibility of other co-existing conditions.

## REFERENCES


1. Vashi NA, Kundu RV. Facial hyperpigmentation: Causes and treatment. Br J Dermatol 2013;169(3):41–56.
2. Khanna N, Rasool S. Facial melanoses: Indian perspective. Indian J Dermatol Venereol Leprol 2011;77:552–564.
3. Nicolaidou E, Antoniou C, Katsambas AD. Origin, clinical presentation, and diagnosis of facial hypermelanoses. Dermatol Clin 2007;25(3):321–326.
4. Vashi NA, Wirya SA, Inyang M, Kundu RV. Facial hyperpigmentation in skin of color: Special considerations and treatment. Am J Clin Dermatol 2017 Apr;18(2):215–230.
5. Pérez-Bernal A, Muñoz-Pérez MA, Camacho F. Management of facial hyperpigmentation. Am J Clin Dermatol 2000;1(5):261–268.
6. Sonthalia S, Sarkar R, Neema S. Maturational hyperpigmentation: Clinico-dermoscopic and histopathological profile of a new cutaneous marker of metabolic syndrome. Pigment Int 2018;5:54–56.
7. Sarkar R, Das A. Periorbital hyperpigmentation: What lies beneath? Indian Dermatol Online J 2018;9:229–230.
8. Singh N, Thappa DM. Pigmentary demarcation lines. Pigment Int 2014;1:13–16.
9. Verma SB, Vasani RJ, Chandrashekar L, Thomas M. Seborrheic melanosis: An entity worthy of mention in dermatological literature. Indian J Dermatol Venereol Leprol 2017;83:285–289.
10. Sachdev D, Kumar P, Debbarman P. A Young Man with Generalized Pigmentation. In: Kothiwala S, Tiwary AK, Kumar P, editors. Clinical Cases in Disorders of Melanocytes. 1st edition. Cham: Springer; 2020. P. 103–110.
11. Bandhlish A, Aggarwal A, Koranne RV. A clinico-epidemiological study of macular amyloidosis from north India. Indian J Dermatol 2012;57(4):269–274.

# E3

# Hyperpigmented macules and patches: Generalized

PC DAS, TALAT FATIMA, NIHARIKA RANJAN LAL

## ABSTRACT

Widespread hyperpigmentation is usually due to increased melanin production or deposition of drugs or heavy metals within the dermis. Generalized hyperpigmentation is seen in a variety of conditions, many of which are associated with other systemic disorders. This chapter discusses a morphological approach that, in conjunction with the clinical history and necessary laboratory tests, allows a definitive diagnosis to be reached.

The text of this chapter is available online at https://routledgetextbooks.com/textbooks/9781032399669/


DOI: 10.1201/9781351054225-8

E4

# Diffuse hyperpigmentation

RAMPAL SHARMA

## ABSTRACT

Increased pigmentation may present in a patchy manner or may cause extensive involvement of a part of or the whole body. A variety of causes, including genetic, metabolic, or inflammatory factors; ultraviolet radiation; drugs; and malignancy, may cause diffuse pigmentation of the skin. This chapter discusses conditions presenting with diffuse pigmentation.

The text of this chapter is available online at https://routledgetextbooks.com/textbooks/9781032399669/

DOI: 10.1201/9781351054225-9

# 4

# Reticulate and mottled pigmentation

SAUMYA PANDA, RASHID SHAHID

## INTRODUCTION

There are many congenital and acquired pigmentary disorders that may present with hyperpigmented macules and/or hypopigmented macules on normal or diffusely hyperpigmented skin with various patterns of distribution. Broadly, these have been categorized into two groups: reticulate and mottled. Their most widely accepted definitions are given in **Box 4.1**. The clinical diagnosis rests on correct identification of the pattern of pigmentation. The clinical differentials of reticulate and mottled pigmentation are listed in **Table 4.1**. Detailed clinical, personal, and family histories, including any exposure to drugs or chemicals, along with comprehensive dermatological and general physical examinations remain crucial diagnostic tools. Clinical clues such as age of onset – early (infantile and/or childhood) and late (adolescence and/or adulthood) – distribution of pigmentation (face, acral, flexures and trunk/generalized) and associated cutaneous as well as systemic findings help in making a clinical diagnosis. The clinical approach to the diagnosis of reticulate and mottled pigmentary disorders is summarized in **Figures 4.1a,b and 4.2a,b**, and salient features of different entities are discussed below.[1–8] This chapter focuses on diseases that typically present with reticulate or mottled pigmentation. Some other pigmentary disorders, such as lichen planus pigmentosus, may sometimes present with reticular pigmentation and are discussed elsewhere.

## RETICULATE HYPERPIGMENTATION

### Kindler syndrome

- Synonyms are Kindler–Weary syndrome, bullous acrokeratotic poikiloderma of Kindler and Weary, congenital bullous poikiloderma, and hereditary acrokeratotic poikiloderma.
- It is a rare autosomal recessive disorder, resulting from mutations in the FERMT1 gene.
- The syndrome is characterized by congenital acral skin blistering, skin fragility, photosensitivity, progressive poikiloderma, and cutaneous atrophy.
- The disease starts occasionally with erosion at birth, followed by prominent traumatic or spontaneous blistering over hands and feet during infancy, which heal without milia formation or scarring. During childhood, the skin fragility and photosensitivity improves significantly; however, reticulated erythematous hypopigmentation within mottled hyperpigmentation and telangiectasia develops in sun-exposed areas and later spreads to non-exposed areas such as chest, abdomen extensor aspects of arms and thighs, and occasionally flexors in adulthood.
- Diffuse poikiloderma appears gradually, becomes more prominent later in life, and persists throughout life. Tissue-paper–like atrophy is present in sun-exposed areas, particularly on the dorsum of hands, feet, knees, and elbows (**Figure 4.3a,b**).
- Other features include erosive gingivitis, dental caries, ectropion, intraoral and corneal scarring, esophageal stricture, rectal and urethral bleeding, palmoplantar hyperkeratosis, and mild webbing of digits.
- There is an increased risk of squamous cell carcinoma (SCC) of lip, oral mucosa, and acral skin.
- DD: Rothmud-Thompson syndrome (poikiloderma associated with sparse hair, short stature, cataract, hypogonadism), Bloom syndrome (telangiectasia, photosensitivity, erythema of the face and sun exposed areas but not true poikiloderma, xeroderma pigmentosum (sparing of acral areas).

### X-linked reticulate pigmentary disorder

- This is an extremely rare X-lined recessive genodermatosis caused by mutation in *POLA1*.
- Female carriers have clinical manifestations limited to skin.
- At birth or within a few weeks of life, female infants develop reticulate hyperpigmentation along the lines of Blaschko. Mild onychodystrophy may be reported sometimes but only in correspondence to pigmentary lesions. During adulthood, hypomelanosis may fade away.


DOI: 10.1201/9781351054225-10

**BOX 4.1: Definitions of terminology used**

- Mottled pigmentation: may have one of the following two presentations
    - Mixture of small hyperpigmented and hypopigmented macules of variable sizes and shapes but with distinct border, on normal looking skin. It is also called "dyschromia."
    - Mottled pigmentation with guttate hypopigmented macules superimposed on generalized/diffuse hyperpigmentation.
- Reticulate hyperpigmentation: Presence of variably pigmented freckle-like hyperpigmented macules with indistinct border on normal-looking skin.

- Between fourth and fifth years of age, male patients may develop asymptomatic, generalized, reticulate hyperpigmentation, with initial involvement of inner thighs, buttocks, and cheeks.
- During the first few months of life, systemic manifestations include recurrent pneumonia and chronic obstructive pulmonary disease. Other systemic manifestations include low birth weight, neonatal colitis, developmental delay, seizures, hemiplegia, severe photophobia, visual impairment, gastroesophageal reflux and intermittent constipation, and kidney stones associated with hypercalciuria.
- Additional features include dental anomalies, hypohidrosis, coarse hair, arched eyebrows, dysmorphic face with upswept frontal hairline, xerosis, delayed bone age, short metacarpals.
- DD: In males – dyskeratosis congenita. In females – stage III incontinentia pigmenti.

Table 4.1 Causes of reticulate and mottled pigmentations

| A. Hyperpigmented macules on normal skin in reticular fashion | B1. Mottled pigmentation with both hypo-and hyperpigmented macules | B2. Mottled pigmentation with Hypopigmented macules superimposed on generalized/diffuse hyperpigmentation |
|---|---|---|
| • Kindler syndrome<br>• Incontinentia pigmenti (3rd stage)<br>• Reticulate acropigmentation of Kitamura (RAPK)<br>• Dermatopathia pigmentosa reticularis<br>• Naegeli–Franceschetti–Jadassohn syndrome (NFJS)<br>• Fanconi anemia<br>a. Progeria/acrogeria syndromes Hutchinson-Gilford syndrome (classic progeria)<br>b. Werner syndrome (adult progeria)<br>c. Nestor-Guillermo progeria syndrome<br>d. Acrogeria<br>• Prurigo pigmentosa<br>• Erythema ab igne<br>• Riehl's melanosis<br>• Lichen planus pigmentosus (LPP)<br>• Erythema dyschromicum perstans (EDP)<br>• Atopic dirty neck<br>• Pigmentation reticularis faciei et colli<br>• Confluent and reticulated papillomatosis of Gougerot and Carteaud (CRP)<br>• Dowling Degos disease (DDD)<br>• Galli-Galli disease<br>• Haber's syndrome<br>• Post-inflammatory hyperpigmentation<br>• Drug induced<br>• X-linked reticulate pigmentary disorder | • Dyschromatosis symmetrica hereditaria (DSH) / (Reticulate acropigmentation of Dohi<br>• Dyschromatosis universalis hereditaria (DUH)<br>• Xeroderma pigmentosum (XP)<br>• Amyloidosis cutis dyschromica<br>• Porphyria cutanea tarda | • Epidermolysis bullosa simplex with mottled pigmentation<br>• Dyskeratosis congenita and its variants:<br>◦ Revesz syndrome<br>◦ Hoyeraal-Hreidarsson (HH) syndrome<br>• Rothmund Thomson syndrome (RTS)<br>• Bloom syndrome<br>• Chediak-Higashi syndrome (CHS)<br>• Griscelli syndrome<br>• Ziprowski-Margolis syndrome<br>• Wende-Baukus (Pegum) syndrome<br>• Berlin syndrome<br>• Progeria and acrogeria<br>• Anonychia with bizarre flexural pigmentation<br>• Chronic arsenicism<br>• Mycosis fungoides<br>• Systemic sclerosis<br>• Secondary syphilis with necklace of Venus<br>• Pinta<br>• Photoleukomelanodermatitis of Kobori (induced by thiazide, afloqualone, tetracycline)<br>• Acromelanosis albo-punctata<br>• Acquired brachial cutaneous dyschromatosis (ABCD)<br>• Photoaging<br>• Vagabond's leukomelanoderma |

## Naegeli-Franceschetti-Jadassohn syndrome (NFJ)

- This is a rare, autosomal dominant form of ectodermal dysplasia resulting from heterozygous mutations in the keratin 14 gene.
- Brown or gray-brown reticulated pigmentation develops by the age of two years, without preceding inflammatory changes, and often fade in puberty.
- Sites involved are abdomen, periocular and perioral regions, with variable involvement of neck, extremities, trunk, axilla, and groin.
- Occasionally some patients develop blistering on their palms and soles.
- Other features include hypohidrosis, lifelong poor heat intolerance, absent or **hypoplastic dermatoglyphics**, non-cicatricial alopecia of scalp, eyebrows, diffuse punctate palmoplantar keratoderma, and dental anomalies.
- There may be nail changes including onychodystrophy, onycholysis, subungual hyperkeratosis, and congenital malalignment of the great toenails.
- DD: Dermatopathia pigmentosa reticularis (lifelong persistence of hyperpigmentation, partial alopecia, absence of dental anomalies), dyskeratosis congenita (X-linked recessive, other features such as alopecia, mucosal leukoplakia, poikiloderma and blood

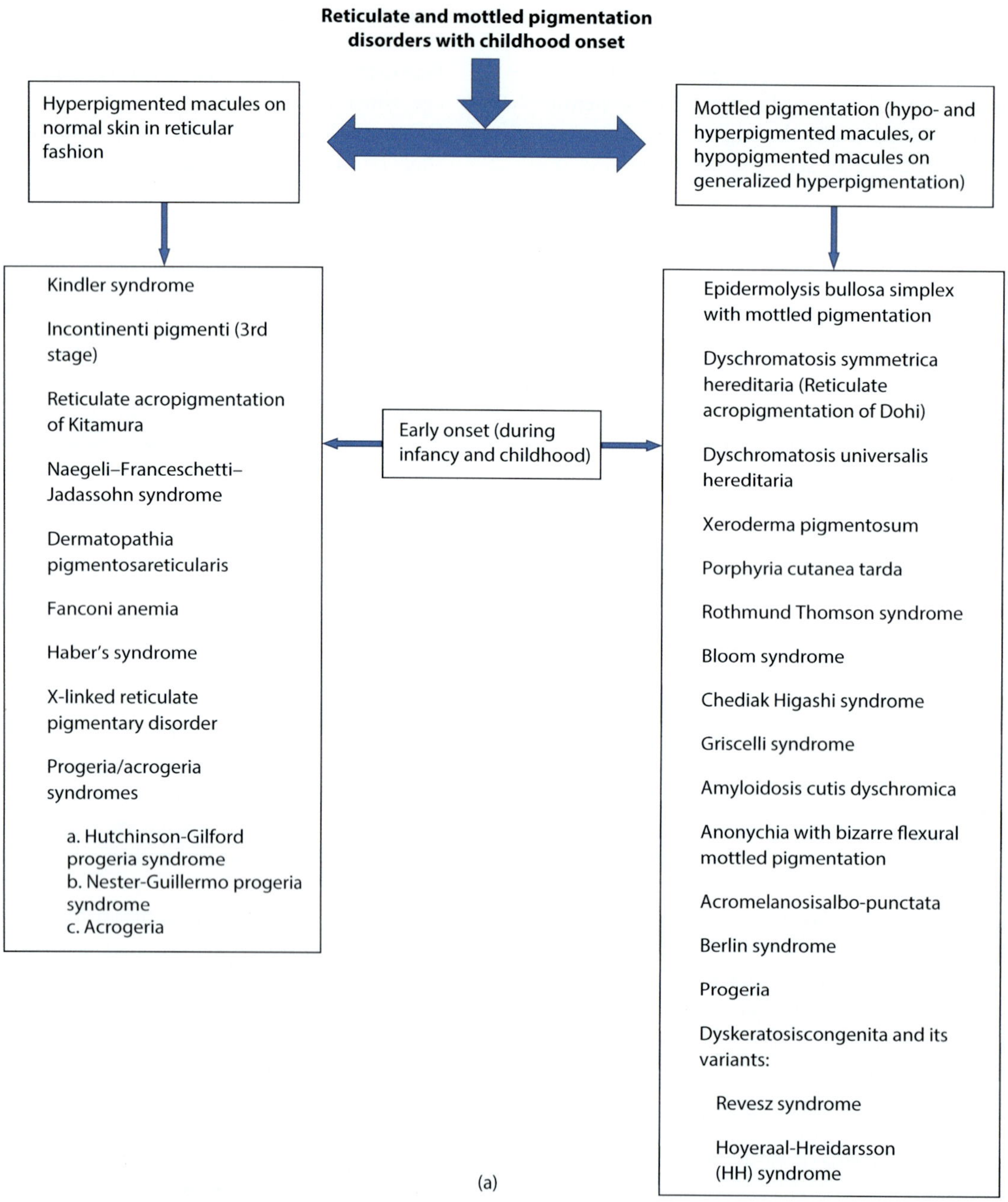


Figure 4.1 **(a)** Disorders causing reticulate and mottled pigmentation- early onset. (*Continued*)

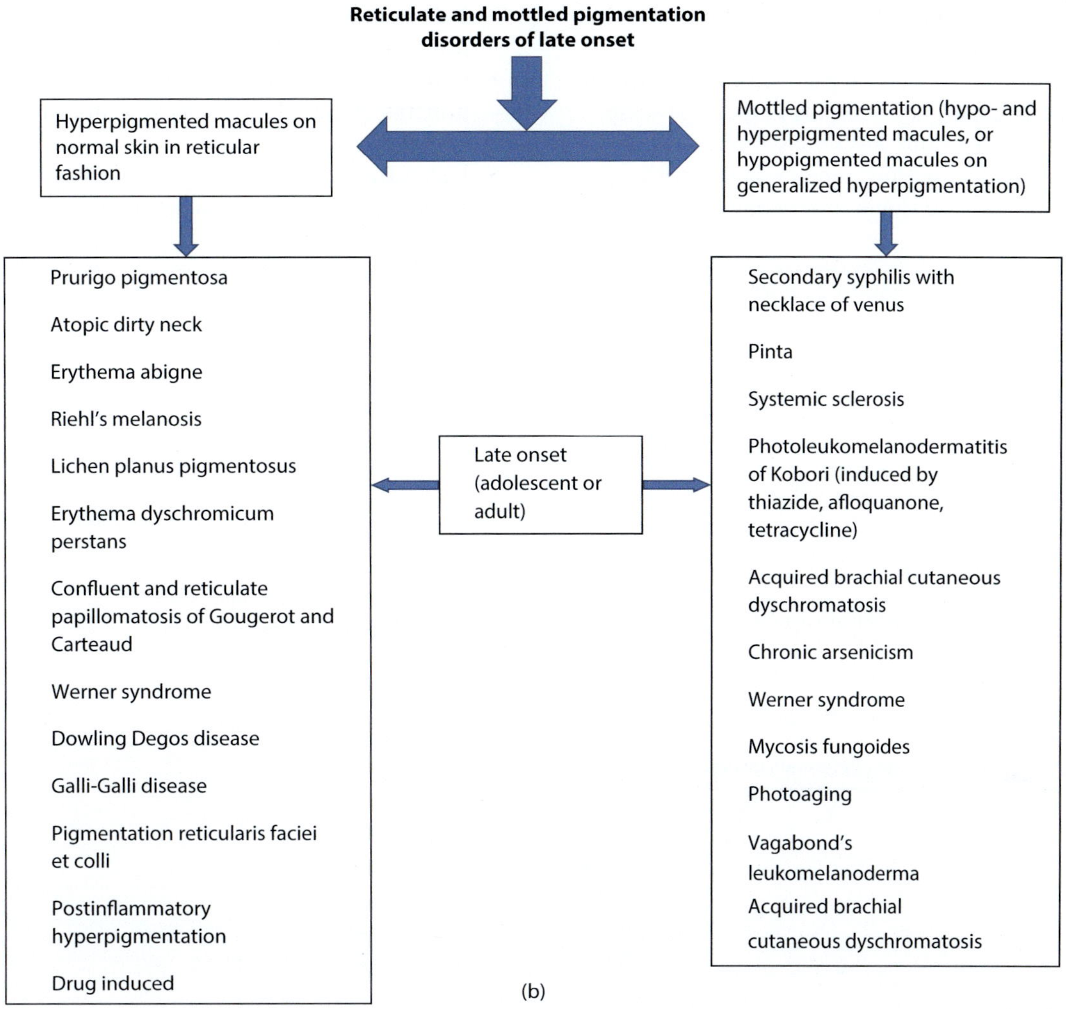


Figure 4.1 (*Continued*) **(b)** Disorders causing reticulate and mottled pigmentation- late onset.

dyscrasias), epidermolysis bullosa simplex (blistering is more prominent), X-linked reticulate pigmentary disorder, Kindler syndrome (poikiloderma present).

## Hidrotic ectodermal dysplasia

- This is also called Clouston syndrome.
- It is an autosomal dominant condition caused by mutation in the *GjB6* gene.
- Nail abnormalities are the most consistent feature and frequently manifest at birth or in early infancy. Nails are typically milky white and smaller, with gradual thickening throughout childhood.
- Slow growth of nail plates, thickening, and spontaneous separation of the nail plate are seen in adults.
- Scalp hairs are slow growing, wiry, pale, fine, and brittle, with patchy alopecia and reduced hair strength. Eyebrows and eyelashes are frequently sparse and axillary, pubic, and body hairs too may be affected.
- Sparse eyelashes may predispose to development of conjunctivitis, blepharitis, cataract, photophobia, and strabismus.
- There is normal sweating and teeth. However, oral leukoplakia may be present.
- Palmoplantar hyperkeratosis may accompany the disease and usually gets worse with age.
- Hyperpigmentation present over bony prominences, joints, axillae, areola, and pubic area. Papules coalescing to form a cobblestone-like pattern may extend from palms and soles onto the dorsal surface of the digits distally.
- DD: Pachyonychia congenita (hypertrophic nail dystrophy, painful palmoplantar keratoderma and blistering, palmoplantar hyperhidrosis, and follicular keratoses on the trunk and extremities, oral leukokeratosis, pilosebaceous cysts), hypotrichosis-deafness syndrome.

## Dermatopathia pigmentosa reticularis (DPR)

- This is an autosomal dominant disorder due to mutation in the keratin 14 gene.
- It usually manifests by the age of two years.
- Reticulated confetti-like hyperpigmented macules develop initially at birth or during infancy before two

years of age, involving trunk and proximal extremities, and persist throughout life.

- Further widespread reticulated pigmentation begins in childhood, along with non-scarring alopecia of scalp, eyebrows and axillae, and onychodystrophy.
- Sparse hair of scalp, eyebrows, and eyelashes with progressive and diffuse alopecia develops.
- Nail changes include onychodystrophy, loss of nail, and pterygium formation.
- Other variable features include hypo- or hyperhidrosis, punctate palmoplantar keratoderma, and adermatoglyphia.
- DD: Naegeli-Franceschetti-Jadassohn syndrome (lacks alopecia, less persistent hyperpigmentation – which fades

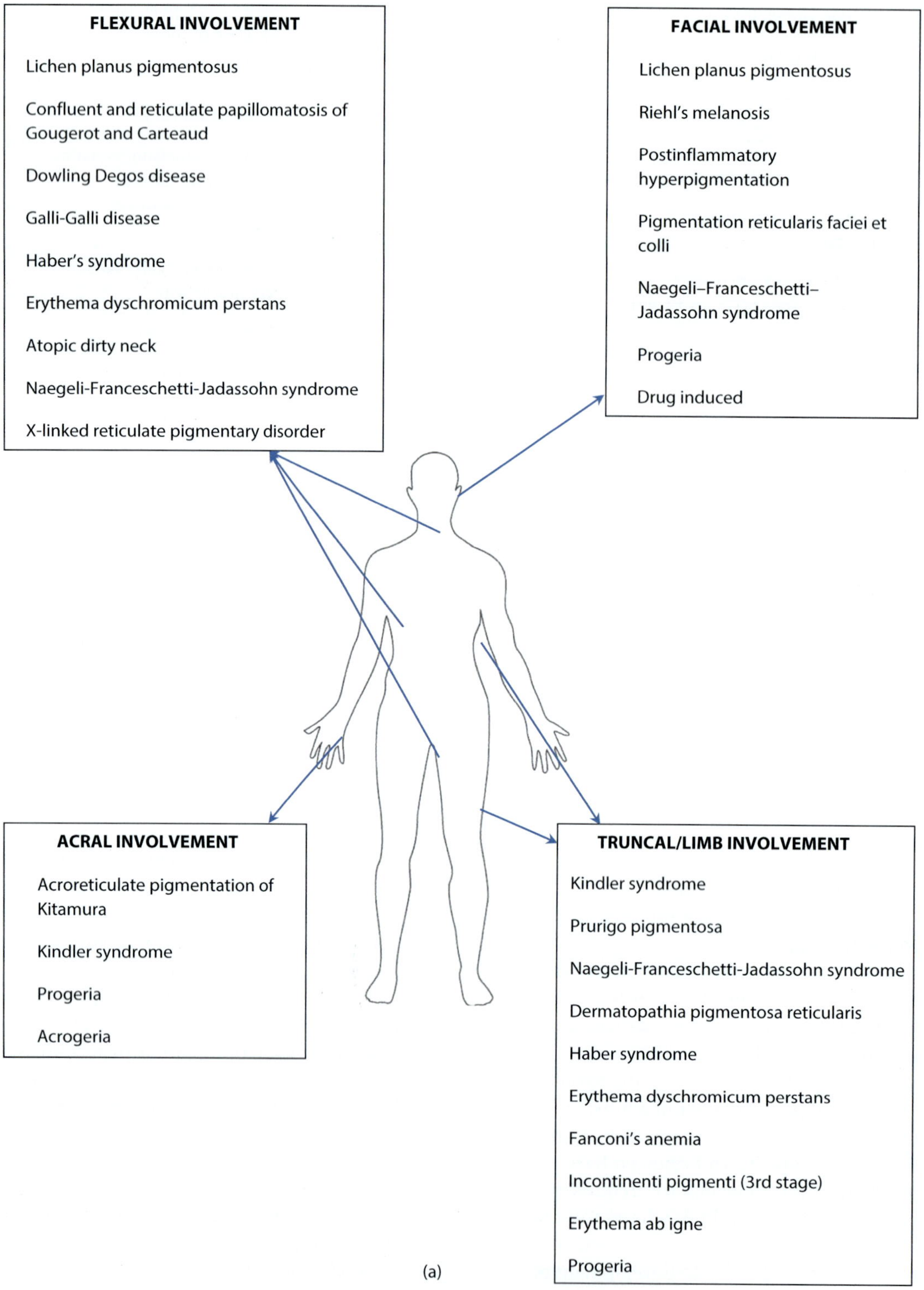


(a)

Figure 4.2 **(a)** Regional distribution of disorders with reticulate pigmentation. (*Continued*)

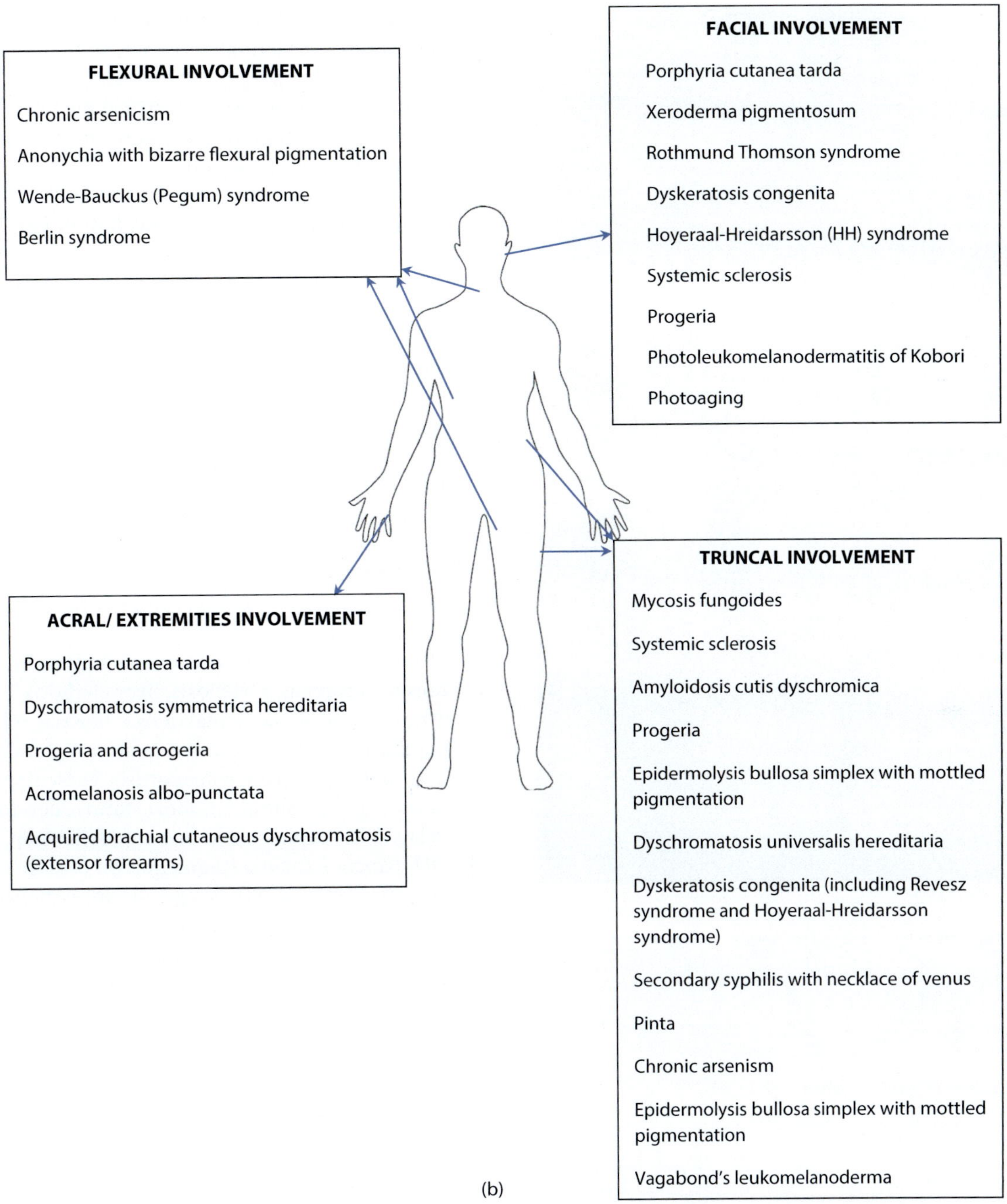


Figure 4.2 (*Continued*) **(b)** Regional distribution of disorders presenting with mottled pigmentation.

after puberty – and dental anomalies), dyskeratosis congenita (X-linked recessive, alopecia, mucosal leukoplakia, poikiloderma, and blood dyscrasias present).

## Dyskeratosis congenita (DKC)

- DKC is also known as Zinsser-Engman-Cole syndrome.
- The most common pattern of inheritance is X-linked recessive. However, a few patients may have autosomal dominant and autosomal recessive forms, which have fewer abnormalities and later onset of symptoms.
- It is caused by *DKC1* gene mutation, and the male-to-female ratio is 3:1.
- The condition is characterized by progressive bone marrow failure and clinically by triad of reticulated hyperpigmentation, nail dystrophy, and leukoplakia.
- During the first decade of life, a lacy reticulated pattern of hyperpigmentation develops, primarily on the neck, upper arms, and upper chest. Occasionally hypopigmented macules are also present.
- Nail changes – such as longitudinal ridging, splitting followed by pterygium formation, flaking or poor

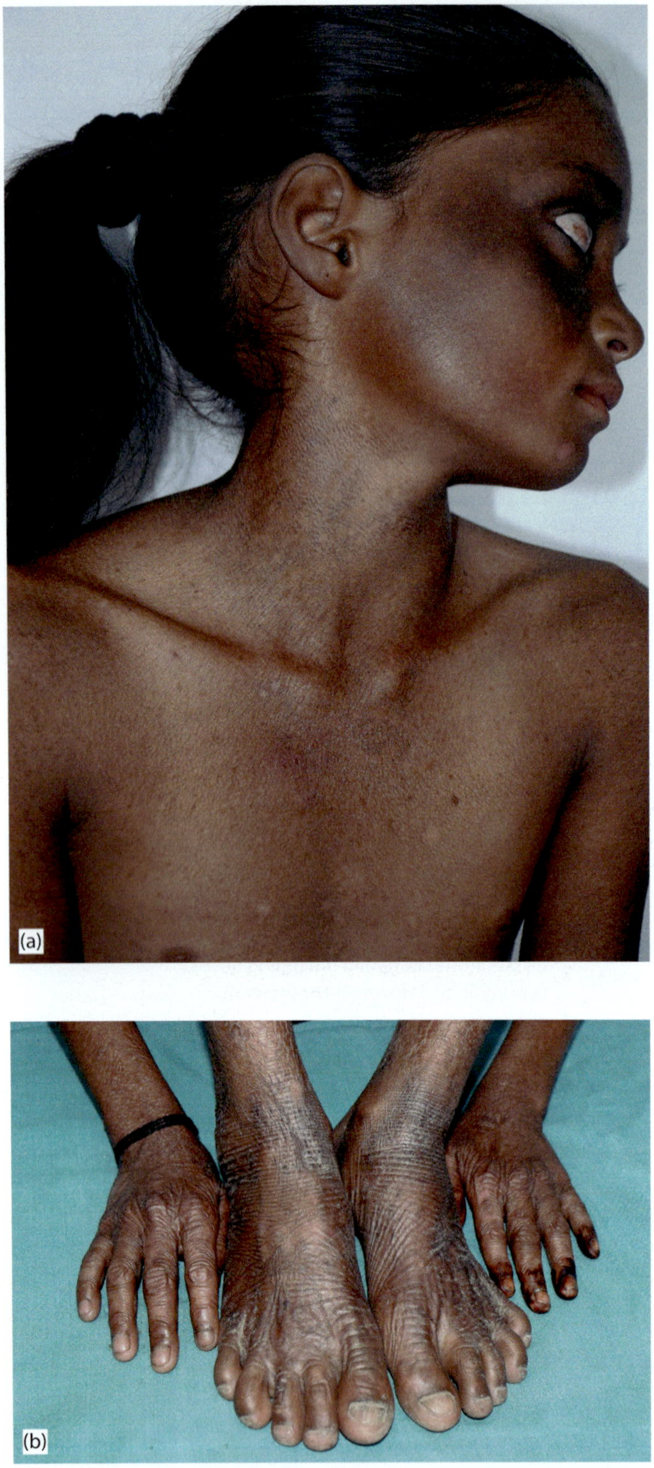


Figure 4.3 **(a)** Poikiloderma on the face and neck in a girl with Kindler syndrome. **(b)** Atrophic scarring on the acral areas in the same patient. (a,b – Courtesy: Dr. Piyush Kumar, Katihar, India.)

growth, and occasionally complete loss of nails – appear during early childhood.
- In the majority of patients, premalignant leukoplakia develops mostly on the lateral portion of the tongue.
- Teeth malformation, extensive caries, decreased root/crown ratio, periodontal disease, and missing teeth are also seen.
- Epiphora due to atresia of lacrimal ductal is common. Blepharitis, ectropion, entropion, and exudative retinopathy may be found.
- Poikiloderma is seen in some patients. Additional features include premature gray hair or hair loss, palmoplantar hyperhidrosis and hyperkeratosis, adermatoglyphia, short stature, acrocyanosis, frictional bullae, wrinkling of extremities, and small genitalia.
- Bone marrow failure is present in most patients during the third or fourth decade, presenting with anemia, thrombocytopenia, or pancytopenia. Pancytopenia may result in pallor, bruising, petechiae, and frequent infections.
- Risk of malignancy, such as squamous cell carcinoma of mouth, anus, vagina, cervix, esophagus, and skin, increases in the fourth or fifth decade. Additionally, there is increased risk of acute myeloid leukemia, myelodysplastic syndrome, and gastrointestinal carcinomas.
- Other systemic manifestations include pulmonary fibrosis, esophageal stenosis, liver cirrhosis, enteropathy, atrial or ventricular septal defect, fibrosis, dilated cardiomyopathy, urethral stenosis, cryptorchidism, male hypogonadism, osteoporosis, avascular necrosis of the hips and shoulder, short stature, developmental delay, microcephaly, and immunodeficiency.
- DD: Fanconi anemia (pigmentation is more generalized, less often reticulated), Naegeli–Franceschetti–Jadassohn (NFJ) syndrome, and dermatopathia pigmentosa reticularis (DPR) (both NFJ and DPR lack leukoplakia and bone marrow involvement).

## Incontinentia pigmenti

- It is X-linked dominant genodermatosis and is embryonically lethal for males.
- Within the first few weeks of life stages 1 and 2 are characterized by erythema, blisters, and verrucous lesions along Blaschko lines.
- Linear reticulate hyperpigmentation (stage 3) develops during infancy, persists during childhood, and fades during adolescence.
- Atrophic hypopigmentation (stage 4) develops during adolescence and persists indefinitely.
- Associated findings include scarring alopecia, nail changes, ophthalmological abnormalities, dental abnormalities, and neurological abnormalities.

## Fanconi anemia

- Primary clinical features include physical features, progressive bone marrow failure, and cancer susceptibility. However, some individuals have neither physical abnormalities nor bone marrow failure.
- Prenatal and/or postnatal short stature is a striking finding.

- It involves abnormal skin pigmentation (40%), generalized hyperpigmentation, café-au-lait macules, and hypopigmentation.
- There may be skeletal malformations (e.g., hypoplastic thumb, hypoplastic radius), microcephaly, ophthalmic anomalies (e.g., microphthalmia, cataracts, astigmatism, strabismus, epicanthal folds, hypotelorism, hypertelorism, ptosis), genitourinary tract anomalies, endocrine irregularities (hypothyroidism, glucose/insulin abnormalities), developmental delay, and/or intellectual disability.
- Incidence of acute myeloid leukemia is 13% by age 50 years. There are solid tumors affecting the head and neck, skin, gastrointestinal tract, and genitourinary tract.
- DD: Neurofibromatosis 1 (because of café-au-lait macules), Nijmegen breakage syndrome (NBS) (short stature, progressive microcephaly with loss of cognitive skills, premature ovarian failure in females, recurrent sinopulmonary infections, and an increased risk for cancer, particularly lymphoma).

## Reticulated acropigmentation of Kitamura (RAK)

- It is a rare autosomal dominant pattern of inheritance (caused by heterozygous mutation in the ADAM10 gene) with high penetrance.
- It is characterized by atrophic, reticulated, slightly depressed, well-demarcated, lentigo-like hyperpigmented macules.
- It is seen commonly on the dorsum of hands and feet during the first decade of life.
- During adulthood, these macules slowly darken over time and spread proximally to the extensor aspect of hand, neck, and face but rarely involve palms and soles (**Figure 4.4a–c**).

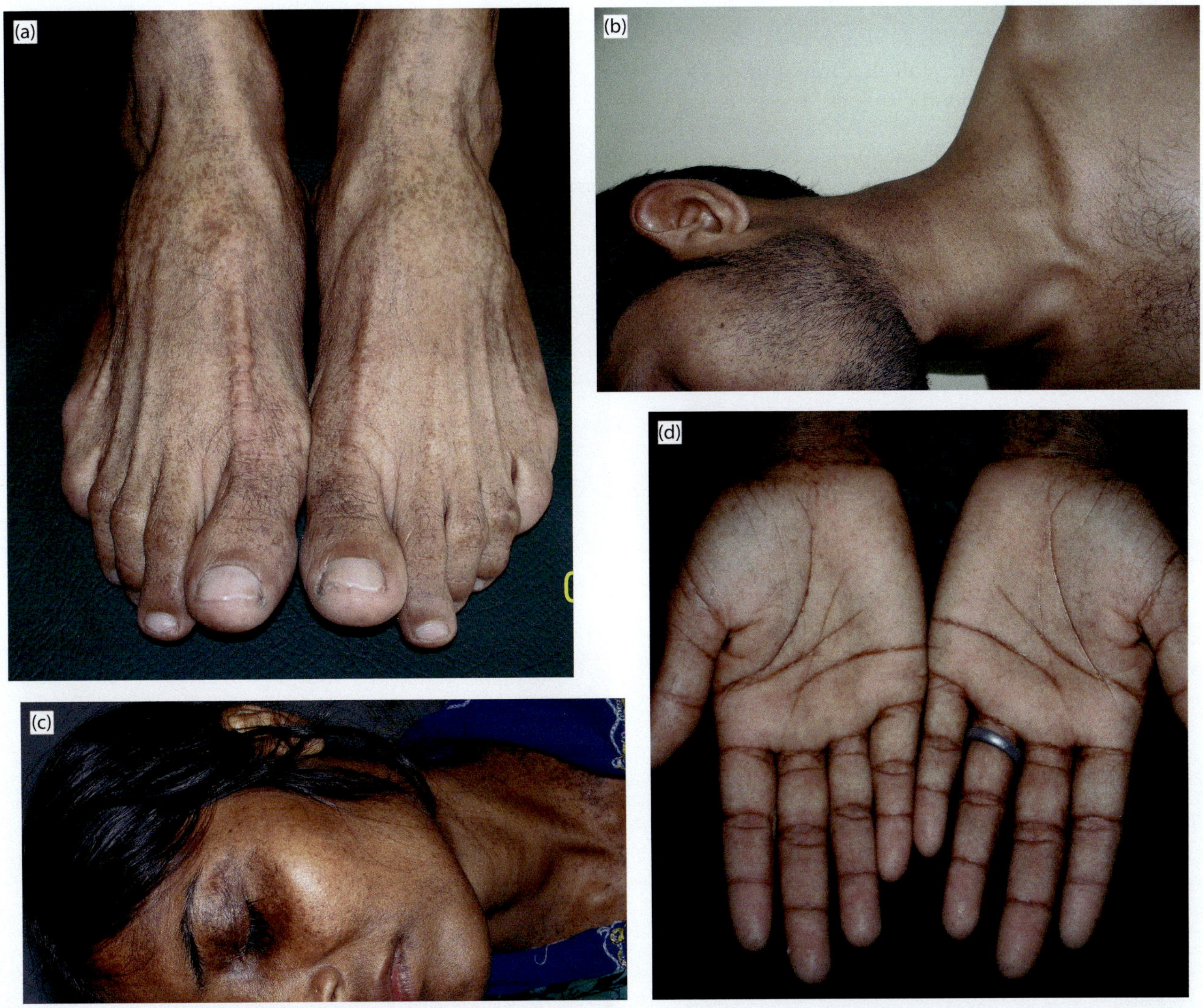


Figure 4.4 **(a)** Pigmented macules in a reticular fashion on the dorsum of feet in a patient with reticulated acropigmentation of Kitamura. **(b)** Discrete pigmented macules on the neck of a young man. **(c)** Coalescing, pigmented macules on the face and neck of a young lady. **(d)** Palmar pits – an important clinical clue to reticulated acropigmentation of Kitamura. (a–d – Courtesy: Dr. Piyush Kumar, Katihar, India.)

- Flexors may occasionally be involved.
- Sunlight may aggravate the condition.
- Other features include pits on palms (**Figure 4.4d**), soles, and dorsal phalangeal surface; dermatoglyphic disruption; partial non-scarring alopecia; and occasionally plantar keratoderma.
- DD: Solar lentigines (hyperpigmented macules are slightly atrophic and develops early in RAK).

## Dowling-Degos disease (DDD)

- This is a rare autosomal dominant disorder caused by mutations in the *KRT5*, *POFUT1*, or *POGLUT1* gene.
- There is no gender predilection.
- Onset is typically during the third or fourth decade of life.
- It is characterized by acquired reticular hyperpigmentation in the intertriginous areas. Reticulated hyperpigmentation with lentigo-like brown macules and small brown papules, sometimes pruritic, begins in flexors such as axillae and groin (**Figure 4.5a–c**). As the disease progresses, it also involves trunk, neck, intergluteal, inframammary areas, and inner aspects of arms and thighs.
- Isolated genital involvement presents in a few patients.
- Mucous membranes are spared.
- Common associated findings include pitted follicular perioral and facial scars, comedones like follicular papules on the back or neck, epidermoid cysts, hidradenitis suppurativa, seborrheic keratosis, pilonidal cysts, SCC, and keratoacanthoma.
- Known variants are Haber's syndrome, Galli Galli disease, and pigmentatio reticularis faciei et colli.
- DD: Acanthosis nigricans (velvety plaques, no follicular involvement), neurofibromatosis type 1 (freckles in axillae and groin), reticulated acropigmentation of Kitamura (RAK) (atrophic hyperpigmented macules on the dorsum of hands and freckles on face appear during childhood, acral involvement).

## Galli-Galli disease

- This is a rare acantholytic variant of Dowling-Degos disease, linked to mutations in the KRT5 gene.
- It is an autosomal dominant with variable penetrance, but it can occur sporadically.
- It is a benign but very pruritic and unaesthetic genodermatosis.

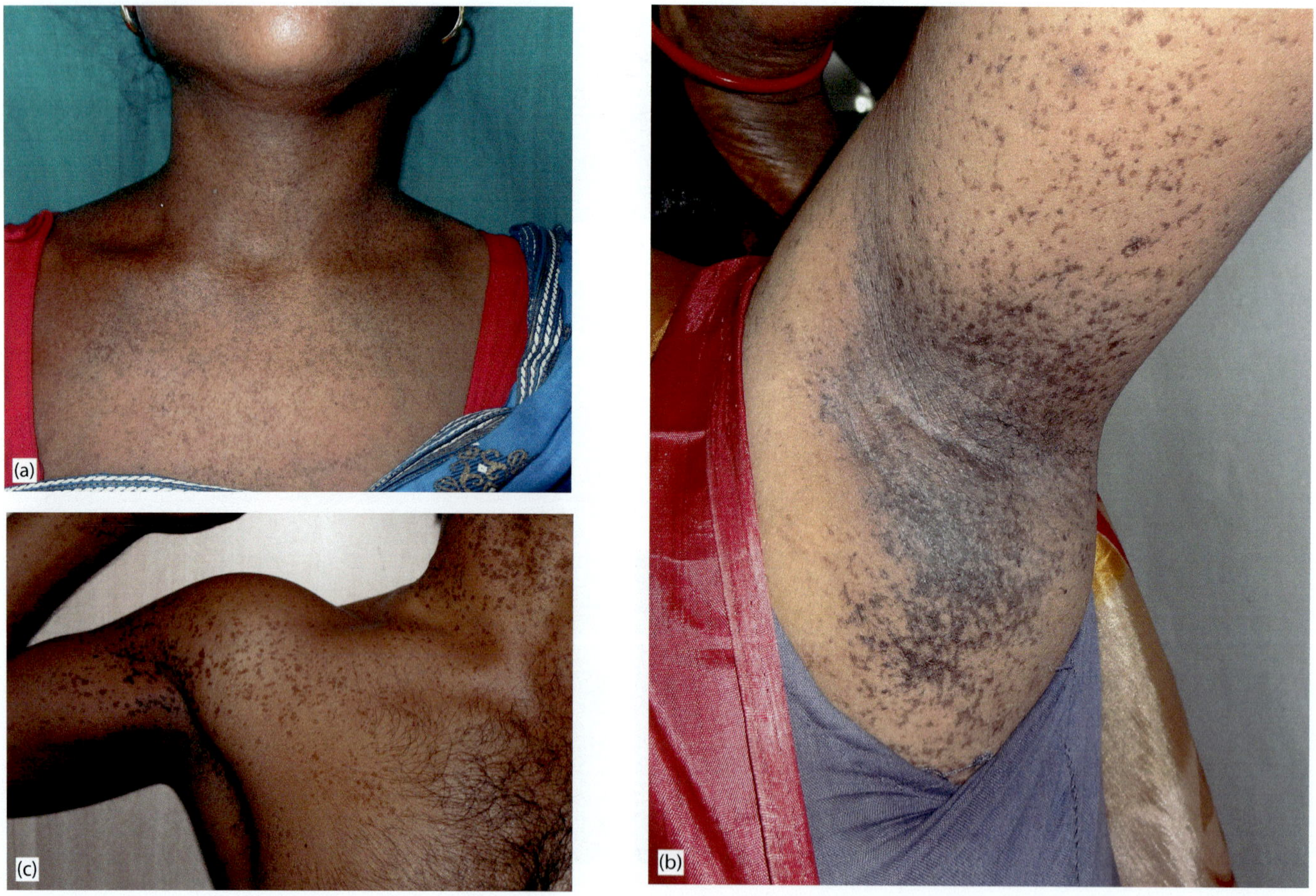


Figure 4.5 **(a)** Pigmented macules on the neck in Dowling Degos disease. **(b)** Axilla showing numerous coalescing pigmented macules in Dowling Degos disease. **(c)** Reticulate pigmented macules affecting neck and axilla. (a,b – Courtesy: Dr. Piyush Kumar, Katihar, India; c – Courtesy: Dr. Dipali Rathod, Mumbai, India.)

- It is clinically characterized by reticulated hyperpigmentation, predominantly affecting the flexures along with pruritic, erythematous, scaly papules, similar to the DDD.

## Confluent and reticulated papillomatosis (CRP)

- This is also known as confluent and reticulated papillomatosis of Gougerot and Carteaud.
- CRP primarily is caused by a bacterium, *Dietzia papillomatosis,* an aerobic gram-positive coccus/rod actinomycete. It may also be caused by endocrinopathies, especially insulin resistance, obesity, pituitary, and thyroid disorders. Others postulated causes are ultraviolet (UV) light, keratinization, and *Malassezia furfur.*
- Occurrence is mostly sporadic, but familial cases are also reported.
- Young women are commonly affected.
- Initial lesions are 1–2 mm papules that enlarge rapidly to 4–5 mm and become brown, hyperkeratotic, verrucous papules, patches, or thin plaques. Lesions first appear in the intermammary area and less frequently in the interscapular and epigastric area.
- Lesions can also involve neck, upper trunk, antecubital fossa, and popliteal fossae (**Figure 4.6a**).
- The papules coalesce to form confluent centrally and reticulated peripherally (**Figure 4.6b**).
- It is largely asymptomatic but rarely mild pruritus may be noted.
- CRP is limited only to the skin, with no systemic involvement. The mucous membranes, palms, and soles are spared.
- DD: Acanthosis nigricans (presence of peripheral reticulation and the absence of mucosal and nail involvement in CRP; in AN there are thicker, more velvety plaques, no scales, lack of reticulation; acanthosis nigricans appears prominently in the axillae and groin area, while CRP presents on the central back and chest), terra firma-forme dermatosis (TFFD) (lesions can easily be removed with alcohol swab), Darier disease (involves seborrheic area, palmoplantar pits, and nail changes, such as blue-red striations and distal

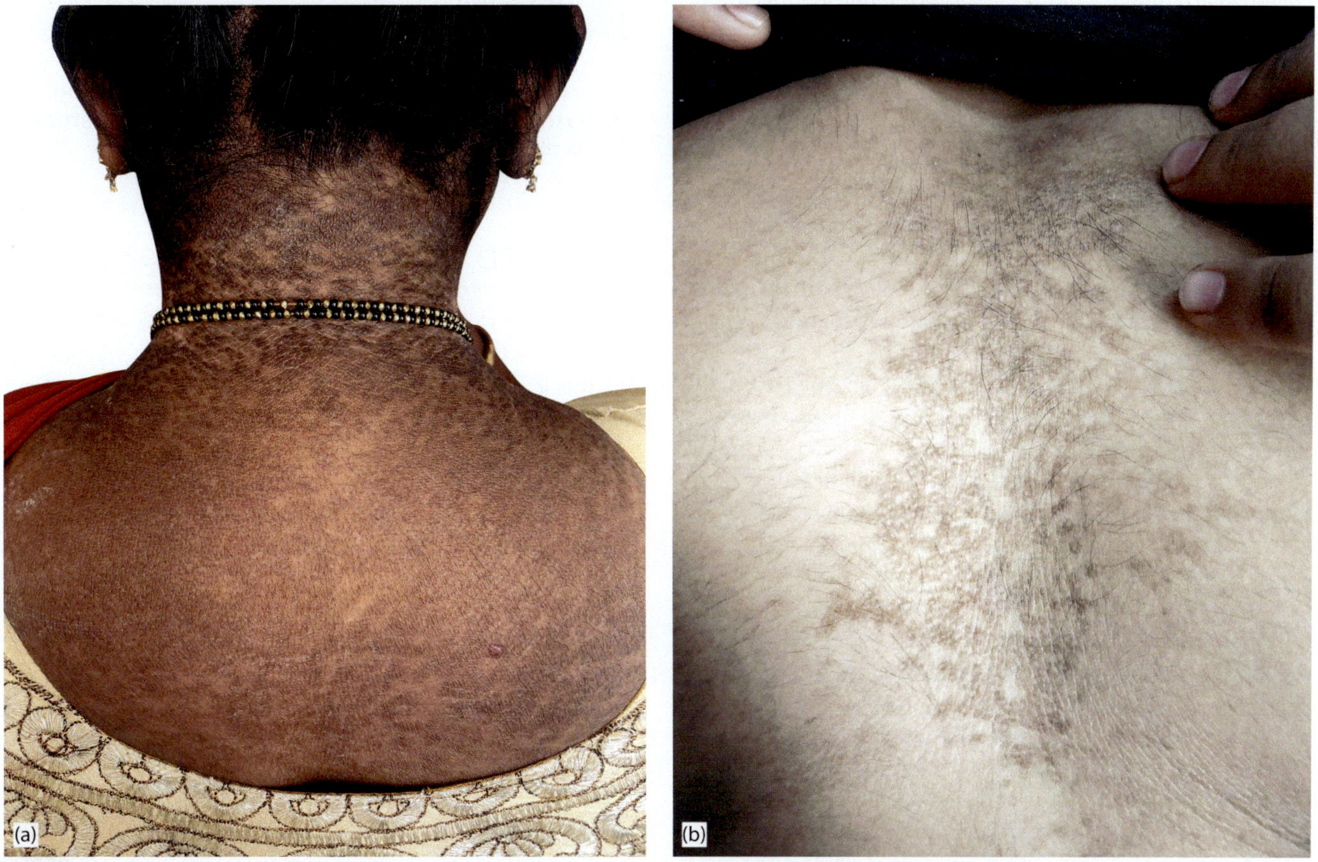


Figure 4.6 **(a)** Confluent and reticulated papillomatosis with reticulated, scaly papules and plaques on the neck and upper back. **(b)** Confluent and reticulated papillomatosis with reticulated, scaly papules and plaques on the central chest. (a – Courtesy: Dr. Neethu Mary George, Sri Siddhartha Medical College, Tumkur, India; b – Courtesy: Dr. Anil Patki, Pune, India.)

V-shaped nicking, may be present), Pityriasis versicolor (brown scales but no reticulation and papillomatosis).

### Prurigo pigmentosa

- This is a rare inflammatory skin disease of unknown pathogenesis.
- Various etiological factors include friction with clothes, sun exposure, physical trauma, contact allergens, *H. pylori* infection, *Borrelia* spirochetes, atopic disease, mechanical stimuli, and drugs such as bismuth subsalicylate containing antacid.
- Females are more commonly affected in third decade of life.
- It is characterized by a sudden onset of symmetrical distribution of pruritic and erythematous macules, urticarial papules, and plaques that may coalesce, then involute within a week to form crusted and scaly red papules leaving a macular reticulated hyperpigmentation.
- There is a predilection for back, neck, and chest. Recurrence occurs at the same site.
- Rarely, pustular and bullous variants present. Often, lesions of different stages are seen.
- DD: Confluent and reticulated papillomatosis (CRP) (central confluence and peripheral reticulation, neck and axilla spared, asymptomatic, no pruritus).

### Erythema ab igne

- This is also known as toasted skin syndrome or fire stains.
- It is a localized skin condition caused by chronic and repeated exposure to infrared radiation in the form of heat insufficient to cause a direct burn.
- Risk factors include heat applied to relieve pain, working near heat exposure, decreased sensation, habitually warming at fire places.
- Heat sources include hot water bottles, heating pads, prolonged hot bathing, infrared lamps, laptops, open fires, etc.
- A lesion starts as transient macular erythematous and blanchable; with repeated exposure to heat, the lesion becomes hyperpigmented and non-blanchable (**Figure 4.7**).
- Epidermal atrophy may overlie the reticulated pigmentation.
- These lesions are usually asymptomatic but can be associated with pain, burning, and itching.
- The bullous form of erythema ab igne is a rare variant. The long-term risk of cutaneous malignancies include squamous cell carcinoma and Merkel cell carcinoma.
- DD: Livedo reticularis (erythema is not persistent, no hyperpigmentation), poikiloderma atrophicans vasculare (no distinct vascular pattern, more atrophic, telangiectatic), Majocchi disease (superficial and annular).

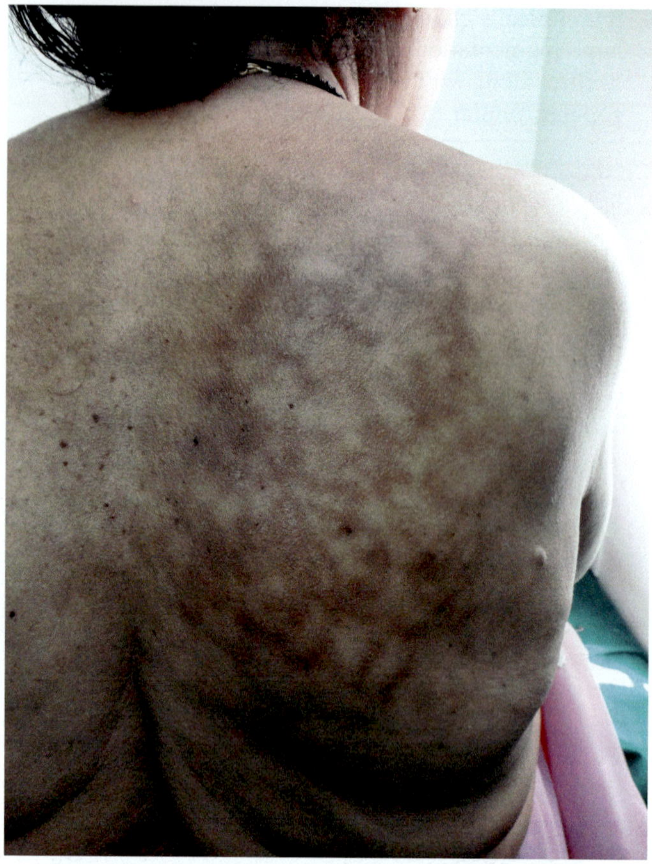

Figure 4.7 Reticulate, persistent hyperpigmentation of erythema ab igne. (Courtesy: Dr. Hiral Shah, Baroda Medical College, Vadodara, India.)

## MOTTLED PIGMENTATION

### Epidermolysis bullosa simplex with mottled pigmentation

- It is a rare autosomal dominant disorder resulting from mutations in either the KRT5 or KRT14 gene. Males and females are affected equally.
- Clinically, it is characterized by mechanically induced hemorrhagic blisters that usually heal without scarring or milia formation. Scarring, when noted, is always atrophic. Sites affected are feet, knees, and hands. Mucous membrane, teeth, and hair are generally spared. Mottled pigmentation appears usually during infancy and persists throughout life. It affects trunk, neck, axilla, and extremities (**Figure 4.8a,b**).
- DD: Autoimmune blistering diseases, staphylococcal scalded skin syndrome.

### Porphyria cutanea tarda

- Porphyrias are photosensitivity disorders due to defects in biosynthesis of heme. Porphyria cutanea tarda is the most common porphyria, which results from decreased activity of uroporphyrinogen decarboxylase,

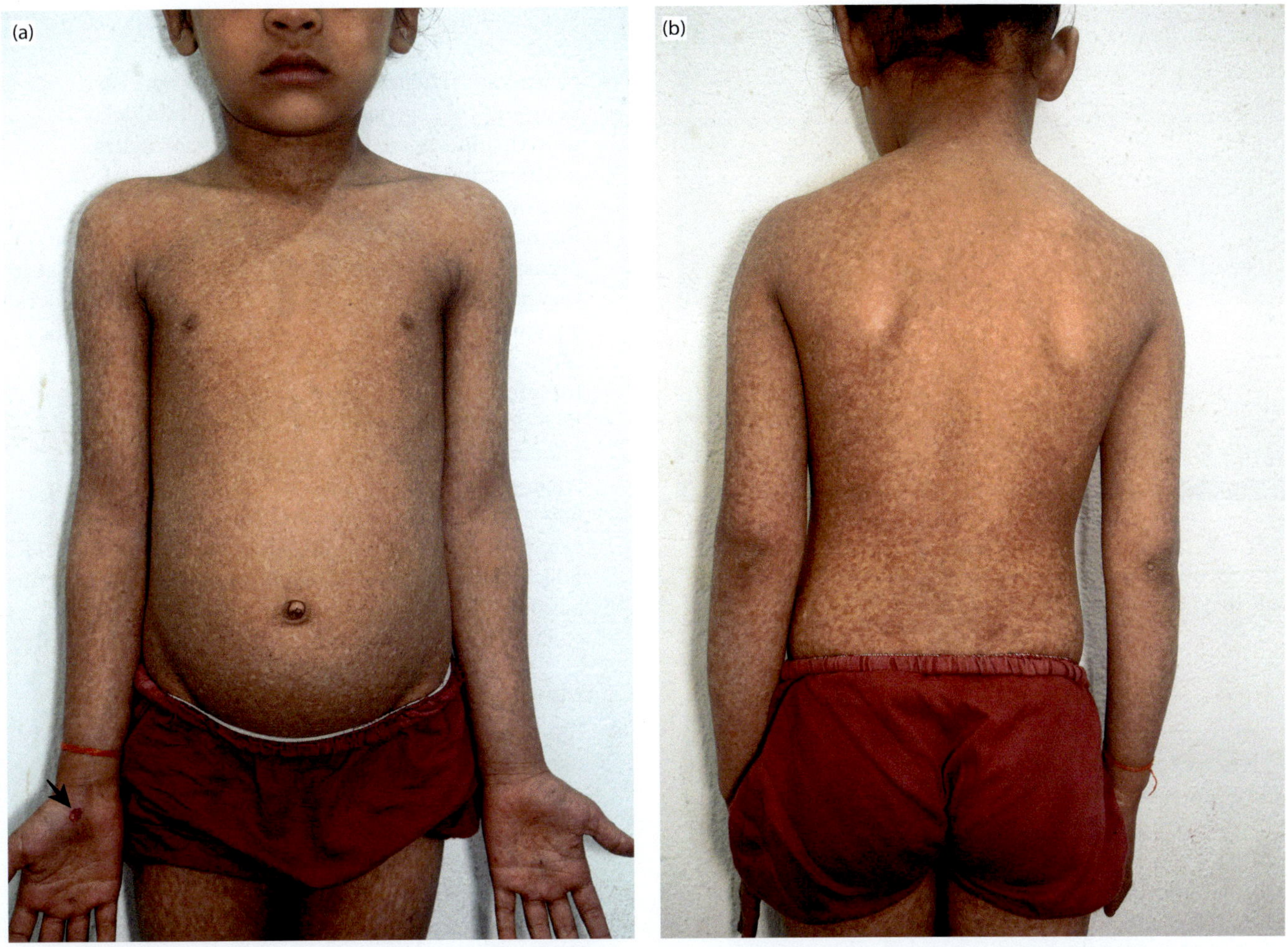


Figure 4.8 **(a)** Epidermolysis bullosa simplex with mottled pigmentation in a child. Note the eroded blister on palm (marked with black arrow). **(b)** Posterior side of same patient. (a,b – Courtesy: Dr. Piyush Kumar, Katihar, India.)

the fifth enzyme in heme biosynthesis. Type 1 PCT is an acquired or sporadic variant; type 2 PCT is an autosomal dominant familial variant.

- It presents with skin fragility, blister formation, erosion, crust, milia formation, thickening of skin and scar in sun-exposed areas. Vesicles and bullae may also develop in sun-exposed areas.
- Mottled pigmentation may also be seen. Pigmentary changes are more frequently present in females on the face (especially periocular).
- Other cutaneous findings include scarring alopecia, hypertrichosis, onycholysis, morpheaform, and sclerodermoid plaque.
- DD: Pseudoporphyria, hepatoerythropoietic porphyria, scleroderma, morphea, bullous pemphigoid, polymorphous light eruption.

## Dyschromatosis symmetrica hereditaria (DSH)

- This is also called acroreticulate pigmentation of Dohi.
- It is a rare skin condition with an autosomal dominant pattern of inheritance, rarely autosomal recessive. Sporadic cases are also known.
- It generally manifests during infancy or early childhood, with hyperpigmented and hypopigmented macules of 3–5 mm that often increases in size and number until adolescence. Sites involved are distal extremities, usually the dorsa of the hands and feet and sometimes forearms and legs. Palms, soles, nails, hair, and mucous membranes are spared (**Figure 4.9**).
- DD: Xeroderma pigmentosum (hyper- and hypopigmented macules are photo-distributed involving face and truck also), Dowling Degos disease (involvement of flexures, dark comedone-like lesions, pitted perioral acneiform scars), reticulate acropigmentation of Kitamura (no hypopigmentation), vitiligo (no hyperpigmentation), dyschromatosis universalis hereditaria (lesions present at birth with truncal involvement).

## Dyschromatosis Universalis Hereditaria (DUH)

- It is a rare disorder of dyschromatosis having both autosomal dominant and recessive patterns of inheritance. Sporadic cases are also seen.

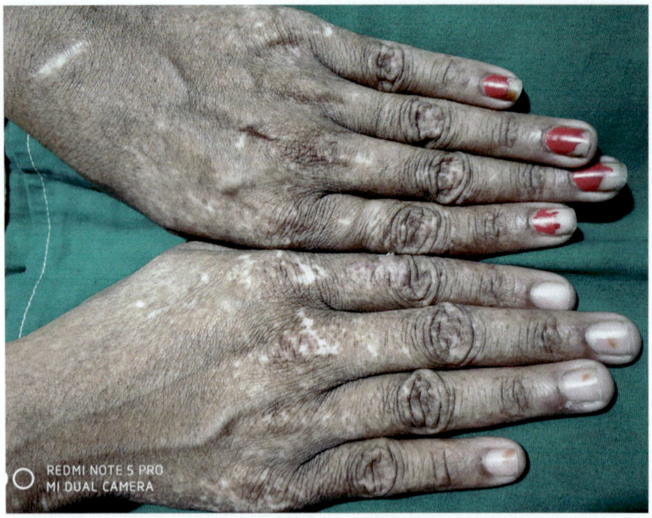


Figure 4.9 Dyschromatosis symmetrica hereditaria with mottled pigmentation of the dorsa of both hands. (Courtesy: Dr. Anil Patki, Pune, India.)

- DUH usually develops dyschromia by the age of 6 years in most of the patients and at birth in few. Hyperpigmented and hypopigmented macules of various sizes usually start on the hands then progress to involve head, neck, trunk. Mottled pigmentation of the tongue and oral mucosa may be seen occasionally.
- Thin, hyperpigmented dystrophic nails with pterygium formation are rarely present.
- Extracutaneous abnormalities include short stature, high tone deafness, neurosensory hearing defects, photosensitivity, glaucoma, cataracts, and seizures.
- DD: Xeroderma pigmentosum (involves photo-exposed areas whereas DUH involves unexposed areas also), acropigmentation of Dohi (localized form involving only the acral areas).

## Xeroderma pigmentosum (XP)

- It is an autosomal dominant disease caused by faulty DNA repair mechanisms.
- The skin is normal at birth, and cutaneous manifestations appear in early childhood, starting with marked photosensitivity and photophobia. Minimal sun exposure can lead to sunburn, manifesting as erythema, blistering, edema, and vesicles. After two years of age, the patient develops solar lentigines and freckles on sun-exposed areas such as face and limbs. Repeated sun exposure results in xerosis, hyper- and hypopigmentation, telangiectasia, atrophy, and scarring of skin (**Figure 4.10a–c**).
- Actinic keratosis, squamous cell carcinoma (SCC), basal cell carcinoma (BCC), and melanoma are other complications that can develop with age.
- Ocular abnormalities include photophobia, conjunctivitis, keratitis, corneal opacification and ulceration, vascularization, ectropion, loss of eyelashes, SCC, and malignant melanoma of sun-exposed part of eyes.
- Neurological deficits include severe progressive neurological degeneration, microcephaly, delayed growth and sexual development, sensorineural deafness, intellectual impairment, peripheral neuropathy, dementia, and ataxia.
- Pigmented xerodermoid is a variant of xeroderma pigmentosum and presents at a later age, with onset in the third or fourth decade of life. The clinical features are similar to those of XP, but the risk of malignancy is much less (compared to XP), and neurological manifestations are rare (**Figure 4.10d**).
- DD: Rothmund-Thomson syndrome (no photosensitivity, absence of pigmentary changes), trichothiodystrophy (absence of ichthyosis, brittle hair and micrognathia, no increase in malignancies), cerebro-oculo-facial syndrome (absence of xerosis, poikiloderma, telangiectasia, and atrophy), porphyrias, basal cell nevus syndrome, UV sensitive syndrome (solar lentigines, photosensitivity, otherwise normal).

## Rothmund-Thomson syndrome

- It is a rare genetic disorder with autosomal recessive inheritance caused by mutations in RECQL4. Consanguinity is reported in few patients.
- Onset of the acute phase is in early infancy, with erythema, edema, vesicles on the cheeks and face, followed by the chronic and persistent phase, which develops gradually over a period of months to years with development of poikiloderma (atrophy, hyperpigmentation and hypopigmentation and telangiectasia) affecting the dorsal aspect of hands and buttocks.
- Other features include sparse eyebrows, eyelashes, and scalp hair; hypoplastic or poorly formed nails; dental anomalies (microdontia, caries, hypoplastic teeth; short stature; mental retardation; speech developmental delay; hyperkeratosis of palms and soles; bilateral juvenile cataracts; chronic vomiting; diarrhea; sensorineural deafness; and pituitary hypogonadism.
- There is increased risk for osteogenic sarcoma, myelodysplastic syndrome, and BCC and SCC.
- DD: Bloom syndrome (no true poikiloderma, recurrent otic and pulmonary infections), Werner syndrome (late onset, initial signs are hoarseness followed by bilateral cataract, type 2 diabetes mellitus), xeroderma pigmentosum (marked photosensitivity, lentigines and freckles on minimal sun exposure, xerosis, keratitis), Kindler syndrome (marked photosensitivity; acral bullae at birth or after minor trauma; keratotic papules of hands, feet, knees, elbows; atrophy of eyelid skin).

## Chronic arsenicism

- Arsenic is a metal that can be ingested through water or medicines or inhaled in occupational exposures. Acute toxicity can be lethal. Chronic arsenic exposure

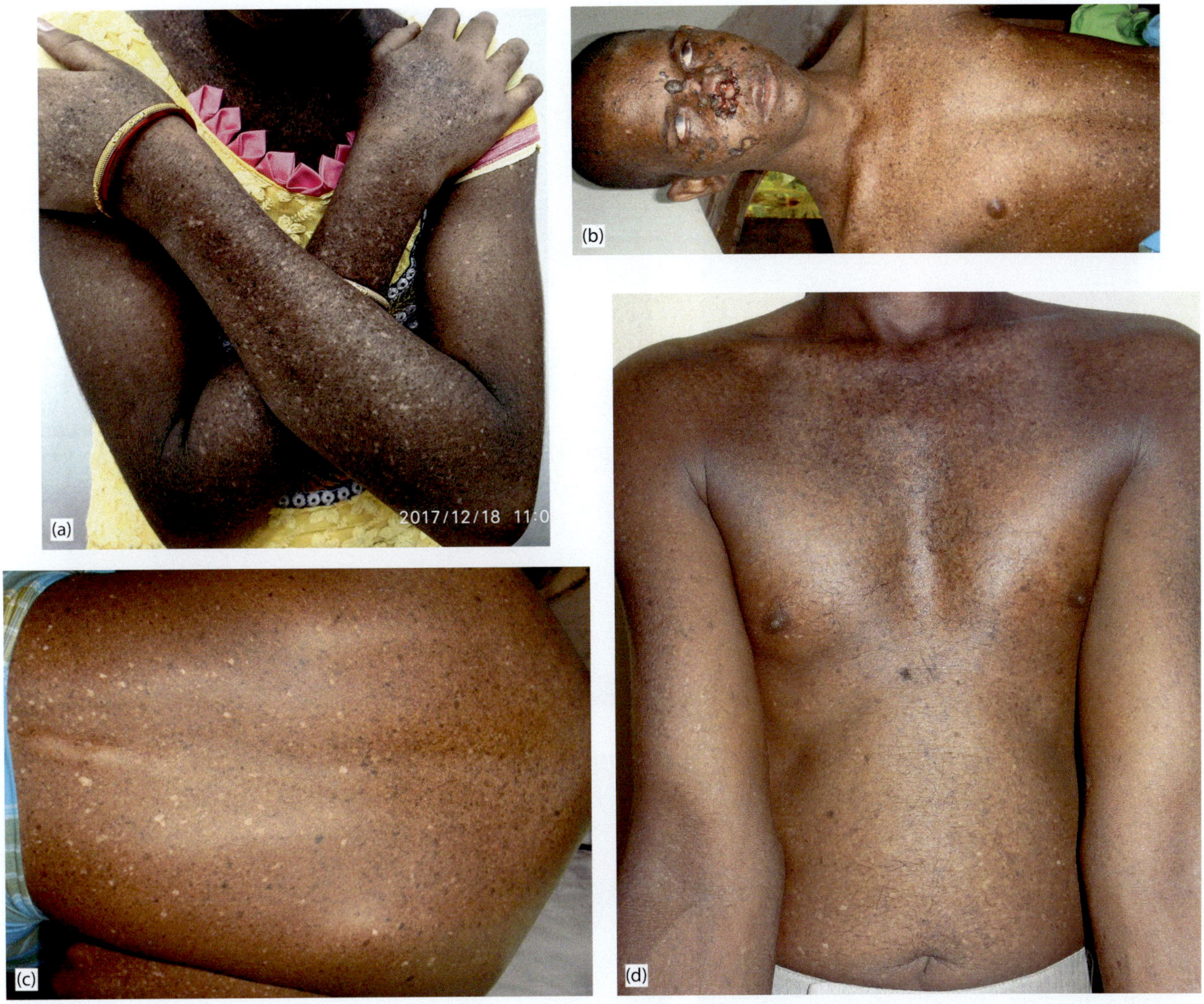


Figure 4.10 **(a)** Mottled pigmentation on the upper extremities in a case of xeroderma pigmentosum. **(b)** Xeroderma pigmentosum with multiple facial malignancies and mottled pigmentation on the trunk. **(c)** Back of the same patient (Figure 4.10b). **(d)** Pigmented xerodermoid with mottled pigmentation on the trunk. (a – Courtesy: Dr. Deverashetti Srinivas, Nizamabad, India; b–d – Courtesy: Dr. Piyush Kumar, Katihar, India.)

is characterized by hyperpigmentation of palms, soles, groin, axilla, nipple, pressure point area with superimposed raindrop-like guttate hypopigmented macules. Arsenical keratosis develops on hands and feet (**Figure 4.11a–d**).

- Other features include peripheral neuropathy, nasal septal perforation, hepatomegaly, liver fibrosis, diabetes mellitus, and diarrhea. Increased risk of malignancies including Bowen's disease, basal cell carcinoma, squamous cell carcinoma, urinary bladder, liver and lung malignancies is noted.
- DD: Dyschromatosis universalis hereditaria.

## Mycosis fungoides (MF)

- MF is the most common type of cutaneous T-cell lymphoma, accounting for around 50% of the all primary cutaneous lymphoma. Males are more commonly affected than females.
- MF has three cutaneous stages. In the **patch stage** lesions are usually flat, non-palpable, erythematous with fine scales and mild pruritus. There is skin atrophy of varying degrees with mottled hyper- and hypopigmentation with telangiectasia present in poikiloderma vasculare atrophicans, a variant of patch phase. Lesions tend to occur initially on covered body areas such as buttocks, trunk, and limb. Unusual shapes, such as annular, polycyclic, or horseshoe, are common. In the **plaque stage** there is erythematous plaque, which may ulcerate and become secondarily infected. Plaque may be hyperpigmented in darkly pigmented skin. The **tumor stage** may consist of patch, plaque, and

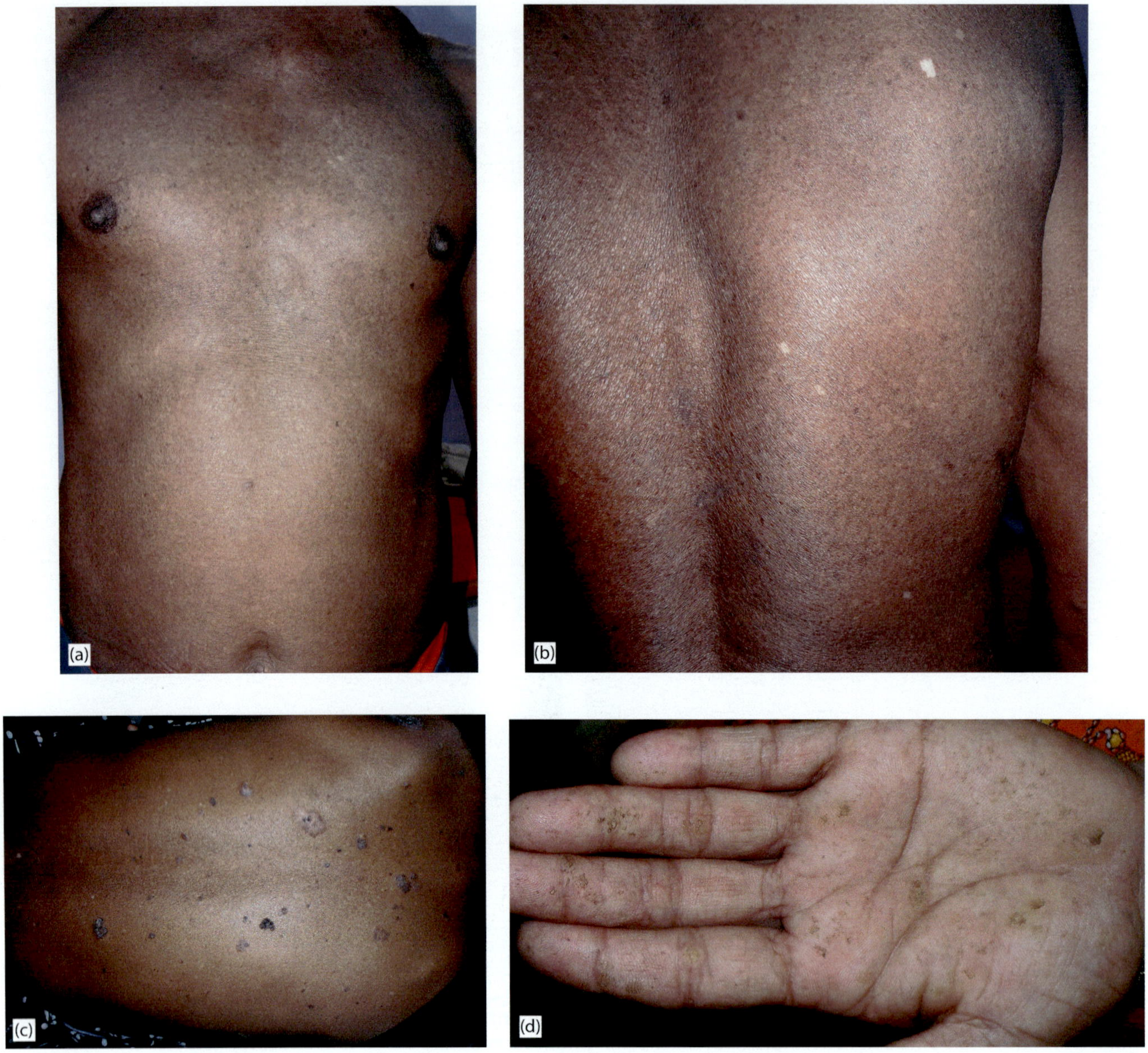


Figure 4.11 **(a)** Increased pigmentation and depigmented macules in chronic arsenicism. **(b)** Back of the same patient (Figure 4.11a). Few pigmented, scaly plaques may be appreciated. **(c)** Another patient with multiple hyperkeratotic scaly plaques on the back in chronic arsenicism. **(d)** Palmar hyperkeratotic papules in chronic arsenicism. (a–d – Courtesy: Dr. Piyush Kumar, Katihar, India.)

tumors. Tumors may arise from pre-existing plaque. Tumor stage tends to ulcerate.

- DD: Patch stage – vitiligo, pityriasis alba, pityriasis versicolor, idiopathic guttate hypomelanosis, leprosy, post-inflammatory hypopigmentation, drug reaction, eczema, large plaque psoriasis. Plaque stage – large plaque psoriasis, lymphomatoid drug reaction, lymphomatoid contact dermatitis. Tumor stage – cutaneous T-cell lymphoma with diffuse pleomorphic infiltrates.

## Amyloidosis cutis dyschromica

- It is a very rare and distinct variant of primary cutaneous amyloidosis. It may have an autosomal dominant inheritance pattern.
- The etiology is unknown, but genetic, environmental and immunological factors have been considered.
- It is characterized by prepubertal onset of mottled pigmentation (mixture of hyper- and hypopigmented and/or depigmented macules of various sizes) primarily affecting sun-exposed areas (**Figure 4.12a–d**).
- DD: Xeroderma pigmentosum (marked photosensitivity, lentigines and freckles on minimal sun exposure, xerosis, keratitis, telangiectasia, atrophy, and scarring of skin, cutaneous malignancies), dyschromatosis universalis hereditaria (lesions present at birth with truncal involvement), reticulate acropigmentation of Dohi (lesions appears during infancy or early childhood, only distal extremities are affected),

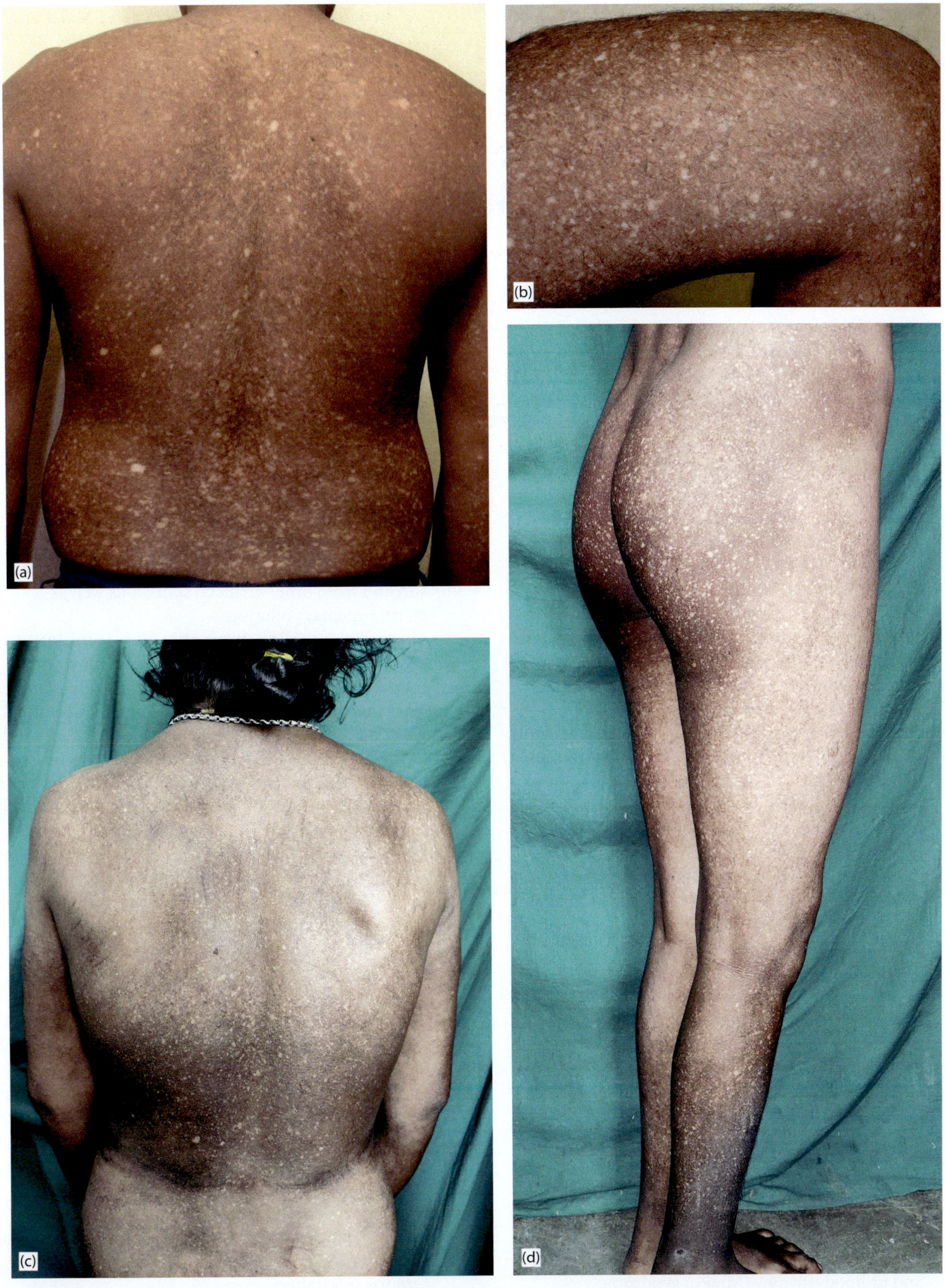


Figure 4.12 **(a)** Amyloidosis cutis dyschromica with both hyperpigmented and hypopigmented macules on the back. **(b)** Close-up of lesions on the thigh. **(c)** Mottled pigmentation on the back in amyloidosis cutis dyschromica. **(d)** Close of lesions on the leg. (a,b – Courtesy: Dr. Piyush Kumar, Katihar, India; c,d – Courtesy: Dr Hiral Shah, Baroda Medical College, Vadodara, India.)

dyskeratosis congenita (progressive bone marrow failure and clinically by triad of reticulated hyperpigmentation, nail dystrophy, leukoplakia).

## Progeria

- **Hutchinson-Gilford syndrome**
  - It is a rare genetic disease caused due to mutation in LMNA gene characterized by accelerated aging that begins during infancy. The patient is usually normal at birth.
  - In the first year, reticulate hyperpigmentation develops on sun-exposed areas, with sclerodermatous skin changes on abdomen, upper thigh, and buttocks. Skin is thin, loose, and wrinkled on hands and feet, with sparse body hair, alopecia of scalp, eyebrows, and eyelashes.
  - Growth failure with rapid infantile fat loss results in prominent superficial veins, perioral cyanosis, small face, beaked nose, protruding eyes and ears, large cranium, frontal bossing and micrognathia giving appearance of "plucked bird."
  - Other findings include dental anomalies, nail dystrophy, high-pitched voice, hearing loss, corneal dryness, insulin resistance, premature atherosclerosis, myocardial fibrosis.
  - Average survival is 12 years.
  - DD: Werner syndrome, Nestor-Guillermo progeria syndrome, Penttinen syndrome.
- **Werner syndrome**
  - It is also called adult progeria or pangeria.
  - It is a rare progeroid syndrome with an autosomal recessive pattern of inheritance caused by mutations in the RECQL2 (WRN) gene. The patient is normal until the beginning of the second decade, when cessation of growth occurs near puberty.
  - Other features of syndrome develop during second or third decade of life. Characteristic features include short stature, beaked nose, prominent eyes, premature graying of hair, alopecia, bird-like facies, high-pitched voice, teeth anomalies, and micrognathia.
  - The cutaneous changes include reticulate hyperpigmentation, skin atrophy, sclerodermatous skin changes, nail dystrophy or hypoplasia, plantar hyperkeratosis, and trophic ulcers of legs.
  - Associated systemic findings include juvenile cataract, hypogonadism, hyperlipidemia, osteoporosis, type 2 diabetes mellitus, and metastatic calcification.
  - There is an increased risk of melanoma, osteosarcoma, and soft tissue sarcoma.
  - DD: Hutchinson Gilford syndrome, Nestor-Guillermo syndrome, Rothmund syndrome, mandibular hypoplasia deafness progeroid features and or lipodystrophy (MDPL) syndrome.
- **Nestor-Guillermo syndrome**
  - It is a rare genetic progeroid syndrome with autosomal recessive pattern of inheritance due to mutation of the AR/BANF1 gene. Males and females are equally affected.
  - Disease onset is usually in the third year of life. It is characterized by reticulate hyperpigmentation, skin atrophy, generalized loss of subcutaneous fat, prominent scalp veins, thin nose and lip, micrognathia, prominent eyes, and short stature.
  - Other findings include nail dystrophy, progressive alopecia, severe osteolysis (notably on mandible, clavicles, ribs, distal phalanges, and long bones), osteoporosis, joint stiffness (mainly of fingers, hands, knees, and elbows), dental anomalies, delayed closure of anterior fontanelle, absence of cardiovascular, atherosclerotic and metabolic complications.
  - Survival is into adulthood.
  - DD: MDPL syndrome, Hutchinson Gilford syndrome, Penttinen syndrome (disease onset is in infancy to childhood with normal stature).

## Photoaging

- It is premature aging of skin caused by repeated exposure to ultraviolet radiation (UV) mainly from sun and from other artificial sources as well as environmental pollution.
- Photoaging usually appears after 50 years of age.
- Pigmentary changes include mottled pigmentation, solar lentigines, freckles, diffuse hyperpigmentation, seborrheic keratoses, and guttate hypopigmentation. It affects mostly sun-exposed areas such as face, neck, back of hands, lips and upper chest and, in women, between knee and ankle.
- Other findings include marked wrinkling around the eyes and mouth, deep creases, forehead frown lines that are visible when not frowning, dry and rough skin, atrophy, inelastic or leathery skin, and telangiectasias. Dark skin tends to have much less pronounced and delayed onset of photoaging.
- Cutis rhomboidalis nuchae (sailor's or farmer's neck) occurs due to chronic sun-exposure. Skin becomes thick, leathery, tough, lichenified on the back of the neck. Favre-Racouchot syndrome presents with nodular elastosis, cysts, and comedones on malar and inferior periorbital, forearm, and helix of ear.
- DD: chronological aging (pigmentary changes are pale, white, hypopigmentation, fine wrinkles, skin is dry and flaky).

## Vagabond's leukomelanoderma

- It is a skin condition characteristically occurring in elderly persons with dietary deficiency in association with poor hygiene and heavy *Pediculus humanus corporis* infestation.
- It presents as hypopigmented macules superimposed on a hyperpigmented background associated with severe itching.

- The lesions can be seen on any site but most commonly affects axilla, groin, wrist, medial side of thigh, and posterior neck.
- DD: Chronic arsenicosis, leucoderma syphiliticum.

### Onchocerciasis

- Onchocerciasis, or river blindness, is caused by the nematode *Onchocerca volvulus*.
- It predominantly affects skin and eyes.
- Cutaneous manifestations include subcutaneous nodules containing adult worms, papular dermatitis, lichenification, and leukoderma.
- Leukoderma is a finding seen in the late stage and is accompanied by sparing of perifollicular skin. This is described as leopard skin and is most often evident on the shins.
- DD: Chronic eczema with post-inflammatory pigmentary changes, leukoderma of scleroderma.

### Treponematoses

- **Pinta**: Hypomelanotic macules occur during late phase of the disease and present as irregular vitiligo-like depigmented areas surrounded by hyperpigmentation over bony prominences. Atrophy, xerosis, and alopecia may also be seen.
- **Yaws**: Symmetric hypomelanotic macules may develop in untreated tertiary yaws over the dorsal aspect of wrists, hands, and metacarpophalangeal and interphalangeal joints. These macules enlarge and coalesce to involve the entire area.
- **Bejel** (Endemic syphilis): Well-defined hypomelanotic macules may occur in late stages of bejel. They are distributed symmetrically over extremities, genitalia, areola, and trunk. Repigmentation occurs on treatment.

### Acquired brachial cutaneous dyschromatosis

- This condition results from sun exposure over a prolonged period of time.
- It presents with bilateral, asymptomatic, brown patches with geographic borders, interspersed with hypopigmented, slightly atrophic macules on the extensor aspect of forearms.
- It may be associated with poikiloderma of Civatte.
- DD: Lentigines.

## REFERENCES


1. Sardana K, Goel K, Chugh S. Reticulate pigmentary disorders. Indian J Dermatol Venereol Leprol 2013;79:17–29.
2. Sinha S, Kulhari A. Reticulate pigmentary disorders: A review. Pigment Int 2019;6:67–76.
3. Vachiramon V. Approach to reticulate hyperpigmentation. Clin Exp Dermatol 2011;36(5):459–466.
4. Zhang J, Li M, Yao Z. Updated review of genetic reticulate pigmentary disorders. Br J Dermatol 2017;177(4):945–959.
5. Baselga E, Esterly NB. Genetic Epidermal Syndromes: Disorders Characterized by Reticulated Hyperpigmentation. In: Nordlund JJ, Boissy RE, Hearing VJ, King RA, Oetting WS, Ortonne JP, editors. The Pigmentary System: Physiology and Pathophysiology. 2nd edition. Oxford: Blackwell Publishing; 2006. P. 780–808.
6. Westerhof W, Dingemans KP. Generalized mottled pigmentation with postnatal skin blistering in three generations. J Am Acad Dermatol 2004;50(5 Suppl):S65–S69.
7. Vachiramon V, Thadanipon K, Chanprapaph K. Infancy- and childhood-onset dyschromatoses. Clin Exp Dermatol 2011;36(8):833–838.
8. Vachiramon V, Thadanipon K, Rattanakaemakorn P. Adult-onset dyschromatoses. Clin Exp Dermatol 2012;37(2):97–103.

5

# Papules: Localized

NIHARIKA RANJAN LAL

## INTRODUCTION

A papule is defined as an elevated, solid lesion of less than 1 cm in diameter. Papules may be localized or distributed in a generalized fashion. They exhibit various morphological characteristics in terms of color (violaceous in lichen planus and lichenoid diseases, red in vascular diseases such as cherry angioma and granuloma pyogenicum, yellow in lipid disorders), surface changes (rough in warts and angiokeratoma, scaly in psoriasis, shiny in molluscum and xanthelasma), and arrangement (coral-bead arrangement in multicentric reticulohistiocytosis) are unique to certain diseases. Regional distribution of localized papules may further help in making a correct diagnosis; for example, syringoma and trichoepithelioma are mostly seen on the face, angiolymphoid hyperplasia and milia en plaque behind the ears. Some papules, such as Gottron papules and xanthomatous papules, may be indicators of systemic illnesses. **Table 5.1** summarizes the common causes of localized papules and their salient diagnostic points are discussed. (Facial papules and follicular papules have not been discussed here.)

### Basal cell carcinoma

- This is the most commonly occurring cancer in the world, a slow-growing tumor for which metastasis is rare.
- Clinical features are flesh-colored or pink pearly papules; these appear on the head or neck in 85% of cases.[1] Patients usually present late when the lesion grows in size and becomes plaque (**Figure 5.1**).
- Ulceration or telangiectatic vessels are also commonly seen.
- The majority occur on areas of skin that are regularly exposed to sunlight or other ultraviolet radiation.
- They can be highly destructive and disfiguring to local tissues when presentation is delayed or treatment is inadequate.
- DD: Acquired melanocytic nevus, Dermatofibroma, skin appendageal tumor.

### Fibrous papule of nose

- Also known as fibrous papule of the face and sporadic angiofibroma, this is a benign angiofibroma affecting the nose most commonly.
- It is mostly seen in the middle-aged patients presenting as a solitary, asymptomatic, flesh-colored, dome-shaped, firm papule seen predominantly on the nose (**Figure 5.2**).

### Psoriasis

- These are well-circumscribed, pruritic, circular, red papules or plaques with silvery-white, dry scales (**Figure 5.3**).[2]
- Removal of scales reveals tiny bleeding spots: Auspitz sign.
- They are mainly distributed on extensor surfaces such as elbows, knees, buttocks, trunk.
- They may develop on sites of trauma: Koebner's phenomenon.
- DD: Lichen planus, tinea corporis, lichen simplex.

### Lichen planus

- Shiny, red/purple-colored, flat-topped papules are present (**Figure 5.4a**).
- Thin, adherent, transparent scale is present.
- Wickham's striae – fine whitish points/lacy lines – may be seen on the surface of well-developed papules.[2]
- A common site is the flexor surfaces of extremities (**Figure 5.4b**).
- It exhibits Koebner phenomenon.
- DD: Psoriasis, lichen simplex chronicus.


DOI: 10.1201/9781351054225-11

Table 5.1 Morphologic characteristics of localized papules

| | | | | |
|---|---|---|---|---|
| A. Single | | • Basal cell carcinoma<br>• Granuloma pyogenicum<br>• Fibrous papule of nose<br>• Steatocystoma simplex<br>• Acquired melanocytic nevus | 5. Yellow papules | • Xanthelasma palpebrarum<br>• Juvenile xanthogranuloma<br>• Benign cephalic histiocytosis<br>• Milia like idiopathic calcinosis cutis |
| B. Multiple | | | 6. White papules | • Milia<br>• Molluscum contagiosum<br>• Calcinosis cutis (milia like) |
| 1. Erythematous | a. Scaly | • Psoriasis<br>• Lichen planus<br>• Subacute cutaneous lupus erythematosus<br>• Discoid lupus erythematosus | 7. Skin-colored papules | • Syringoma<br>• Trichoepithelioma<br>• Eccrine hidrocystoma<br>• Pearly penile papules<br>• Lichen nitidus<br>• Lichen scrofulosorum<br>• Skin tags<br>• Acne keloidalis nuchae<br>• Piezogenic pedal papules<br>• Steatocystoma multiplex<br>• Neurofibroma<br>• Localized papular mucinosis |
| | b. Non-scaly | • Papular sarcoidosis<br>• Lupus vulgaris<br>• Granuloma annulare<br>• Lupus miliaris disseminatus faciei (LMDF)<br>• Jessner's lymphocytic infiltrate<br>• Granuloma faciale<br>• Multicentric reticulohistiocytosis | 8. Follicular papules | • Lichen spinulosus<br>• Keratosis pilaris<br>• Pityriasis rubra pilaris<br>• Follicular lichen planus |
| 2. Papules mixed with vesicles or pustules | | • Rosacea (with pustules)<br>• Acne vulgaris (with pustules)<br>• Gianotti-Crosti syndrome (with vesicles) | 9. Linear papules | • Linear psoriasis<br>• Linear lichen planus<br>• Linear verrucous epidermal nevus<br>• Inflammatory linear verrucous epidermal nevus<br>• Lichen striatus<br>• Linear porokeratosis<br>• Nevus comedonicus |
| 3. Hyperpigmented | | • Granular parakeratosis<br>• Darier disease<br>• Dermatosis papulosa nigra<br>• Reactive perforating collagenosis<br>• Lichen amyloidosis<br>• Adenoma sebaceum<br>• Bowenoid papulosis<br>• Prurigo nodularis<br>• Acquired melanocytic nevi<br>• Eruptive vellus hair cyst<br>• Gottron papules (violaceous) | 10. Vascular papules | • Lobular capillary hemangioma<br>• Angiokeratomas<br>• Bacillary angiomatosis<br>• Cherry angioma<br>• Tufted angioma<br>• Targetoid hemosiderotic hemangioma<br>• Angiolymphoid hyperplasia with eosinophilia |
| 4. Verrucous surface | | • Verruca vulgaris<br>• Acrokeratosis verruciformis<br>• Seborrheic keratosis<br>• Nevus sebaceous | 11. Papules with necrotic center | • Papulonecrotic tuberculid<br>• Lymphomatoid papulosis |

## Subacute cutaneous lupus erythematosus, papulosquamous variety

- This presents as erythematous, scaly papules and plaques (**Figure 5.5**).[2]
- It occurs in sun-exposed areas, including the upper thorax (V distribution), upper back, and the extensor surfaces of arms and forearms.
- Lesions are not indurated, and heal without scarring; vitiligo-like hypopigmentation may occur.
- DD: Psoriasis, nummular eczema, pemphigus foliaceus.

## Discoid lupus erythematosus (DLE)

- These are the most common lesions of chronic cutaneous lupus erythematosus (CCLE).

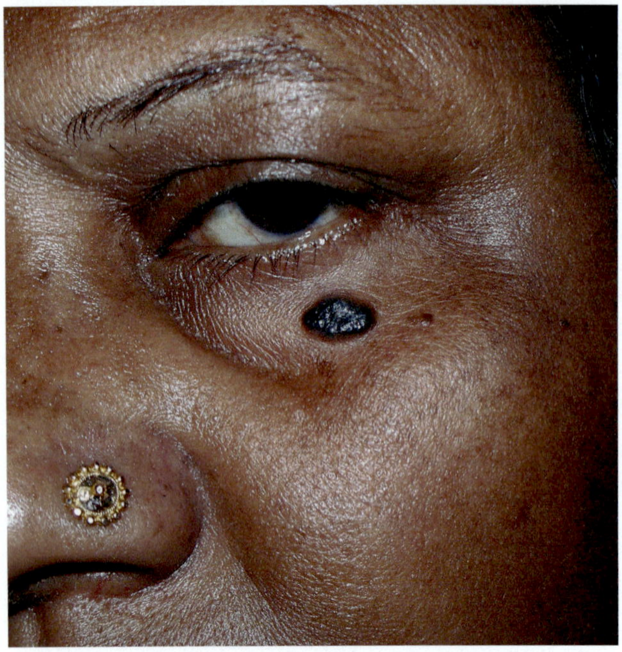

Figure 5.1 Hyperpigmented annuar plaque on face in basal cell carcinoma. (Courtesy: Dr. Piyush Kumar, Katihar, India.)

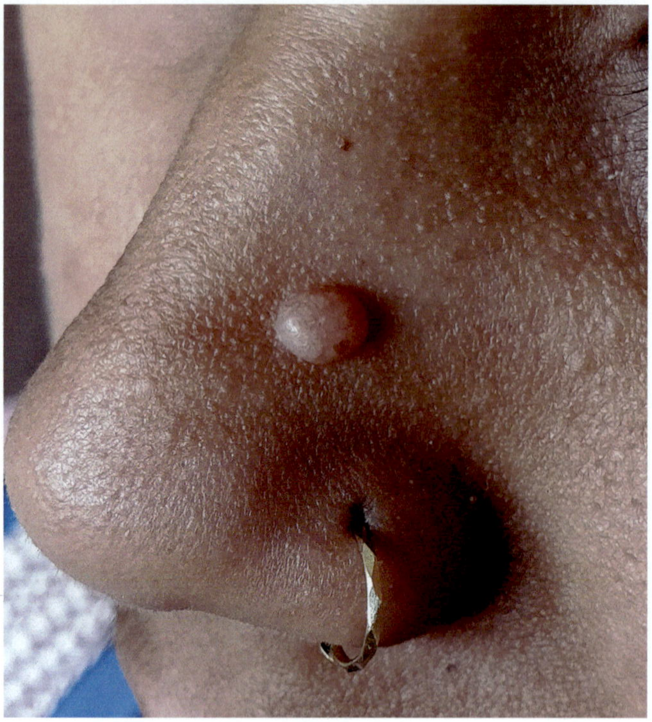

Figure 5.2 Fibrous papule of nose. Solitary, firm, skin-colored papule. (Courtesy: Dr. Swetalina Pradhan, AIIMS Patna, India.)

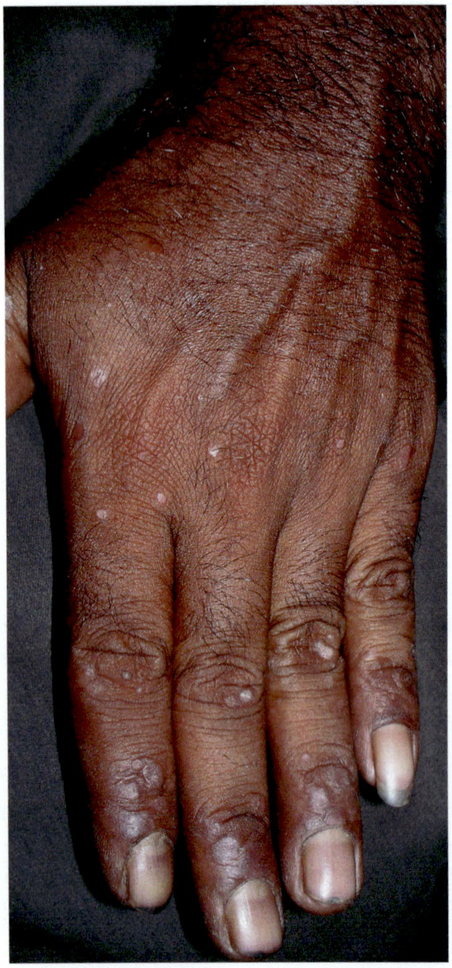

Figure 5.3 Erythematous scaly papules of psoriasis.

- Clinical features are well-demarcated, scaly, erythematous macules or papules.
- It gradually develops into an indurated discoid (coin-shaped) plaque with an adherent scale that is painful to remove (**Figure 5.6**).[3]
- There may be extension into the hair follicle, result in scarring alopecia.
- Through time, lesions typically become atrophic, with hyperpigmentation peripherally and depigmentation centrally.
- Localized DLE commonly involves the head and neck, in particular scalp and ears.
- DD: Psoriasis, lichen planus.

## Papular sarcoidosis

- This presents as asymptomatic, red-brown/purple papules < 1 cm in diameter[4] (**Figure 5.7**).
- It often affects the eyelids, periorbital area, and nasolabial folds.
- It may herald the onset of systemic disease.
- It may heal spontaneously with/without scarring.
- DD: Acne, rosacea, lupus miliaris disseminatus faciei (LMDF), lupus vulgaris.

## Lupus vulgaris

- This presents as soft reddish-brown papules with apple-jelly nodules on diascopy (**Figure 5.8a,b**).

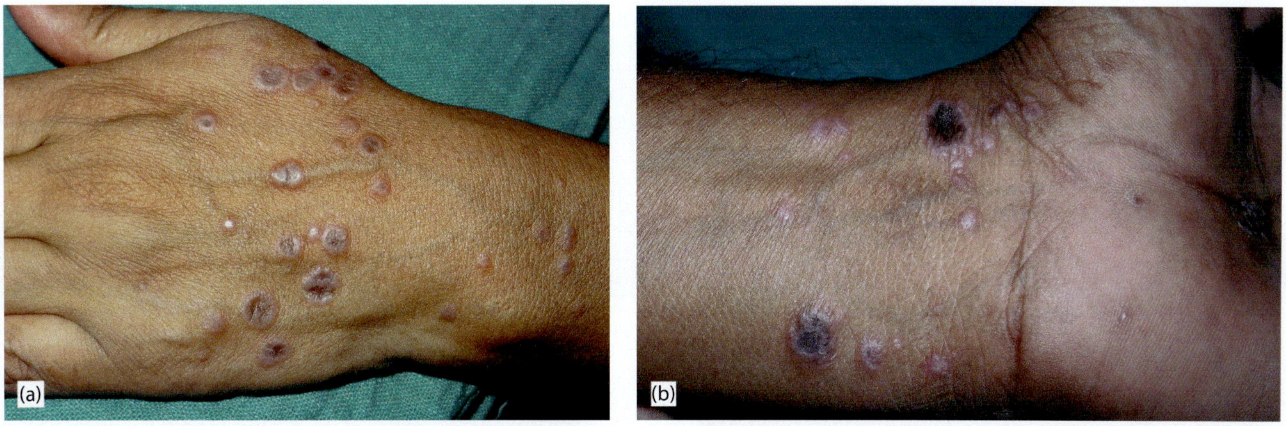


Figure 5.4 **(a)** Violaceous, flat-topped papules in lichen planus. **(b)** Lichen planus, flexor distribution. (a,b – Courtesy: Dr. Piyush Kumar, Katihar, India.)

- A lesion starts as a papule, but patients usually present late when the lesion reaches plaque stage.
- DD: Sarcoidosis, Jessner's lymphocytic infiltration.

## Granuloma annulare

- This is a common, benign, chronic inflammatory disorder of unknown cause.
- It is characterized by grouped papules in an enlarging annular shape (**Figure 5.9**).[1]

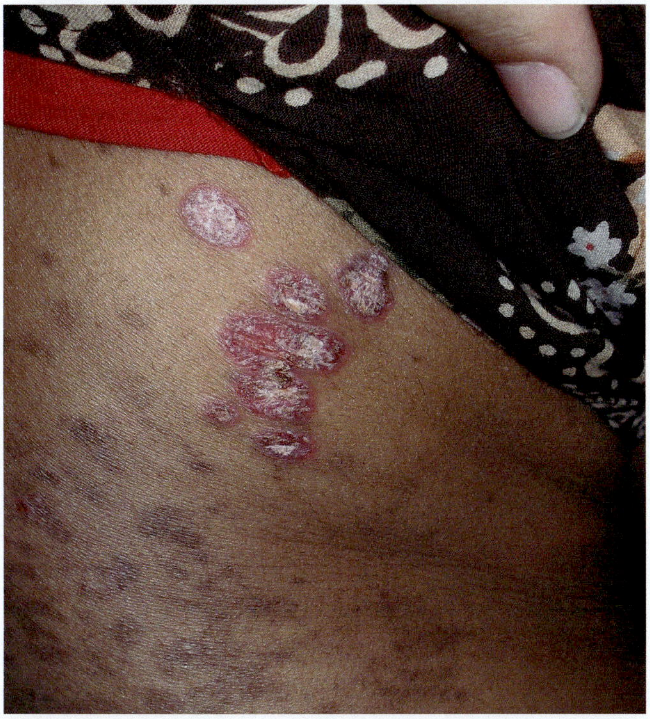

Figure 5.5 Psoriasiform papules in subacute lupus erythematosus on back. (Courtesy: Dr. Piyush Kumar, Katihar, India.)

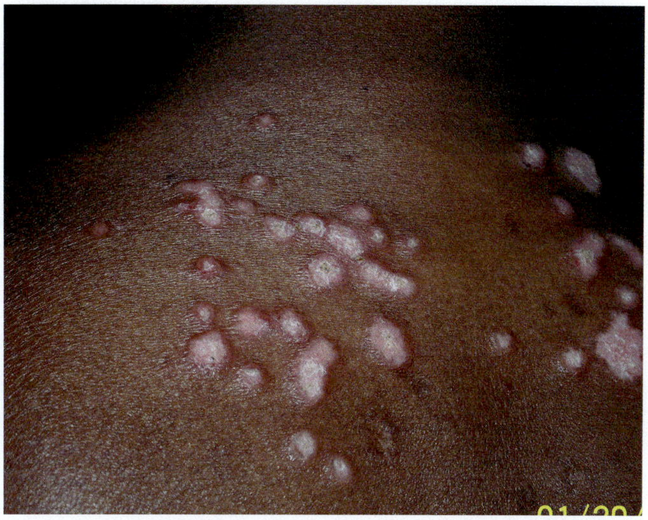

Figure 5.6 Erythematous papules with adherent scales on the back in DLE. (Courtesy: Dr. Piyush Kumar, Katihar, India.)

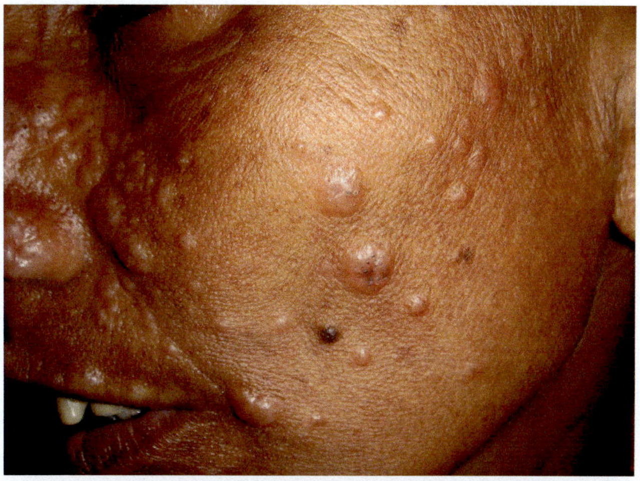

Figure 5.7 Papular sarcoidosis. (Courtesy: Dr. Piyush Kumar, Katihar, India.)

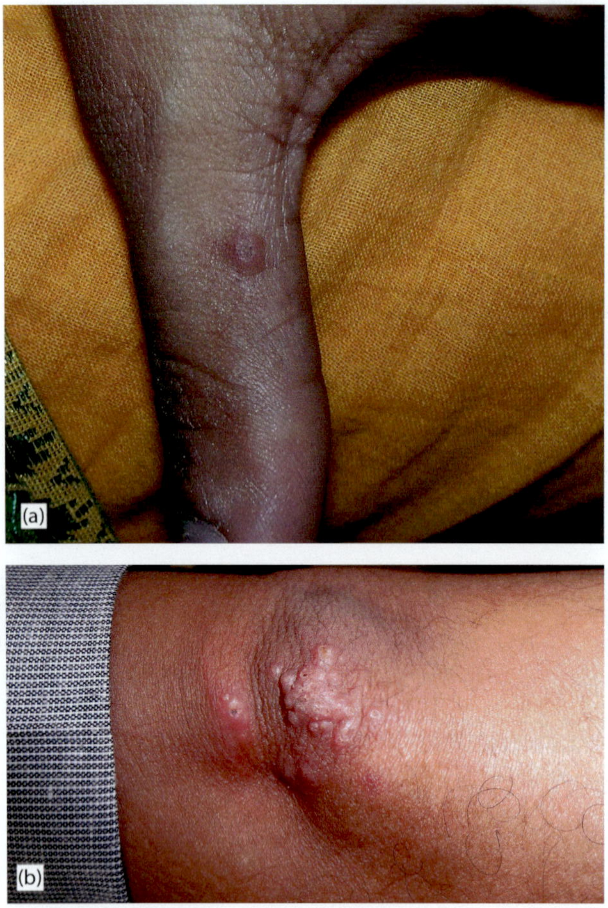


Figure 5.8 **(a)** Papular lesion of lupus vulgaris. **(b)** Grouped, coalescing erythematous papules on the knee in Lupus vulgaris. (a – Courtesy: Dr. Piyush Kumar, Katihar, India.)

- The most common presentation is plaque; uncommon forms are subcutaneous, perforating, patch, linear, and rarely acute painful papules.
- A small percentage of cases are associated with autoimmune diseases, systemic diseases, infections, and malignancies.
- D/D: Lupus vulgaris, sarcoidosis, Hansen's disease.

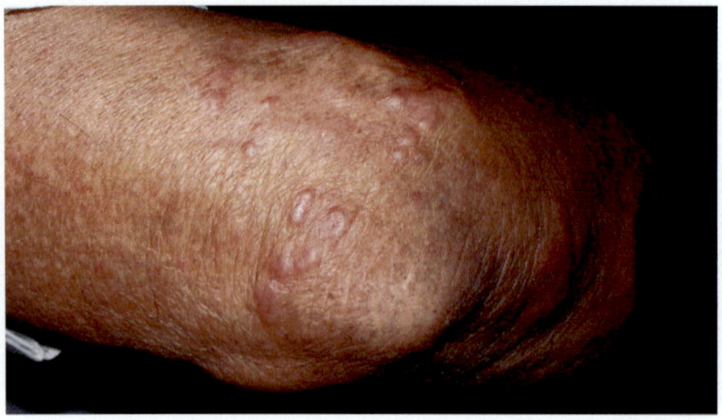

Figure 5.9 Erythematous shiny papules in granuloma annulare. Annular plaque is also seen on forearm. (Courtesy: Dr. Piyush Kumar, Katihar, India.)

### Lupus miliaris disseminatus faciei (LMDF)

- Granulomatous eruption characterized by monomorphic, reddish-brown papules and nodules (**Figure 5.10a,b**).[5]
- It is predominantly localized on the face (chin, forehead, cheeks, eyelids).

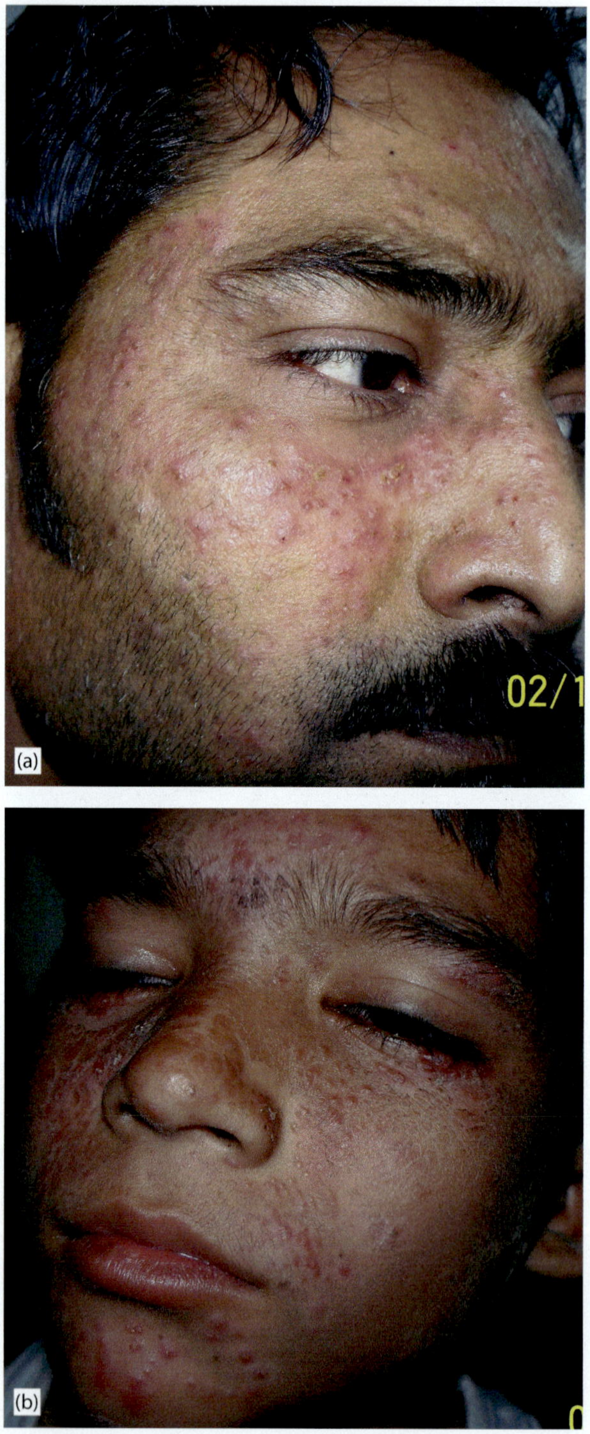


Figure 5.10 **(a)** Erythematous, monomorphic papules distributed symmetrically on face in lupus miliaris disseminatus faciei. **(b)** Lupus miliaris disseminatus faciei. The scaling seen on the face is due to retinoid application. (a,b – Courtesy: Dr. Piyush Kumar, Katihar, India.)

- Diascopy often reveals an apple-jelly nodule-like appearance.
- It is self-limiting and heals with pock-like scars.
- DD: Sarcoidosis, acne, lupus vulgaris.

### Jessner's lymphocytic infiltration

- This presents with asymptomatic, erythematous papules/plaques that tend to take an annular or horseshoe-like configuration.
- The face is the most common site.
- Some degree of photosensitivity may be associated.
- DD: Pseudolymphoma, papular sarcoidosis, tumid LE, PMLE.

### Papulopustular rosacea

- This is a chronic inflammatory skin disease commonly affecting the face.
- It is characterized by flushing, redness, papules, pustules, and dilated blood vessels (**Figure 5.11**).
- It is symmetrically distributed on central face.
- Triggering factors are spicy/caffeinated food, sunlight, stress, strenuous exercise, and some types of cosmetics.
- DD: Acne vulgaris, steroid dermatitis, demodicosis.

### Acne vulgaris

- This is a common skin condition starting in puberty.
- The face is the most common site; the back and chest may be affected.

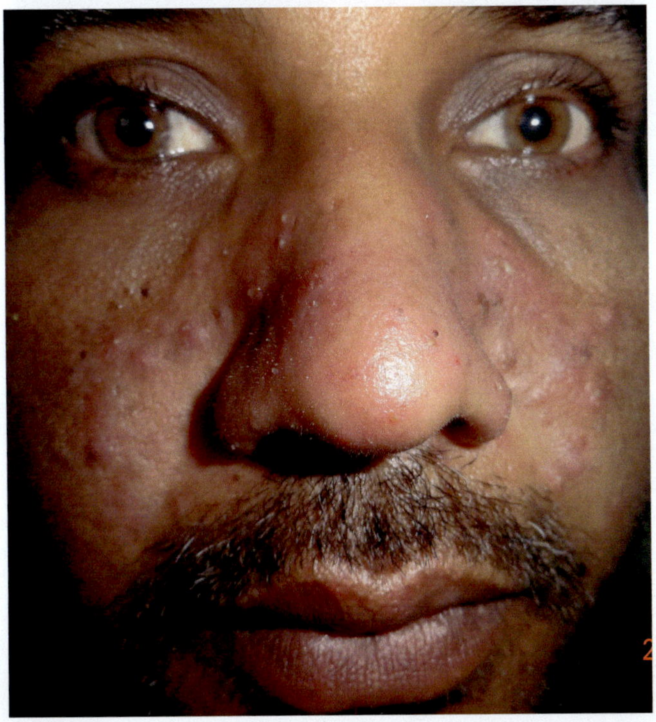

Figure 5.11. Erythema, papules, and few pustules are symmetrically distributed over the face in rosacea. (Courtesy: Dr. Piyush Kumar, Katihar, India.)

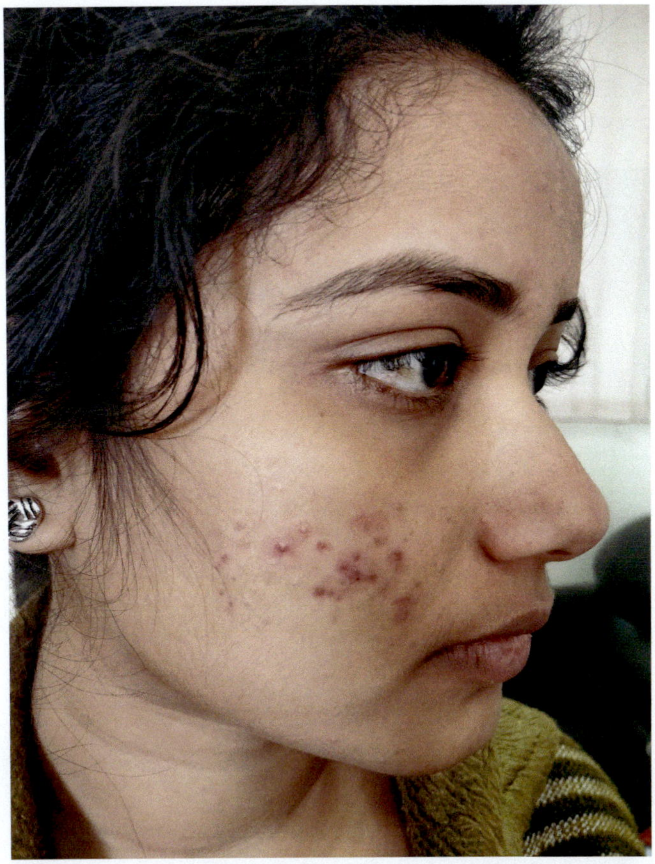

Figure 5.12 Erythematous papules on cheek in a teenager with acne.

- Preadolescent acne mainly occurs on forehead, adolescent acne on cheeks, and adult acne on jaw.[6]
- A lesion begins with a microcomedo that may evolve into a papule/nodule (**Figure 5.12**).
- Other morphologies seen are comedones, pustules, nodules, cysts, scars, and hyperpigmentation.
- DD: Bacterial folliculitis, rosacea, LMDF.

### Granular parakeratosis

- This is a rare, idiopathic, benign skin condition.
- Erythematous to brown, scaly, crusted, hyperkeratotic papules coalesce to form plaques.
- Intertriginous sites are most commonly affected, especially the axilla.[7]
- No definitive cause is known; it may be because of physical irritation/contact allergy, or it could be a disorder of cornification rather than contact dermatitis.
- DD: Darier disease, Hailey-Hailey disease (HHD), pemphigus vegetans.

### Darier disease

- This is genodermatosis with autosomal dominant inheritance.
- Distribution is on seborrheic and intertriginous areas.

- Coalescence of the papules produces irregular warty plaques that, in flexures, become hypertrophic and malodorous with painful fissures (**Figure 5.13a,b**).[8]

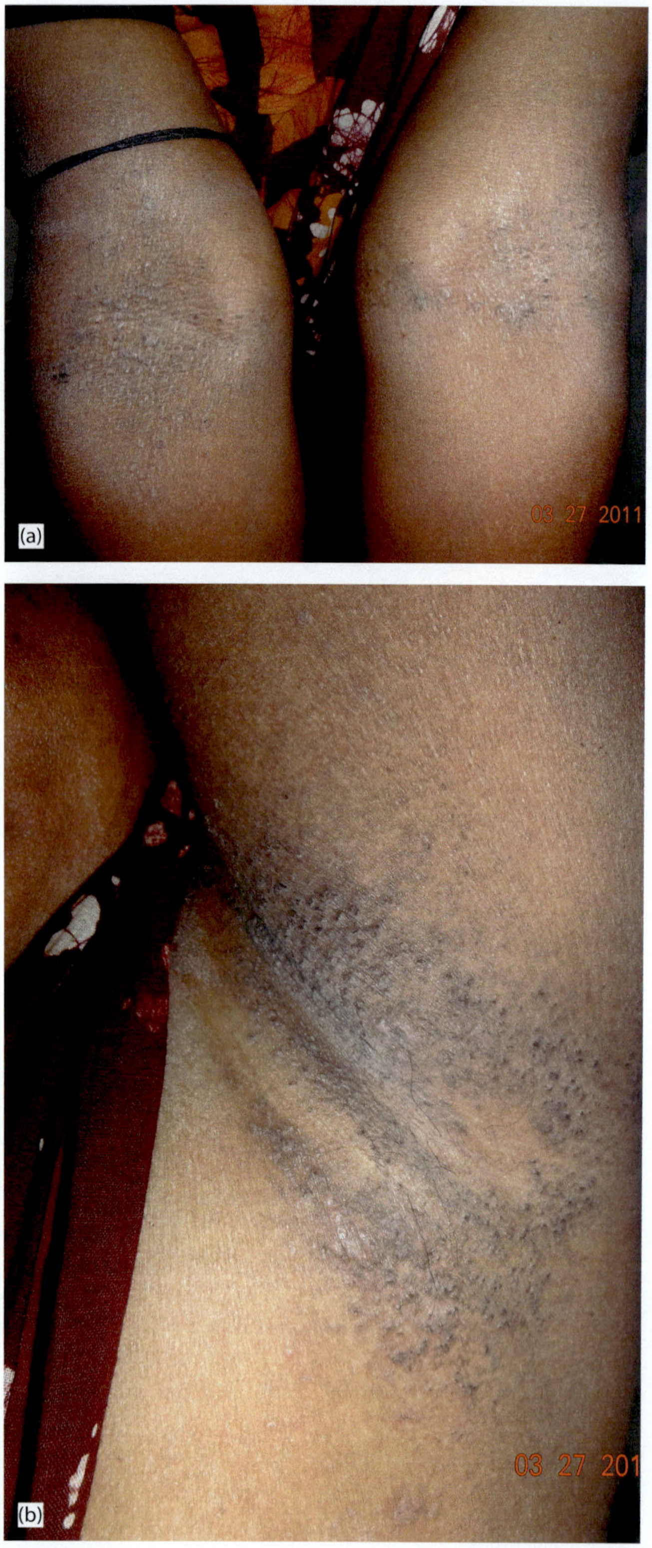

Figure 5.13 **(a)** Darier disease presenting as dirty, warty papules in elbow flexures. **(b)** Darier disease affecting axilla.

- Oral mucosa is involved in 50% of cases; white/red papules appear on palatal/alveolar mucosa (cobblestone appearance).
- Associated nail abnormalities include nail fragility, red and white longitudinal stripes, and V-shaped notches at the free margin of nails.
- DD: HHD, seborrheic dermatitis, acanthosis nigricans, pemphigus vegetans.

### Dermatosis papulosa nigra (DPN)

- This is considered a variant of seborrheic keratosis, more common in black people.
- Sun exposure plays major role.
- Multiple small, 1–5 mm, hyperpigmented, asymptomatic papules appear (**Figure 5.14**).
- It is mostly seen on the face (malar regions and forehead, followed by chin) and less commonly over the neck, upper back, and chest.
- It develops during puberty and increases with age.
- DD: Skin tags, plane warts.

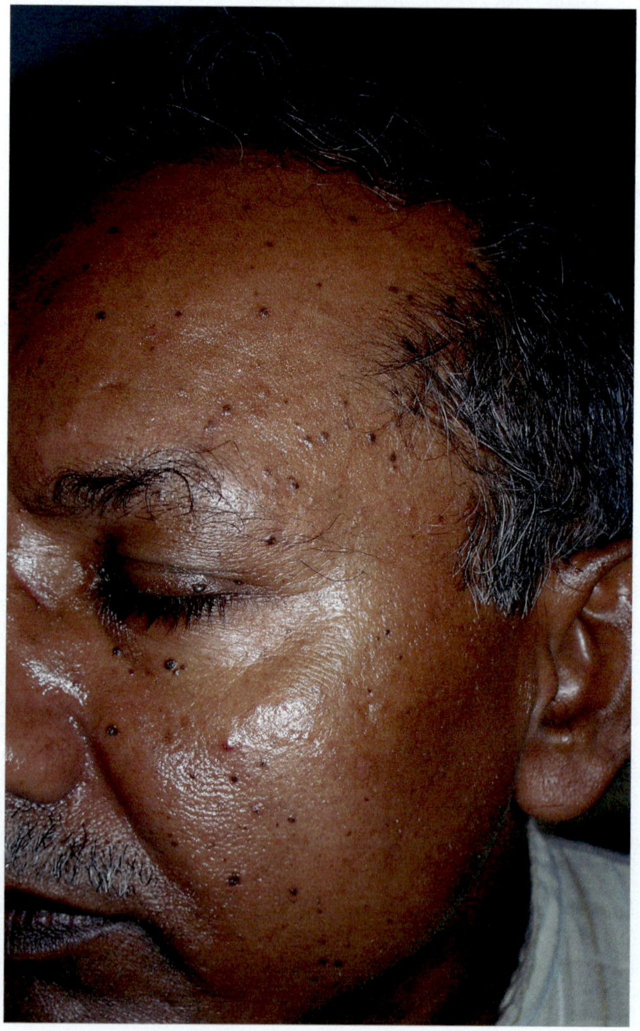

Figure 5.14 Dermatosis papulosa nigra seen as multiple, hyperpigmented, small papules on face. (Courtesy: Dr. Piyush Kumar, Katihar, India.)

## Reactive perforating collagenosis

- It is a type of transepidermal elimination disorder in which altered collagen is extruded from the dermis.
- It may be inherited or acquired.
- The acquired form is associated with trauma, insect bites, diabetes, or chronic renal failure.
- It manifests as isolated papules with keratotic plugs in the center (**Figure 5.15a,b**).[9]
- It occurs mostly on the extremities and back, sometimes on the face and neck.
- Extremely pruritic Koebnerization is seem in **Figure 5.15c**.
- It is usually self-healing in six to eight weeks without any therapy but often recurs.
- DD: Prurigo nodularis, Kyrle's disease.

## Lichen amyloidosis

- This is the most common form of primary localized cutaneous amyloidosis.
- The cause is unknown, maybe induced by scratching.
- Clinical features include multiple pruritic, firm, hyperpigmented, hyperkeratotic papules on the shins that later coalesce to give the appearance of a rippled pattern (**Figure 5.16**).
- DD: Prurigo nodularis, lichen planus.

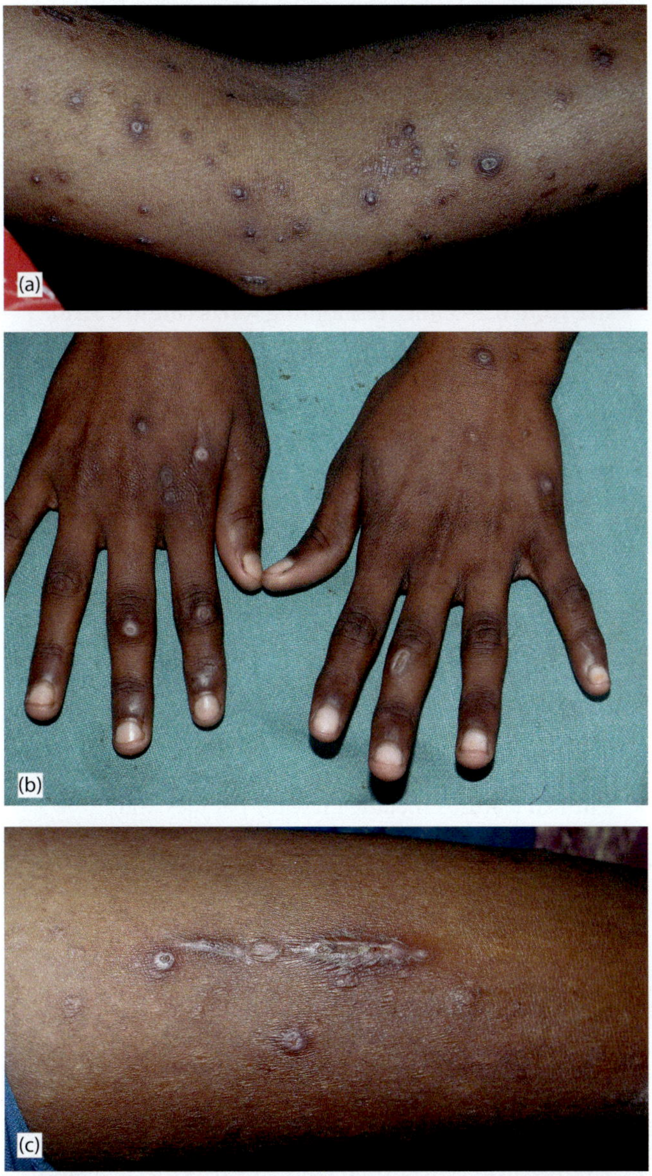


Figure 5.15 **(a)** Reactive perforating collagenosis presenting as multiple papules with a central keratotic plug. **(b)** Reactive perforating collagenosis. **(c)** Koebnerization seen in reactive perforating collagenosis. (a–c – Courtesy: Dr. Piyush Kumar, Katihar, India.)

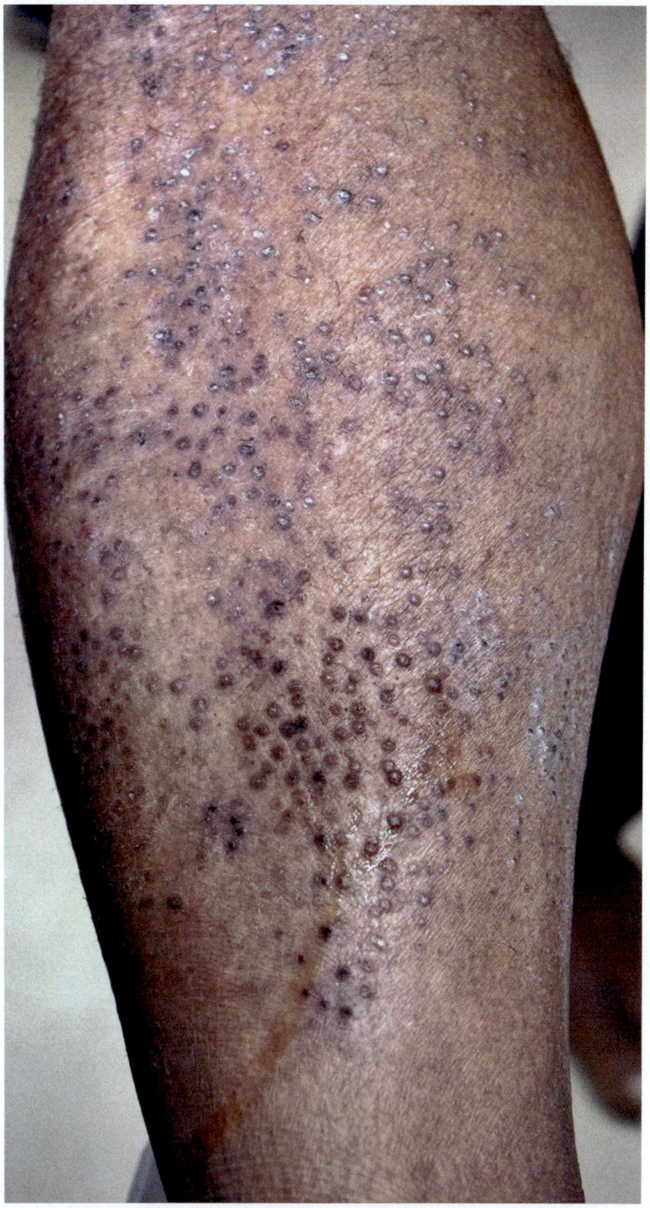

Figure 5.16 Hyperpigmented, keratotic papules on shin in lichen amyloidosis. (Courtesy: Dr. Piyush Kumar, Katihar, India.)

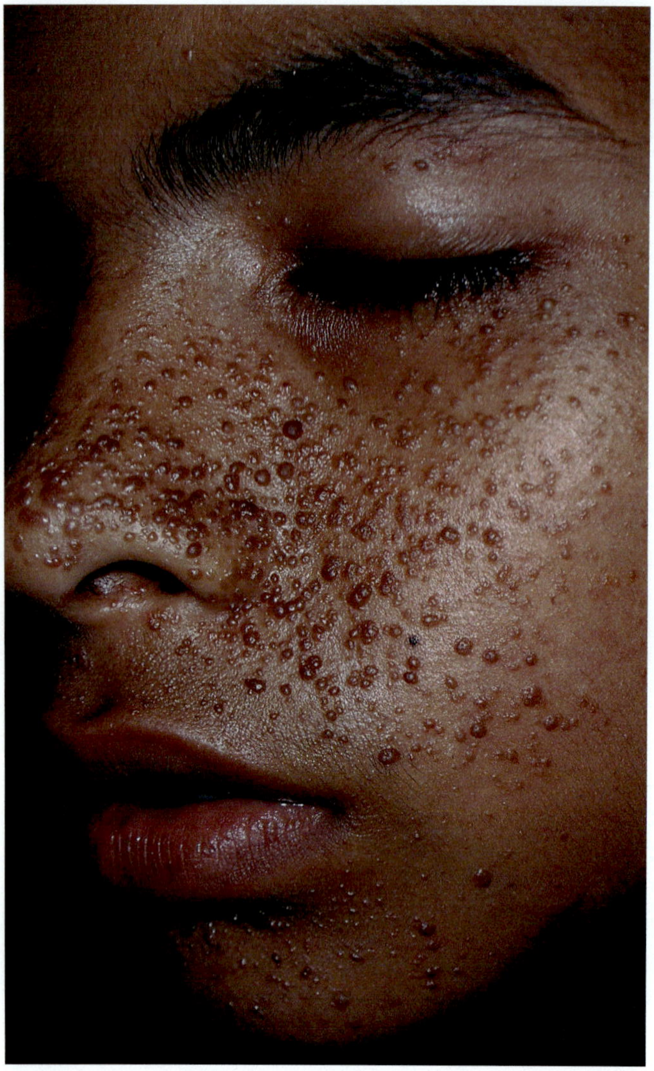

Figure 5.17 Red-brown papules on the central face in facial angiofibroma. (Courtesy: Dr. Piyush Kumar, Katihar, India.)

## Adenoma sebaceum (facial angiofibroma)

- This is a benign tumor with both angiomatous and fibrous components.
- It is one of the cutaneous hallmarks of tuberous sclerosis.
- It starts appearing by 5–10 years of age and gradually increases till puberty.
- Skin-colored to hyperpigmented papules commonly involve the central face, bilaterally and symmetrically covering the glabellar area, the dorsum of nose, adjoining cheeks, upper lip, and chin (**Figure 5.17**).[10]
- DD: Trichoepithelioma, acrochordons, intradermal nevi, acne, syringoma.

## Bowenoid papulosis

- This is caused by the human papilloma virus (HPV) in the sexually active age group.
- The causative agent is HPV 16; HPV serotypes such as 18, 31, 33, 39, and 52 have also been implicated.

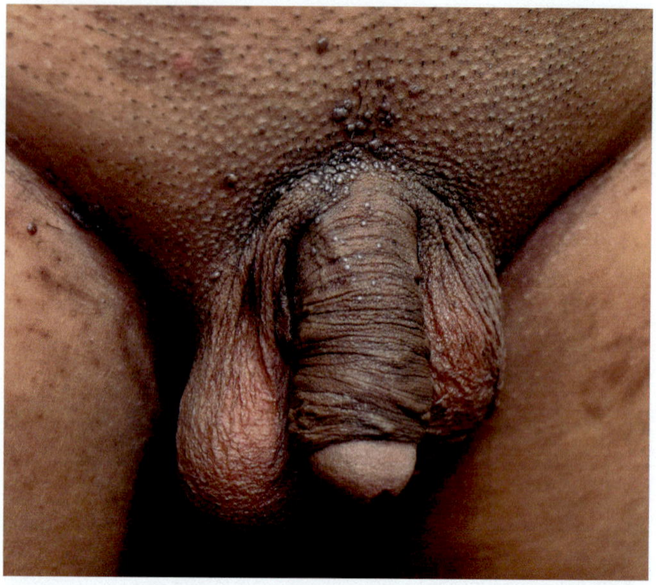

Figure 5.18 Smooth-surfaced, pigmented papules of bowenoid papulosis. (Courtesy: Dr. Piyush Kumar, Katihar, India.)

- Clinical features include pigmented papules ranging in size from 0.2–3 mm, resembling warts (**Figure 5.18**).
- Frequent sites are the penis and vulva; other areas such as oral, periungual, and neck region may be affected.
- In females, it is referred to as multifocal vulvar intraepithelial neoplasia.
- DD: Genital warts, lichen planus, molluscum contagiosum, seborrheic keratosis, and Bowen's disease.

## Acne keloidalis

- This is a chronic inflammatory condition seen in dark-skinned races with curly or kinky hair.
- Males are predominantly affected, usually after puberty.
- Androgen may play an important role; skin injuries from irritation, occlusion, trauma, friction, and hair-cutting practices are contributing risk factors.
- Clinical features include multiple papules and/or pustules on nuchal and/or occipital areas (acne keloidalis nuchae). Other sites, such as the upper trunk, too may be affected (**Figure 5.19a,b**).
- It is extremely pruritic; bleeding may occur.
- Secondary bacterial infection by *Staphylococcus aureus* is common.
- Recurrent episodes lead to scarring alopecia.
- DD: Keloid, tufted folliculitis.

## Prurigo nodularis

- This is chronic-relapsing, highly pruritic dermatosis.
- It is characterized by several to hundreds of hyperkeratotic, pruritic papules and nodules, sometimes excoriated or ulcerated, with a tendency to symmetrical distribution on the shoulders, on the back, the buttocks, and the upper and lower limbs (**Figure 5.20a,b**).

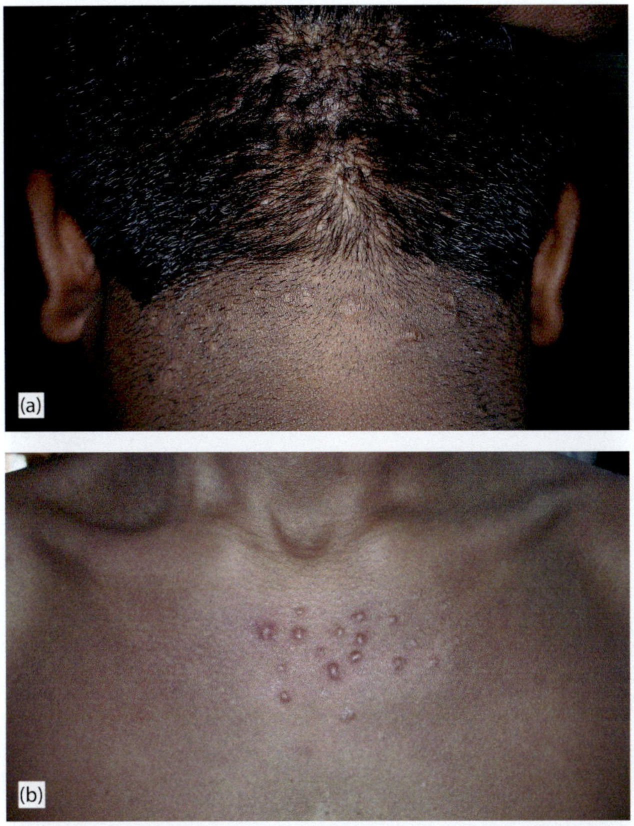


Figure 5.19 **(a)** Acne keloidalis nuchae seen as keloid-like papules on the nuchal area. **(b)** Acne keloidalis lesions on the chest. (a,b – Courtesy: Dr. Piyush Kumar, Katihar, India.)

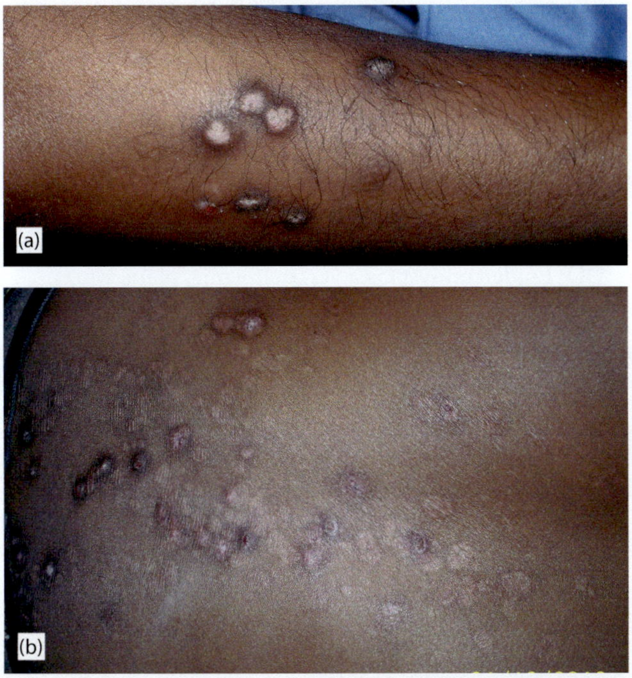


Figure 5.20 **(a)** Prurigo nodularis. **(b)** Hyperpigmented, excoriated papules in prurigo nodularis. Older lesions have healed with scarring. (a,b – Courtesy: Dr. Piyush Kumar, Katihar, India.)

- Sparing of the upper mid back, known as "butterfly sign," is distinctive.
- It may be associated with atopy, type 2 diabetes mellitus, thyroid disorders, HCV infection, non-Hodgkin lymphoma and psychiatric disorders, particularly depression and anxiety.
- DD: Lichen planus, nodular amyloidosis.

## Acquired melanocytic nevus

- Common acquired melanocytic nevi (CAMN) is a common, largely acquired, condition resulting from benign proliferation of nevus cells.
- It may appear as macules, papules, and nodules.[1]
- It is typically less than 1 cm (often < 6 mm) in diameter, with smooth and regular borders (**Figure 5.21**).
- Compound melanocytic nevi are elevated in relation to adjacent uninvolved skin and present as papules or nodules and are often lighter in color, ranging from tan to light brown.
- Intradermal melanocytic nevi often display no significant pigmentation, presenting as a flesh-colored papule or nodule.
- DD: Basal cell carcinoma, solar lentigo, melanoma, seborrheic keratosis.

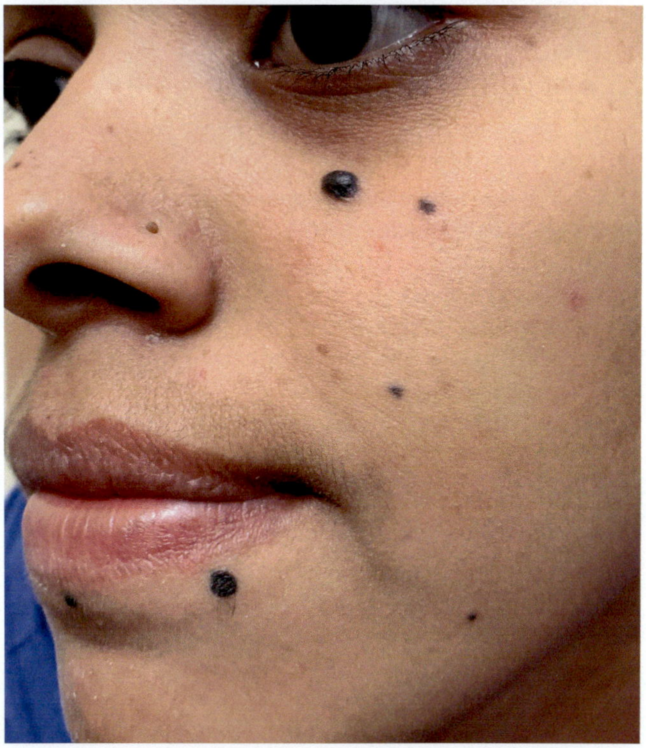

Figure 5.21 Shiny, smooth, hyperpigmented papules in acquired melanocytic nevus. (Courtesy: Dr. Piyush Kumar, Katihar, India.)

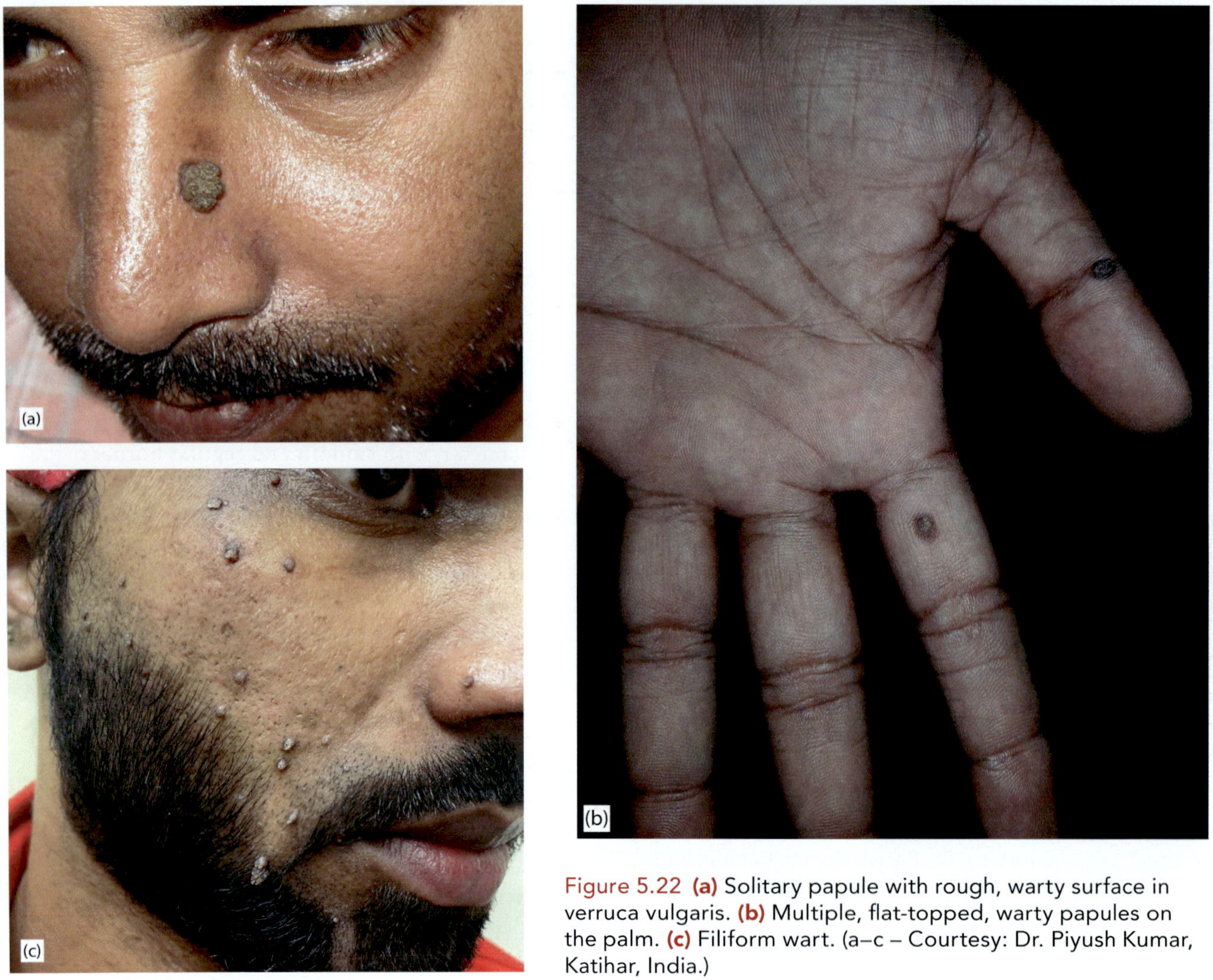

Figure 5.22 **(a)** Solitary papule with rough, warty surface in verruca vulgaris. **(b)** Multiple, flat-topped, warty papules on the palm. **(c)** Filiform wart. (a–c – Courtesy: Dr. Piyush Kumar, Katihar, India.)

## Eruptive vellus hair cyst

- This is a rare follicular developmental abnormality of the vellus hair follicles.
- Clinical features include multiple small normochromic or hyperpigmented, dome-shaped papules, soft to firm in consistency, ranging from 1 to 5 mm in diameter.
- It may be topped with central puncta or a umbilicated or hyperkeratotic crust.
- Common sites are the chest and extremities, rarely abdomen, neck, axillae, face, and groin.
- DD: Comedones, keratosis pilaris, infundibular cysts.

## Verruca vulgaris

- These are hyperkeratotic, exophytic, and dome-shaped papules or nodules (**Figure 5.22a–c**).
- They are located on fingers, hands, knees, elbows, or any other sites of trauma.
- They exhibit pseudo Koebnerization.
- DD: lichen planus, seborrheic keratosis, epidermal nevus.

## Acrokeratosis verruciformis

- This is rare genodermatosis with autosomal dominant inheritance.
- Clinical features include flat-topped, polygonal, brownish to skin-colored papules and verrucous plaques (**Figure 5.23**).
- Sites are the back of the proximal and distal interphalangeal joints of the hands and feet.
- Punctate keratosis on the palms and soles may also be seen.
- DD: Epidermodysplasia verruciformis, plane warts.

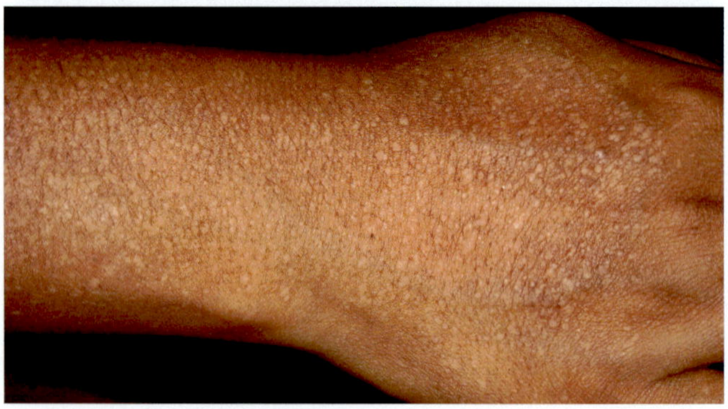

Figure 5.23 Flat-topped, skin-colored papules on dorsum of hand in acrokeratosis verruciformis. (Courtesy: Dr. Piyush Kumar, Katihar, India.)

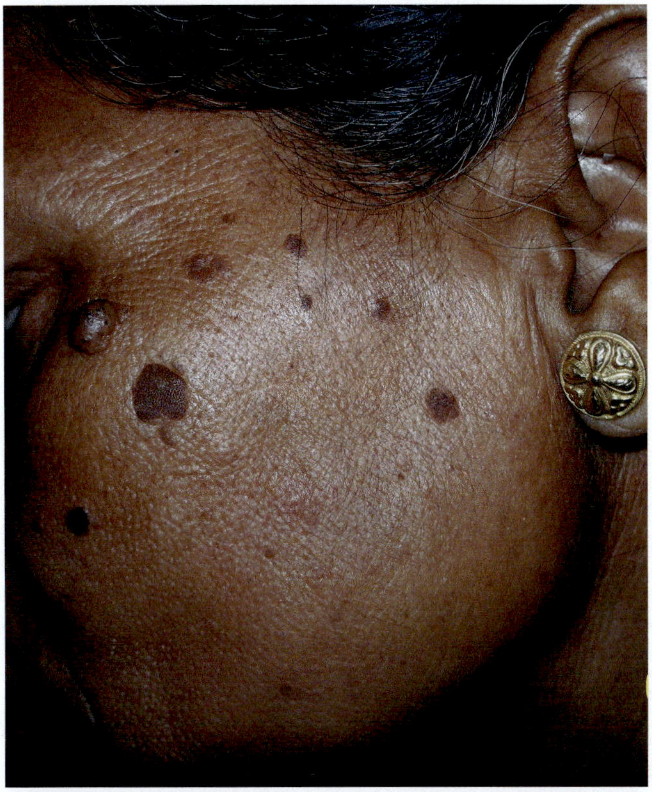

Figure 5.24 Flat-topped, hyperpigmented papules with a stuck-on appearance in seborrheic keratosis. (Courtesy: Dr. Piyush Kumar, Katihar, India.)

## Seborrheic keratosis

- These are the most common benign epidermal tumors that are associated with increased age.
- Clinical features include solitary or multiple well-demarcated brownish papules or plaques with a verrucous surface (**Figure 5.24**).
- Common sites are the head, neck, and trunk.
- DD: Actinic keratoses, verruca vulgaris, lentigines.

## Nevus sebaceous

- This is a congenital hamartomatous lesion with an epithelial and adnexal origin.
- It is present in approximately 0.3% of newborns.
- It may contain any component of skin, including sebaceous and apocrine glands or hair follicles.
- It appears as smooth or velvety yellow-orange well-circumscribed grouped papules and plaques (**Figure 5.25**).[11]
- Hormonal changes at puberty may lead to verrucous changes.
- The most common site is the vertex of the scalp.
- It may be associated with syndromic features such as mental retardation, central nervous system abnormalities, oculocardiac defects, or skeletal abnormalities (linear nevus sebaceous syndrome, or Schimmelpenning syndrome).
- Malignant changes may occur.
- DD: Warts, syringocystadenoma papilliferum.

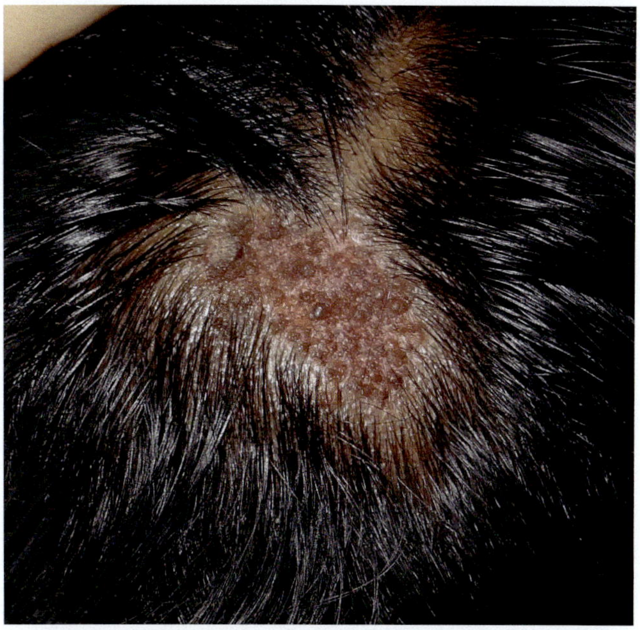

Figure 5.25 Brown papules on scalp coalescing to form plaque in nevus sebaceous. Note verrucous surface changes, indicating post-pubertal growth. (Courtesy: Dr. Piyush Kumar, Katihar, India.)

## Juvenile xanthogranuloma

- This condition belongs to the group of non-Langerhans cell histiocytosis.
- It affects infants and small children.
- It usually appears as yellow-brown papules and nodule, often on the head and neck (**Figure 5.26**).[11]

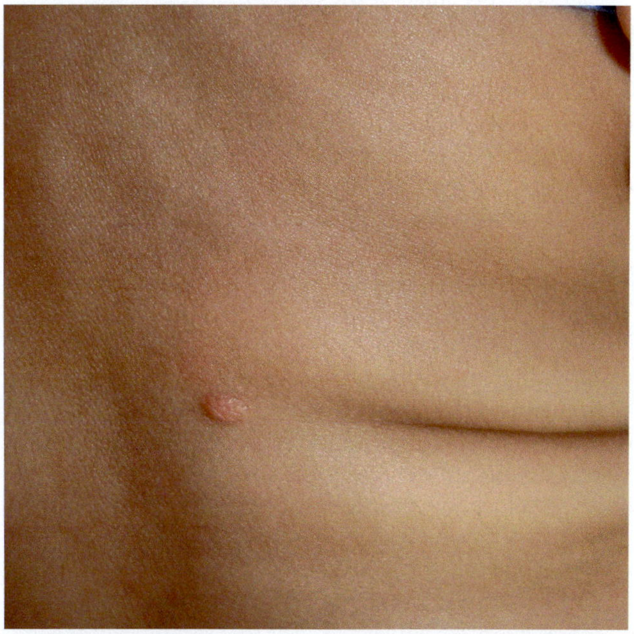

Figure 5.26 Yellow-orange solitary papule on trunk in juvenile xanthogranuloma. (Courtesy: Dr. Santosh Rathod, Smt. NHL Municipal Medical College, V.S. Hospital Ahmedabad, India.)

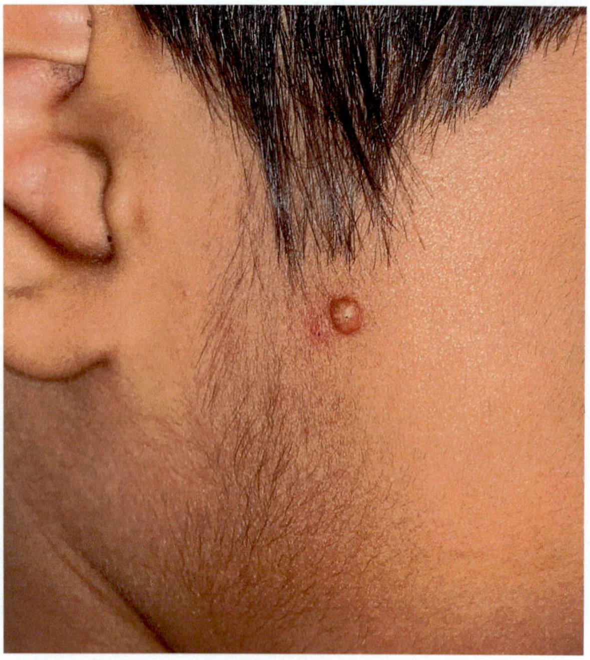

Figure 5.27 Papule of benign cephalic histiocytosis. (Courtesy: Dr. Piyush Kumar, Katihar, India.)

- Sporadically, internal organs may get affected, including eyes, lungs, liver, central nervous system, and bones.
- DD: Urticaria pigmentosa, xanthoma.

## Benign cephalic histiocytosis

- This is also known as papular histiocytosis of the head.
- It is a rare self-limiting non-Langerhans histiocytosis that typically starts at the end of first year of life.
- Clinical features include asymptomatic eruption of yellow to brown papules on the head and neck of infants and young children (**Figure 5.27**).
- Subsequently it spontaneously regresses, leaving atrophic pigmented macules.
- DD: Plane warts, multiple Spitz nevi, juvenile xanthogranuloma, Langerhans cell histiocytosis, urticaria pigmentosa, generalized eruptive histiocytosis, and lichenoid sarcoidosis.

## Milia-like idiopathic calcinosis cutis

- Milia-like idiopathic calcinosis cutis (MICC) is a peculiar subtype of idiopathic calcinosis cutis.
- The lesions appear as multiple, round, whitish papules resembling milia (**Figure 5.28a,b**).
- The predilection sites are the hands and feet, but it can occur on the any part of the body.
- Calcified sweat ducts have been described in some patient as the pathogenesis; another theory is that the lesions represent micro epidermal cysts that secondarily generate an inflammatory reaction and calcium deposition.
- May heal spontaneously, with or without scarring.
- DD: Warts, epidermal cysts, molluscum contagiosum, and syringomas.

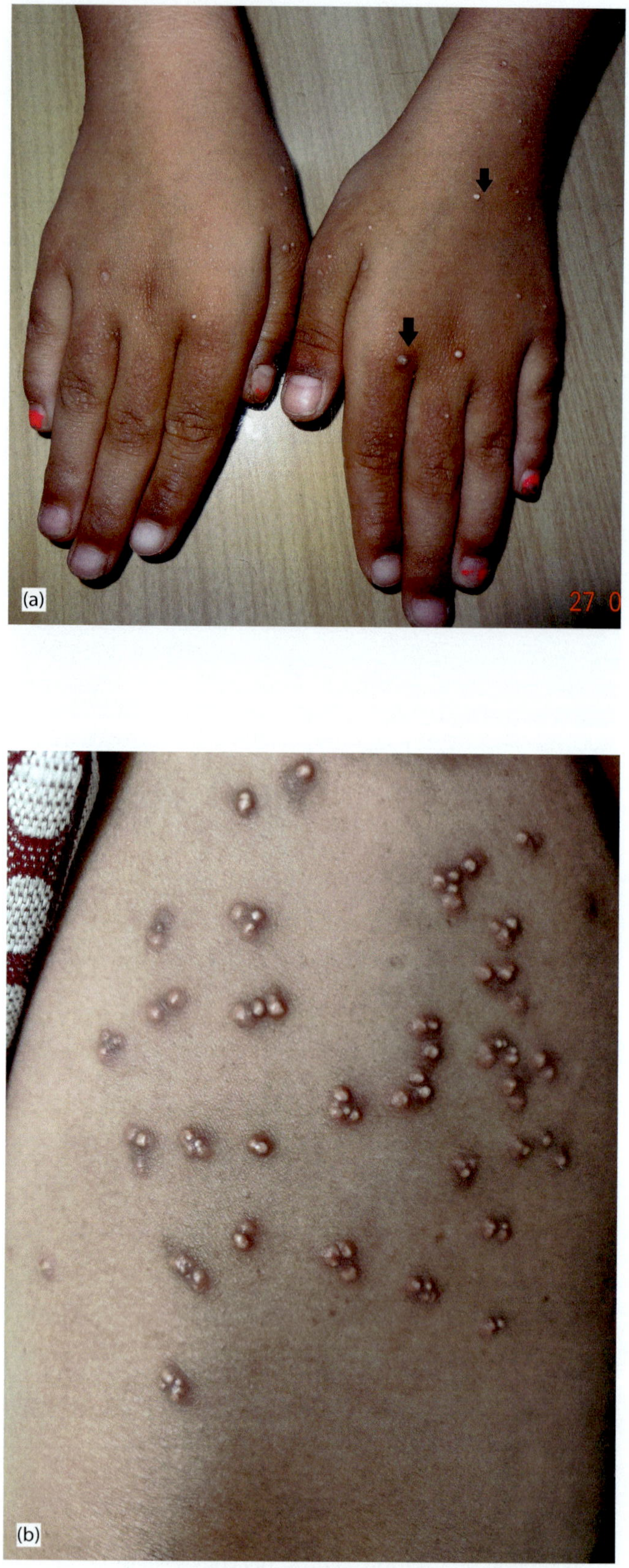


Figure 5.28 **(a)** Milia-like calcinosis cutis in a child with Down syndrome. **(b)** Papules of calcinosis cutis. (a – Courtesy: Dr. Piyush Kumar, Katihar, India; b – Courtesy: Dr. Dependra Kumar Timshina, Remedy Clinics, Siliguri, India.)

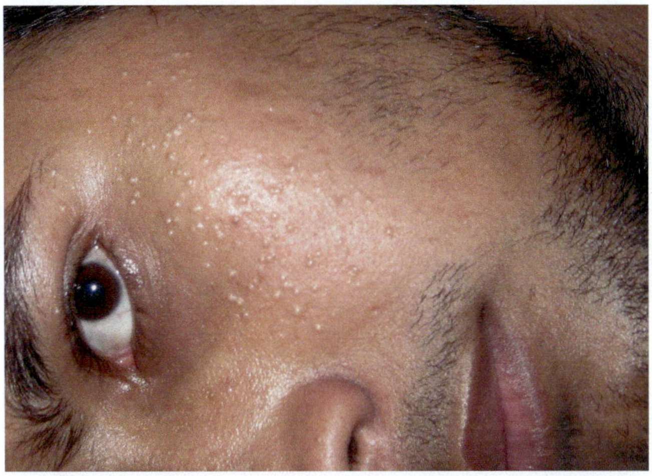

Figure 5.29 Milia seen as white papules on the cheek. (Courtesy: Dr. Piyush Kumar, Katihar, India.)

## Milia (singular: milium)

- Milia are tiny white keratin-containing cysts.
- They present as 1–2 mm asymptomatic, umbilicated, white or yellowish, spherical subepidermal keratin cysts occurring primarily on the face in all ages.
- In neonatal milia many newborns have milia on face, hard palate (Bohn nodules), and gum margin (Epstein pearls). The lesions resolve spontaneously.
- Primary milia is common in children and young adults, and are usually found around eyes, cheeks, and genitalia. They arise from an infundibular portion of the hair (**Figure 5.29**).
- Secondary milia may occur over the area of trauma or skin injury as in second degree burn, epidermolysis bullosa, porphyria cutanea tarda, bullous lichen planus, radiotherapy, chronic steroid use, cosmetic procedure like dermabrasion, etc. They arise from the eccrine sweat ducts.
- Milia en plaque present as numerous, grouped milia on erythematous and oedematous base. The lesions are mostly seen in the post-auricular area, on eyelid, or cheek.

## Molluscum contagiosum

- Molluscum contagiosum is caused by Molluscum contagiosum virus (MCV) (MCV strain 1-4).
- It is characterized by firm, white to flesh-colored, dome-shaped, pearly papules, having a central umbilication from which one can express a cheesy material (**Figure 5.30a,b**).[12]
- In children it commonly affects face, axilla, and extremities.
- In the sexually acquired form (usually in adults) lesions occur on the genitalia and inner thighs (**Figure 5.30c**).
- In immunocompromised patients, lesions may be atypical (like giant MC more than 1.5 cm) and may involve mucosal surface.
- DD: Acne, milia, warts, trichoepithelioma.

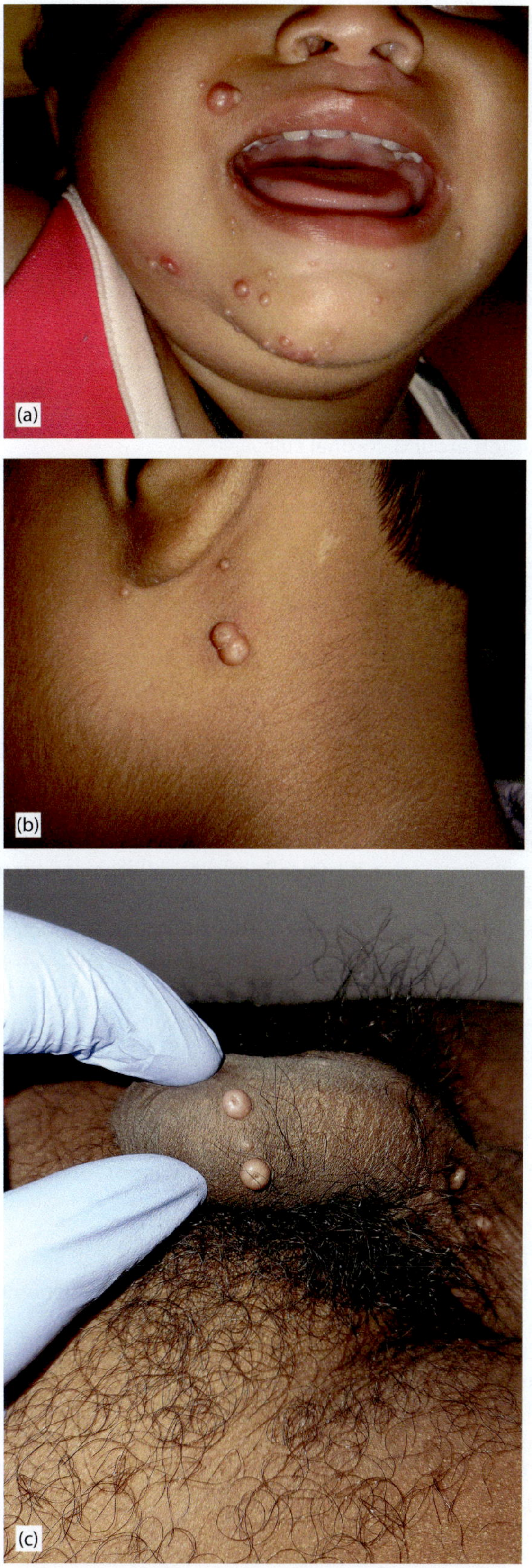


Figure 5.30 **(a)** Pearly white, umbilicated, dome-shaped papules in molluscum contagiosum. Some of the bigger lesions appear erythematous. **(b)** Molluscum contagiosum. **(c)** Umbilicated papules of molluscum contagiosum affecting the penis. (a–c – Courtesy: Dr. Piyush Kumar, Katihar, India.)

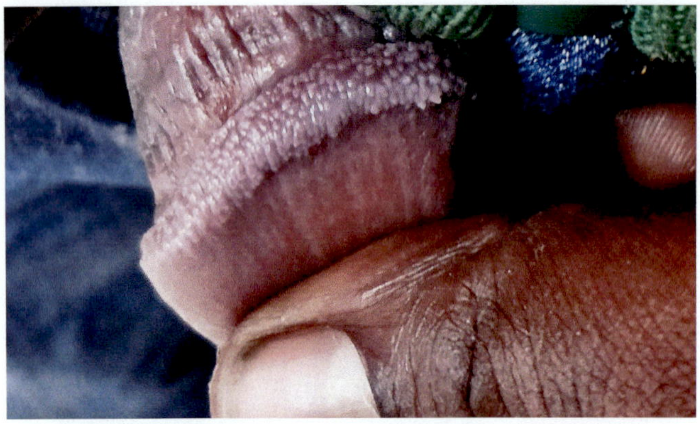

Figure 5.31 Pearly penile papules. Pink, small papules arranged around coronal sulcus.

## Pearly penile papules

- These are common, benign lesions that appear on the corona of the glans penis during adolescence or early adulthood.
- Clinical features include uniform, skin-colored, dome-shaped papules that orient in one to two rows around the glans penis (**Figure 5.31**).
- DD: Condyloma acuminata, molluscum contagiosum.

## Lichen nitidus

- Lichen nitidus is an inflammatory skin eruption of unknown cause; it typically affects children and young adults.
- It presents as shiny, flat-topped, skin-colored, pinhead-sized papules (**Figure 5.32**).[4]
- These are typically arranged in groups on the chest, abdomen, genitalia, and upper extremities.
- Koebner phenomenon are seen.
- Oral mucosa (white papules) and nail lesions (thickening, ridging, pitting) may be seen.
- There is spontaneous resolution.
- DD: Lichen spinulosus, papular mucinosis, plane warts.

## Lichen scrofulosorum

- This is a rare tuberculid.
- Tiny, skin-colored, perifollicular papules are arranged in groups.[13]
- They are normally smooth; they may have spiny projections with fine scales.
- Usually, they appear on the abdomen, chest, back, and proximal parts of the limbs.
- The condition shows as a strongly positive tuberculin test.
- DD: Lichen nitidus, keratosis pilaris, lichen spinulosus.

## Skin tags

- These are also known as fibroepithelial polyps, or acrochordons.
- A common benign skin condition, it consists of a bit of skin projecting from the surrounding skin (**Figure 5.33**).[1]

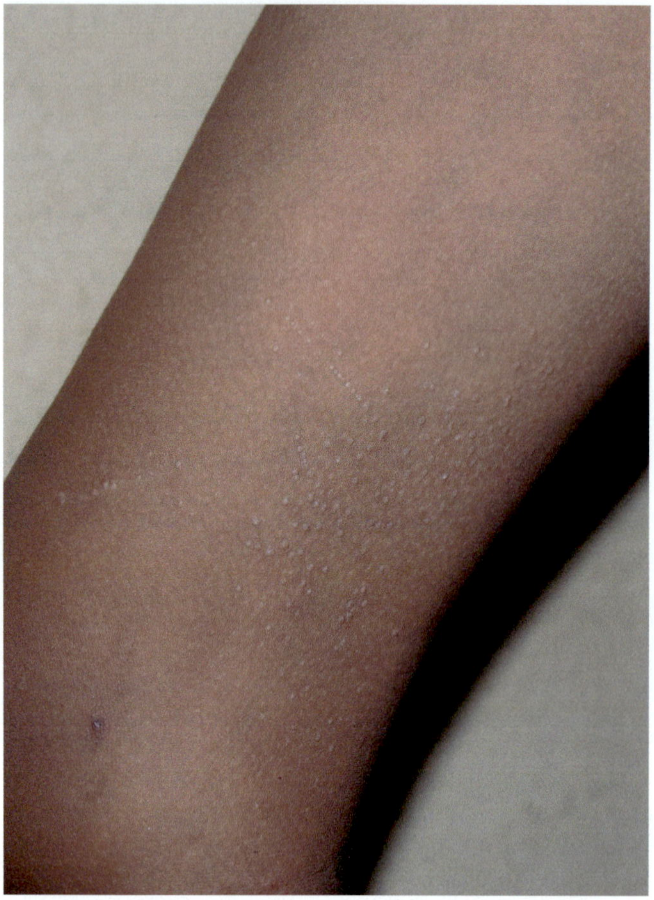

Figure 5.32 Shiny, pinpoint papules in lichen nitidus exhibiting Koebner phenomenon. (Courtesy: Dr. Piyush Kumar, Katihar, India.)

- They often develop at sites of friction.
- They are reported to be associated with many diseases, including type 2 diabetes mellitus (DM) and obesity.
- DD: Verruca plana, DPN.

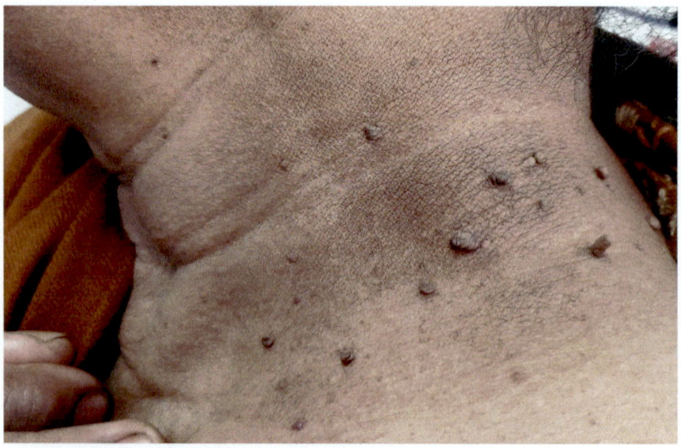

Figure 5.33 Skin tag. Skin-colored, soft sessile, and pedunculated papules on neck.

### Piezogenic pedal papules

- Skin-colored asymptomatic papules are observed in usually healthy individuals, especially athletes and marathon runners.
- They are constituted of herniations of fat tissue into weight-carrying connective tissue of the heels (**Figure 5.34a,b**).
- They occur as a result of continuous pressure on the heels from lifting excessive weight, jumping, running, or carrying heavy loads.
- A few cases have been reported to occur in patients with rheumatic heart disease and Ehler Danlos syndrome.
- DD: Xanthoma, gouty tophi.

### Steatocystoma multiplex

- This is a hamartomous malformation of the pilosebaceous duct junction.
- Clinical features include dome-shaped, asymptomatic papules; early lesions are translucent and change to a yellowish color with age (**Figure 5.35a,b**).

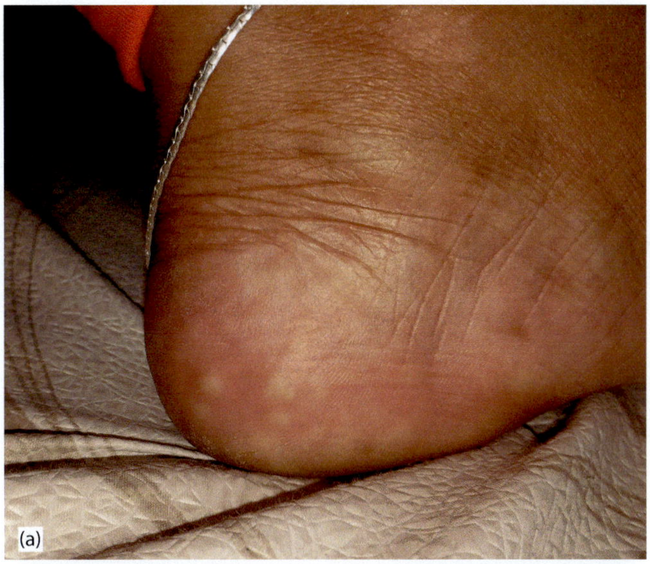

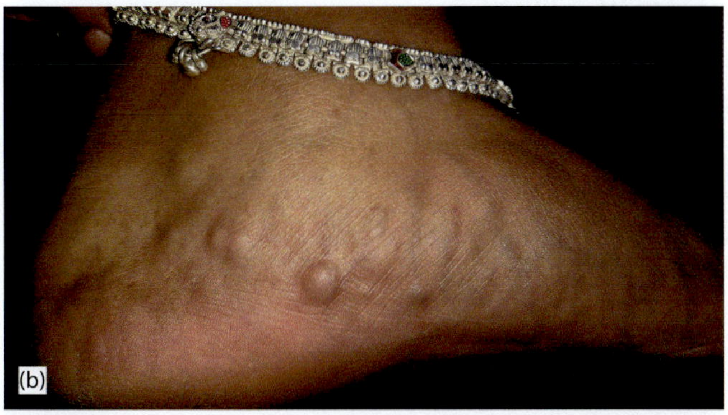

Figure 5.34 **(a)** Piezogenic pedal papules. **(b)** Piezogenic pedal papules (a – Courtesy: Dr. Sunil Patwardhan, Pune, India; b – Dr. Anup Kumar Tiwary, Consultant Dermatologist, Yashoda Hospital and Research Center, Ghaziabad, India.)

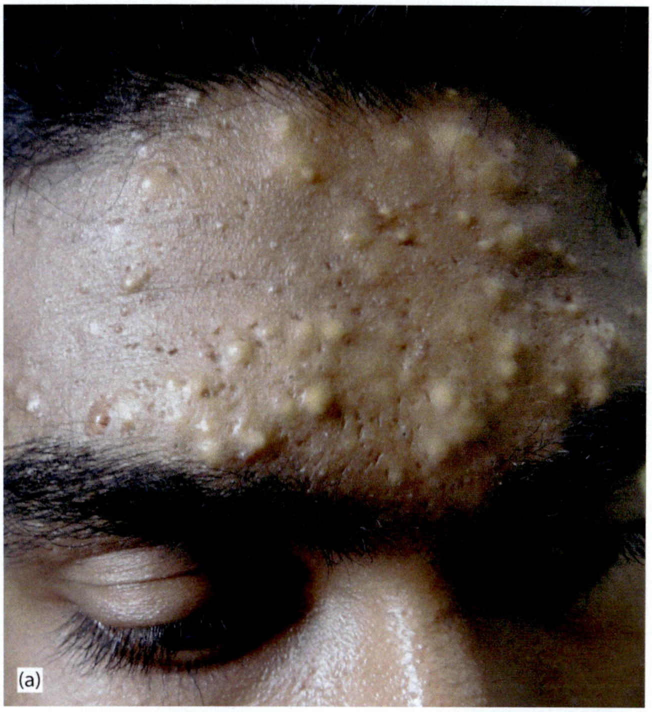

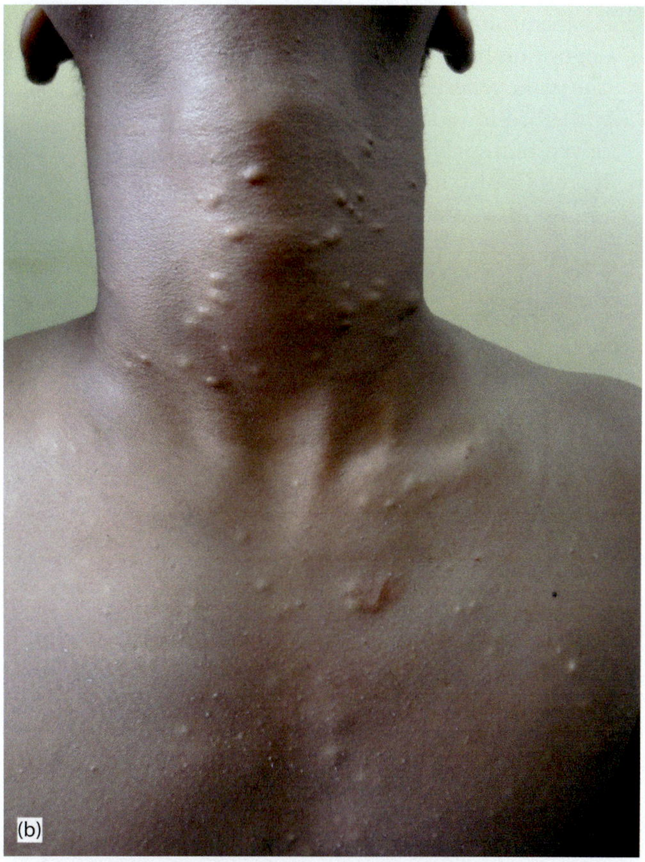

Figure 5.35 **(a)** Yellow, dome-shaped papules on forehead in steatocystoma multiplex. **(b)** Steatocystoma multiplex over chest. (b – Courtesy: Dr. Piyush Kumar, Katihar, India.)

- Common sites are axilla, groin, trunk, scrotum, and the proximal extremities. The sternal region is commonly affected in males.
- A solitary lesion is known as steatocystoma simplex.
- DD: Eruptive vellus hair cyst, milia, trichilemmal cyst.

## Neurofibromas

- Neurofibromas are benign tumors that arise from Schwann cells.
- Dermal tumors are soft dome-shaped tumors but can also present as pedunculated, nodular, or plaque-like (**Figure 5.36**).[1]
- They demonstrate a buttonhole sign.
- Histologically, they are made of mixed cells like Schwann cells, perineural cells, and fibroblasts.
- They are associated with other features like café-au-lait macules, Crowe's sign, plexiform neurofibroma in neurofibromatosis-1 (NF1), and with schwannomas and meningioma in NF2.
- DD: Lipoma, dermal melanocytic nevus, acrochordons.

## Localized papular mucinosis

- Also called lichen myxedematosus, this is a primary cutaneous mucinosis characterized by dermal mucin deposition in absence of thyroid disorder.
- The pathogenesis is a proliferation of fibroblasts with fibrosis and excessive deposition of mucin (glycosaminoglycans) in the dermis.
- It is clinically characterized by a few to multiple, 2–5-mm, skin-colored, firm, waxy, dome-shaped papules that may coalesce to form plaque, causing thickening and hardening of the skin.
- DD: Lichen nitidus, scleromyxedema, eruptive LP, mucinous LE.

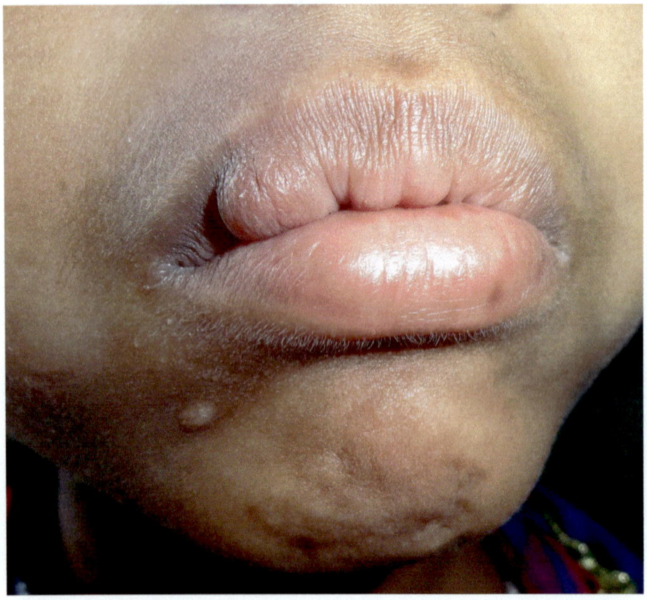

Figure 5.36 Small, soft, skin-colored papule of neurofibroma on the chin and a nodule over upper lip.

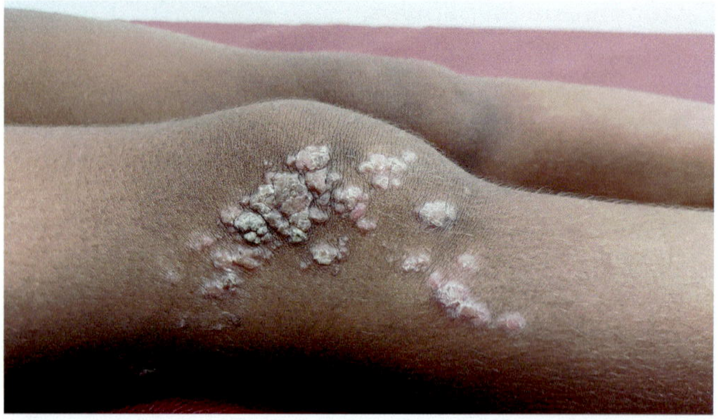

Figure 5.37 Psoriatic papules and plaques arranged linearly along Blaschko's line. (Courtesy: Dr. PC Das and Dr. Piyush Kumar, Katihar, India.)

## Linear psoriasis

- This is a rare form of psoriasis.
- It is characterized by late onset and rapid progression.
- There is linear distribution of psoriatic lesions along Blaschko's lines (**Figure 5.37**).
- DD: Linear LP, inflammatory linear verrucous epidermal nevus (ILVEN) (no response to antipsoriatic treatment).

## Linear lichen planus

- The etiology is unknown; however, it is associated with HIV and hepatitis C infection.
- It is much more common in children than adults.
- Pruritic violaceous papules follow lines of Blaschko (**Figure 5.38**).
- It may co-exist with classic LP lesions.
- Rarely, it may have zosteriform/dermatomal distribution following herpes zoster infection.
- DD: Linear Blaschkitis, lichen striatus, linear porokeratosis.

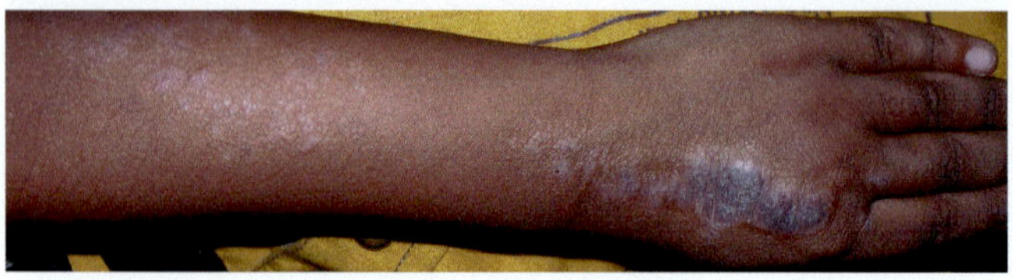

Figure 5.38 Linear lichen planus. (Courtesy: Dr. Piyush Kumar, Katihar, India.)

### Linear verrucous epidermal nevus (linear VEN)

- This is present at birth or in infancy.
- Lesions are flat, velvety, papillomatous in the newborn.
- They are keratotic and verruciform in adolescence.
- Color may range from skin color to brown.
- Lesions are arranged in streaks or swirls along Blaschko lines (**Figure 5.39a,b**).[14]
- When generalized, it is known as "systematized epidermal nevus."
- Multiple lesions may be associated with defects in the skeletal and central nervous system; this is known as "epidermal nevus syndrome."
- DD: Linear psoriasis, linear porokeratosis, lichen striatus.

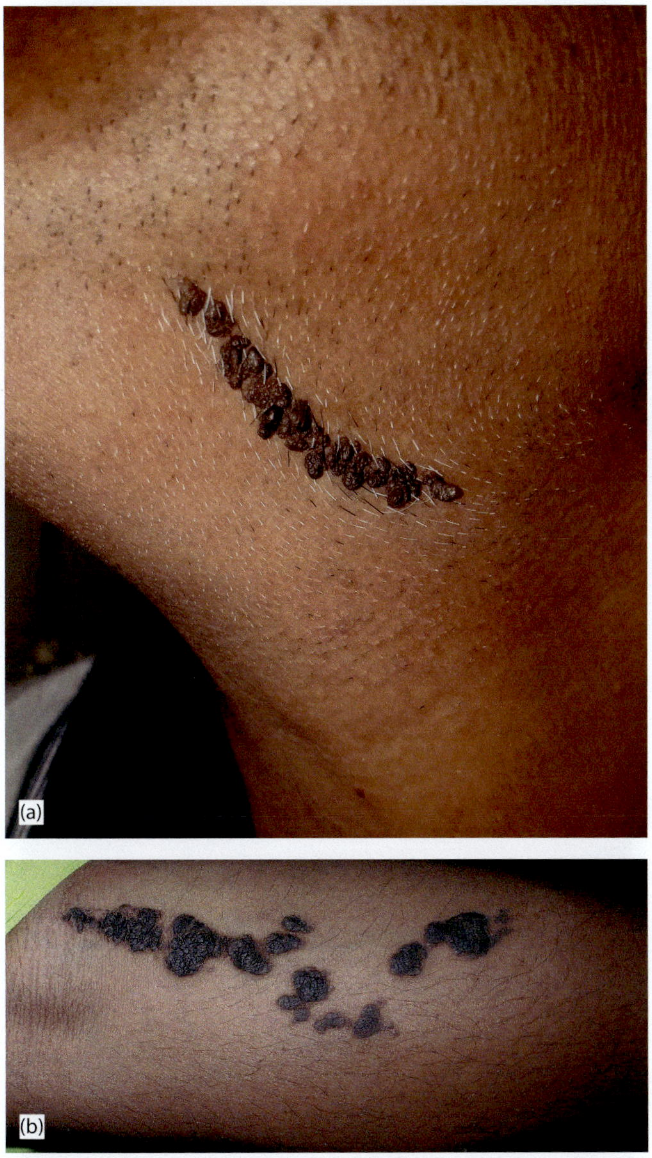

Figure 5.39 **(a)** Linear verrucous epidermal nevus on the neck. **(b)** Linear verrucous epidermal nevus on the calf. (b – Courtesy: Dr. Piyush Kumar, Katihar, India.)

### Inflammatory linear verrucous epidermal nevus (ILVEN)

- This is characterized by early onset and slow progression.
- It is extremely pruritic.
- Erythematous and hyperkeratotic verrucous/lichenoid/psoriasiform papules appear along lines of Blaschko[15] (**Figure 5.40**).
- DD: Linear psoriasis, linear VEN.

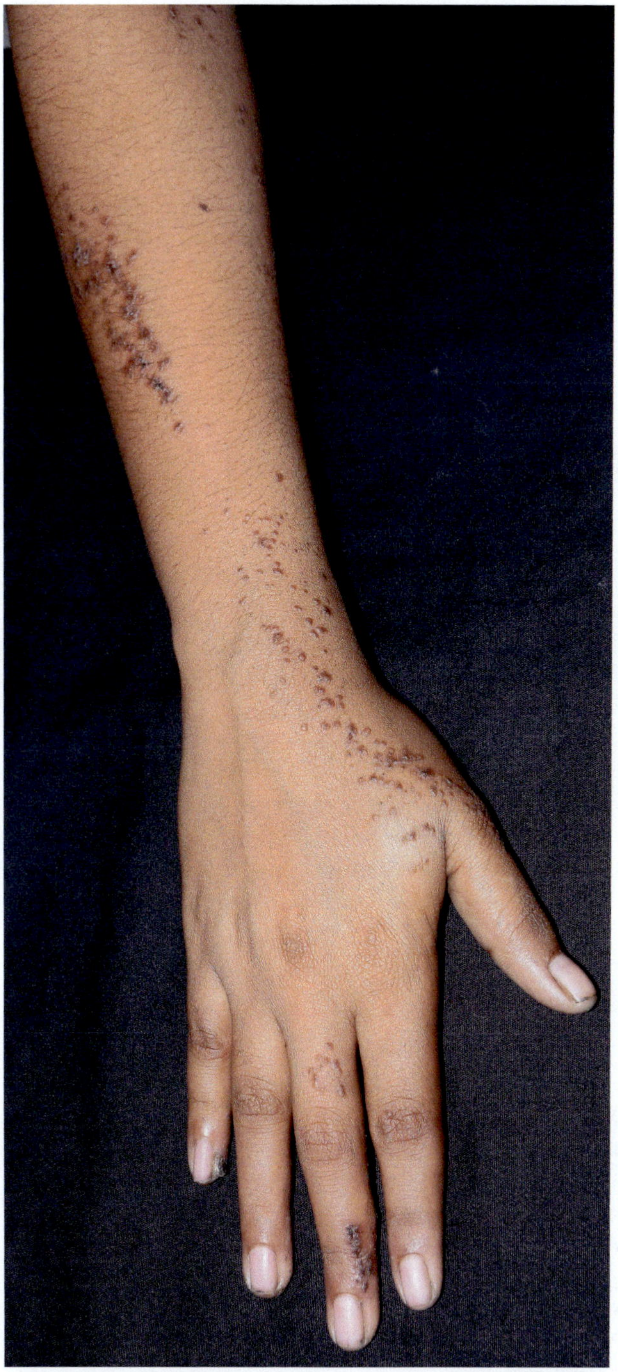

Figure 5.40 Grouped erythematous scaly and crusted papules along the lines of Blaschko. (Courtesy: Dr Piyush Kumar, Katihar, India.)

### Lichen striatus

- This is usually seen in young children with female preponderance.
- Affects the age range between 5 and 15 years.
- Tiny 1- to 2-mm flat-topped scaly erythematous papules appear along Blaschko's lines.
- It is commonly seen on limbs.
- It is asymptomatic or mildly pruritic.
- It will spontaneously regress in about one year.
- DD: Linear LP, linear VEN, linear psoriasis.

### Linear porokeratosis

- Porokeratosis is a disorder of keratinocyte growth and differentiation.
- It presents as sharply demarcated scaly papules with a distinctive hyperkeratotic ridge containing thread-like grooves (**Figure 5.41**).
- It follows Blaschko's lines.
- DD: Linear lichen planus, linear psoriasis, linear VEN.

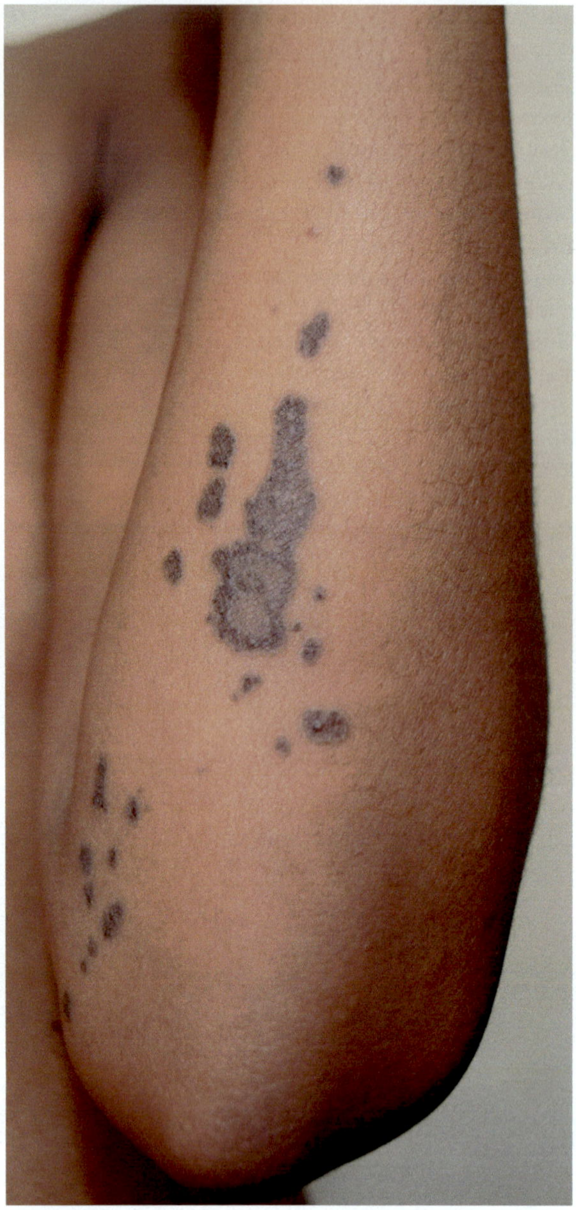

Figure 5.41 Linear porokeratosis. (Courtesy: Dr. Piyush Kumar, Katihar, India.)

### Nevus comedonicus

- Nevus comedonicus is a rare hamartoma of the pilosebaceous unit.
- In most cases, it has been present since birth, but it may also develop later.
- It features bundles of papules and dilated follicular openings containing epidermal residues and firm pigmented horny plugs, similar to comedones (**Figure 5.42**).
- It typically presents a linear or zosteriform distribution, but extensive areas have also been described.
- The most frequently affected sites are the face, trunk, neck, and upper limbs.
- It is a part of nevus comedonicus syndrome, which also consists of ocular, ostial, and neurological defects.
- DD: Nevus sebaceous, familial dyskeratotic comedones.

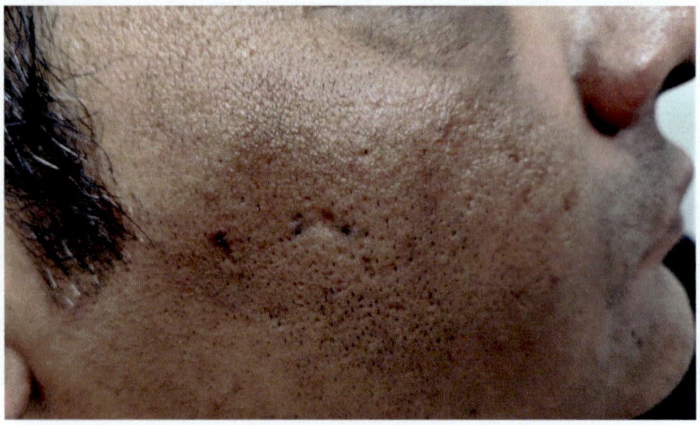

Figure 5.42 Nevus comedonicus. (Dr. Anup Kumar Tiwary, Consultant Dermatologist, Yashoda Hospital and Research Center, Ghaziabad, India.)

### Lobular capillary hemangioma (granuloma pyogenicum)

- Also known as lobular capillary hemangioma, this is a benign vascular tumor that occurs on the skin and mucous membranes.
- It can arise spontaneously, in sites of injury, or within capillary malformations.
- It is associated with medications such as oral contraceptives, retinoids, gefitinib, capecitabine, and afatinib.
- Clinical features include small or large, smooth or lobulated, reddish exophytic vascular nodules that can grow rapidly (**Figure 5.43a,b**).[16]
- They tend to bleed profusely.

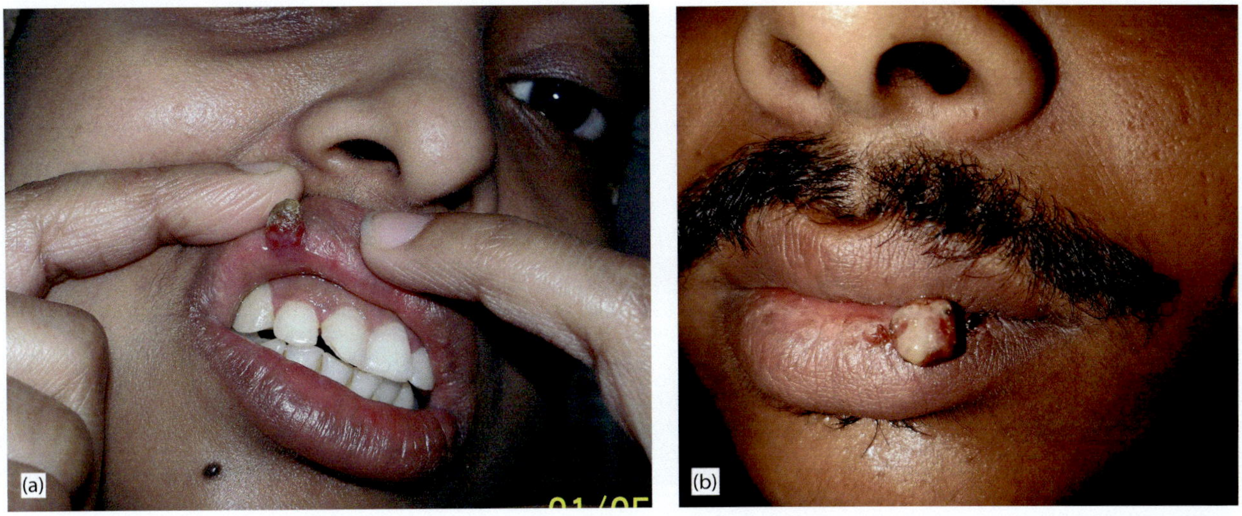


Figure 5.43 **(a)** Lobular capillary hemangioma presenting as vascular papule with hyperkeratotic surface on lip mucosa. **(b)** Infected lobular capillary hemangioma. (a – Courtesy: Dr. Piyush Kumar, Katihar, India.)

- Common sites are hands, lower lips and gingiva most frequently affected; intraoral lesions may occur during pregnancy.
- DD: Cherry angioma, Kaposiform hemangioendothelioma, hemangioma.

## Angiokeratomas

- These are ectasias of dermal capillaries with an acanthotic and hyperkeratotic overlying epidermis.
- Clinical features include red to brown verrucous papules that may bleed.[16]
- There are four types of localized angiokeratomas.
- Solitary papular angiokeratoma typically occurs on the lower extremities.
- Localized angiokeratoma appears on the scrotum and vulva (Fordyce type) (**Figure 5.44a**).
- Angiokeratoma circumscriptum naeviforme presents as multiple hyperkeratotic papular and plaque-like lesions, usually unilaterally on the lower leg, foot, thigh, and buttock (**Figure 5.44b**).
- Bilateral angiokeratomas occur on the dorsa of the fingers and toes (Mibelli).
- DD: Verruca vulgaris, hemangioma, Spitz nevus, pigmented basal cell carcinoma (BCC).

## Bacillary angiomatosis

- This is an infection with *Bartonella henselae* or *B. quintana* presenting as vaso-proliferative lesions, mostly in immunocompromised hosts, including advanced HIV patients.
- Clinical features include single or multiple bright-red to deep-purple, dome-shaped papules, nodules, or plaques.
- Lesions may bleed profusely with trauma.
- DD: Cherry angioma, Kaposi sarcoma.

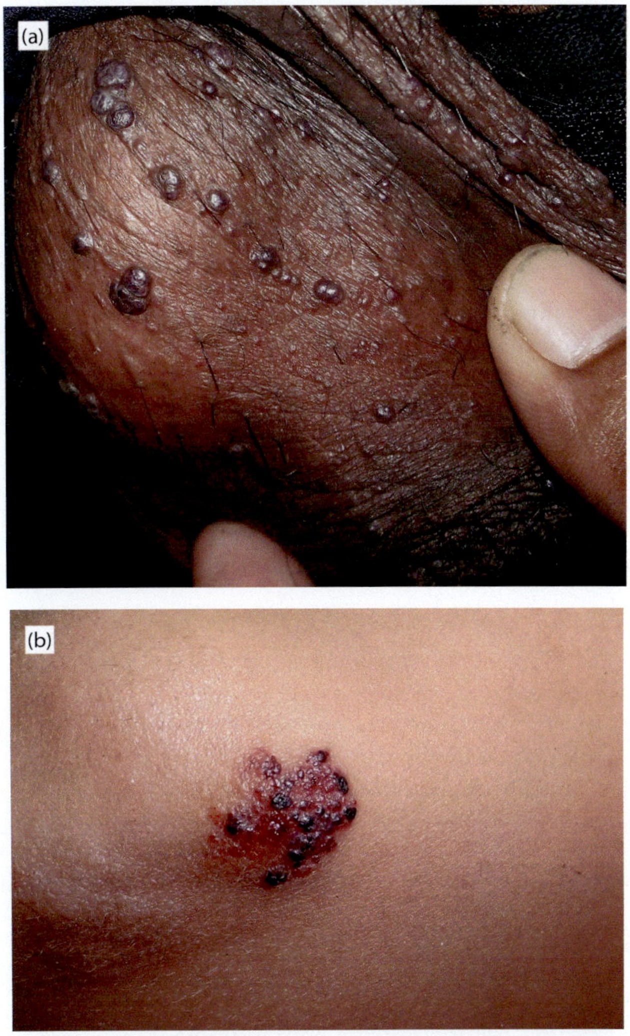


Figure 5.44 **(a)** Multiple vascular papules on scrotum in angiokeratoma of Fordyce. **(b)** Multiple hyperkeratotic vascular papules coalescing to form plaque in angiokeratoma circumscriptum naeviforme. (a – Courtesy: Dr. Piyush Kumar, Katihar, India.)

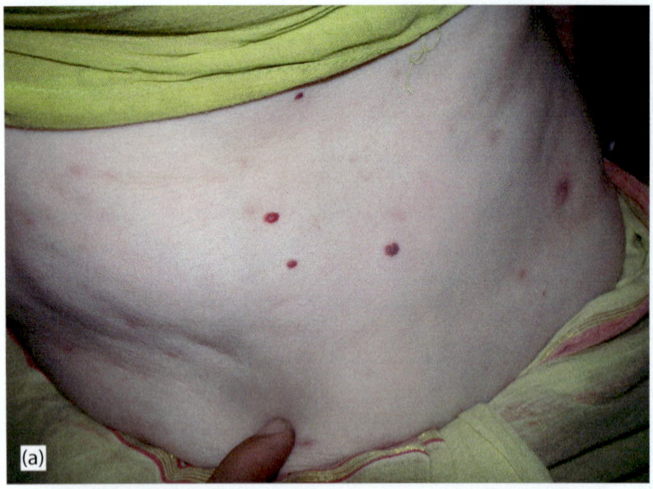


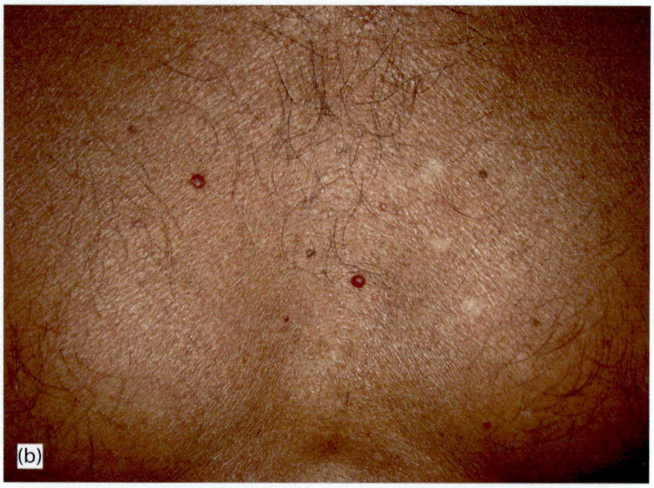


Figure 5.45 **(a)** Multiple bright-red papules in cherry angioma. **(b)** Cherry angioma in a middle-aged man. (a,b – Courtesy: Dr. Piyush Kumar, Katihar, India.)

## Cherry angioma

- This is the most common type of acquired vascular proliferation of the skin.
- It is also known as senile angioma or Campbell de Morgan spots.
- It usually develop after the third decade; the number of lesions increases with increasing age.
- Eruptive cherry angioma is seen in pregnancy, malignancy, mustard gas poisoning, and immunosuppression with cyclosporine.
- Clinical features include early lesions that appear as flat, red macules, resembling petechiae (**Figure 5.45a,b**).[16]
- As the lesions develop, they become 1- to 5-mm red papules.
- They are usually asymptomatic but may bleed with trauma.
- They most commonly occur on the trunk or proximal extremities.
- DD: Angiokeratoma, pyogenic granuloma.

## Tufted angioma

- This rare, benign angiomatous condition is also called angioblastoma of Nagakawa.
- Lesions usually arise between the ages of one and five years; occasionally they may be present at birth.
- Clinically characterized by erythematous papules, plaques, and nodules, most commonly involving the neck, upper trunk, and proximal part of extremities.
- It may show increased sweating or growth of fine lanugo hair.
- DD: Kaposi sarcoma, Kaposiform hemangioendothelioma, and low-grade angiosarcoma.

## Targetoid hemosiderotic hemangioma

- This is also known as hobnail hemangioma.
- It presents as a vascular, benign solitary lesion of unknown origin, probably lymphatic, affecting young or middle-aged people.
- Clinical features include a small violaceous papule surrounded by a pale, thin area and a peripheral ecchymotic ring.
- It is commonly located on the trunk or extremities.
- DD: Hemangioma, dermatofibroma, melanoma.

## Angiolymphoid hyperplasia with eosinophilia (ALHE)

- This is a rare, benign vascular tumor.
- It is clinically manifested by 2- to 3-cm light brown to pink dermal papules or nodules.
- Lesions occur preferentially on the face, scalp, auricular region, and neck (**Figure 5.46a,b**).[17]
- DD: Kimura disease, pleomorphic adenoma (**Figure 5.46c**), pyogenic granuloma, hemangioma.

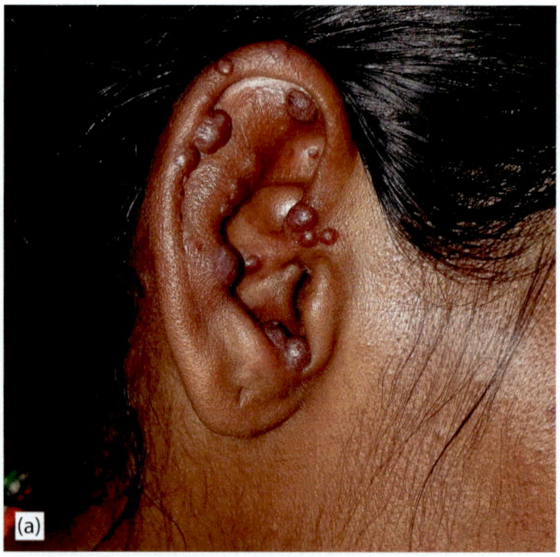


Figure 5.46 **(a)** Erythematous papules on pinna in angiolymphoid hyperplasia with eosinophilia. (*Continued*)

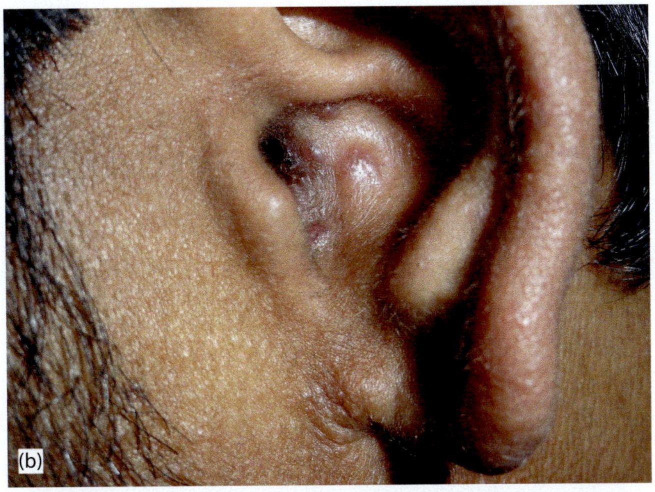

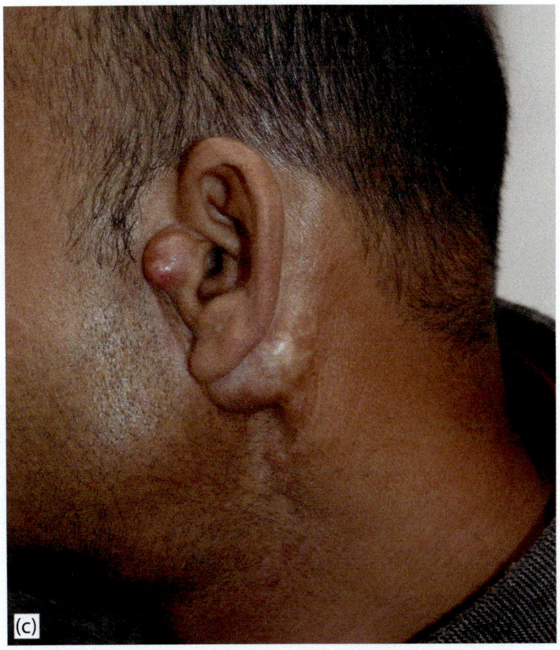

Figure 5.46 (*Continued*) **(b)** Angiolymphoid hyperplasia with eosinophilia. **(c)** Pleomorphic adenoma. A close differential of angiolymphoid hyperplasia with eosinophilia. (a – Courtesy: Dr. RR Madhukar, Patna, India; c – Courtesy: Dr. Piyush Kumar, Katihar, India.)

## Lymphomatoid papulosis

- This is a continuous self-healing, papular eruption.
- It is clinically benign and histologically malignant.
- Erythematous papules and/or nodules progress to form esicular/crusted/hemorrhagic lesions.
- They undergo spontaneous healing with scarring.
- They usually occur over the trunk and limbs.
- DD: Pityriasis lichenoides et varioliformis acuta (PLEVA), guttate psoriasis, insect dermatitis.

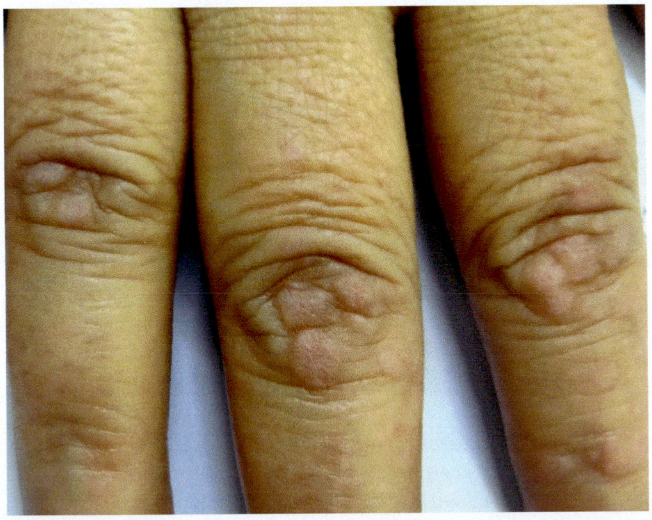

Figure 5.47 Flat-topped, slightly erythematous papules on interphalangeal joints in dermatomyositis.

## Gottron papules

- These are small purple/red flat papules on extensor surfaces, particularly the elbows and joints of the hand (**Figure 5.47**).
- They are pathognomonic for dermatomyositis.[18]
- Other features for dermatomyositis must be looked for: heliotrope rash, muscle weakness.
- DD: Psoriasis, lupus erythematosus, lichen planus.

## Multicentric reticulohistiocytosis

- This is a rare systemic granulomatous disorder.
- Cutaneous features are pink/red/brown/papules the dorsum of hand and face.
- Papules often occur in a periungual distribution, producing a characteristic "coral beads" appearance.
- Mucosa are involved in one-third of cases.
- This is often associated with severe and rapidly destructive arthritis.
- DD: lichen planus, dermatomyositis.

## Gianotti-crosti syndrome

- Also known as papular acrodermatitis of childhood, this is a rare and self-limited dermatosis.
- The cause is herpesvirus type B, EBV.
- Peak incidence occurs in infants between one and six years of age.
- Clinical features include symmetrical and multiple, monomorphic and erythematous papular eruption with acral distribution; the torso generally remains intact (**Figure 5.48a**).

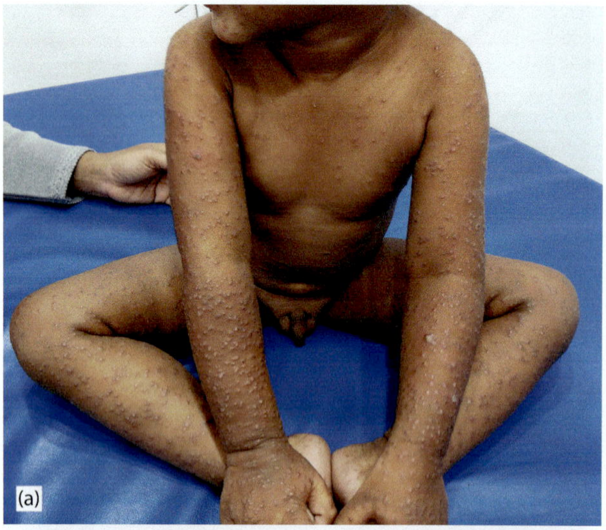

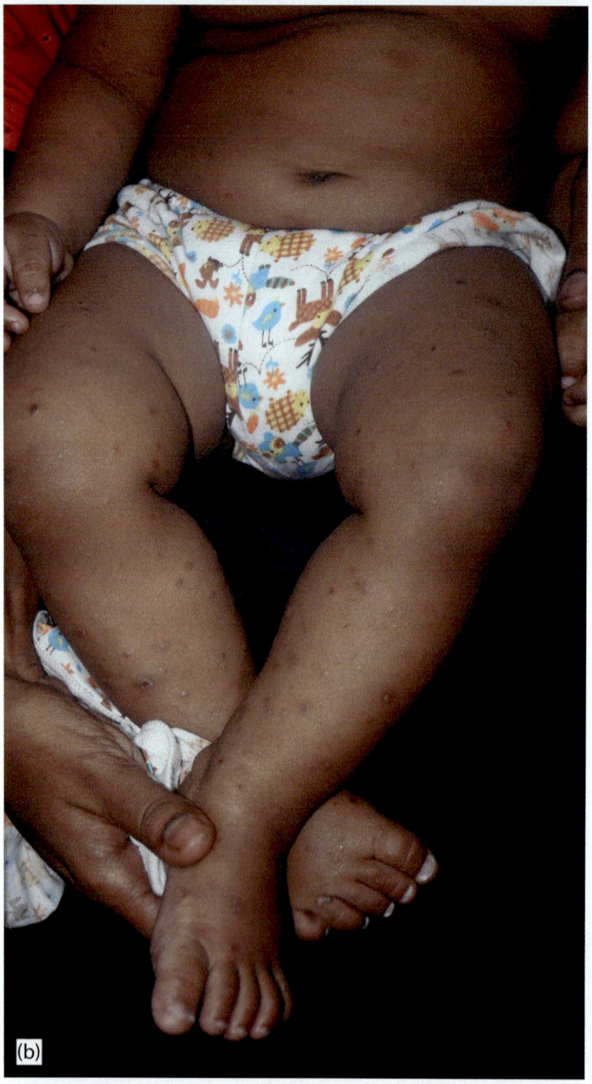

Figure 5.48 **(a)** Gianotti-crosti syndrome with monomorphic papulovesicles on the extremities. **(b)** Papular urticaria with papulovesicles on the lower extremities. Prior lesions have healed with hyperpigmentation and scarring. (a – Courtesy: Dr. Deverashetti Srinivas, Nizamabad, India; b – Courtesy: Dr. Piyush Kumar, Katihar, India.)

- Systemic manifestations are unusual and include low-grade fever, generalized lymphadenopathy, hepatomegaly, and splenomegaly.
- DD: insect dermatitis, scabies, papular urticaria (**Figure 5.48b**).

## Additional image – Figure 5.49

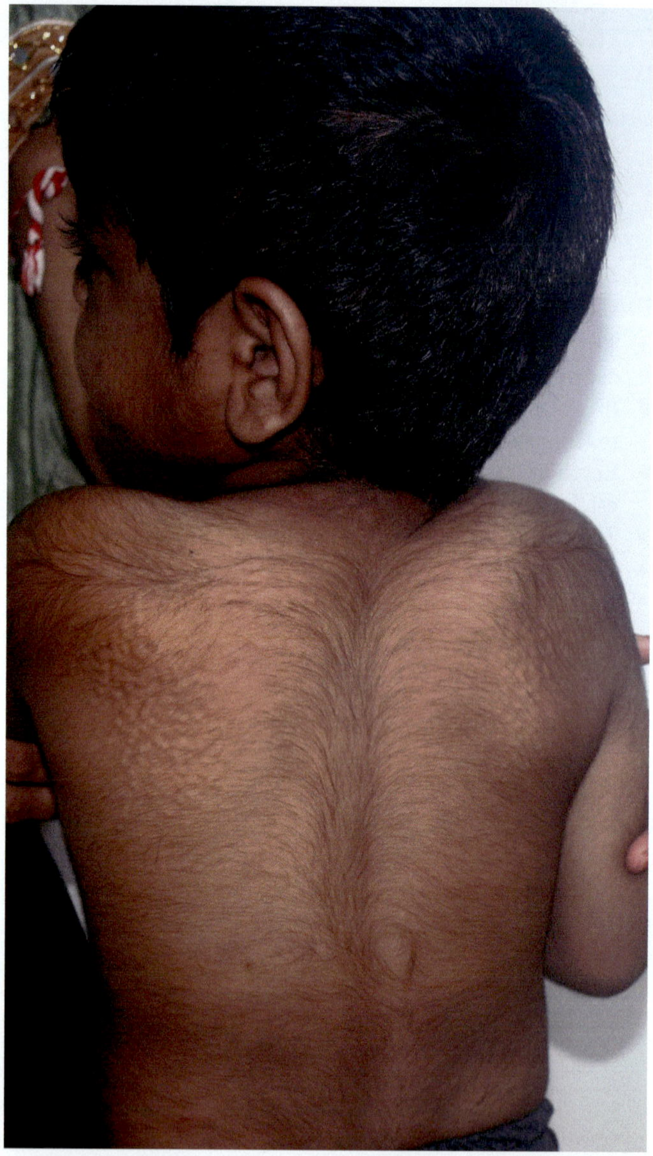

Figure 5.49 Bilateral, grouped, skin-colored papules on the scapular area in a child with Hunter syndrome. "Pebbly papules with a cobblestone appearance" present on the upper trunk and shoulder are a characteristic feature of Hunter syndrome. Note short neck and hypertrichosis in the child. (Courtesy: Kumar P, Das PC, Das A. Hunter syndrome. JAMA Dermatol 2022;158(12):1438.)

## REFERENCES


1. Fitzpatrick JE, High WA, Kyle WL. Urgent Care Dermatology: Symptom-Based Diagnosis. 1st ed. Philadelphia: Elsevier; 2018. Chapter 6. Papular Eruptions: No Scale. p. 83–96.
2. Fitzpatrick JE, High WA, Kyle WL. Urgent Care Dermatology: Symptom-Based Diagnosis. 1st ed. Philadelphia: Elsevier; 2018. Chapter 7. Scaly Papular Lesions. P. 97–112.
3. Lee HJ, Sinha AA. Cutaneous lupus erythematosus: Understanding of clinical features, genetic basis, and pathobiology of disease guides therapeutic strategies. Autoimmunity 2006;39:433–444.
4. Ely JW, Stone MS. The Generalized Rash: Part I. Differential Diagnosis. Am Fam Physician 2010;81(6):726–734.
5. Nath AK, Sivaranjini R, Thappa DM, Basu D. Lupus miliaris disseminates faciei with unusual distribution of lesions. Indian J Dermatol 2011;56:234–236.
6. Fitzpatrick JE, High WA, Kyle WL. Urgent Care Dermatology: Symptom-Based Diagnosis. 1st ed. Philadelphia: Elsevier; 2018. Chapter 23. Follicular Disorders. P. 375–384.
7. Ramesh A, Sampath V, Kasiviswanathan P, RajanBabu D. Overview of axillary dermatoses: Case series in a tertiary care institution. Int J Res Dermatol 2019;5(4):784–791.
8. Tüzün Y, Wolf R. Commentary: Fold (intertriginous) dermatoses: When skin touches skin. Clin Dermatol 2015;33(4):411–413.
9. Tiwary AK, Mishra DK, Chaudhary SS. A rare case of familial reactive perforating collagenosis. Indian J Paediatr Dermatol 2017;18:230–233.
10. Curatolo P, Bombardieri R, Jozwiak S. Tuberous sclerosis. Lancet 2008;372(9639):657–668.
11. Fitzpatrick JE, High WA, Kyle WL. Urgent Care Dermatology: Symptom-Based Diagnosis. 1st ed. Philadelphia: Elsevier; 2018. Chapter 33. Yellow Lesions. P. 553–564.
12. Bubna AK. Umbilicated lesions in dermatology. Clin Dermatol Rev 2019;3:99–103.
13. Santos JB, Figueiredo AR, Ferraz CE, Oliveira MH, Silva PG, Medeiros VL. Cutaneous tuberculosis: Epidemiologic, etiopathogenic and clinical aspects - Part I. An Bras Dermatol 2014;89(2):219–228.
14. Fitzpatrick JE, High WA, Kyle WL. Urgent Care Dermatology: Symptom-Based Diagnosis. 1st ed. Philadelphia: Elsevier; 2018. Chapter 17. Linear and Serpiginous Lesions. P. 289–300.
15. Tiwary AK. Adult onset of inflammatory linear verrucous epidermal nevus: Truly a rare experience. J Pak Assoc Dermatol 2019;29(2):253–256.
16. Fitzpatrick JE, High WA, Kyle WL. Urgent Care Dermatology: Symptom-Based Diagnosis. 1st ed. Philadelphia: Elsevier; 2018. Chapter 32. Vascular Tumors. P. 535–552.
17. Tiwary AK, Kumar P. Report of two cases of angiolymphoid hyperplasia with eosinophilia and review of literature. Int J Health Sci Res 2017;7(8):503–506.
18. DeWane ME, Waldman R, Lu J. Dermatomyositis part I: Clinical features and pathogenesis. J Am Acad Dermatol 2019;82(2):267–281.

# 6

# Facial papules

PIYUSH KUMAR, RIZWANA BARKAT

## INTRODUCTION

The etiopathological processes causing facial papules can be diverse, ranging from benign (infective, inflammatory, or neoplastic) to malignant conditions. The list of clinical differentials of facial papules can be overwhelming, but a careful consideration of the number of lesions, age of presentation, relative distribution on the face, presence or absence of other lesions and scars, and clinical characteristics of the individual papule often helps in arriving at a clinical diagnosis in majority of cases (**Figures 6.1** and **6.2**, **Tables 6.1** and **6.2**). This chapter discusses a clinical approach to the diagnosis of facial papules, followed by a brief description of some important conditions presenting as papules on the face.[1–4]

### Acne vulgaris

- Acne vulgaris (AV) is a common condition caused by follicular blockage (due to hyperkeratinization) and/or inflammation of pilosebaceous units. Acne can present as non-inflammatory lesions (comedones), inflammatory lesions (papules, pustules, and nodules), or a mixture of both.
- AV is most commonly seen in adolescents and less commonly in adults. Of note, AV shows male predilection in adolescent population and female preponderance in adult population. Female patients may have features of polycystic ovarian syndrome (PCOS).
- AV is most common on the face but affects the back and chest too. Lesions on the face are most severe

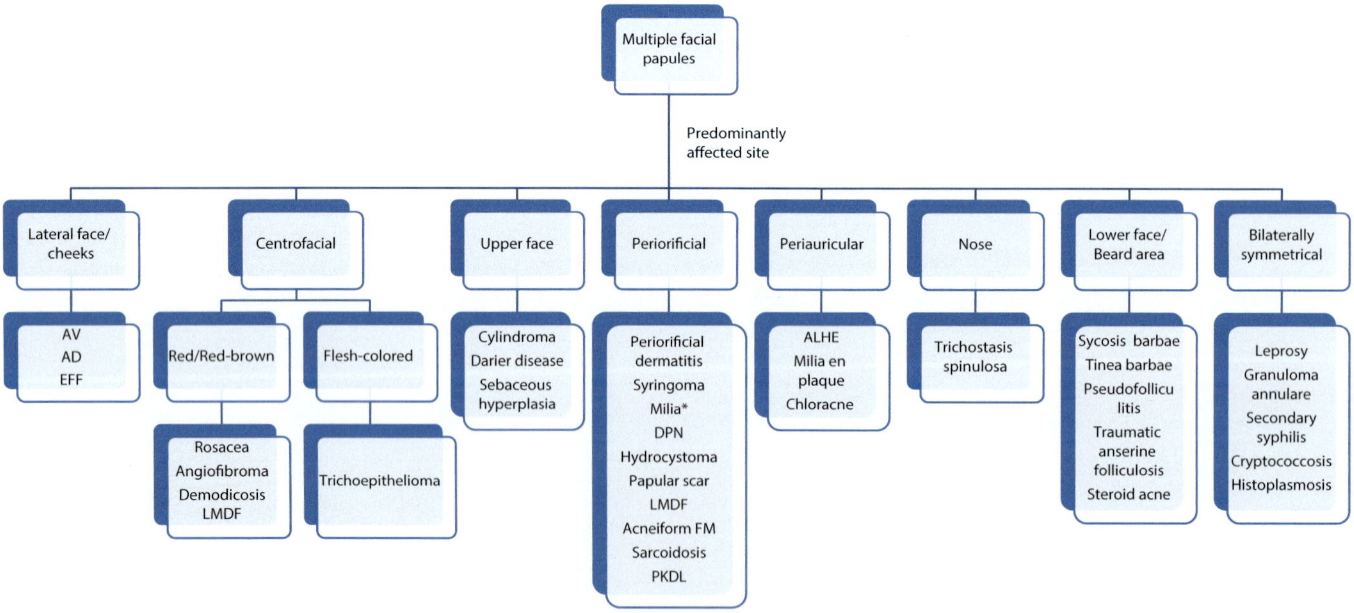


Figure 6.1 Clinical approach to multiple facial papules (AV – acne vulgaris, AD – atopic dermatitis, EFF – erythromelanosis follicularis faciei, LMDF – lupus miliaris disseminatus faciei, DPN – dermatosis papulosa nigra, FM – follicular mucinosis, PKDL – post-kala azar dermal leishmaniasis, ALHE – angiolymphoid hyperplasia with eosinophilia).


DOI: 10.1201/9781351054225-12

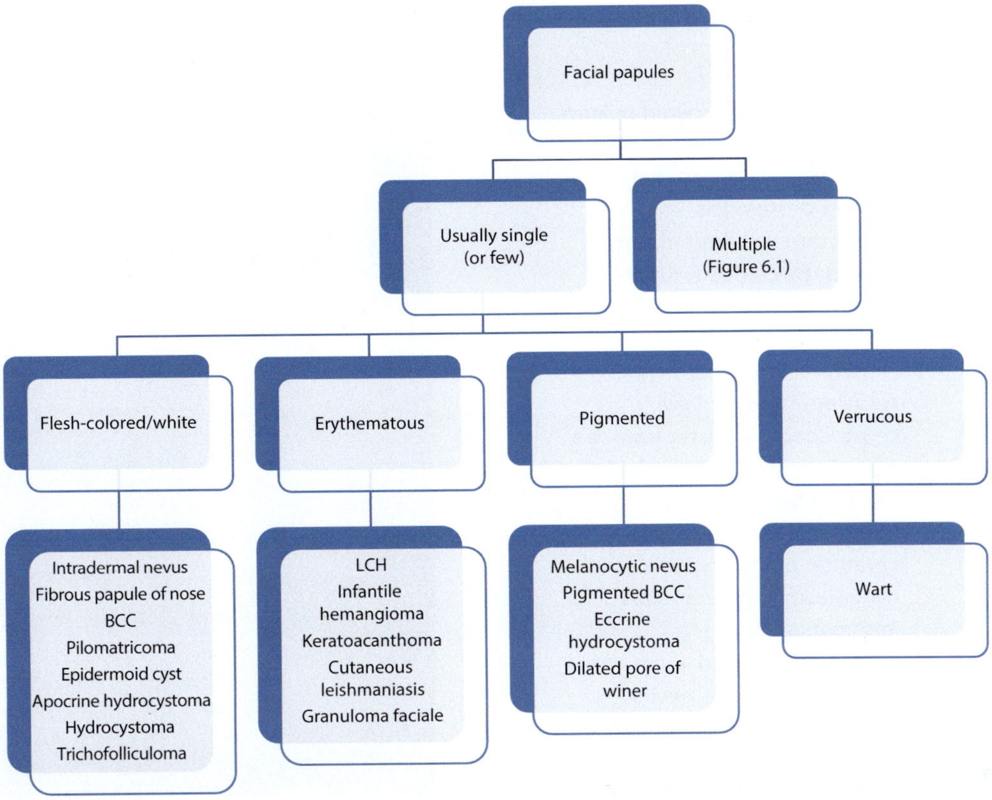


Figure 6.2 Clinical approach to solitary facial papule (BCC – basal cell carcinoma, LCH – langerhans cell histiocytosis).

on the cheeks. However, in women with PCOS, perioral, or jawline, areas are affected with increased frequency.

- The disease is clinically characterized by non-inflammatory and skin lesions, mainly in the sebum-rich areas, such as face, back and chest. There may be associated soreness, itching, and pain.
  - Comedones – These are the pathognomonic lesions of AV and may be a whitehead (closed comedone) (**Figure 6.3a,b**) or a blackhead (open comedone) (**Figure 6.3c**) without any clinical signs of inflammation.
  - Inflammatory lesions are characterized by erythematous papules and pustules (**Figure 6.3d,e**). In severe cases, nodules and cysts too may be seen (**Figure 6.3f,g**).
- Post-inflammatory hyperpigmentation and atrophic or hypertrophic scars are the sequelae of acne.
- Neonatal cephalic pustulosis – acne lesions may be present in the first few weeks of life too (because of maternal hormones) and tend to resolve spontaneously.
- DD:
  - For inflammatory lesions – seborrheic dermatitis (yellowish greasy scales), rosacea (photosensitivity, telangiectasia, central face affection), demodicosis, bacterial folliculitis (**Figure 6.3h**).

Table 6.1 Facial papules and usual age of presentation

| Age of presentation | Diseases |
|---|---|
| Infancy/ early childhood | Infantile hemangioma, neonatal cephalic pustulosis, common acquired melanocytic nevus (CAMN), childhood granulomatous periorificial dermatitis (CGPD), Darier disease, keratosis follicularis spinulosa decalvans (KFSD), inherited cylindroma, lipoid proteinosis (with vesicobullous lesions) |
| Adolescence | Acne vulgaris, verruca plana, trichoepithelioma, angiofibroma, neurofibromas, traumatic anserine folliculosis, erythromelanosis follicularis faciei, dermatosis papulosa nigra |
| Adults/ elderly | • Solitary – basal cell carcinoma (BCC), solitary cylindroma, hydrocystoma, pilomatricoma<br>• Multiple – sebecous hyperplasia, rosacea, demodicosis, trichostasis spinulosa, lymphoma-associated FM |

Table 6.2 Clinical characteristics of facial papules

| Clinical features | Diseases |
|---|---|
| Waxy papules | • Solitary – BCC, colloid milium, keratoacanthoma<br>• Multiple – trichoepithelioma, lipoid proteinosis |
| Translucent papules | Hidrocystoma, colloid milium, papular sarcoidosis, lupus miliaris disseminatus faciei (LMDF) |
| Umbilicated papules | Molluscum contagiosum (MC), sebaceous hyperplasia, cryptococcosis, histoplasmosis |
| Ulcerated /crusted papules | Atopic dermatitis, BCC, lobular capillary hemangioma, keratoacanthoma (central keratotic plug), cryptococcosis, histoplasmosis, cutaneous leishmaniasis |
| Verrucous/ keratotic papules | • Linearly arranged – verrucous epidermal nevus, nevus sebaceous (in post-pubertal life), warts<br>• Randomly arranged – seborrheic keratosis, Darier disease, keratosis follicularis spinulosa decalvans |
| Linearly arranged papules | Molluscum contagiosum, verruca plana and common wart, verrucous epidermal nevus |
| Papulopustular lesions | Acne vulgaris, rosacea, sycosis barbae, pseudofolliculitis barbae, tinea barbae, tinea faciei, periorificial dermatitis, demodicosis, secondary syphilis, cryptococcosis, histoplasmosis, chloracne, acneiform follicular mucinosis |
| Expressed contents | • White solid material – MC<br>• Cheesy, smelly, semisolid material – epidermoid cyst<br>• Oily material – steatocystoma multiplex<br>• Gelatinous – colloid milium |
| Papules healing with scarring | Acne vulgaris, LMDF, sycosis barbae, tinea barbe, keratoacanthoma, infantile hemangioma, lipoid proteinosis, KFSD, chloracne, cutaneous leishmaniasis |

- For comedones – syringoma (skin-colored or lightly pigmented angulated papules), sebaceous hyperplasia (yellowish papules in elderly), trichoepithelioma, steatocystoma multiplex, milia, molluscum contagiosum (**Figure 6.3i**).

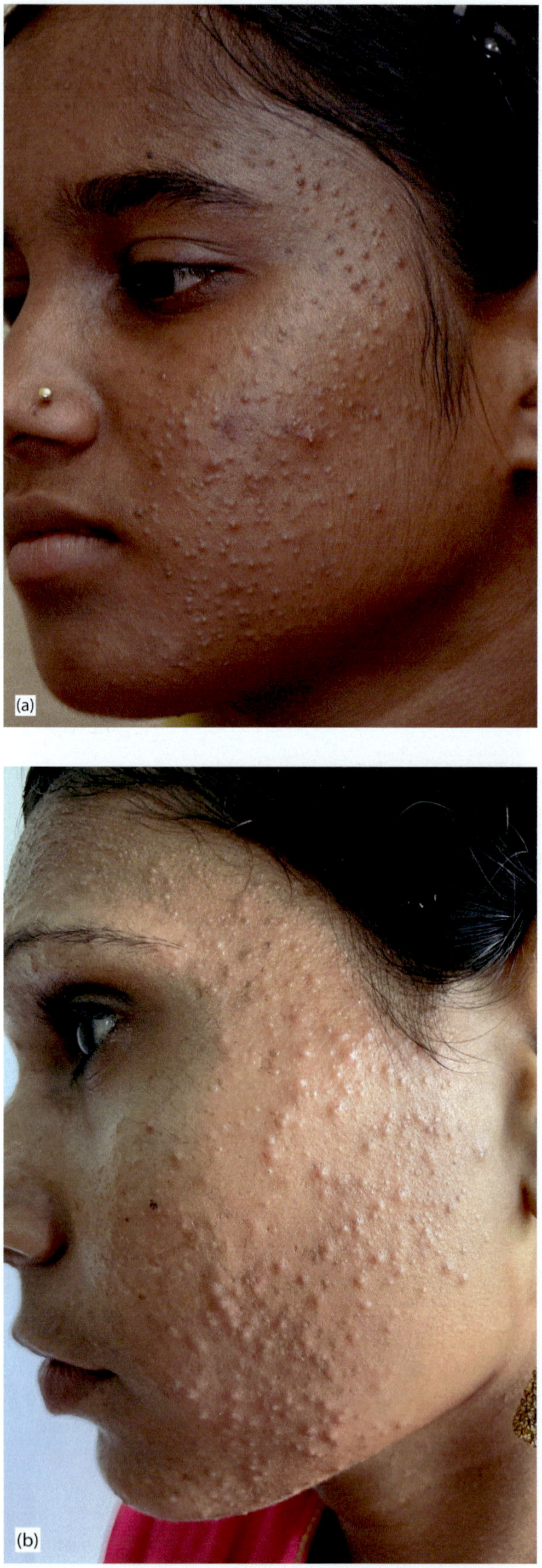

Figure 6.3 **(a)** Closed comedones seen as discrete, skin-colored papules on the face. Few isolated inflammatory papules and papulopustules are seen. **(b)** Closed comedones. (*Continued*)

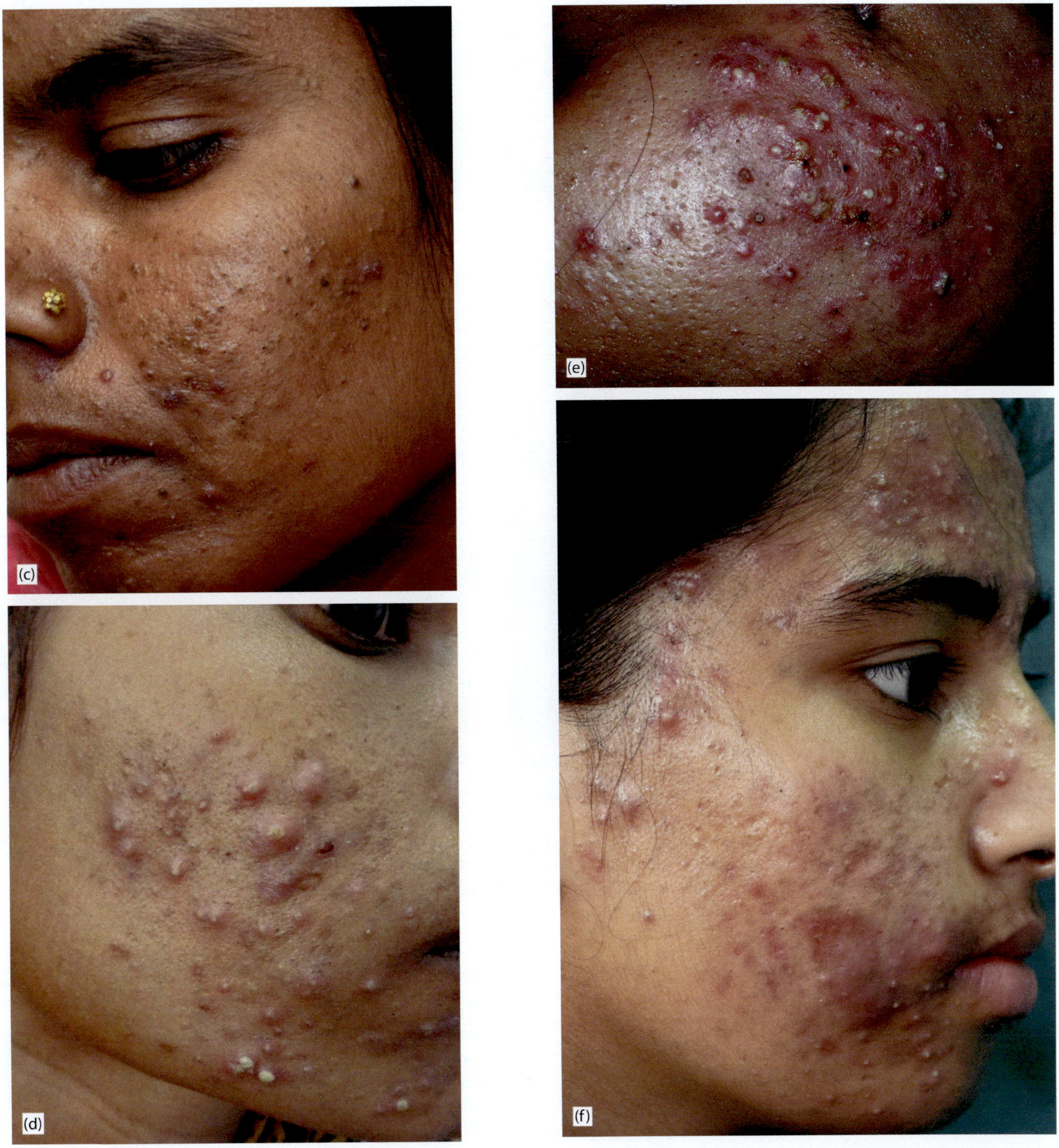


Figure 6.3 (*Continued*) **(c)** Open comedones seen as skin-colored papules with dilated follicular opening and central pigmented, keratotic material. **(d)** Erythematous papules and pustules in acne vulgaris. **(e)** In severe cases, lesions tend to become confluent. **(f)** Soft nodules and cystic in a young girl. (*Continued*)

## Atopic dermatitis

- Facial atopic dermatitis is usually seen in babies and children. The cheeks and forehead are often affected.
- Skin is dry, red, itchy, and irritable. Patients may have erythematous papules and plaques, or vesicular, oozing, crusted lesions (**Figure 6.4**). Other body parts are often affected.
- DD: Scabies, seborrheic dermatitis, contact dermatitis.

## Erythromelanosis follicularis faciei (EFF)

- EFF is an under-recognized condition of unknown etiology, characterized by a triad of follicular papules, well-demarcated erythema, and hyperpigmentation.

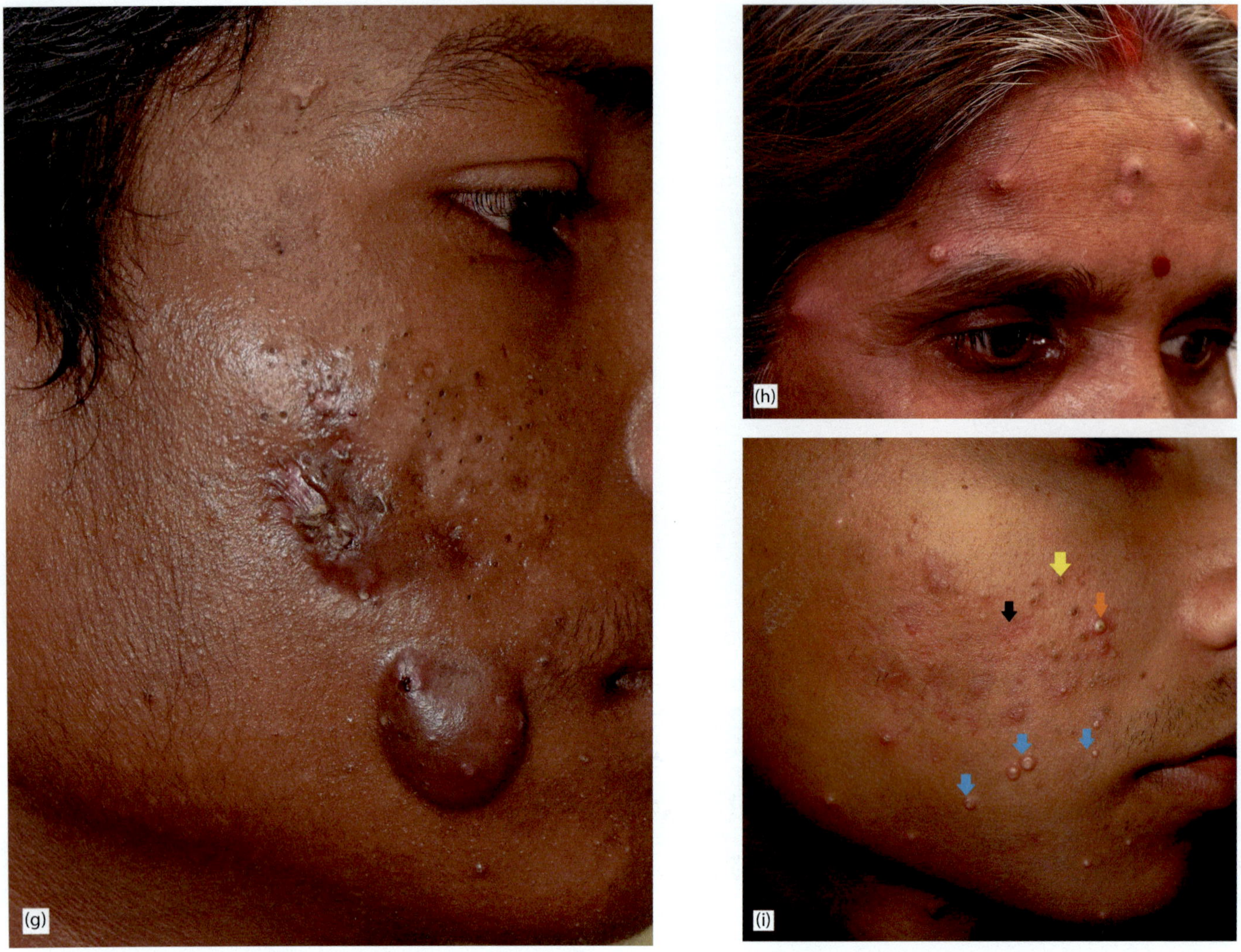


Figure 6.3 (*Continued*) **(g)** Nodulocystic lesions on face. Note presence of open comedones and scarring. **(h)** Erythematous papules, pustules, and nodules of bacterial folliculitis. **(i)** This particular patient has both acne vulgaris – mid face pustule (orange arrow), open comedones (yellow arrow), post-acne erythema (black arrow) – and molluscum contagiosum (lower face, blue arrow). (i – Courtesy: Dr. PC Das, Katihar, India.)

- The condition is mostly seen in adolescents of Asian ancestry and typically affects lateral face and preauricular areas. When it affects the neck too, it is called erythromelanosis follicularis faciei et colli (EFFC).
- Patients present with grouped, tiny follicular papules over a background of well-defined erythema and hyperpigmentation (**Figure 6.5**). Telangiectasia too may be observed at times.
- Patients may have associated keratosis pilaris over extremities.
- DD: Poikiloderma of Civatte, Riehl's melanosis, and pigmented peribuccal erythrosis of Brocq.

## Rosacea

- Rosacea is a chronic, idiopathic, inflammatory facial condition showing periodic remission and relapses.
- Middle-aged women with fair skin, blue eyes, and blonde hair are more commonly affected.
- Various triggers, such as sunlight, heat, cold, wind, spicy food, alcohol, and stress, aggravate the disease.
- The condition is characterized by varying degrees of erythema, flushing and telangiectasia, and inflammatory lesions, and is divided into four subtypes. In many patients, different types may coexist, and one type may progress another type.
  - **Erythematotelangiectatic rosacea** – It is the earliest change in rosacea and is initially transient, later becoming persistent. Clinically it is characterized by flushing and persistent central facial erythema (sparing the periocular area) and is accompanied by a burning or stinging sensation. At times, the surface may be scaly because of low-grade

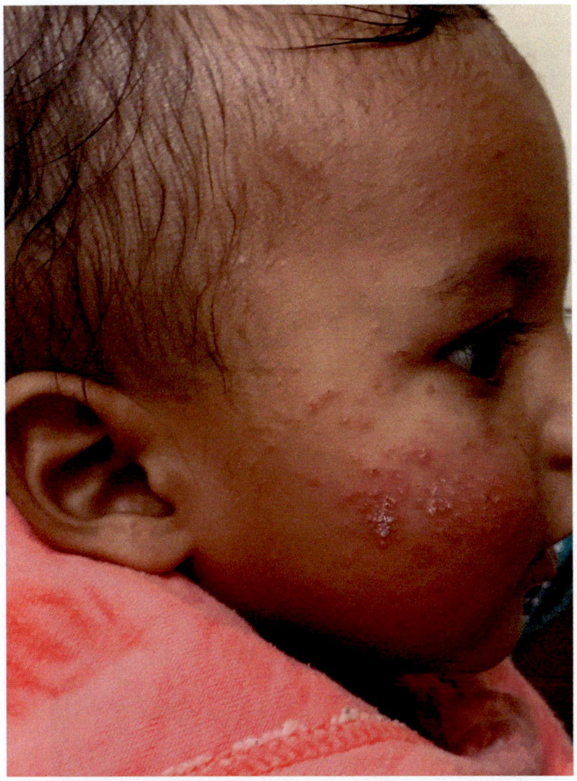

Figure 6.4 Erythematous scaly papules on the face in atopic dermatitis.

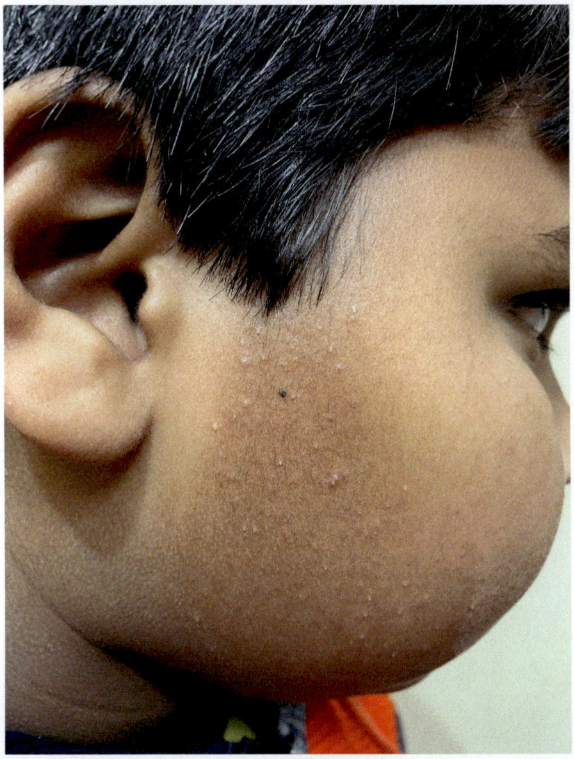

Figure 6.5 Erythromelanosis follicularis faciei presenting as multiple tiny follicular papules over a background of well-defined erythema and hyperpigmentation present over the right cheek.

dermatitis. Patients often complain of exacerbation of a burning or stinging sensation when topical agents are applied.

- **Papulopustular rosacea** – This stage is characterized by persistent erythema (> 3 months), and erythematous papules and pustules in the central area of face are associated with burning and stinging (**Figure 6.6**).
- **Phymatous rosacea** – This is an end stage of the disease, seen in patients with long-standing disease, and is clinically characterized by thickened skin with irregular nodular surface. The condition usually affects the nose (rhinophyma), chin (gnathophyma), forehead (metophyma), cheeks, and ears. One particular patient may or may not develop phymatous changes of all sites.
- **Ocular rosacea** – Ocular rosacea may precede or may develop concurrently with skin lesions. Patients with ocular rosacea complain of eye stinging or burning, dryness, irritation with light, or foreign body sensations. Ocular findings include blepharitis, conjunctivitis, inflammation

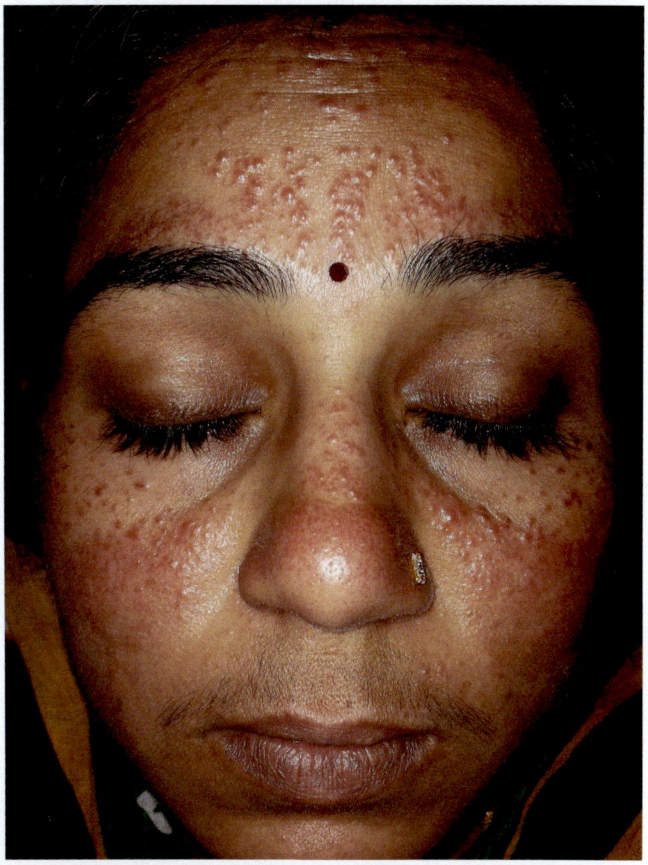

Figure 6.6 Persistent erythema with erythematous papules and pustules over the bilateral cheek, nose, and forehead. (Courtesy: Dr. Hiral Shah, Baroda Medical College, Vadodara, India.)

of the lids and meibomian glands, interpalpebral conjunctival hyperemia, and conjunctival telangiectasias.
- DD: Acne vulgaris.

## Facial angiofibroma

- Cutaneous angiofibroma refers to a group of clinically different lesions with the same histologic findings – proliferation of stellate and spindled cells, thin-walled blood vessels, and concentric collagen bundles. The clinical presentations include facial angiofibromas, fibrous papule of nose, pearly penile papules, and Koenen tumors.
- Facial angiofibromas, previously known as adenoma sebaceum (a misnomer), are cutaneous hallmarks of tuberous sclerosis complex (TSC). Multiple facial angiofibromas are also seen in multiple endocrine neoplasia type 1 (MEN-1) and Birt-Hogg-Dubé syndrome.
- Facial angiofibromas appear in childhood, increase in number and size until adolescence, and then become stable.
- Clinically, it manifests as multiple symmetrical, reddish-brown, dome-shaped papules with smooth surface occurring over the central face, which often concentrates around alar grooves, nose, cheeks, nasal opening, and chin with relative sparing of upper lip and lateral face (**Figure 6.7a,b**). The lesions may coalesce to form plaques (**Figure 6.7c**).
- A few cases of unilateral, nevoid facial angiofibroma have also been reported (**Figure 6.7d**).[5]

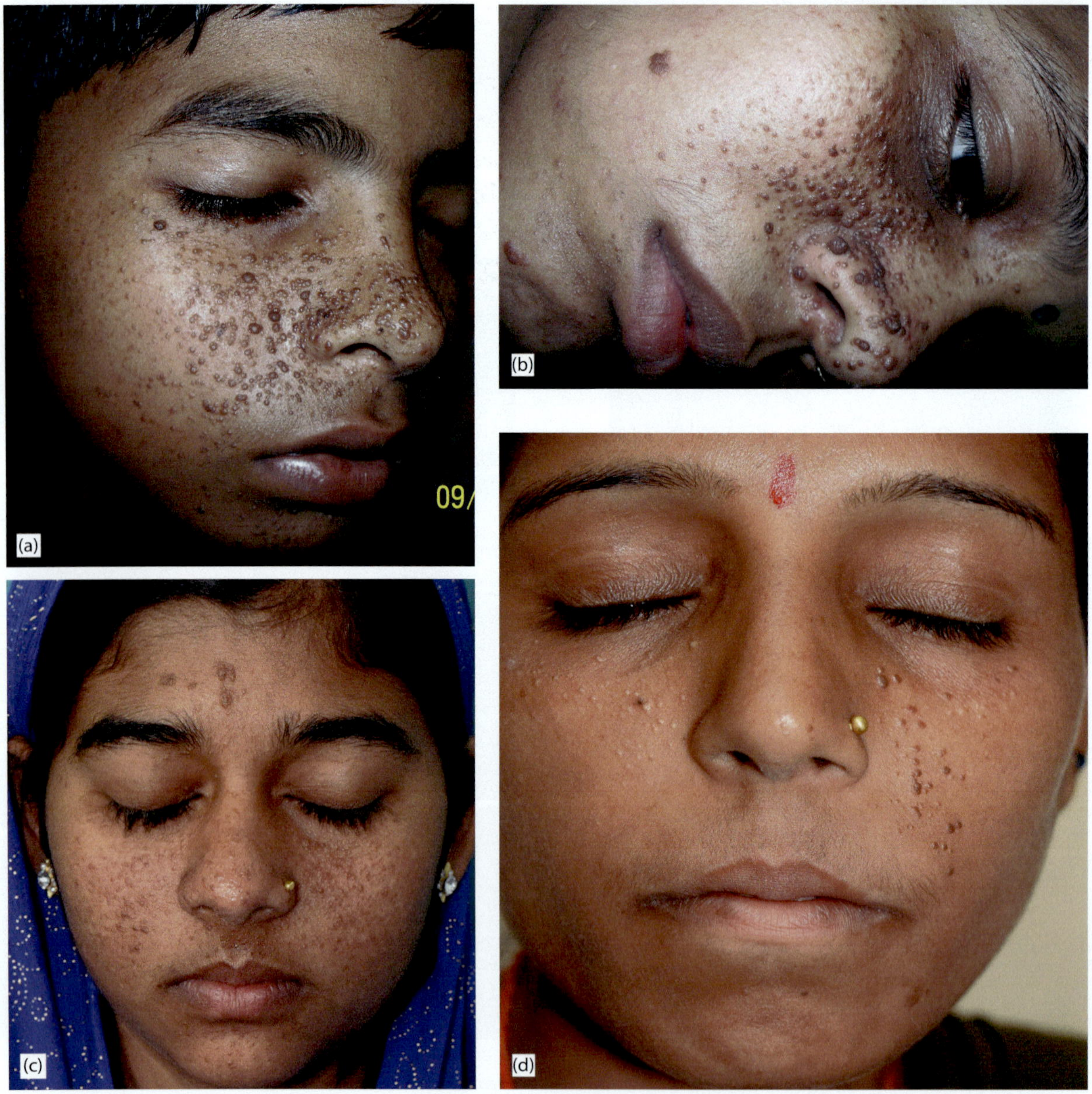


Figure 6.7 **(a)** Facial angiofibroma seen as multiple dome-shaped, red-brown papules on the cheeks and nose. **(b)** Numerous facial angiofibromas in a young lady. **(c)** Plaques of facial angiofibroma on the forehead. **(d)** Unilateral facial angiofibroma.

- DD: Verruca plana (pseudo koebnerization, randomly distributed), rosacea, acne vulgaris.

## Demodicosis[6]

- Demodicosis is a cutaneous infestation caused by *Demodex folliculorum* and *Demodex brevis* (collectively known as Demodex), a saprophytic mite that is a commensal organism of pilosebaceous units. *D. folliculorum* infestation is more common and is usually localized to the face, while *D. brevis* is found on the neck and chest.
- It can occur as a primary disease or may develop secondary to immunosuppression or topical glucocorticoids/calcineurin inhibitors use.
- Primary demodicosis presents in middle-aged to elderly populations and has facial involvement, typically affecting periorificial areas. On the other hand, secondary demodicosis has an early onset and is characterized by more diffuse facial distribution or truncal involvement.
- Primary demodicosis may have one of these presentations:
  - Pityriasis folliculorum-like (spinulate demodicosis) – Patients develop discrete fine, whitish or yellowish, spiky changes involving sebaceous hair follicles (**Figure 6.8a**). It may have associated faint erythema and little inflammation.
  - Rosacea-like (rosaceiform; papulopustular demodicosis) – Patients have papulopustular lesions in perioral, periorbital, and periauricular regions (**Figure 6.8b**).
  - Demodicosis gravis (nodulocystic demodicosis) – Patients develop nodular lesions, pus formation, and/or abscess-like lesions.
- DD: Acne vulgaris (comedones, not periorificial localization), seborrheic dermatitis (yellow greasy scales), rosacea (photosensitivity, telangiectasia).

## Lupus miliaris disseminatus faciei (LMDF) (Facial idiopathic granulomas with regressive evolution [FIGURE])

- LMDF is an uncommon, benign, granulomatous, inflammatory skin disease of unknown etiology affecting mainly the central area of face showing a characteristic tendency to involve the eyelids.
- The exact prevalence is not known, but the disease may be more common in Asians.
- Both the sexes can be affected with LMDF; however, young males in their twenties are predominantly affected.
- The skin lesions are multiple, monomorphic, smooth, discrete, reddish-brown or brown to yellowish dome-shaped translucent papules, nodules, and tiny pustules which are symmetrically distributed in the central area of the face (lower area of forehead, lower portions of eyelid, nasolabial folds, cheeks, and the

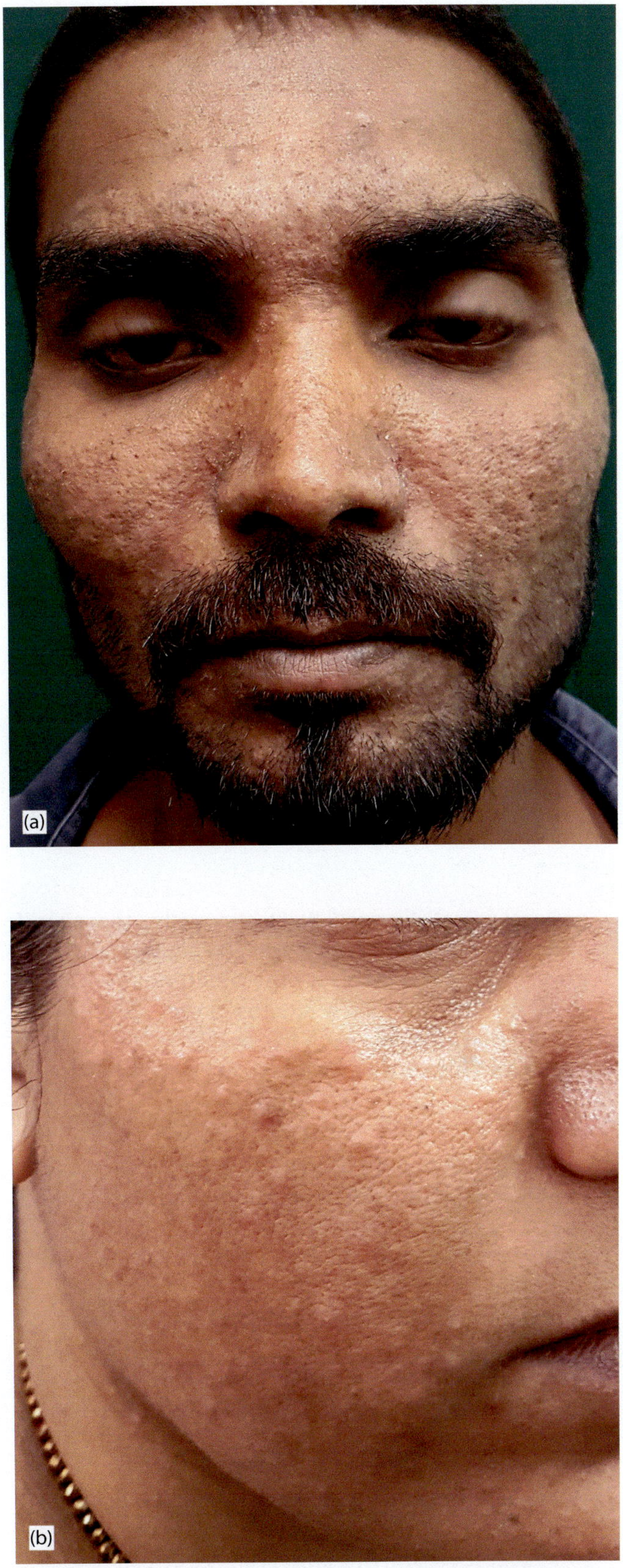


Figure 6.8 **(a)** Demodicosis presenting as erythema and whitish projections from the follicles. **(b)** Multiple erythematous papules present over the cheek and forehead in demodicosis. (a,b – Courtesy: Dr. Shekhar Neema, Armed Forces Medical College Pune, India.)

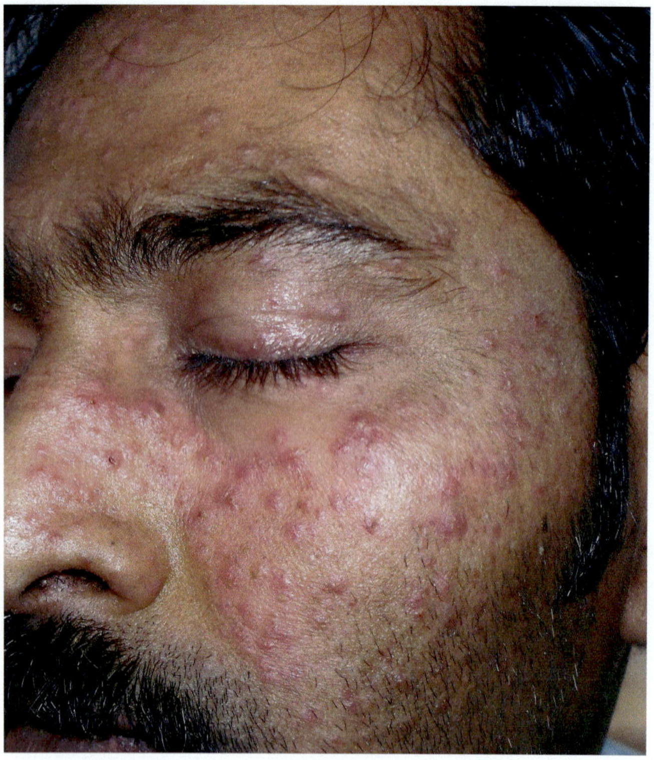

Figure 6.9 Lupus miliaris disseminatus faciei seen as multiple, monomorphic, discrete, reddish dome-shaped translucent papules on the face. Note involvement of lower eyelids.

perioral areas) (**Figure 6.9**). Occasionally other sites, such as axillae, chest, neck, arms, hand, legs, and groin, can also be involved. The condition resolves spontaneously over a few months to years, leaving behind characteristic pock-like scars.

- DD: Acne vulgari, rosacea, secondary syphilis.

## Trichoepithelioma

- Trichoepithelioma is a benign hamartomatous tumor of pilosebaceous follicle usually occurring in childhood or early adolescence as solitary or multiple types. Multiple trichoepithelioma is usually transmitted as an autosomal dominant trait.
- Females are more commonly affected than males.
- The lesion mainly occurs on the central face – nasolabial folds, nose, upper lip, forehead, and eyelids. It may occasionally involve the scalp, neck, and upper trunk.
- The lesions present as skin-colored to pink, firm, rounded, shiny, translucent, well-demarcated papulonodular lesions with slightly depressed center (**Figure 6.10a,b**). Rarely, multiple lesions may coalesce to form large lesions, giving an appearance of leonine facies.
- Rarely, dermatomal distribution may be noted.
- Syndromes associated are Brooke-Spiegler syndrome, Rombo syndrome, and Bazex syndrome.
- DD: BCC (usually solitary, hyperpigmented lesion, mainly confined to sun-exposed area), closed comedones, steatocystoma multiplex.

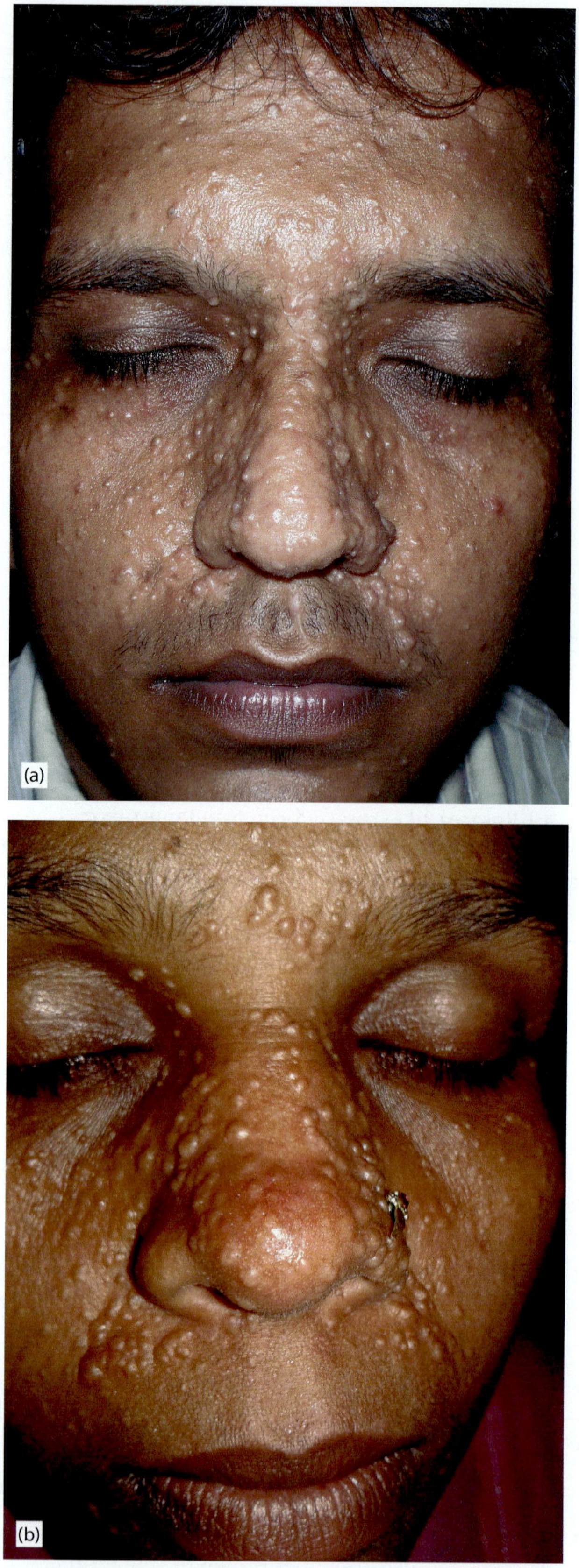


Figure 6.10 **(a)** Trichoepithelioma seen as multiple skin-colored, round, shiny, translucent papules with a slightly depressed center over the central face. **(b)** Grouped yellowish papulonodular lesions of trichoepithelioma on central face. (b – Courtesy: Dr. PC Das, Katihar, India.)

## Cylindroma

- Cylindroma is a benign skin-appendageal tumor, originating from the sweat glands. It can be solitary (sporadic) or multiple (autosomal dominant inheritance).
- Solitary cylindroma is usually seen in middle-aged and elderly individuals; inherited cylindroma has its onset in childhood. The tumor is more prevalent among females.
- The lesions are mostly seen on head and neck region.
- The patient presents with asymptomatic, solitary or multiple, firm, rubbery, smooth, pink to red hairless papules, nodules, and/or tumors. Multiple lesions over scalp can cover the entire scalp giving an appearance of disfiguring turban, hence named "turban tumor."
- Rarely, there may be a malignant transformation to cylindrocarcinoma.
- Brooke-Spiegler syndrome is an autosomal dominant syndrome with multiple skin-adnexal neoplasms, including cylindroma, trichoepitheliomas, and rarely spiradenomas (**Figure 6.11**).

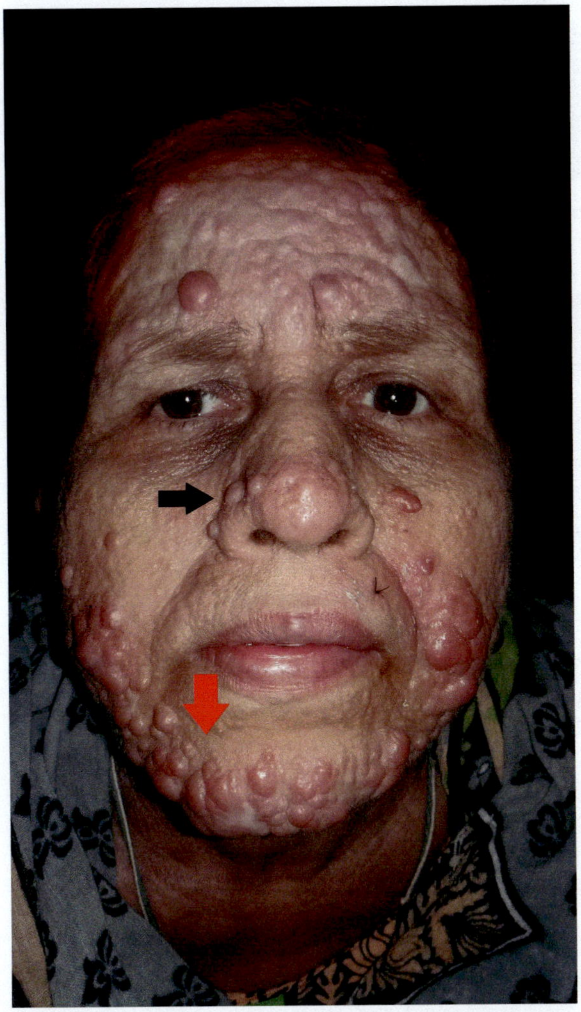

Figure 6.11 A lady with Brooke-Spiegler syndrome. Cylindromas are seen as erythematous papulonodular lesions (red arrow) on the lower face and forehead, and trichoepitheliomas are seen as flesh-colored papulonodular lesions (black arrow) on the central face, in perinasal area. (Courtesy: Dr. Hiral Shah, Baroda Medical College, Vadodara, India.)

- DD: Keloid, pleomorphic adenoma, trichilemmal cyst (pilar cyst), trichoepithelioma.

## Darier disease (Keratosis follicularis, Darier-White disease)

- Darier disease is a rare autosomal dominant genodermatosis that occurs as a result of mutation in the ATP2A2 gene.
- The onset of disease is usually in childhood or adolescence, with no sexual predilection.
- There is a history of disease aggravation by heat, sweat, humidity, sunlight, UVB exposure, mechanical trauma, and pregnancy.
- Clinically, the lesions are symmetrically distributed hyperkeratotic, greasy papules that coalesce to form irregular warty plaque or papillomatous masses mainly involving the seborrheic areas and intertriginous areas (**Figure 6.12a,b**). The lesions may become malodorous, with painful fissures.
- Zosteriform, or linear vesiculobullous, isolated acral hemorrhagic, acrokeratosis verruciformis of Hopf, comedonal and hypopigmented/leukodermic macules are its rare morphological variants.
- Pitting or punctate keratosis may be seen on palms and soles.
- The oral lesions are seen in 50% of cases as asymptomatic, multiple white or red firm papules that may coalesce, giving an appearance of "cobblestones," and affect primarily the alveolar and buccal mucosa.
- Associated nail findings include nail fragility, red and white longitudinal bands, and V-shaped notches at the free margins of the nails.
- Neuropsychiatric abnormalities include mild mental retardation and epilepsy.
- DD: Seborrheic dermatitis, acne vulgaris, confluent and reticulated papillomatosis.

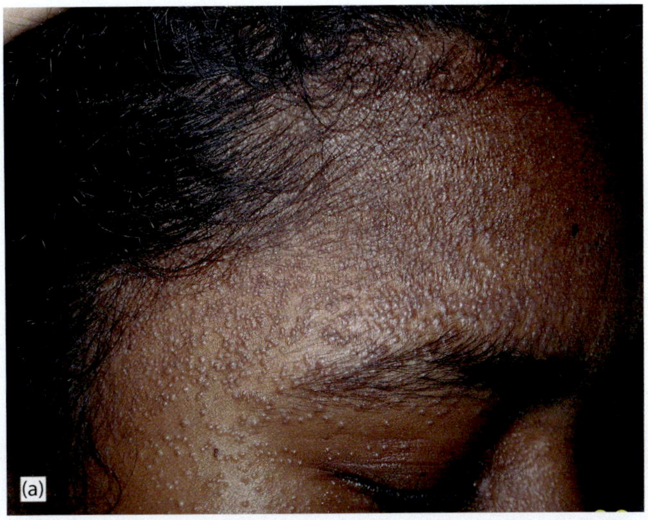


Figure 6.12 **(a)** Dirty-looking, hyperkeratotic papules on the face in Darier disease. (*Continued*)

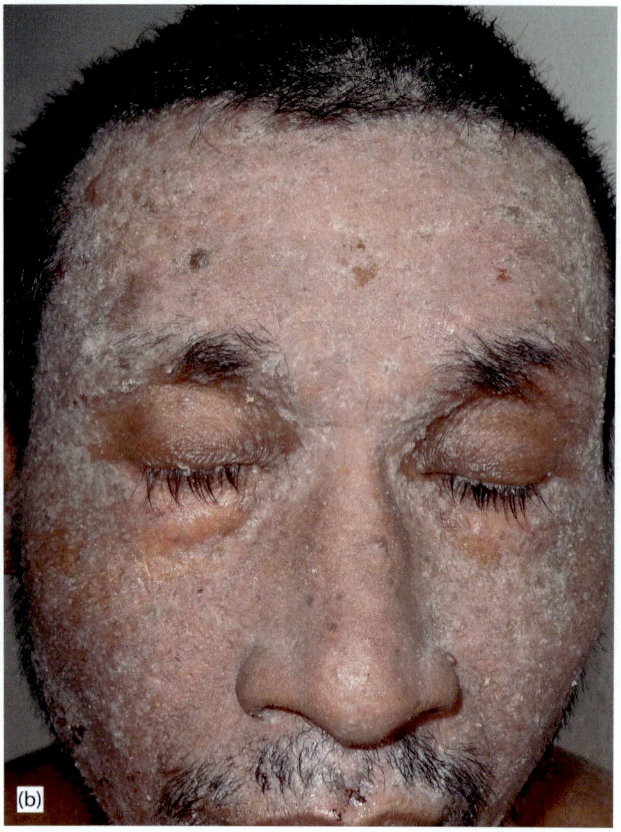


Figure 6.12 (*Continued*) **(b)** Lesions tend to get confluent to form plaques in summer. Also, the surface may get macerated.

## Sebaceous hyperplasia

- Sebaceous gland hyperplasia (SH) is a benign hamartomatous condition characterized by presence of ≥4 sebaceous lobules attached to the infundibulum of each pilosebaceous unit.
- It starts appearing by middle age and increases in number with age. Familial cases may have an earlier onset and widespread lesions.
- Most commonly, it affects the face (forehead, cheeks, and nose), but occasionally it may involve chest, areola, mouth, scrotum, foreskin, shaft of penis, and vulva. The lesion consists of single or multiple, asymptomatic, small, yellowish papules with a central dell (**Figure 6.13a,b**). Surface may show telangiectasia.
- Variants include giant form, linear or zosteriform arrangement, diffuse form, familial form.
- **Juxtaclavicular beaded lines** are another unique clinical presentation of SH and present as closely placed, tiny, papules arranged in parallel rows on the neck, around the clavicle.
- DD: Epidermoid cyst, vellus hair cyst, steatocystoma multiplex, basal cell carcinoma.

## Periorificial dermatitis (perioral dermatitis)

- Perioral dermatitis ("air hostess" dermatitis) is a chronic eczematous facial dermatitis of an unknown etiology,

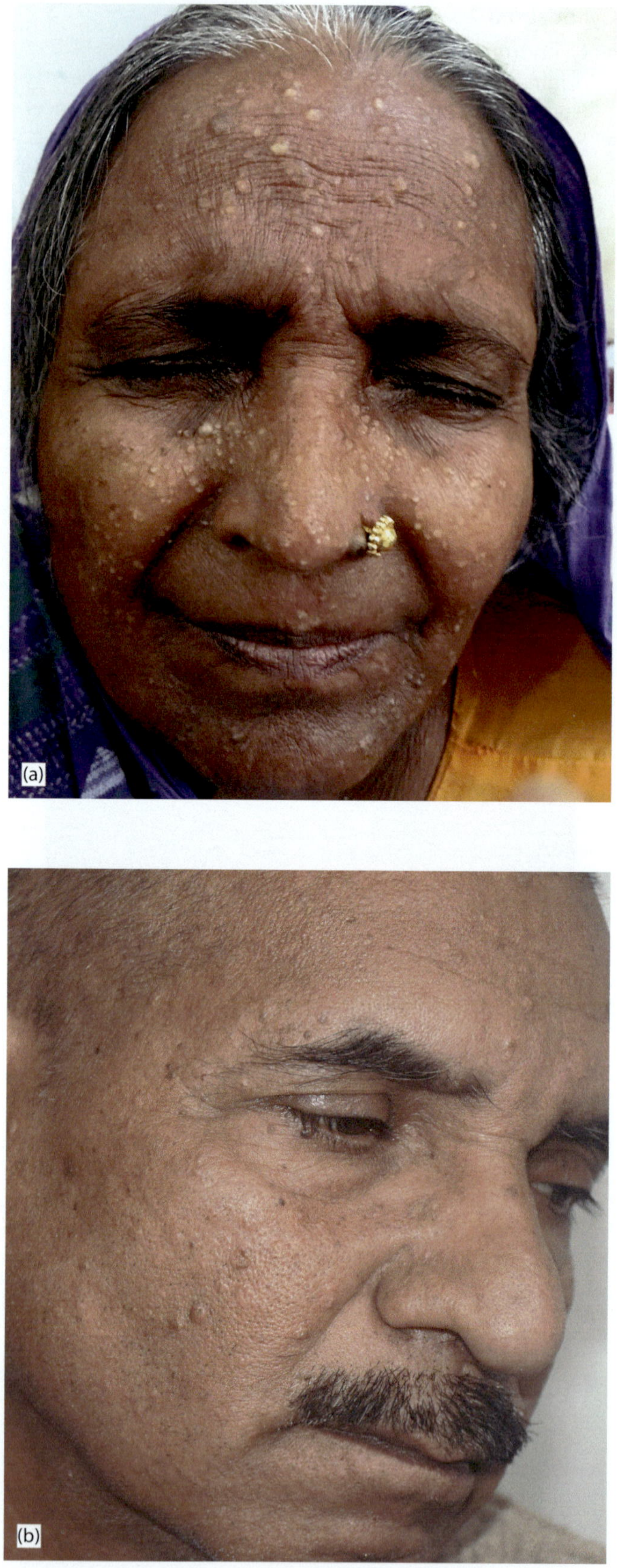


Figure 6.13 **(a)** Multiple small, yellow papules on the face in an elderly lady with sebaceous hyperplasia. **(b)** Multiple small, skin-colored papules of sebaceous hyperplasia on the face.

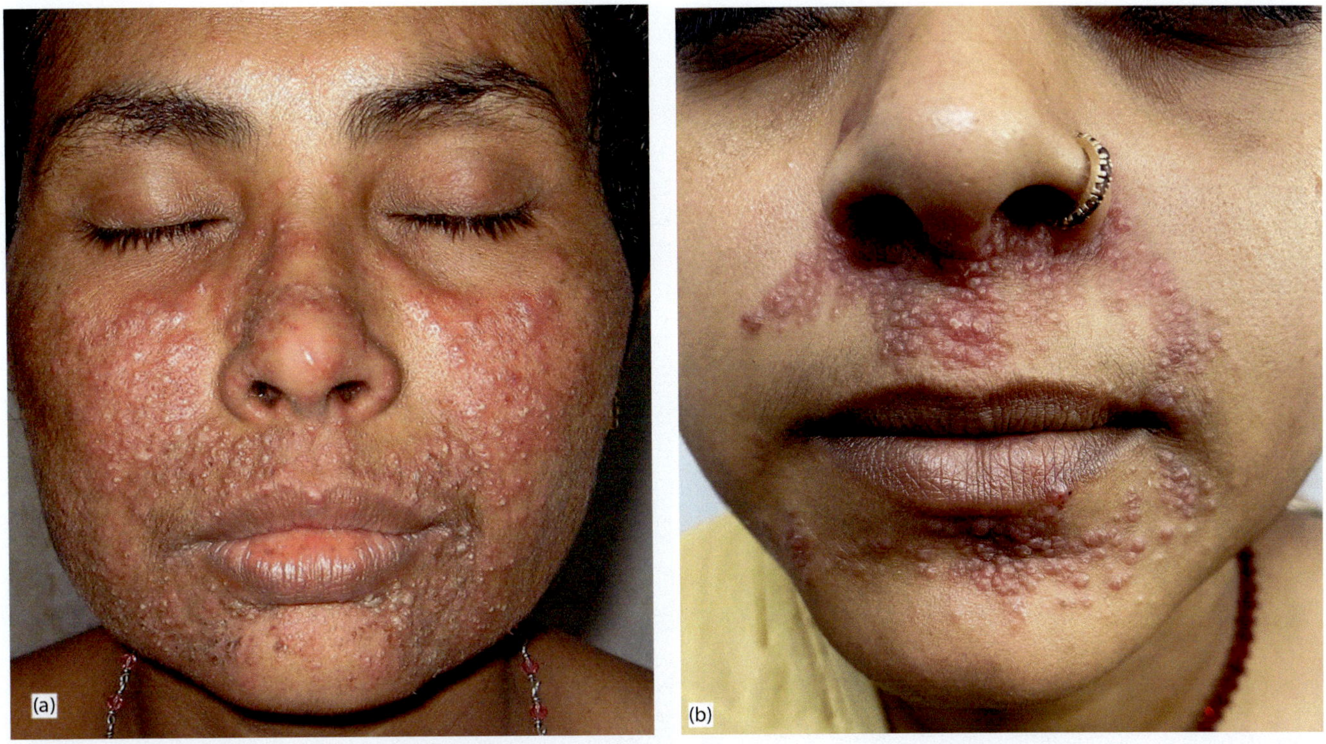


Figure 6.14 **(a)** Papulopustules of periorificial dermatitis on an erythematous base over the perioral area, nose, bilateral cheek, and chin, with sparing of vermilion border of lips. **(b)** Periorifical dermatitis presenting as closely set erythematous papules around the lips. (b – Courtesy: Dr Esther Nimisha, Jamshedpur, India.)

typically affecting the skin around the eyes, the nostrils, and the mouth. The disease runs a chronic course.

- It is common in children and in women aged 20–45 years.
- Prior history of use of topical application or inhalation of corticosteroids, fluorinated toothpaste, paraffin-based skin care ointments and cosmetics, physical sunscreens, and sunlight exposure may be observed.
- The characteristic lesions are monomorphic, dome-shaped, skin-colored to yellowish-brown papules, papulovesicles, and papulopustules on an erythematous base with or without scales affecting the perioral area, periorbital area, nasolabial folds, and chin. When the perioral area is involved, classical sparing of vermilion border of lips is noted (**Figure 6.14a,b**). The condition is associated with a burning or stinging sensation and rarely pruritus. Patients may develop unilateral lesions too.
- Extra-facial sites, such as neck, trunk, extremities, and genital areas, have also been reported.
- It usually heals without scarring, though in some cases atrophic pits and scarring are noted.
- **Childhood granulomatous periorificial dermatitis (CGPD)/facial Afro-Caribbean childhood eruption (FACE)** is the granulomatous variant that presents with flesh-colored to erythematous to yellow-brown papules and plaques in the same distribution. It typically affects prepubertal children and is more common in males and possibly in colored skin. It differs from periorificial dermatitis by absence of pustules and absence of erythema and scaling. CGPD may persist for months and then resolve spontaneously without any sequelae.
- DD: Rosacea, seborrheic dermatitis, atopic dermatitis, steroid induced rosacea (periorificial dermatitis spares cheeks, and forehead).

## Syringoma

- Syringoma is a benign adnexal tumor originating from intraepidermal eccrine duct.
- The disease usually occurs during puberty or during third and fourth decade of life, with female preponderance.
- There may be a history of summer aggravation.
- Lesions typically involve the periorbital area. Other commonly involved sites are axillae, chest, abdomen, penis, and vulva.
- The lesions are characteristically seen as multiple, small, ill-defined to well-defined, angulated, smooth-surfaced, skin-colored, yellowish, or brownish papules (**Figure 6.15a,b**). The surface may be flat or rounded. The lesions are usually bilaterally symmetrical.
- The eruptions are usually asymptomatic, although pruritus has been reported in some cases.
- Four major clinical variants are
    - Localized
    - Generalized
    - Down syndrome associated
    - Familial form

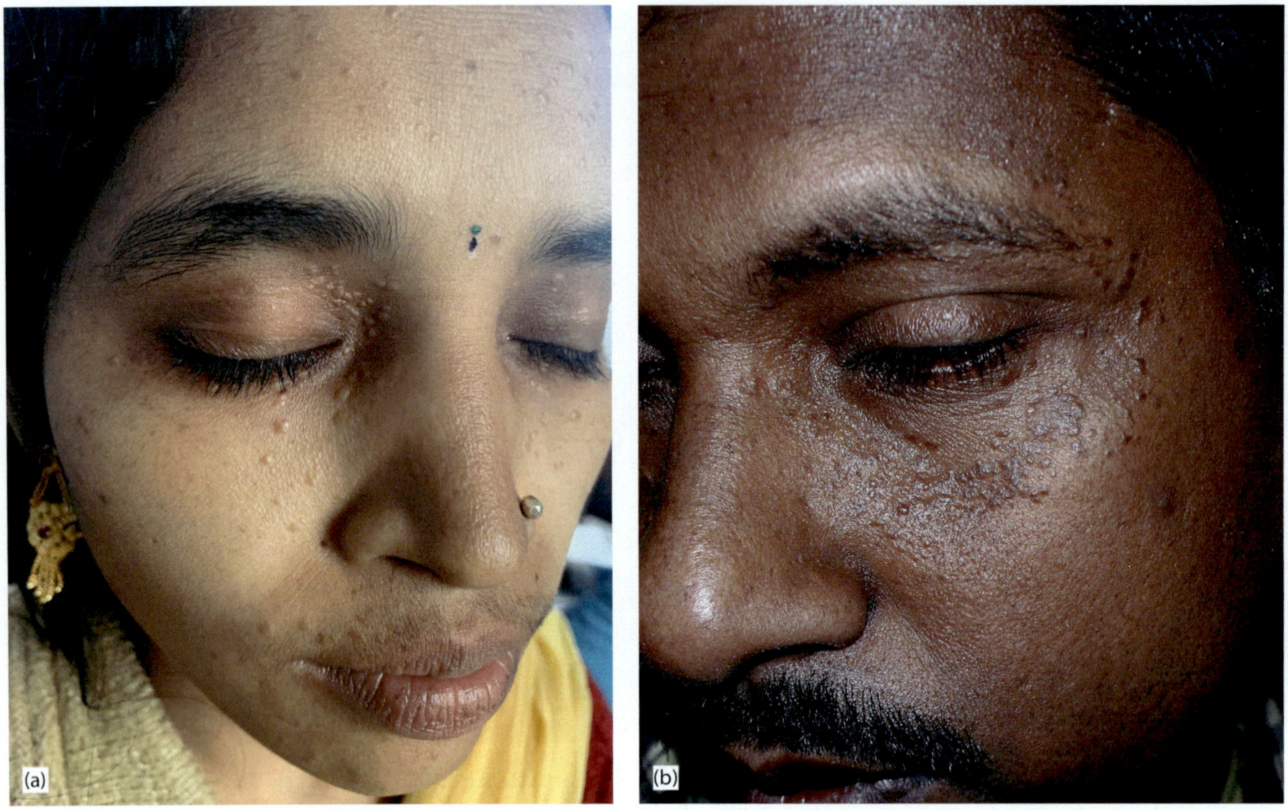

Figure 6.15 **(a)** Syringoma seen as multiple aggregated, small, brownish papules present over the periorbital areas. **(b)** Pigmented lesions of syringoma in periorbital area. (a – Courtesy: Dr. Rashid Shahid, Katihar Medical College, Katihar.)

- Morphologically, uncommon variants include lichen planus-like, milium-like, and plaque-like syringoma.
- Associated diseases include
  - Down syndrome
  - Diabetes mellitus
  - Ehlers-Danlos syndrome
  - Marfan syndrome
  - Hyperthyroidism.
  - Nicolau-Balus syndrome – syringoma in association with milia and atrophoderma vermiculata
  - Brooke-Spiegler syndrome
- DD: Verruca plana (pseudo Koebnerization can be seen), eruptive xanthoma (yellowish lesions), lichen planus (pruritic, violaceous lesions, often showing Koebnerization).

## Milia

- Milia (singular: milium) are small, benign, keratin-filled cysts and may be primary with spontaneous onset or secondary appearing after trauma, some inflammatory skin diseases, or use of certain topical or systemic drugs. Primary milia are believed to originate from obstruction of vellus hair (lower infundibulum), while secondary milia are derived from eccrine sweat ducts mostly.
- Milia are seen in all age groups; even congenital milia are known.
- The lesions are clinically seen as asymptomatic, single or multiple, randomly arranged, discrete, pearly white, dome-shaped papules measuring 1–2 mm in diameter (**Figure 6.16a**).
- Congenital milia are common on face (especially nose) and scalp and show spontaneous resolution within a couple of weeks (**Figure 6.16b**).
- Primary milia of children and adults favor cheeks and eyelids, and tend to persist.
- Secondary milia arise as a cutaneous reaction to traumatic stimuli and are localized to the involved body site.
- Milia en plaque is a rare variant of primary milia, characterized by numerous tiny milia within an erythematous base, arising spontaneously on a healthy skin. It commonly affects the head and neck region, especially periauricular and periorbital areas and on the nasal bridge.
- Multiple eruptive milia refer to the appearance of numerous milia over weeks to months. The lesions affect head and neck, upper trunk, and upper extremities.
- Genodermatoses associated with extensive milia include Bazex-Dupre-Christol syndrome, Rombo syndrome, Brooke-Spiegler syndrome, pachyonychia congenita type II and basal cell nevus syndrome.
- Drugs precipitating development of milia include topical corticosteroid, fluorouracil, penicillamine, cyclosporine, dovitinib, sorafenib, benoxaprofen, and acitretin.

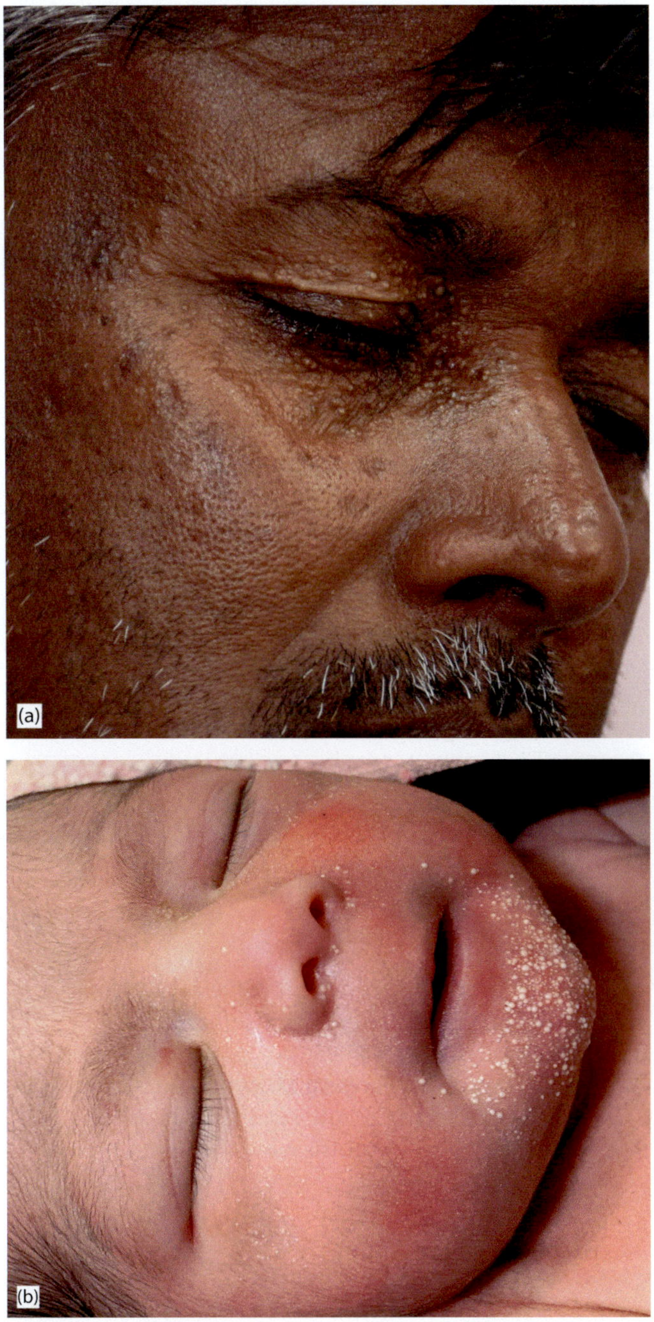

Figure 6.16 **(a)** Milia seen as multiple, discrete, pearly white, dome-shaped papules present over periocular areas. **(b)** Numerous pearly white papules of congenital milia on the face more prominent over the chin.

- DD: Molluscum contagiosum (central umbilication), vellous hair cyst (flesh-colored papule), miliary calcinosis cutis.

## Dermatosis papulosa nigra (DPN)

- DPN, a clinical variant of seborrheic keratosis (SK), is a benign epidermal growth, common in Asians and Africans.
- In contrast to SK, DPN has its onset in adolescence and the number of lesions peaks in sixth decade.
- Women are more frequently affected. There is often a family history of DPN.
- DPN presents as multiple, asymptomatic, small (1–5 mm), dome-shaped, smooth-surfaced, black papules over sun-exposed areas, including the face. Lesions on the face are symmetrically distributed over malar areas, temples, and forehead (**Figure 6.17a,b**). The size

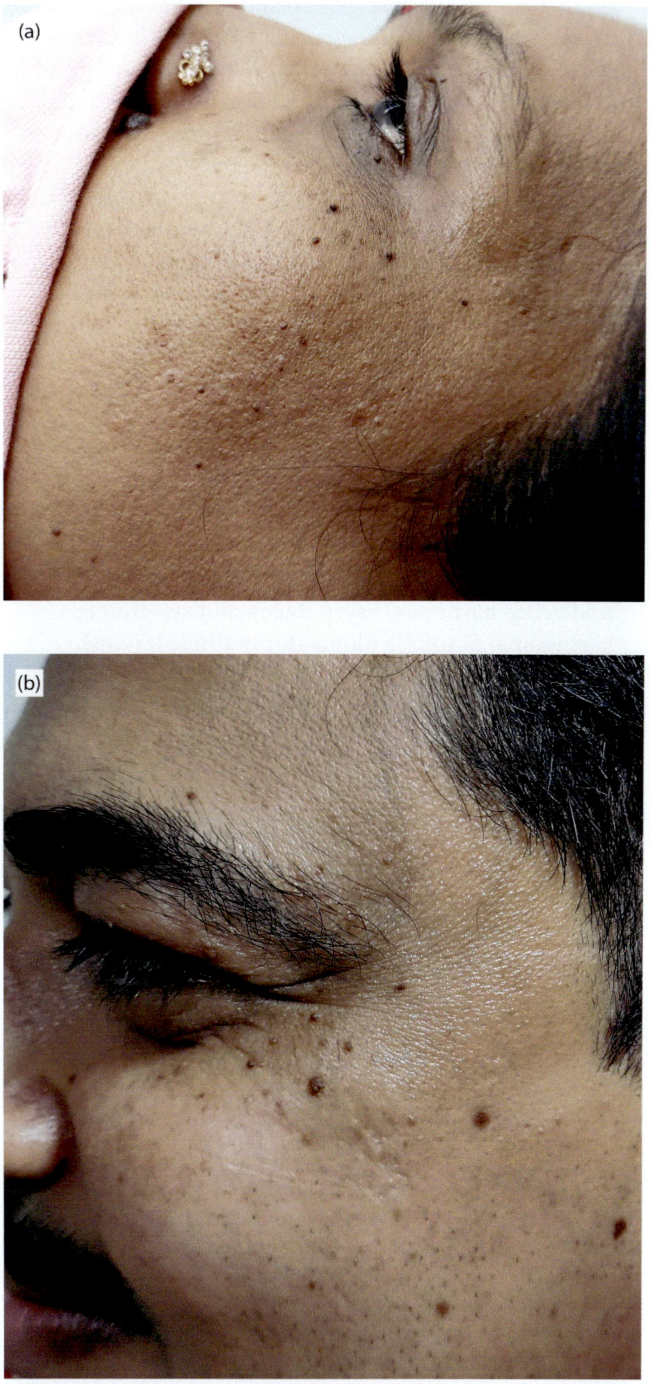

Figure 6.17 **(a)** Dermatosis papulosa nigra seen as multiple dome-shaped, hyperpigmented papules randomly distributed over the face. **(b)** Dermatosis papulosa nigra as pigmented dome-shaped papules. Patient has junctional and compound melanocytic nevi too.

and number of papules usually increase over time. The lesions do not resolve spontaneously.
- DD: Verruca plana, syringoma, angiofibroma.

## Hidrocystoma

- Hidrocystoma are benign cystic dilatations of the glandular or ductal part of sweat glands and are classified into two types depending on the origin – apocrine (cystic proliferation of apocrine glands) and eccrine (cystic dilatation of intradermal sweat ducts) types. The eccrine type is further classified into two groups – the Smith and Chernosky type (solitary) and the Robinson type (multiple).
- Hidrocystomas are mostly seen in middle-aged to elderly persons.
- Hidrocystomas present as dome-shaped, translucent, smooth-surfaced lesions in the head and neck region (**Figure 6.18**). The clinical features of eccrine and apocrine hidrocystoma are summarized in **Table 6.3**.
- Eccrine hidrocystoma typically appears in the periorbital area, but does not affect eyelid margin. Apocrine hidrocystoma is mainly seen on the eyelid margin near the inner canthus rather than periorbital area.
- Multiple apocrine hidrocystomas have been described in Goltz-Gorlin syndrome and Schopf-Schultz-Passarge syndrome.
- DD: Intradermal nevus, epidermoid cyst, appendageal tumor, basal cell carcinoma (for solitary lesion) and vellus hair cysts, Favre-Racouchot syndrome, syringoma, fibrofolliculoma (for multiple lesions).

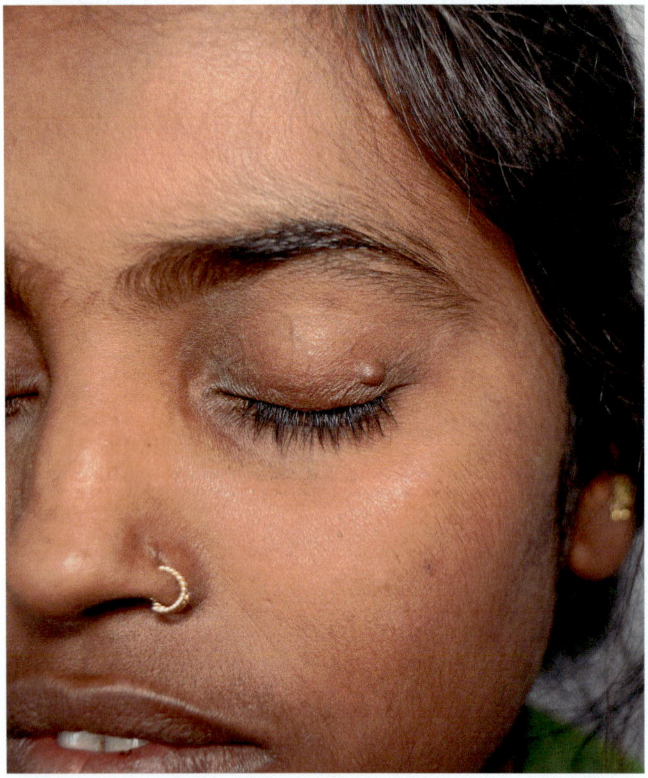

Figure 6.18 Single, skin-colored cyst of hidrocystoma present over the left upper eyelid.

Table 6.3 Apocrine and eccrine hidrocystoma

| Features | Apocrine hidrocystoma | Eccrine hidrocystoma |
|---|---|---|
| Number | Single (rarely, multiple) | Single (Smith and Chernosky type) or multiple (Robinson type) |
| Size | Large (3–15 mm) | Small (1–6 mm) |
| Color | Flesh-colored to brown and light-blue tint | Dark-blue tint to black |
| Typical site | Eyelid margin, inner canthus (cysts of Moll's glands) | Periorbital area |
| Other sites | Chest, shoulder, axilla, umbilicus, foreskin, penal shaft, vulva, and fingers | Ear, trunk, scalp, and upper limbs |
| Gender predilection | None | Females (specially Robinson type) |
| Summer aggravation | No | Yes<br>May disappear completely in cooler weather |

## Papular scar

- Scarring is one of the persistent sequelae of various inflammatory processes, and it assumes a different morphology.
- Papular scars on face present as asymptomatic multiple non-scaly, skin-colored, soft, small fibrous papules, distributed typically over the nasal skin and the chin (**Figure 6.19**).

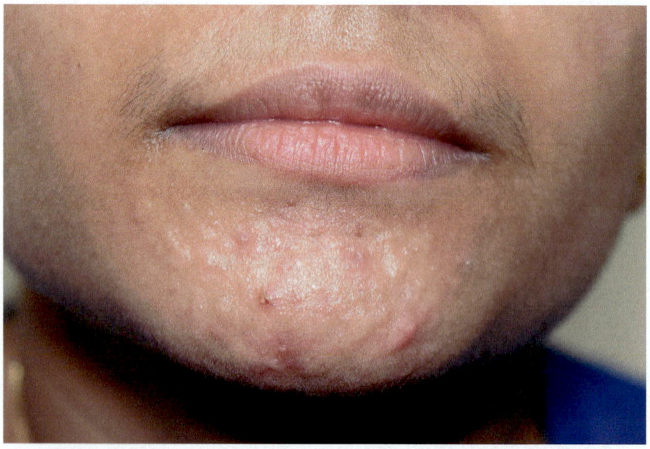

Figure 6.19 Multiple skin-colored papular scars interspersed with a few erythematous papules on the chin in gnathophyma.

- Papular scars usually follow acne vulgaris and rosacea.[7] Other types of scars may be associated.
- DD: Trichoepithelioma, open comedones.

## Follicular mucinosis (FM)

- Follicular mucinosis is characterized by mucinous degeneration of follicles on histopathology and clinically presents as follicular papules, alopecia of hairy areas, and/or erythematous infiltrated plaques.
- FM may present as a benign primary disorder or be associated with malignant lymphoproliferative processes such as cutaneous T- and B-cell lymphomas.
- Primary FM is seen in the younger population and shows spontaneous resolution. The most common presentation is a solitary (or a few) papule in the head and neck region.
- Acneiform FM has been described as a rare variant of primary FM that presents with erythematous-to-skin-colored papules on the face (**Figure 6.20**). The disease runs a chronic course, and the lesions may persist for months to years.[8]
    - DD: Perioral dermatitis (reddish papules, vesicles, and pustules on an erythematous base with a tendency to coalesce), granulomatous periorificial dermatitis (yellow-to-brown papular lesions over perioral, perinasal and periocular regions, common in children), sarcoidosis.
- Lymphoma-associated FM is typically seen in the older population and does not resolve spontaneously. Lesions are often multiple, spread over the trunk and extremities.

## Sarcoidosis

- Sarcoidosis is a multisystem granulomatous disease of an unknown etiology characterized by non-caseating epithelioid cell granuloma with few or no inflammatory cells ("naked granuloma"). It commonly affects the lungs, lymph nodes, liver, eyes, bones, and skin.
- The disease occurs more commonly in second to fourth decades of life, though it can be seen in any age group showing female predominance.
- Papular sarcoidosis is common on the face but may affect any site. It clinically presents as multiple scattered or confluent, indurated papules of various colors, including red, reddish-brown, violaceous, translucent, or hyperpigmented (**Figure 6.21**). Most lesions exhibit little or no surface changes.
- Lupus pernio – Patients present with chronic, indurated papules or plaques that affect the mid-face, particularly the alar rim of the nose and are more likely to have more severe systemic involvement.
- Associated erythema nodosum and alopecia may be seen.
- Diagnosed cutaneous sarcoidosis requires a work-up for systemic involvement, followed by periodic monitoring.
- DD: Leprosy, PKDL, LMDF.

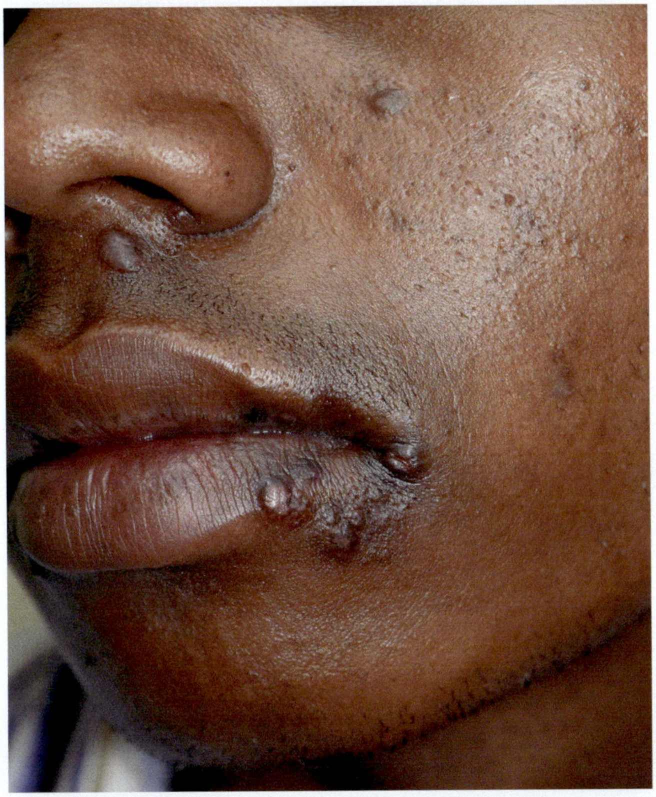

Figure 6.20 Acneiform follicular mucinosis.

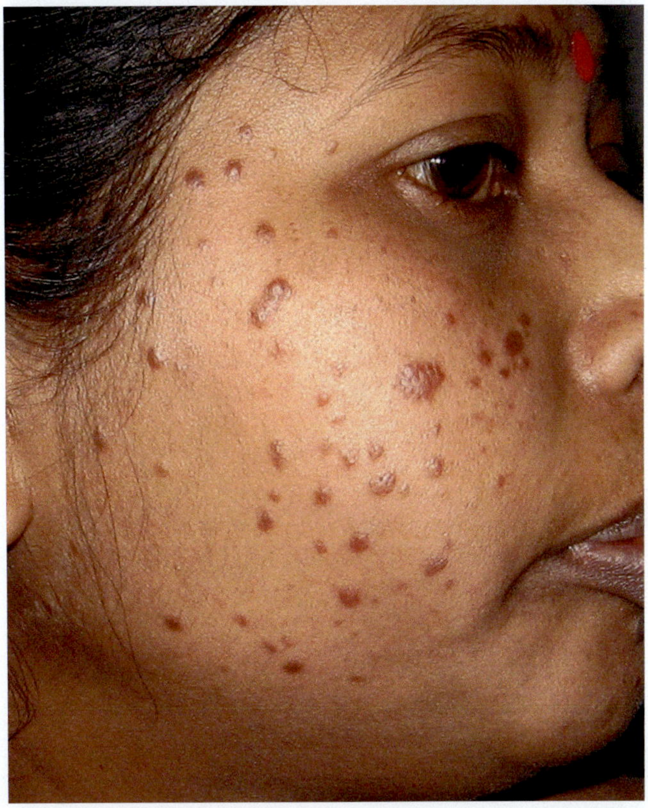

Figure 6.21 Red-brown papules and plaques of sarcoidosis on the face.

## Post-Kala azar dermal leishmaniasis (PKDL)

- PKDL presents as hypopigmented macules and erythematous, juicy papules, first appearing on the face, especially the muzzle area of the face. Over time, lesions coalesce with each other and grow in size to form papulonodular lesions (**Figure 6.22a,b**).

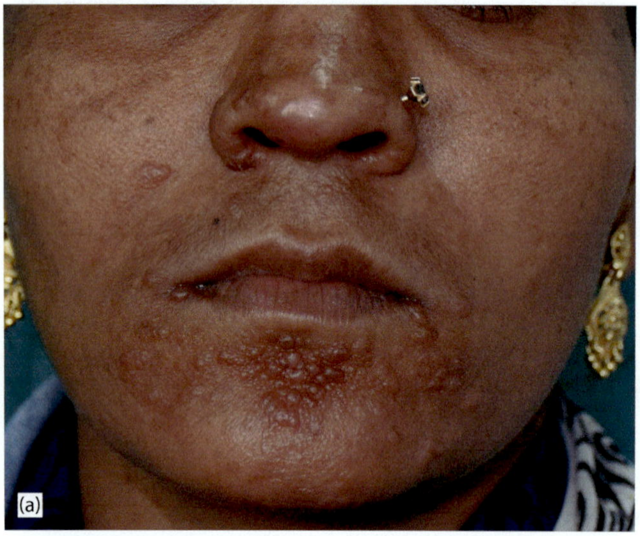


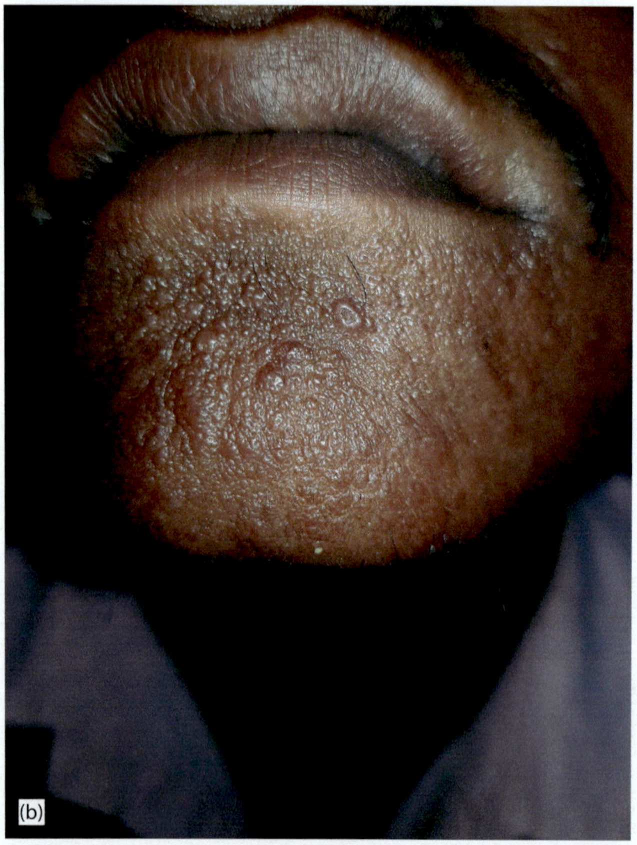


Figure 6.22 **(a)** Post-kala azar dermal leishmaniasis presenting as multiple confluent, shiny, erythematous papules present over the muzzle area of the face. **(b)** Post-kala azar dermal leishmaniasis presenting as multiple confluent, shiny, erythematous papules over the chin.

- Lesions progress to involve the trunk and upper extremities.
- DD: Lepromatous leprosy, sarcoidosis.

## Angiolymphoid hyperplasia with eosinophilia (ALHE)

- ALHE is a rare, benign, idiopathic skin tumor characterized by vascular proliferation and eosinophil invasion. The condition appears to be common in Asians and is uncommon in colored skin.
- The condition usually affects young to middle-aged adults, with a slight female predominance.
- The classical site of affection is the preauricular region. The lesion is mostly seen in the head and neck region (forehead or scalp) but may affect hands, shoulders, breasts, penis, oral mucosa, and the scrotum too.
- It presents with solitary or multiple, flesh-colored to erythematous or hyperpigmented, dome-shaped, smooth-surfaced, grouped dermal papules or nodules clustered on a normal-appearing skin. The condition is usually asymptomatic but can be associated with pain or pruritus in a few cases. Uncommon symptoms include bleeding, pulsation, ulceration, and lymphadenopathy.
- DD: Kimura's disease (the lesions are broad subcutaneous masses and is more deep), eruptive lobular capillary hemangioma (pyogenic granuloma), bacillary angiomatosis.

## Chloracne (metabolizing acquired dioxin-induced skin hamartomas/MADISH)

- Chloracne is a systemic toxic disease caused by exposure to halogenated aromatic hydrocarbons either by inhalation, ingestion, or direct contact, affecting the skin and internal organs such as eyes, central nervous system, and liver.
- Chloracnegens include polychlorinated naphthalenes, polychlorinated biphenyls, polychlorinated phenols, etc., and are commonly found in fungicides, insecticides, herbicides, and wood preservatives.
- The lesions usually affect the cheeks, retroauricular areas, axillae, and groin.
- The disease starts clinically as erythema and edema of the affected area followed by formation of fine comedones involving almost every follicle giving a slate-gray pigmentation. Soon, lesions progress to open and closed comedones, nodules, and cysts. Lesions heal with scarring (**Figure 6.23a,b**).
- Additional findings include hyperpigmentation of nails, hypertrichosis, hyperhidrosis, and porphyria cutanea tarda.
- Systemic features are anemia, fatigue, anorexia, arthritis, peripheral neuropathy, impotence, hyperlipidemia, and ophthalmopathy.
- DD: Steroid acne, acne vulgaris.

## Trichostasis spinulosa

- TS results from hyperkeratosis of the infundibulum and subsequent retention of numerous vellus hairs surrounded by a keratinous sheath, in a dilated follicle.

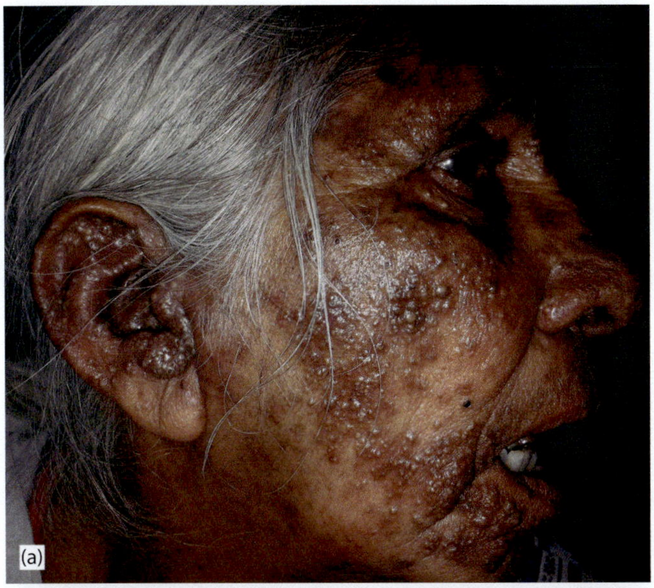

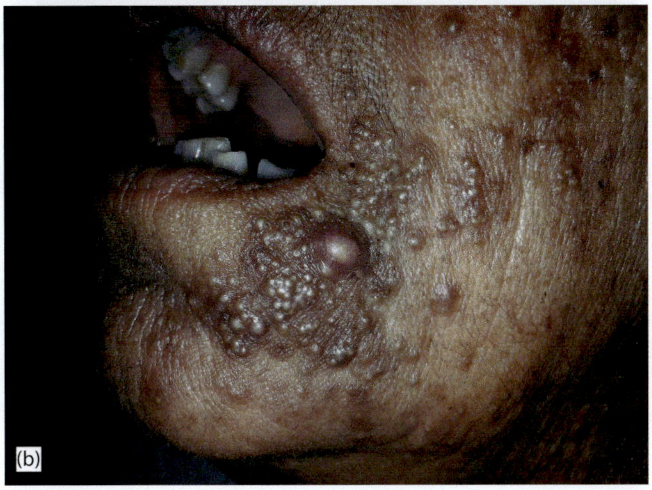

Figure 6.23 **(a)** Chloracne presenting as numerous closed and a few open comedones, erythematous nodules with slate-gray pigmentation present over the face and ear. **(b)** Chloracne with erythematous nodules. (a,b – Courtesy: Dr. Hiral Shah, Baroda Medical College, Vadodara, India.)

- Elderly males are mostly affected, and the nose and interscapular areas are most commonly affected sites.
- The patients present with typical 1-mm or smaller, black follicular papules or plugs. The lesions may have protruding tufts of fine hairs, which may not be visible to naked eye and may require a hand lens or dermatoscope for visualization. These tufts of hairs can be easily removed without causing any discomfort to the patient (**Figure 6.24**).
- DD: Open comedones, keratosis pilaris.

## Sycosis barbae

- Sycosis barbae is a bacterial infection of the hair follicle of the beard area, usually caused by *Staphylococcus aureus*.
- The disease affects the men who shave irregularly. Those who shave daily or not at all rarely experience the disease.
- It occurs more commonly in males 20–40 years of age.

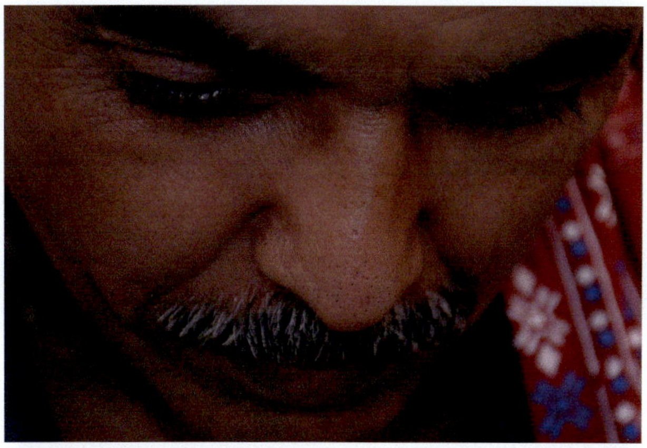

Figure 6.24 Multiple black papules on nose in trichostasis spinulosa.

- The clinical lesions are itchy or painful, erythematous, grouped, follicular papules and pustules appearing predominantly on the upper lip and below the angles of the mouth (**Figure 6.25a,b**). If left untreated, the lesions may progress to abscess formations and may leave scars on healing. Recurrence is common.
- DD: Tinea barbae, acne vulgaris.

## Tinea barbae

- Tinea barbae is dermatophytic infection of the beard and moustache areas of the face and generally affects only adult men.
- It clinically presents as follicular erythematous papules, nodules, pustules, and crusting around the hairs

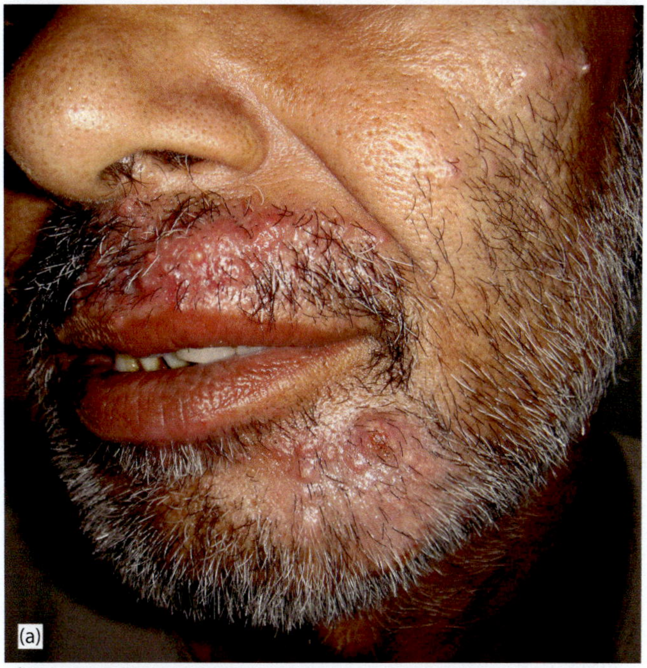

Figure 6.25 **(a)** Sycosis barbae seen as multiple grouped erythematous papules and pustules over an erythematous nodular base present over the upper lip and below angles of mouth. Note satellite pustules. *(Continued)*

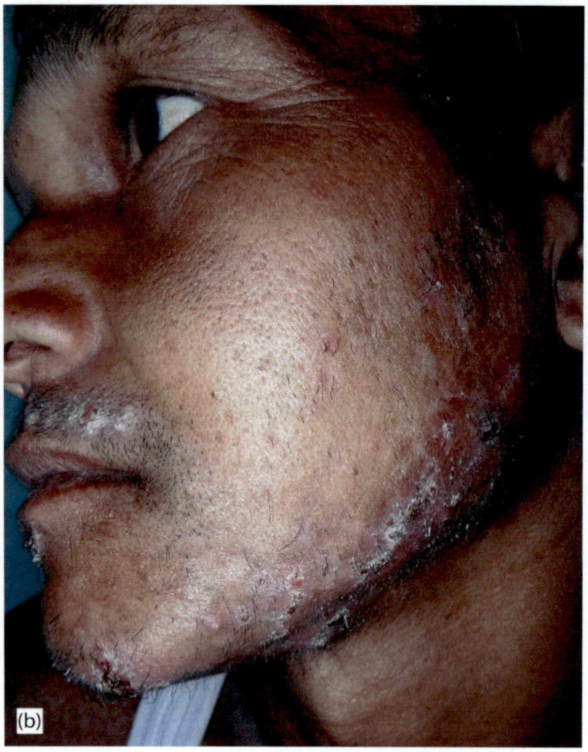

Figure 6.25 (*Continued*) **(b)** Severe cases may show involvement of other hair-bearing areas. Note scarring and alopecia from previous lesions.

(kerion). The hairs from the affected areas can be pulled out easily without any pain.

- Involvement of upper lip is rare.
- DD: Sycosis barbae.

## Pseudofolliculitis barbae (PFB) (shaving bumps)

- PFB is a foreign-body inflammatory reaction against the hair keratins that have entered the dermis through extrafollicular or transfollicular penetration.
- The condition is mostly seen in post pubertal males with thick curly hairs and in populations with dark-colored skin. Hirsute females too can develop pseudofolliculitis barbae after shaving. The sites common to both sexes include axillary and pubic areas.
- History of improper shaving techniques (e.g., against the grain) is common.
- The patients present with painful, flesh-colored or erythematous papules with a hair shaft in the center, and lesions usually appear after shaving. The hair shaft can be gently lifted up to free the free end of hair embedded in the dermis (**Figure 6.26**).
- The condition may progress to pustules and abscess formation. Long-standing cases develop post-inflammatory hyperpigmentation, scarring, and keloid formation.
- DD: Folliculitis.

## Traumatic anserine folliculosis

- Traumatic anserine folliculosis is thought to result from friction and trauma, and is more common in children and adolescents.

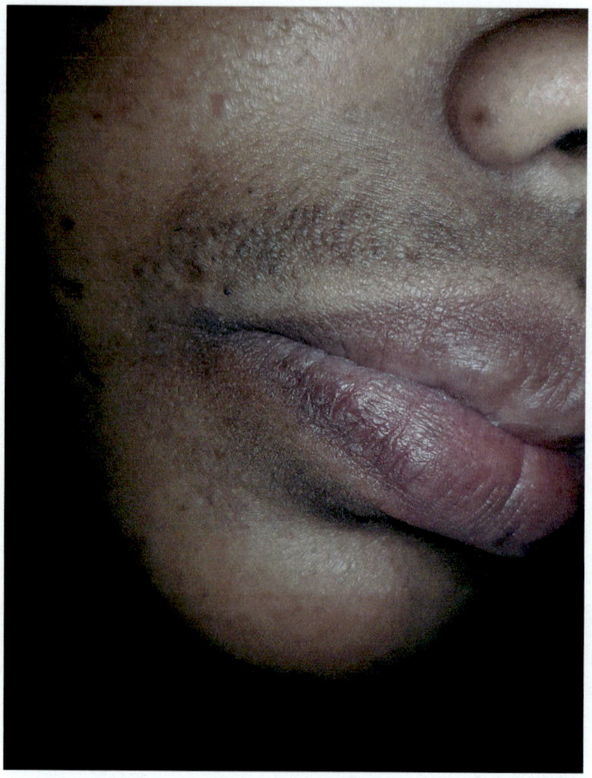

Figure 6.26 Pseudofolliculitis barbae seen as multiple firm hyperpigmented papules present over the moustache area.

- Chin, jaws, and neck are the most commonly affected sites.
- It is characterized by multiple closely set grouped follicular papules with anserine (goose skin-like) appearance (**Figure 6.27a–c**).

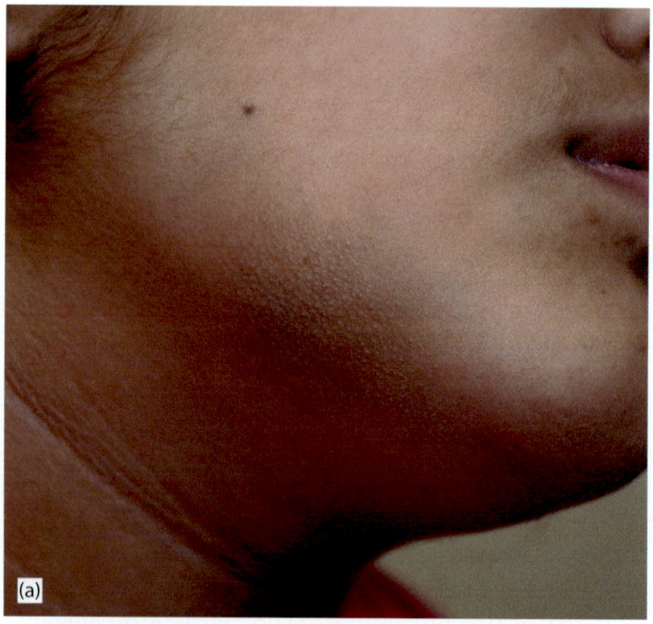

Figure 6.27 **(a)** Traumatic anserine folliculosis seen as multiple grouped follicular papules localized to an area over the right jaw. Note clear-cut demarcation between lesional and non-lesional skin. (*Continued*)

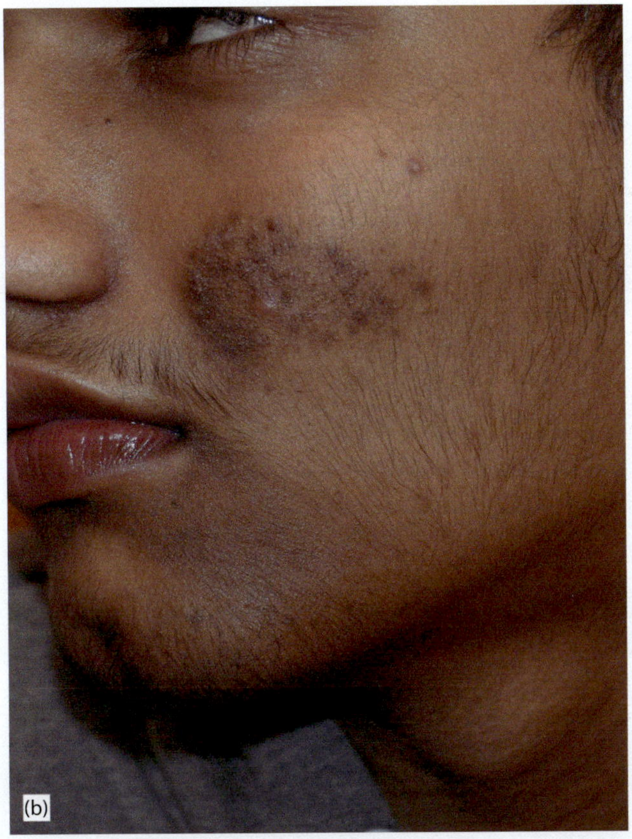

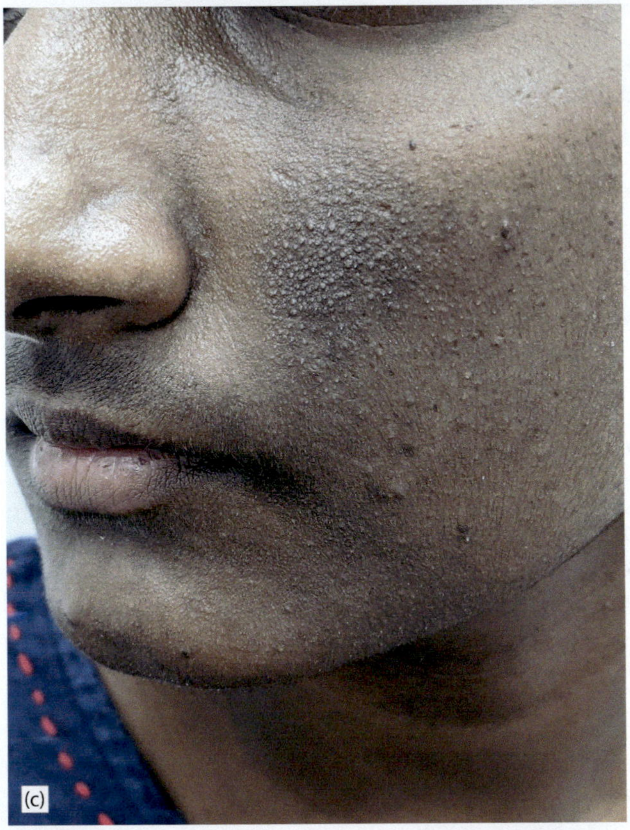

Figure 6.27 (*Continued*) **(b)** Localized grouped follicular papules in traumatic anserine folliculosis. **(c)** Traumatic anserine folliculosis in an adolescent. (c – Courtesy: Dr. Deverashetti Srinivas, Nizamabad, India.)

- DD: Keratosis pilaris, lichen spinulosus, disseminate and recurrent infundibular folliculitis.

## Steroid acne

- It is an acneiform eruption seen after corticosteroid therapy (systemic, topical, or intravenous).
- No age is spared, but most patients are young adults. Steroid acne is less common in colored skin.
- The lesions are characterized by monomorphic, papulopustular eruptions at the same stage of development. Comedones are absent in the acute inflammatory stage but may appear later on (**Figure 6.28a–c**).
- The face and trunk are commonly affected. In the case of inhaled steroids, lesions occur in and around the nose and mouth.
- DD: Acne vulgaris, chloracne.

## Lepromatous leprosy

- Leprosy (Hansen's disease) is a chronic infectious disease caused by *Mycobacterium leprae* and affects mainly the skin and peripheral nervous system.

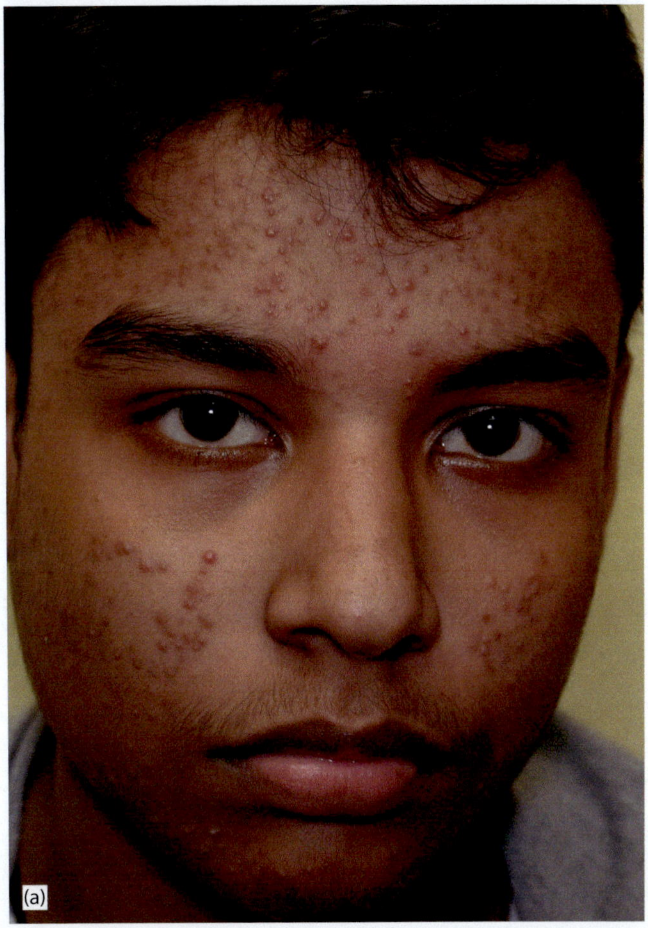

Figure 6.28 **(a)** Erythematous monomorphic papules in steroid-induced acne. (*Continued*)

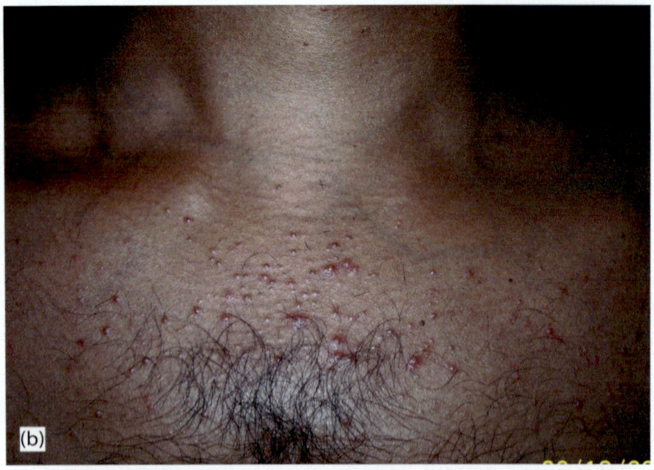


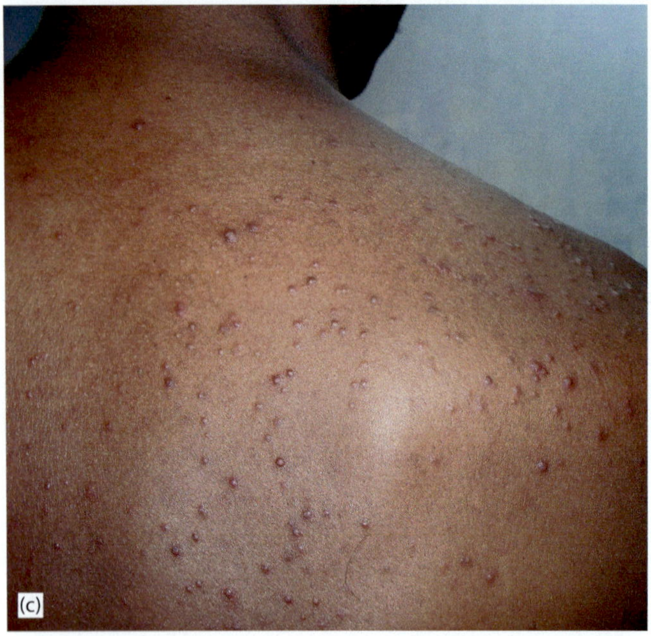


Figure 6.28 (*Continued*) **(b)** Chest involvement in steroid-induced acne. **(c)** Upper back involvement in steroid-induced acne.

- Lepromatous leprosy presents with generalized hypopigmented macules, erythematous papulonodular lesions, erythematous plaques, and diffuse infiltration, including facial involvement. The lesions are bilaterally symmetrical (**Figure 6.29**). In severe cases, the face may assume the appearance of leonine facies. Other associated findings include madarosis, infiltration of ear lobules with papulonodular lesions, and blocked nose with occasional bleeding. Late cases may have saddle-nose deformity and Buddha ears.
- Nerve trunks on the face and peripheral nerve trunks are thickened, with sensory loss in gloves-and-stockings pattern.

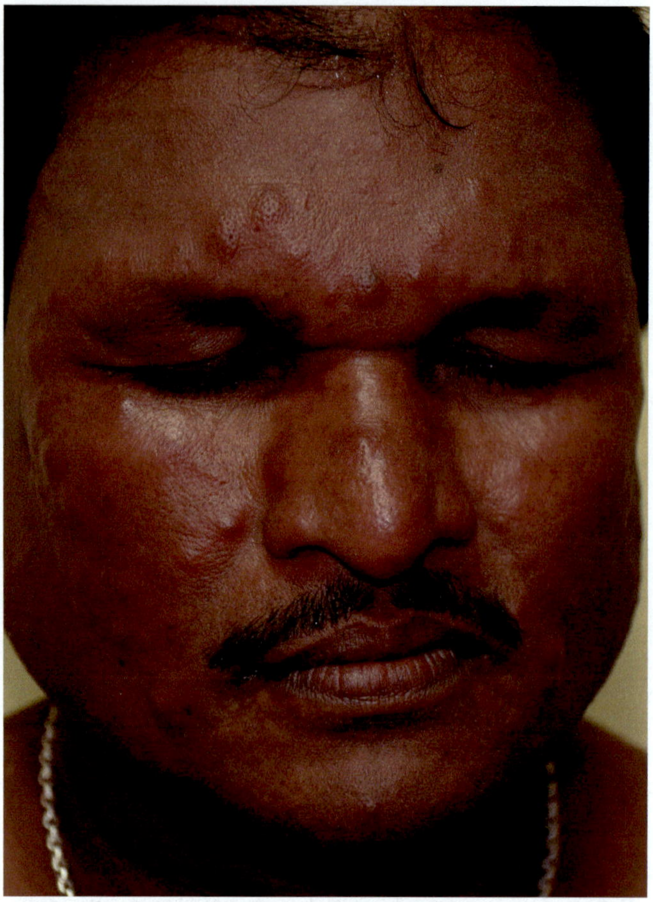

Figure 6.29 Multiple erythematous papulonodules over the face in lepromatous leprosy.

- DD: Post-kala azar dermal leishmaniasis, sarcoidosis, secondary syphilis, lymphoma.

## Granuloma annulare

- It is an idiopathic dermatosis characterized by annular lesions with asymptomatic, skin-colored papules at the periphery and central clearing (**Figure 6.30a,b**).
- It is usually asymptomatic in nature; however, occasional pruritus has been reported.
- The central part is slightly depressed and skin colored/ hyperpigmented.
- Although the face can be involved, the dorsal hands, feet, and extensor aspect of upper and lower limbs are the commoner sites.
- There are several variants:
  - Localized
  - Generalized (diabetes mellitus, thyroid disease)
  - Perforating
  - Patch type
  - Subcutaneous
  - Acute-onset, painful
- DD: Closed comedones, Tinea faciei, molluscum contagiosum, deep fungal infections.

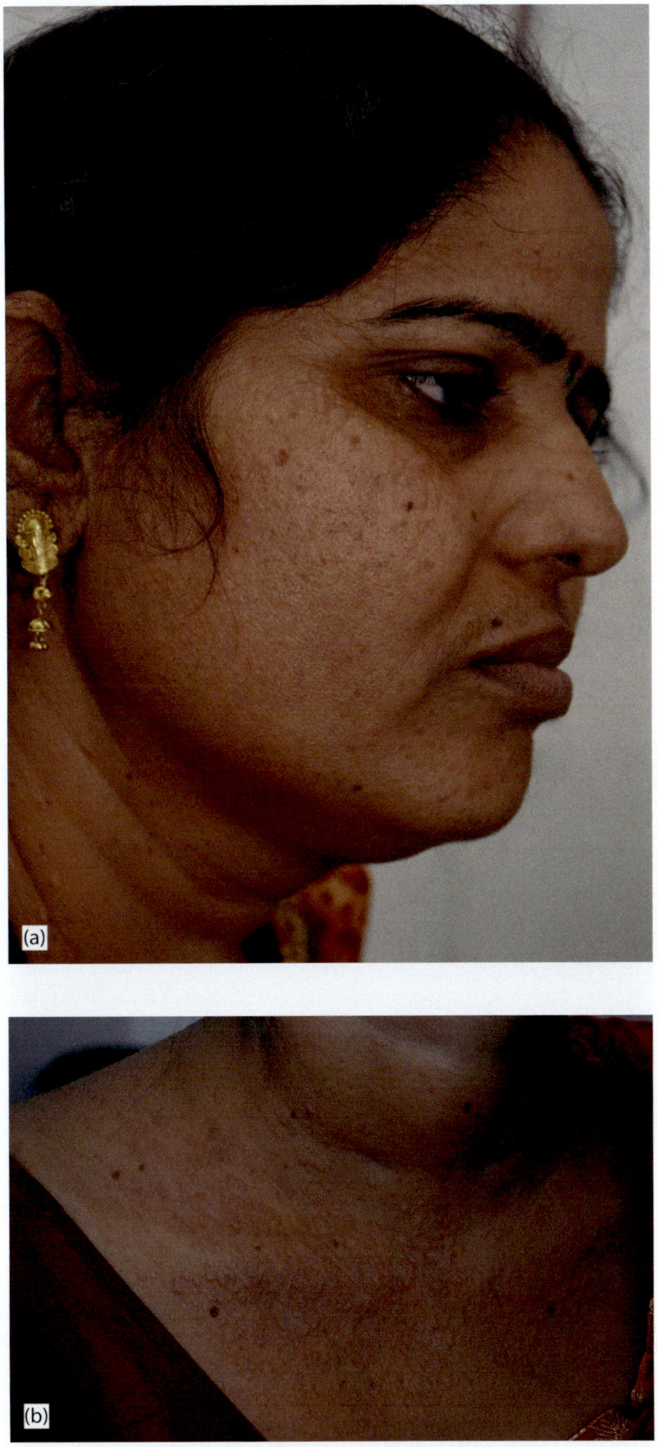

Figure 6.30 **(a)** Multiple skin-colored papules on face in granuloma annulare. **(b)** Similar papules on neck.

## Secondary syphilis[9]

- Syphilis is a sexually transmitted disease caused by the spirochete *Treponema pallidum,* occurring in primary, secondary, and tertiary stages, with a long and chronic course in the untreated patients.
- The secondary stage (secondary syphilis) appears three weeks after the appearance of primary lesion (chancre) with a normal duration of two to ten weeks but can last for up to 12 months.
- The cutaneous manifestations of secondary syphilis are variable, classically comprising four major types of rashes: macular, papular, papulosquamous, or pustular.
- Papular lesions are the most prominent cutaneous manifestation of the secondary syphilis that follow an evanescent coppery-red macular rash. The lesions are usually asymptomatic, erythematous, or brownish-red, discrete, papules, often showing a collarette of scales (**Figure 6.31a,b**). The eruption is generalized, involving both skin and mucous membrane, is bilaterally symmetrical and more prominent on upper extremities followed by the abdomen and lower extremities, with a

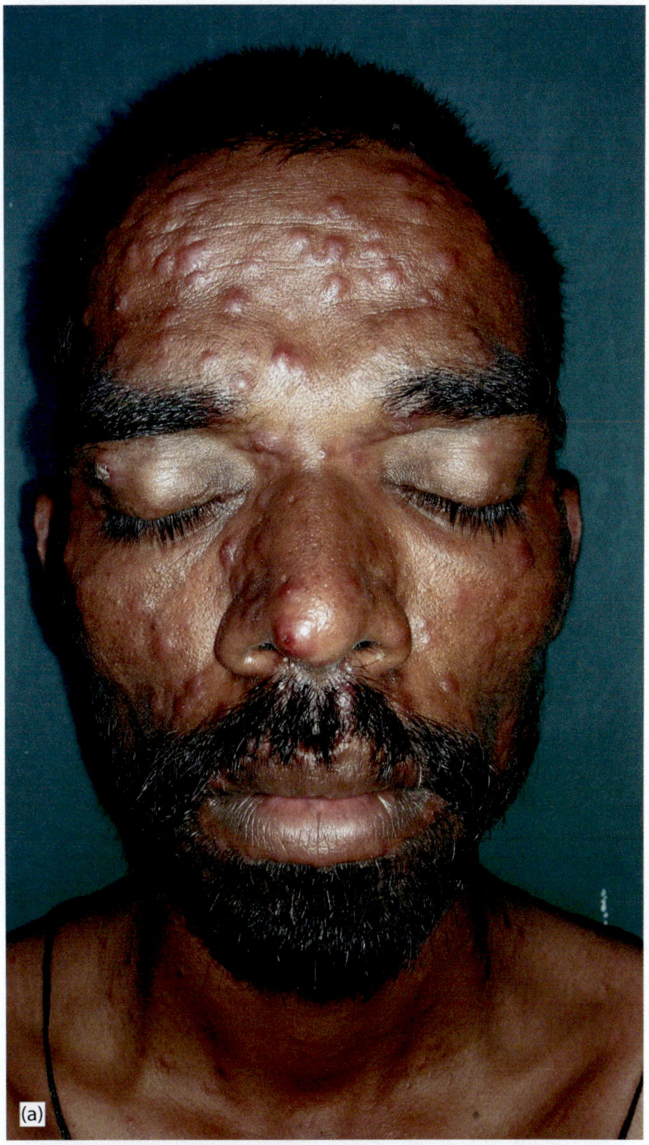

Figure 6.31 **(a)** secondary syphilis seen as multiple erythematous, shiny papulonodular lesions with crust over few lesions. (*Continued*)

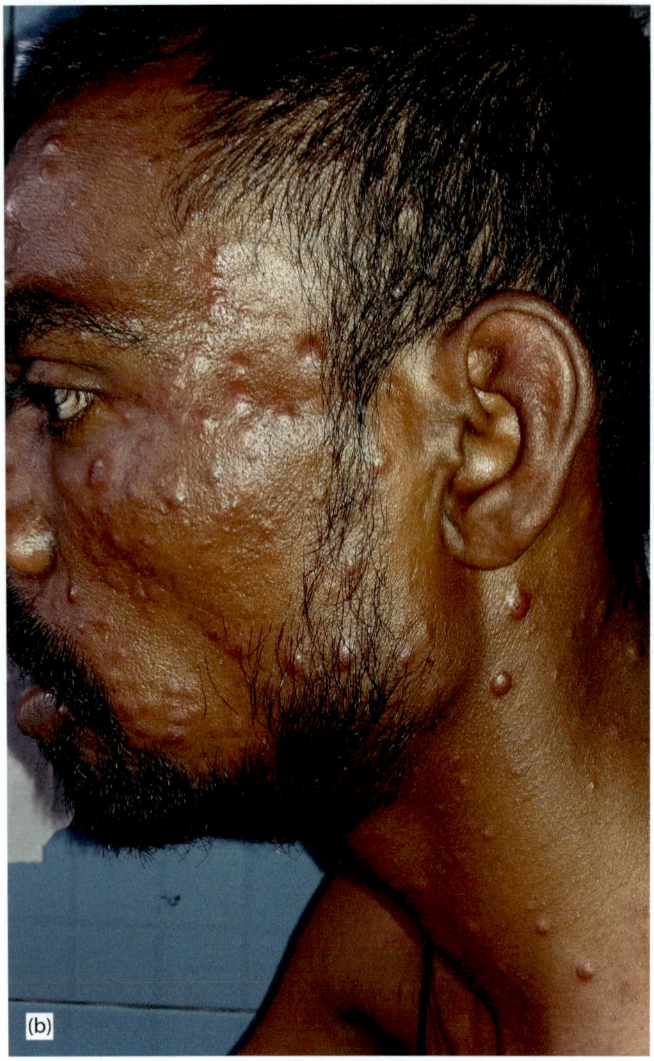


Figure 6.31 (*Continued*) **(b)** Same patient – side profile. (a,b – Courtesy: Dr. Hiral Shah, Baroda Medical College, Vadodara, India.)

predilection for the palms and soles. Large papular and nodular lesions on the face are also seen.

- Lesions may have a lichenoid or psoriasiform appearance and may assume annular configuration.
- Patients often have condylomata lata – flat, moist papules and plaques in groin and perianal region.
- Systemic features include low-grade fever, generalized lymphadenopathy, headache, and malaise.
- DD: Leprosy, sarcoidosis, psoriasis.

## Cryptococcosis

- Cryptococcosis is an opportunistic infection caused by the encapsulated yeast *Cryptococcus neoformans*. The infection is mostly seen in immunocompromised, but immunocompetent patients too may develop the disease.
- Cutaneous cryptococcosis can be primary (through direct inoculation) or secondary (through dissemination).
- Primary cutaneous cryptococcosis develops at the site of trauma, and the lesion is usually solitary and on the exposed parts. The lesion starts as a papule, grows to become a nodule, and then ulcerates, accompanied by regional lymphadenopathy.
- Disseminated cutaneous cryptococcosis is common in immunocompromised patients. Though lesions may be generalized, they are predominant on the head and neck region. The most common presentation is umbilicated papules and nodules of varying size that develop a central hemorrhagic crust (**Figure 6.32**). Other presentations include acneiform papules or pustules, warty crusted plaques, and ulcers.
- Cutaneous lesions in disseminated disease precede other symptoms of disseminated disease by two to eight months. Central nervous system (CNS) involvement is common and manifestations include meningeal signs, nerve palsies, vertigo etc.

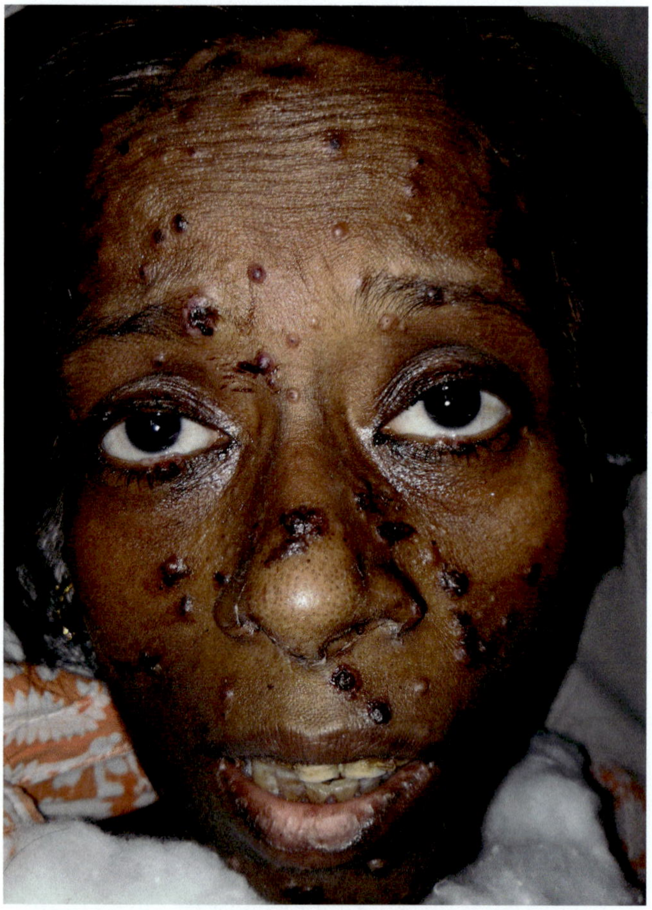

Figure 6.32 Cryptococcosis in an immunocompromised lady, seen as multiple umbilicated papules and nodules of varying sizes with central hemorrhagic crust. (Courtesy: Dr. Hitesh Khatri, Gauhati Medical College and Hospital, India.)

- DD: Basal cell carcinoma and molluscum contagiosum (for single lesions), molluscum contagiosum, acne vulgaris, secondary syphilis, and histoplasmosis (for multiple lesions).

## Histoplasmosis (Darling disease, reticuloendotheliosis, Ohio Valley disease, bat disease, caver's and miner's fever)

- Histoplasmosis is a deep mycosis caused by *Histoplasma capsulatum* and is prevalent in tropical countries. Infection is acquired after inhalation of conidia, and lungs (followed by spleen and liver) are the most commonly affected organ. Immunocompromised persons may develop disseminated disease.
- People at risk are miners, engineers, farmers, archeologists, guano collectors, anthropologists, builders, and persons with certain interests, such as cavers, birders, etc.
- Mucocutaneous lesions are usually seen in disseminated histoplasmosis; primary cutaneous histoplasmosis (painless ulcer with regional lymphadenopathy) is very rare.
- Generalized involvement with the face and mucosae (oral, perianal, and genital) affection is common in disseminated disease.
- The range of cutaneous lesions is diverse and includes, but is not limited to, papules (umbilicated, with hemorrhagic crusts), acneiform eruptions, erythematous papules, plaques with or without crusts, keratotic plaques, pustules, and nodules. Mucosa may show painful nodules, erosions or ulcers. There may be an associated erythema multiforme or erythema nodosum.
- DD: Acne vulgaris, molluscum contagiosum, cryptococcosis, lymphoma.

## Common acquired melanocytic nevus (CAMN) (mole)

- CAMN is a benign proliferation of a type of melanocyte known as a "nevus cell" (which forms nests and lacks dendrites).
- Based on the location of nests of nevus cells, CAMN is further classified into three types – junctional (nests at the dermo-epidermal junction [DEJ]), compound (nests at DEJ and in dermis), and intradermal (nests in dermis). Junctional CAMN presents as macules; both compound and intradermal CAMN present as facial papules.
- No race is spared, but the mean number of CAMN is lower in people with colored skin.
- It starts appearing after the first six months of life, increases in number during childhood and adolescence, and then slowly regresses with age.
- Compound nevus presents as smooth-surfaced, dome-shaped, round to oval pigmented papules with sharply demarcated border and homogenous pigmentation. The color varies from tan to dark brown to black (**Figure 6.33a–c**). In smaller lesions the elevation is subtle.

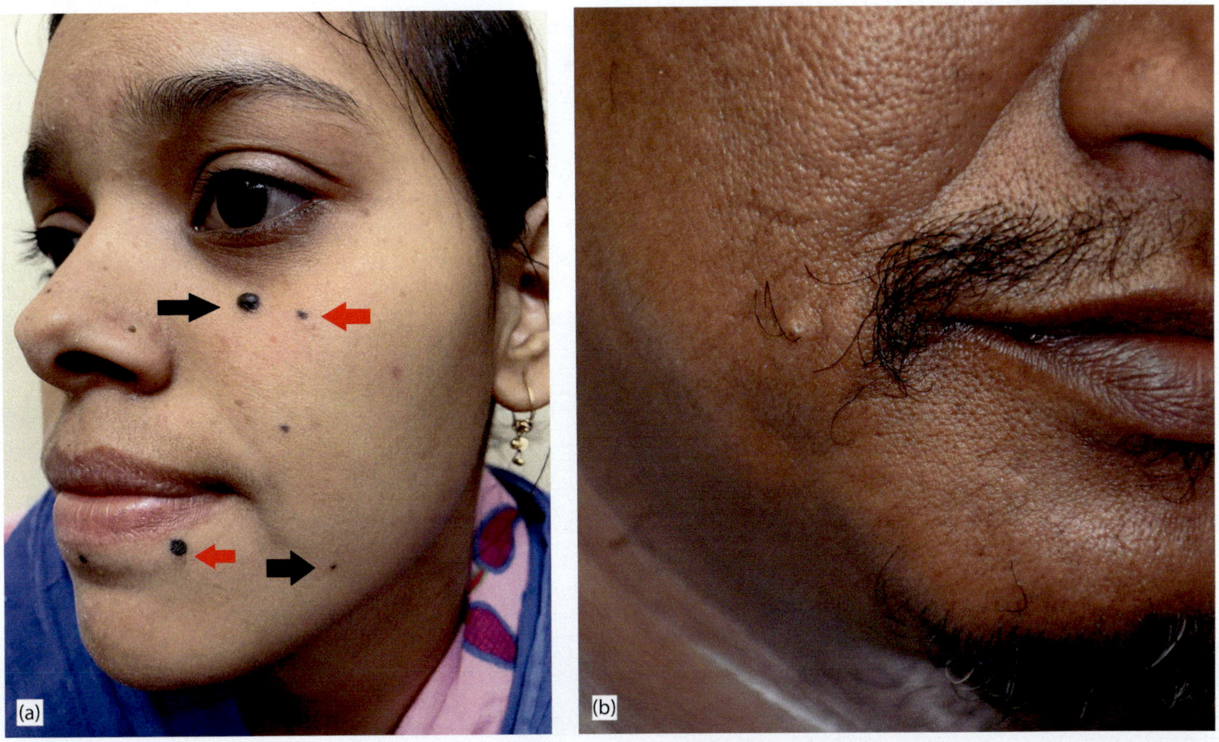


Figure 6.33 **(a)** Compound nevus seen as dome-shaped, black papules (black arrow) of varying sizes. Additionally, the patient has pigmented macules of junctional melanocytic nevus (red arrow). **(b)** Gradually the lower part of compound nevus may lose pigment and become skin-colored. (*Continued*)

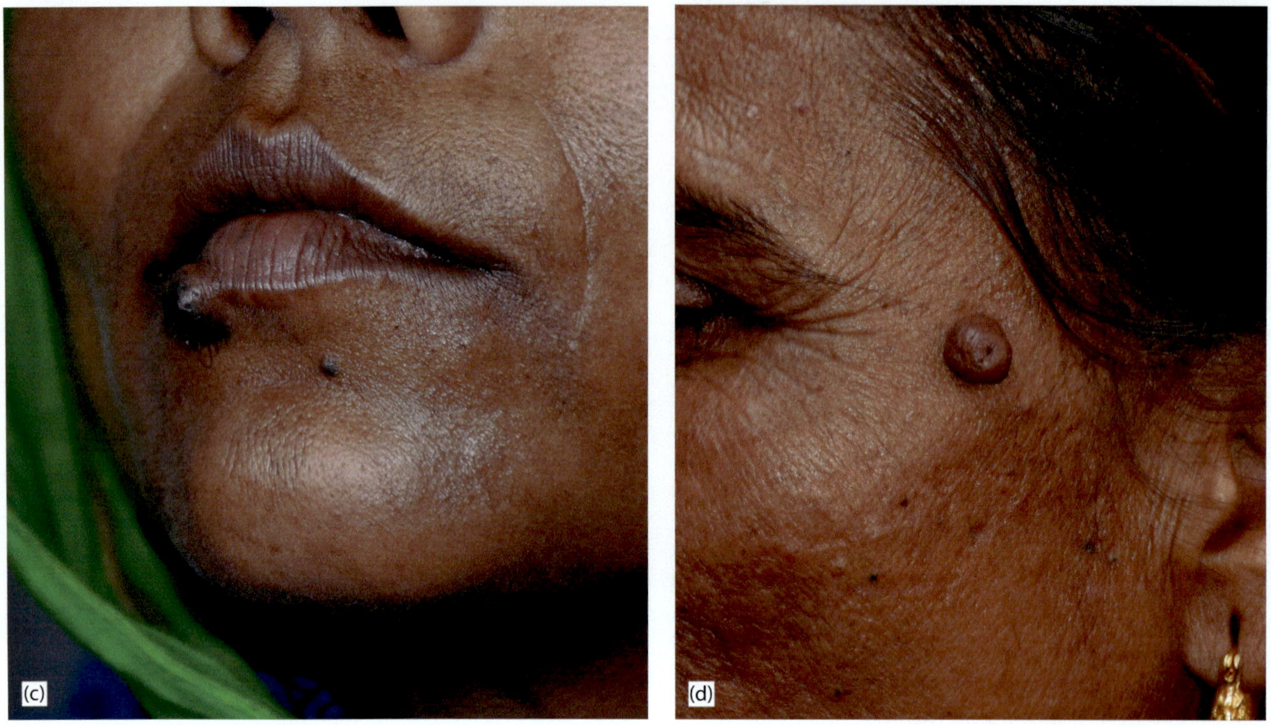


Figure 6.33 (*Continued*) **(c)** Large compound nevus with partly pigmented and non-pigmented skin. **(d)** Soft to firm skin-colored papulonodule of intradermal melanocytic nevus.

- Intradermal nevus presents as skin-colored to tan, dome-shaped papules with a soft, rubbery texture (**Figure 6.33d**). Sometimes lesions may be papillomatous, pedunculated, or cerebriform.
- Cerebriform intradermal nevus may occur in association with various syndromes such as Noonan syndrome, Beare-Stevenson syndrome, Ehlers-Danlos syndrome, Michelin tire baby syndrome, Turner syndrome, and fragile X syndrome.
- DD: Pigmented basal cell carcinoma, melanoma (for compound nevus), osteoma, basal cell carcinoma, fibrous papule of nose, appendageal tumor (for intradermal nevus).

## Fibrous papule of nose

- Fibrous papule of the nose (fibrous papule of the face, sporadic angiofibroma) is a benign angiofibroma affecting the nose most commonly, hence the name.
- It is mostly seen in the middle-aged patients.
- It usually presents as solitary asymptomatic, flesh-colored, dome-shaped, firm papule seen predominantly on the nose (mainly over ala, alar groove, and tip of the nose) (**Figure 6.34**). Also, it may occur over the chin, cheeks, forehead, and neck. Sometimes, a central hair may be seen. It persists lifelong unchanged.
- Rarely, multiple lesions may be noted.
- DD: Intradermal melanocytic nevus, warts, nodular basal cell carcinoma.

## Basal cell carcinoma (BCC)

- BCC is the most common non-melanoma skin cancer, arising from the pluripotential cells in the basal layer of the epidermis or follicular structures. It is a slow-growing, locally destructive tumor of the epidermis, having a metastatic rate $\leq 0.1\%$.
- BCC is common in elderly males and in light-skinned individuals.

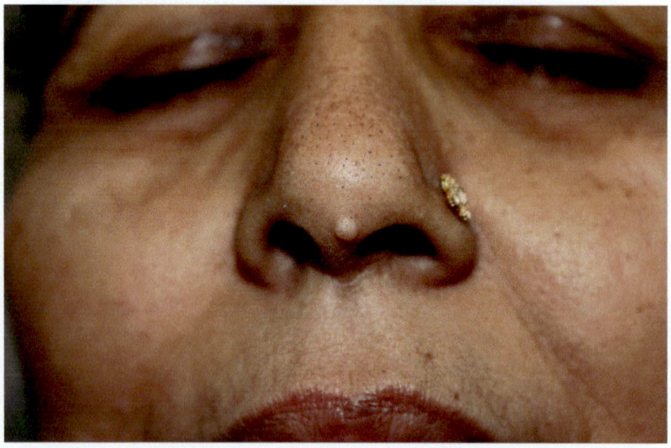

Figure 6.34 Fibrous papule of the nose. Note trichostasis spinulosa on the tip of nose. (Courtesy: Dr. Divya Sachdev, Raipur, India.)

- It is usually seen on the face, head (scalp included), and neck.
- Nodular BCC is the most common form and presents as a solitary asymptomatic, round, shiny, flesh-colored papule with telangiectasia. The lesion grows very slowly, and central ulceration may develop, leaving a rolled, pearly border with telangiectasia (a valuable clinical clue) (**Figure 6.35a**).
- Pigmented BCC appears to be very common in colored skin and is characterized by partial or complete pigmentation of the tumor. The lesion mimics melanoma, and the presence of a rolled, pearly border allows clinical differentiation from the latter.
- As the BCC is mostly pigmented in our experience and the pigmented papule of BCC mimics many common conditions such as acquired melanocytic nevus and DPN (and seborrheic keratosis) **(Figure 6.35b)**, we do not see many cases with BCC in the papule stage. Patients usually present late with plaque or noduloulcerative lesions.
- Lack of awareness among the population is another reason for late diagnosis. We have diagnosed BCC incidentally in patients presenting with less serious conditions, such as tinea corporis or miliaria rubra.
- The clinical variants are superficial, morphoeic (sclerosing), micronodular, and fibroepithelioma of Pinkus.
- DD: For non-pigmented BCC – intradermal nevus, keratoacanthoma, appendageal tumor, fibrous papules of the face, solitary trichoepithelioma, molluscum contagiosum; for pigmented BCC – CAMN (compound type), melanoma, seborrheic keratosis.

## Dilated pore of Winer

- It is a benign adnexal tumor showing follicular differentiation.
- It is clinically characterized by an asymptomatic, solitary, enlarged pore with a central keratin plug, surrounded by normal skin.
- The most common sites are the face and neck; however, truncal distribution has been reported in middle-aged subjects (males more than females).
- The exact etiology remains unknown; some consider it to be an epidermal inclusion cyst with epithelial hyperplasia, while others consider it to be a variant of nevus comedonicus.
- DD: Epidermal inclusion cyst, melanocytic nevus.

## Pilomatricoma (pilomatrixoma, or calcifying epithelioma of Malherbe)

- Pilomatricoma is a benign tumor with differentiation toward the matrix of the hair follicle.
- It can develop at any age, showing bimodal peak presentation during first and sixth decades of life and affects women more commonly than men.
- The most commonly affected sites are the head and neck, followed by upper extremity, trunk, and lower extremity.
- The lesion is usually an asymptomatic (sometimes tender), firm, deeply seated papule, nodule, or tumor, adherent to the skin but not to the underlying tissue. The color of overlying skin varies from flesh-colored to red to bluish-purple (**Figure 6.36**).
- Stretching of the skin over the tumor shows multiple facets and angles known as "tent sign." Additionally, applying pressure over one edge of the lesion causes the opposite

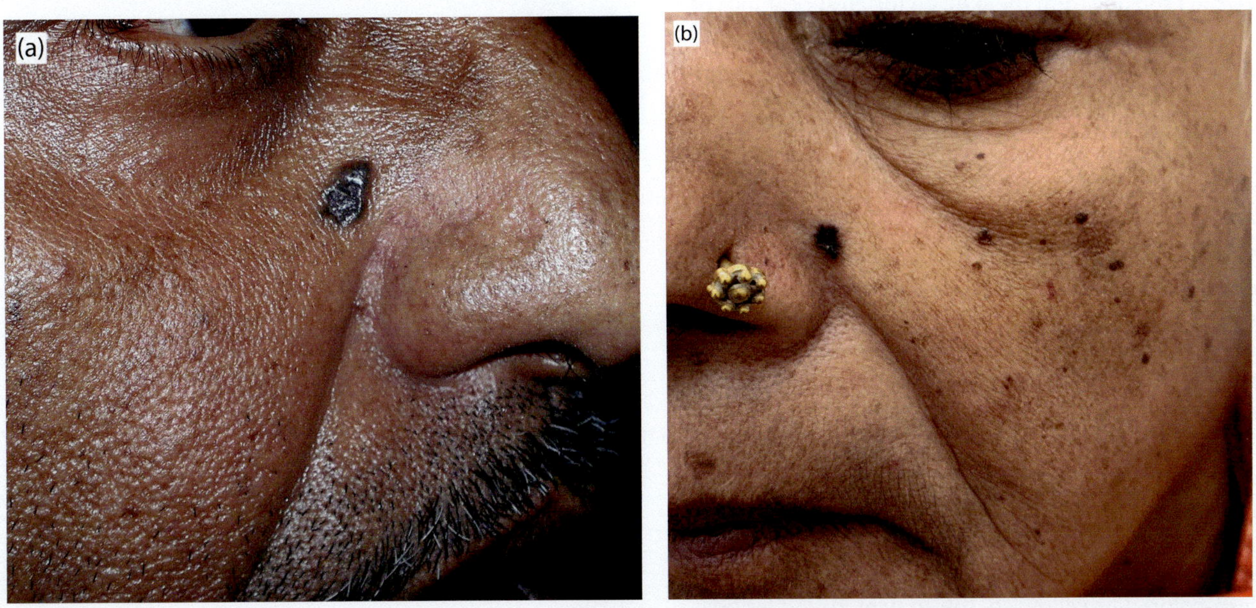


Figure 6.35 **(a)** Small basal cell carcinoma seen as solitary shiny, hyperpigmented papule with an annular plaque with rolled, pearly border. **(b)** small annular plaque of basal cell carcinoma near ala nasi. Note multiple acquired melanocytic nevi on the cheek.

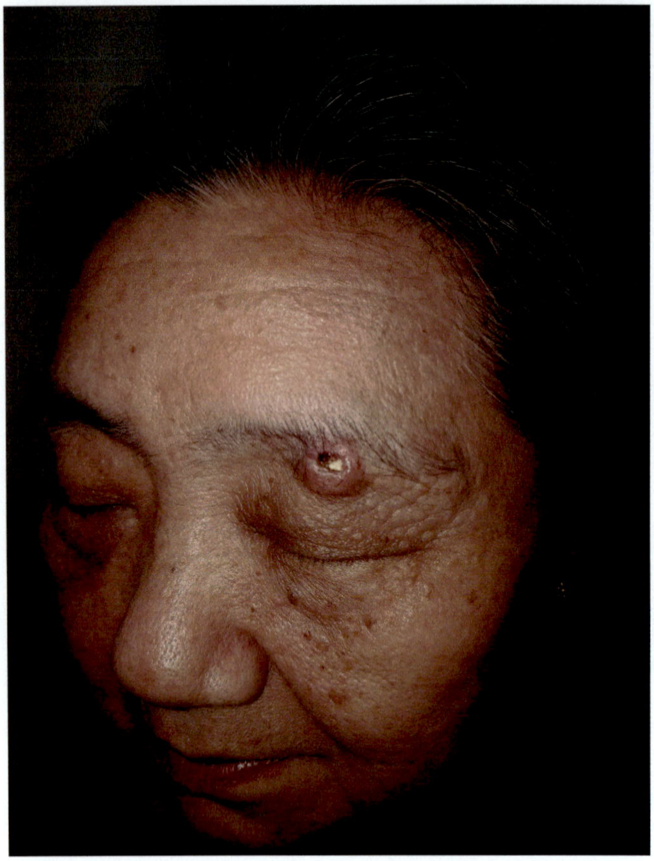

Figure 6.36 Pilomatricoma seen as flesh-colored nodule with central ulceration over the left eyebrow. (Courtesy: Dr. Raghuraj Hegde, Ophthalmic plastic surgery and Ophthalmology Oncology, Manipal Hospital, Bangalore, India.)

edge to protrude from the skin, giving an appearance of a teeter totter. Both these signs are pathognomonic and relate to calcification within the lesion.

- DD: Appendageal tumor, epidermoid cyst, foreign bodies granuloma.

## Epidermoid cyst (epidermal inclusion cyst, sebaceous cyst)

- An Eepidermoid cyst (EC) is a benign encapsulated lesion filled with keratin and has its origin in infundibular portion of pilosebaceous unit. The preferred term for this entity is epidermoid cyst. Sebaceous cyst is a misnomer. Very small, superficial epidermoid cysts are called milia.
- EC appears to be more common in men and in third and fourth decades of life.
- There may be a history of discharge of foul-smelling, "cheese-like," semi-solid material.
- EC presents as asymptomatic, single or multiple, flesh-colored or yellowish, soft to firm, round lesions of variable size. The most characteristic feature is a central, dark, punctum (**Figure 6.37a,b**) that may not be obvious in smaller lesions.

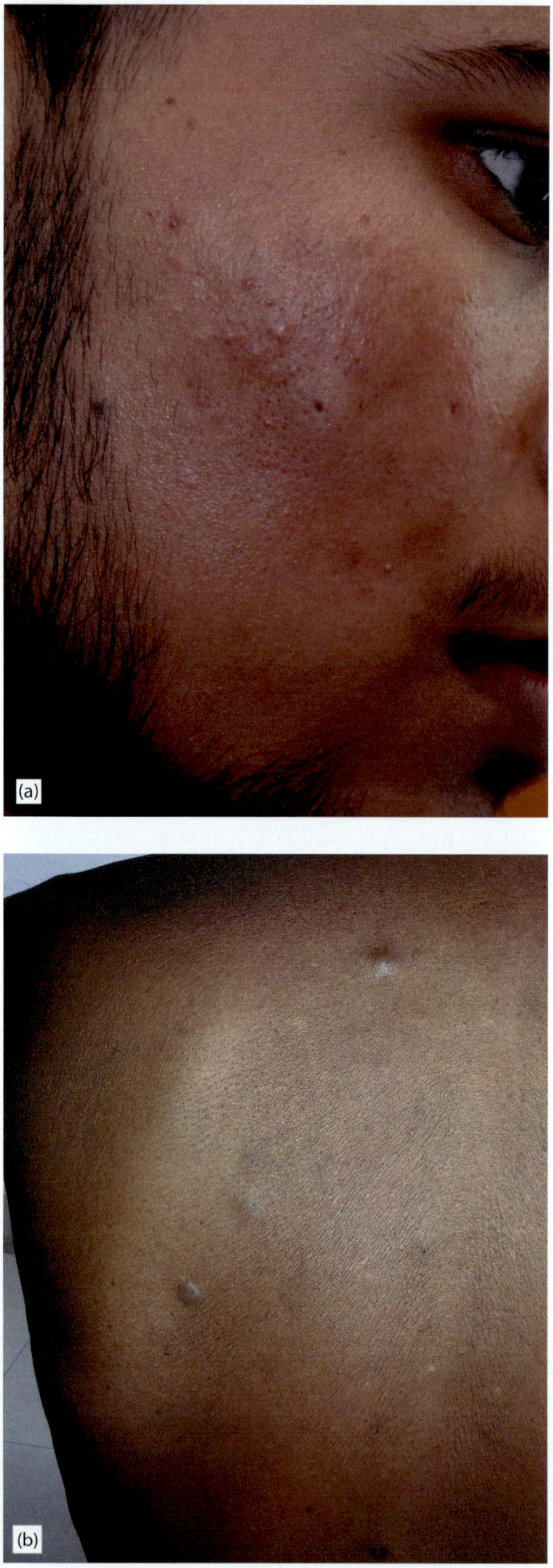


Figure 6.37 **(a)** Epidermoid cyst seen as single, flesh-colored round cyst with central, dark, punctum over the right cheek. **(b)** Multiple bluish cysts with central punctum.

Table 6.4 Clinical characteristics of appendageal tumor

| | Onset | Clinical features | Sites | Comments |
|---|---|---|---|---|
| Trichofolliculoma (**Figure 6.38a,b**) | Adulthood | Solitary flesh-colored papule or nodule<br>Clinical hallmark is tuft of white hair emerging from the central pore | Face (specially around the nose) | |
| Dilated pore of Winer | Adulthood | Enlarged solitary comedo<br>A keratotic plug can be expressed. This allows further removal of caseous, white keratin. | Face – mostly on the upper lip, cheek, or forehead | Common in light -skinned people<br>Male predilection |
| Trichodiscoma/ fibrofoliculoma | Young adults | Solitary or multiple small (2–4 mm), flesh-colored, smooth-surfaced, dome-shaped papules | Face – chin, nose, cheeks, ears, and eyebrows | Multiple lesions may occur in isolation or may be a part of Birt-Hogg-Dubé syndrome – triad of multiple fibrofolliculomas, trichodiscomas, and acrochordons |
| Trichoadenoma of Nikolowski | Adulthood | Solitary skin-colored papule or nodule | Face is most commonly involved site followed by buttock | |
| Trichilemmoma | Adulthood | Single or multiple small, flesh-colored papules that are 1–5 mm in diameter<br>As the lesion grows, it develops a hyperkeratotic surface. | Face, neck | May arise within nevus sebaceous<br>Multiple lesions are a part of Cowden syndrome |
| Tumor of follicular infundibulum | Elderly patients | Solitary form – scaly papule or nodule<br>Eruptive form – sudden onset of multiple variably scaling, hypopigmented macules and papules | Head and neck | Slight female preponderance |

- The lesions are mostly asymptomatic but may get ruptured/infected and then become red and painful.
- Malignancy may develop in long-standing cases.
- Multiple EC are seen in Gardner syndrome, Gorlin syndrome, basal cell nevus syndrome, and pachyonychia congenita.
- DD: Trichilemmal cyst, dermoid cyst, pilomatricoma, lipoma, BCC.

## Trichofolliculoma

See **Table 6.4** and **Figure 6.38a,b**.

## Lobular capillary hemangioma (LCH) (pyogenic granuloma)

- LCH (pyogenic granuloma, or granuloma pyogenicum, granuloma telangiectaticum – a misnomer) is a common, usually solitary, lobulated, benign vascular proliferation of skin and mucous membranes.
- The disease usually occurs in the second decade of life but may affect any age group and has a predilection for males. Mucosal lesions are more common in females.
- There is a history of repeated bleeding from the lesion.
- Clinically it appears as an asymptomatic, usually solitary, bright-red to brownish-red, vascular papule

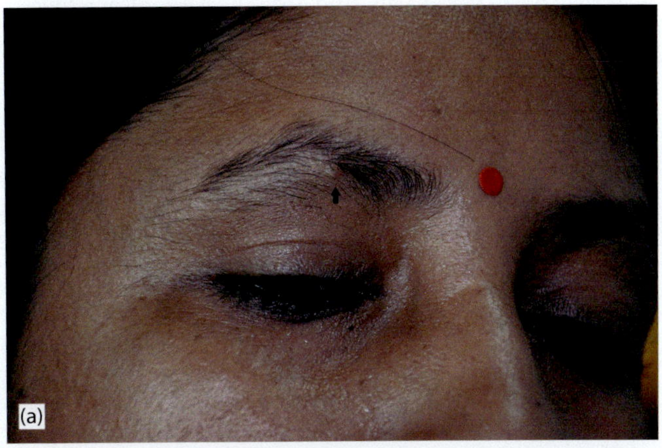


Figure 6.38 **(a)** Trichofolliculoma seen as a skin-colored papule. (*Continued*)

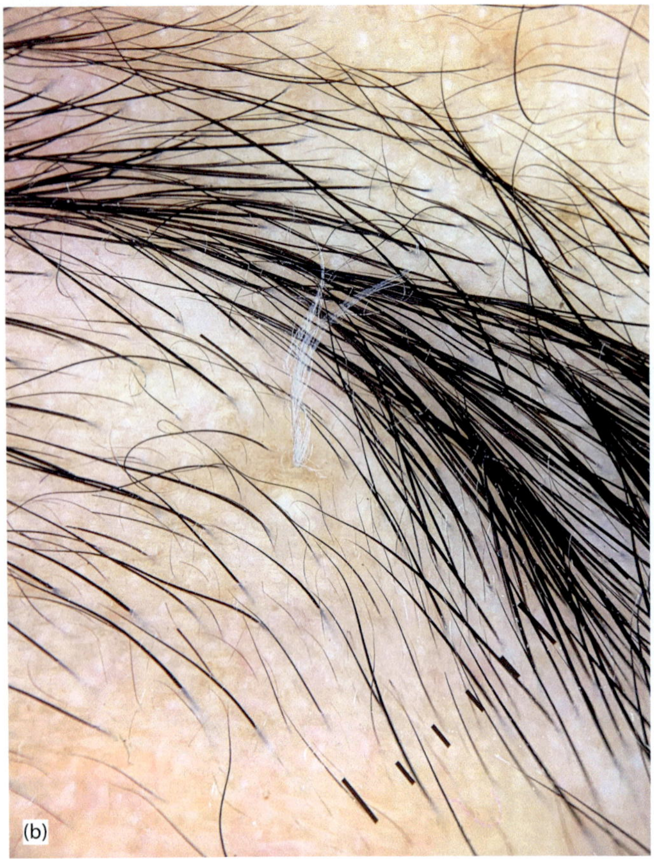

Figure 6.38 (*Continued*) **(b)** Dermoscopy image showing a wisp of white hairs emerging from the central part of the lesion.

or nodule with a glistening surface (**Figure 6.39a,b**). The lesion is partially compressible without any pulsation, rapidly growing, and friable and may be sessile, or pedunculated. A surrounding collarette of scales is seen at the base of the lesion in the majority of cases. Bleeding, erosion, ulceration, and crusting are frequent.

- It may bleed very easily, and growth ceases after a few weeks of an initial phase of rapid evolution, rarely showing spontaneous resolution.
- DD: Angiolymphoid hyperplasia with eosinophilia, infantile hemangioma, basal cell carcinoma.

## Infantile hemangioma

- Infantile hemangioma (IH) is a true neoplasm of endothelial cells and is the most common benign soft-tissue tumor of infancy and childhood. It is well known for its rapid growth during the first few weeks to months of a child's life, followed by a spontaneous but slow involution. Most infantile hemangiomas resolve by the age of nine years.
- It occurs in greater frequency in girls, whites, premature infants, twins, and children born to mothers of high maternal age.

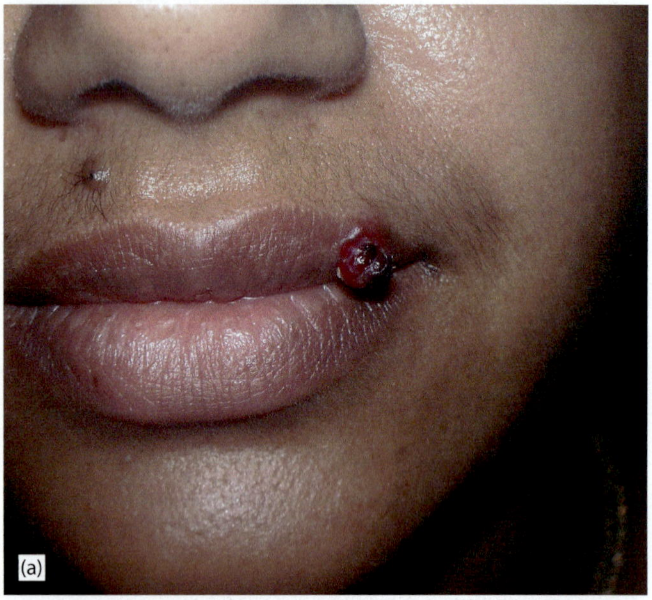

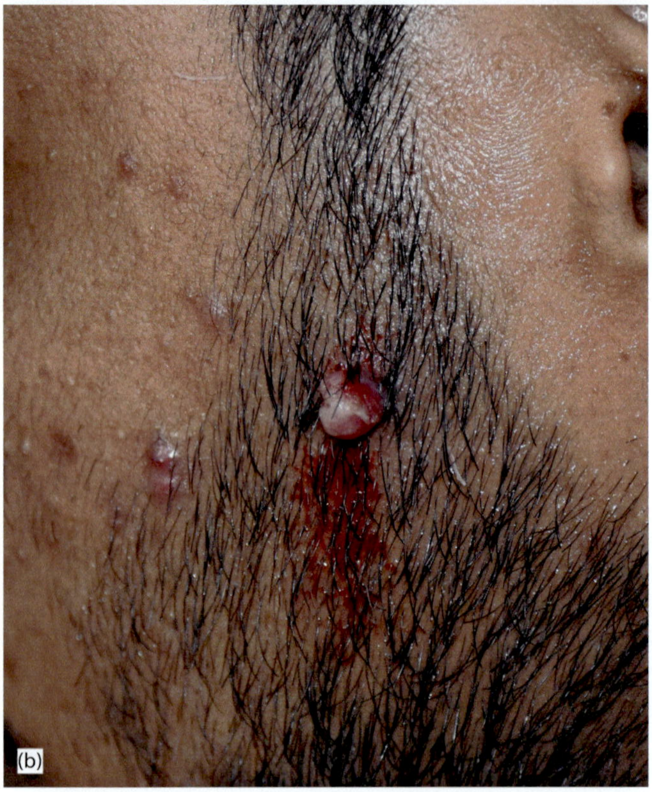

Figure 6.39 **(a)** Lobular capillary hemangioma seen as a solitary bright-red vascular papule over the lower lip. **(b)** A solitary lesion of lobular capillary hemangioma on the cheek. The lesion often bleeds spontaneously.

- It is most commonly seen in the head and neck region.
- IH may be present at birth or appear in the first few weeks after birth and usually manifests as a solitary, asymptomatic pale patch that grows rapidly to an erythematous papule. As it grows, it may assume a dome-shaped, bosselated, plaque-like, or tumoral

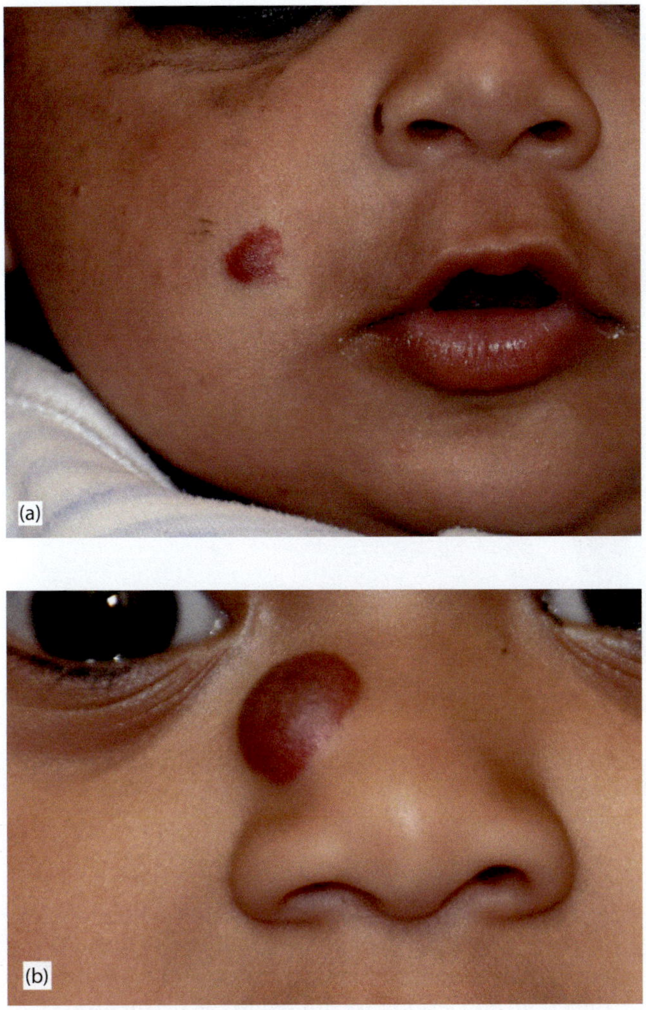


Figure 6.40 **(a)** Infantile hemangioma seen as solitary dome-shaped erythematous papule present over the face. **(b)** Infantile hemangioma over the nose.

appearance (**Figure 6.40a,b**). The lesion may be firm, rubbery, and tense.

- Involution starts at the center and spreads centrifugally. With involution, the lesion becomes less red and assumes a flesh-colored appearance. Also, the lesion becomes softer and more compressible. Finally, the lesion may resolve completely with no evidence of a previous pathologic process.
- However, about 50–60% of lesions resolve incompletely, and residual changes like telangiectasia, stippled scarring, anetoderma or epidermal atrophy, hypopigmentation, and redundant skin with fibrofatty tissue may persist.
- DD: For popular IH – lobular capillary hemangioma (granuloma pyogenicum), angiokeratoma.

## Keratoacanthoma

- Keratoacanthoma mostly occurs on sun-exposed sites, such as the face, neck, and dorsum of the upper extremities, and is less common in darker-skinned individuals.
- Keratoacanthoma originates as a solitary, firm, dome-shaped, skin-colored or reddish papule. It grows rapidly, achieving a size of 1–2 cm within weeks and assumes the morphology of a dome-shaped nodule with a smooth shiny surface and a central crateriform ulceration or keratin plug (**Figure 6.41a,b**). The surface may show telangiectatic

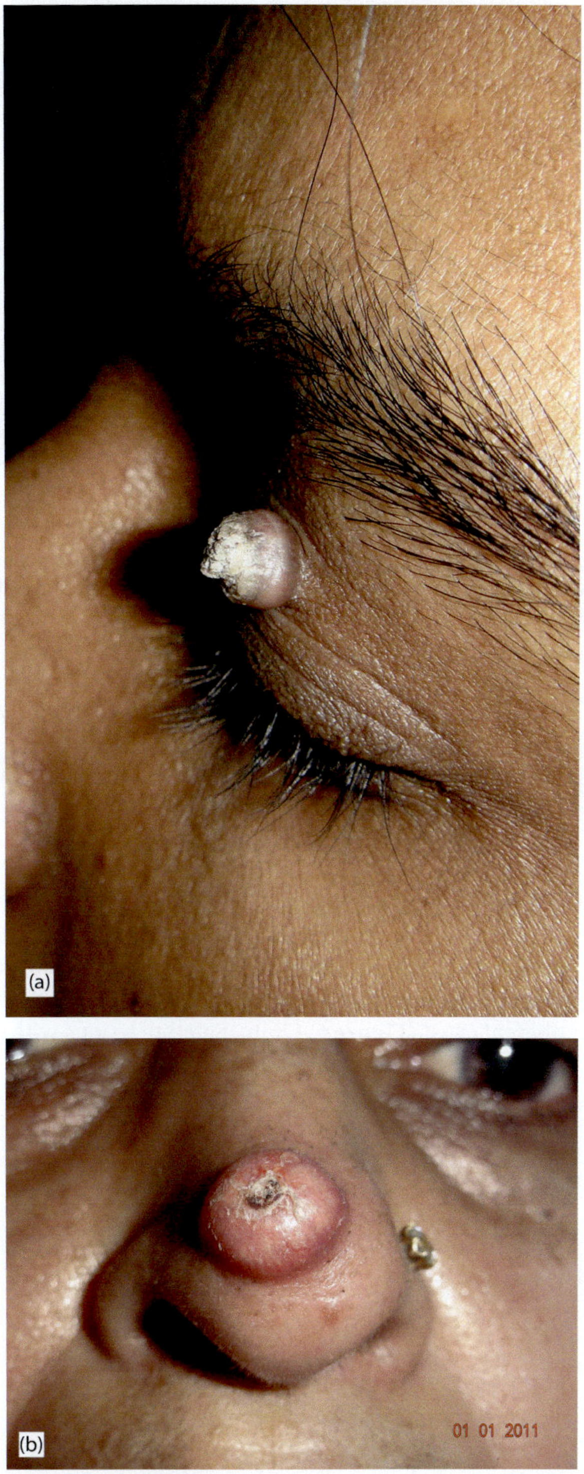


Figure 6.41 **(a)** Keratoacanthoma seen as a solitary dome-shaped nodule with central keratin plug over the left upper eyelid. **(b)** Solitary keratoacanthoma over nose. (Courtesy: Dr. Niharika Ranjan Lal, ESIPGIMSR, Kolkata, India.)

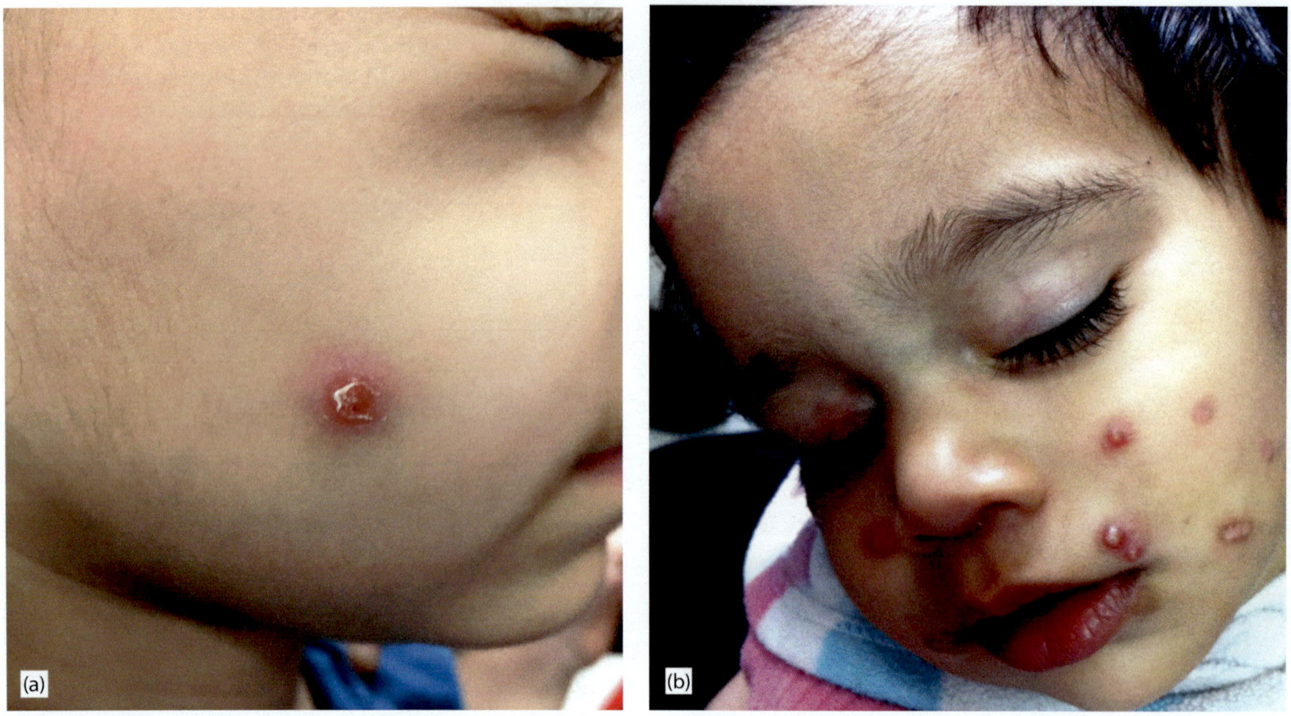


Figure 6.42 **(a)** Cutaneous leishmaniasis seen as a solitary erythematous papule with central adherent crust over the right cheek. **(b)** Cutaneous leishmaniasis presenting as multiple erythematous papules with satellite lesions over the face. (a,b – Courtesy: Prof. Reza Yaghoobi, Ahvaz Jundishupor University of Medical Sciences, Iran.)

blood vessels, and the keratin plug may grow to form a cutaneous horn.

- The lesion may remain static for months and then may heal with atrophic scarring. It may rarely progress to invasive or metastatic carcinoma.

## Cutaneous leishmaniasis (CL)

- CL starts as an erythematous papule at the site of a bite on exposed parts, including face. The papule increases in size, becomes a nodule, and finally ulcerates with an adherent crust (**Figure 6.42a,b**). Satellite lesions with a nodular lymphangitis may develop.
- Lesions may show spontaneous resolution over months to years and heal with atrophic scarring.
- Immunosuppressed patients may develop disseminated lesions.
- DD: Lupus vulgaris

## Granuloma faciale

- Granuloma faciale presents with multiple or solitary, soft, well-circumscribed papules, plaques, or nodules (**Figure 6.43**). The surface of the lesion is smooth and may show prominent follicular openings. Extrafacial lesions may occur.
- DD: Hansen's disease, sarcoidosis, PKDL.

## Molluscum contagiosum (MC)

- Molluscum contagiosum (water warts) is an infection of skin and mucosa, caused by a DNA poxvirus molluscum contagiosum virus (MCV).
- Facial MC is commonly seen in children and immunosuppressed patients. In immunocompetent adults, MC usually presents as a sexually transmitted infection, and lesions are limited to the perineum, genitalia, lower abdomen, or buttocks.

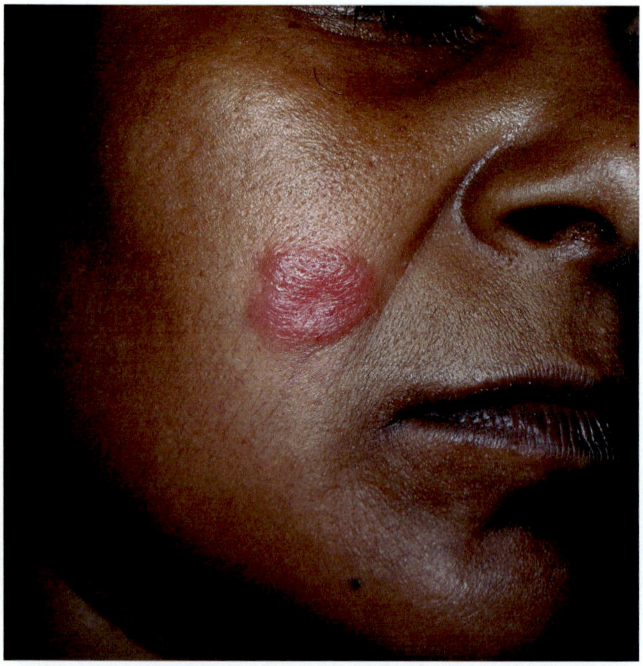

Figure 6.43 Granuloma faciale presenting as erythematous edematous plaque over the right cheek. Surface is remarkable for follicular prominence and telangiectasia.

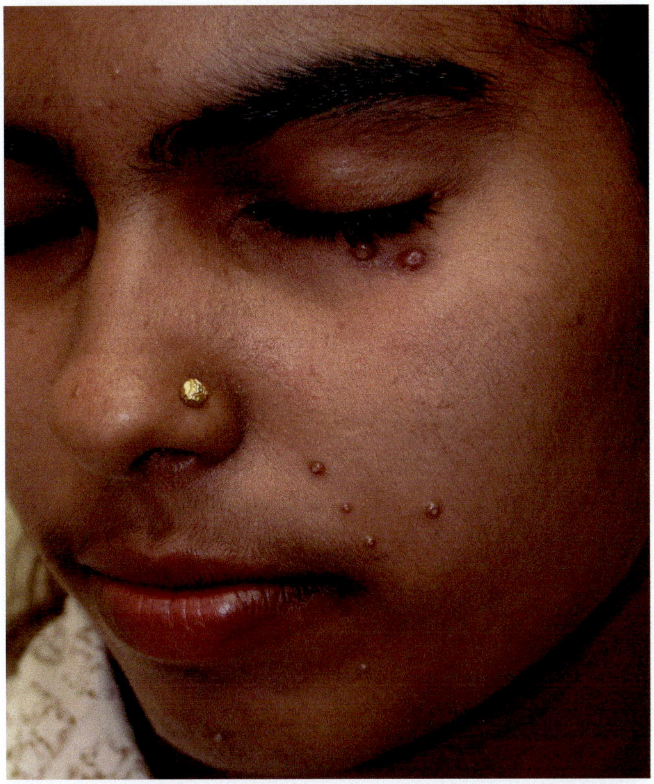

Figure 6.44 Multiple discrete, dome-shaped, pearly white, umbilicated papules molluscum contagiosum over the face.

- In children and immunocompetent patients, the lesion usually presents as asymptomatic, single or multiple, discrete, dome-shaped, pearly white papules of variable size, with central umbilication and usually resolves spontaneously over weeks or months (**Figure 6.44**). Pseudo-Koebnerization may be observed and, when present, is a valuable clinical clue.
- In immunosuppressed patients, atypical variants such as giant molluscum (> 1.5 cm), mucosal lesions, molluscum presenting as an abscess, molluscum without an umblication, tender molluscum, nodular molluscum, or rarely agminate type have been reported.
- DD: Milia (absence of umblication), closed comedones, vellus hair cyst, epidermoid cyst, cryptococcosis (in immunosuppressed patients).

## Neurofibroma

- Patients with neurofibromatosis type 1 (NF1) may develop facial neurofibromas, along with generalized neurofibromas and other features of NF1.
- Facial neurofibromas present as asymptomatic, soft, skin-colored to pigmented, papulonodular lesions which may be sessile, or pedunculated (**Figure 6.45a,b**).
- DD: PKDL, lymphoma, lepromatous leprosy.

## Nevus sebaceous

- Nevus sebaceous may present on the face. Initially the lesion starts as hairless, solitary, linear or round, slightly raised, yellow, orange or tan plaque since birth or soon

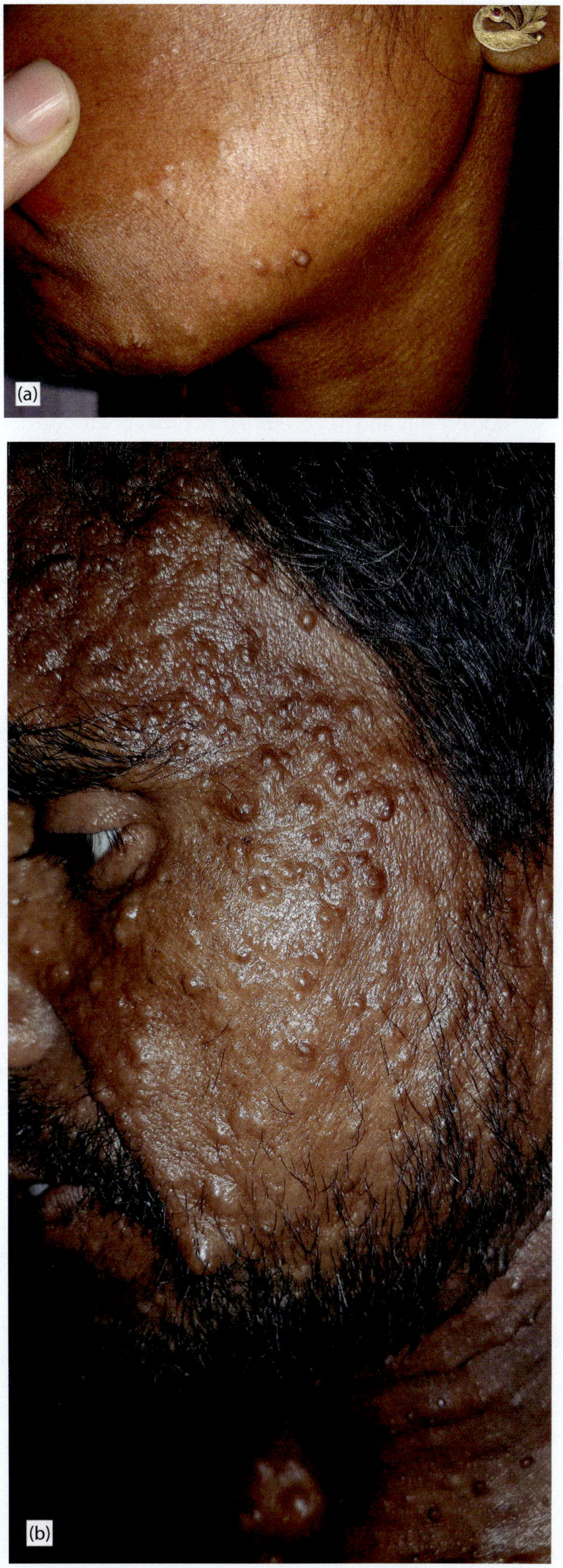



Figure 6.45 **(a)** Skin-colored papules of neurofibromatosis type 1. **(b)** Neurofibromatosis type 1 with multiple, slightly pigmented, papulonodular lesions over the face. (b – Courtesy: Dr. PC Das, Katihar, India.)

after. At puberty, the lesion starts growing and develops papulonodular lesions with a verrucous surface or mammillated appearance (**Figure 6.46**).

- Later in life, the lesion may develop various appendageal tumors; syringocystadenoma papilliferum and trichoblastoma are most common tumors developing in nevus sebaceous.
- DD: Wart, verrucous epidermal nevus.

## Viral warts

- **Verruca plana** (plane warts) are benign skin tumors caused by infection with human papillomavirus, type 3, and less commonly, 10, 27, and 41.
    - The disease is more common in children and adolescents and has no sexual or racial predisposition. Immunocompromised individuals and those who are on immunosuppressant treatment are at risk of developing large, extensive, and resistant warts.
    - The lesions are smooth, flat-topped, round or polygonal in shape, varying from 1–5 mm or more in diameter, usually skin-colored or may be pigmented, and affecting mainly the face, neck, and extremities (**Figure 6.47a–c**). Pseudo Koebnerization is seen in most of the cases.
    - DD: Syringoma, pityriasis versicolor.
- **Filiform warts** are digitate papules with verrucous tops. These warts are particularly common on the face (**Figure 6.47d**).
- DD: Skin tag.
- **Verruca vulgaris** (common warts)
    - These are hyperkeratotic papules with an irregular surface.
    - They can occur on any part of body, hands being the commonest site. They can be seen on face too (**Figure 6.47e**)
    - DD: Seborrhoeic keratosis, lichen planus, keratoacanthoma.

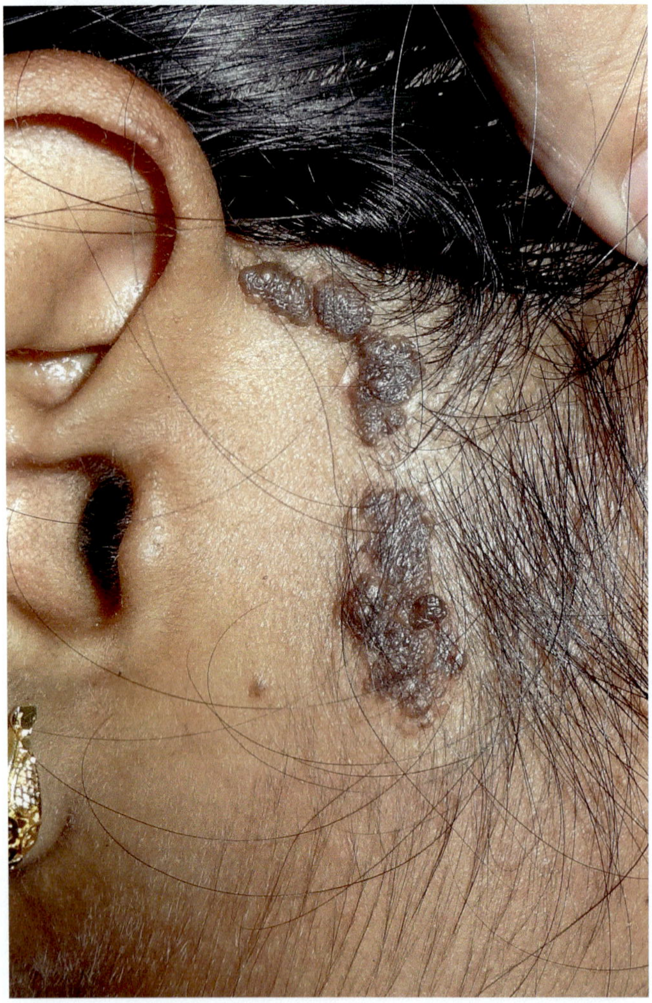

Figure 6.46 Nevus sebaceous presenting as multiple linear tan plaque and grouped papulonodular lesions with verrucous surface over the right auricular area.

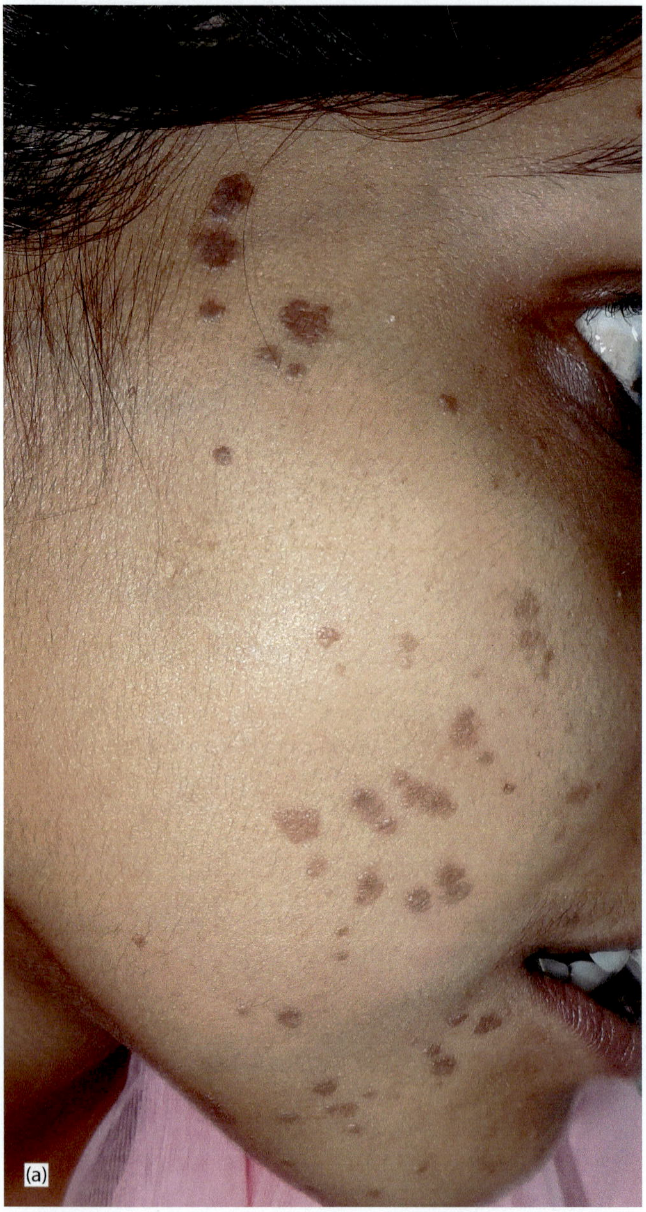


Figure 6.47 **(a)** Multiple flat-topped, round or polygonal, slightly pigmented papules of verruca plana. *(Continued)*

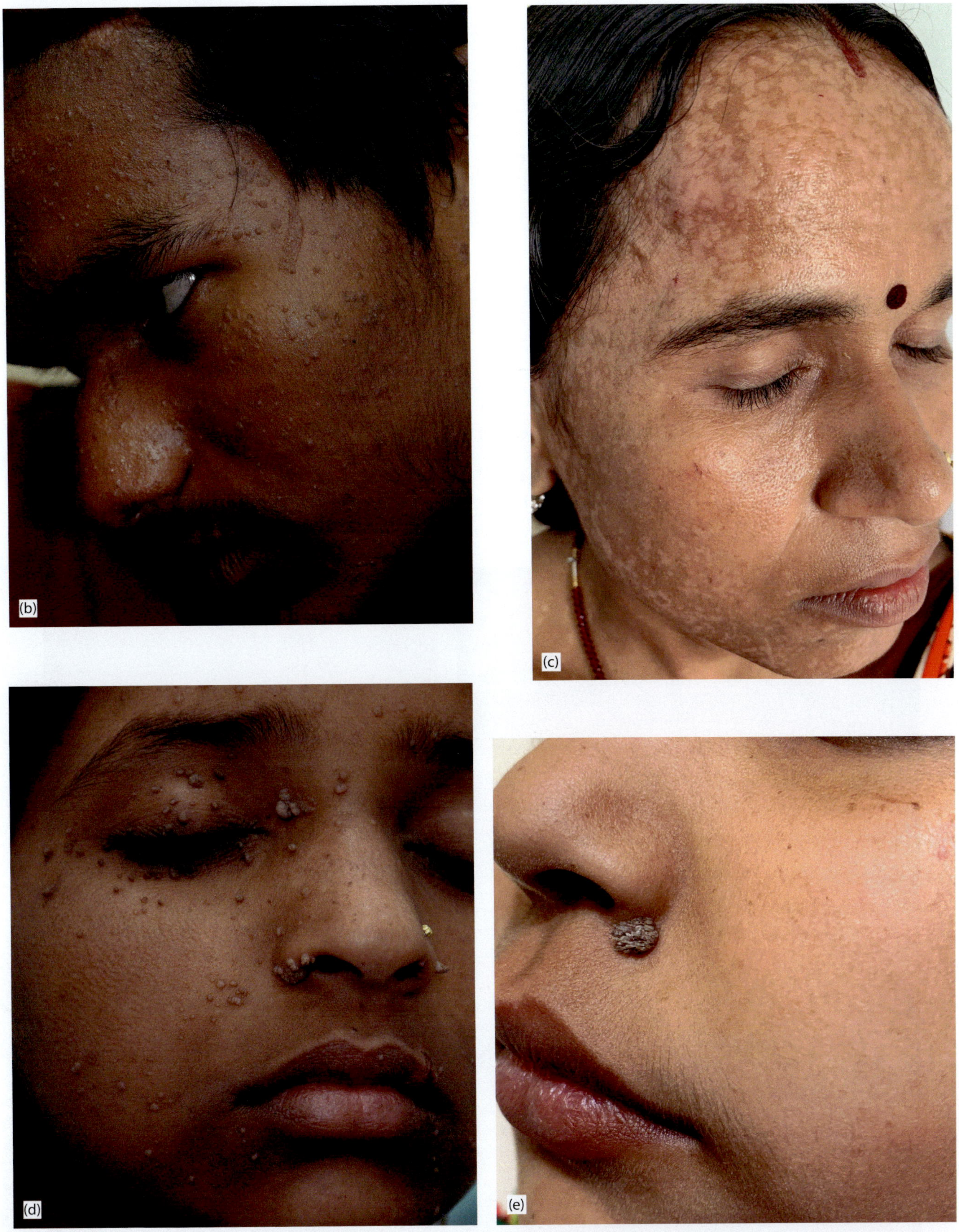

Figure 6.47 (*Continued*) **(b)** Skin-colored papules of verruca plana. Note linear arrangement of lesions (pseudo-Koebnerization, black arrow). **(c)** Multiple coalescing hypopigmented papules of verruca plana. **(d)** Multiple digitate papules of filiform warts on face. **(e)** Solitary verrucous papule of common wart on face.

## Seborrheic keratosis (SK)

- SK is the most common benign epidermal tumor, resulting from a clonal expansion of a mutated epidermal keratinocyte and appearing on hair-bearing areas. Mucosa, palms, and soles are spared.
- SK is more common in Caucasian populations with no gender predilection. They start to appear in middle age and increase in number throughout life.
- SK presents as multiple asymptomatic (sometimes pruritic), well-circumscribed, light-tan to dark-brown or black, round to oval macules, patches, papules, or plaques with a keratotic (rough) or waxy surface. Lesions have a "stuck-on" appearance, a valuable clinical clue for diagnosis (**Figure 6.48a,b**). Many lesions develop keratotic plugging of the surface and become thicker over time.
- Manipulation might lead to swelling, oozing or bleeding, crusting and darkening of the lesion (irritated SK).
- Sign of Leser-Trélat (eruptive SK) is known as a sign of internal malignancy, most commonly associated with adenocarcinoma of gastrointestinal tract. But it may be rarely seen with non-cancerous conditions such as inflammatory dermatoses and drug reactions.
- Clinical variants of SK:
  - Stucco keratosis (keratosis alba) – superficial gray to light-brown flat keratotic lesions over acral areas (dorsa of the hands and feet, the ankles, forearms).
  - Melanoacanthoma – deeply pigmented SK.
  - Polypoid lesions – small polypoidal lesions at the site of friction (neck, under the breast, or in the axillae). They mimic skin tags but have furrowed rough surfaces.
  - Dermatosis papulosa nigra.
- DD: Verruca vulgaris, junctional nevus, compound nevus.

## Verrucous epidermal nevus

- This is clinically characterized by skin-colored to dirty-brown or black irregular/verrucous papules distributed along the lines of Blaschko.

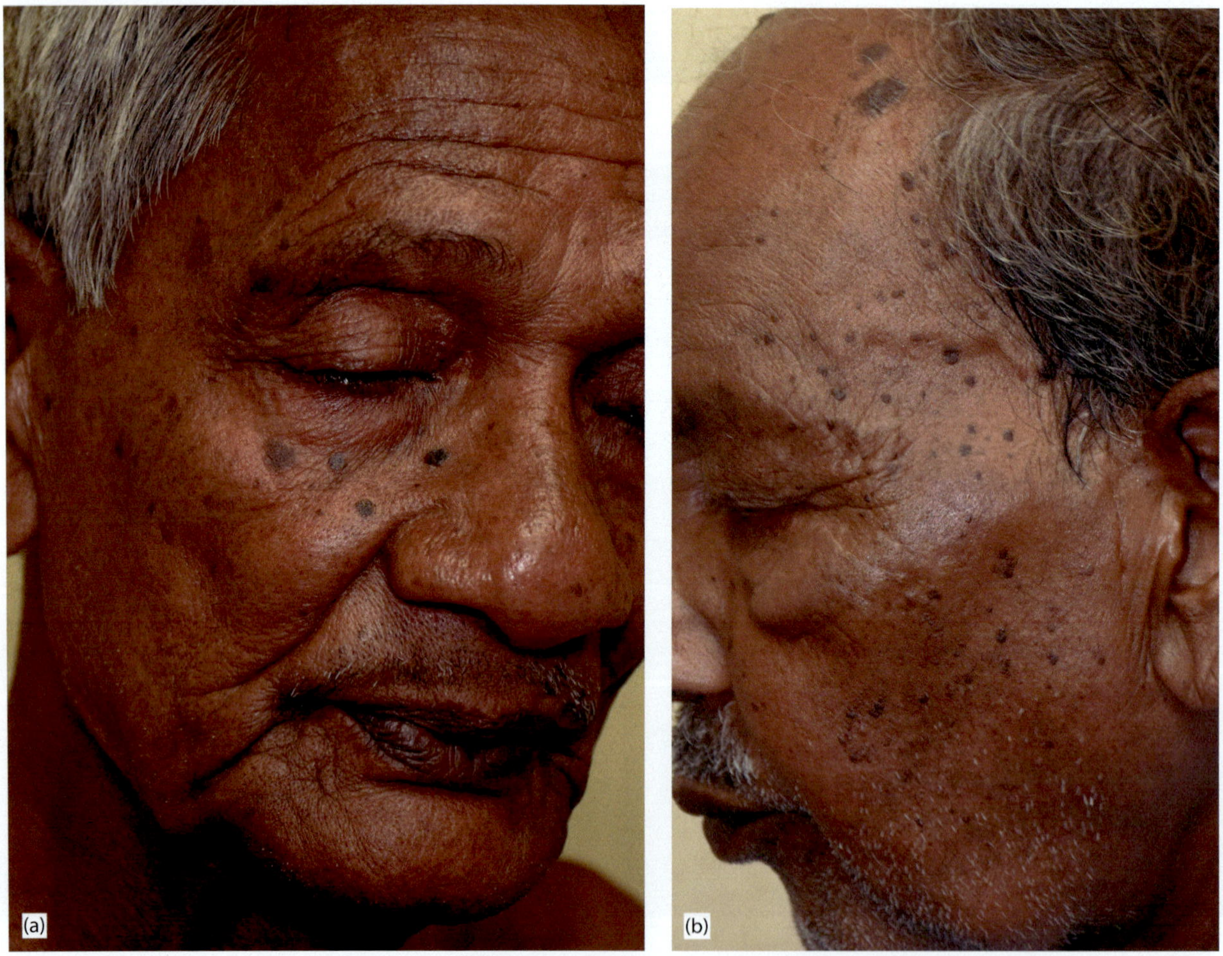


Figure 6.48 **(a)** Multiple pigmented papules and plaques of seborrheic keratosis. Note stuck-on appearance of lesions. **(b)** Seborrheic keratosis seen as sharply demarcated, pigmented, papules and plaques with a keratotic surface over the face.

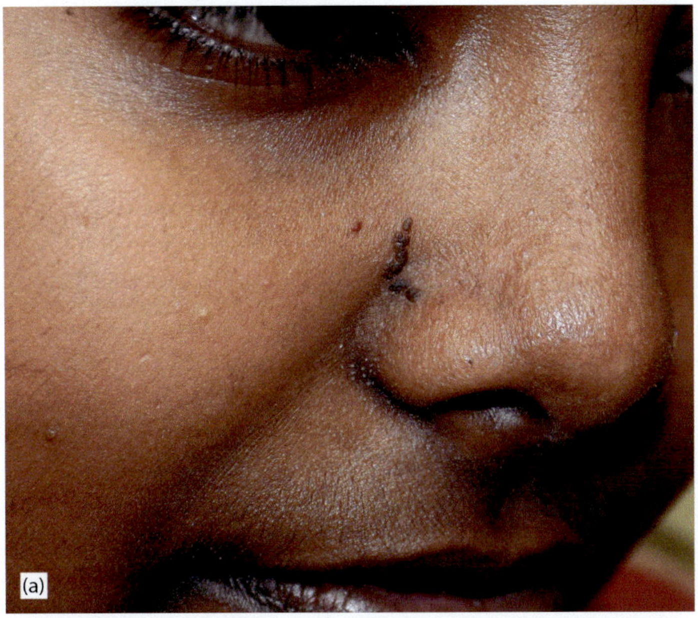

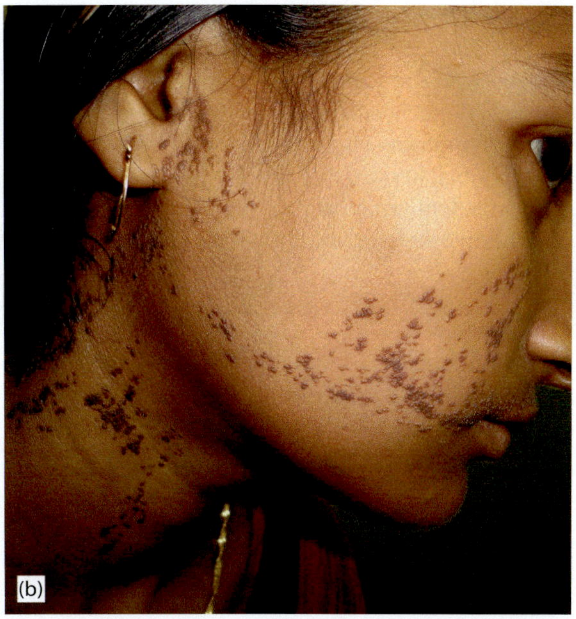

Figure 6.49 **(a)** Verrucous epidermal nevus seen as dirty-looking, pigmented, verrucous papules distributed along the lines of Blaschko. **(b)** Multiple linear bands of verrucous epidermal nevus along the lines of Blaschko.

- They often coalesce to form linear plaques (**Figure 6.49a,b**).
- They usually appear at birth or in childhood.
- They can occur on any part of body, unilaterally or bilaterally.
- DD: Nevoid psoriasis, linear lichen planus, Blaschkitis.

## Basaloid follicular hamartoma (BFH)

- BFH is a rare, benign neoplasm of the hair follicle, caused by mutation of the PTCH gene.
- BFH usually presents as single or multiple 1- to 2-mm brown to dark-colored papules on the face, scalp, and neck.
- Five clinical forms are recognized:
    - Solitary or multiple papules
    - Localized linear papules/plaques (linear unilateral basaloid follicular hamartoma (LUBFH) or linear unilateral basal cell nevus)
    - Localized papules with associated alopecia
    - Generalized papules associated with myasthenia gravis and alopecia (Brown-Crounse syndrome)
    - Generalized autosomal dominant familial type without associated disorder, but with other associated findings including milia, comedone-like lesions, palmar pitting, hypohidrosis, and hypotrichosis
- Multiple BFH are also noted in nevoid basal cell carcinoma syndrome (Gorlin syndrome or basal cell nevus syndrome) and Bazex-Dupré-Christol syndrome.

## Keratosis follicularis spinulosa decalvans

- KFSD is a disorder of epidermal differentiation caused by impaired cholesterol and lipid metabolism in epidermis. It is an X-linked condition, and males are mostly affected. It is one of the entities included under the umbrella term keratosis pilaris atrophicans (KPA) (**Box 6.1**).

### BOX 6.1: Keratosis pilaris atrophicans (KPA)

KPA is characterized by follicular keratotic papules that heal by atrophy and/or alopecia. Additional findings common to this group of disorders are an atopic tendency and keratosis pilaris on the extensor surfaces of the extremities. It includes the following:

- Keratosis pilaris atrophicans faciei (KPAF)/ulerythema ophryogenes – onset in first few months of life; common in boys; presents with erythema and follicular keratotic papules on the lateral third of the eyebrows. Disease progresses to atrophy and alopecia, which may extend to the cheeks and forehead.
- Atrophoderma vermiculatum (AV) – usually in children (before puberty); erythematous follicular keratotic papules that slowly progress to the characteristic reticular atrophy; described as worm-eaten, reticular, or honeycomb atrophy. Occurs on the cheeks, preauricular area, and forehead.
- Keratosis follicularis spinulosa decalvans (KFSD).

- The skin lesions develop within the first month of life and are characterized by follicular keratotic papules, especially on the scalp and face, associated with scarring alopecia of the scalp, eyelashes, and eyebrows.
- Ocular symptoms are prominent and include photophobia, keratitis, conjunctivitis, congenital glaucoma, lenticular cataract, and corneal dystrophy.
- DD: Ichthyosis follicularis alopecia photophobia (IFAP) syndrome.

## Histiocytoses

- The histiocytoses are a group of disorders characterized by abnormal proliferation and accumulation of cells of the mononuclear phagocytic system consisting of Langerhans cells, macrophages, and dendritic cells.
- Histiocytoses are broadly grouped into Langerhans cell histiocytoses (LCH) and non-LCH, based on predominant infiltrating cells – Langerhans cell in LCH and dermal dendritic cells (and cells with phenotype of other than Langerhans cells and dermal dendrocytes) in non-LCH.
- The major histiocytoses that may present with or develop facial papules are summarized in **Table 6.5**.

## Colloid milium

- Colloid milium refers to a group of degenerative, cutaneous deposition disorders related to excessive sun exposure (and hydroquinone use) and is characterized by amorphous, hyaline-like deposits in the dermis.

Table 6.5 Facial papules in histiocytoses

| Disease | Onset | Cutaneous features | Predominantly affected sites | Extracutaneous/ Systemic features |
|---|---|---|---|---|
| **Langerhans cell histiocytosis** | | | | |
| **Letterer-Siwe Disease** (**Figure 6.50a,b**) | Children 2-3 years | Yellow-brown scaly papules, petechiae and crust | Seborrheic area, intertriginous areas | Fever, anemia, thrombocytopenia, pulmonary infiltrates, hepatosplenomegaly, lymphadenopathy. |
| **Hashimoto-Pritzker disease** | At birth or Infancy | Multiple, red-brown papules, nodules, or vesicles<br>Spontaneous resolution is noted | Generalized | Lymph nodes, bones, liver, and lungs involvement |
| **Non-Langerhans cell histiocytosis** | | | | |
| **Juvenile xanthogranuloma (Figure 6.50c,d)** | Infants and young children | Solitary or multiple firm rubbery, yellow brown papules and nodules | Head and neck (including face) | Eye, lungs, central nervous system, and bone lesions |
| **Benign cephalic histiocytosis** | Infants and young children | Yellow to red-brown macules and papules<br>Lesions heal with hyperpigmentation and may vanish completely over months or years. | Face (cheeks, forehead, ears), and neck | Diabetes insipidus (rare) |
| **Generalized eruptive histiocytosis** | Adults | Recurrent crops of red to brown papules<br>Lesions resolve with hyperpigmented macules or small scars | Generalized – face, trunk, proximal extremities<br>Flexures are spared | None |
| **Papular xanthoma** | Adults | Yellow or yellow-red papulonodular lesions with no tendency to coalesce<br>Lesions may heal with anetoderma-like scarring | Head, back | Patients are normolipemic<br>No systemic involvement |
| **Progressive nodular histiocytosis (Figure 6.50e)** | Adults | Superficial yellow-orange papules | Random | Oral cavity, larynx, and conjunctival mucosa involvement |
| **Xanthoma disseminatum (Figure 6.50f,g)** | Young children | Round to oval, orange to yellow-brown papules and nodules occurring over flexures | Flexures – neck, axilla, antecubital fossa, perianal area, and groins<br>Mucosal involvement | Diabetes insipidus |

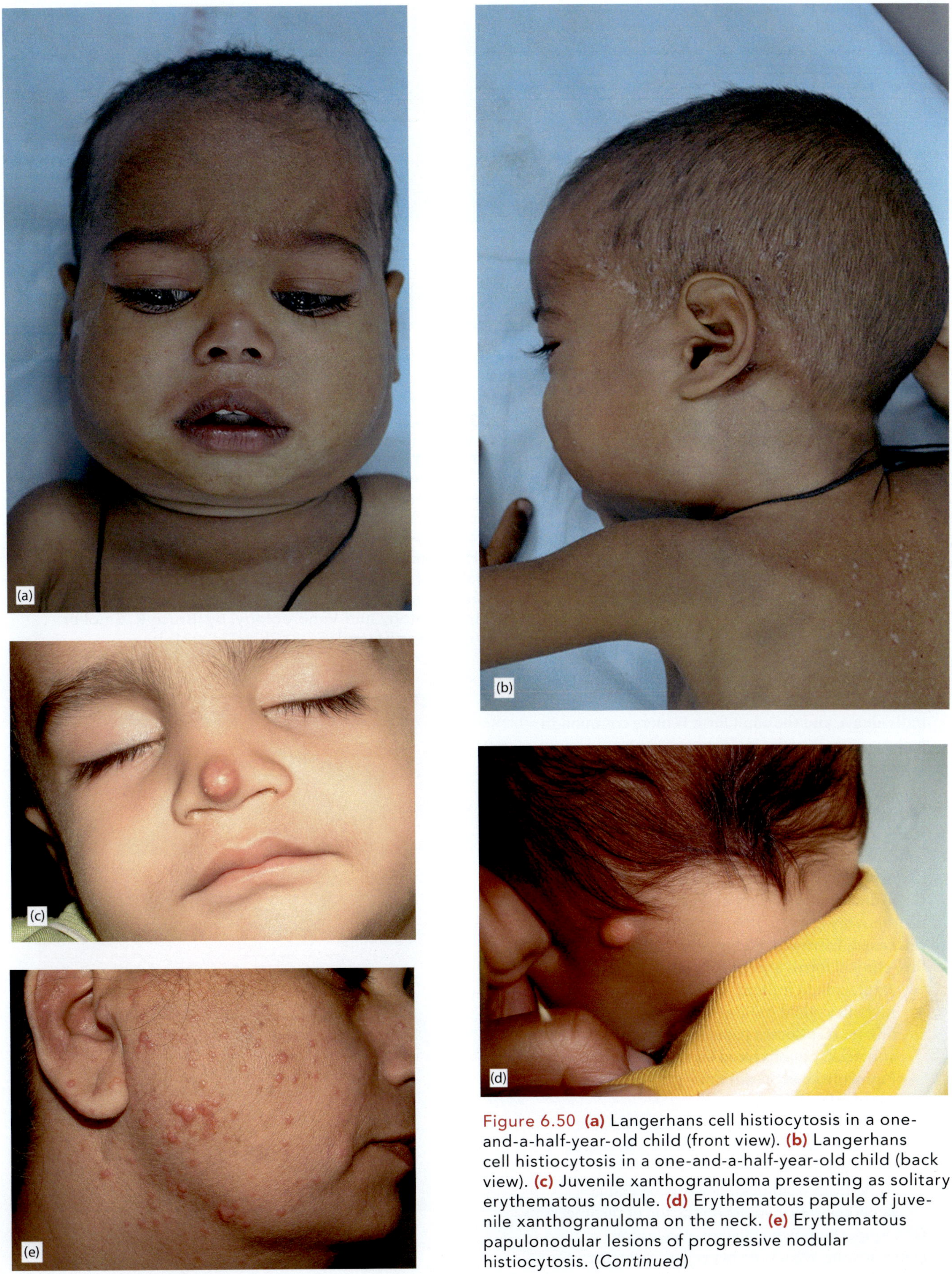


Figure 6.50 **(a)** Langerhans cell histiocytosis in a one-and-a-half-year-old child (front view). **(b)** Langerhans cell histiocytosis in a one-and-a-half-year-old child (back view). **(c)** Juvenile xanthogranuloma presenting as solitary erythematous nodule. **(d)** Erythematous papule of juvenile xanthogranuloma on the neck. **(e)** Erythematous papulonodular lesions of progressive nodular histiocytosis. (*Continued*)

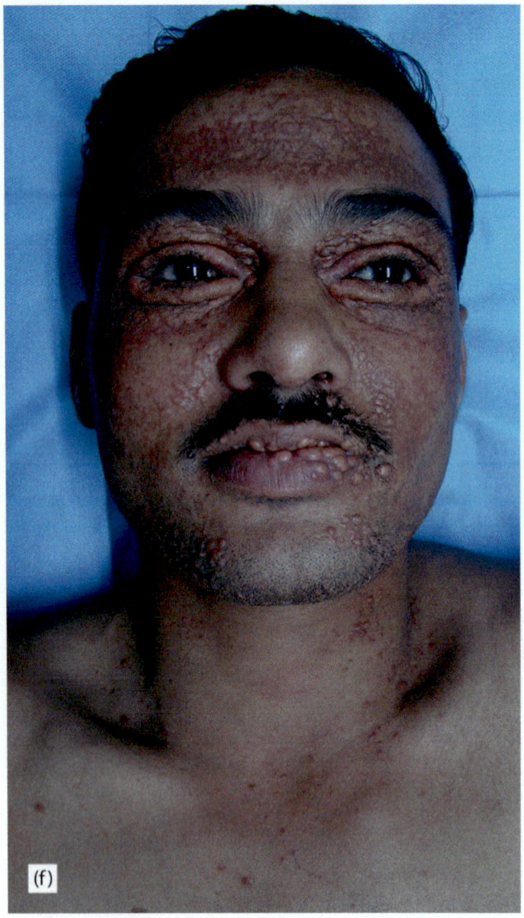


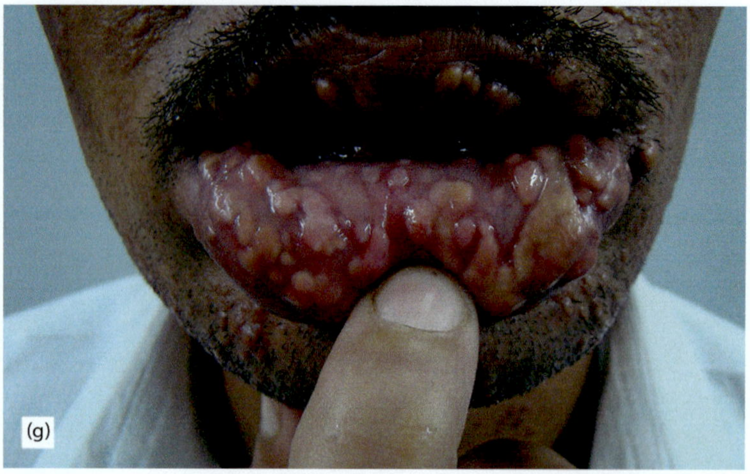


Figure 6.50 (*Continued*) **(f)** Yellow-orange confluent papules, plaques, and nodules in Xanthoma disseminatum in a young man. **(g)** Mucosal lesions in Xanthoma disseminatum. (a,b,f – Courtesy: Dr. Sudhir Singh, Department of Dermatology and Venereology, Jawahar Lal Institute of Medical Sciences, Nagpur, India; c,e – Courtesy: Dr. Neena Khanna, Department of Dermatology and Venereology, All India Institute of Medical Science, New Delhi, India; d – Courtesy: Dr. Santosh Rathod, SVPIMSR, Smt. NHL Municipal Medical College, V.S. Hospital, Ahmedabad.) [a–c, e–g: Reprinted by permission from Springer International Publishing [Atlas of Dermatology, Dermatopathology and Venereology] by [Bruce R. Smoller and Nooshin Bagherani] [COPYRIGHT] (2021).]

- The condition is more common in light-skinned individuals, and the adult form is more common in males.
- Lesions on the face are common on the cheeks, periorbital area, nose, and ears. Other commonly affected sites are the neck, hands, and forearms.
- Clinically, it is characterized by waxy, partially translucent, firm papules ranging from 1–5 mm in diameter (**Figure 6.51**). The lesions appear in crops. Gelatinous material can be expressed. The underlying skin shows signs of actinic damage and may be thickened, furrowed, and hyperpigmented.
- Five clinical forms are recognized:
  - Adult colloid milium – described above.
  - Juvenile colloid milium – clusters of small, yellow-brown, translucent papules and plaques on the face and neck. Lesions bleed on minor trauma.
  - Pigmented colloid milium – gray-black clustered papules on the face.
  - Nodular colloid milium – solitary nodule or plaque on chronically sun-exposed skin, particularly the face.
  - Acral form – painless, slowly progressive, hyperkeratotic papules on the top of the fingertips.
- DD: Epidermal inclusion cyst, molluscum contagiosum, sebaceous hyperplasia, steatocystoma multiplex.

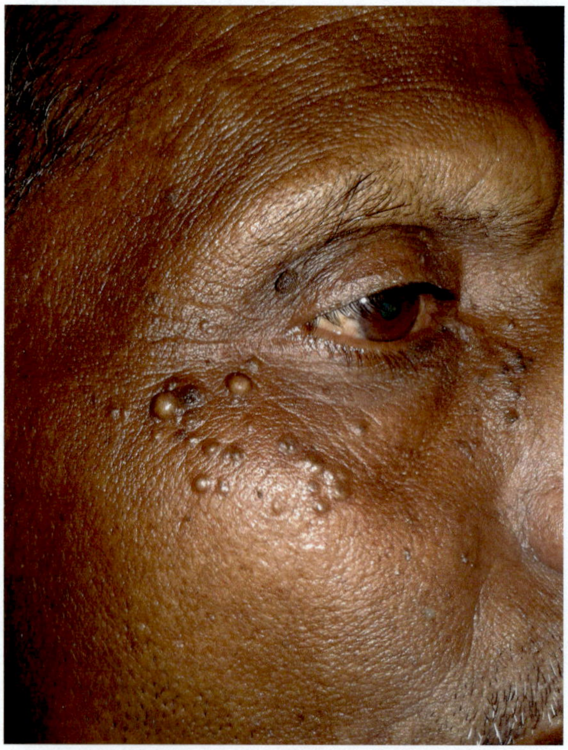

Figure 6.51 Colloid milium seen as multiple waxy, firm, yellowish papules below the right lateral canthus. (Courtesy: Dr. PC Das, Katihar, India.)

## Lipoid proteinosis

- Lipoid proteinosis is a rare autosomal recessive genodermatosis caused by mutations in the gene encoding extracellular matrix protein 1 (ECM1) and is characterized by the deposition of an amorphous hyaline material in the skin, mucosa, and viscera.
- There is no racial or sex predilection. Patients usually present in infancy and early childhood. The pathognomonic feature is a hoarse cry due to laryngeal infiltration.
- The earliest skin findings are vesicobullous lesions, erosions, and crusts on skin and mucosa. Face and extremities are most commonly involved, and lesions heal with pox-like atrophic scarring.
- As the child grows, there is dermal infiltration resulting in thickened, waxy, yellowish skin and the appearance of papules, plaques, and nodules on the face. Moniliform blepharosis (multiple papules along the eyelid margins, resembling a string of pearls) is considered a cutaneous hallmark of the disease (**Figure 6.52**).
- Patients may develop hyperkeratotic plaques on sites of trauma – elbows, knees, and dorsum of the hands.
- Associated findings are woody firmness and impaired mobility of the tongue, cobblestone appearance of mucosa, and patchy or diffuse hair loss.
- CNS features include seizures, behavioral changes, learning difficulties, and rage attacks may be observed.
- DD: Colloid milium, Lichen myxedematosus.

## Tinea faciei

- Tinea faciei is a dermatophytic infection that occurs over the face in women and prepubertal boys, and non-bearded areas of men.
- It can affect all age groups, with two peaks – children between 2 and 14 years, and adults 20–40 years of age.

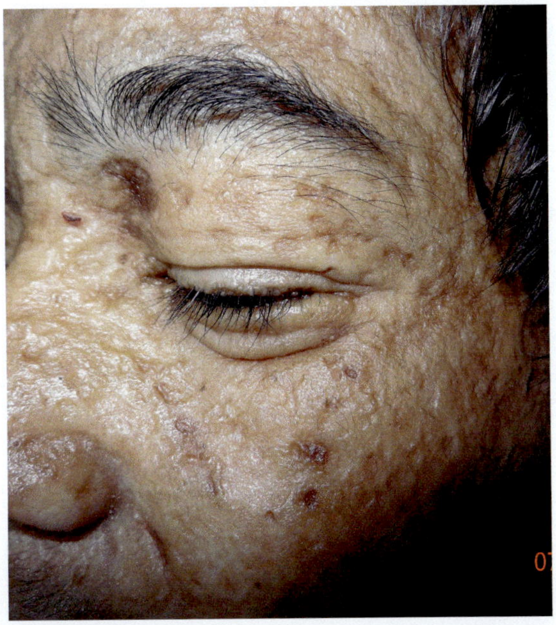

Figure 6.52 Papules on the eyelid margin in lipoid proteinosis. Note waxy, yellowish thickened skin and pock-like scars at places.

- Clinically it appears as single or multiple erythematous, scaly, annular, or polycyclic plaque with papules, pustules, and crusting at the margin. The lesion spreads centrifugally, with a clear, hypopigmented center (**Figure 6.53a,b**). It may be associated with itching, burning, or photosensitivity.

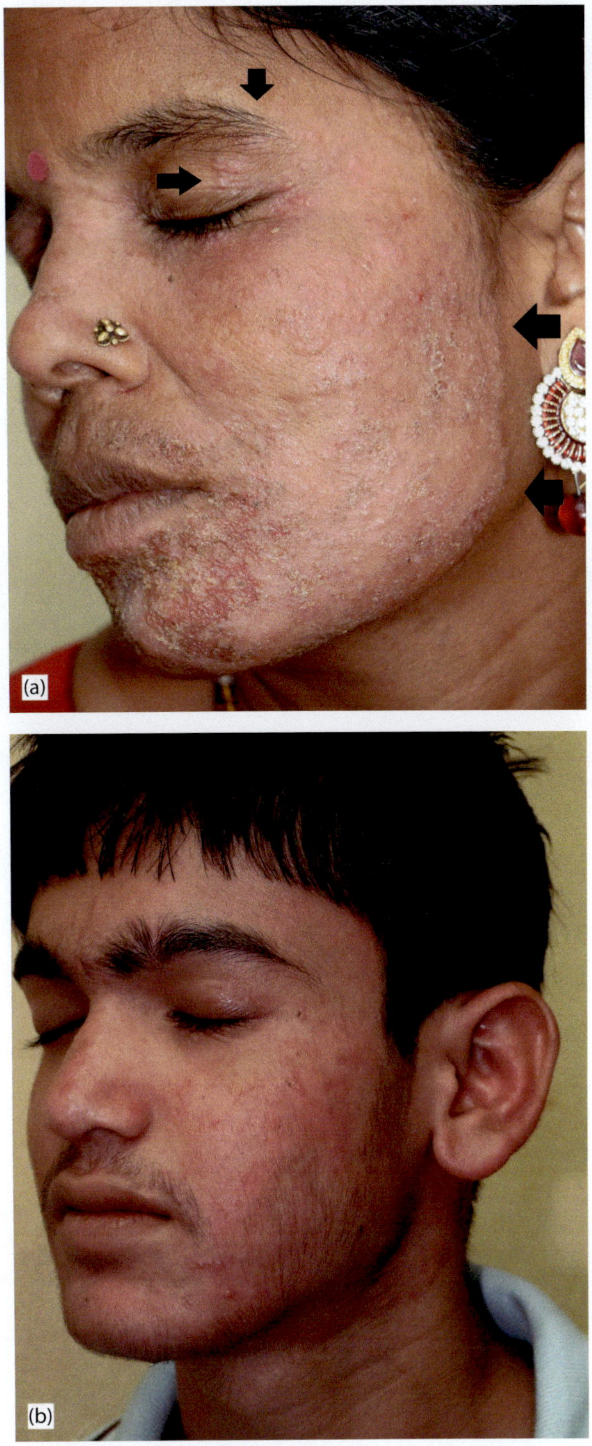


Figure 6.53 **(a)** Steroid-modified tinea presenting as erythematous scaly papules, erosions, and crusts on a background of erythematous skin. Note the margin of the lesion (black arrow), a clue to the diagnosis. **(b)** Erythematous papules on an erythematous face in steroid-modified tinea.

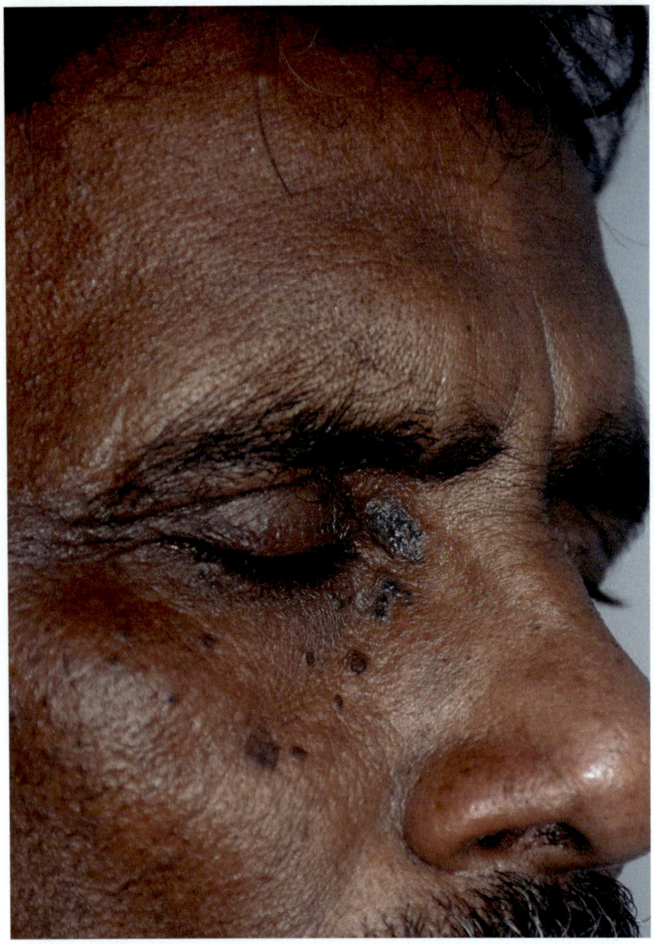

Figure 6.54 Senile comedones – clustered and confluent open comedones near the medial canthus of eye.

- In steroid-modified lesions, central clearing is not obvious. The diagnosis rests on a high index of suspicion.
- DD: Seborrheic dermatitis, atopic dermatitis, contact dermatitis.

Additional image – Figure 6.54

## REFERENCES


1. Marks R. Facial Skin Disorders. 1st edition. Oxford: Informa Healthcare; 2007. P. 1–164
2. Zeichner JA. Acneiform Eruptions in Dermatology A Differential Diagnosis. 1st edition. New York: Springer; 2014. P. 3–404.
3. Ubriani R, Grossman ME. Facial papules as a marker of internal malignancy. Med Clin North Am 2009;93(6):1305–1331.
4. Foreman RK, McDivitt Duncan L. Appendage Tumors of the Skin. In: Kang S, Amagai M, Bruckner AL, Enk AH, Margolis DJ, McMichael AJ, Orringer JS, editors. Fitzpatrick's Dermatology in General Medicine. 9th edition. New York: McGraw Hill; 2019. P. 1820–1856.
5. Basu D, Kumar P, Das A. Unilateral Facial Angiofibromas. Skinmed 2019;17(1):52–53.
6. Chen W, Plewig G. Human demodicosis: Revisit and a proposed classification. Br J Dermatol 2014;170(6):1219–1225.
7. Kumar P, Das A. Gnathophyma. Skinmed 2018;16(1):45.
8. Kumar P, Das A, Barkat R. Persistent perioral papules in a young man. Indian J Dermatol Venereol Leprol 2019;85:407–409.
9. Baughn RE, Musher DE. Secondary Syphilitic Lesions. Clin Microbiol Rev 2005;18(1):205–216.

E5

# Papules: Generalized

NIHARIKA RANJAN LAL

## ABSTRACT

Many conditions may present as generalized papular rash. Various clinical characteristics, such as surface features (scaling, crusting, necrosis), associated vesicular or pustular lesions, and systemic features, are helpful in arriving at clinical diagnosis. This chapter discusses common and uncommon causes of generalized papular rash on the basis of presence/absence of constitutional symptoms and other morphological characteristics.

The text of this chapter is available online at https://routledgetextbooks.com/textbooks/9781032399669/

DOI: 10.1201/9781351054225-13

# E6

# Follicular papules

RAMESH CHANDRA GHARAMI

## ABSTRACT

Follicular papules are centered on the pilosebaceous units. They may present with or without inflammation and have variable clinical features. Often these lesions present a diagnostic challenge due to their similar clinical appearance. This chapter discusses the different conditions presenting with follicular papules and appendageal tumors along with their salient features. Dermatologists need to be aware of these entities for early and accurate diagnosis.

The text of this chapter is available online at https://routledgetextbooks.com/textbooks/9781032399669/

 DOI: 10.1201/9781351054225-14

7

# Plaques: Localized

ANIRBAN DAS

## INTRODUCTION

Conditions presenting as plaques may be localized or generalized in distribution, and may be infective, inflammatory, genetic, or neoplastic in nature. Important clinical pointers include duration of lesions, color, presence or absence of surface changes (scales, follicular plugging, scarring, verrucosity), and consistency of the lesions (succulent, hard). Also, distribution of lesions gives us important input in making a clinical diagnosis. For example, tuberculosis verrucosa cutis is mostly seen on trauma-prone sites, whereas plaques of erythrokeratodermia variabilis are seen over joints, such as knees. This chapter discusses the clinical approach to the diagnosis of localized plaques, outlined in **Table 7.1**, and salient clinical features of different entities are discussed below.[1–7]

## ERYTHEMATOUS PLAQUES

### Psoriasis

- It is a common, chronic, inflammatory, and proliferative condition of the skin.
- Psoriasis presents with well-demarcated, erythematous scaly plaques. Scales are loosely attached and have a typical silvery/micaceous character (**Figure 7.1a,b**).
- Auspitz phenomenon – Repeated scratching with a glass slide results in a wet surface with characteristic pinpoint bleeding (Auspitz sign) on removal of the scaly membrane. Demonstration of Auspitz sign is considered diagnostic (**Figure 7.1c**).
- Koebnerization may be seen (**Figure 7.1d**).
- The lesions may be localized (affecting any part of the body) or generalized, with striking involvement of extensor aspects of the extremities (**Figure 7.1e**).
- Occasionally, a white blanching ring around the lesion, known as the Woronoff ring, may be seen.
- Palmoplantar psoriasis – a notable localized form of psoriasis. May remain localized or may be associated with a widespread disease.
    - Typically scaly patches on which a fine silvery scale can be evoked by scratching.
    - DD: lichen simplex chronicus, hyperkeratotic eczema (less-defined margin, history of vesicles).
- Scalp psoriasis – another notable localized form of psoriasis.
    - Whole scalp may be diffusely involved, or multiple discrete plaques of varying size may be seen (**Figure 7.1f**).
    - Usually restricted to hair-bearing areas, extending a short distance beyond the hairline and around the ear.
    - DD: Pityriasis amiantacea, seborrheic dermatitis.
- Genital psoriasis – a notable localized form of psoriasis.
    - Males: The glans penis is the most affected part. In circumcised men, lesions are similar to appearance at other sites. In the uncircumcised, the plaques lack the scale but the color and well-defined edge are usually distinctive (**Figure 7.1g**). DD: Erythroplasia of Queyrat, plasma cell balanitis.
    - Females: The most common presentation is a symmetrical, non-scaly, well-demarcated thin plaque affecting the labia majora, associated with marked pruritus.
    - DD: chronic erythematous vulvitis without vaginitis.

### Leprosy[8]

- Varied manifestations depending on underlying cell-mediated immunity and degree of proliferation of *Mycobacterium leprae.*
- Tuberculoid pole (TT and BT leprosy) has a few lesions and a few thickened peripheral nerve trunks. Lesions in tuberculoid pole show lesional hypo/anesthesia, loss of hairs and loss of sweating, and appear dry.
- The lesions in lepromatous pole (BL and LL leprosy) are smaller and numerous, consisting of macules, papules, plaques, and nodules arranged in a bilateral symmetric manner (especially in LL leprosy). The lesions may not show lesional hypoaesthesia (rather, sensory loss in a gloves-and-stockings pattern is seen) and appear shiny and infiltrated (in contrast to tuberculoid pole). Multiple peripheral nerve trunks may be affected in a symmetrical manner, again more so in lepromatous leprosy.

DOI: 10.1201/9781351054225-15

Table 7.1 Clinical approach to localized plaque

| Onset | Striking feature | Additional clues | Diseases |
|---|---|---|---|
| Acquired | Erythematous | Scaly plaques | • Silvery scales – psoriasis<br>• Greasy scales – seborrheic dermatitis<br>• Ichthyotic – pityriasis rotunda, erythrokeratodermia variabilis, progressive symmetric erythrokeratoderma<br>• Scales on active margin – tinea corporis<br>• Collarette of scales – pityriasis rosea<br>• Adherent scales – actinic keratosis, discoid lupus erythematosus<br>• Violaceous – lichen planus |
| | | Associated with hair loss | Leprosy, alopecia mucinosa |
| | | Loss of sensation | Leprosy |
| | | Sun-exposed area | Discoid lupus erythematosus, polymorphous light eruption, Jessner's lymphocytic infiltration, tumid lupus erythematosus |
| | | Acral | • Scaly – psoriasis (extensors), secondary syphilis<br>• Firm, around joints – xanthoma (yellowish lesions), erythema elevatum diutinum<br>• Pagetoid reticulosis |
| | | Peau d'orange appearance | Sweet syndrome, erysipelas, cellulitis, urticaria* |
| | | Annular, skin-colored | Granuloma annulare |
| | | Miscellaneous | Sarcoidosis, granuloma multiforme, cutaneous lymphoid hyperplasia |
| | Hyperkeratotic | Itchy | Lichen simplex chronicus, lichen planus hypertrophicus, |
| | | Usually multiple | Verruca vulgaris (pseudo-Koebnerization seen) |
| | | Usually solitary | • Healing with scarring – lupus vulgaris<br>• Lymphatic spread (in case of multiple lesions), sporotrichosis, cutaneous leishmaniasis<br>• Trauma prone areas – tuberculosis verrucosa cutis, chromomycosis<br>• Mycobacterium marinum<br>• Verrucous xanthoma<br>• Benign lichenoid keratosis |
| | | Annular | Porokeratosis (see Chapter 23) |
| | Non-scaly plaques | Pigmented | Seborrheic keratosis, melanocytic nevus |
| | | Skin/pale-colored | Mastocytoma, shagreen patch, granuloma annulare (annular) |
| | | Erythematous | Mastocytoma, polymorphic eruption of pregnancy, urticaria* |
| | Atrophic | | Morphea, lichen sclerosus et atrophicus (prominent follicular openings) |
| | Ulcerated plaques | Erythematous | Necrobiotic lipoidica, Bowen's disease, Paget's disease, extramammary Paget's disease |
| | | Pigmented | Basal cell carcinoma |
| | | Macerated | Pemphigus vegetans |
| Congenital | Yellow/pale-colored | | Milia en plaque, nevus sebaceous, nevus lipomatosus superficialis, collagen nevus |
| | Hyperpigmented | | Verrucous epidermal nevus, verrucous hemangioma |
| | Erythematous | | Hemangioma (vascular), inflammatory linear verrucous epidermal nevus (linear) |

* The lesion in urticaria is a wheal. It has been included here for clinical similarity with plaque.

- Tuberculoid leprosy (TT) – The lesions consist of one or a few erythematous/hypopigmented patch or plaque. The lesions have a well-defined, elevated margin and are dry, and hairless with complete loss of sensation. Over time, the center of the lesion may get atrophic, giving an annular appearance (**Figure 7.2a**).
- Borderline tuberculoid leprosy (BT) – Lesions of BT leprosy mimic those of TT leprosy but are more in number and larger in size, with less-defined margin. In fact, lesions can be large enough to cover a big part of the extremity. Another characteristic feature is the margin being ill-defined at places, with finger-like

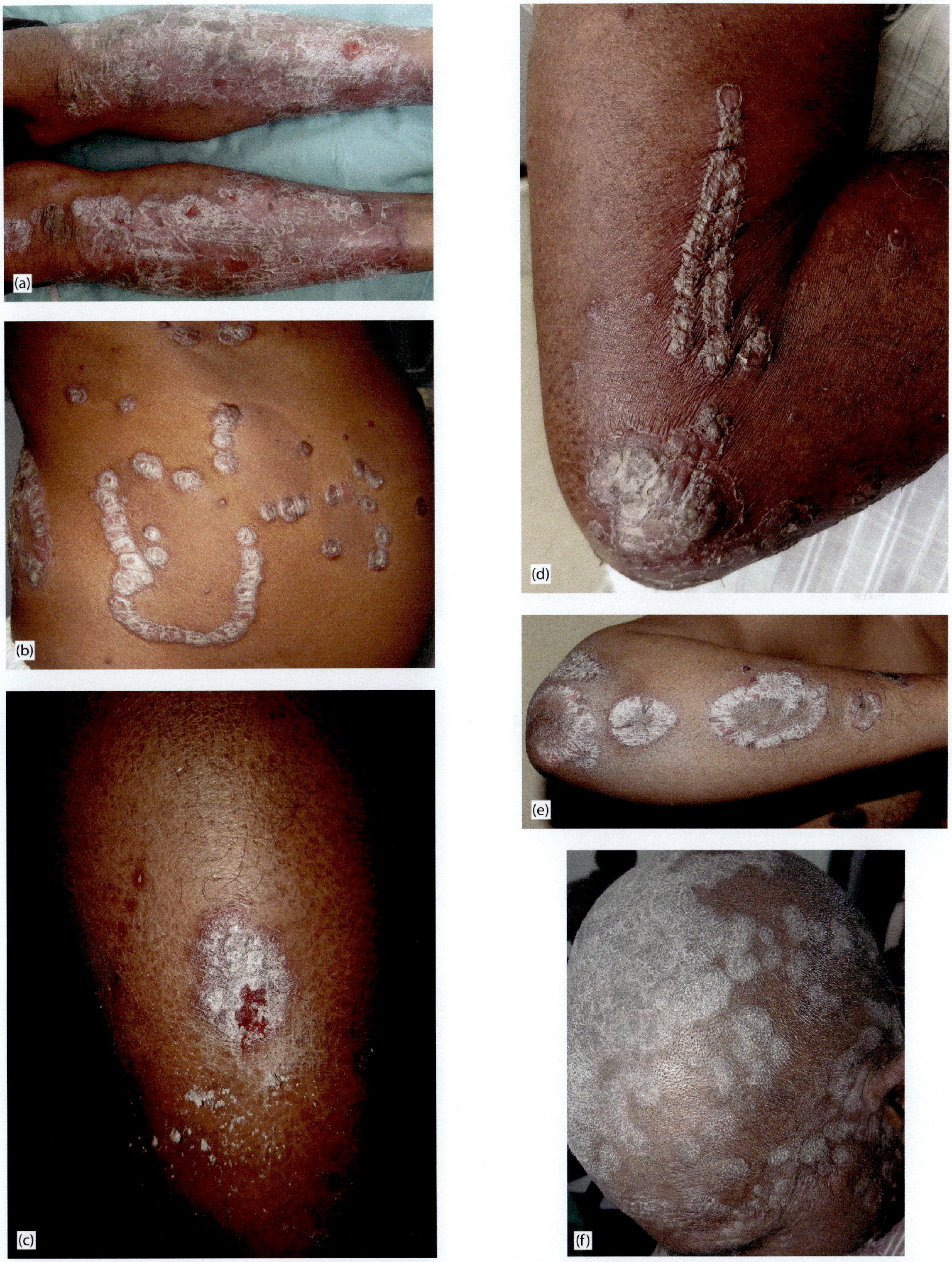


Figure 7.1 **(a)** Silvery scales in psoriasis. **(b)** Arcuate lesions of chronic plaque psoriasis. **(c)** Auspitz sign – pinpoint bleeding on the removal of scales. **(d)** Koebnerization in psoriasis. **(e)** Annular plaques of psoriasis over extensor aspect of the forearm. **(f)** Scalp involvement in psoriasis. (*Continued*)

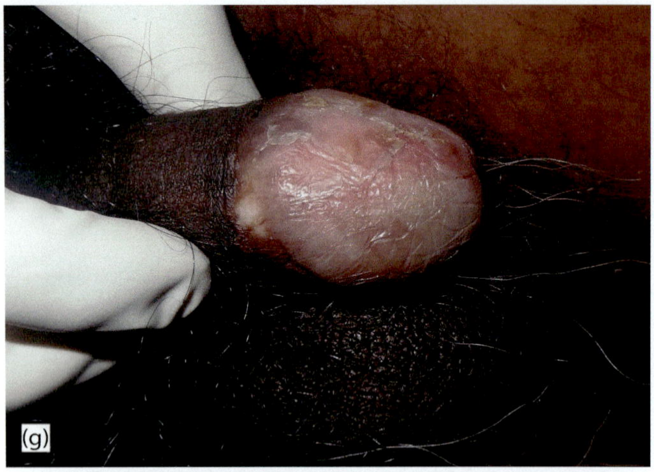

Figure 7.1 (*Continued*) **(g)** Psoriasis over glans penis. (a,b,e–g – Courtesy: Dr. Piyush Kumar, Katihar, India; c,d – Courtesy: Dr. Niharika Ranjan Lal, ESIPGIMSR, Kolkata, India.)

pseudopodia and satellite lesions. The lesions show typical features of leprosy (i.e., hypoaesthesia, hair loss, and loss of sweating) (**Figure 7.2b–g**).

- Localized lepromatous leprosy – A relatively rare presentation of lepromatous leprosy is the solitary lesion with a high bacterial count. This can present as erythematous plaque and may be tender to touch; it is mostly localized over the face (cheek, preauricular region, bridge of nose, and upper eyelid) (**Figure 7.2h**).

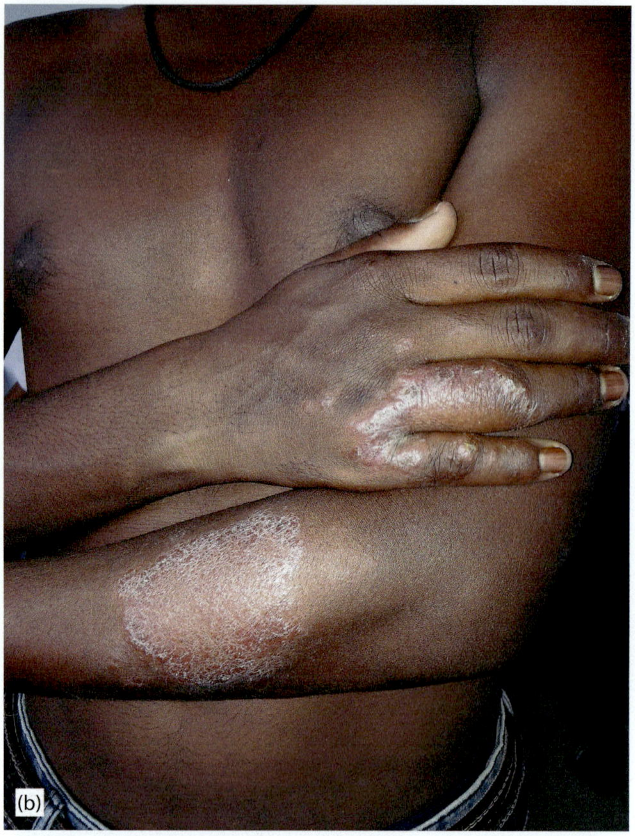

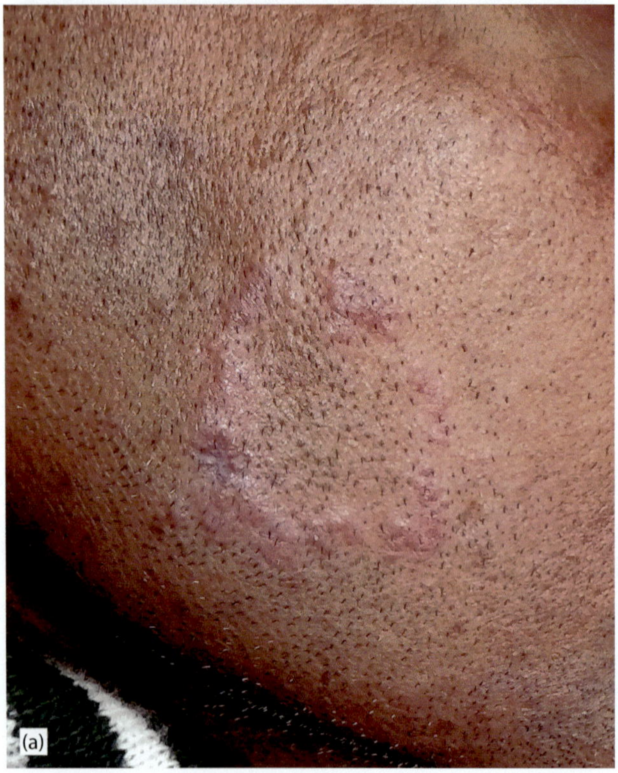

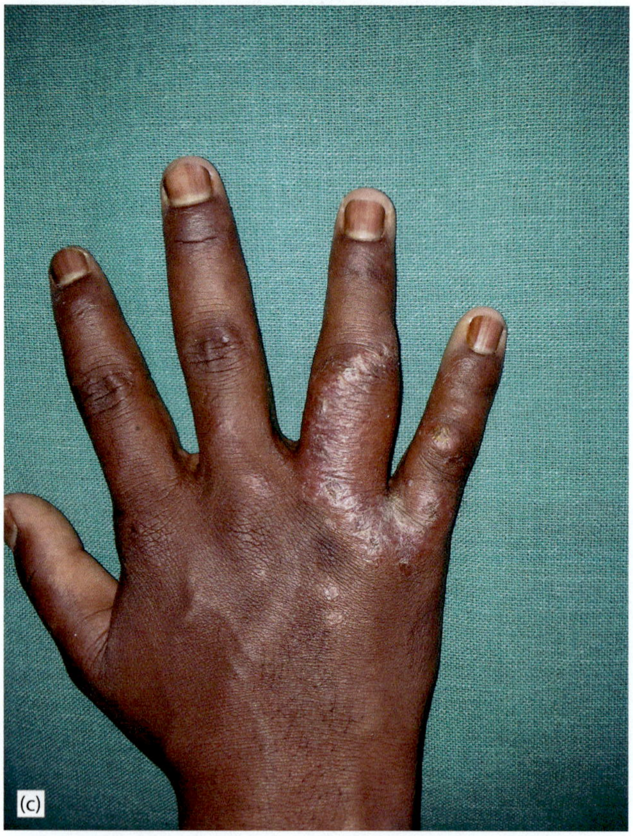

Figure 7.2 **(a)** Annular, erythematous plaque in TT leprosy. **(b)** Two annular plaques of BT leprosy. **(c)** BT leprosy with lesion over dorsum of right hand. (*Continued*)

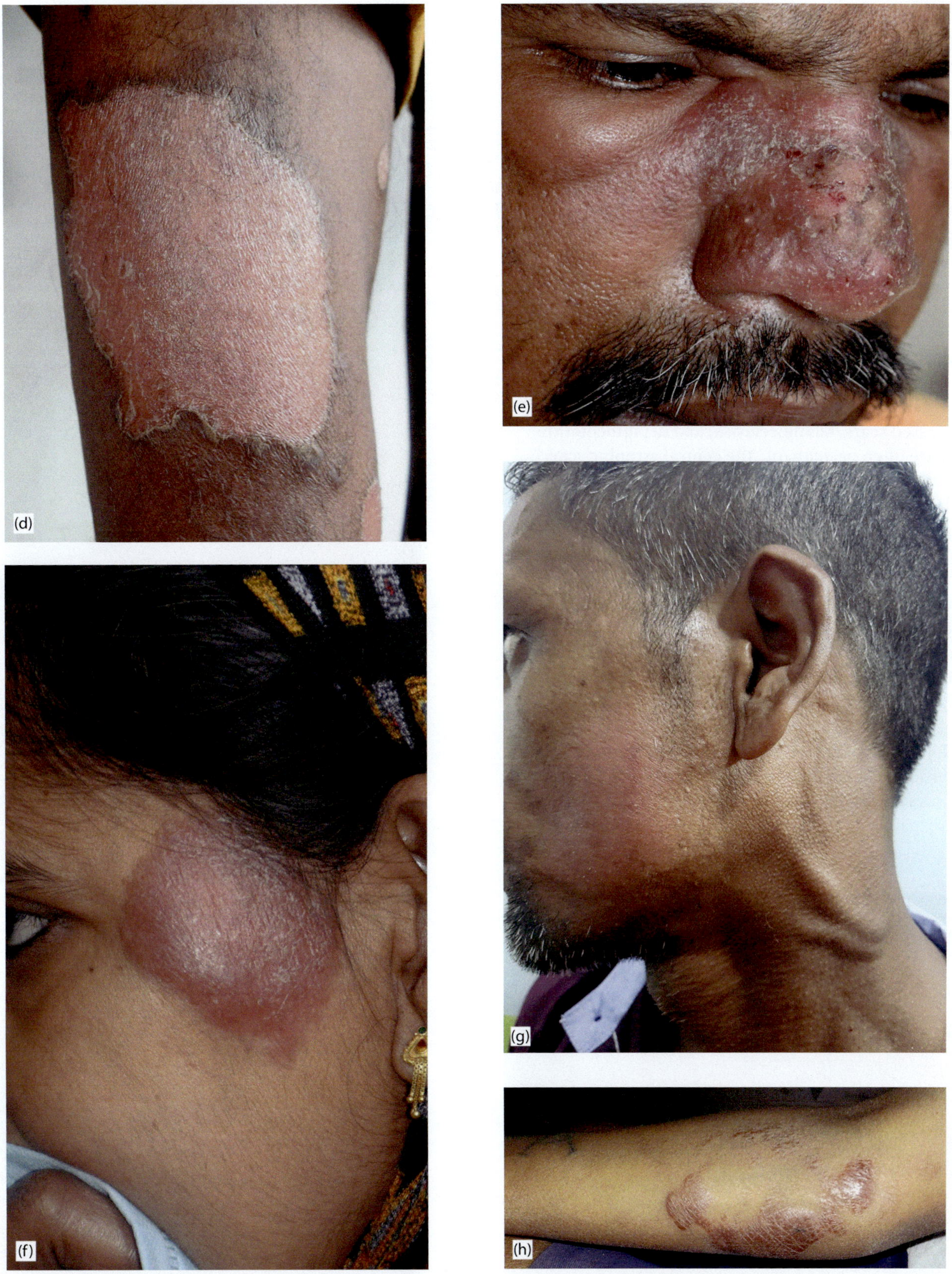


Figure 7.2 (*Continued*) **(d)** Large plaque of BT leprosy with type 1 lepra reaction. **(e)** Erythematous edematous scaly plaque of BT leprosy type 1 lepra reaction. **(f)** BT leprosy with type 1 lepra reaction. Note edema of surrounding areas. **(g)** Erythematous scaly plaque of borderline tuberculoid leprosy with grossly thickened greater auricular nerve. **(h)** Localized lepromatous leprosy. Localized plaques. (a – Courtesy: Dr. Niharika Ranjan Lal, ESIPGIMSR, Kolkata, India; b–f,h – Courtesy: Dr. Piyush Kumar, Katihar, India. g – Courtesy: Dr PC Das, Katihar, India.)

- DD: Sarcoidosis (red or tan brown), psoriasis, tinea corporis (itchy, central clearing, peripheral papules, pustules, and scales), granuloma annulare (annular plaque, margin has discrete papules).

## Discoid lupus erythematosus (DLE)[9]

- The term localized DLE is used to describe patients who have lesions only on the head or neck.
- Early and well-developed lesions are well-defined, erythematous plaques with adherent scale, seen over sun-exposed areas mostly (**Figure 7.3a,b**). Sometimes, the lesions may develop into a verrucous plaque.
- Follicular plugging is a characteristic feature accounting for keratotic spikes under the scales (carpet-tack sign) and wide follicular pits in ears.
- In the evolution of lesion the plaques slowly expand, with active indurated erythema at the periphery, leaving depressed scars, telangiectasias, and depigmentation that are often permanent. The central atrophic scarring is very characteristic (**Figure 7.3c,d**).
- In late lesions or after healing they appear with hyperpigmented border and atrophic depigmented center (**Figure 7.3e**).
- On scalp, it may cause cicatricial alopecia.
- These lesions occur most often on the head and neck areas; in particular the ear canal and scalp should always be examined. Mucosal involvement is common. Lips may have focal or diffuse involvement (**Figure 7.3f,g**).
- Linear DLE is a rare variant (**Figure 7.3h**).
- DD: Psoriasis (micaceous scales, Auspitz sign, extensors), lichen planus (pruritic, purplish flat-topped papules and plaques, flexures), seborrheic dermatitis (scaly patches and plaques, scalp, face, upper back).

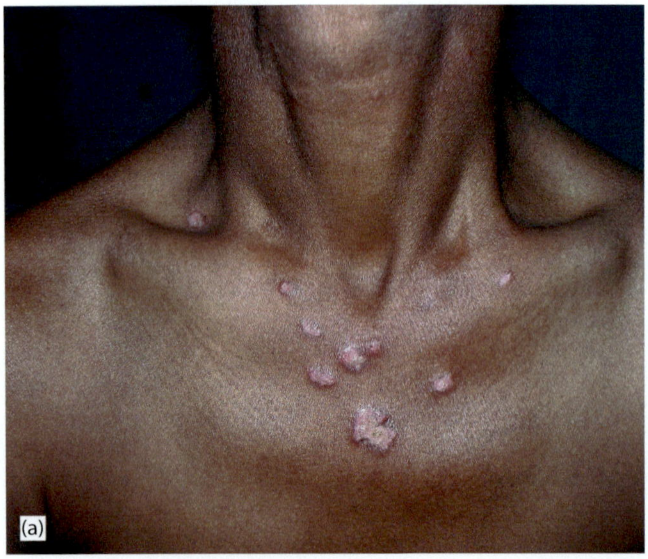
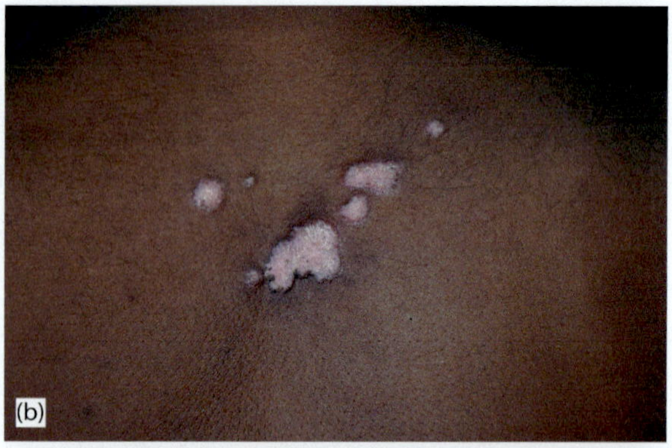
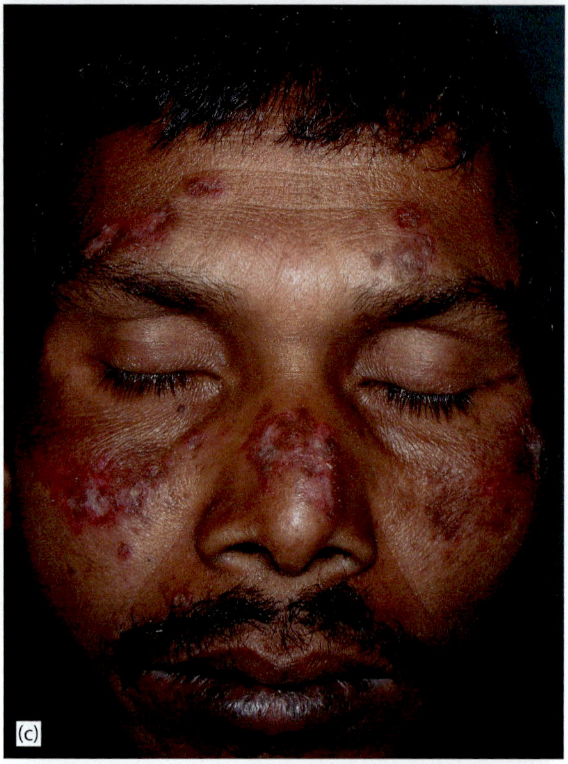
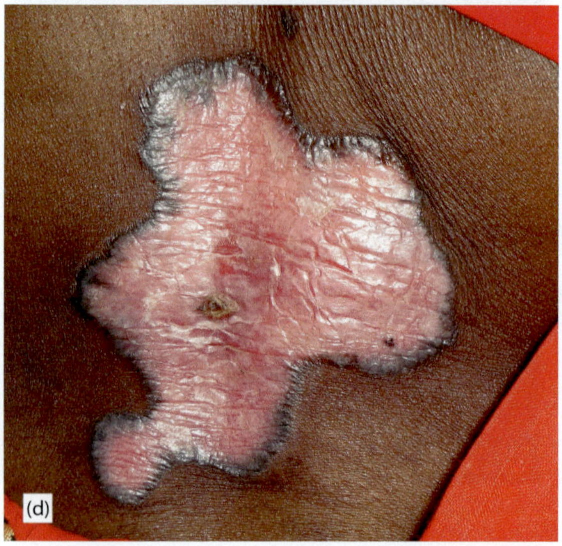

Figure 7.3 **(a)** Erythematous, scaly papules and plaques of discoid lupus erythematosus on the chest. **(b)** Early DLE lesions on the upper back. **(c)** Well-developed lesion of DLE – bilaterally symmetrical large erythematous scaly plaque with well-defined margin. **(d)** DLE lesions may grow to a large size and may have a pigmented margin. *(Continued)*

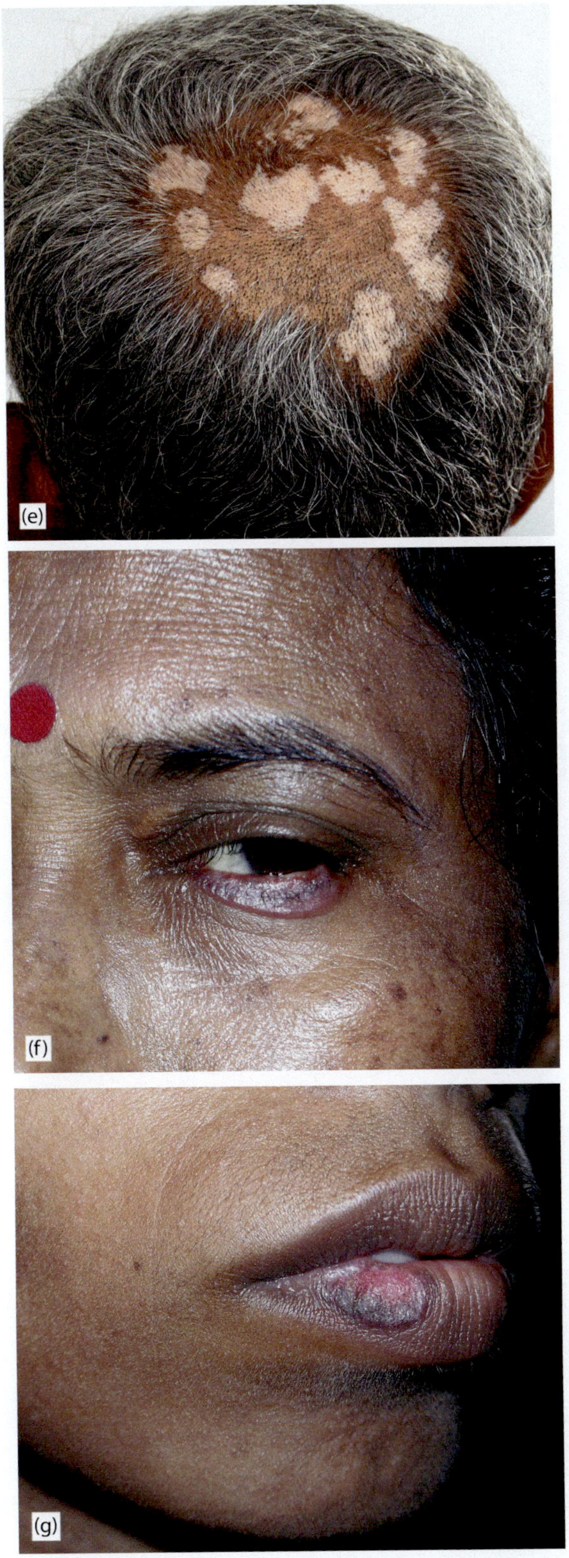

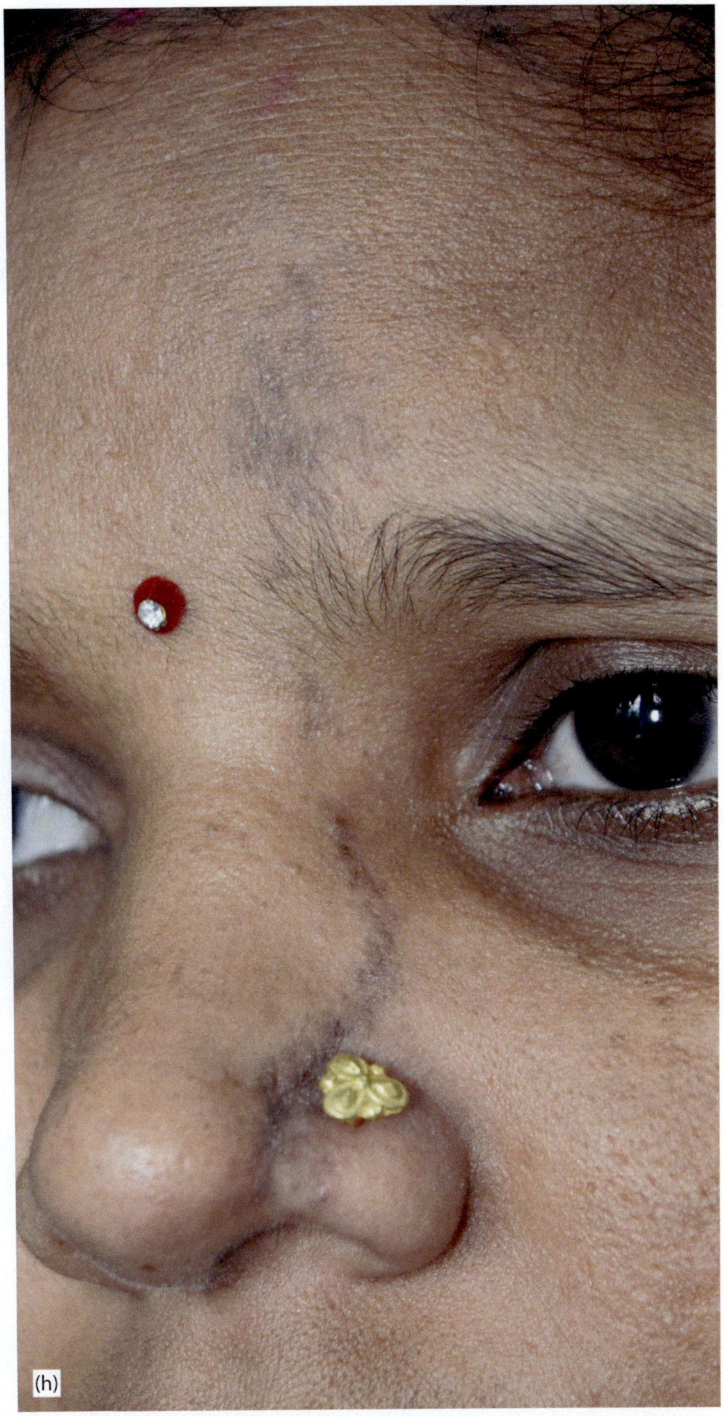

Figure 7.3 (*Continued*) **(e)** Healed lesion of DLE – depigmented patches on the scalp. **(f)** DLE. Erythematous plaque over left lower eyelid. **(g)** Well-defined plaque of DLE on lip. **(h)** Linear lesion of DLE. (a–h – Courtesy: Dr. Piyush Kumar, Katihar, India.)

## Polymorphic light eruption (PLE)

- Polymorphic light eruption is an idiopathic photosensitivity disorder.
- PLE most commonly presents as itchy, closely set, pinpoint papules, and lesions may coalesce to form a scaly plaque. Tiny papules can be seen near the margin of the plaque and are important clinical clues (**Figure 7.4a–c**).
- Another common presentation is erythematous plaques over face, sides of the neck, and sun-exposed areas of arms and hands, appearing a few hours after intense sun exposure (**Figure 7.4d**).

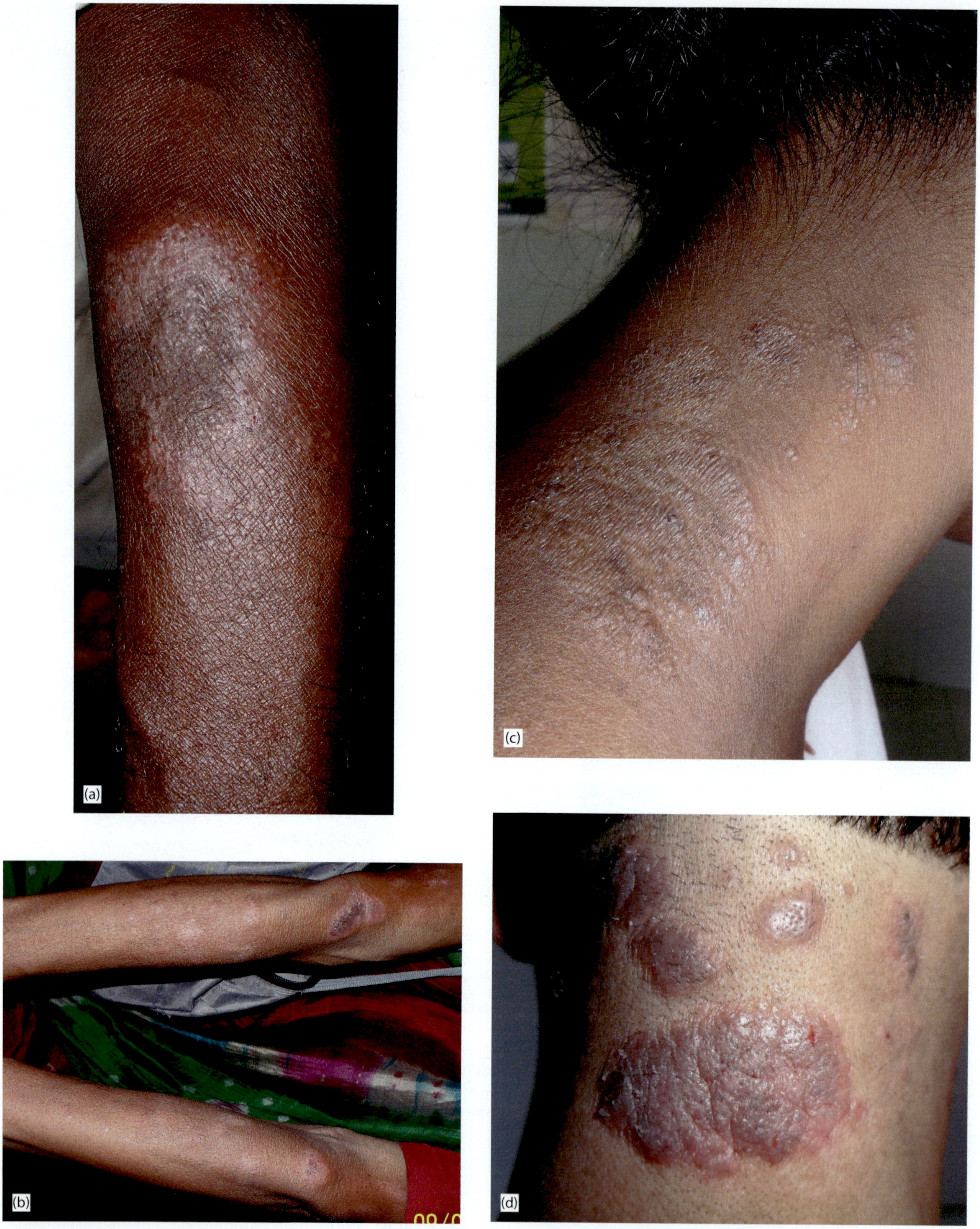


Figure 7.4 **(a)** Polymorphous light eruption seen as scaly plaque with tiny, hypopigmented papules around its margin. **(b)** The lesions typically involve extensor aspect of forearms bilaterally. **(c)** PLE lesions on the neck. **(d)** Erythematous plaques of PLE on the nape of the neck. (*Continued*)

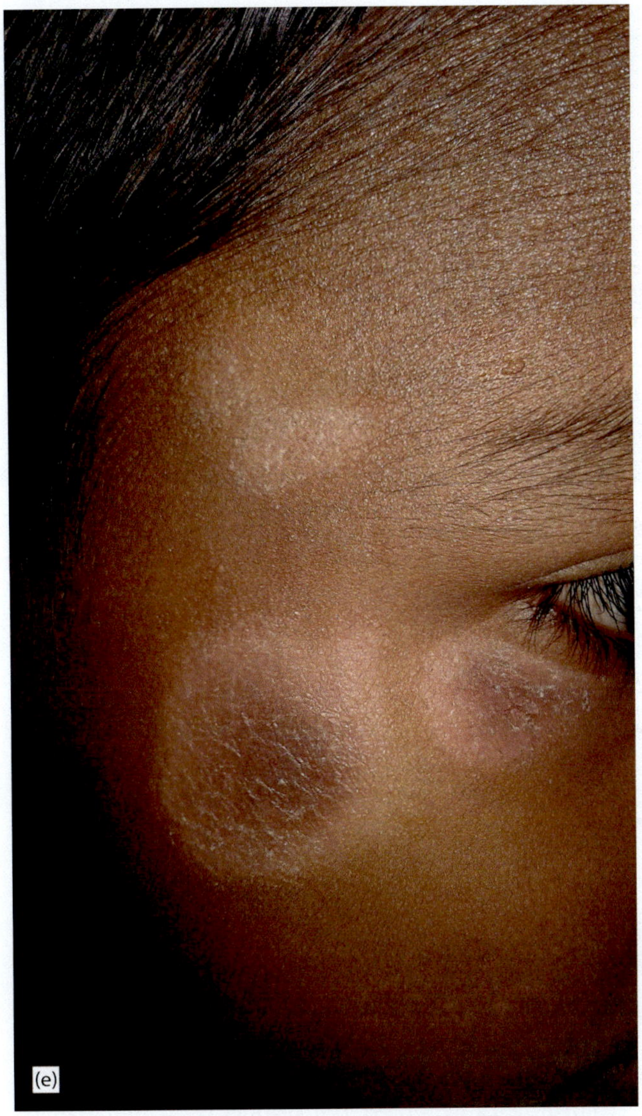


Figure 7.4 *(Continued)* **(e)** Facial lesion of PLE in a child. (a,b – Courtesy: Dr. Piyush Kumar, Katihar, India; c–d, Courtesy: Dr. Niharika Ranjan Lal, ESIPGIMSR, Kolkata, India; e – Courtesy: Dr. PC Das, Katihar, India.)

- Common sites are the upper back and extensor arms.
- Face involvement is commonly seen in children. The lesions commonly involve skin near the lateral canthus (**Figure 7.4e**).
- Clinical variants are lichenoid plaque, targetoid lesions, eczematous, vesicles, and prurigo like lesions.
- Recurrence in spring is common.
- DD: Jessner's lymphocytic infiltration (non-scaly plaques on face), seborrheic dermatitis (scaly ill-defined patches over face, scalp), psoriasis (micaceous scales, Auspitz sign, extensors).

## Jessner's lymphocytic infiltrate[10]

- This is an idiopathic benign lymphocytic proliferation.
- Characteristically lesions are single or multiple, small, non-scaly, solid, pink or red plaques or nodules associated with photosensitivity. The lesions may remain unchanged for several years and then spontaneously disappear, leaving no scars.
- They commonly appear on the face, neck, and back.
- DD: Lymphocytoma cutis (plum-colored plaques, lymphoid follicles in histopathology), sarcoidosis (red or tan-brown plaques, naked granuloma), polymorphic light eruption (micropapules coalesced to form plaques, extensors, sun-exposed area).

## Sarcoidosis[11]

- Cutaneous lesions in sarcoidosis exhibit many different morphologies.
- Plaques in sarcoidosis occur due to coalescence of papules and appear as yellow, brown, red, or tan, with or without mild scaling (**Figure 7.5a**). There is apple-jelly appearance on diascopy.
- Lesions may assume an annular shape because of peripheral evolution and central clearing, with hypopigmentation, atrophy, or scarring (**Figure 7.5b,c**).

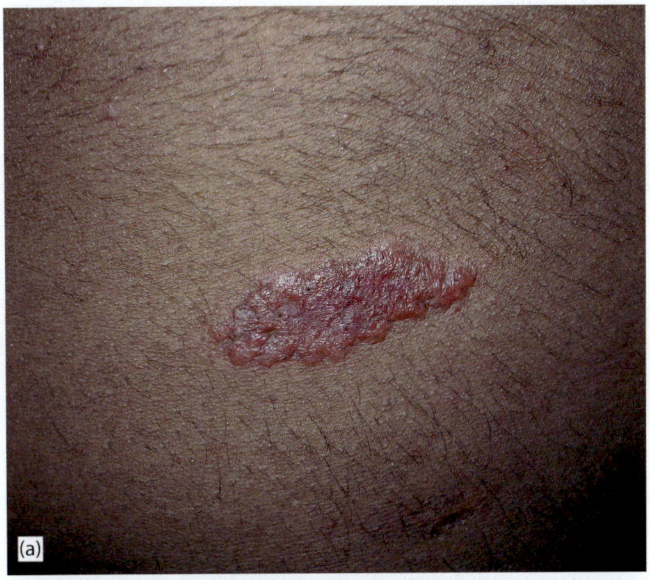


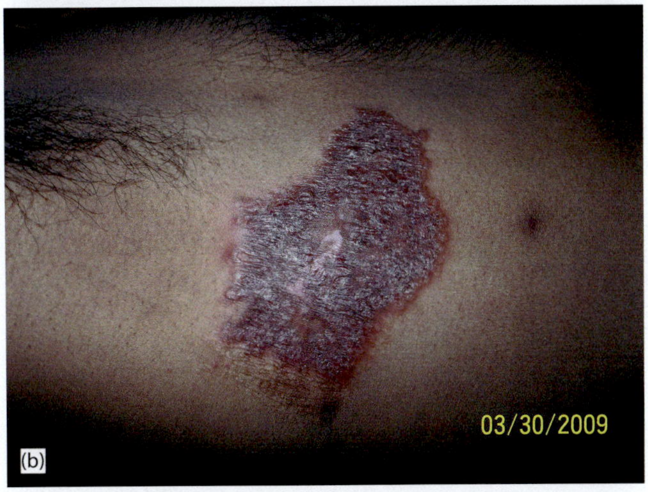


Figure 7.5 **(a)** Erythematous, shiny plaque in sarcoidosis. **(b)** Annular lesion of the sarcoidosis with central depigmented, atrophic scarring. *(Continued)*

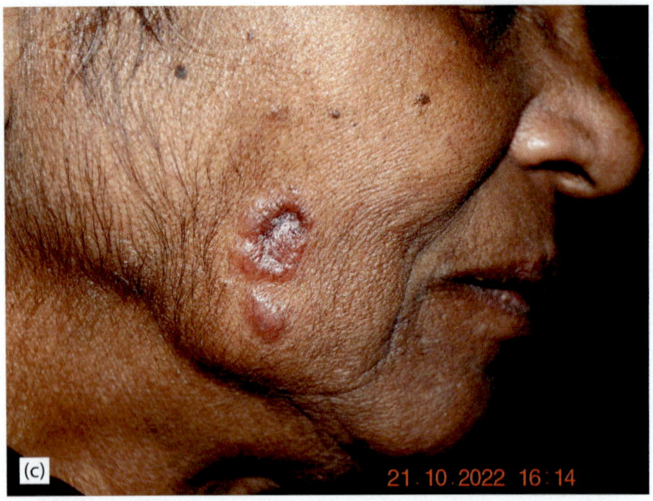


Figure 7.5 (*Continued*) **(c)** Plaques of sarcoidosis on the face. (a,b – Courtesy: Dr. Piyush Kumar, Katihar, India; c – Courtesy: Prof. Sanjay Khare, MGM Medical College, Indore, India.)

- They occur mainly on the face, shoulder, and lower limbs in irregular shapes.
- There is a history of very slow progression or remaining static over many months.
- Lupus pernio: chronic, red-purple indurated papules or plaques that affect the mid-face, particularly the alar rim of the nose, cheeks, ears, fingers and toes; nasal lesions may be associated with granulomatous infiltration of nasal mucosa.
- Angiolupoid type: a type of plaque psoriasis characterized by prominent telangiectasia; solitary, on the bridge of nose and central face.
- Other variants include papular, annular, subcutaneous, lichenoid, hypopigmented, ichthyosiform, psoriasiform, verrucous.
- DD: Leprosy (hypopigmented, hypoesthetic patches), psoriasis (micaceous scales, Auspitz sign, extensors), Jessner's lymphocytic infiltration (non-scaly erythematous plaques on face).

## Cutaneous lymphoid hyperplasia/lymphocytoma cutis[10]

- It is a benign, cutaneous B-cell lymphoproliferative condition.
- It consists of solitary or grouped, erythematous or violaceous papules, nodules or plaques that enlarge slowly and may reach a diameter of 3–5 cm; they can be occasionally translucent and are mostly asymptomatic but sometimes photosensitive lesions over the face, chest, and upper extremities (**Figure 7.6**).
- DD: Jessner's lymphocytic infiltration (non-scaly erythematous plaques on face), sarcoidosis (red or tan-brown plaques, naked granuloma), TT leprosy with reaction (hypopigmented, hypoesthetic, tenderness, swelling), tumid lupus erythematosus, polymorphic light eruption.

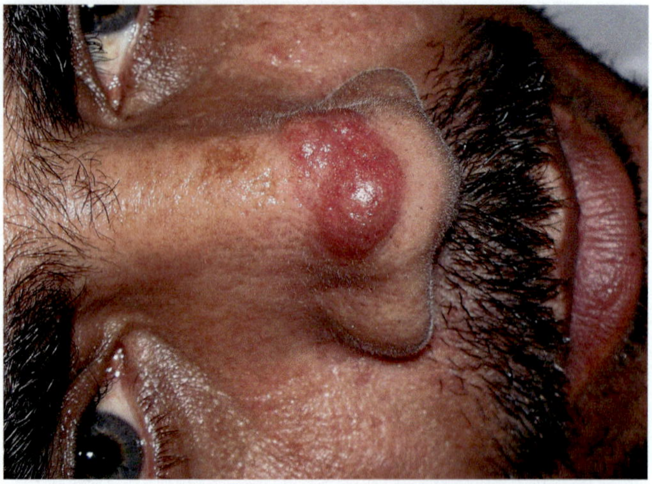

Figure 7.6 Erythematous, translucent, plaque over the nose in cutaneous lymphoid hyperplasia. (Courtesy: Dr. Piyush Kumar, Katihar, India.)

## Erythema elevatum diutinum

- This is a rare, chronic, cutaneous eruption characterized by fibrosing plaques with histological evidence of leukocytoclastic vasculitis.
- It presents with multiple, red-violaceous, red-brown, or orange-yellow plaques over elbows, knees, and small joints of the hands and feet in symmetrical manner. Initially, the lesions are soft, but eventually they fibrose and leave atrophic scars. Lesions are mostly asymptomatic but may be painful at times.
- DD: Xanthoma (yellow plaques and nodules, joints and fingers, hyperlipidemia), gouty nodulosis, rheumatoid nodules (joint pain), lichen planus hypertrophicus (bluish-black hyperkeratotic plaques shin, follicular papules in surroundings), Sweet's syndrome (lesions are acute, more often asymmetrical and located on the arms, face and neck).

## Erysipelas

- Erysipelas is an acute β-hemolytic group A streptococcal infection of the skin.
- There is local redness, heat, swelling, and a characteristic red, raised, erythematous plaque with an indurated border that spreads rapidly over the skin with constitutional symptoms like high fever and joint pain (**Figure 7.7a,b**).
- DD: Cellulitis (margin is not well defined), erysipeloid (polygonal plaques, central clearing, peripheral extension, fingers), urticaria (itchy, transient, evanescent edematous hives/wheals).

## Alopecia mucinosa[12]

- In alopecia mucinosa, malignant T cells are highly concentrated in and about hair follicles. There are often mucinous deposits in follicles, which are then destroyed, producing alopecia.

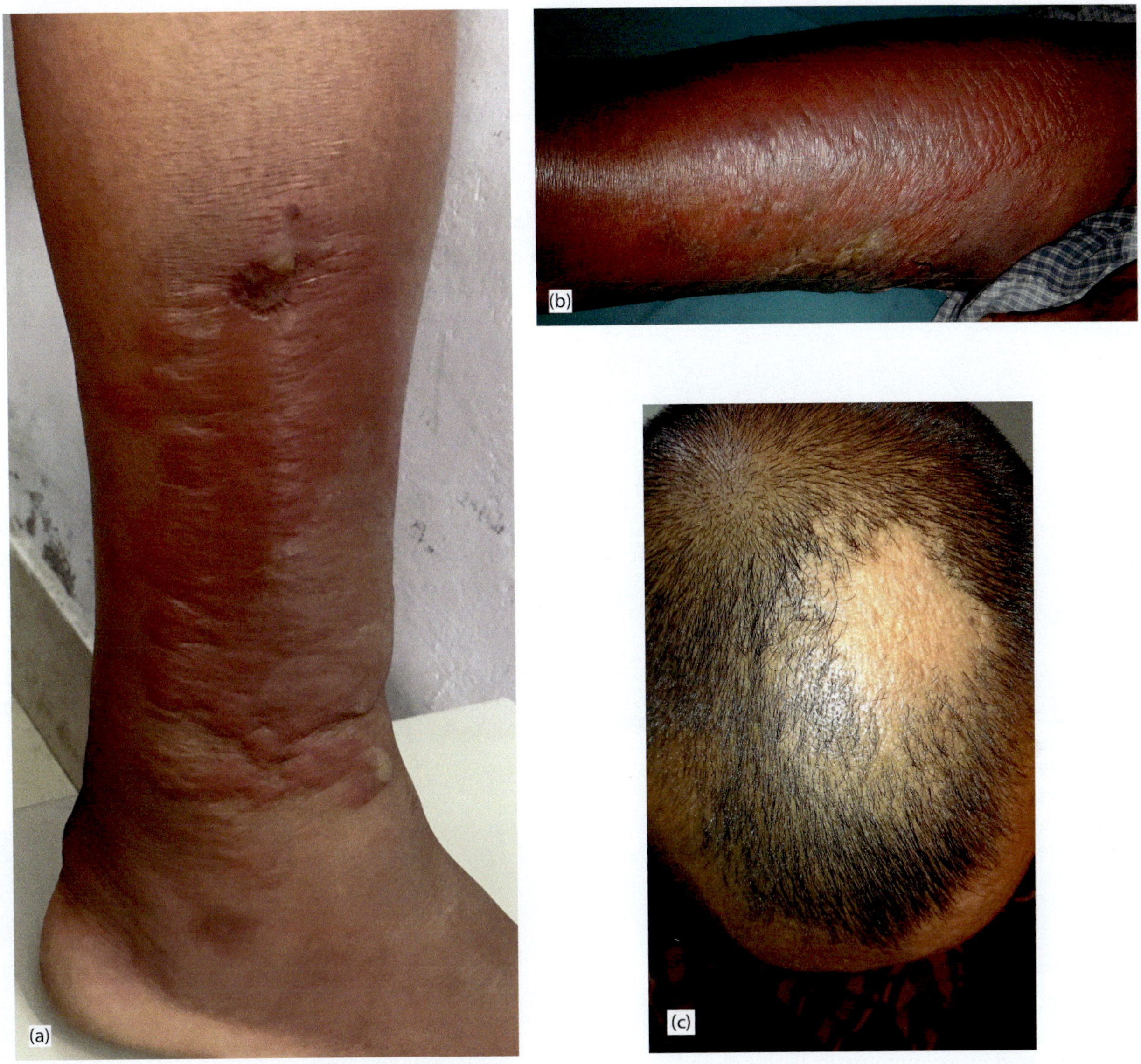

Figure 7.7 **(a)** Erysipelas seen as erythematous, shiny plaque with a palpable border over the left leg. **(b)** Erysipelas with edematous surface. **(c)** Coalescing papules and plaque with hair loss in follicular mucinosis. (a – Courtesy: Dr. Piyush Kumar, Katihar, India; b – Courtesy: Dr. Niharika Ranjan Lal, ESIPGIMSR, Kolkata, India; c – Courtesy: Tanumay Raychaudhury, The Skin Hospital, Westmead Skin and Cancer Foundation, Australia.)

- Clinically, follicular papules and plaques are often associated with severe pruritus and with a predilection for the face and scalp. Prominent giant comedones are often a prominent feature with acneiform lesions, and rarely mucinorrhoea may also be present.
- Follicular papules and plaques with hair loss occur, typically over the face, neck, and scalp, rarely on the trunk and limbs associated with hair loss (**Figure 7.7c**).
- DD: Psoriasis (micaceous scales, Auspitz sign, extensors), leprosy with type 1 reaction (hypopigmented and erythematous tender plaque +/– sensory loss), nevus sebaceous (smooth hairless plaque, verrucous in puberty, areas-scalp, face and neck).

## Pagetoid reticulosis

- Pagetoid reticulosis has two clinical patterns.
- Classic Woringer–Kolopp pagetoid reticulosis – one or few acral plaques that are sharply bordered, scaly, and stable.
    - Solitary persistent, hyperkeratotic, erythematous plaque on acral area, mainly on palm/sole
    - Localized variant of cutaneous T cell lymphoma
    - DD: Palmoplantar psoriasis (hyperkeratotic plaques with fissures), hyperkeratotic eczema (diffuse plaques, deep-seated vesicles, side of the fingers), lichen planus (yellowish hyperkeratotic plaques over palms and soles)
- Disseminated Ketron–Goodman pagetoid reticulosis – described in Chapter 8.

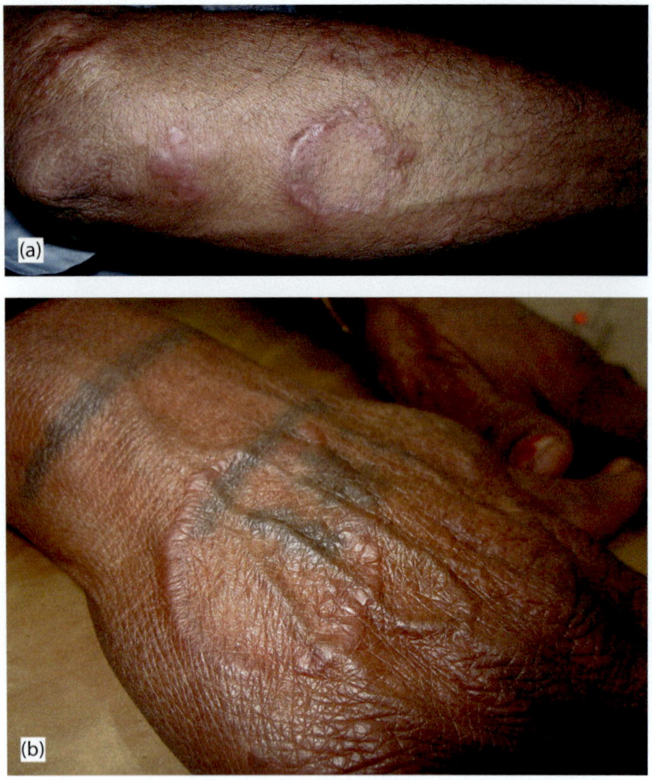


Figure 7.8 **(a)** Erythematous, annular plaque in granuloma annulare. Note that the margin appears beaded with papules. **(b)** Granuloma annulare. (a – Courtesy: Dr. Piyush Kumar, Katihar, India; b – Courtesy: Dr. PC Das, Katihar, India.)

## Granuloma annulare

- It is a benign, usually self-limiting, cutaneous disease that presents as arciform-to-annular plaques.
- It is characterized by asymptomatic, flesh-colored, smooth, shiny, well-defined annular plaques, bordered by closely set small papules (beaded appearance) (**Figure 7.8a,b**).
- The center may be slightly hyperpigmented and depressed.
- Plaques commonly appear on dorsal hands, feet, and fingers and extensor arms and legs.
- Variants include localized, generalized, perforating, patch-type, subcutaneous, acute onset painful acral.
- DD: Tinea corporis (itchy, central clearing, peripheral papules, scales), leprosy (hypopigmented hypoesthetic plaque).

## Granuloma multiforme

- This is a reactive skin disorder of unknown etiology, characterized clinically by confluent annular plaques and histologically by focal necrobiosis and histiocytic granuloma.
- Small papules evolve into round/oval plaques with raised active margin and depressed and hypopigmented centers.
- They occur mainly on sun-exposed skin and in adult African women.
- DD: Granuloma annulare (annular plaque, discrete papules in periphery), tinea corporis (central clearing, peripheral papules, scales), leprosy (hypopigmented hypoesthetic plaque).

## Xanthoma

- Xanthoma is a local deposition of lipid-laden macrophages mainly due to hyperlipidemia.
- It is localized to typical sites: xanthelasma palpebrum, tuberous xanthoma, and tendinous xanthoma.
- Generalized forms of xanthomas include eruptive xanthoma and generalized plane xanthoma.
- Xanthelasma palpebrum appears as bilateral and occasionally symmetrical, soft papules and plaques present on the eyelids (**Figure 7.9a–c**).
    - The upper eyelid and region around the medial canthus are the most common sites of involvement.
    - It may present as associated conditions such as localized cutaneous phenomenon or systemic hyperlipidemia.
- Tuberous xanthoma are yellowish nodules on bony prominences (i.e., elbow and knee) and on knuckles and buttocks (**Figure 7.9d**).

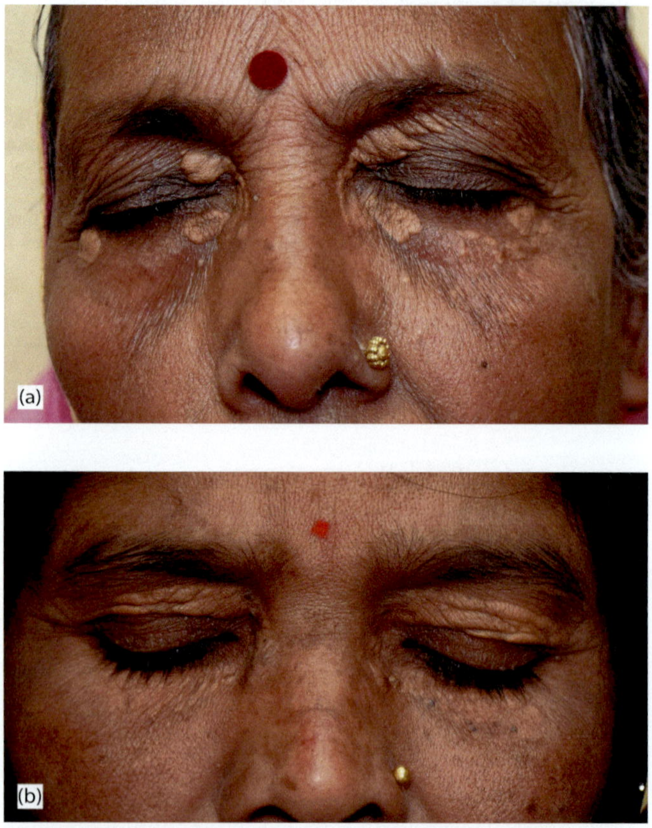


Figure 7.9 **(a)** Yellow, shiny plaques on upper and lower eyelids in xanthelasma palpebrarum. **(b)** Bilaterally symmetrical lesions in xanthelasma palpebrarum. *(Continued)*

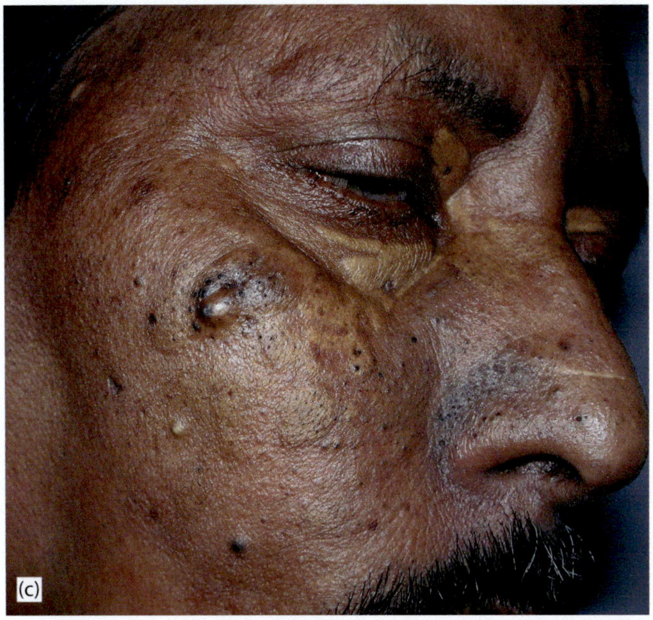

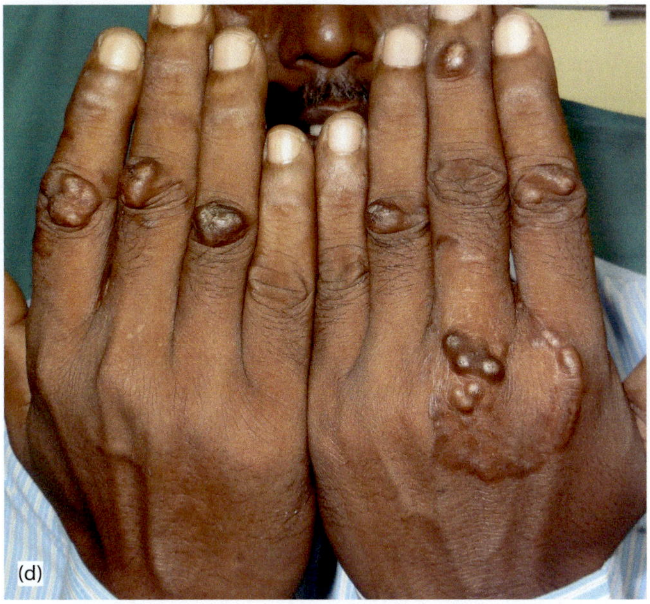

Figure 7.9 (*Continued*) **(c)** Extensive lesion of xanthelasma palpebrarum extending beyond periocular area. Note the presence of extensive senile comedones. **(d)** Tuberous xanthomas on knuckles. (a–c – Courtesy: Dr. Piyush Kumar, Katihar, India; d – Courtesy: Dr. Niharika Ranjan Lal, ESIPGIMSR, Kolkata, India.)

- Tendinous xanthoma is seen particularly on the Achilles tendon and the dorsa of hands and feet.
- Palmar xanthomas are plaques over the palm and flexures of fingers, also yellow streaks along palmar creases. They usually start as macules or slightly palpable plaques; the condition is pathognomonic of type III/familial dysbetalipoproteinemia.
- DD: Erythema elevatum diutinum (yellow-orange plaques appearing on elbow, knee, small joints of hands, with leukocytoclastic histopathology), juvenile xanthogranuloma (yellow papules/plaques, head-neck region, histiocytic proliferation), nevus lipomatosus cutaneous superficialis (soft, yellowish plaques, mainly over buttocks/thighs).

## Tumid lupus erythematosus[9]

- This presents with single or multiple succulent, non-scarring, erythematous plaques (**Figure 7.10**).
- There is no follicular plugging as with discoid lupus erythematosus (DLE).
- Areas such as the face, neck, upper back, and forearms are predominantly involved.
- It heals spontaneously without atrophy, scarring, or pigmentation.
- DD: Lupus vulgaris (apple-jelly nodules, scarring at one end and progression on another), sarcoidosis (red/tan-brown plaques with naked granuloma), Jessner's lymphocytic infiltrate (erythematous plaques over face).

## Cellulitis

- Predisposing factors include diabetes mellitus, HIV infection/AIDS, chronic kidney disease, chronic liver disease, and presence of foreign bodies, including surgical devices.
- It may develop after a trauma or may complicate a pre-existing dermatosis.

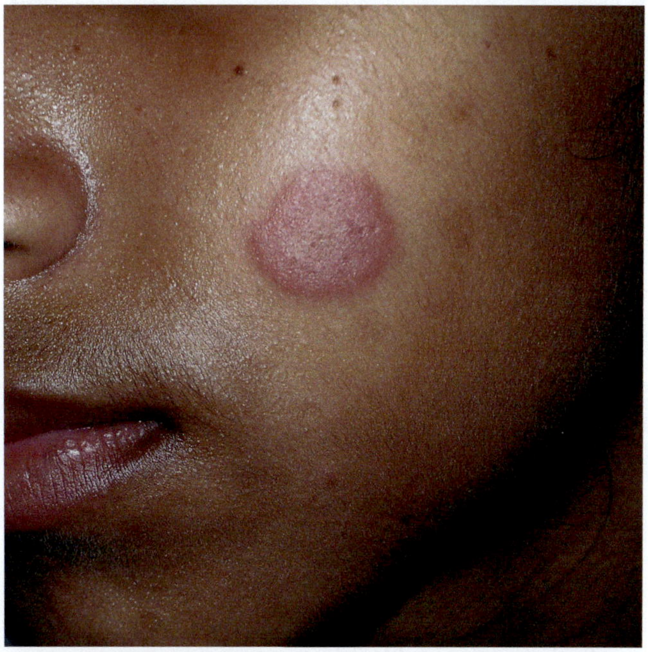

Figure 7.10 Erythematous, juicy plaque on face in tumid lupus erythematosus. (Courtesy: Dr. Piyush Kumar, Katihar, India.)

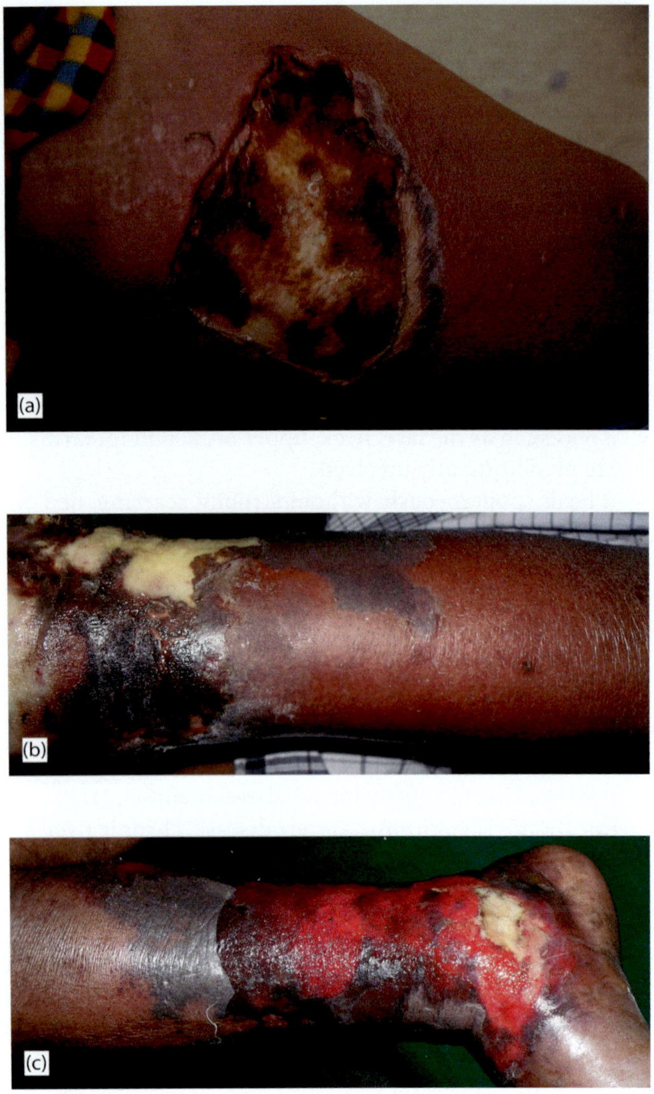

Figure 7.11 **(a)** Ulcerated plaque in cellulitis in localized plaque. **(b)** Severe case of cellulitis skin hemorrhage and necrosis. **(c)** Another case of severe cellulitis with eroded surface. (a–c – Courtesy: Dr. Piyush Kumar, Katihar, India.)

- Patients may have malaise, chills, and fever. Lesions are most commonly located on the lower extremity.
- It presents as a painful ill-defined swelling of the affected part. The skin appears erythematous and warm. Regional lymphadenopathy is common (**Figure 7.11a–c**).
- Clinical signs of severe disease include violaceous hue, presence of hemorrhage and bullae, skin sloughing, sensory loss over the lesion, lymphatic spread, rapid progression, and hemodynamic instability.
- DD: Erysipelas (**Table 7.2**), erysipeloid (polygonal plaques, central clearing, peripheral extension, fingers), urticaria (itchy, transient, evanescent edematous hives/wheals).

Table 7.2 Differentiating cellulitis from erysipelas

| Cellulitis | Erysipelas |
|---|---|
| Presents with low-grade fever with a less abrupt onset. | There is abrupt onset of fever accompanied by chills. |
| The skin appears brownish-black in dark-skinned individuals and dull red in Caucasians. | Dark-skinned people may have brownish-gray skin, while Caucasians may have bright-red skin. |
| The border of the infected area is less well defined and fades into the surrounding skin. | The infected area is hot and tender and spreads; the border is well-defined, and the surface is shiny. |
| Blisters are uncommon. | There are vesicles and bullae (subcutaneous edema). |
| Cause is multibacterial, such as staphylococci, streptococci, haemophilus. | Group A haemolytic streptococci is the main organism. |

## HYPERKERATOTIC PLAQUES

### Tuberculosis verrucosa cutis[13]

- this is a localized form of cutaneous tuberculosis due to inoculation of organisms into the skin of a previously infected patient who usually has a moderate or high degree of immunity.
- Lesions are mostly seen on trauma-prone areas (e.g. feet, knees, buttocks, etc.).
- A lesion starts as an asymptomatic, indurated, warty papule and progresses to verrucous plaque with finger-like projections (**Figure 7.12a–c**).
- Color is purplish, red, or brown. Consistency is generally firm, but there may be areas of relative softening.
- The center may progress to massive, papillomatous excrescences or, uncommonly, may involute to leave a white atrophic scar.
- The disease runs a chronic progressive course.

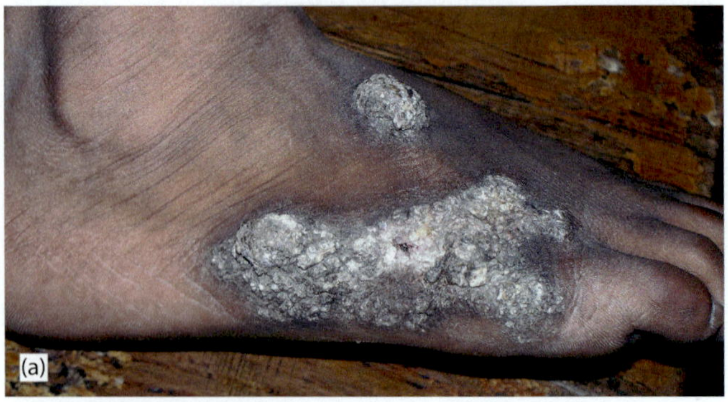

Figure 7.12 **(a)** Verrucous plaque in tuberculosis verrucosa cutis. *(Continued)*

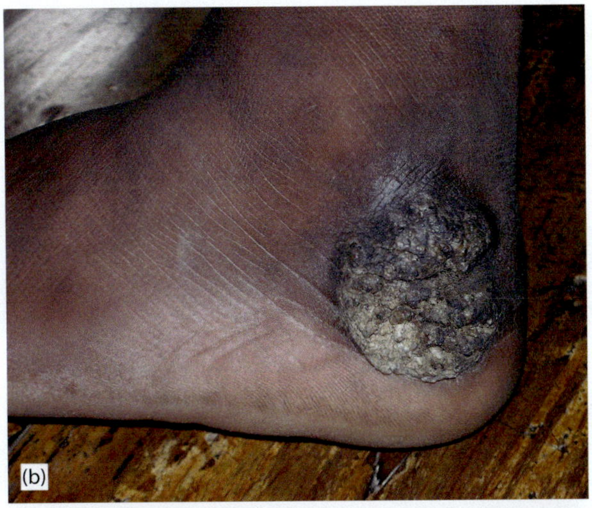

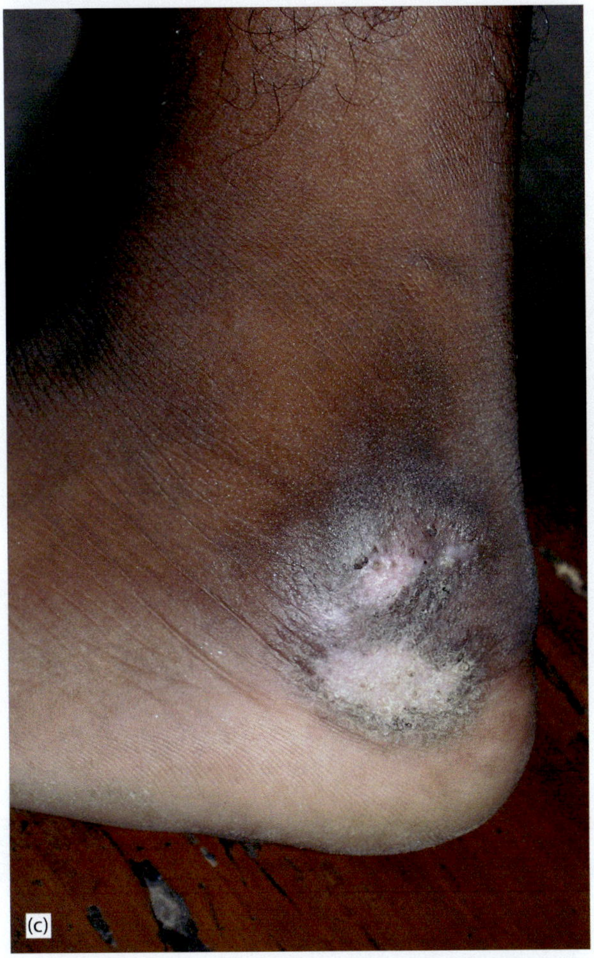

Figure 7.12 (*Continued*) **(b)** Solitary verrucous plaque of tuberculosis verrucosa cutis. **(c)** Resolution of lesion with antitubercular treatment. (a–c – Courtesy: Dr. Piyush Kumar, Katihar, India.)

- DD: Verruca vulgaris (multiple plaques, pseudo Koebnerization), sporotrichosis (oozy plaque, lymphatic spread), psoriasis (micaceous scales, fissures, Auspitz sign, well-marginated), lupus vulgaris (gradual extension at one margin, scarring in another margin).

## Lupus vulgaris[14]

- This is a chronic progressive primary form of cutaneous tuberculosis
- It consists of flat plaque composed of soft, reddish-brown papules (**Figure 7.13a**) with irregular edges. The surface of the lesion may be smooth or covered with psoriasiform scale (**Figure 7.13b–d**).
- There is apple-jelly appearance on diascopy.

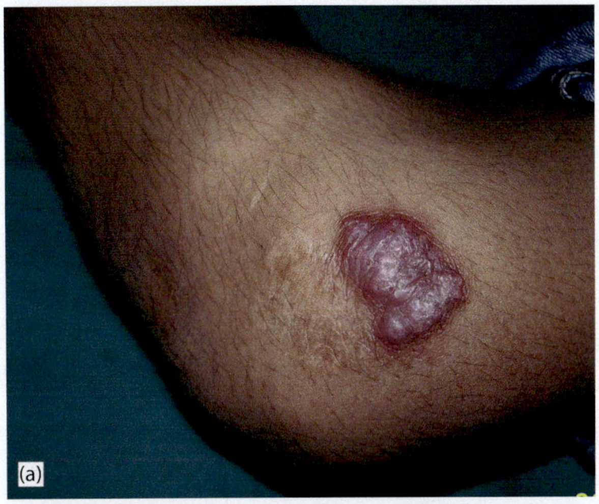

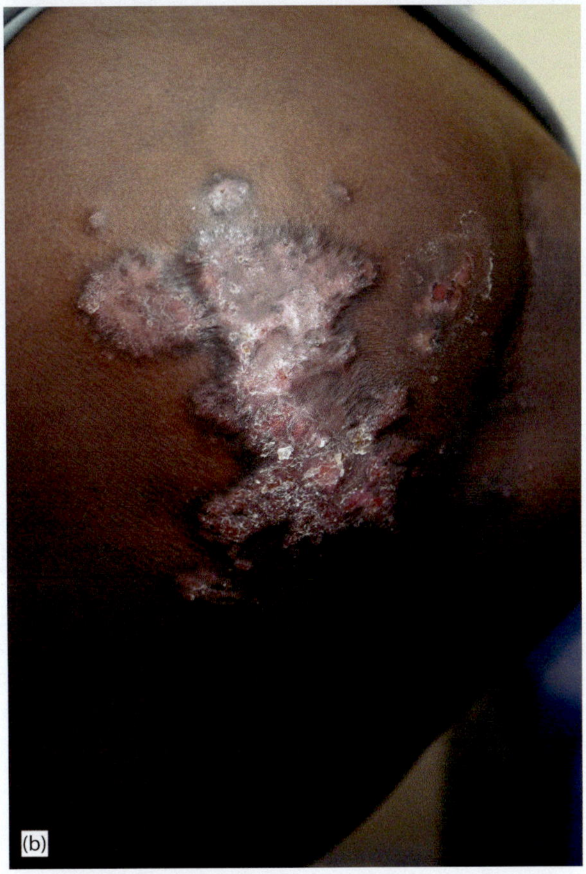

Figure 7.13 **(a)** Lupus vulgaris presenting as erythematous scaly plaque. Note scarring in the vicinity. **(b)** Erythematous, scaly plaque of lupus vulgaris on the buttock. (*Continued*)

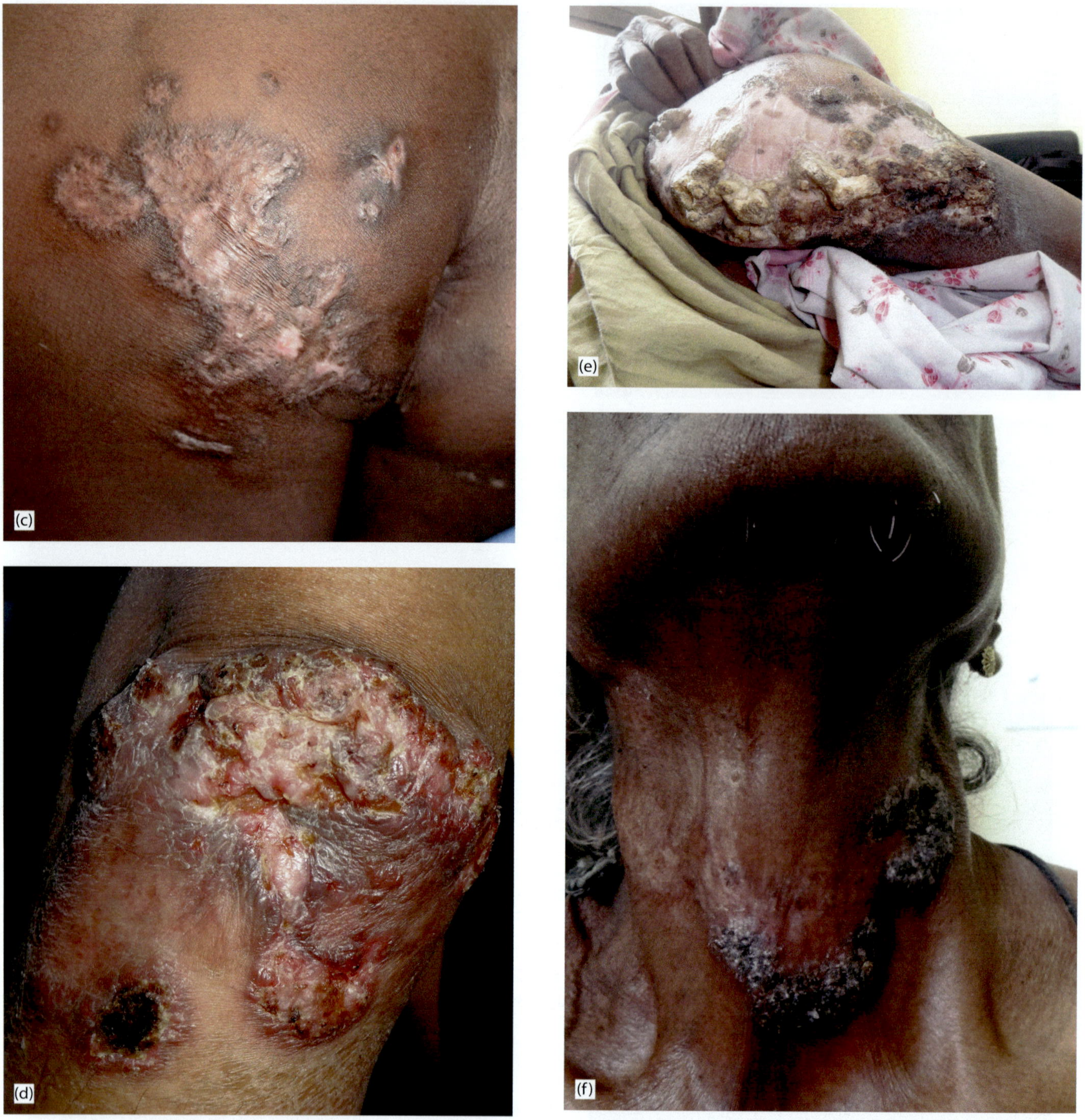

Figure 7.13 (*Continued*) **(c)** Clinical resolution of lesion with treatment. Residual scarring is seen. **(d)** Erythematous scaly plaque with crusting at places. **(e,f)** Lupus vulgaris with advancing edge showing hyperkeratotic plaque; inactive edge healed with scarring. (a–d – Courtesy: Dr. Piyush Kumar, Katihar, India; e,f – Courtesy: Dr. Niharika Ranjan Lal, ESIPGIMSR, Kolkata, India.)

- There is gradual extension in some areas and healing with scarring in other areas; it may cause tissue destruction and deformity. Large plaques show irregular areas of scarring with islands of active lupus tissue (**Figure 7.13e,f**).
- It is seen over face, extremities and trunk.
- Morphological variants include ulcerative and mutilating forms, vegetating forms, tumor like forms and papular-nodular forms.
- DD: Tuberculosis verrucosa cutis (oozy plaque, areas – sole, buttocks), sporotrichosis (lymphatic spread), sarcoidosis (red/brown plaque, naked granuloma).

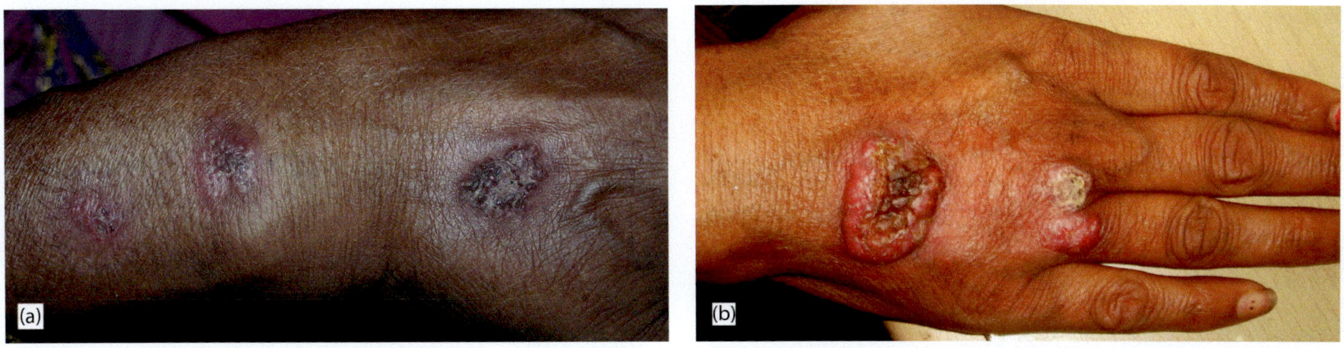


Figure 7.14 **(a)** Erythematous crusted plaques in lymphocutaneous sporotrichosis. **(b)** Crusted plaques of sporotrichosis localized to the dorsum of the hand. (a – Courtesy: Dr. Piyush Kumar, Katihar, India.)

## Sporotrichosis[14]

- Sporotrichosis is an acute or chronic fungal infection caused by *Sporothrix schenckii.*
- Commonly affected populations include agriculturists, foresters, gardeners, florists, and nursery workers handling plants or plant material.
- Traumatic inoculation is the typical mode for acquisition of skin infection in immunocompetent hosts.
- Clinically sporotrichosis manifests as 1) lymphocutaneous (most common type), 2) fixed cutaneous, 3) multifocal or disseminated cutaneous, and 4) extracutaneous or systemic sporotrichosis.
- The lymphocutaneous type is characterized by a nodulo-ulcerative lesion (sporotrichotic chancre) at the inoculation site and strings of similar lesions along the lymphatics proximal to the initial lesion (**Figure 7.14a**).
- Fixed cutaneous sporotrichosis is less common and occurs as localized, asymptomatic, erythematous, papulo-plaque, papulo-pustules, nodules or verrucous plaque and occasionally, a non-healing ulcer or a small abscess at the inoculation site (**Figure 7.14b**).
- Multifocal (disseminated) cutaneous sporotrichosis (≥3 lesions involving two different anatomical sites) and extracutaneous (systemic, osteoarticular, pulmonary, meningeal) forms are very rare.
- DD: Chromomycosis (warty papules, satellite lesions, copper-penny bodies in histopathology), tuberculosis verrucosa cutis (oozy plaque, appears on soles and buttocks), verruca vulgaris (warty plaque/papules, pseudo-Koebnerization), leishmaniasis, atypical mycobacterial infection.

## Chromomycosis (chromoblastomycosis)[14]

- This is subcutaneous mycosis caused by traumatic implantation of dematiaceous fungi.
- Warty papules slowly enlarge to form painless hyperkeratotic plaque, often with central scarring; some forms may appear like psoriasiform plaques (**Figure 7.15a–c**).
- Satellite lesions and lymphatic spread to adjoining areas. Large verrucous swellings and lymphedema develop in later stages.
- Lesions are usually found on exposed sites, particularly feet, legs, arms, face, and neck.
- DD: Sporotrichosis (warty plaques, lymphatic spread), tuberculosis verrucosa cutis (oozy plaque, appears on soles, buttocks), verruca vulgaris (warty plaque/papules, pseudo-Koebnerization), blastomycosis (by the absence of sharp border containing minute abscesses).

## Cutaneous Leishmaniasis (CL)

- Leishmaniasis is a group of diseases caused by several species of the genus *Leishmania.*
- Most of the cases are from hot and dry areas like deserts of North and South America, the Mediterranean basin,

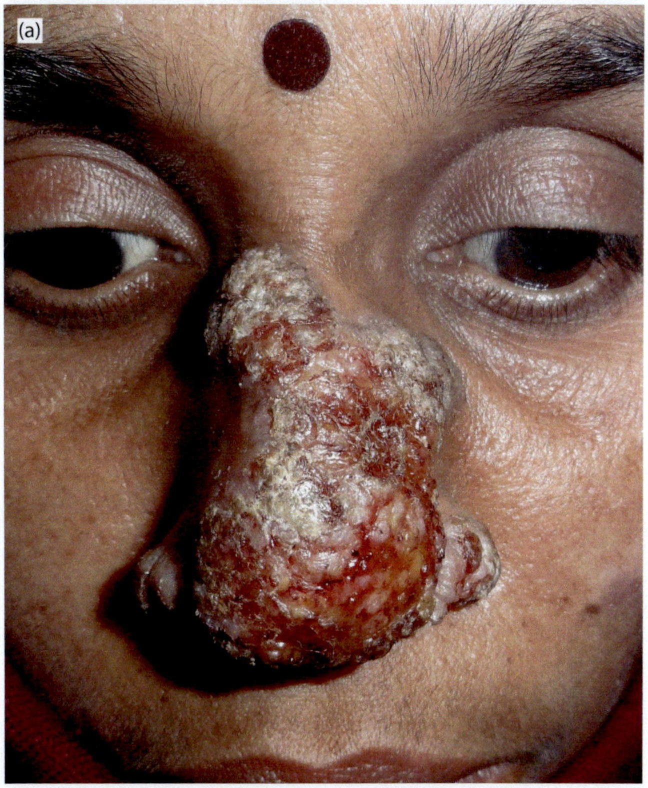


Figure 7.15 **(a)** Chromoblastomycosis. Warty plaque. (*Continued*)

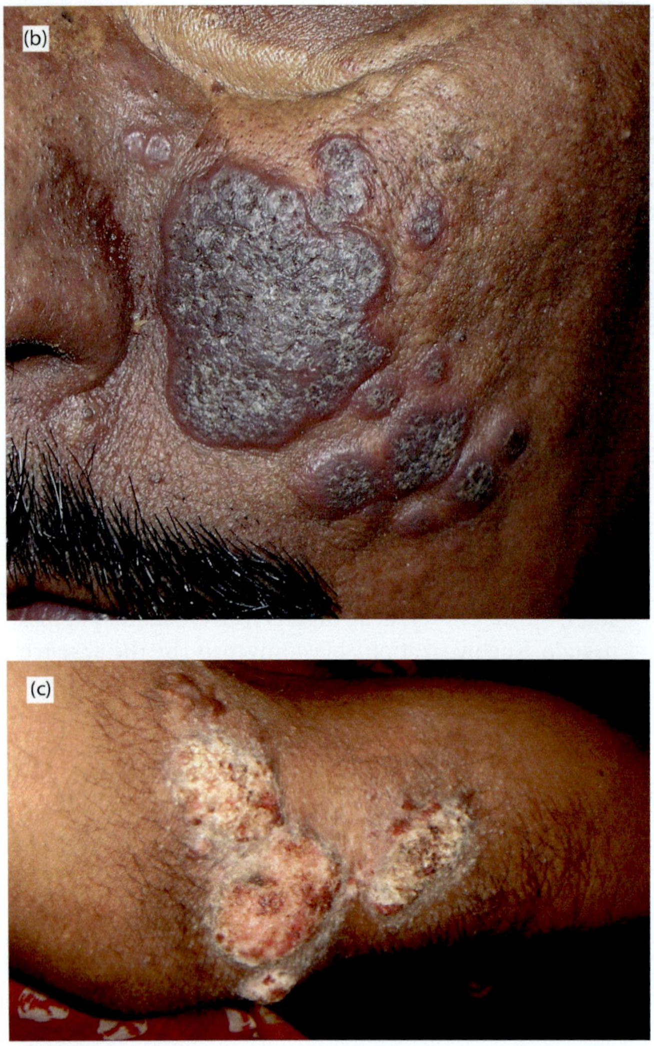


Figure 7.15 (*Continued*) **(b)** Chromoblastomycosis. **(c)** Verrucous plaque of chromomycosis on the thigh and leg. (a,b – Courtesy: Dr. Niharika Ranjan Lal, ESIPGIMSR, Kolkata, India.)

the Middle East, and Central Asia. In India, CL is endemic to the Thar desert and neighboring areas of Rajasthan.

- Non-tender firm plaques or nodules form central ulceration and crusting and a raised border (**Figure 7.16a–c**). Lesions are wet or dry. The lesions heal with fibrosis.
- Variants include cutaneous, diffuse cutaneous, mucocutaneous, leishmaniasis recidivans, and post kala-azar dermal leishmaniasis.
- In leishmaniasis recidivans (lupoid leishmaniasis) brown-red or brown-yellow papules appear, usually close to a scar of an old lesion of cutaneous leishmaniasis or actually in the scar; these papules coalesce and form a plaque closely resembling lupus vulgaris.
- DD: Tuberculosis verrucosa cutis (oozy plaque, appears on soles and buttocks), sporotrichosis (warty plaques, lymphatic spread), lupus vulgaris (gradual extension at one margin, scarring in another margin).

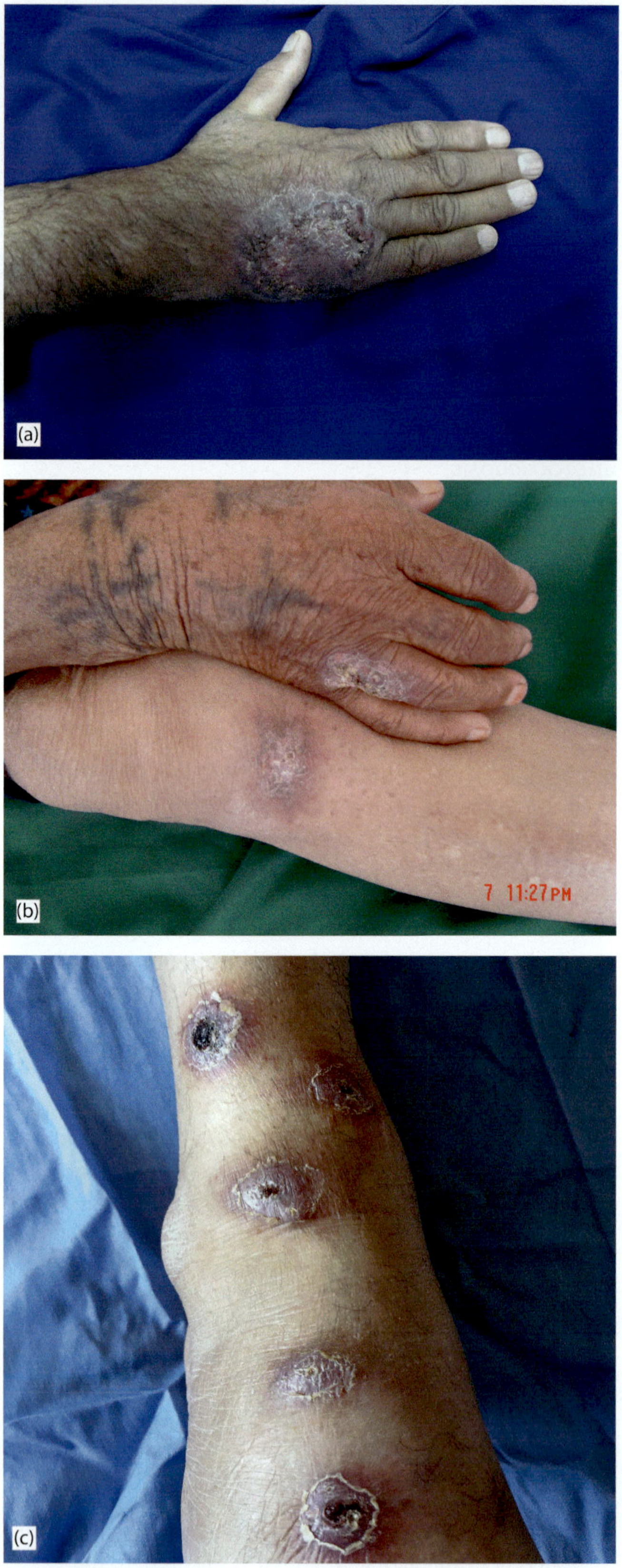


Figure 7.16 **(a)** Well -defined, erythematous crusted plaque of cutaneous leishmaniasis on the hand. **(b)** Two plaques of cutaneous leishmaniasis on exposed sites. **(c)** Sporotrichoid spread of lesions in cutaneous leishmaniasis. (a–c – Courtesy: Prof. Reza Yaghoobi, Department of Dermatology, Ahvaz Jundishupor University of Medical Sciences, Iran.)

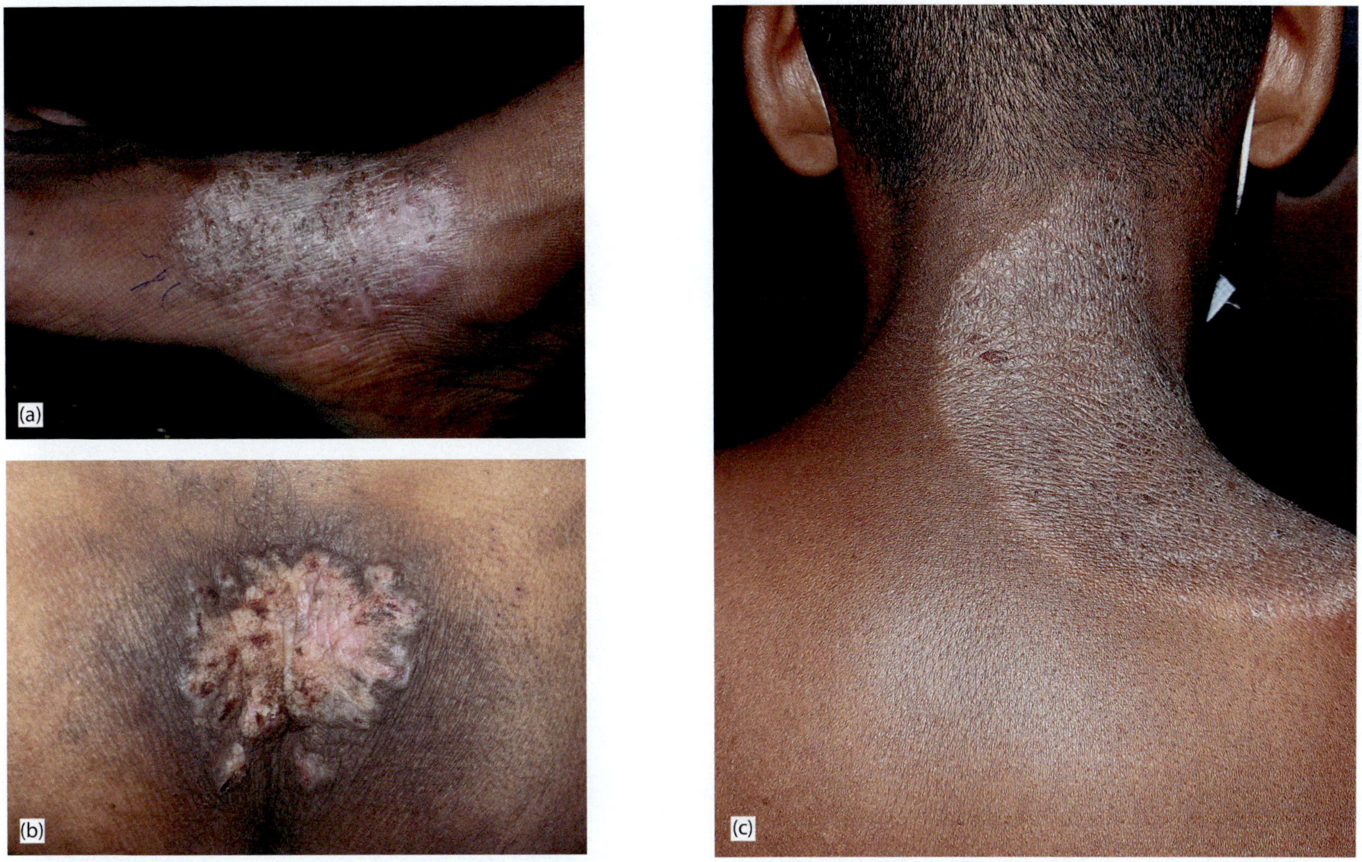


Figure 7.17 **(a)** Erythematous, thick plaque on the dorsum of the foot, with prominent skin markings and excoriations in lichen simplex chronicus. **(b)** Lichen simplex chronicus on the sacral area. Note lichenification of the surrounding skin. **(c)** Lichen simplex chronicus over the nape of the neck. (a–c – Courtesy: Dr. Piyush Kumar, Katihar, India.)

## Lichen simplex chronicus

- Also known as neurodermatitis circumscripta, lichen simplex chronicus is a chronic skin disease characterized by lichenified plaques that occur as result of constant scratching or rubbing of the skin.
- The typical presentation of LSC is a circumscribed, lichenified, pruritic plaque. Scales and excoriation are often present (**Figure 7.17a–c**).
- Typically located over the dorsum of the foot, nape of the neck, wrist, and back.
- DD: Tuberculosis verrucosa cutis (oozy plaque that appears on soles and buttocks), sporotrichosis (warty plaques, lymphatic spread), lichen planus hypertrophicus (verrucous plaque with scaling on the shins, with follicular papules in surroundings).

## Lichen planus hypertrophicus

- This is typically present as extremely pruritic red, yellow-gray, or red-brown papules and verrucous, flat-topped plaques. They are firm to palpation and display a verrucous or hyperkeratotic surface (**Figure 7.18a–c**).
- In dark skinned people, they often appear pigmented with purplish to black in color.
- They may be surrounded by follicular papules – an important clinical clue, when present.
- Most often they appear on the pretibial area of the lower extremity and the ankles. Lesions can also appear on other areas of the lower limbs, upper limbs, trunk, or in a generalized fashion.

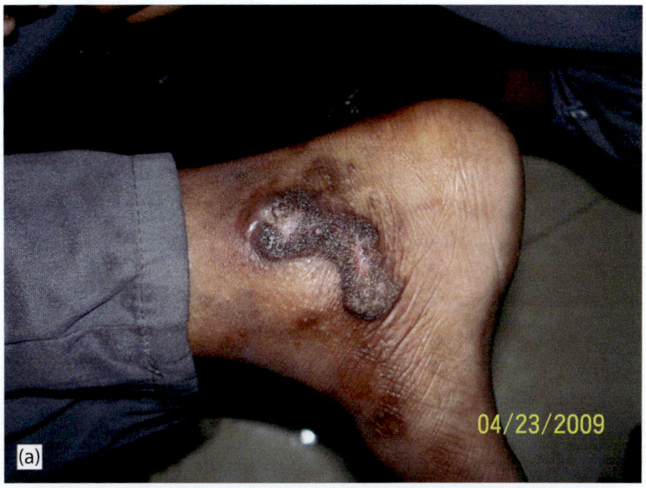


Figure 7.18 **(a)** Hyperkeratotic verrucous plaque in lichen planus hypertrophicus. *(Continued)*

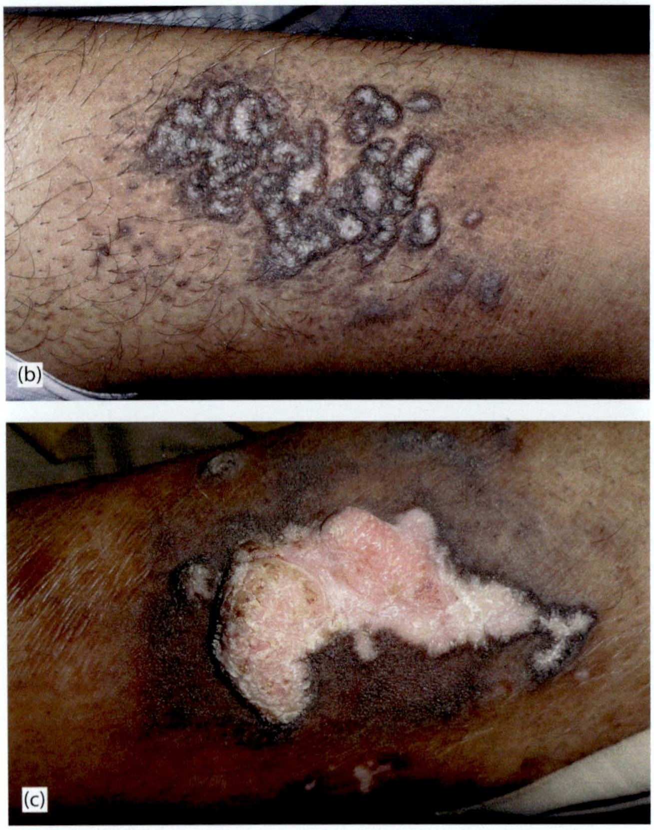

Figure 7.18 (*Continued*) **(b)** Lichen planus hypertrophicus. **(c)** Lichen planus hypertrophicus. (a,b – Courtesy: Dr. Piyush Kumar, Katihar, India; c – Courtesy: Dr. Niharika Ranjan Lal, ESIPGIMSR, Kolkata, India.)

- DD: Prurigo nodularis, verruca vulgaris (warty plaques, pseudo-Koebnerization), tuberculosis verrucosa cutis (oozy plaque on the soles and buttocks), chronic plaque psoriasis (micaceous scales, fissures, Auspitz sign, well-marginated), pretibial epidermolysis bullosa pruriginosa.

## Verruca vulgaris

- This has a viral etiology caused by human papilloma virus (HPV).
- Hyperkeratotic papules/plaques with an irregular rough surface occur on any part of the body (**Figure 7.19a,b**) as solitary or multiple, endophytic, or exophytic lesions (**Figure 7.19c,d**).
- Although the lesions are usually 2–10 mm in diameter, they can grow up to a giant verruca vulgaris, whose size is larger than 1 cm.
- Commonly found on the hands, acral areas, and trauma-prone areas.
- Pseudo-Koebnerization involves the spread of lesions to the site of trauma (**Figure 7.19e**).
- DD: Tuberculosis verrucosa cutis (oozy plaque on the soles and buttocks), verrucous carcinoma (destructing surroundings, warty surface, bulldozing effect in histopathology), lichen simplex chronicus (lichenified plaque, caused by excoriations, occurring on the dorsum of hands and feet, nape of neck).

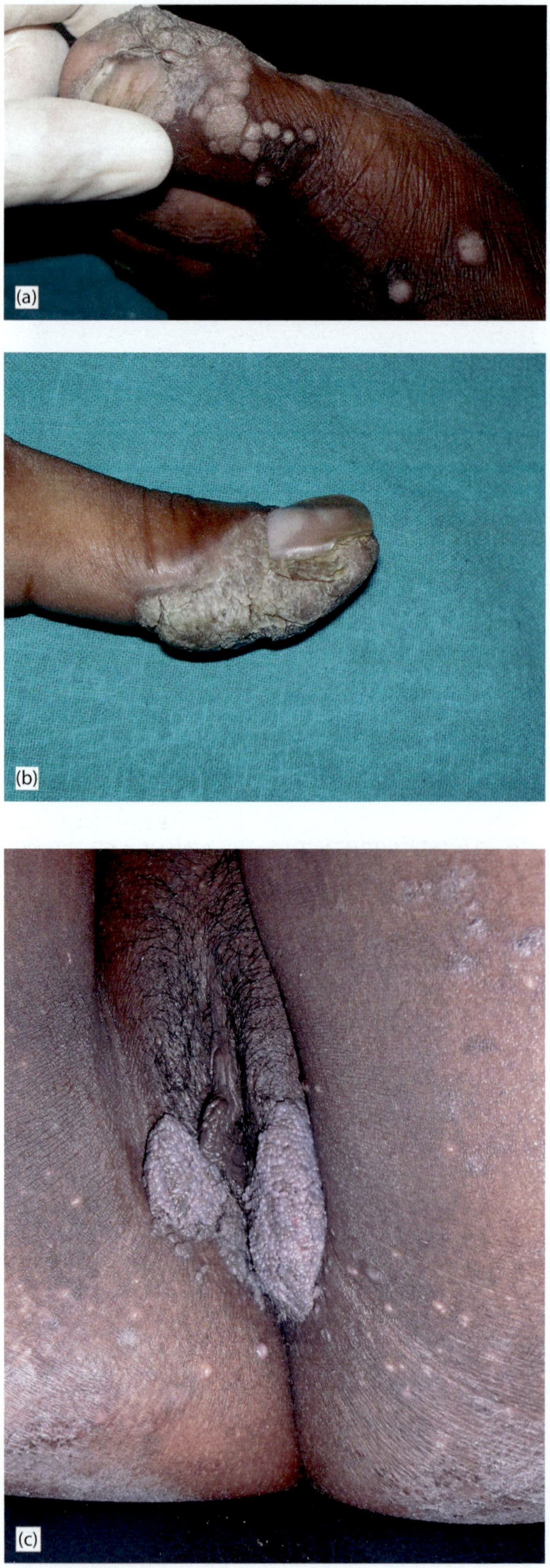

Figure 7.19 **(a)** Verrucous flat-topped papules coalescing to form plaque on the great toe in verruca vulgaris. **(b)** Verrucous plaque on the thumb in verruca vulgaris. **(c)** Exophytic plaque on labia in condyloma acuminata. (*Continued*)

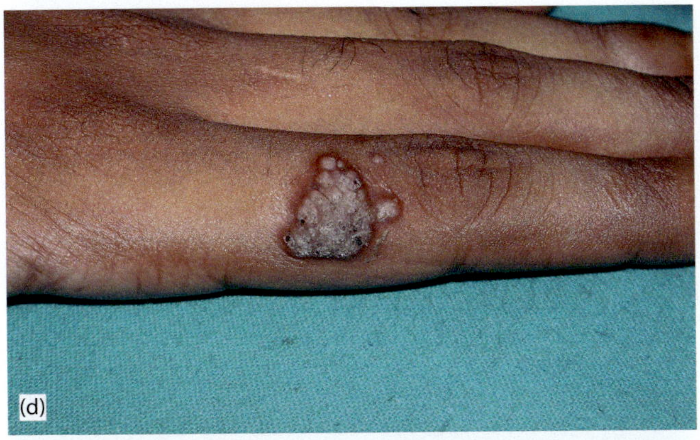


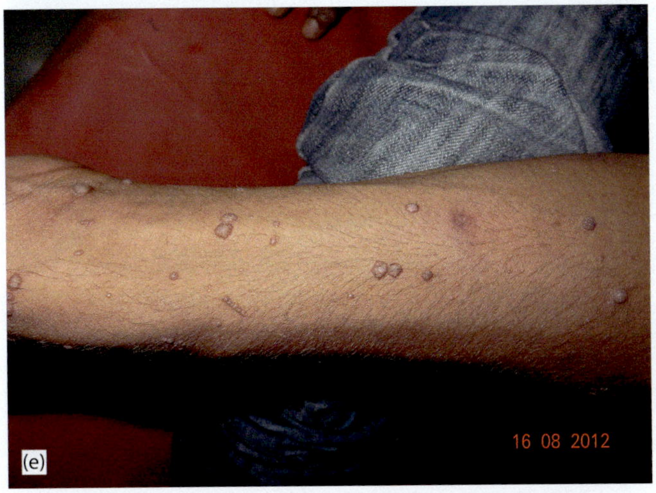


Figure 7.19 (*Continued*) **(d)** Flat-topped, verrucous plaque showing pinpoint hemorrhagic points. **(e)** Warts presenting multiple papules and plaques. Note pseudo-Koebnerization. (a,b,d,e – Courtesy: Dr. Piyush Kumar, Katihar, India; c – Courtesy: Dr. Niharika Ranjan Lal, ESIPGIMSR, Kolkata, India.)

## Benign lichenoid keratosis (lichen planus-like keratosis)

- This is a common benign neoplasm of the skin.
- Solitary, dusky-red to violaceous scaly patches occur on the head and neck, trunk, or distal extremities; on the face it may present as a solitary asymptomatic round lesion.
- It may be rough or scaly in texture and can transition from pink to violaceous to hyperpigmented as it regresses. Multiple regression phases may be present within the lesion.
- DD: Verruca vulgaris (warty plaques, pseudo-Koebnerization), tuberculosis verrucosa cutis (oozy plaque on the soles and buttocks), lichen planus hypertrophicus (verrucous plaque with scaling on the shins, with follicular papules in surroundings).

## Keloids/hypertrophic scar

- Keloids and hypertrophic scars are the result of aberrant wound healing after injury to the reticular dermis (**Table 7.3**).
- Keloids are flesh-colored to reddish brown, firm nodules (**Figure 7.20a**) and plaques with peripheral claw-like projections at sites of trauma or inflammation (**Figure 7.20b**).

Table 7.3 Keloid and hypertrophic scar

| Keloid | Hypertrophic scar |
|---|---|
| Firm, smooth growth over original wound but extends beyond wound area | Firm, red growth over scar but does not cross the original wound area |
| Itchy and claw-like projections; extends beyond months of wound | Non-itchy and confined within scar and no projections; proliferates up to six months |
| Happens in genetically predisposed individual, mainly over chest and shoulders | Happens when there is lot of tension on healing wound |
| Does not reduce on its own; rather itching and projections increase | Over several months scar becomes pale and flat |

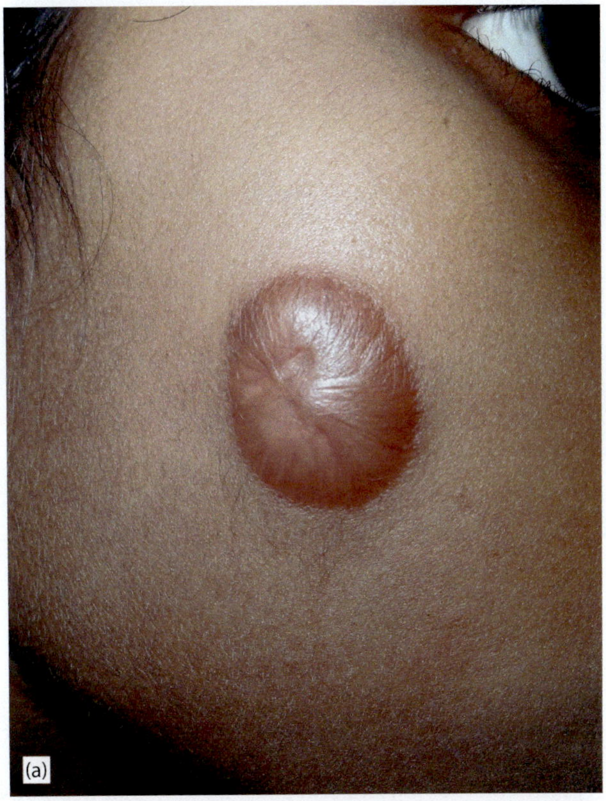


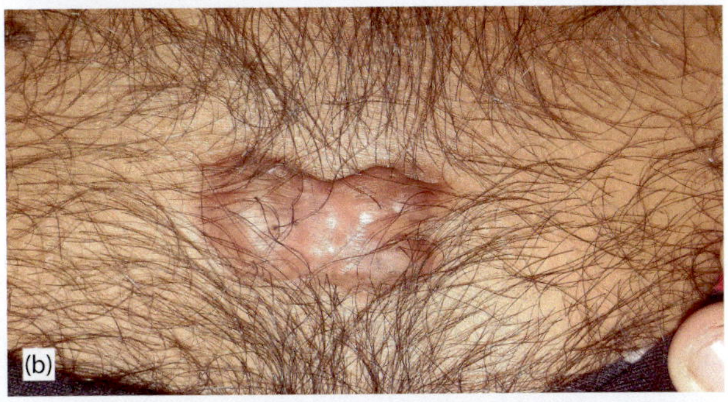


Figure 7.20 **(a)** Keloid. Smooth, shiny plaque on the face. **(b)** Keloid. Claw-like projections extending beyond plaque margin. (*Continued*)

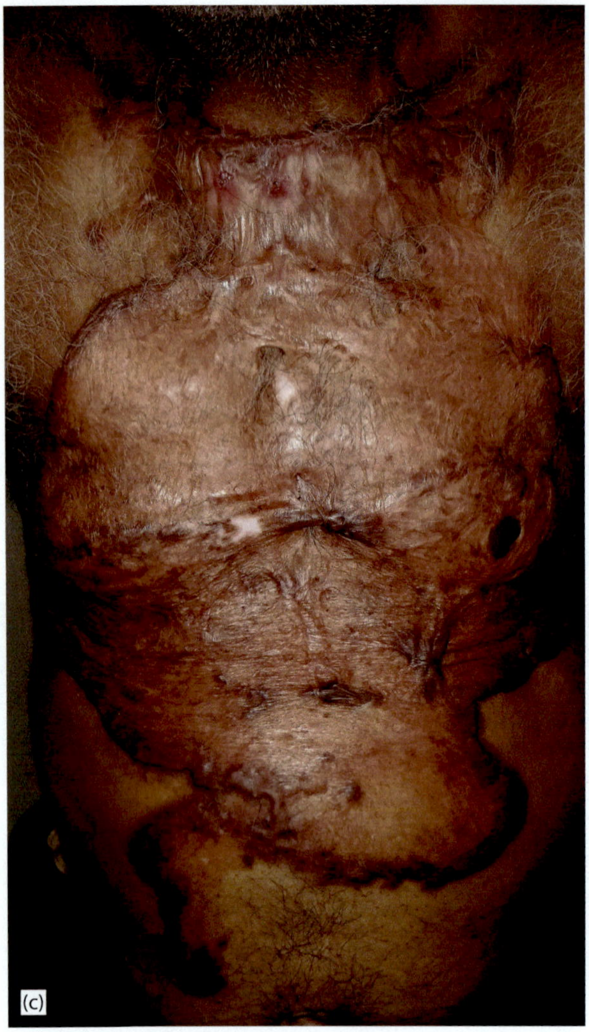


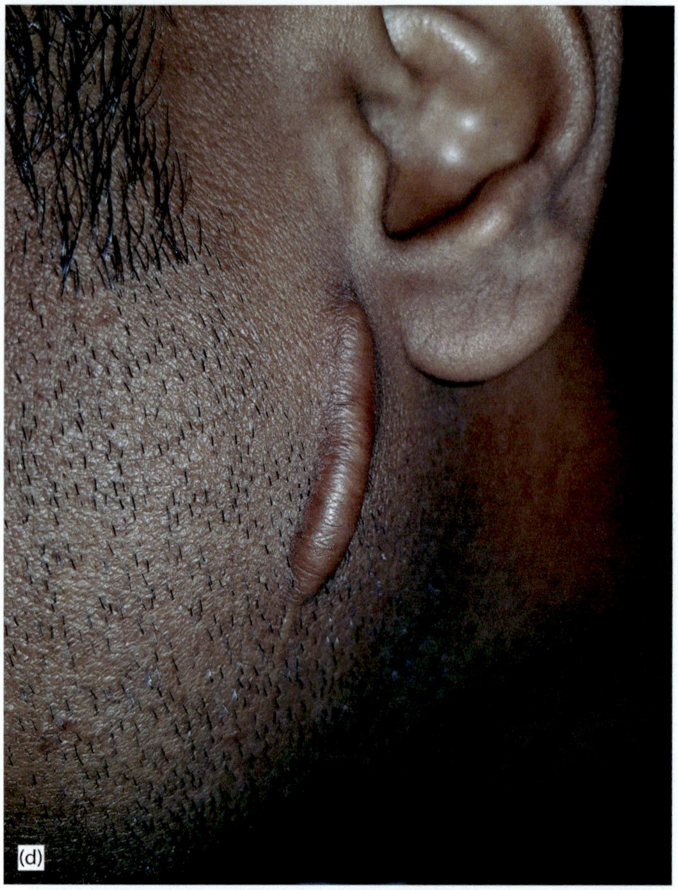


Figure 7.20 (*Continued*) **(c)** Keloid. **(d)** Hypertrophic scar at the site of trauma. (a–c – Courtesy: Dr. Niharika Ranjan Lal, ESIPGIMSR, Kolkata, India; d – Courtesy: Dr. PC Das, Katihar, India.)

- Keloids spread beyond the margins of inciting trauma even six months after the onset (**Figure 7.20c**).
- In hypertrophic scarring there is also proliferation of scar tissue but within six months of onset, and it doesn't spread beyond the margin of scar. It doesn't have claw-like extensions (**Figure 7.20d**).
- DD: Lobomycosis (keloidal plaque/nodule, child's pop-beads–like arrangement of fungi), B-cell lymphoma (plum-colored nodules and plaques, follicular histology with atypia and mitoses).

## ATROPHIC PLAQUES

### Morphea

- Morphea is a localized form of scleroderma.
- It is characterized by oval or linear well-circumscribed sclerotic lesions of varying sizes.
- Morphea-en-plaque looks like circumscribed, indurated, oval/round plaques surrounded by a lilac-colored border that progresses to form sclerotic, smooth, shiny, ivory-colored plaques, with loss of hair follicles and hyperpigmentation (**Figure 7.21a–c**).
- It is commonly seen over the trunk and extremities.
- Other variants include morphea profundus, guttate morphea, keloidal morphea, linear morphea, pansclerotic morphea, and generalized morphea.
- DD: Lichen sclerosus et atrophicus (ivory/white depressed papules, coalesced to form plaque, genital and back), scar (wrinkled depressed surface, collagen loss).

### Lichen sclerosus et atrophicus (LSA)

- Whitish polygonal papules coalesce to form plaques with follicular plugs on surface (**Figure 7.22a**).
- Older lesions are porcelain white and shiny (**Figure 7.22b**).
- Purpuric lesions may develop on the surface in active lesions.
- It is asymptomatic, but genital lesions may itch.

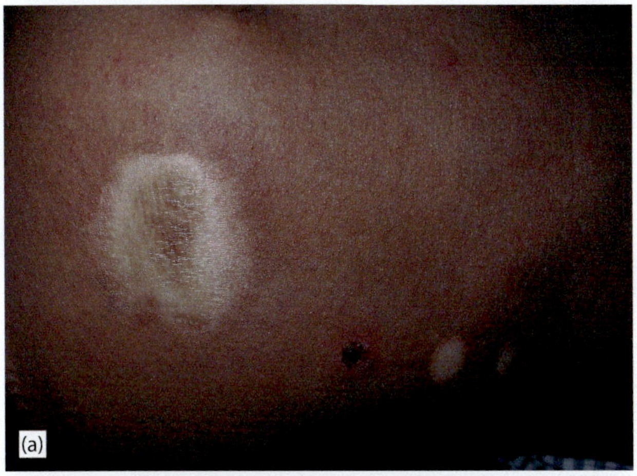

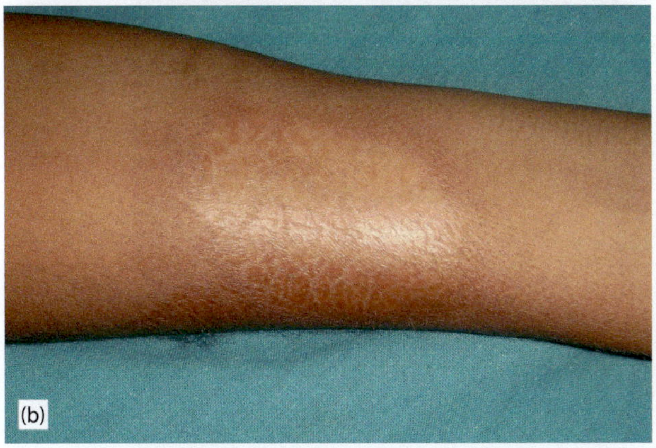

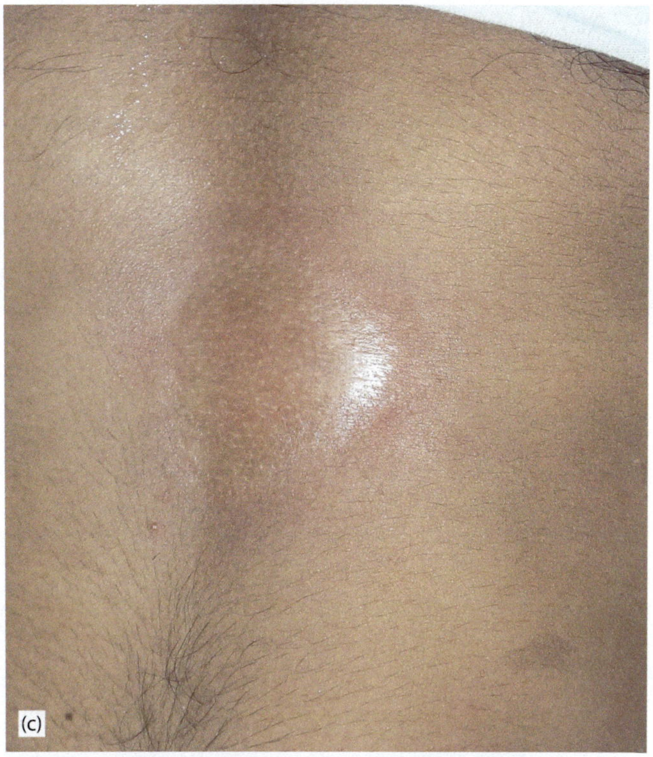

Figure 7.21 **(a)** Morphea. Shiny, depigmented patch with wrinkled surface. **(b)** Well-defined lesion of morphea on the forearm. **(c)** Morphea lesion on the chest. (a–c – Courtesy: Dr. Piyush Kumar, Katihar, India.)

- Variants include genital and extragenital.
- Extragenital LSA is most commonly seen on the back and shoulders.
- DD: Morphea (atrophic patch, shiny, wrinkled, tough skin), pityriasis versicolor (hypopigmented scaly patches, perifollicular area, appears on the back, neck, and side of face), malignant atrophic papulosis (depressed porcelain-white papules with livid red periphery, telangiectasia, ischemic infarcts in intestines, kidney).

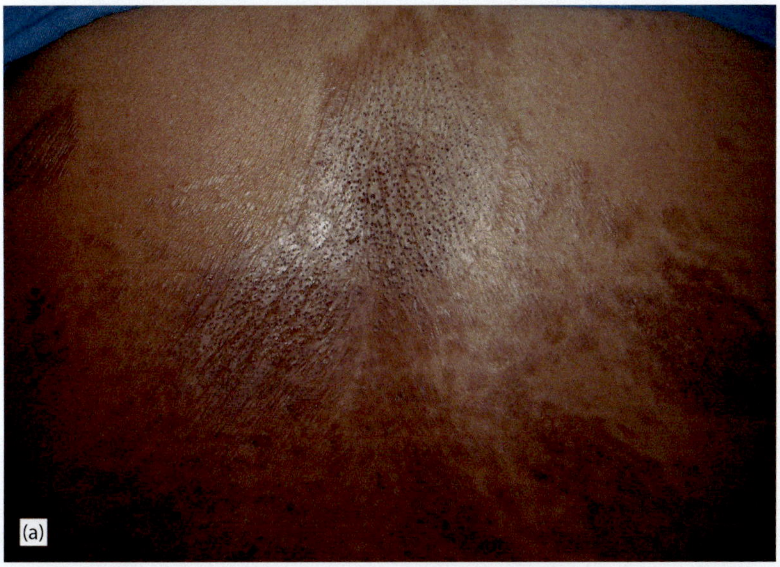

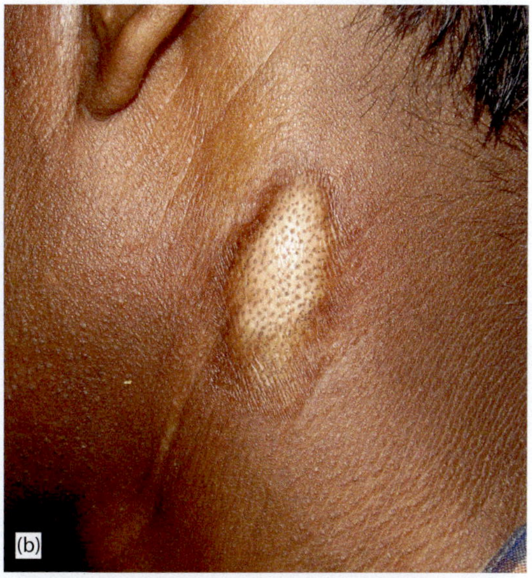

Figure 7.22 **(a)** Shiny, atrophic plaque with prominent follicular opening in lichen sclerosus atrophicus. **(b)** Porcelain white plaque with follicular prominence in lichen sclerosus atrophicus. (a,b – Courtesy: Dr. Piyush Kumar, Katihar, India.)

## SCALY PLAQUES

### Seborrheic dermatitis (SD)[15]

- This is a common inflammatory condition that affect the seborrheic areas of the body.
- SD often presents as well-delineated erythematous plaques (or patches) with greasy, yellowish scales of varying extents in regions rich in sebaceous glands, such as the scalp (**Figure 7.23a**), the retro-auricular area (**Figure 7.23b**), face (nasolabial folds, upper lip, eyelids **Figure 7.23c** and eyebrows), and the upper chest. Distribution of the lesions is generally symmetrical. Truncal lesions may be oval and petaloid scaly plaques.

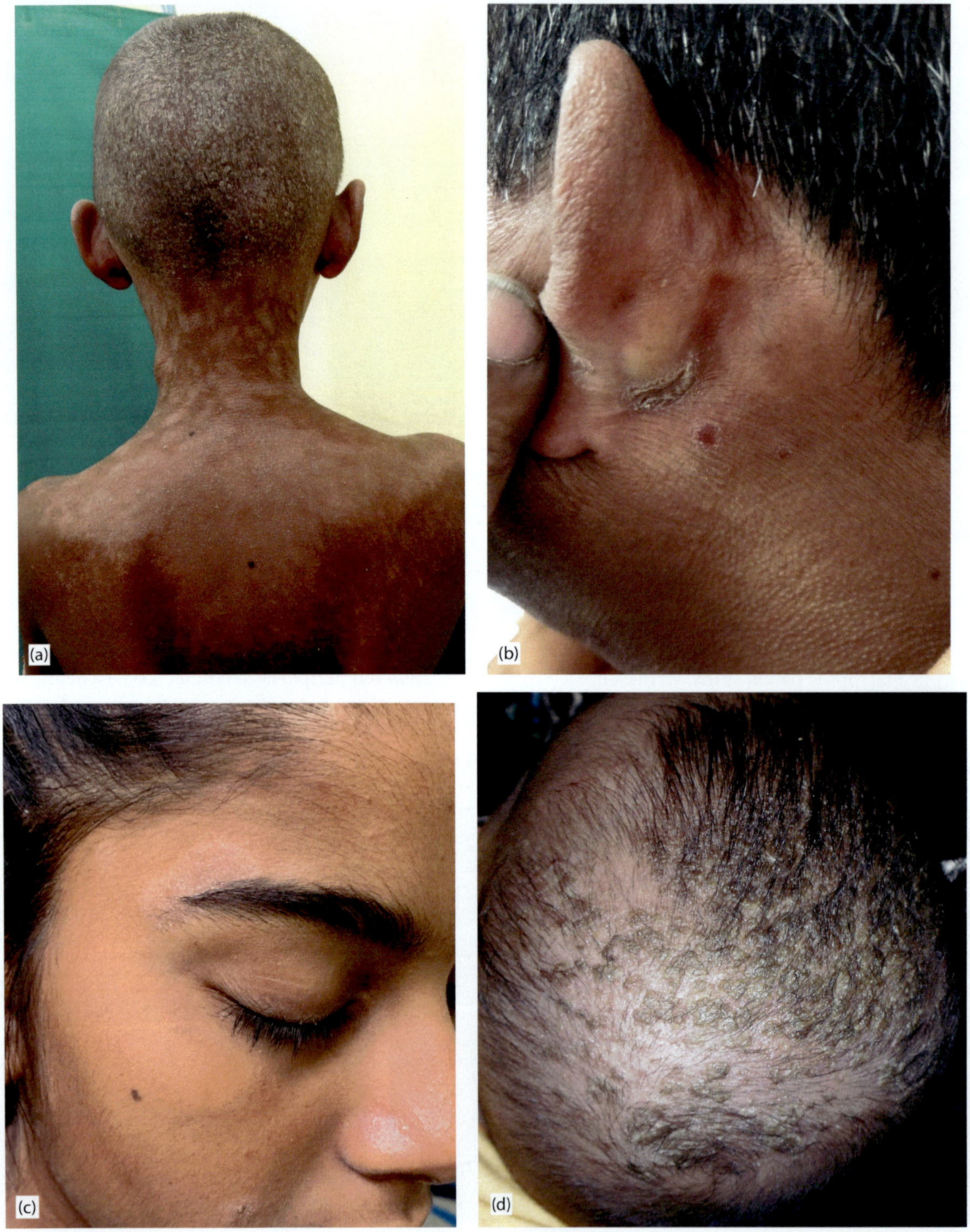


Figure 7.23 **(a)** Greasy, yellow scales on the scalp in seborrheic dermatitis. **(b)** Scaling in the retroauricular area in seborrheic dermatitis. **(c)** Seborrheic dermatitis presenting as scaling and erythema over the eyelid margin and a scaly plaque near the eyebrow. **(d)** Greasy, crusted scales over the vertex of the scalp in an infant (cradle cap). (a,b,d –Courtesy: Dr. Niharika Ranjan Lal, ESIPGIMSR, Kolkata, India; c – Courtesy: Dr. Piyush Kumar, Katihar, India.)

Table 7.4 Differential diagnosis of seborrheic dermatitis

| Diagnosis | Diagnostic Clues |
|---|---|
| Psoriasis | Usually involves extensor, palmar, plantar, nails, and extensor areas. Thick plaques sharply limited with silvery white scales. Positive family history. Arthritis is present in 10% of patients. Uncommon in children. |
| Atopic Dermatitis | First appearance after three months of age; pruritus and restlessness are common. Frequently involves scalp, cheeks, and extensor areas. Flexures involvement is more frequent in older ages. Family history of atopy such as eczema, allergic rhinitis, and asthma. Self-resolves by age 12. |
| Tinea Capitis | Commonly seen in children, frequently accompanied by hair-loss patches with "black dots" (broken hair). Highly contagious. KOH examination of the hair shaft and fungal culture confirm the diagnosis. Household members of patient should be examined. |
| Rosacea | Usually targets the face. Papulopustules and telangiectasias on the malar, nose, and perioral regions with slight desquamation. Recurrent edema and flushing. |
| Systemic Lupus Erythematosus (SLE) | In acute stage, a butterfly rash on the face that spares the nose bridge or nasolabial folds. Photosensitivity is common. Skin lesions are generally associated with other clinical signs of SLE. Histology and serologic tests, such as antinuclear autoantibodies, confirm the diagnosis. |
| Pemphigus Foliaceus | Erythema, scaling, and crusting that first present on the scalp and face can expand to the chest and back. Histology, direct immunofluorescence with anti-desmoglein antibodies confirm diagnosis. |
| Pityriasis Rosea | Abrupt onset, appearance of herald patch, and resolution within weeks. |
| Secondary Syphilis | Peripheral lymphadenopathy, mucosal lesions, and palmoplantar maculo-papules. Serology tests such as VDRL/ RPR, FTA-ABS confirm diagnosis. |
| Diaper Dermatitis | Occurs on convex skin surfaces in contact with diaper, such as lower abdomen, genitalia, buttocks, and upper thighs. Spares skin folds. Pustules are common. |
| Langerhans Cell Histiocytosis | Multisystem disease. Brown to purplish papules prone to coalesce on the scalp, retro-auricular areas, axillae, and inguinal folds. Possible lytic bone lesions, liver, spleen, and lung involvement. Histology confirms diagnosis. |

- In infants the most common form of SD is cradle cap. It appears as red-yellow plaques coated by thick, greasy scales on the vertex, appearing within three months of birth (**Figure 7.23d**).
- DD – **Table 7.4**.

## Herald patch of pityriasis rosea

- This is an acute, asymptomatic or mildly pruritic eruption.
- It appears as single or multiple 2- to 5-cm oval plaque with a fine collarette of scale inside the periphery of the lesion (**Figure 7.24**).
- Crops of similar but smaller lesions appear several days to weeks later, arranged along the lines of cleavage ("Christmas tree" appearance).
- It resolves spontaneously after four to eight weeks.
- DD: Small plaque parapsoriasis (scaly plaques, digitate lesions over trunk), seborrheic dermatitis (scaly plaques, seborrheic areas), secondary syphilis (palmoplantar scaly lesions, VDRL +ve, rebound phenomenon).

## Actinic keratosis (AK)

- Actinic keratosis occurs as multiple, small, discrete keratotic papules/plaques on sun-damaged skin (**Figure 7.25a–c**).
- It is mainly seen in tropical countries like Australia, New Zealand, and South Africa (skin color is lighter and the UV rays are more intense).
- Diseases like vitiligo and albinism with loss of protective melanocytes predispose the patient to develop AK.
- It is commonly seen over the nose, lips, bald scalp, and extremities.

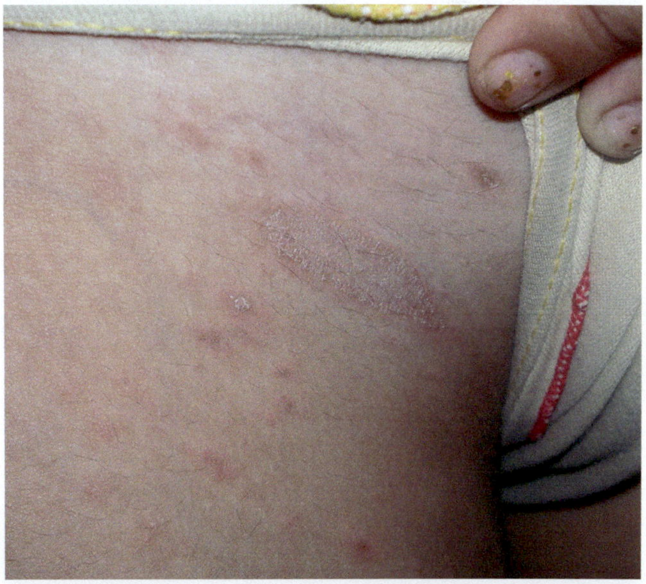

Figure 7.24 Herald patch of pityriasis rosea with collarette of scales surrounded by multiple daughter lesions. (Courtesy: Dr. Piyush Kumar, Katihar, India.)

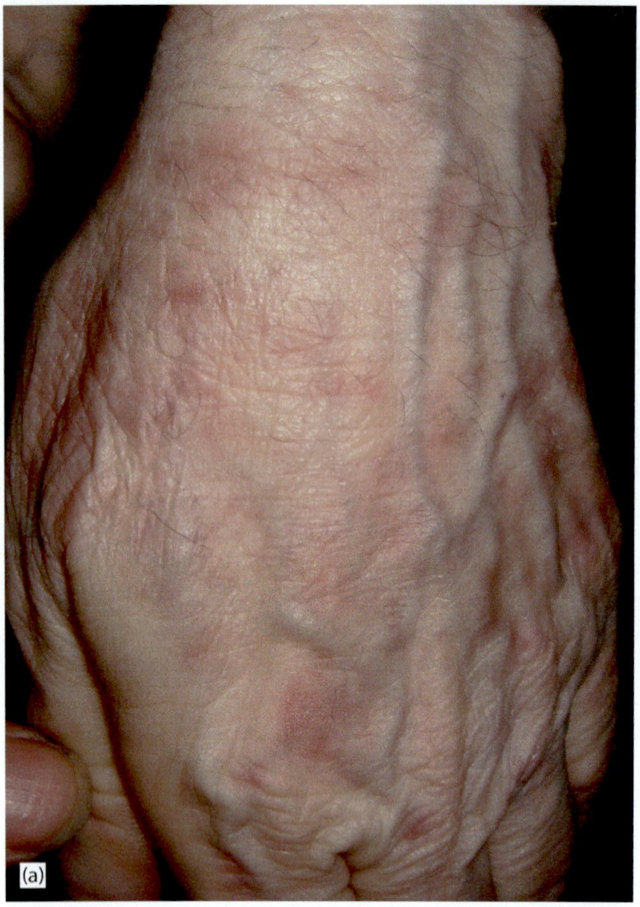


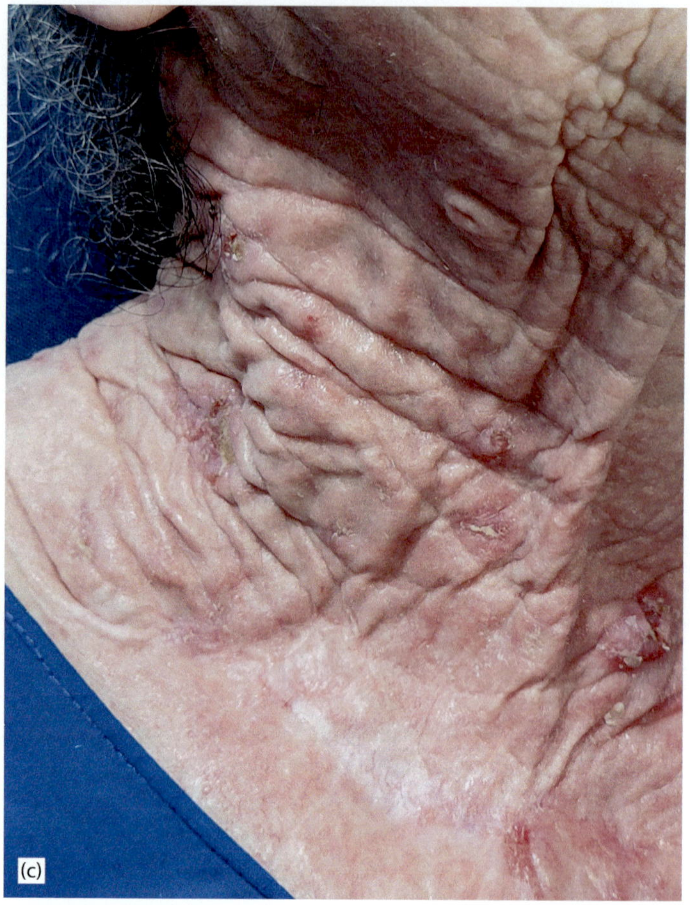


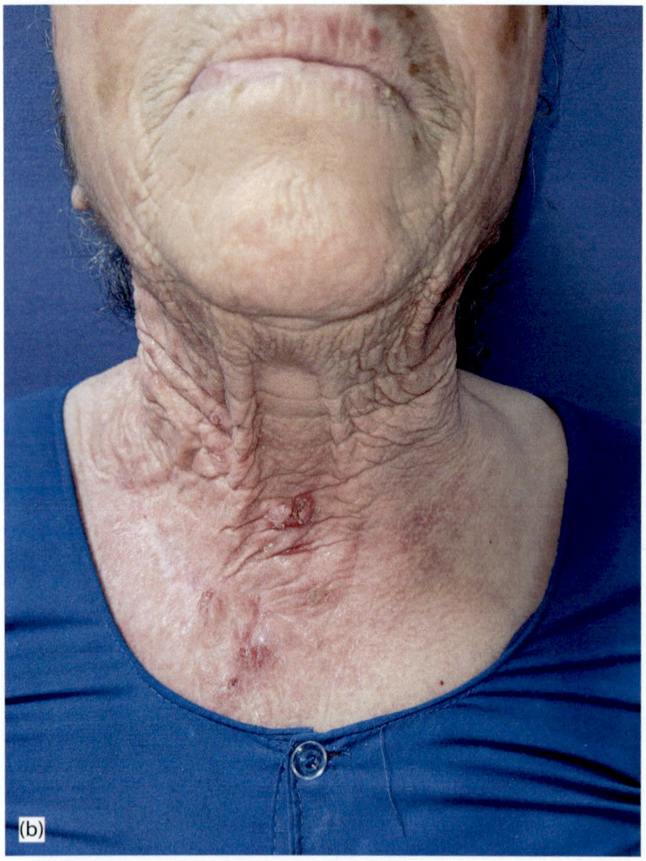


- DD: Bowen's disease (oozy, scaly plaque, wind-blown appearance, atypical cells), squamous cell carcinoma (fungating mass, atypical cells, mitoses).

## Pityriasis rotunda

- Pityriasis rotunda is disorder of keratinization characterized by geometrically perfect circular sharply defined patches of dry ichthyosiform scaling.
- Circular/oval, fixed, well-defined, scaly hypopigmented or hyperpigmented plaques occur on the trunk and extremities.
- It is often associated with neoplasia (hepatocellular carcinoma) and systemic diseases.

Figure 7.25 **(a)** Pink papules and plaques in early actinic keratosis in an albino. **(b)** Multiple lesions of actinic keratosis on a background of chronic photodamaged skin. Note the relative absence of lesions on the left chest which was usually covered by saree. **(c)** Closeup of the lesions in the same patient. Note yellowish, thickened photoaged skin on the right side of the neck. (a – Courtesy: Dr. Piyush Kumar, Katihar, India; b,c – Courtesy: Dr. Shekhar Neema, Associate Professor, Armed Forces Medical College, Pune, India.)

- DD: Tinea corporis (itchy, annular, scaly plaques with peripheral papules), parapsoriasis (digitate lesions, trunk), pityriasis rosea (collarette of scales, inverted fir tree appearance).

## PLAQUES WITHOUT SCALING

### Pruritic urticarial papules and plaques of pregnancy

- This condition is usually seen in primigravida in the third trimester of pregnancy.
- Erythematous, urticarial papules and plaques occur on the abdomen around the umbilicus.
- 1- to -2mm lesions appear within abdominal striae.
- DD: Urticaria (transient, evanescent, edematous plaque).

### Seborrheic keratosis[16]

- Seborrheic keratoses are common, benign, pigmented epidermal tumors.
- The condition is commonly seen in middle-aged to elderly people, especially of colored skin.
- Round to oval hyperpigmented macules evolve toward stuck-on brownish to black warty plaques with a greasy smooth surface showing plugged follicular orifices (**Figure 7.26a,b**). The lesions typically have a "stuck on" appearance.
- They typically occur over the face and upper trunk.
- Variants include the following:
  - Solar lentigo: flat, circumscribed, pigmented patches seen on sun-exposed areas.
  - Dermatosis papulosa nigra: small, sessile, black lesions on the head and neck. Common in colored skin.
  - Stucco keratoses: Multiple gray or white papules on the dorsal aspect of lower extremities.
  - Melanoacanthoma: Large, pigmented variant.
- DD: Verrucous epidermal nevus (congenital, verrucous, usually linear), verruca vulgaris (pseudo-Koebnerization, warty plaque and papules), Bowenoid papulosis (genital, warty papules and plaques, HPV infection, precancerous).

### Mastocytoma

- Mastocytosis is a group of disorders characterized by abnormal proliferation and accumulation of mast cells, involving the skin only (cutaneous mastocytosis) or the bone marrow and other extracutaneous organs (systemic mastocytosis).
- Mast cells produce mediators histamine, heparin, tryptase, proteases, chymase, cytokines (tumor necrosis factor and interleukins), chemokines to name a few. These mediator-related symptoms are flushing, itching, blistering, diarrhea, abdominal pain, vomiting, hypotension, headache, and bone pain.
- Cutaneous mastocytosis presents as solitary or multiple skin-colored to yellowish papules or plaques, often with a peau d'orange appearance of the surface.
- Stroking or rubbing of lesions produces wheals (Darier's sign).
- Lesions occur most commonly on trunk, arm or neck.
- Bullae may occur over lesions (bullous mastocytosis).
- Most lesions appear before one year of age and involute over several months to years.
- DD: Erysipelas (peau d'orange, erythema, edema, vesicles over limbs), urticarial wheals (transient, evanescent, edematous plaque), papular urticaria/insect bite hypersensitivity (erythema, papules and plaques, extremities).

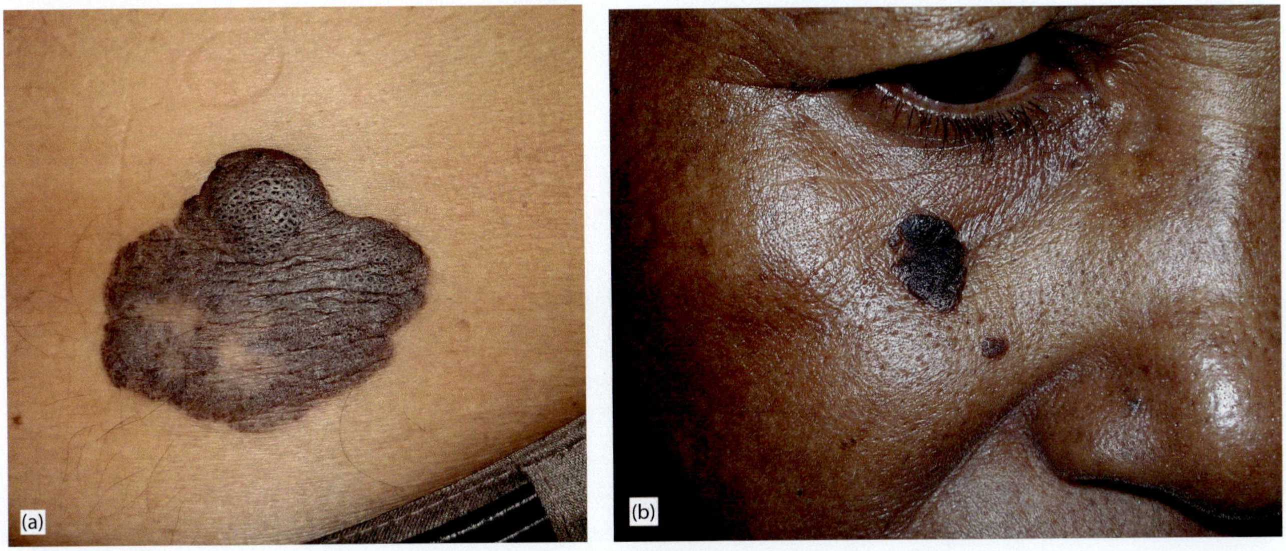


Figure 7.26 **(a)** Seborrheic keratosis presenting as hyperkeratotic plaque showing plugged follicular orifices. **(b)** Seborrheic keratosis on face. (a – Courtesy: Dr. Niharika Ranjan Lal, ESIPGIMSR, Kolkata, India; b – Courtesy: Dr. Piyush Kumar, Katihar, India.)

## Melanocytic nevus

- It can be congenital or acquired.
- Macules/plaques are dark-brown to black and may be hairy (**Figure 7.27a**).
- They can be small (<2 cm), medium (2–20 cm), or large (>20 cm) (**Figure 7.27b,c**). Giant hairy nevi mostly occur on the trunk.
- DD: Becker's nevus (shoulder, hypertrichosis, after puberty, hyperpigmentation, acneiform eruption), acquired smooth-muscle hamartoma (elliptical, lumbosacral area, hypertrichosis, smooth muscle bundles at different angles), nevoid acanthosis nigricans (verrucous, velvety, diffuse plaque).

## Shagreen patch

- It is a connective tissue hamartoma, found in approximately half the patients with tuberous sclerosis complex.
- It presents as elevated pink to yellow-brown plaques with an orange-peel–like texture, ranging from several millimeters to several centimeters in length (**Figure 7.28**).
- Shagreen patches are asymmetric and usually appear on dorsal surfaces, such as the back and the lumbosacral regions, but occasionally occur on the chest or the abdomen.
- They typically develop during the first decade of life.
- Other features of tuberous sclerosis, such as angiofibroma and ash-leaf macules, are also seen.
- DD: Collagenoma (trunk/buttocks, linear or zosteriform, single/multiple), xanthoma (yellow, hyperlipidemia).

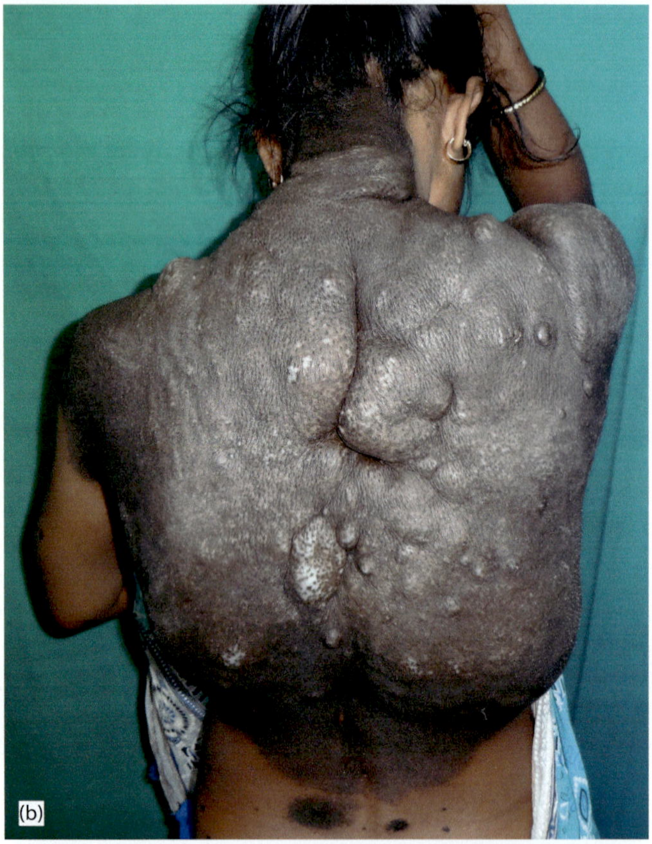


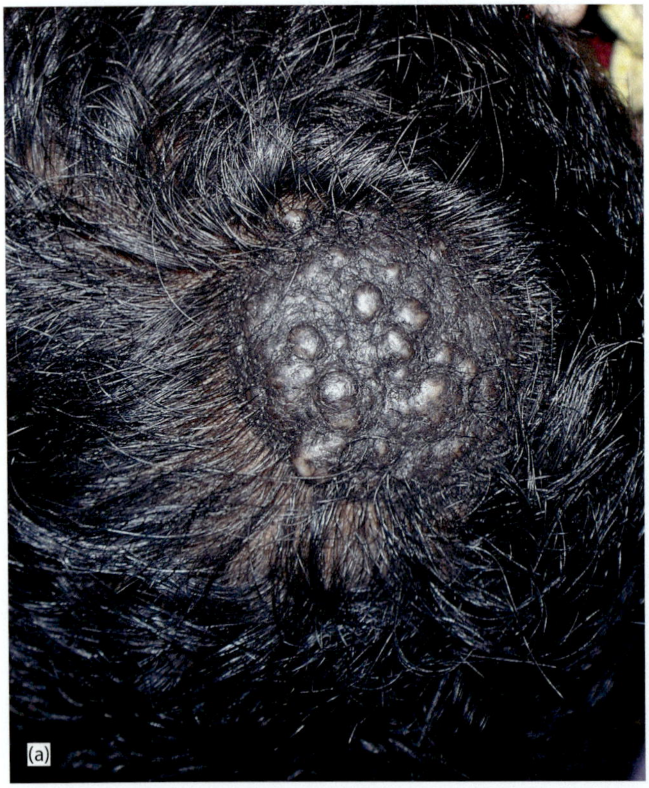


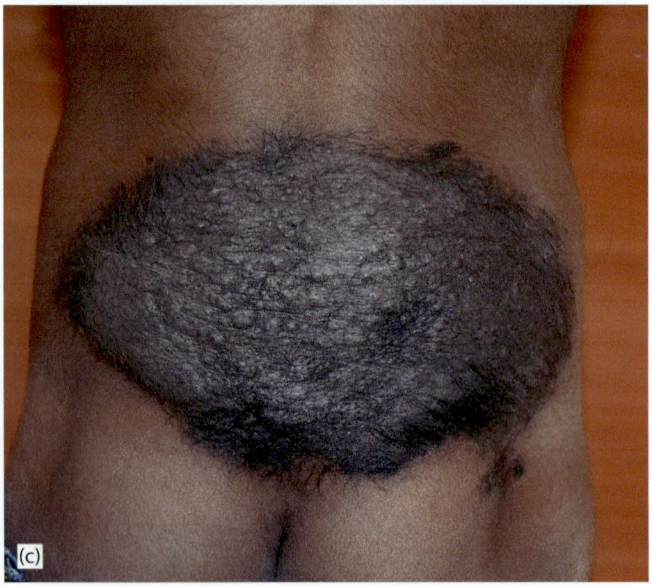


Figure 7.27 **(a)** Congenital melanocytic nevus on scalp. **(b)** Giant congenital melanocytic nevus on trunk. **(c)** Large congenital melanocytic nevus on the lower back. Note lesional hypertrichosis and nodularity. (a,c – Courtesy: Dr. Piyush Kumar, Katihar, India; b – Courtesy: Dr. Niharika Ranjan Lal, ESIPGIMSR, Kolkata, India.)

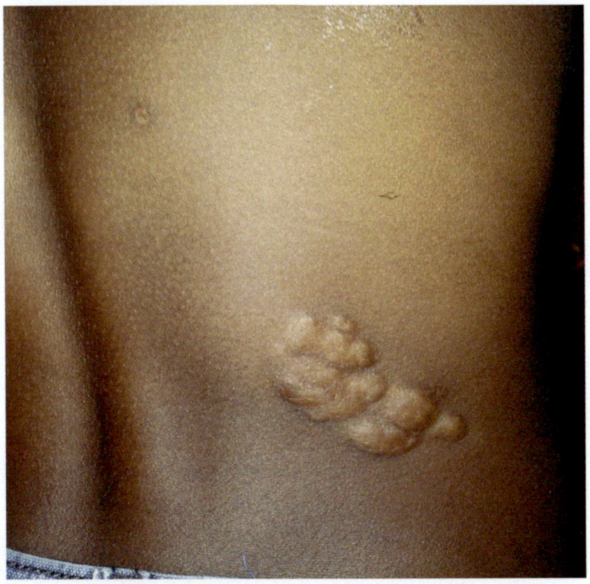

Figure 7.28 Yellow soft plaque on the lumbosacral area in tuberous sclerosis. (Courtesy: Dr. Piyush Kumar, Katihar, India.)

## ULCERATED PLAQUE

### Basal cell carcinoma

- Basal cell carcinoma (BCC) is the most commonly occurring cancer in the world, generally a slow-growing tumor for which metastases is rare.
- Clinical features are dependent on the subtype of BCC. Nodular or cystic BCCs present as raised red, pearly, translucent lesions with peripheral telangiectasia. Superficial BCC may mimic discoid eczema or Bowen's disease, while morphoeic BCC presents as a subtle scar-like plaque.
- It is a slow-growing wavy, translucent nodule with central ulceration (**Figure 7.29a,b**).
- Pigmentation is a common finding (**Figure 7.29c**).
- Crusting/bleeding may be seen.
- Usually it is a solitary lesion.

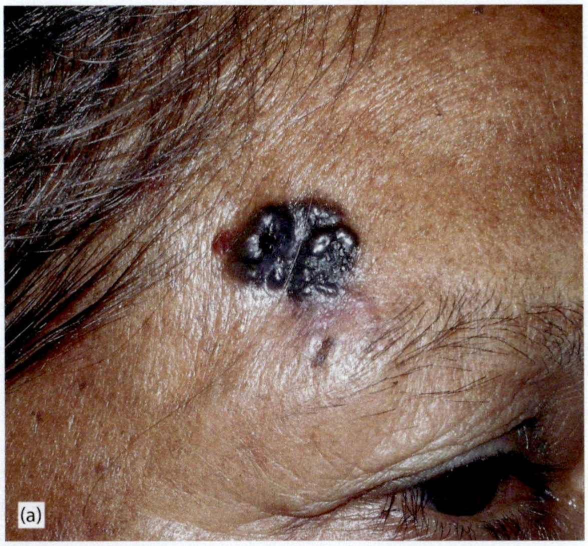


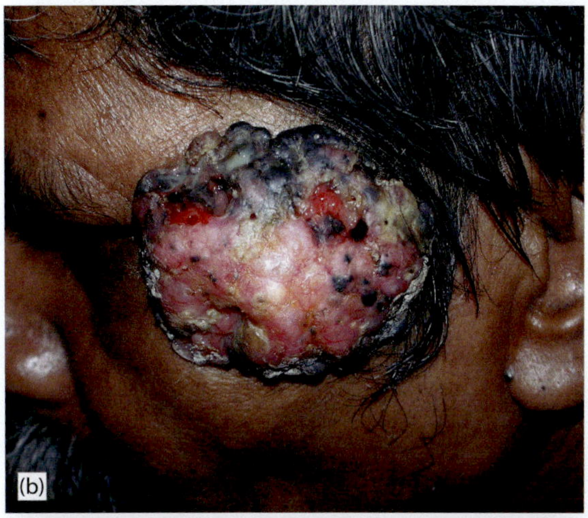


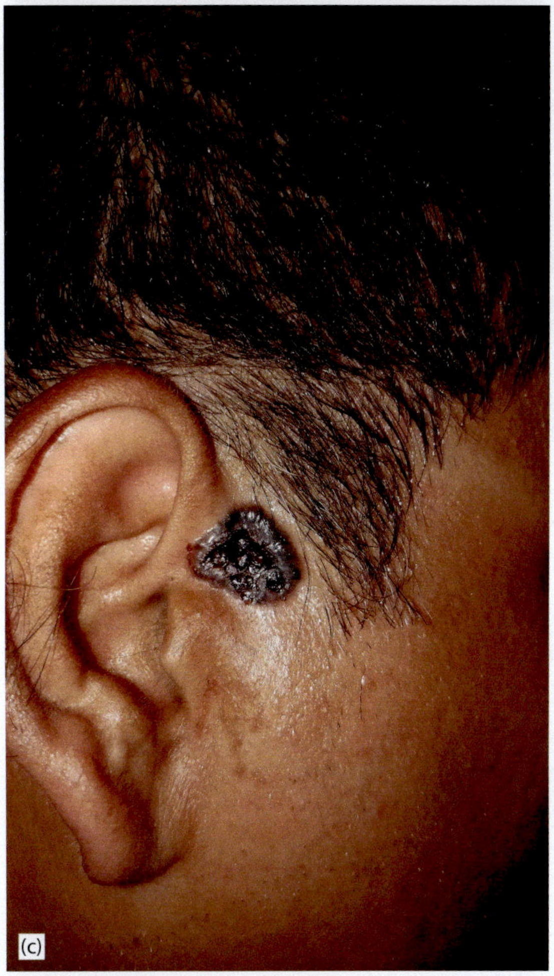


Figure 7.29 **(a)** Pigmented, smooth-surfaced plaque of basal cell carcinoma with waxy, rolled border. **(b)** Large plaque of basal cell carcinoma with central smooth surfaced, erythematous area and telangiectasia. The margin is typically pigmented, waxy, and rolled. **(c)** Pigmented basal cell carcinoma with central ulceration and hemorrhagic crust. (a–c – Courtesy: Dr. Piyush Kumar, Katihar, India.)

- Typically appears over the head and neck region, such as nose, forehead, cheeks, periocular area, and ears.
- It has a characteristic rolled border, and telangiectasia is seen over the lesion.
- Variants include nodular, superficial spreading, morphoeic, fibroepithelioma of pinkus.
- DD: Porokeratosis (double-ridge with central crater, annular plaque, column parakeratosis), melanoma (darkly pigmented, ulceration, mainly over feet in the Indian subcontinent), seborrheic keratosis (verrucous, pedunculated/stuck on, pigmented).

## Necrobiosis lipoidica diabeticorum

- Necrobiosis lipoidica diabeticorum is a chronic granulomatous dermatitis of unknown cause that is most often associated with diabetes mellitus.
- The lesions appear as yellow-brown, telangiectatic plaques with central atrophy and raised violaceous borders. They occur most frequently on the shins or the dorsa of the feet. Ulcers, which exist in about 30% of lesions, are often induced by trauma. In rare cases squamous-cell carcinomas develop, typically in older, ulcerated lesions.
- DD: Psoriasis (micaceous scaly plaque, Auspitz sign, extensors), morphea (atrophic, sclerosis, thickened surface).

## Bowen's disease

- It is an in situ squamous cell carcinoma (SCC).
- Clinically a typical case of Bowen's disease is a slowly enlarging erythematous patch or plaque (**Figure 7.30a**) that is well demarcated and has a scaling or crusted

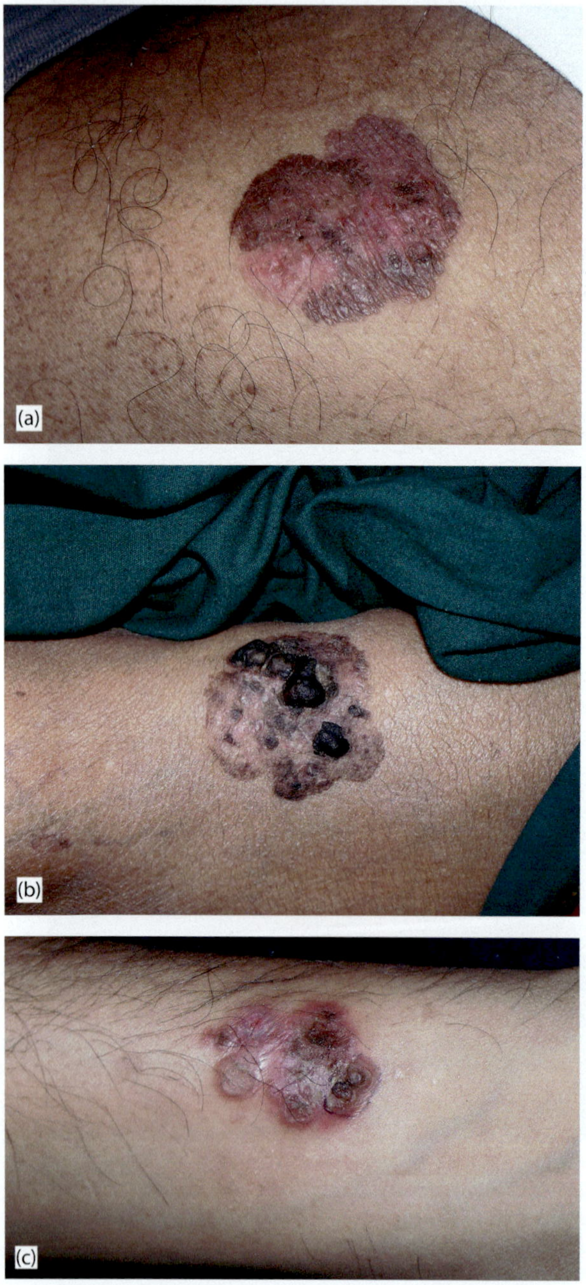


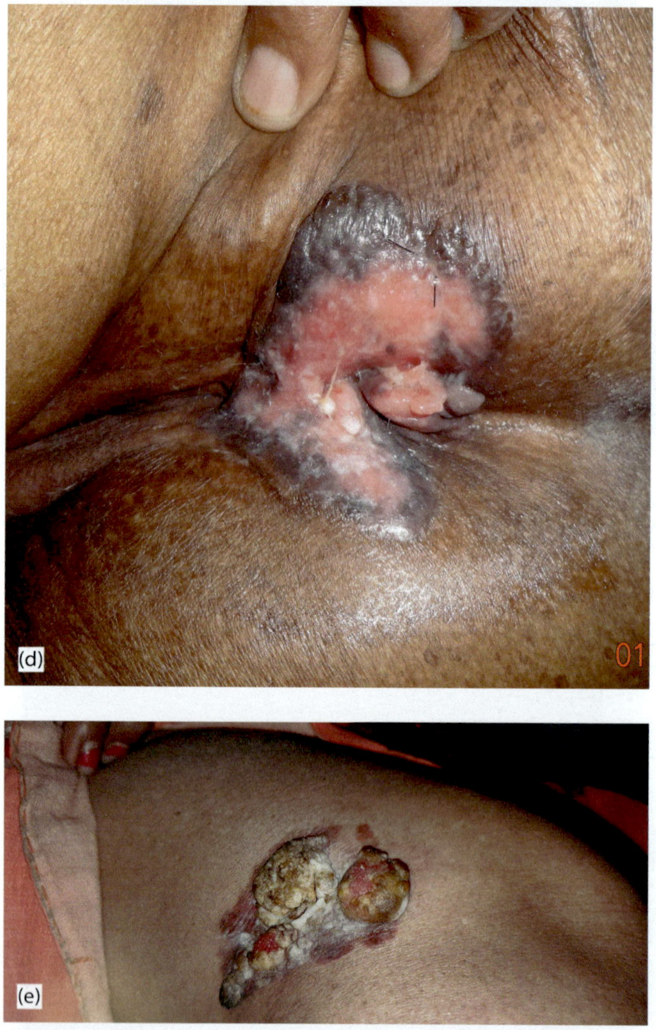


Figure 7.30 **(a)** Erythematous scaly plaque in Bowen's disease. **(b)** Well-demarcated, crusted, erythematous plaque in Bowen's disease. **(c)** Bowen's disease on the forearm. **(d)** Perianal Bowen's disease. **(e)** Nodules of squamous cell carcinoma developing within the lesion of Bowen's disease. (a–c – Courtesy: Dr. Piyush Kumar, Katihar, India; d – Courtesy: Dr. Niharika Ranjan Lal, ESIPGIMSR, Kolkata, India; e – Courtesy: Dr. Ashutosh Ranjan, Consultant Dermatologist, Chhapra, India.)

surface (**Figure 7.30b,c**). In some cases it can be pigmented or verrucous.
- It is commonly located on the lower limbs and on the head and neck; it may also be seen subungual or periungual, palmar, genital, and perianal (**Figure 7.30d**).
- Frank SCC may develop (**Figure 7.30e**).
- Multiple lesions are seen in association with chronic arsenicosis.
- DD: Psoriasis (micaceous scales, Auspitz sign, extensors), Paget's disease (oozy plaques, crusting, breasts, vulva).

## Pemphigus vegetans

- Vesicles or bullae evolve into hypertrophic granulating, fissured plaques with erosions. Edges studded with pustules (**Figure 7.31**).
- Seen mainly in flexures (i.e., axilla, groin). Mucosal erosions and hyperkeratotic tongue are seen.
- DD: Darier-White disease (dirty, warty papules, flexures, dyskeratosis), intertrigo (ill-defined plaques, itchy, bacterial-fungal-dermatitis etiology), Hailey-Hailey disease (oozy, crusts over flexures, dilapidated brick wall, dyskeratosis).

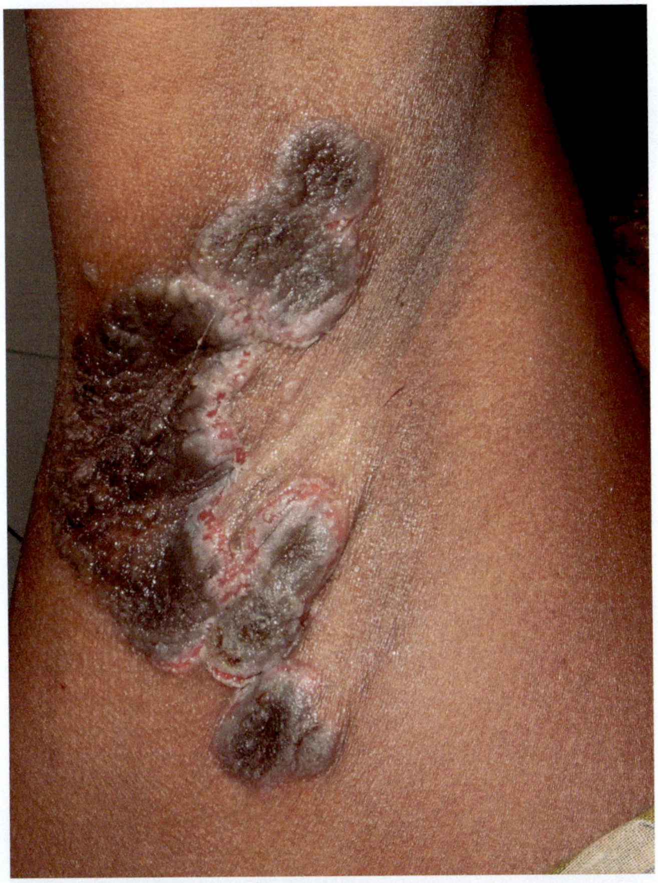

Figure 7.31 Macerated plaques with fissures in axilla in pemphigus vegetans. (Courtesy: Dr. Piyush Kumar, Katihar, India.)

## Paget's disease

- Paget's is an uncommon cutaneous intraepithelial adenocarcinoma involving the epidermis and extending into the dermis.
- There are slow-growing well-defined, erythematous plaques with crusting resembles eczema (**Figure 7.32a,b**).
- An irregular, slightly raised border is unilaterally seen on nipple, areola, and adjoining skin of the breast.
- It may cause retraction or destruction of nipple.

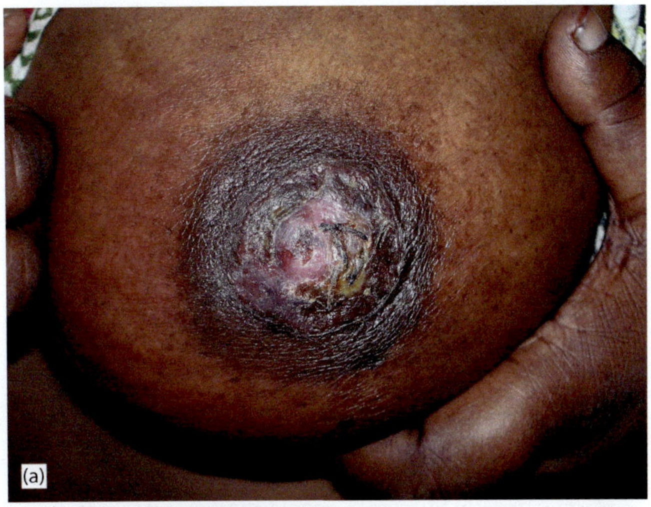

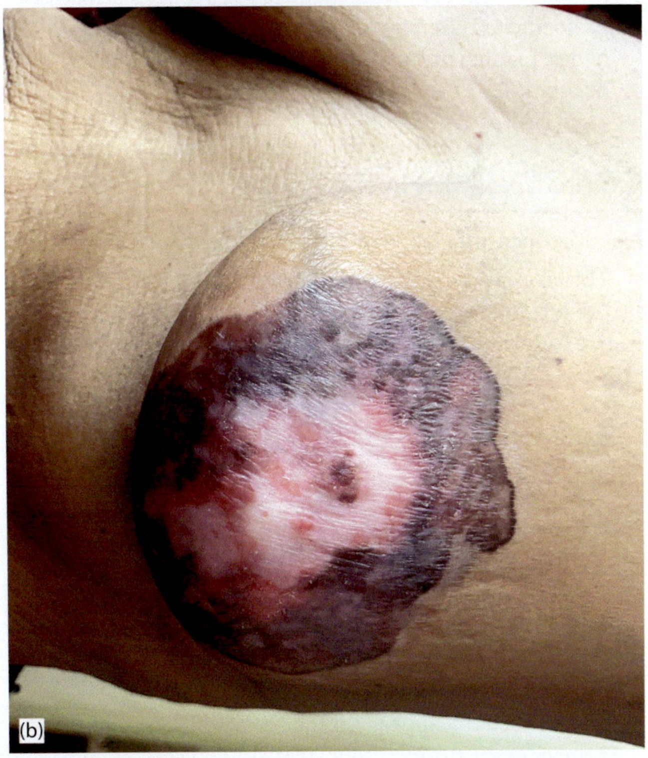

Figure 7.32 **(a)** Paget's disease presenting as crusted plaque on the nipple. Note partial destruction of the nipple. **(b)** Large lesion of Paget's disease with complete loss of nipple. (*Continued*)

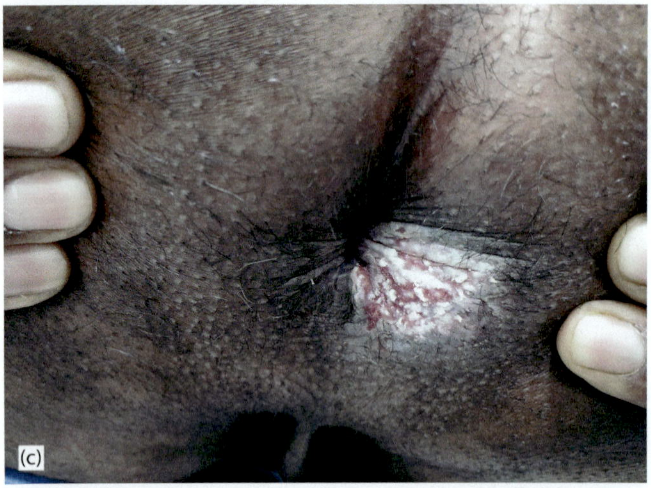

Figure 7.32 (*Continued*) **(c)** Extramammary Paget's disease in perianal area. (a – Courtesy: Dr. Piyush Kumar, Katihar, India; b – Courtesy: Dr Rajeev Ranjan, Ara, India; c – Courtesy: Dr. Santoshdev Rathod, SVPIMSR, Smt. NHL Municipal Medical College, V.S. Hospital, Ahmedabad, India.)

- Subjacent breast lump may be palpated.
- Extramammary cases can be seen on vulva, perianal area (**Figure 7.32c**), scrotum, penis, and axilla.
- DD: Bowen's disease (well-defined plaques, crusts, oozing, disarray of atypical cells), nipple eczema (diffuse plaque, usually bilateral), nevoid hyperkeratosis of nipple (congenital, scaly plaques), neurodermatitis, periorificial tuberculosis, lichen simplex, psoriasis, lichen planus, mycosis fungoides, and seborrheic dermatitis.

## CONGENITAL PLAQUES

### Milia-en-plaque

- This appears as plaques of keratin-filled cysts in the preauricular or periorbital area.
- There is superficial, pearly white/yellowish, dome-shaped, 1–2 mm papular coalescence.
- DD: Nevus sebaceous (verrucous at puberty, sebaceous proliferation).

### Nevus sebaceous[17, 18]

- It is a congenital hamartomatous lesion with an epithelial and adnexal origin.
- Solitary, hairless, linear or rounded, slightly elevated yellowish plaques with a velvety surface (**Figure 7.33**) occur.
- It becomes verrucous at puberty.
- Plaques usually appear on the scalp or face.
- Appendageal tumors, such as syringocystadenoma papilliferum, may develop in later life.
- DD: Verrucous epidermal nevus (verrucous from onset, hairs inside the structure), seborrheic keratosis (verrucous, brown/black, sun-exposed area).

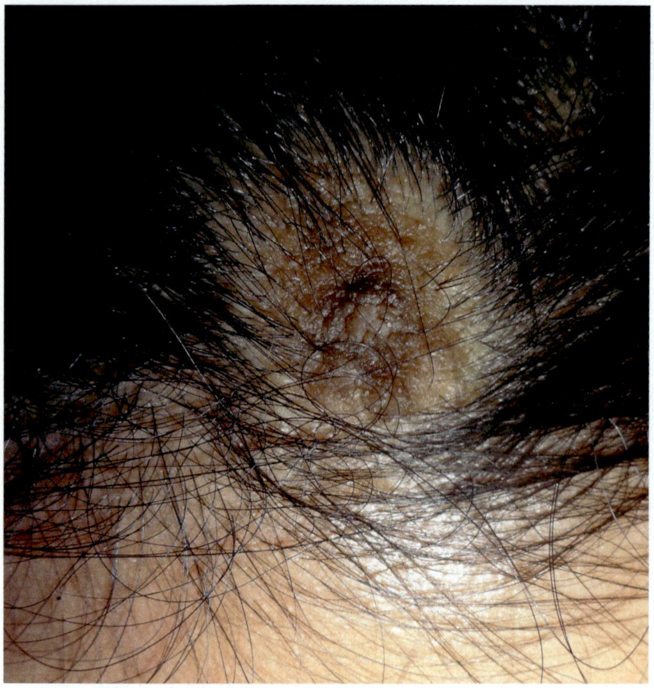

Figure 7.33 Nevus sebaceous presenting as yellow-brown alopecic plaque on scalp with velvety surface. (Courtesy: Dr. Niharika Ranjan Lal, ESIPGIMSR, Kolkata, India.)

### Verrucous epidermal nevus[17, 18]

- Verrucous epidermal nevi (VEN) are non-inflammatory keratinocytic hamartomas composed of keratinocytes
- Skin-colored to dirty-brown or black verrucous papules coalesce to form linear plaques along the lines of Blaschko (**Figure 7.34a,b**).
- They usually appear at birth or early childhood.
- In systematized VEN, many linear lesions are limited to one side of the body (Nevus unius lateris, **Figure 7.34c**) or have a bilateral symmetrical distribution (ichthyosis hystrix).

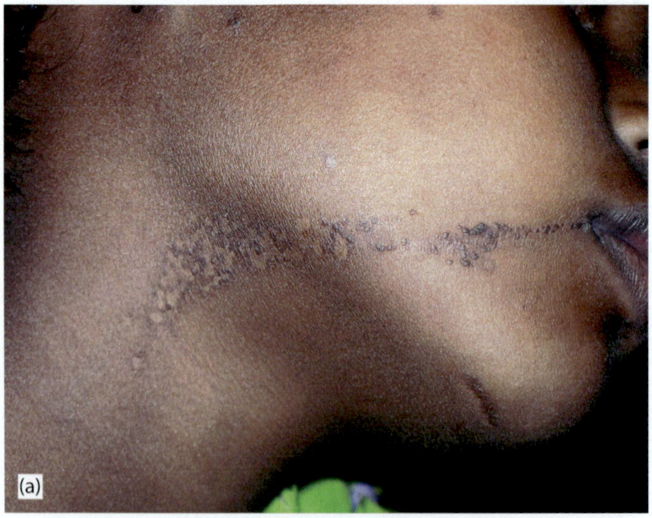

Figure 7.34 **(a)** Hyperpigmented verrucous papules coalescing to form plaque in verrucous epidermal nevus. (*Continued*)

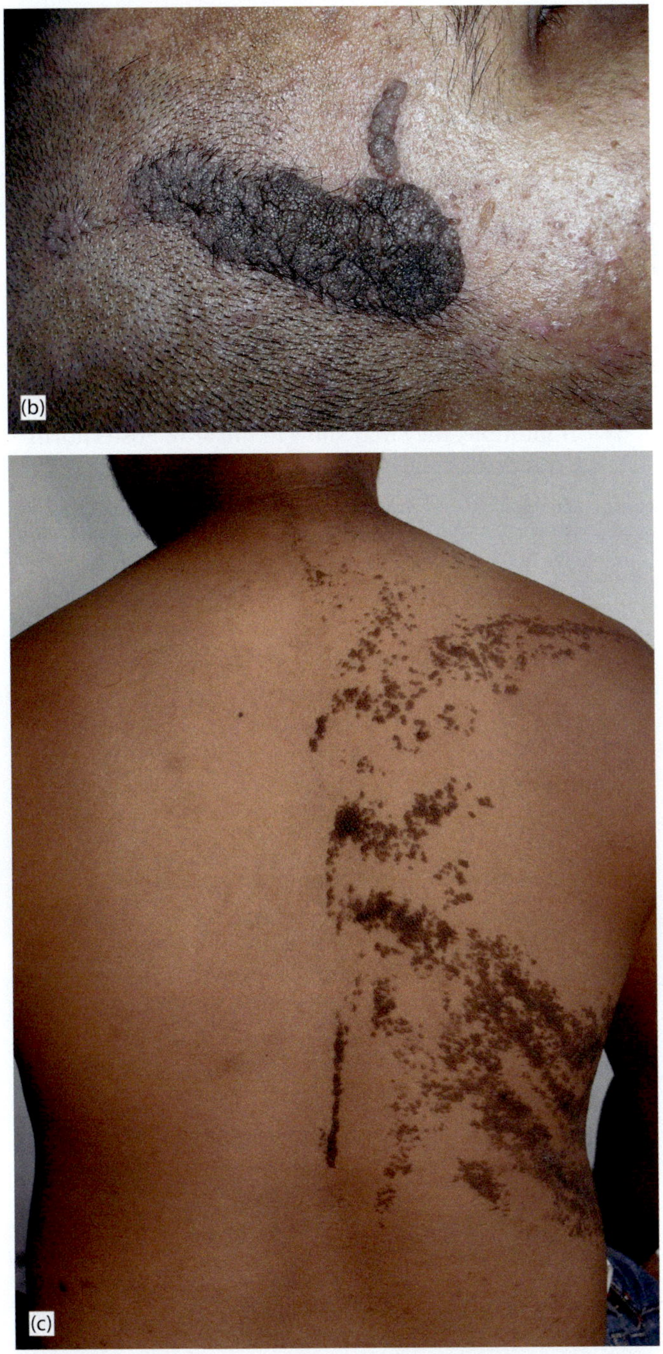


Figure 7.34 (*Continued*) **(b)** Verrucous epidermal nevus along the lines of Blaschko. **(c)** Nevus unius lateralis. (a–c – Courtesy: Dr. Piyush Kumar, Katihar, India.)

- DD: Nevus sebaceous (verrucous at puberty, sebaceous proliferation), linear Darier, linear verruca vulgaris, verrucous stage of incontinentia pigmenti.

## Nevus lipomatosis superficialis

- It is a rare hamartoma of adipose tissue.
- It is divided into classical form and solitary form. It usually presents as a clustered group of soft, fleshy, skin-colored or yellowish nodules, which are either sessile or pedunculated growths with a smooth, wrinkled or cerebriform surface (**Figure 7.35a,b**).

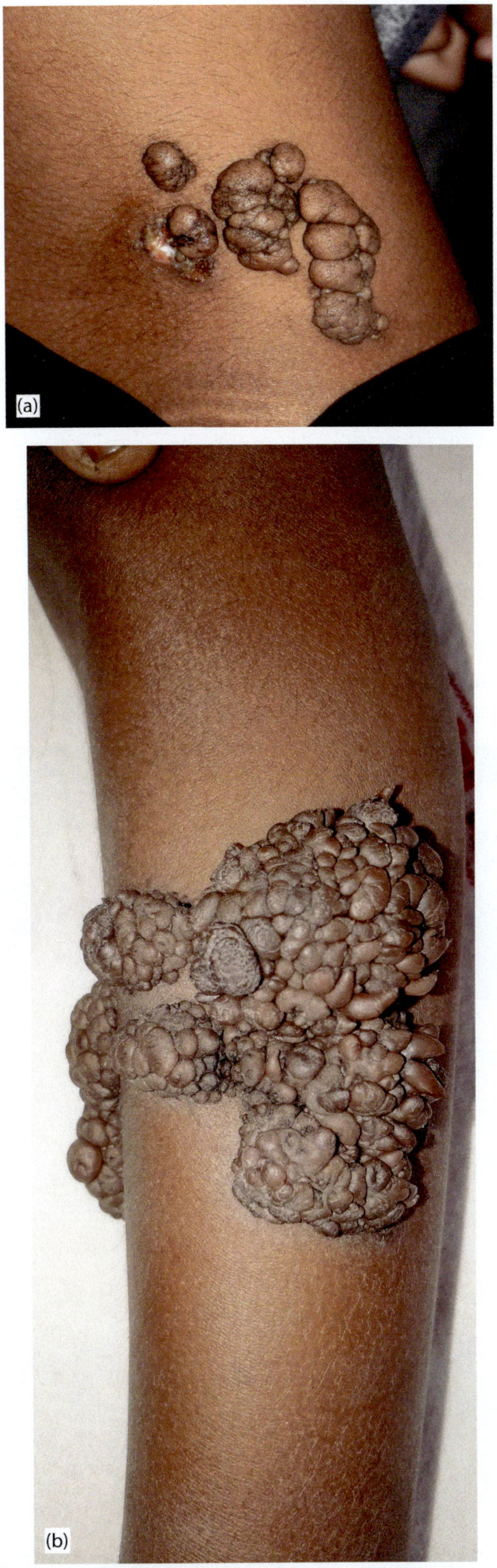


Figure 7.35 **(a)** Grouped, smooth-surfaced, yellowish plaques and papulonodules in a case of nevus lipomatosus superficialis. **(b)** Large lesion of nevus lipomatosus superficialis on the forearm. (a – Courtesy: Dr. Piyush Kumar, Katihar, India; b – Courtesy: Dr. Niharika Ranjan Lal, ESIPGIMSR, Kolkata, India.)

- The most common sites are pelvic girdle, buttocks, back or abdomen. They are usually present at birth or emerge during the first two decades of life.
- DD: Connective tissue nevus (light yellow-orange plaques, congenital, lumbosacral area, linear or zosteriform, shagreen leather appearance), xanthoma (yellowish plaques, lipid laden macrophages, hyperlipidemia).

## Inflammatory linear verrucous epidermal nevus (ILVEN)[17, 18]

- Extremely pruritic papules occur in linear streaks along Blaschko's lines (**Figure 7.36**).
- They appear mainly on the lower extremities.
- They are more common in girls; they may be congenital or occur later.
- They are resistant to therapy.
- DD: Verrucous epidermal nevus (non-itchy, verrucous plaques), nevus sebaceous (head and neck region, verrucous after puberty), seborrheic keratosis (verrucous, brown/black, sun-exposed area).

## Connective tissue nevus[19]

- Connective tissue nevus are circumscribed hamartomatous malformations in which one or more components of dermis are altered. Based on the predominant tissue involved, these may be classified as collagenomas (collagen), elastomas (elastin), or nevus mucinosis (proteoglycans).
- Collagenomas may be acquired (eruptive and sporadic type) or inherited (dermatofibrosis lenticularis disseminata in the Buschke-Ollendorf syndrome, familial cutaneous collagenoma (FCC), and shagreen patches seen in tuberous sclerosis).
  - The nevus is 1–15 cm diameter, light-yellow to orange, with the surface resembling shagreen leather (**Figure 7.37**).
  - Present on trunk, mainly lumbosacral area.
  - If multiple, they may show in linear or zosteriform arrangement.
  - The histopathology of collagenoma shows increased amount of collagen fibers, with either normal or decreased elastic tissue.
  - DD: nevus lipomatosus (plaques or tumoral mass, back/buttocks, peau d'orange appearance), xanthoma (yellowish plaques, lipid laden macrophages, hyperlipidemia).
- Certain elastic tissue nevi that may present as localized plaque are cutaneous features in Buschke Ollendorff syndrome and inherited pseudoxanthoma elasticum.

## Verrucous hemangioma

- It is a rare form of vascular malformation that is usually congenital.
- The lesions appear as well-circumscribed erythematous bluish macules that increase in size with time, acquiring an erythematous violet color and the surface becoming verrucous and hyperkeratotic (**Figure 7.38**).
- They usually occur over the lower extremities.
- They may bleed on trauma.
- DD: Angiokeratoma circumscriptum neviforme (congenital, hyperkeratotic, bluish-red, well-defined,

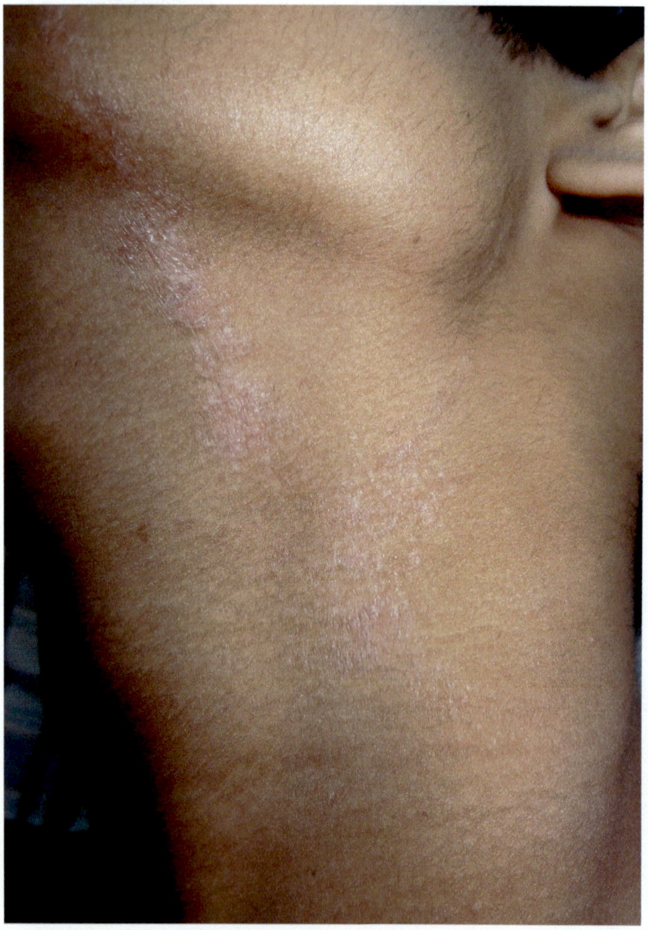

Figure 7.36 Linear erythematous scaly plaque on the neck in a case of inflammatory linear verrucous epidermal nevus. (Courtesy: Dr. Piyush Kumar, Katihar, India.)

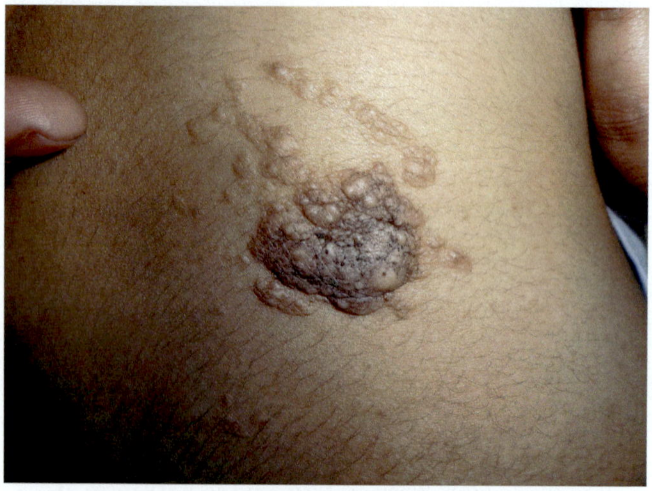

Figure 7.37 Grouped, firm, plaques and papules of collagenoma. (Courtesy: Dr. Niharika Ranjan Lal, ESIPGIMSR, Kolkata, India.)

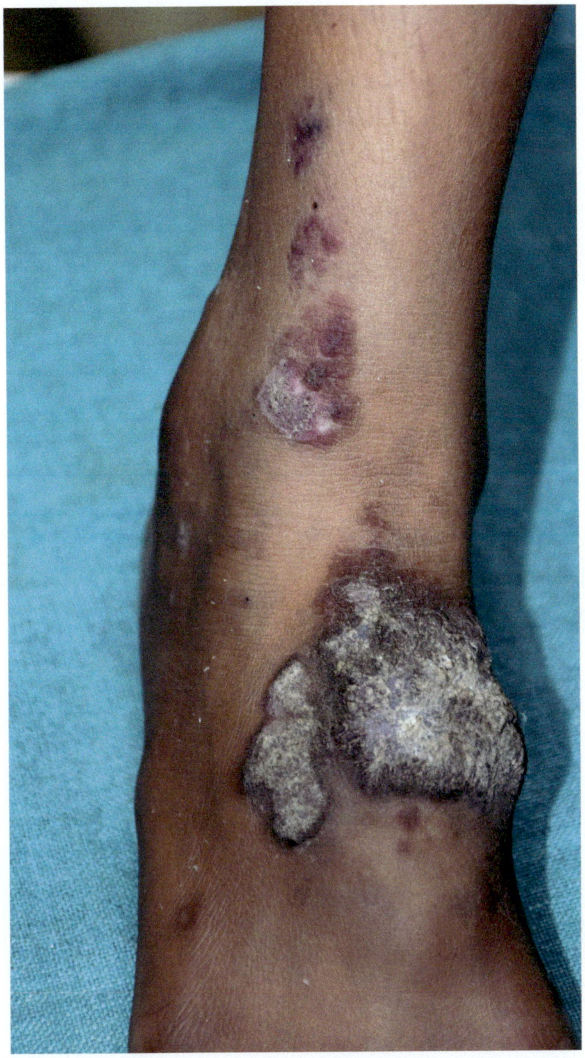

Figure 7.38 Violaceous, hyperkeratotic plaque in verrucous hemangioma. (Courtesy: Dr. Piyush Kumar, Katihar, India.)

capillary/venous proliferation in dermal or subcutaneous planes), lichen simplex, prurigo nodularis.

## Hemangioma[20]

- Hemangiomas are vascular neoplasms caused by the abnormal proliferation of endothelial cells and aberrant blood vessels architecture.
- In infantile hemangioma (IH) risk factors include female gender, prematurity, low birth weight, multiple pregnancies, advanced maternal age, and in vitro fertilization.
    - They mostly affect the head and neck region; they can be classified into superficial, deep, and mixed.
    - Superficial hemangiomas, when fully formed, are characterized by bright-red vascular plaques or nodules. Deep haemangiomas manifest as partially compressible, subcutaneous, bluish vascular swellings. Mixed haemangiomas have both superficial and deep components (**Figure 7.39a,b**).
    - Ulceration, bleeding may occur.
    - They may cause life-threatening complications if they occur over vital organs or dangerous areas like the eye, ear, nose, or throat (**Figure 7.39c,d**).

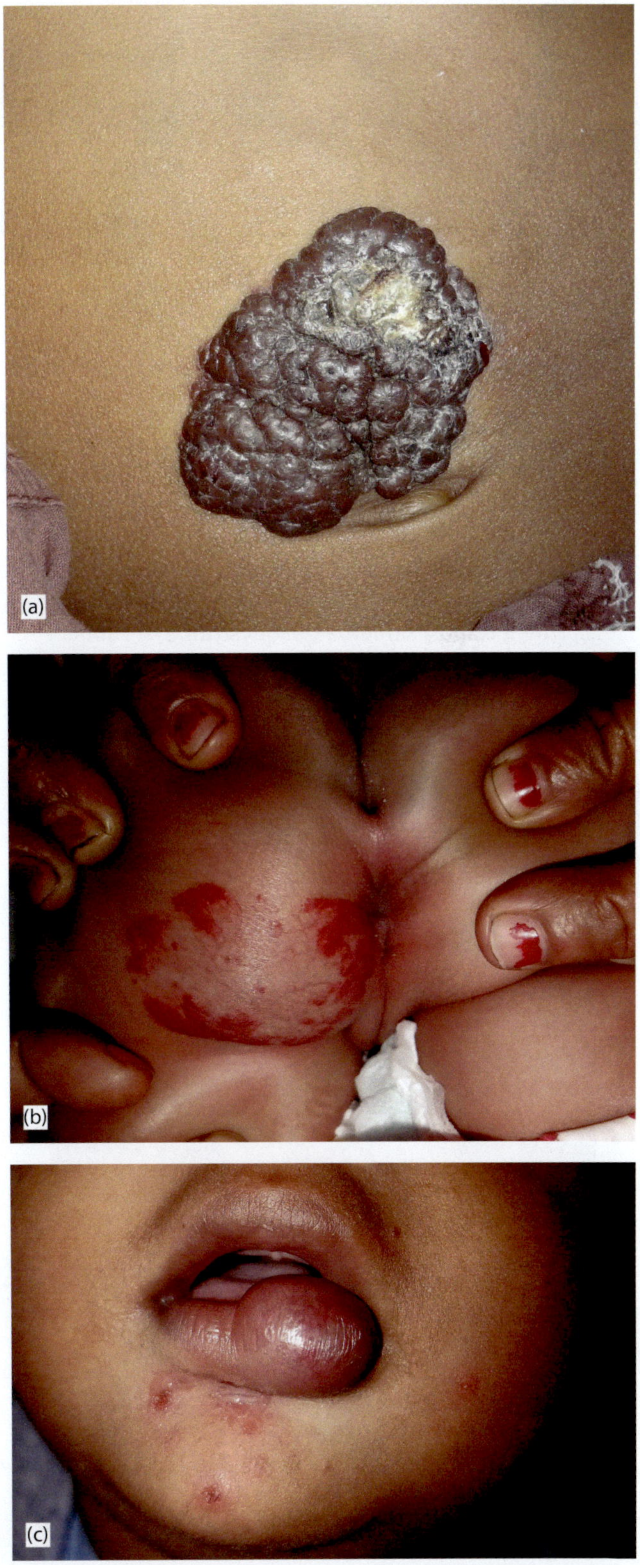


Figure 7.39 **(a)** Infantile hemangioma on abdomen. **(b)** Hemangioma. **(c)** Hemangioma over the lip. *(Continued)*

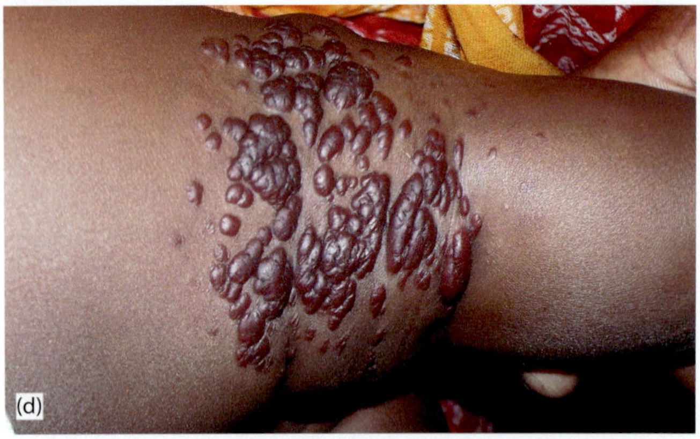

Figure 7.39 (*Continued*) **(d)** Grouped, smooth-surfaced erythematous papules and plaques in infantile hemangioma. (a,d – Courtesy: Dr. Piyush Kumar, Katihar, India; b,c – Courtesy: Dr. Niharika Ranjan Lal, ESIPGIMSR, Kolkata, India.)

- IH has a characteristic natural course: a rapid proliferative phase in infancy that is followed by a gradual involutional phase over the next several years of life.
- DD: Congenital hemangioma, venous malformation (congenital, red/bluish-red, does not change over time), Kaposi sarcoma (plaques/tumors, rubbery consistency, brawny edema over the leg, may be associated with AIDS).

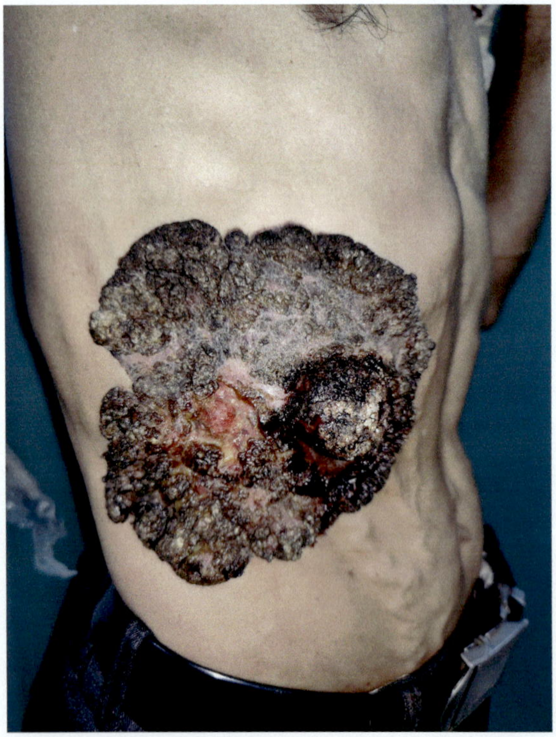

Figure 7.40 Squamous cell carcinoma (SCC) presenting as giant, pigmented verrucous plaque with focal ulcerations. This SCC developed in a pre-existing lesion neglected for years. The pre-existing lesion could not be determined, and the patient was lost to follow-up. (Courtesy: Dr. Rajesh Kumar Mandal, North Bengal Medical College, Darjeeling, India.)

- Congenital hemangiomas are present and fully formed at birth; they do not exhibit the postnatal proliferative phase characteristic of IH. The two variants are the noninvoluting congenital hemangioma (NICH) and rapidly involuting congenital hemangioma (RICH).
  - They usually present with exophytic masses or plaques on different parts of the body, such as the head, limbs, or neck.
  - Noninvoluting congenital hemangiomas (NICHs) present as well-circumscribed, oval, plaque-like masses containing overlying telangiectasias with a rim of pallor; they remain stable without growth or involution.
  - Rapidly involuting congenital hemangiomas (RICHs) undergo a rapid involution phase beginning in the first year of life; they typically occur within the head, neck, and lower extremity regions.
  - DD: infantile hemangioma (histology shows lack of glucose transporter 1 in congenital hemangioma).

Additional image – Figures 7.40 and 7.41.

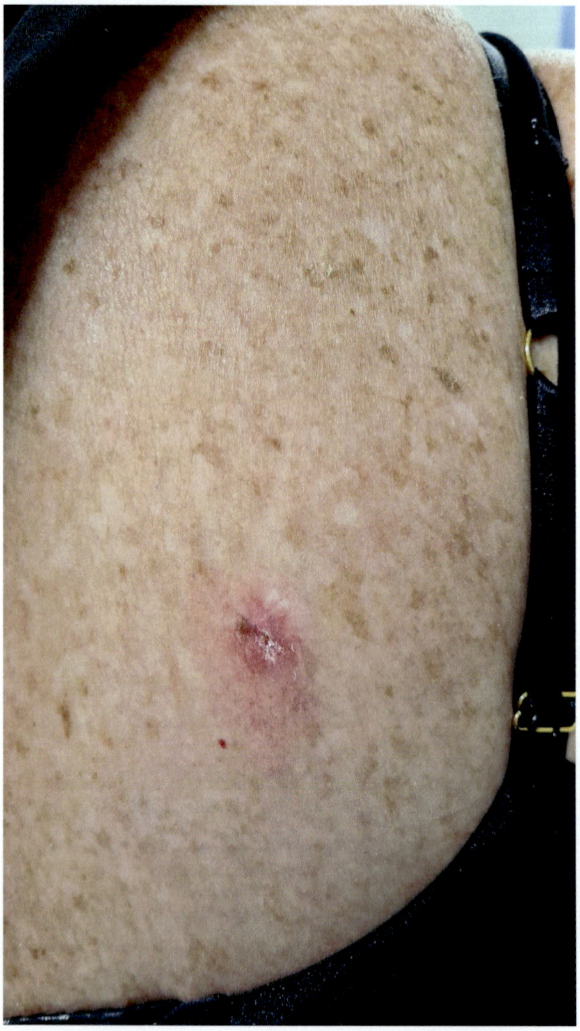

Figure 7.41 Amelanotic melanoma seen as erythematous scaly and crusted plaque. (Courtesy: Dr. Tanumay Raychaudhury, Skin and Cancer Foundation, The University of Sydney, Australia.)

## REFERENCES


1. Lipsker D. Clinical Examination and Differential Diagnosis of Skin Lesions. 1st edition. France: Springer-Verlag; 2013. Chapter 35. Palpable Erythematous Lesions. P. 195–200.
2. Lipsker D. Clinical Examination and Differential Diagnosis of Skin Lesions. 1st edition. France: Springer-Verlag; 2013. Chapter 31. Skin-Colored Palpable Lesions. P. 185–188.
3. Lipsker D. Clinical Examination and Differential Diagnosis of Skin Lesions. 1st edition. France: Springer-Verlag; 2013. Chapter 32. Brown, Black, Blue, or Gray Palpable Lesions. P. 189–190.
4. Lipsker D. Clinical Examination and Differential Diagnosis of Skin Lesions. 1st edition. France: Springer-Verlag; 2013. Chapter 33. White Palpable Lesions. P. 191–192.
5. Lipsker D. Clinical Examination and Differential Diagnosis of Skin Lesions. 1st edition. France: Springer-Verlag; 2013. Chapter 34. Yellow Palpable Lesions. P. 193–194.
6. Fitzpatrick JE, High WA, Kyle WL. Urgent Care Dermatology: Symptom-Based Diagnosis. 1st ed. Philadelphia: Elsevier; 2018. Chapter 8. Plaques with Scale. P. 113–122.
7. Fitzpatrick JE, High WA, Kyle WL. Urgent Care Dermatology: Symptom-Based Diagnosis. 1st ed. Philadelphia: Elsevier; 2018. Chapter 28. Papillomatous and Verrucous Lesions. P. 461–476.
8. Talhari C, Talhari S, Penna GO. Clinical aspects of leprosy. *Clin Dermatol* 2015;33(1):26–37.
9. Filotico R, Mastrandrea V. Cutaneous lupus erythematosus: Clinico-pathologic correlation. *G Ital Dermatol Venereol* 2018;153(2):216–229.
10. Mitteldorf C, Kempf W. Cutaneous Pseudolymphoma. *Surg Pathol Clin* 2017;10(2):455–476.
11. Karadağ AS, Parish LC. Sarcoidosis: A great imitator. *Clin Dermatol* 2019;37(3):240–254.
12. Rudikoff D. Differential diagnosis of round or discoid lesions. *Clin Dermatol* 2011;29(5):489–497.
13. Chen Q, Chen W, Hao F. Cutaneous tuberculosis: A great imitator. *Clin Dermatol* 2019;37(3):192–199.
14. La Hoz RM, Baddley JW. Subcutaneous fungal infections. *Curr Infect Dis Rep* 2012;14(5):530–539.
15. Sampaio AL, Mameri AC, Vargas TJ, Ramos-e-Silva M, Nunes AP, Carneiro SC. Seborrheic dermatitis. *An Bras Dermatol* 2011;86(6):1061–1074.
16. Hafner C, Vogt T. Seborrheic keratosis. *J Dtsch Dermatol Ges* 2008;6(8):664–677.
17. Garcias-Ladaria J, CuadradoRosón M, Pascual-López M. Epidermal nevi and related syndromes – Part 1: Keratinocytic nevi. *Actas Dermosifiliogr* 2018;109(8):677–686.
18. Garcias-Ladaria J, CuadradoRosón M, Pascual-López M. Epidermal nevi and related syndromes – Part 2: Nevi derived from adnexal structures. *Actas Dermosifiliogr* 2018;109(8):687–698.
19. Arora H, Falto-Aizpurua L, Cortés-Fernandez A, Choudhary S, Romanelli P. Connective tissue nevi: A review of the literature. *Am J Dermatopathol* 2017;39(5):325–341.
20. Johnson EF, Davis DM, Tollefson MM, Fritchie K, Gibson LE. Vascular tumors in infants: Case report and review of clinical, histopathologic, and immunohistochemical characteristics of infantile hemangioma, pyogenic granuloma, noninvoluting congenital hemangioma, tufted angioma, and kaposiform hemangioendothelioma. *Am J Dermatopathol* 2018;40(4):231–239.

# 8

# Plaques: Generalized

DHIRAJ KUMAR

## INTRODUCTION

Generalized plaques are seen in a wide range of dermatological diseases. Clinical clues that aid in diagnosis include symptoms (e.g., systemic features such as fever and malaise are seen in Sweet syndrome, lepra reaction, erythema multiforme and urticarial vasculitis to name a few), color of the lesions (erythematous, violaceous, yellow, hyperpigmented), surface changes (scaly, verrucous, velvety, edematous, ulcerated, etc.), nature of scales (silvery, greasy, fine, coarse), and shape of lesions (linear, annular), among others. Also, it is important to recognize plaques developing because of dermal changes including infiltration. Very often, such plaques have thin, stretched, shiny epidermis and are better felt than seen. Notable examples include granuloma annulare, sarcoidosis, Hansen's disease, hypertrophic scar, morphea, lichen sclerosus et atrophicus, etc. This chapter discusses the clinical approach to diseases presenting with generalized plaques (outlined in **Table 8.1**), followed by a brief description of entities.[1–7]

### Chronic plaque psoriasis

- Chronic plaque psoriasis presents with well-defined, erythematous, circumscribed, dry scaly plaques of various size with easily detachable, silvery white lamellate scales on the surface (**Figure 8.1a**). Removal of scales may reveal bleeding points (Auspitz sign).
- The eruption is usually symmetrical. It shows a predilection for the scalp, umbilical region, sacrum, and extensor aspect of extremities (**Figure 8.1b**). Nail involvement shows pitting, oil spot, salmon patch, subungual hyperkeratosis.
- DD: Pityriasis rubra pilaris (peculiar yellow and salmon-colored papules and plaques with moderate scale, nutmeg-grater feel, small islands of normal skin), small plaque parapsoriasis (fine scaly, finger-like plaques on flanks), psoriasiform syphilid (copper-colored papules, rebound tenderness, condyloma lata, VDRL positive, mucosal lesions), Reiter's disease (reactive arthritis) (**Figure 8.1c**).

### Rupioid psoriasis

- The term rupioid has been used to describe well-demarcated, cone-shaped plaques with thick, dark, lamellate, and adherent crusts on the skin that somewhat resemble oyster or limpet shells.
- DD: reactive arthritis, disseminated histoplasmosis, secondary syphilis, and photosensitive skin lesions in association with aminoaciduria.

### Pityriasis rubra pilaris

- Classical adult-onset PRP
  - This is characterized by salmon-colored follicular hyperkeratosis on an erythematous base, often prominent on the backs of fingers.
  - There is a predilection for the side of neck, trunk, and extensor aspect of extremities.
  - It classically manifests first by scaling and erythema of the scalp; it spreads in a cephalocaudal direction.
  - Papules are acuminate, reddish-brown with a central horny plug, giving a nutmeg-grater feel.
  - These papules coalesce to form large red-to-orange-red plaques that are often weeping, with distinctive "islands of sparing" (*nappes claires*) (**Figure 8.2a,b**).
  - It is associated with palmoplantar hyperkeratosis (yellow-orange waxy palmoplantar keratoderma).
  - DD: Psoriasis (micaceous scales, Auspitz sign, extensors), progressive symmetric erythrokeratoderma (autosomal dominant, sparing of trunk), subacute cutaneous lupus erythematosus (common in females, sun-exposed areas, and polycyclic annular lesion with thin scales.).
- Juvenile-onset PRP
  - This can be classical (generalized) or circumscribed.
  - Generalized form: The appearance is similar to adults with prominent thickening of the skin of the palms and soles.
  - Circumscribed form: The most common features are well-circumscribed plaques of erythema and follicular hyperkeratosis occurring on elbows and knees.


DOI: 10.1201/9781351054225-16

Table 8.1 Clinical approach to diseases presenting with generalized plaques

| Feature | Additional clues | Diseases |
|---|---|---|
| Erythematous | Scaly | • Profuse silvery scales – psoriasis vulgaris<br>• Heaped up scales – rupioid psoriasis<br>• Adherent scales (predominantly photo distributed) – generalized chronic cutaneous lupus erythematosus, subacute lupus erythematosus<br>• Mild scales with follicular hyperkeratosis – pityriasis rubra pilaris<br>• Others – Papulosquamous syphilid, parapsoriasis, progressive symmetric erythrokeratoderma |
| | Non-scaly | • Edematous plaques – urticaria, urticarial vasculitis, urticaria pigmentosa, urticarial phase of bullous pemphigoid, pruritic polymorphous papules and plaques of pregnancy (PUPPP)<br>• Infiltrative plaques – sarcoidosis, lepromatous leprosy, borderline lepromatous leprosy |
| Annular plaques | Scaly | Figurate erythema, tinea corporis |
| | Non-scaly | Annular urticaria, disseminated granuloma annulare, erythema marginatum |
| Atrophic | | Generalized morphea, generalized lichen sclerosus et atrophicus |
| Hyperkeratotic | Warty plaques | Darier disease, epidermodysplasia verruciformis (EDV) |
| | Along lines of Blaschko | Systemized verrucous epidermal nevus, verrucous stage of incontinentia pigmenti |
| | Velvety soft | Generalized acanthosis nigricans |
| | Others | Seborrheic keratosis |
| Ulcerated | | Kaposi sarcoma, vegetative pyoderma gangrenosum, necrotic erythema nodosum leprosum, mycosis fungoides, disseminated leishmaniasis |
| Yellow | | Necrobiotic xanthogranuloma |
| Crusted plaques | | Norwegian scabies, Sulzberger-Garbe disease |

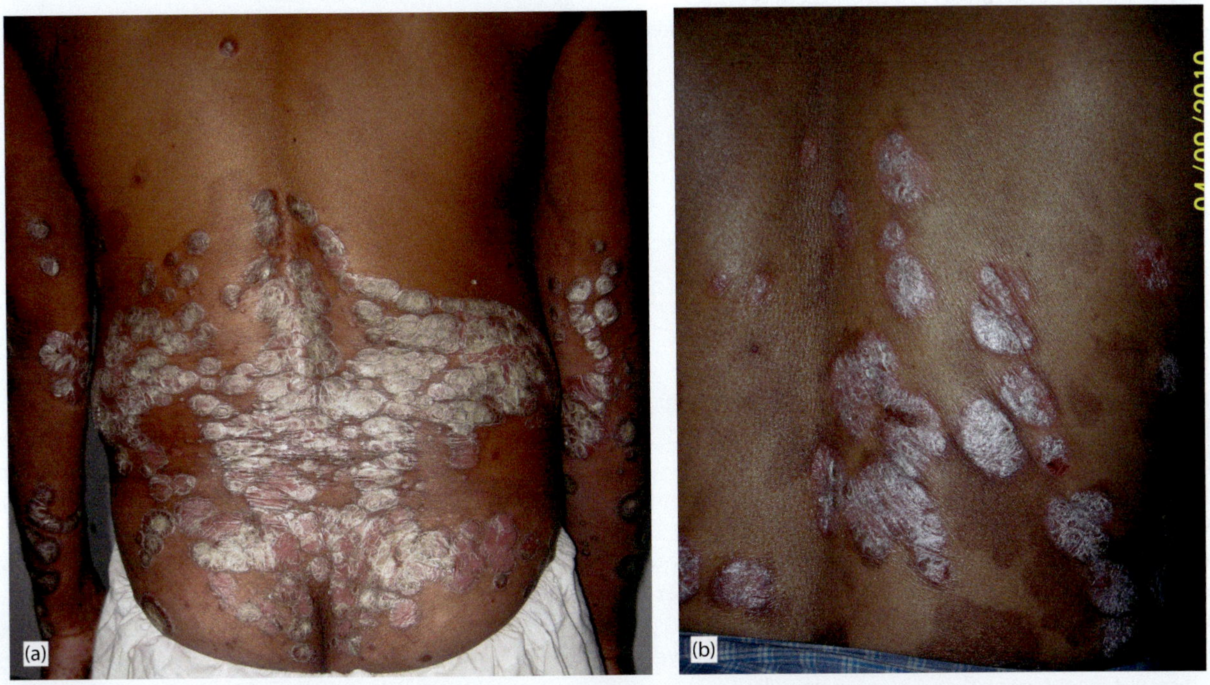


Figure 8.1 **(a)** Erythematous plaques with silvery scales in psoriasis vulgaris. **(b)** Psoriasis vulgaris lesions on the back. (*Continued*)

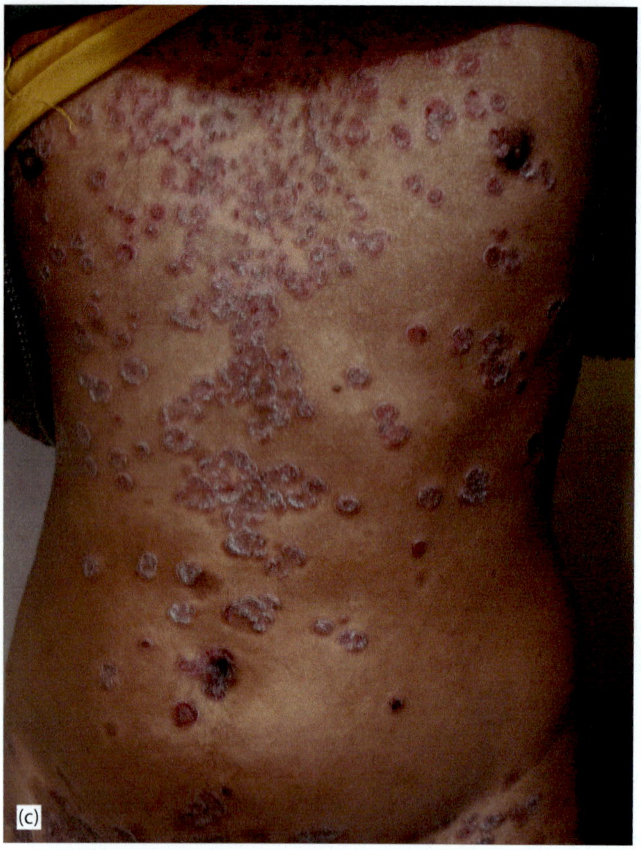

Figure 8.1 (*Continued*) **(c)** Erythematous, scaly and crusted, papules and plaques in reactive arthritis. (a–c – Courtesy: Dr. Piyush Kumar, Katihar, India.)

- Atypical Juvenile PRP
    - Follicular hyperkeratosis is a prominent feature with keratoderma. Erythema with scleroderma like changes of hands and feet are seen.
    - Onset is in the first years of life.

## Leprosy

- Leprosy has varied manifestations depending on the underlying cell-mediated immunity and degree of proliferation of *Mycobacterium leprae*.
- Borderline tuberculoid (BT) leprosy: There are a few, asymmetrical, usually well-demarcated lesions with a somewhat dry surface. They may be annular in shape, with a clearly defined outer border (**Figure 8.3a**). The surface may be scaly, with marked sensory impairment and hair loss. Peripheral nerve involvement is widespread or asymmetrical.
- Mid-borderline (BB) leprosy: Presents with some, asymmetrical, less-well–demarcated, somewhat shiny lesions, often annular with a characteristic, punched-out appearance. (The outer border is vague, while the inner border is clearly defined.) There is moderate sensory impairment and hair loss over lesions. Peripheral nerve involvement is widespread and asymmetrical.
- Borderline lepromatous (BL) leprosy: There are many, roughly symmetrically distributed macules, papules, nodules, and plaques with sloping edges. Sensation and sweating over individual lesion are slightly affected. The nerve is enlarged and symmetrical (**Figure 8.3b**).
- Lepromatous (LL) leprosy: There are multiple, poorly defined, erythematous macules, papules, nodules, and plaques. They are symmetric in distribution, and common sites of involvement are the face, buttocks, and lower extremities, with gloves-and-stocking anesthesia. Additional late signs are madarosis, saddle nose, and mega lobule of ear (**Figure 8.3c,d**).

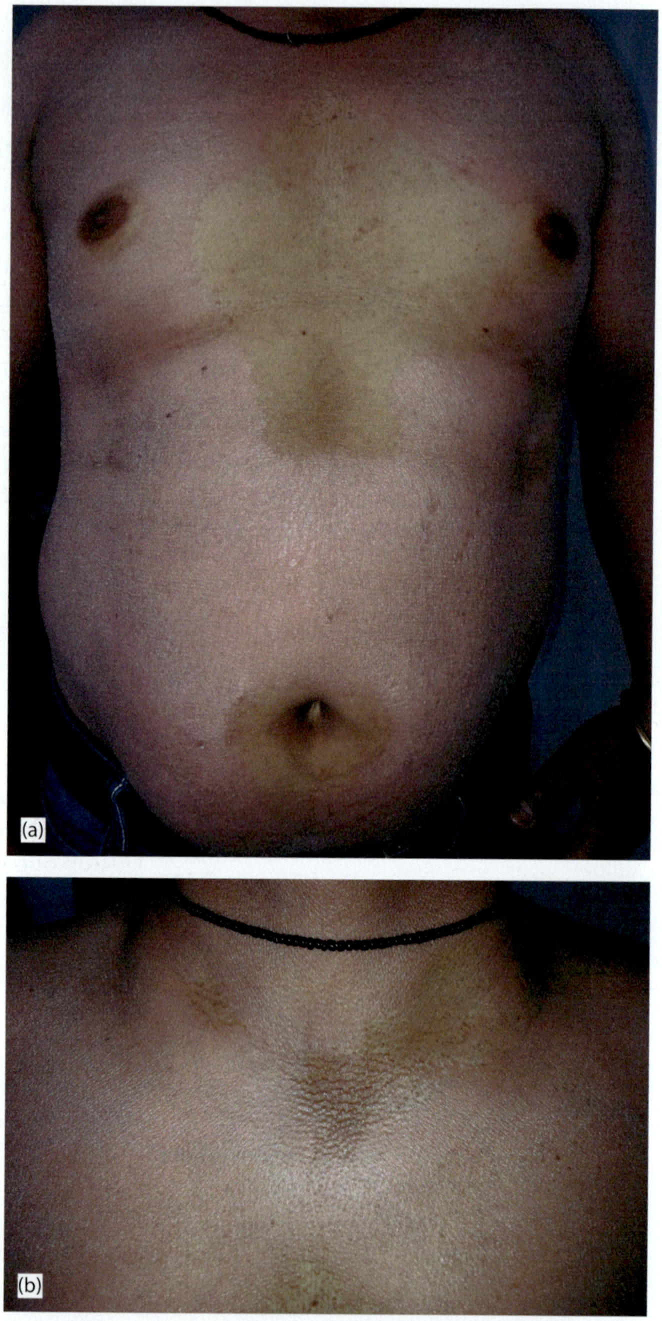

Figure 8.2 **(a)** Generalized pityriasis rubra pilaris with skin areas. **(b)** Close-up of lesions showing discrete keratotic papules near the margin of erythematous plaque. (a,b – Courtesy: Dr. Piyush Kumar, Katihar, India.)

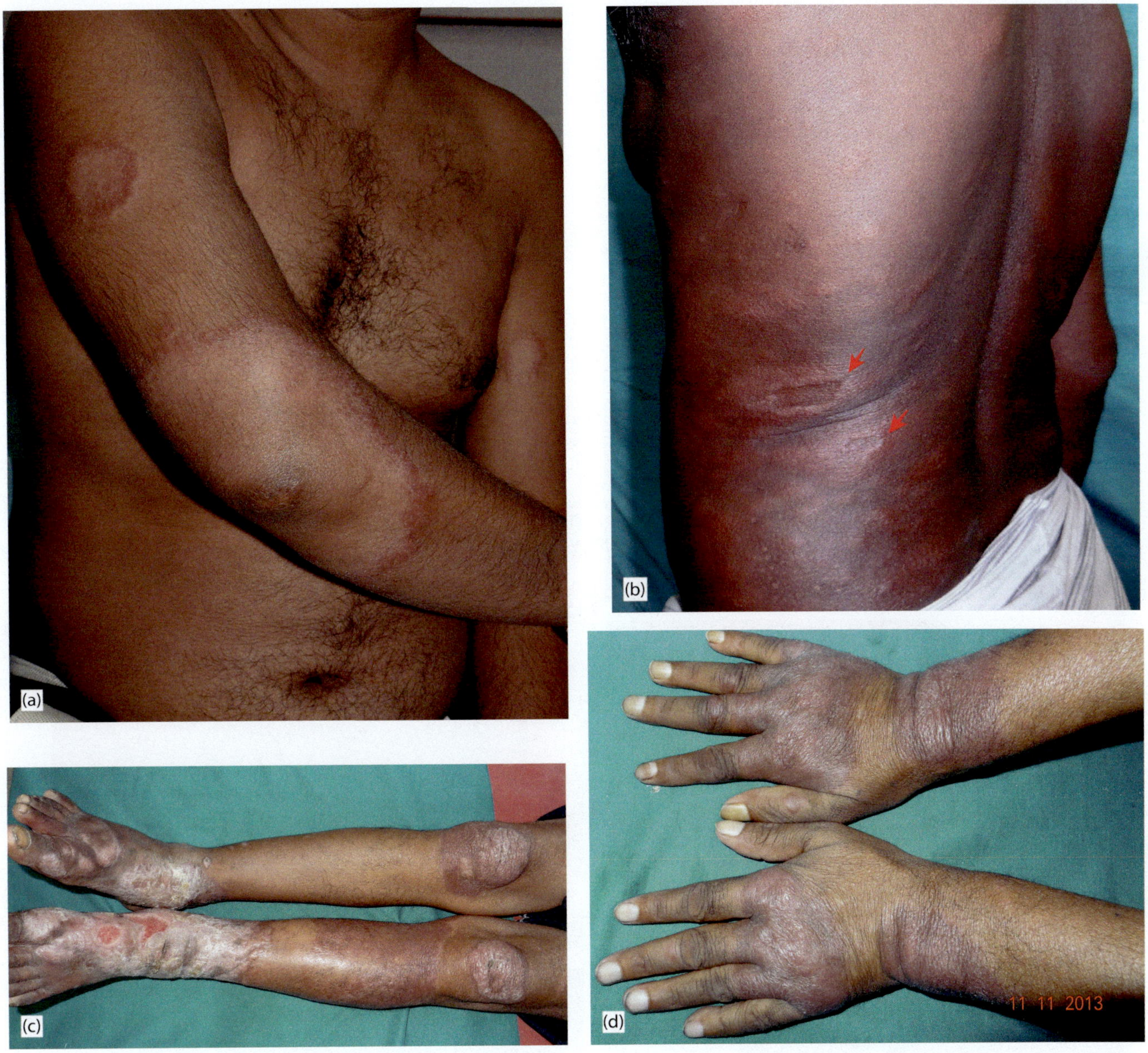


Figure 8.3 **(a)** Generalized papules and plaques in borderline tuberculoid leprosy. Plaques are erythematous, annular, and dry with visible hair loss. **(b)** Copper-colored infiltrative plaques in borderline lepromatous leprosy. Annular punched-out lesions resembling "inverted saucer" (marked with an arrow). **(c)** Erythematous, mildly scaly, infiltrative plaques with ulceration in lepromatous leprosy. **(d)** Lepromatous leprosy with infiltrative plaques on hands. (a – Courtesy: Dr. Piyush Kumar, Katihar, India; b – Courtesy: Dr. Niharika Ranjan Lal, ESIPGIMSR, Joka, Kolkata, India; c–d – Courtesy: Dr. Piyush Kumar, Katihar, India.)

- DD: Sarcoidosis (red or tan-brown, naked granuloma in histopathology), tinea corporis (central clearing, peripheral papules and scales), granuloma annulare (annular plaque, peripheral discrete papules).

### Chronic cutaneous lupus erythematosus (discoid lupus erythematosus)

- This condition presents well-defined, erythematous plaques with follicular hyperkeratotic surface, telangiectasias and adherent scales that heal with scarring, peripheral hyperpigmentation, and central hypopigmentation (**Figure 8.4a–f**).
- It involves follicular plugging, keratotic spikes under the scales (carpet-tack sign), and wide follicular pits in ears.
- It results in cicatricial alopecia when the scalp is involved.
- Sites of predilection include chronic sun-exposed areas: scalp, forehead, cheeks, ears, nose, upper lip, and chin. In generalized chronic cutaneous lupus erythematosus, lesions are present below the head and neck.
- DD: Psoriasis (micaceous scales, Auspitz sign, extensors), lichen planus (pruritic, purplish, flat-topped papules and plaques, flexures).

## Subacute cutaneous lupus erythematosus

- Photosensitive dermatosis commonly noted in females.
- Two types can present with generalized plaques: papulosquamous and annular.
- Papulo-squamous type: May be psoriasiform or eczematous.
- There are symmetrical widespread non-scarring erythematous patches and plaques with a tendency to confluence (psoriasiform). The lesions vary from pink to red, covered with thin scales (**Figure 8.5a**).
- It usually appears on light-exposed areas such as the trunk and arms.

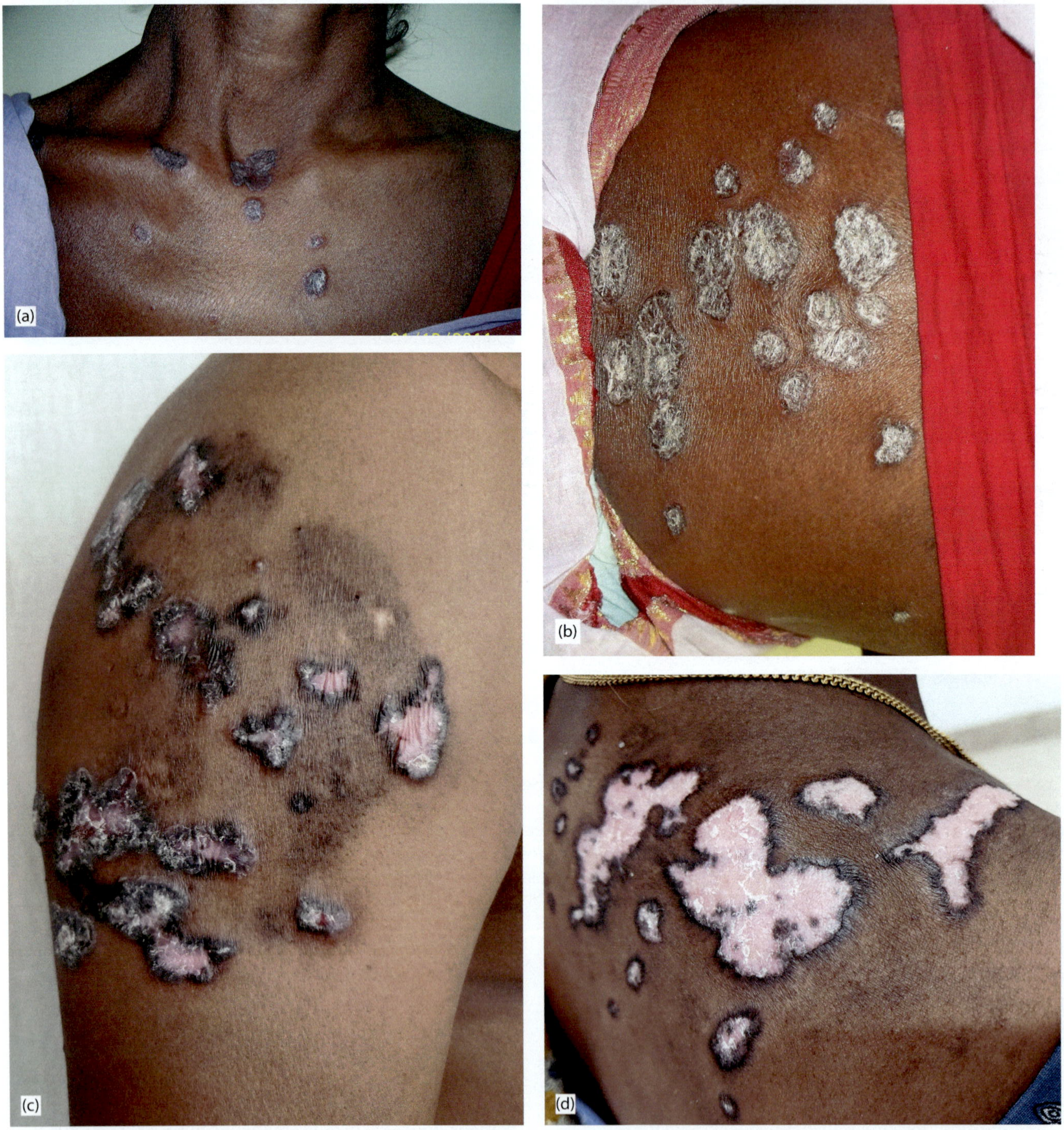


Figure 8.4 **(a)** Generalized chronic cutaneous lupus erythematosus. Lesions extending below head and neck. Violaceous plaques with adherent scales. **(b)** Generalized chronic cutaneous lupus erythematosus. **(c)** Erythematous plaques with central adherent scales and hyperpigmented borders in chronic cutaneous lupus erythematosus. Central atrophy characterized by wrinkled surface. **(d)** Well-developed lesions of discoid lupus erythematosus. (*Continued*)

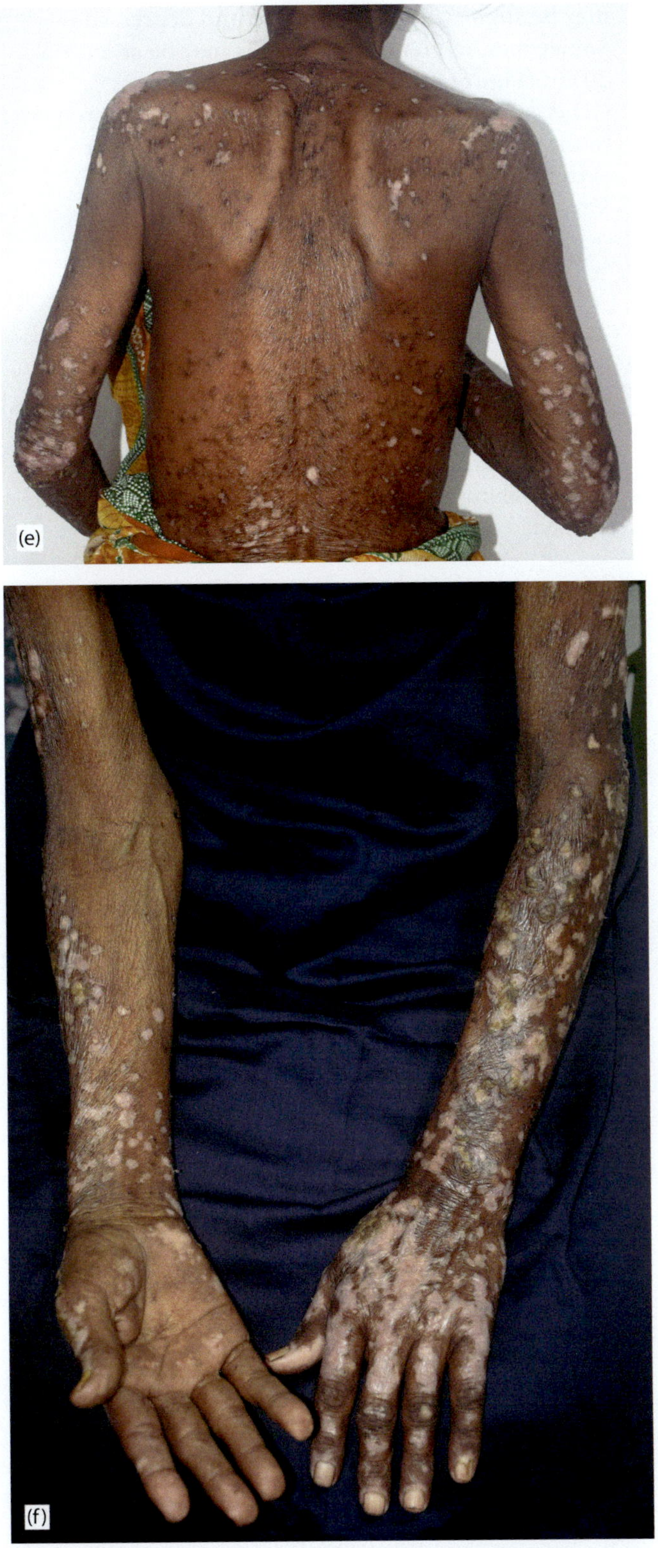


Figure 8.4 *(Continued)* **(e)** Generalized pigmented, scaly papules and plaques of generalized discoid lupus erythematosus in an elderly female. **(f)** Preferential involvement of extensor surface of upper extremities in discoid lupus erythematosus; some lesions have verrucous surface. (a,b – Courtesy: Dr. Piyush Kumar, Katihar, India; c – Courtesy: Dr. Niharika Ranjan Lal, ESIPGIMSR, Joka, Kolkata, India; d – Courtesy: Dr. Deverashetti Srinivas, Nizamabad, India; e–f – Courtesy: Dr. Piyush Kumar, Katihar, India.)

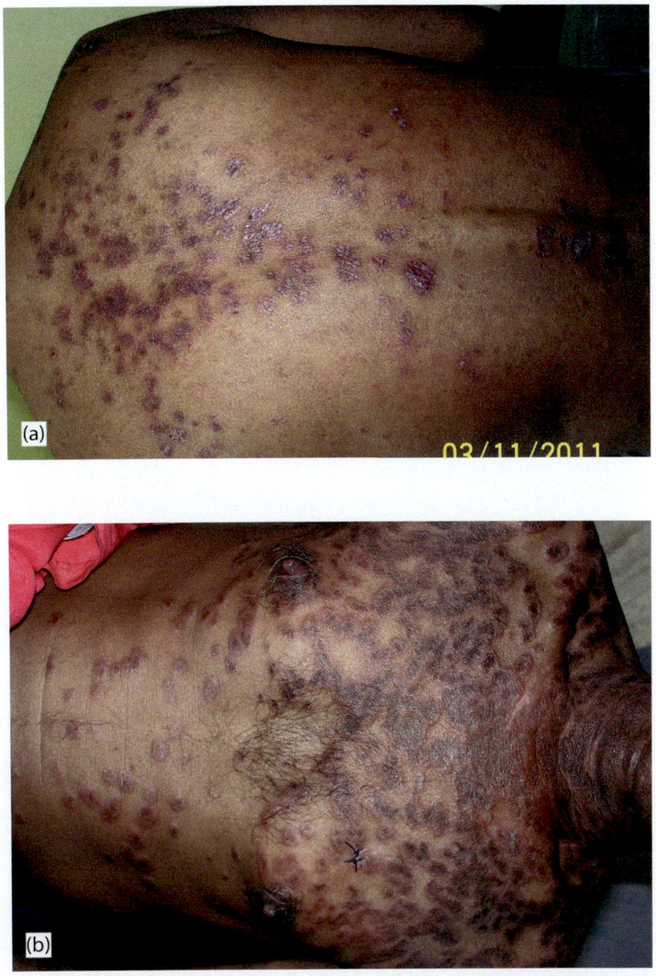


Figure 8.5 **(a)** Psoriasiform lesions of subacute lupus erythematosus. **(b)** Annular erythematous plaques with mild scales in subacute lupus erythematosus. (a,b – Courtesy: Dr. Piyush Kumar, Katihar, India.)

- Annular or target-like type: The plaques are annular in configuration, with raised pink-red borders and central clearing; rarely they may be erythema multiforme-like with blisters (Rowell Syndrome) (**Figure 8.5b**).
- Photosensitivity and arthritis are frequently associated.
- DD: Photosensitive eczema (pruritus, lichenification), tinea corporis (center clearing, peripheral papules, scales), psoriasis (micaceous scales, Auspitz sign, extensors), photolichenoid drug eruption.

## Sweet syndrome

- Sweet syndrome is an uncommon disease having a female preponderance.
- The association with infections, autoimmune diseases, inflammatory bowel disease and malignancies, as well as the greater incidence in women, suggests a hypersensitivity reaction.
- An upper respiratory tract infection or flu-like illness frequently precedes the development of the syndrome.

- It shows succulent plaques, as large as 10–15 cm, with irregular borders also known as rocky island pattern; sometimes there is an illusion of vesiculation – plaques look vesicular but are solid when pressed; they may be dotted with pustules.
- Face, neck, upper trunk, and extremities are common sites; oral lesions are seen in 20% of cases; more common in drug-related cases.
- It includes systemic symptoms such as fever, arthralgia, and myalgia.
- It involves peripheral leukocytosis and elevated ESR.
- DD: Erythema multiforme (target lesion, oral lesion), erythema nodosum, leukemic infiltrates, erythema elevatum diutinum (more chronic).

## Sarcoidosis

- Sarcoidosis is a systemic granulomatous disorder of unknown origin that most commonly involves the lungs; cutaneous manifestations are seen in up to one-third of patients and may be the first clinical sign of disease.
- Red-brown to violaceous papules and plaques appear most often on the face, in particular the nose, neck, upper back and extremities. Upon diascopy, lesions show the color of "apple jelly."
- The plaque form shows characteristically diffuse lesions and are of irregular shape with more superficial nodules superimposed, sometimes having a crescentic or serpiginous outline, chiefly involving shoulders and lower limbs.
- Individual plaques can develop central clearing, leading to an annular configuration, or they can contain prominent telangiectasias (angiolupoid form).
- Specific cutaneous lesions are mostly asymptomatic.
- In lupus pernio, large bluish-red and dusky violaceous nodules and plaques occur symmetrically on the nose, cheeks, ears, fingers, hands, and toes; the lesions may feel soft, doughy, or indurated. The surface of the lesion is often glistening. Ulceration and mutilation are rare. Involved ear lobes may become massive ("turkey ears").
- Lichenoid, hypopigmented, ichthyosiform, psoriasiform, and verrucous variants of sarcoidosis present as plaque.
- DD: Leprosy (hypopigmented, hypoesthetic patches), psoriasis (micaceous scales, Auspitz sign, extensors), granulomatous secondary syphilis (erythematous non-scaly plaque, mucosal lesion, positive VDRL test).

## Generalized granuloma annulare (GA)

- Granuloma annulare is a benign, usually self-limiting, cutaneous disease that presents as arciform or annular plaques.
- The plaques may be skin-colored, pink, or violaceous in color and are formed by small papules measuring a few millimeters in diameter. The center of the lesion may be slightly hyperpigmented and depressed. Sometimes, in giant form, lesions may be as large as 20 cm (**Figure 8.6**).
- Generalized GA has a later age of onset, poorer response to therapy, and predilection for the trunk and/or extremities.
- Variants
  - Localized: papules
  - Perforating: papules
  - Patch-type: patches
  - Subcutaneous: nodules
- DD: Sarcoidosis (red or tan-brown plaques, naked granuloma), mycosis fungoides, lichen planus (pruritus, violaceous plaque, Wickham's striae), tinea corporis (central clearing, peripheral papules, scales, KOH mount), leprosy (hypopigmented hypoesthetic plaque, thickened nerve, AFB present).

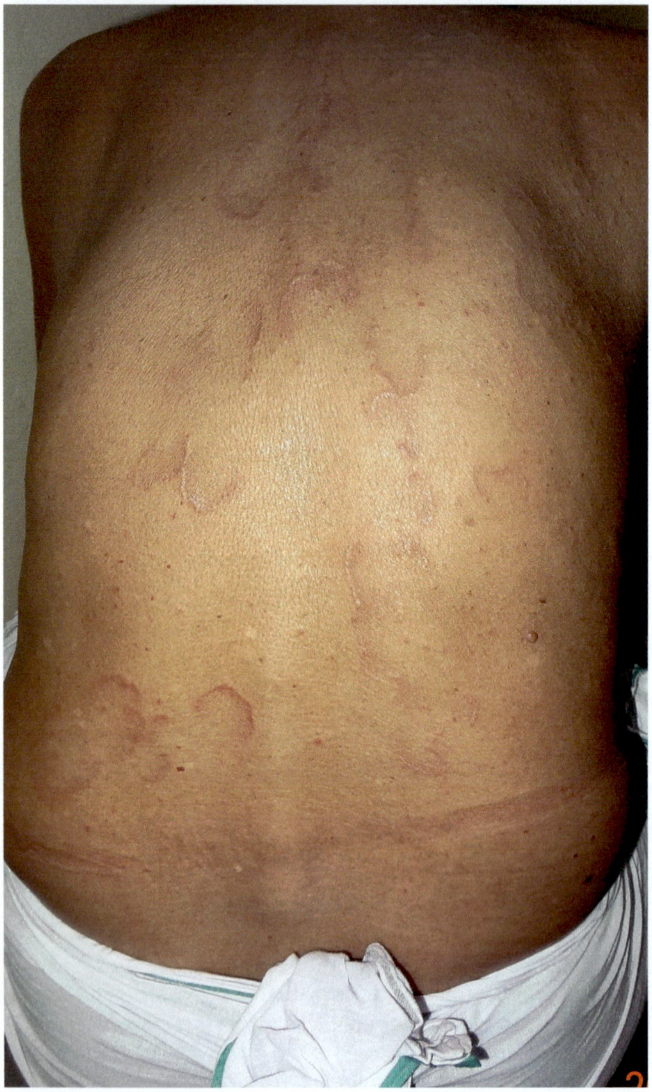

Figure 8.6. Annular, arcuate erythematous plaques on the back in disseminated granuloma annulare. (Courtesy: Dr. Piyush Kumar, Katihar, India.)

## Granuloma multiforme

- This is a reactive skin disorder of unknown etiology, characterized clinically by confluent annular plaques and histologically by focal necrobiosis and histiocytic granuloma.
- The initial lesions are papules that soon evolve to form annular and polycyclic lesions with papular or nodular edges. Elevated plaques may also occur. The lesions tend to last for months or years, extend with central healing, and often leave hypopigmented macules in most cases.
- Sun-exposed sites of upper trunk and arms are predominantly affected.
- DD: Granuloma annulare (annular plaque, discrete papules in periphery), tinea corporis (central clearing, peripheral papules, scales, KOH mount), leprosy (hypopigmented hypoesthetic plaque, thickened nerve, AFB), sarcoidosis, necrobiosis lipoidica diabeticorum.

## Necrobiotic xanthogranuloma

- This is a rare, progressive multisystem histiocytic disease characterized by destructive cutaneous and subcutaneous lesions affecting men and women equally.
- The classic skin lesion is an asymptomatic indurated papule, nodule, or plaque with a yellow "xanthomatous" hue. Plaques are firm and indurated, with an active red border and atrophic center.
- The most common site affected is the periorbital area, trunk, and proximal extremities; the condition begins at around 50 years of age.
- Lesions are yellow plaques and nodules that are deep, firm, and indurated with active an red border and atrophic center.
- DD: Granuloma annulare (annular plaque, discrete papules in periphery), sarcoidosis (red or tan-brown plaques, naked granuloma, borderline leprosy (multiple patches, nodules, and plaques with sensory impairment, thickened nerves, AFB present), xanthoma (yellow plaques and nodules affecting joints and fingers, hyperlipidemia).

## Mycosis fungoides (plaque stage)

- It is an epidermotropic cutaneous T cell lymphoma characterized by a proliferation of small- to medium-sized CD4+ T cells with cerebriform nuclei. More commonly seen in elderly males.
- Lesions are macular to start with and gradually become more infiltrated to form plaques and nodules.
- Plaques are slightly erythematous and scaly, often with a cigarette-paper surface (wrinkled appearance, also called pseudo-atrophy); sites of predilection include buttocks, trunk, upper thighs, and upper arms. Less often, involvement of flexures, scalp, and palms is seen. If confronted with erythematous scaly plaques with varying shades of color, always think of mycosis fungoides (**Figure 8.7a–f**).
- Pagetoid reticulosis has two clinical patterns:
    - Classic Woringer–Kolopp pagetoid reticulosis: One or few acral plaques sharply bordered, scaly, stable.
    - Disseminated Ketron–Goodman pagetoid reticulosis: Widespread plaques without patch stage lesions or pruritus; most do not distinguish this form from mycosis fungoides.

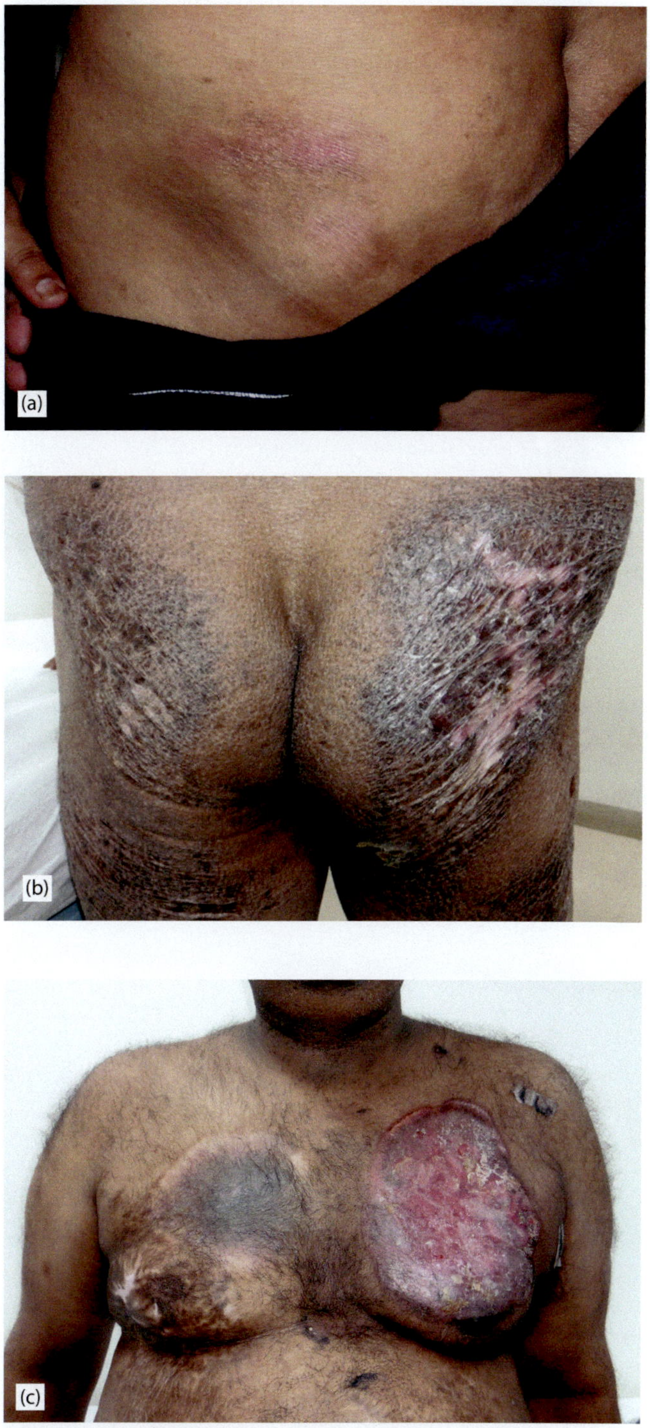

Figure 8.7 **(a)** Erythematous scaly plaque of mycosis fungoides. **(b)** Hyperpigmented, atrophic, scaly plaques in mycosis fungoides. **(c)** Large erythematous scaly plaque with erosions at places. (*Continued*)

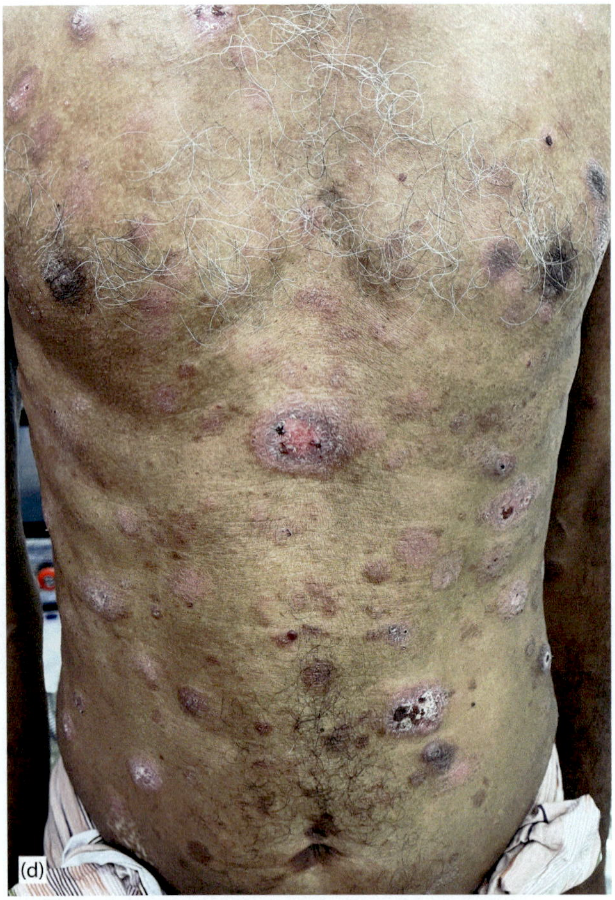

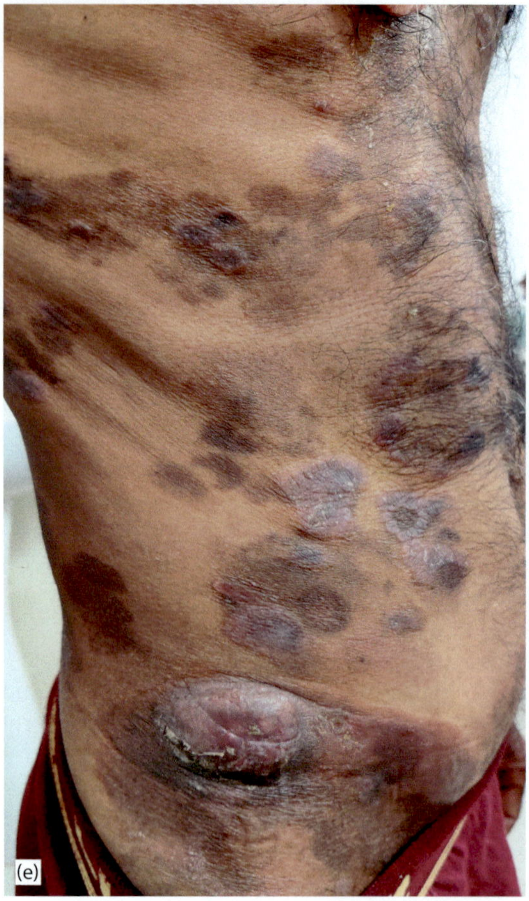

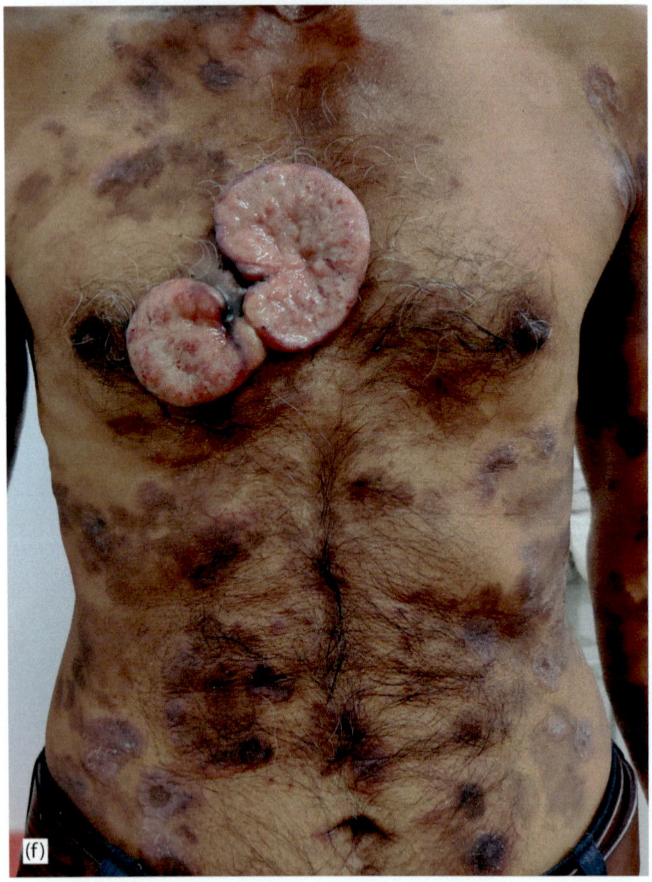

- Any patient with persistent polymorphic plaques involving the pelvic girdle area should have a skin biopsy. Early stages of MF may mimic allergic contact dermatitis, atopic dermatitis, and fungal infection.
- DD: Chronic plaque psoriasis (micaceous scales, Auspitz sign, extensors), granuloma annulare (annular plaque, discrete papules in periphery, no lymphadenopathy), sarcoidosis (red or tan-brown plaques, naked granuloma).

Figure 8.7 (*Continued*) **(d)** Mycosis fungoides presenting as multiple, erythematous scaly plaques of varying sizes. Some of these plaques are ulcerated and crusted. **(e)** Violaceous, scaly plaques healing with dyspigmentation and atrophy in mycosis fungoides. **(f)** Classic reniform ulcerated plaques of mycosis fungoides on the chest in the same patient. (a–c – Courtesy: Dr Tanumay Raychaudhury The Skin Hospital, Westmead Skin and Cancer Foundation, Australia; d – Courtesy: Dr. Soumyajit Roychoudhury, Berhampore, India; e,f – Courtesy: Dr. Bhuvaneshwari Dewangan, Dr. Naveen Keshwani, Dr. Monica Jain, and Dr. Siddhartha Dash. Shri Shankaracharya Institute of Medical Sciences, Chattisgarh, India.)

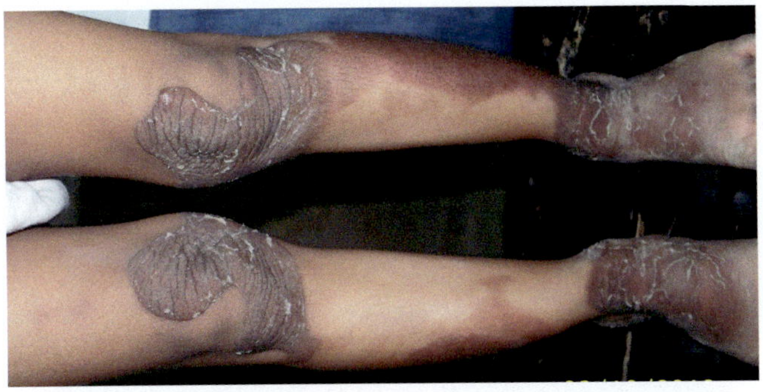

Figure 8.8. Well-circumscribed, thick, erythematous areas of scaling in a child in progressive symmetric erythrokeratoderma. (Courtesy: Dr. Piyush Kumar, Katihar, India.)

## Progressive symmetric erythrokeratoderma (PSEK)

- This is a rare, autosomal dominantly inherited genodermatosis condition presenting early in childhood.
- Cutaneous lesions in PSEK start early in infancy and present as well-circumscribed, non-migratory areas of erythema with scaling distributed symmetrically on the knees, elbows, buttocks, head, and dorsal surfaces of the hand and feet. Gradually the scaling progresses to become hyperkeratotic plaques and becomes stable after puberty (**Figure 8.8**). The trunk is spared.
- DD: Erythrokeratodermia variabilis (EKV; lesions in EKV fluctuate in their extent, and they can be induced by external mechanical pressure and show seasonal variation), chronic plaque psoriasis (seasonal variation, micaceous scales, Auspitz sign, trunk), pityriasis rubra pilaris (nutmeg-grater feel, island of normal skin).

## Urticaria

- Urticaria (or "hives" or "nettle rash") consists of itchy, blanchable wheals (**Figure 8.9a,b**).
- These wheals vary in size from 1 mm to many centimeters.
- They are caused by vasoactive mediators, predominantly histamine, released from mast cells.
- In the vast majority of cases the wheals are transient, lasting for only a few hours in any one place, but with new wheals appearing in other places.
- Etiology: lesions may be precipitated by physical factors (cold, heat, sweating, exercise, pressure, sunlight, water and vibration), food (salicylates in food/additives, preservatives, colors), drugs (aspirin, NSAIDS, infections (*Helicobacter pylori*, dental infections), autoimmune conditions (systemic lupus erythematosus, Sjogren syndrome) to name a few.
- DD: urticarial vasculitis, urticaria pigmentosa.

## Urticarial vasculitis

- This is a chronic disease that presents as urticarial lesions that persist for more than 24 hours, often demonstrate purpura, and leave behind post-inflammatory hyperpigmentation.

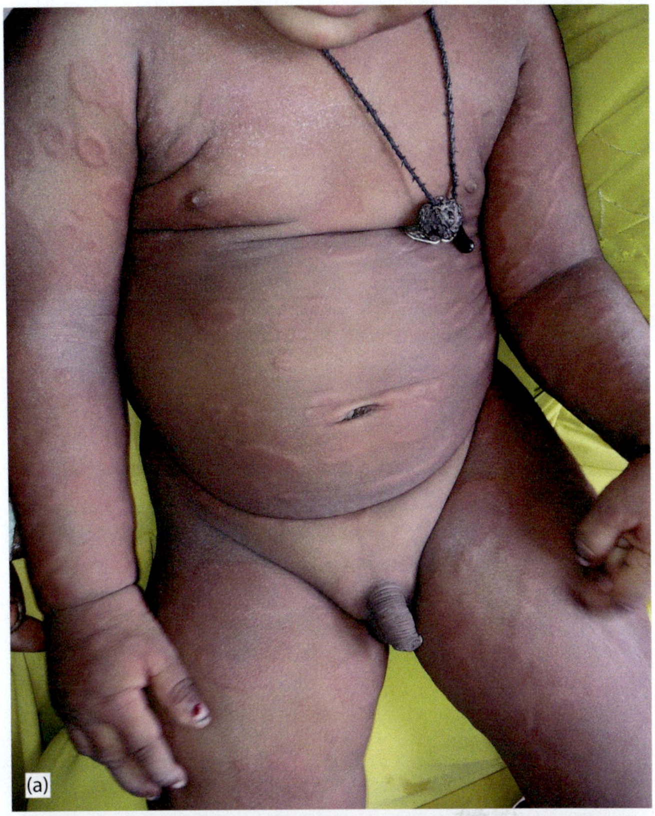

(a)

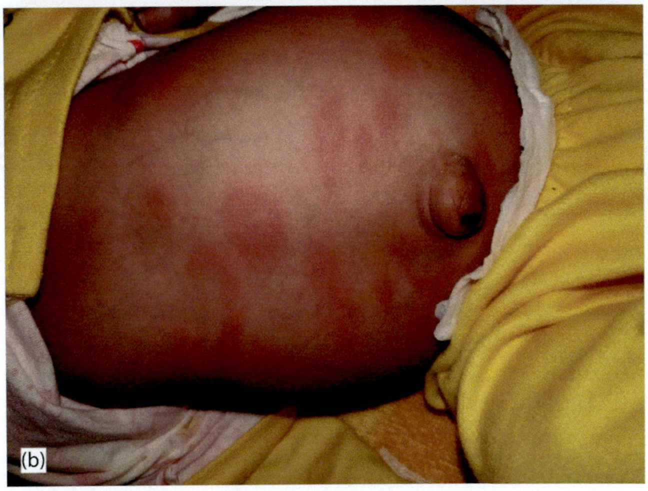

(b)

Figure 8.9 **(a)** Annular, erythematous, edematous plaques in generalized urticaria in a child. **(b)** Generalized urticarial plaques in a child. (a – Courtesy: Dr. Piyush Kumar, Katihar, India; b – Courtesy: Dr. Niharika Ranjan Lal, ESIPGIMSR, Kolkata, India.)

- Clinically, erythematous indurated wheals with purpuric foci mostly occur on the trunk and proximal limbs, with symptoms of pain rather than itch.
- The condition is thought to be mediated via a type III/immune complex hypersensitivity reaction, in which antigen/antibody complexes deposit in vessel walls.
- DD: Urticarial phase of bullous pemphigoid (persistent, vesicle formation), erythema multiforme (associated with herpes infection, target lesion).

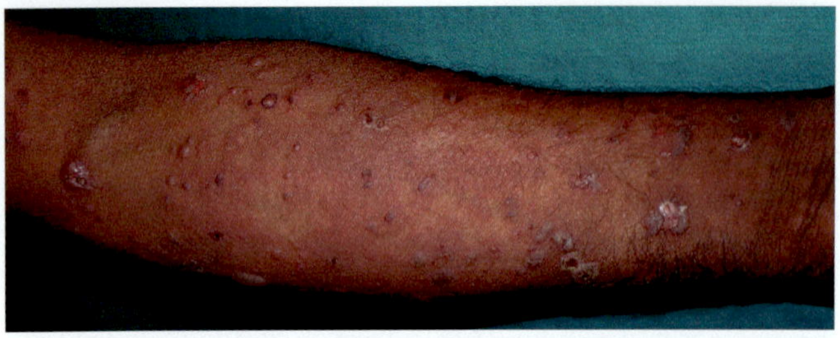

Figure 8.10. Urticarial phase bullous pemphigoid. (Courtesy: Dr. Piyush Kumar, Katihar, India.)

## Bullous pemphigoid (urticarial phase)

- Bullous pemphigoid is a common immunobullous disorder that mostly occurs in elderly people.
- Bullous pemphigoid commonly starts with itching and a non-specific rash on the limbs that may be either urticaria-like or occasionally eczematous (**Figure 8.10**).
- Commonly affected sites are lower abdomen, inner thighs, and flexor of forearm.
- The urticarial prodrome usually lasts one to three weeks before blisters occur.
- Mucosal lesions are less common and less severe compared to pemphigus vulgaris.
- DD: Urticaria (transient, evanescent, edematous plaque), erythema multiforme (associated with herpes infection, target lesion), dermatitis herpetiformis (intensely pruritic, extensors, gluten hypersensitive enteropathy, dramatic response to dapsone.)

## Generalized morphea

- This is a rare condition in which idiopathic sclerosis of the skin occurs in a widespread manner.
- Classic morphea presents as well-circumscribed sclerotic plaques with ivory center and red-violet periphery (lilac ring), starting as an erythematous patch that slowly spreads, attaining size of 5–20 cm, in which spontaneous or therapy-induced regression occurs (**Figure 8.11a,b**).
- The main areas involved are the upper trunk, breasts, abdomen, and upper thighs.
- It is more common in females and appears at the age of 30 to 40 years. Systemic findings are not common; rarely it includes malaise or Raynaud's phenomenon. It is most common on the trunk in young girls.
- It resolves with atrophy and hyperpigmentation.
- DD: Pseudo-scleroderma (porphyria cutanea tarda and graft versus host disease), drug-induced sclerosis (Bleomycin), systemic sclerosis (Raynaud's phenomenon, face and extremities are more common, worsen with age, systemic disease), eosinophilic fasciitis (acute onset, pain and edema, more in male), generalized lichen sclerosus (papule, follicular plugging).

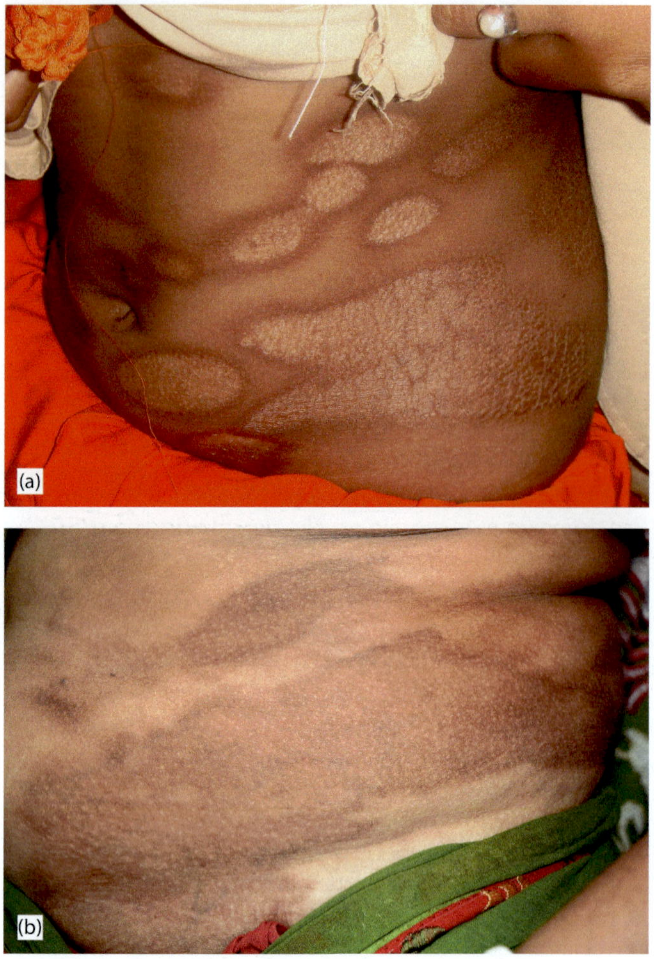


Figure 8.11 **(a)** Multiple, shiny, atrophic, indurated plaques on abdomen and flank in generalized morphea. **(b)** Large indurated plaques of morphea on the abdomen in a middle-aged lady. (a,b – Courtesy: Dr. Piyush Kumar, Katihar, India.)

## Generalized lichen sclerosus et atrophicus (LSA)

- This is a dermatosis that presents with either porcelain-white papules and plaques or atrophy and classic histological picture.
- The etiology is not clear, but immunoglobulin G (IgG) antibodies against extracellular matrix protein 1 (EMP 1) have been identified.
- Typical cutaneous lesions are small, ivory or porcelain-white, shiny round macules or papules that are semi-translucent, resembling mother of pearl. These lesions get aggregated into plaques that are slightly raised or level with the surface of the skin; typically their surface shows prominent dilated sweat ducts or pilosebaceous orifices containing yellow or brown horny plugs (**Figure 8.12a–c**).
- The lesions on the skin are symptomless, and extragenital lesions occur on the trunk, particularly on the upper part and around the umbilicus, the neck, the axillae, and the flexor surfaces of the wrists. Genital lesions may itch.

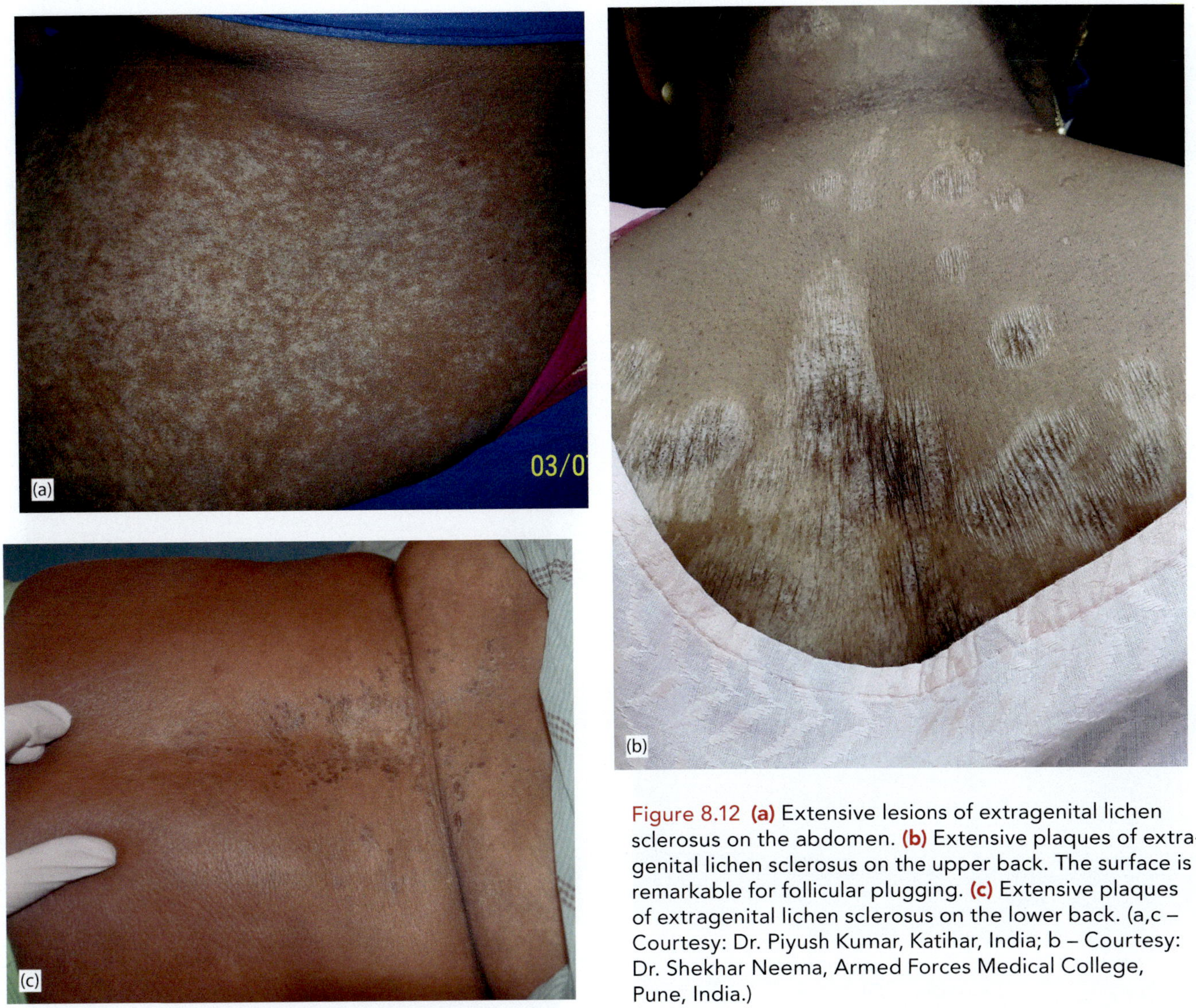


Figure 8.12 **(a)** Extensive lesions of extragenital lichen sclerosus on the abdomen. **(b)** Extensive plaques of extragenital lichen sclerosus on the upper back. The surface is remarkable for follicular plugging. **(c)** Extensive plaques of extragenital lichen sclerosus on the lower back. (a,c – Courtesy: Dr. Piyush Kumar, Katihar, India; b – Courtesy: Dr. Shekhar Neema, Armed Forces Medical College, Pune, India.)

- DD: Generalized morphea (lacks characteristic papules of LSA), atrophic lichen planus (extremely pruritic, raised, violaceous), annular atrophic plaque type of DLE.

## Darier disease

- Darier disease is an autosomal dominant disorder with primarily follicular keratoses and distinct histology.
- It occurs due to mutation in a calcium channel regulating gene ATP2A2, encoding SERCA2; that leads to disturbance in calcium homeostasis and is thought to interfere with desmosome stability.
- Early lesions are discrete or confluent, rough, greasy, skin-colored or yellowish brown papules that coalesce particularly in the axillae, perineum, groin, and natal cleft to form irregular, warty, fissured plaques, sometimes becoming vegetating and malodorous (**Figure 8.13a–c**).
- White painless palatal papules appear as cobblestone in the oral cavity.

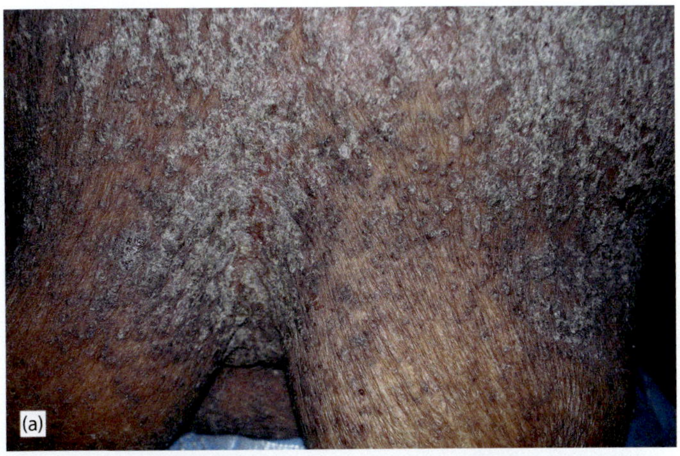

Figure 8.13 **(a)** Hyperpigmented, dirty, warty papules coalescing to form generalized plaques in Darier disease. *(Continued)*

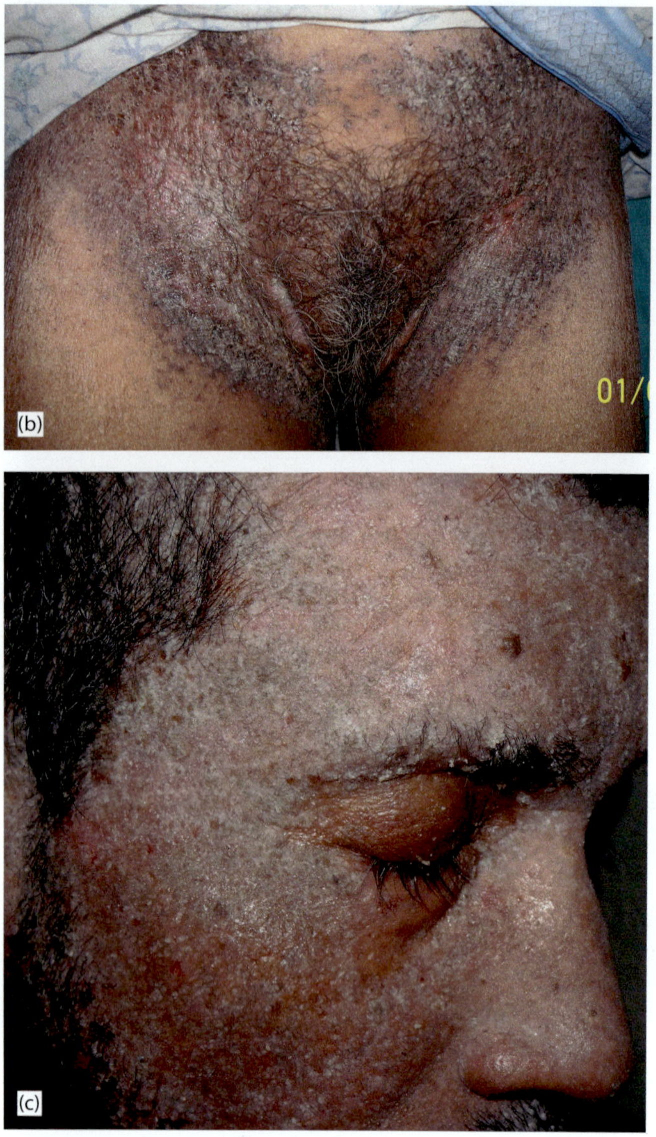

Figure 8.13 (*Continued*) **(b)** Macerated plaques and keratotic papules of Darier disease. **(c)** Severe facial involvement in Darier disease in summer. (a–c – Courtesy: Dr. Piyush Kumar, Katihar, India.)

- Nails show longitudinal red and white bands, subungual hyperkeratosis, and triangular nicking of the free edges.
- DD: Seborrheic dermatitis (absence of family history, spares mucosa and nails, appears less on acral area), acanthosis nigricans, pemphigus vegetans, transient acantholytic dermatosis (discrete, intertriginous area).

## Tinea corporis

- Tinea corporis is a dermatophyte infection of the skin of trunk and extremities, excluding the palms, soles, and inguinal region.
- The infection spreads centrifugally, resulting in annular scaly plaques of various shapes and sizes with pustules at the active border (**Figure 8.14a,b**).

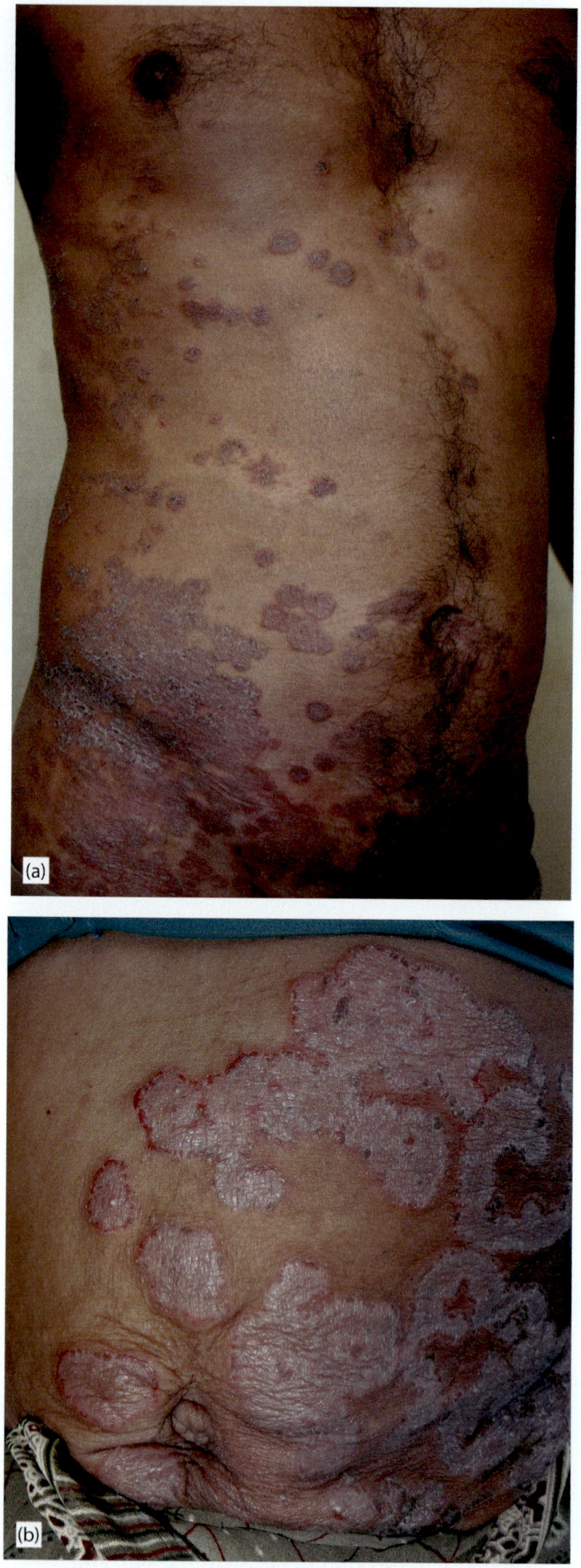

Figure 8.14 **(a)** Erythematous, annular and polycyclic plaques with scales on active border in extensive tinea corporis. **(b)** Annular and polycyclic erythematous scaly plaques in extensive tinea corporis. (a,b – Courtesy: Dr. Piyush Kumar, Katihar, India.)

- Lesions start as erythematous flat, scaly spots and then develop a raised border that expands in all directions, with healing in the center, giving the classical "ring-like" appearance.
- There are variable degrees of inflammation, in some instances with pustule formation, depending on nature of dermatophyte and host response.
- Unjustified medications can obscure central clearing and cause tinea incognito.
- Early lesions usually present as red papules or plaques and develop into extremely itchy scaly plaques anywhere on the body.
- DD: Granuloma annulare (annular plaque, discrete papules in periphery, central depression), borderline tuberculoid leprosy (hypoesthesia, hypopigmentation, thickened nerves), psoriasis (micaceous scales, Auspitz sign, extensor aspect of limbs), nummular eczema (oozy plaque, no central clearing, no peripheral papules).

## Figurate erythemas

- These are patterned erythemas, often annular in shape and occasionally migratory. Various patterns and forms have been described.
- Erythema annulare centrifugum begins as pink papules that expand centrifugally to develop central clearing; they can reach sizes up to 6–10 cm in diameter over a period of one to two weeks. In the superficial form lesions are minimally elevated, with desquamation at the inner margin (trailing scale) (**Figure 8.15**); in deep gyrate erythema, advancing edges are obviously elevated without associated scale or pruritus.
  - The usual affected sites are the trunk and proximal parts of limbs, rarely if ever involving palms, soles, scalp, or mucus membranes.
  - It is associated with *Borrelia* infection.
- In erythema gyratum repens (EGR), patients usually have multiple annular or polycyclic erythematous lesions that develop scale at their edges; they advance at a rapid rate (up to 1 cm/day) to develop a wood-grain or Zebra-like pattern due to development of rings within rings on trunk.
  - It is a paraneoplastic sign of internal malignancy (EGR is commonly seen in association with the malignancies of lung, breast, esophagus, and stomach).
- In erythema marginatum (rheumaticum), lesions begin as erythematous macules that spread peripherally and become patches or plaque with no scale. They may be arranged polycyclically. Sites affected are the trunk, axillae, and proximal extremities, with sparing of the face. It is associated with the active phase of rheumatic fever and is generally seen in conjunction with carditis.
- DD: Granuloma annulare (annular plaque, discrete papules in periphery, central depression), urticaria (transient, evanescent edematous hives/wheals), tinea corporis (rarely wide spread, central clearing, KOH), secondary syphilis (scaly plaques, rebound tenderness, VDRL positivity).

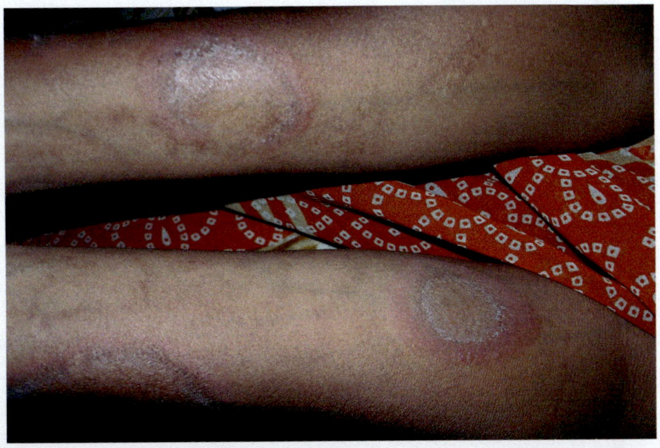

Figure 8.15 Annular erythematous plaques with fine trailing scales in erythema annulare centrifugum. (Courtesy: Dr. Piyush Kumar, Katihar, India.)

## Parapsoriasis

- Parapsoriasis is broadly divided into small and large plaque variants.
- Small-plaque parapsoriasis
  - A chronic asymptomatic condition mostly benign in nature.
  - Characterized by asymptomatic scaly patches or slightly raised papules and plaques over trunk and proximal extremities. Individual lesions are monomorphic round or oval erythematous patches, 2.5–5 cm in diameter, with slight scaling and waxy, yellow tinge.
  - Usually occurs at middle age and evolves gradually over months to years; there is sparing of the pelvic girdle area.
- Large-plaque parapsoriasis
  - Associated with development of definite mycosis fungoides, so long-term follow up of these cases is required.
  - Characterized by presence of persistent, large, yellow-orange atrophic patches and thin plaques on the trunk and limbs.
- If plaques show striking polymorphism and poikiloderma, this suggests mycosis fungoides.
- DD: Pityriasis rosea (pruritus, herald patch, collarette of scale, hanging curtain sign), pityriasis lichenoides (young adults, necrosis and varioliform scar, lateral trunk, spontaneous resolution), guttate psoriasis (sudden onset, pharyngitis, thicker plaque).

## Papulosquamous syphilids

- Syphilis is a chronic infection caused by *Treponema pallidum* and characterized by florid clinical manifestations interspersed with periods of asymptomatic latency; it has primary, secondary, and tertiary stages as well as a latent period of variable length.

- Papulosquamous syphilids are the most common clinical presentation of secondary syphilis. Typically they do not itch, are coppery-red in color, and are symmetric in distribution.
- Generalized, nonpruritic, papulosquamous eruptions range in size from 1–2 mm to 15–20 mm, and they vary in color from pink to violaceous to red-brown. Psoriasiform plaques of the palms and soles are common in black people, as are annular and circinate papular rashes (**Figure 8.16**).
- Mucosal lesions range from small, superficial ulcers that resemble painless aphthae to large gray plaques.
- DD: Pityriasis rosea (pruritus, lesions along the cleavage line, herald patch, collarette of scale, hanging curtain sign), scaly varieties of tinea corporis, parapsoriasis (elderly, necrosis absent, no lymphadenopathy, absent prodromal symptoms), drug eruptions (scarlatiniform or morbilliform, pruritic), psoriasis (thick scale, absence of lymphadenopathy and mucous patches).

## Norwegian scabies

- Human scabies is a pruritic condition caused by infestation by the host specific mite *Sarcoptes scabiei var. hominis.*
- Typically, small erythematous papules with a variable degree of excoriation present symmetrically on the finger web, wrist, axilla, umbilical, and genital regions. Severe eczematous changes are common and may be widespread, with severe and extensive secondary infection.
- Crusted scabies (Norwegian or hyperkeratotic scabies) is found in immunocompromised or debilitated patients.
- In these patients, the infestation assumes a heavily scaling and crusted appearance (**Figure 8.17a–c**).
- DD: Atopic dermatitis (chronic, history of atopy, white dermatographism, seasonal variation, raised immunoglobulin E level), allergic contact dermatitis (confined to area of contact, erythematous plaque with oozing and crusting, patch test), dermatitis herpetiformis (papulovesicles, extensor site, gluten sensitivity), psoriasis (micaceous scales, Auspitz sign, extensors).

## Sulzberger-Garbe disease

- This is also known as exudative discoid and lichenoid chronic dermatitis.
- This is an extremely pruritic condition characterized by discoid lesions with "lichenoid" and exudative phases, which either coexist or alternate rapidly with each other.
- There may be showers of round, erythematous, oozy plaques.

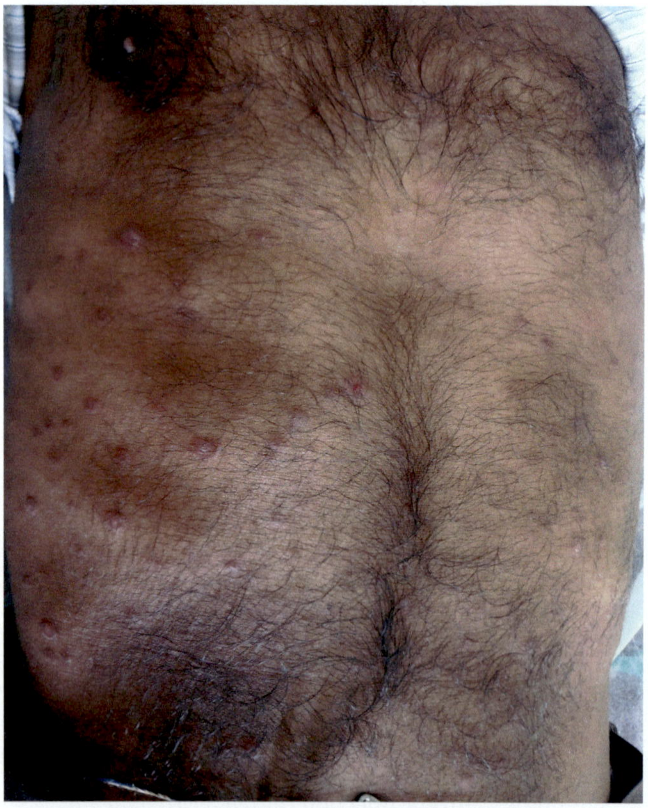

Figure 8.16 Scaly papules and plaques of secondary syphilis. (Courtesy: Dr. Santoshdev Rathod, SVPIMSR, Smt. NHL Municipal Medical College, V.S. Hospital, Ahmedabad, India.)

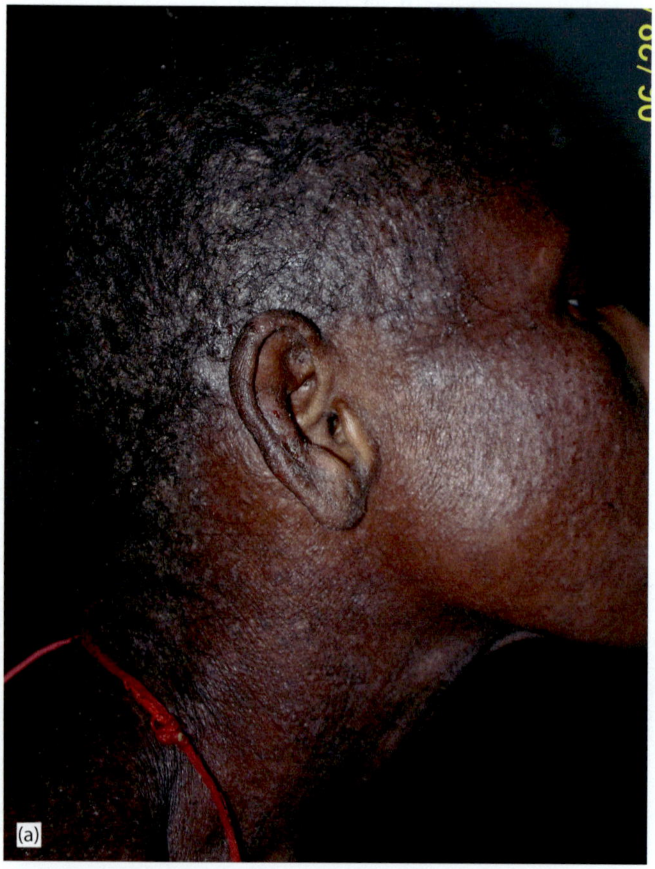

Figure 8.17 **(a)** Crusted, scaly plaque in Norwegian scabies. (*Continued*)

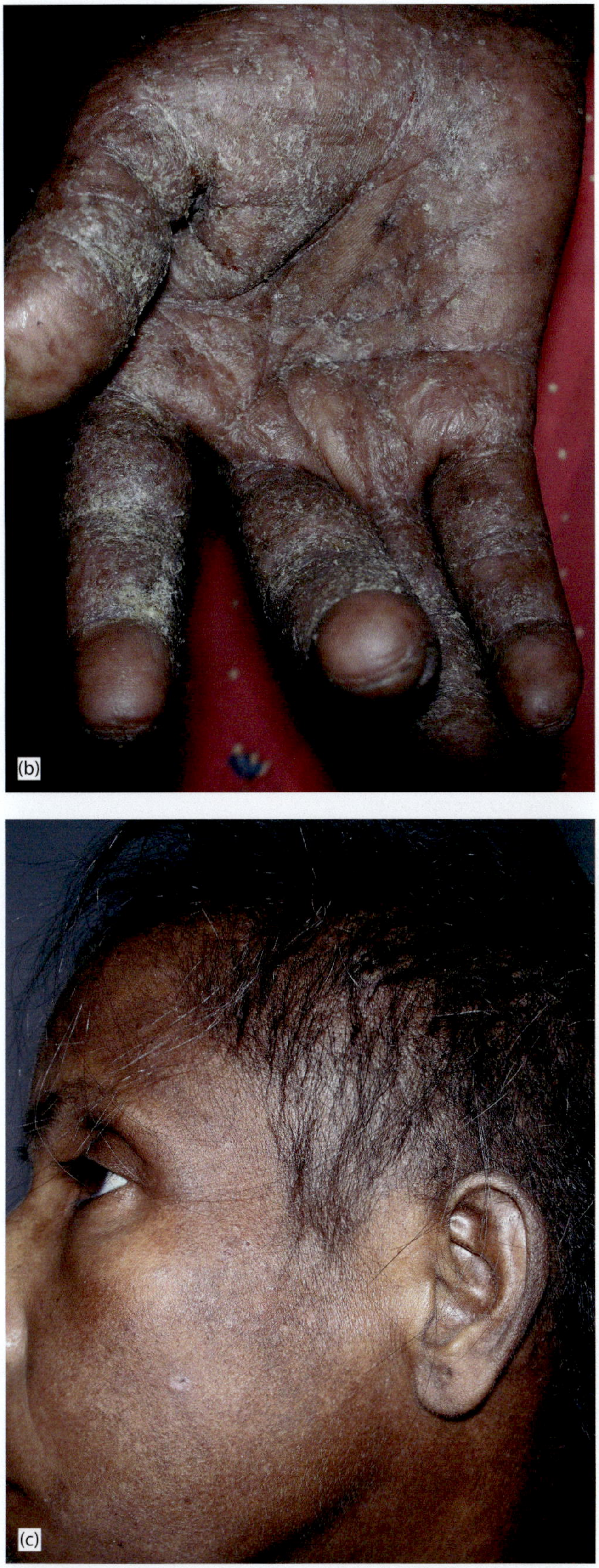


Figure 8.17 (*Continued*) **(b)** Palm involvement in Norwegian scabies. **(c)** Resolution of lesions with anti-scabies treatment. (a–c – Courtesy: Dr. Piyush Kumar, Katihar, India.)

- Penile and scrotal lesions are common and are almost pathognomonic.
- DD: Mycosis fungoides (mildly itchy, generalized, epidermotropism, atypical cells), contact dermatitis (localized, asymmetrical, patch test), dermatitis herpetiformis (papulovesicles, extensor site, gluten sensitivity).

## Generalized seborrheic keratosis

- Generalized seborrheic keratosis presents as oval, slightly raised, tan/light-brown to black, sharply demarcated papules or plaques, rarely more than 3 cm in diameter (**Figure 8.18**).
- Mostly present on the trunk, face, and extremities.
- Palms and soles are usually spared.
- The sudden appearance of numerous seborrheic keratosis may be a cutaneous sign of internal malignancy (Leser-Trelat sign).
- DD: Verruca vulgaris (pseudo-Koebnerization, warty plaque, and papules), post-pemphigus acanthoma.

## Pruritic urticarial papules and plaques of pregnancy (PUPPP)

- This eruption is characterized by erythematous papules and plaques that begin as 1- or 2-mm lesions within the abdominal striae.
- It spreads within a day to involve the abdomen, thighs, buttocks, and extremities.

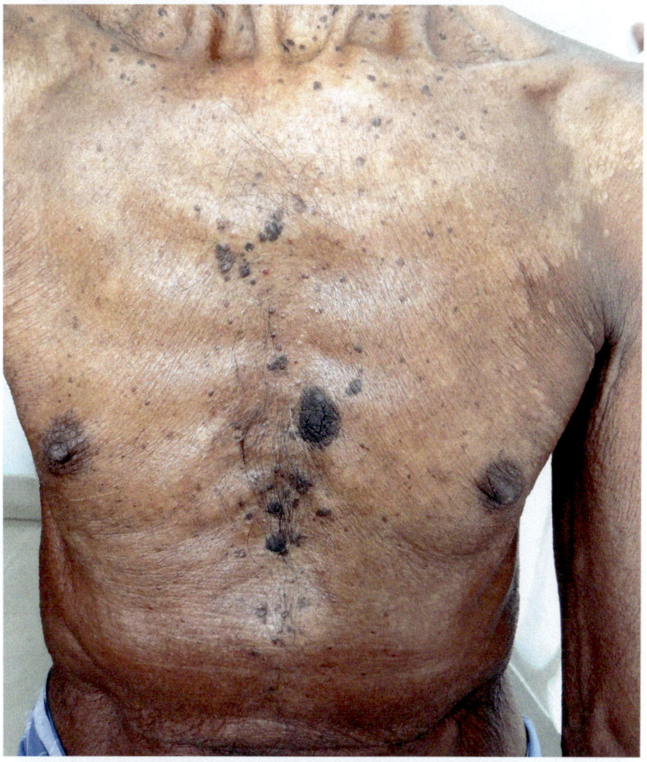

Figure 8.18 Multiple hyperpigmented papules and plaques on chest in seborrheic keratosis. Central larger plaques show hyperkeratotic surface. (Courtesy: Dr. Piyush Kumar, Katihar, India.)

- It spares the periumbilical area, face, palm, soles, and mucosa.
- It is most common in primigravida in the later part of pregnancy.
- DD: Pemphigoid gestationis (early part of pregnancy, involves umbilical area, no relation with striae), contact dermatitis (scaly, weeping plaque, hyperkeratotic), urticaria (transient, evanescent, edematous plaque).

## Urticaria pigmentosa

- This is the most common pattern of cutaneous mastocytosis.
- Urticaria pigmentosa develops in the first year of life.
- Adult onset urticaria pigmentosa is present most commonly at 20 to 40 years of age.
- Numerous reddish-brown or pale, pruritic, monomorphic maculopapules, plaques or nodules appear in a symmetrical distribution, mainly on the trunk and thighs (**Figure 8.19a,b**).

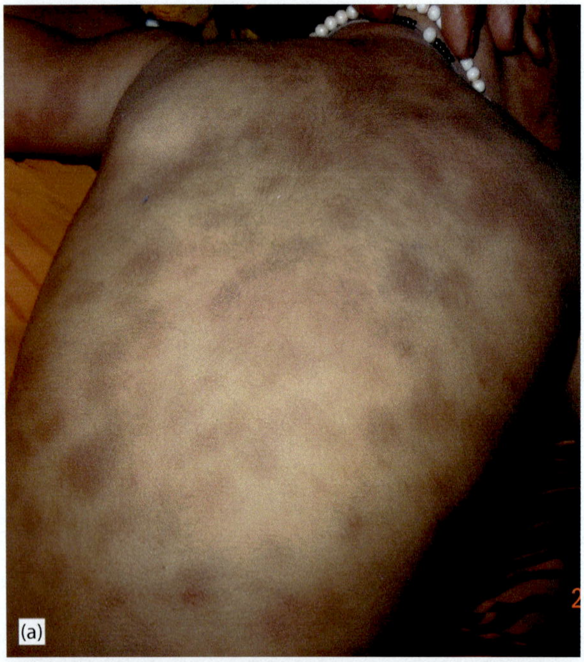


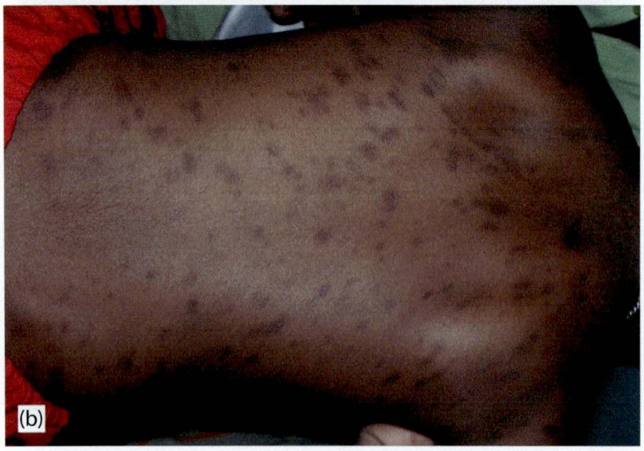


Figure 8.19 **(a)** Pigmented plaques of urticaria pigmentosa on the back. **(b)** Another case of urticaria pigmentosa. (a,b – Courtesy: Dr. Piyush Kumar, Katihar, India.)

- Face, head, palms, and soles are spared.
- The edges of the lesions are not completely sharp.
- They become edematous within a few minutes of gentle rubbing (Darier sign).
- DD: Urticaria (transient, evanescent, edematous plaque), juvenile xanthogranuloma (asymptomatic, rubbery in consistency, head and neck are is the most common site).

## Kaposi sarcoma (KS)

- Kaposi sarcoma is formed by the proliferation of abnormal vascular endothelial cells.
- It is A multifocal systemic disease with four principal clinical variants:
  - Classic Kaposi sarcoma
  - African endemic KS
  - KS due to iatrogenic immunosuppression
  - AIDS-related epidemic KS
- Cutaneous lesions can vary from pink patches to dark violet plaques, nodules, or polyps.
- The process usually begins on the extremities, most commonly on (**Figure 8.20**) the feet and occasionally on the hands, ears, or nose.
- The lesions may involute to leave pigmented scars or may become eroded, ulcerated, or fungating.
- Different stages of lesions are found in the same patient.
- There is predilection for the head, neck, trunk, and mucous membrane.
- DD: Pseudo-Kaposi's sarcoma (non-progressive, spindle-cell proliferation in histopathology), angiosarcoma (localized, lymphedema).

## Erythema nodosum leprosum (ENL)

- ENL is encountered during therapy of patients with lepromatous leprosy or borderline leprosy.
- Classic ENL is characterized by the appearance of crops of tender, painful subcutaneous nodules with associated constitutional symptoms (**Figure 8.21a–c**). Acute lesions appear in crops and heal over several days. Commonly affected sites are the face and extensor surfaces of the limbs.

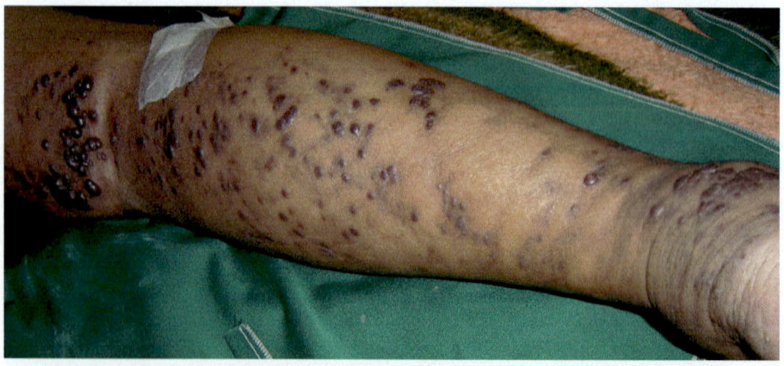

Figure 8.20 Numerous violaceous plaques and nodules in Kaposi sarcoma. (Courtesy: Prof. Reza Yaghoobi, Department of Dermatology, Ahvaz Jundishupor University of Medical Sciences, Iran.)

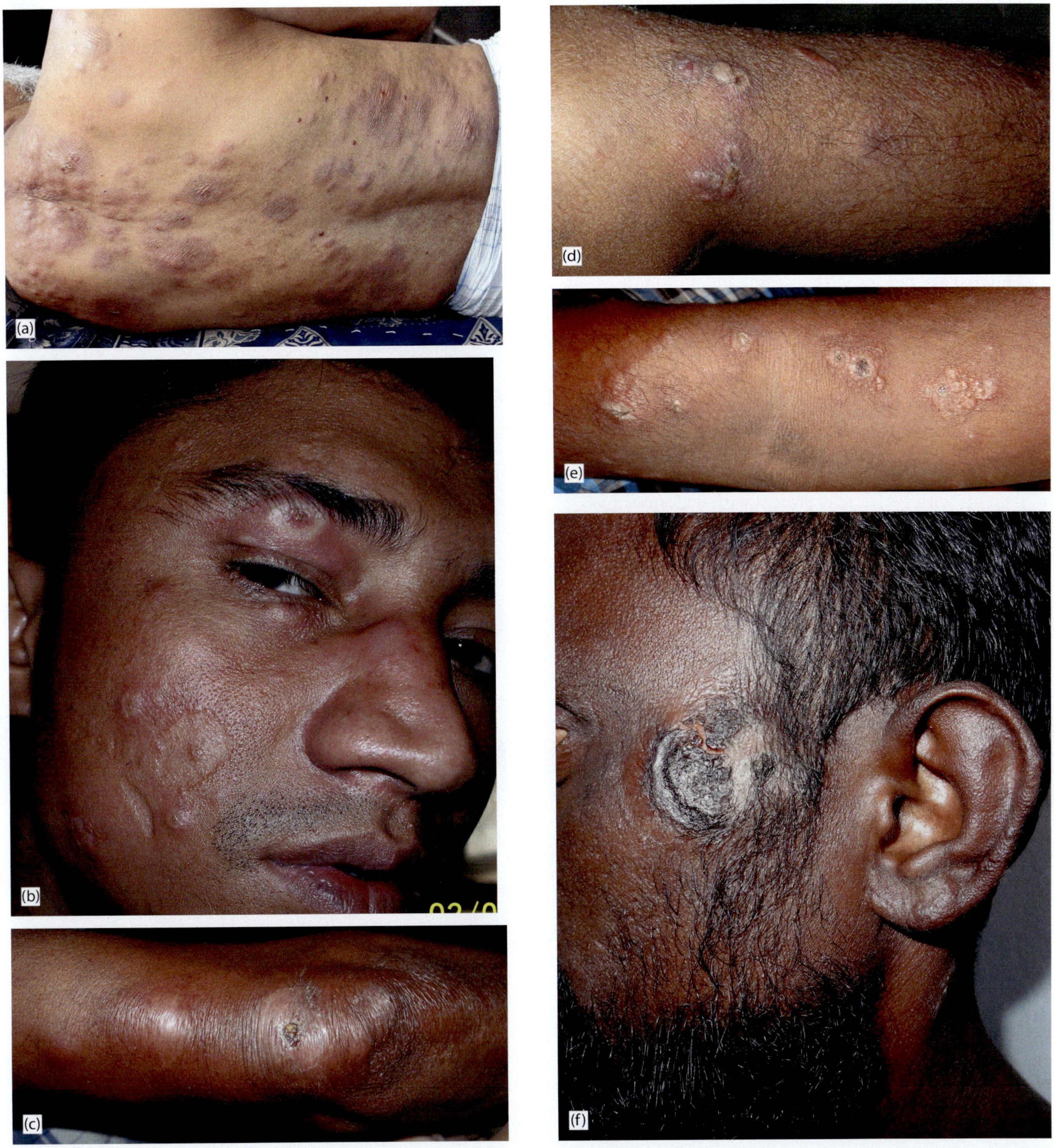


Figure 8.21 **(a)** Multiple erythematous edematous plaques and nodules of erythema nodosum leprosum. **(b)** Erythematous, edematous plaques of erythema nodosum leprosum (ENL) on the face. Prior lesions have healed with atrophic scarring. **(c)** Erythematous, edematous plaque and nodules in ENL. **(d)** Pustular ENL. **(e)** Erythema multiforme like lesions in ENL. **(f)** Eschar covering an ulcerated plaque in ENL. (a–f – Courtesy: Dr. Piyush Kumar, Katihar, India.)

- Ulceration may occur that heals with scarring.
- The Lucio reaction occurs in patients with lucio leprosy. Clinically, it appears as irregularly shaped erythematous patches that become dark, sometimes forming bullae and becoming necrotic, leaving deep painful ulcers that are slow to heal. It is due to infarction consequent upon deep cutaneous vasculitis.
- Other clinical variants of ENL are vesicobullous, pustular, hemorrhagic, and erythema multiforme-like (**Figure 8.21d–f**).

- DD: Cutaneous necrotizing vasculitis (mucous membrane involvement, no sensory complaints, no nerve thickening, negative slit skin smear), Lucio leprosy (extremities, erythematous patch, superficial scar).

## Disseminated cutaneous leishmaniasis

- Disseminated cutaneous leishmaniasis may be seen in both New and Old World diseases.
- Multiple non-ulcerated papules and plaques, chiefly on exposed surfaces, characterize this type.
- The disease begins with a single ulcer, nodule, or plaque from which satellite lesions may develop and disseminate to cover the entire body (**Figure 8.22**).
- DD: Lepromatous leprosy (gloves-and-stockings anaesthesia, thick peripheral nerve, AFB positive), malignant lymphoma.

## Post-kala azar dermal leishmaniasis (PKDL)

- Patients with PKDL may present with widespread papules, plaques, and nodules in addition to hypopigmented patches.
- These plaques and nodules usually develop over existing hypopigmented patches, and the lesions are usually distributed over the face, trunk, and upper extremities (**Figure 8.23a,b**).
- Sometimes, plaques and nodules develop de novo, and such lesions show a predilection for acral areas, especially over the joints (**Figure 8.23c**).

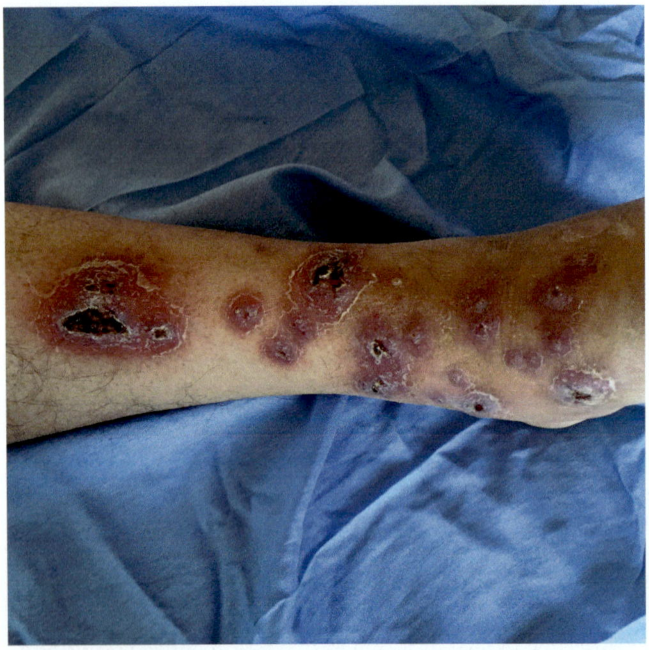

Figure 8.22 Multiple crusted plaques and ulcers in cutaneous leishmaniasis. (Courtesy: Prof. Reza Yaghoobi, Department of Dermatology, Ahvaz Jundishupor University of Medical Sciences, Iran.)

## Diffuse acanthosis nigricans

- Acanthosis nigricans (AN) is characterized by hyperpigmentation and velvet-textured plaques, symmetrically distributed.

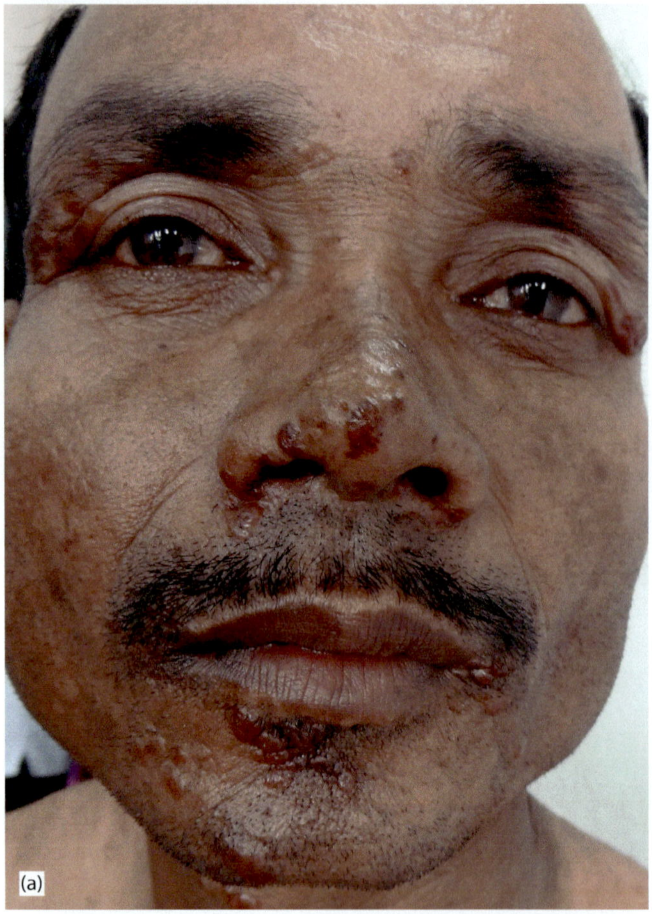

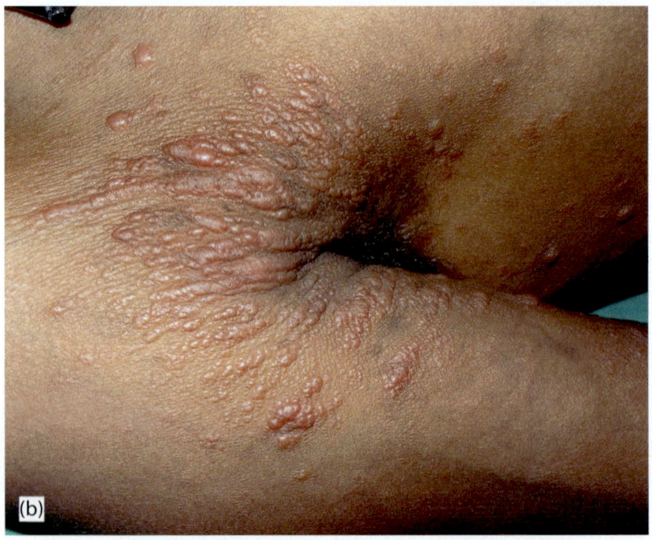

Figure 8.23 **(a)** Erythematous, smooth-surfaced papules and plaques on the face in post-kala azar dermal leishmaniasis (PKDL). **(b)** Typical erythematous, succulent papules and plaques of PKDL. (*Continued*)

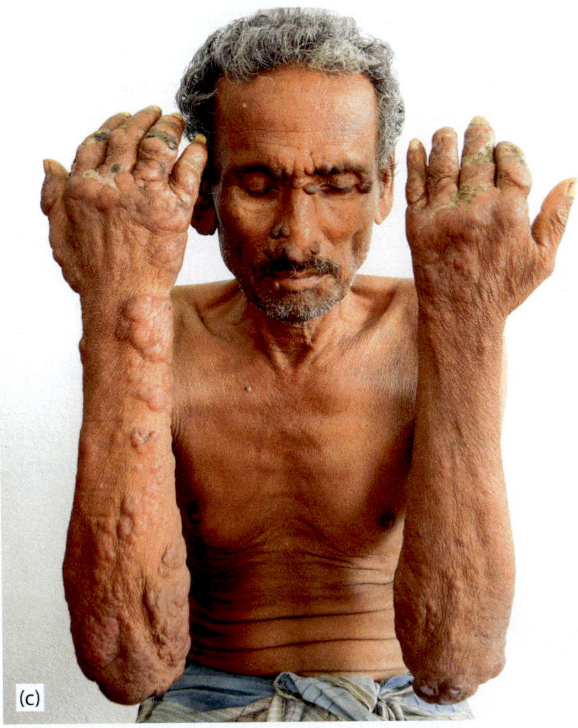


Figure 8.23 (*Continued*) **(c)** Erythematous and skin-colored infiltrative plaques and nodules in post-kala azar dermal leishmaniasis. (a–c – Courtesy: Dr. Piyush Kumar, Katihar, India.)

- Clinically, it presents as brown to gray-black papillomatous cutaneous thickening in the flexural areas, including the postero-lateral neck, axillae, groin, and abdominal folds (**Figure 8.24a,b**).

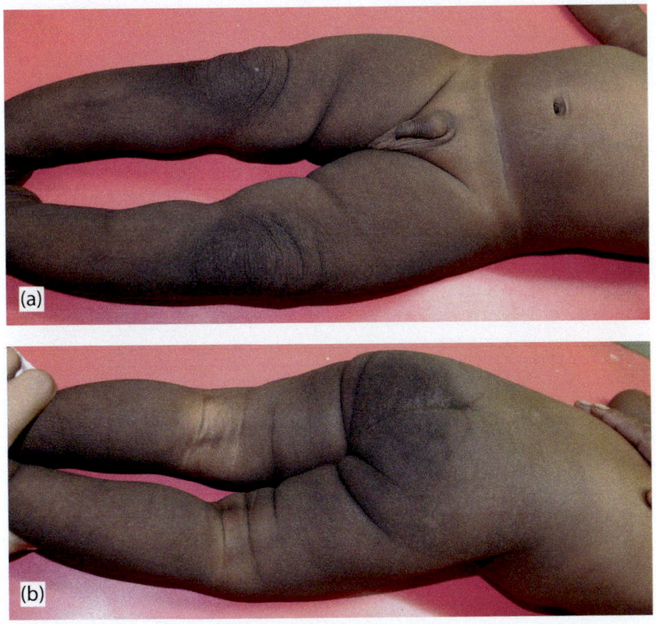


Figure 8.24 **(a)** Hyperpigmented, grayish-black velvety patch in generalized acanthosis nigricans. **(b)** Generalized acanthosis nigricans. (a,b – Courtesy: Dr. Piyush Kumar, Katihar, India.)

- Palms and soles may show thickening of the palmar skin, with exaggeration of the dermatoglyphics (tripe palms).
- DD: Addison's disease (pigmentary change, mucosal involvement), epidermolytic hyperkeratosis (blisters, spine like scales).

## Epidermodysplasia verruciformis

- Epidermodysplasia verruciformis (EV) is a rare, inherited disorder characterized by widespread HPV infection and cutaneous SCCs.
- EV usually manifests in childhood with persistent and often widespread warts.
- Individual lesions typically have either the appearance of flat warts or flat scaly red-brown macules that resemble pityriasis versicolor (**Figure 8.25a,b**).
- On the trunk are lesions that are red, tan, or brown patches/plaques or hypopigmented, very slightly scaly plaques resembling tinea versicolor. Plaques on the elbows may resemble psoriasis (**Figure 8.25c**).
- Later Bowen disease and squamous cell carcinoma develop, primarily in sun-exposed skin.

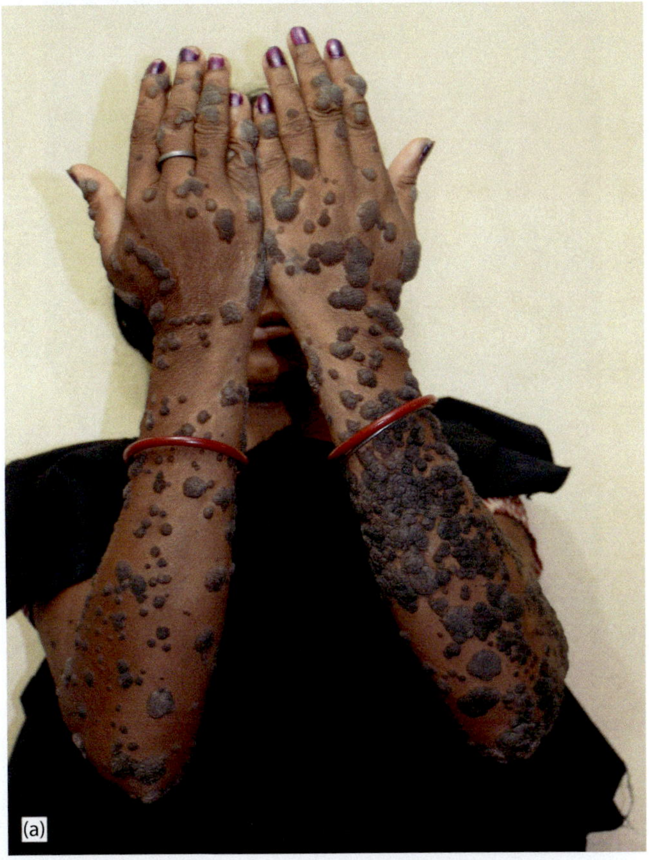


Figure 8.25 **(a)** Numerous pigmented and verrucous plaques in a middle-aged lady with epidermodysplasia verruciformis. (*Continued*)

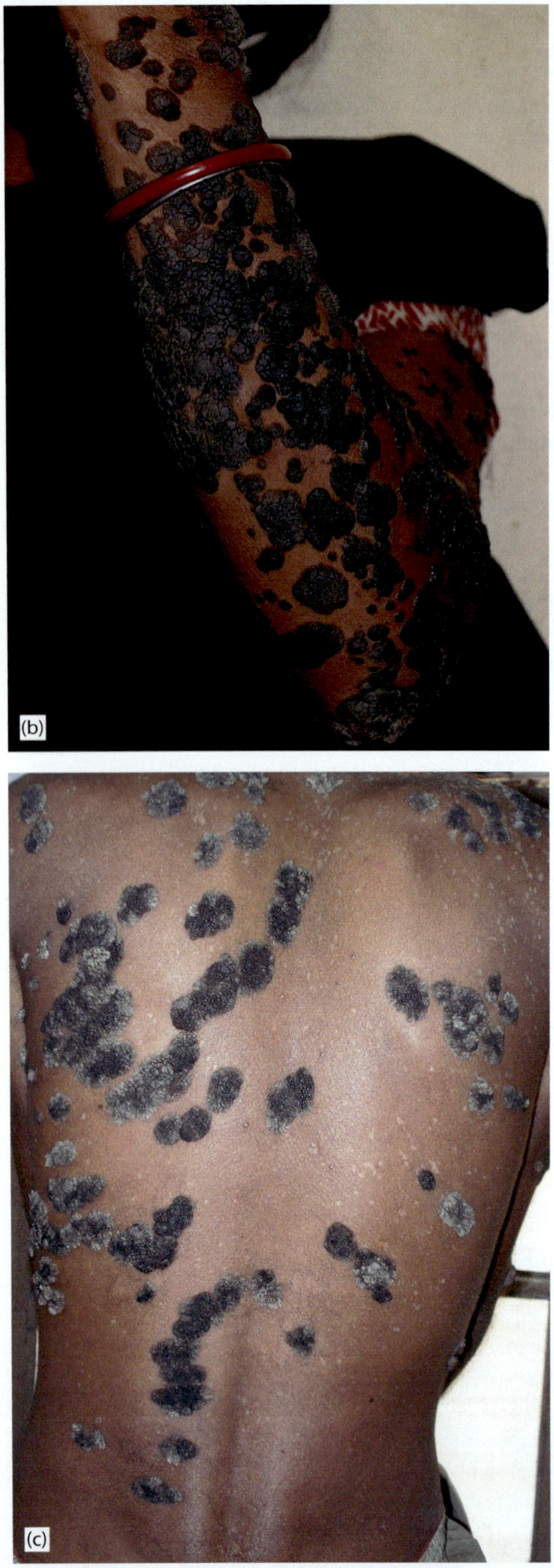

Figure 8.25 (*Continued*) **(b)** Plaques may coalesce to form larger lesions. **(c)** Hyperpigmented, verrucous, keratotic plaques in epidermodysplasia verruciformis. (a,b – Courtesy: Dr. PC Das and Dr. Piyush Kumar, Katihar, India; c – Courtesy: Dr. Piyush Kumar, Katihar, India.)

- DD: Widespread warts (pseudo-Koebner, immunocompromised patient), pityriasis versicolor (scaly, perifollicular, spaghetti-and-meatball appearance).

## Systematized verrucous epidermal nevus

- Verrucous epidermal nevi are congenital, non-inflammatory cutaneous hamartomas composed of keratinocytes following Blaschko's lines.
- When two or more linear lesions are present, the term "systematized" is used.
- At birth they have a whitish or macerated appearance that becomes velvety pigmented streaks or plaques within few days (**Figure 8.26a,b**).
- They may involve adjacent mucosal surfaces and nail folds.

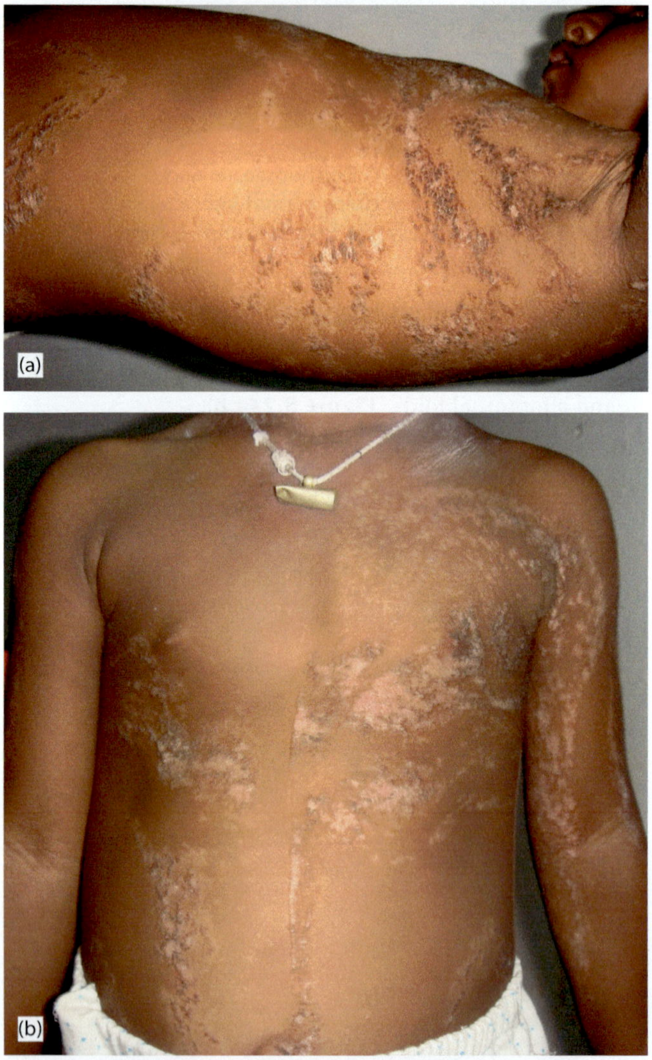

Figure 8.26 **(a)** Hyperpigmented, mildly scaly papules coalescing to form plaques distributed linearly along Blaschko's lines in systemized verrucous epidermal nevus. **(b)** Systemized verrucous epidermal nevus. (a,b – Courtesy: Dr. Piyush Kumar, Katihar, India.)

- DD: Incontinentia pigmenti (mostly in female, four distinct clinical stages), ichthyosis bullosa of Siemens (non-Blaschkoid pattern, Mauserung phenomenon).

### Incontinentia pigmenti (verrucous stage)

- This is an X-linked dominant condition caused by NEMO gene mutation and clinically characterized by spattered pigmentation on the trunk, preceded by vesicular and verrucous changes.
- There are four phases of lesions, all following a peculiar linear and streaked pattern, starting with the vesicular phase and gradually changing into the verrucous and pigmentary phase.
- The verrucous phase has smooth red nodules or plaques, often irregularly linear, along Blaschko's lines on the limbs and trunk. The plaques, bluish-purple in color, may be extensive and precede the bullae and may ulcerate to heal with characteristic, bizarre "Chinese letter pattern" pigmentation.
- The most commonly involved extracutaneous organ is the teeth followed by bone and CNS.
- DD: Verrucous epidermal nevi (no vesicular phase, males can be affected).

### Erythema multiforme (EM)

- EM is an acute, self-limited skin disease characterized by the abrupt onset of symmetrical fixed red papules and plaques.
- Erythematous plaques, typically 1–3 cm in diameter, evolve into pathognomonic "target lesions" or "iris lesions" consisting of a central zone of dusky erythema or vesicle, surrounded by a rim of pallor and a third zone of erythema commonly seen over distal extremities (**Figure 8.27**).
- It rarely becomes bullous or urticarial. It heals spontaneously over weeks, sometimes with residual hyperpigmentation.
- Sites of predilection are the palms, dorsa of hands, soles, peri-oral area and face, and genital areas.
- It is accompanied by febrile prodrome and arthralgias.
- Variants are EM minor and EM major, mostly EM minor because of recurrent HSV infection, while EM major is associated with mycoplasma.
- DD: Stevens-Johnson syndrome (10–30% skin involvement with epidermal loss and mucosal erosions, drug causation), erythema multiforme-like lupus erythematosus (Rowell syndrome), secondary syphilis (scaly plaques, rebound tenderness, VDRL positivity), Sweet syndrome (true target lesion absent, papillary dermal edema, response to steroid).

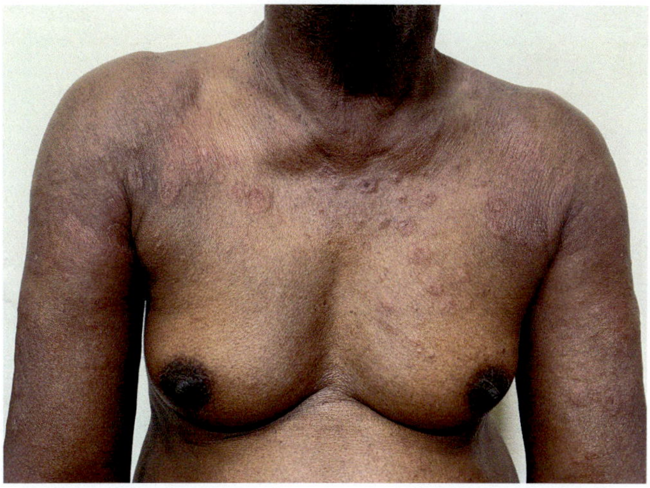

Figure 8.27 Generalized plaques in erythema multiforme characterized by central vesiculation, zone of edematous plaque and erythema at periphery. (Courtesy: Dr. Piyush Kumar, Katihar, India.)

## REFERENCES


1. Lipsker D. Clinical Examination and Differential Diagnosis of Skin Lesions. 1st edition. France: Springer-Verlag; 2013. Chapter 35. Palpable Erythematous Lesions. P. 195–200.
2. Lipsker D. Clinical Examination and Differential Diagnosis of Skin Lesions. 1st edition. France: Springer-Verlag; 2013. Chapter 31. Skin-Colored Palpable Lesions. P. 185–188.
3. Lipsker D. Clinical Examination and Differential Diagnosis of Skin Lesions. 1st edition. France: Springer-Verlag; 2013. Chapter 32. Brown, Black, Blue, or Gray Palpable Lesions. P. 189–190.
4. Lipsker D. Clinical Examination and Differential Diagnosis of Skin Lesions. 1st edition. France: Springer-Verlag; 2013. Chapter 33. White Palpable Lesions. P. 191–192.
5. Lipsker D. Clinical Examination and Differential Diagnosis of Skin Lesions. 1st edition. France: Springer-Verlag; 2013. Chapter 34. Yellow Palpable Lesions. P. 193–194.
6. Fitzpatrick JE, High WA, Kyle WL. Urgent Care Dermatology: Symptom-Based Diagnosis. 1st ed. Philadelphia: Elsevier; 2018. Chapter 8. Plaques with Scale. P. 113–122.
7. Fitzpatrick JE, High WA, Kyle WL. Urgent Care Dermatology: Symptom-Based Diagnosis. 1st ed. Philadelphia: Elsevier; 2018. Chapter 28. Papillomatous and Verrucous Lesions. P. 461–476.

# 9

# Nodules: Localized

ASEEM SHARMA, TRUPTI AGARWAL, MANISH KHANDARE, MADHULIKA MHATRE

## INTRODUCTION

Localized nodules pose a diagnostic dilemma owing to the sheer number of differentials encountered. The clinical features that help in evaluating a nodular growth are listed in **Table 9.1**. The authors have, with the view to reduce the diagnostic challenge, adopted a color-based classification (**Table 9.2**). Needless to say, the entities under each color code should be considered as differential diagnoses for each other. Other useful clinical clues are listed in **Table 9.3**, and their salient features are discussed below.[1–5] While evaluating a nodule, one must look for ominous signs. The presence of nodules in the pediatric age group and indurated nodules in an adult, especially progressive or exhibiting surface changes, is ominous, and warrants a biopsy to rule out malignancy or metastasis. Other ominous presentations include a nodule developing in an existing mole, an elderly patient with a lesion in a sun-exposed area, and a middle-aged or elderly patient who develops widespread skin nodules over a period of a few weeks especially if they are unwell and losing weight, etc.

### Cavernous hemangioma

- It is a slow-flowing venous malformation present at birth, though it may not always be evident.
- It presents as non-proliferating vascular birthmarks composed of anomalous ectatic venous channels.

Table 9.1 Clinical characteristics of a nodule

- Age of onset
- Duration
- Site
- Distribution
- Color
- Surface anatomy
- Fixity to underlying skin
- Texture
- Symptomatology – pruritus, tenderness
- Evolution – tumor (size, rate of growth), surface changes (pigmentation, excoriation, necrosis, ulceration)

- They are soft, compressible blue masses that enlarge when the affected area is in a dependent position or with physical activity.
- The blue color is pathognomonic and caused by the presence of ectatic anomalous venous channels within the dermis.
- There is no increase in local skin temperatures or thrill on palpation of the lesion.

### Blue rubber bleb nevus syndrome

- It is a rare vascular anomaly syndrome consisting of multifocal venous malformations (VM). The malformations are most prominent in the skin, soft tissues, and gastrointestinal (GI) tract but may occur in any tissue.
- They are characterized by soft, elevated lesions on the skin or just under the skin that are dark blue, red, purple-red, or black (**Figure 9.1**).

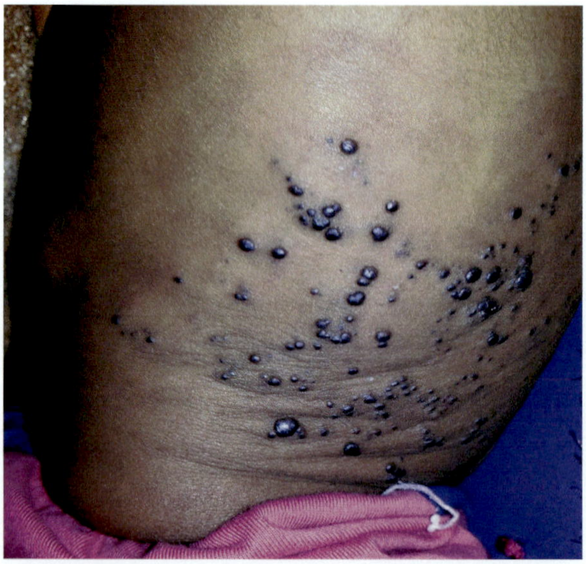

Figure 9.1 Multiple, clustered blue-black nodules of blue rubber bleb nevus syndrome. The background skin is erythematous. (Courtesy: Dr. Anup Kumar Tiwary, Consultant Dermatologist, Yashoda Hospital and Research Center, Ghaziabad, India.)



DOI: 10.1201/9781351054225-17

Table 9.2 Clinical approach to localized nodules

| Color | Diseases |
|---|---|
| **Blue** | • **Compressible** – cavernous hemangioma, blue rubber bleb nevus<br>• **Firm** – pigmented histiocytoma/dermatofibroma, blue nevus, pilomatricoma, glomus tumor |
| **Red** | • **Painful:**<br>  • Fingers: glomus tumor, Osler nodes<br>  • Face and trunk: acne conglobata<br>  • Face/extremity: sporotrichosis<br>  • Ear: chondrodermatitis nodularis helicis<br>  • Axilla: hidradenitis suppurativa<br>  • Anywhere: furunculosis, leiomyoma<br>• **With systemic features:** erythema nodosum, erythema nodosum leprosum, localized Sweet's syndrome, cutaneous lymphoma, leukemia cutis<br>• **Vascular lesions**<br>  • Infant: hemangioma<br>  • Adult near ear: angiolymphoid hyperplasia with eosinophilia<br>  • Anywhere: pyogenic granuloma<br>• Itchy: prurigo nodularis, nodular scabies<br>• Associated with edema<br>  • eosinophilic cellulitis<br>  • acroangiodermatitis of Mali<br>• Ulcerated nodules: scrofuloderma, atypical mycobacterial infections, nodular vasculitis, cutaneous polyarteritis nodosa<br>• Occupational contact with cattle: orf, milker's nodule<br>• Surface telangiectasia: keloid<br>• Others: Giant molluscum contagiosum, amelanotic melanoma, clear cell acanthoma, eccrine poroma, Kaposi sarcoma, Merkel cell tumor, cylindroma, Spitz nevus, granuloma faciale (lever type), Spitz nevus, cutaneous leishmaniasis, schwannoma |
| **Yellowish** | • Children – juvenile xanthogranuloma<br>• Head and neck region – sebaceous hyperplasia (yellow-white), necrobiotic xanthogranuloma (around eyes), chondroid syringoma, steatocystoma multiplex<br>• Around joints – xanthoma (tendinous, tuberous), tophi<br>• Central punctum – dilated pore of Winer<br>• Ulcerative: tertiary syphilis (gumma)<br>• Soft, cerebriform surface: nevus lipomatosus |
| **Brown** | • Children – mastocytoma, melanocytic nevi (compound)<br>• Elderly – malignant melanoma, dermatofibrosarcoma protuberans<br>• Immunosuppressed/ ill patients – deep mycoses |
| **Black** | • Smooth surface – melanocytic nevi (compound), pigmented dermatofibroma<br>• Ulcerated surface – malignant melanoma<br>• Keratotic surface – cutaneous horn |
| **Skin-colored** | • Soft, anywhere – neurofibroma, macro acrochordon<br>• Scalp: cylindroma<br>• Over bony prominences: rheumatoid nodules<br>• Face: sebaceous hyperplasia<br>• Mobile: lipoma<br>• Miscellaneous: subcutaneous granuloma annulare, melanocytic nevi (intradermal), histoid leprosy |
| **White and Translucent nodules** | • Hard – cutaneous calcinosis, tophus, osteoma cutis<br>• Multiple, elderly population – sebaceous hyperplasia (yellow-white) |

- They may be tender, contain blood and be easily compressed, and are usually located on the upper limbs, trunk, and soles of the feet but can occur anywhere.
- DD: Kaposi sarcoma, angiosarcoma, vascular anomalies associated with congenital or systemic diseases (Klippel-Trenaunay-Weber, Ehlers-Danlos, the CREST variant of scleroderma, and Osler-Weber-Rendu syndrome).

Table 9.3 Clinical clues to diagnose localized nodules

| Clue | Dermatoses |
|---|---|
| **Pruritic nodules** | Prurigo nodularis, nodular scabies, pseudolymphoma (arthropod-bite), mastocytosis, lymphoma cutis, leukemia cutis |
| **Painful nodules** | "Blend an egg"<br>• **B**lue rubber bleb nevus<br>• **L**eiomyoma<br>• **E**ccrine spiradenoma<br>• **N**eurofibroma<br>• **D**ercum disease<br>• Chondrodermatitis nodularis helicis<br>• **A**ngiolipoma<br>• **N**euroma<br>• **N**eurilemmoma<br>• **E**ndometriosis<br>• **E**rythema nodosum<br>• **G**lomus tumor<br>• **G**ranular cell tumor<br>• Foreign body **G**ranuloma |
| **Consistency** | • **Hard** – osteoma cutis, calcinosis cutis, pilomatricoma<br>• **Firm** – dermatofibroma, chondroid syringoma, keloid, prurigo nodularis, trichoepithelioma, rheumatoid nodule, juvenile xanthogranuloma, leukemia cutis, connective tissue nevi<br>• **Soft** – neurofibroma, angiolipoma, lipoma |
| **Rapidly growing nodules** | Hemangioma, Kaposi sarcoma, keratoacanthoma, malignant granular cell tumor, Merkel cell tumor, cutaneous metastases, nodular melanoma, pilomatricoma, pyogenic granuloma, subcutaneous granuloma annulare |

## Dermatofibroma

- Dermatofibroma is a benign, dermal, and superficial subcutaneous myofibroblastic proliferation microscopically mimicking fibromatosis.
- It is more commonly seen in young adults, and females are more commonly affected.
- It is commonly seen on the lower extremities.
- It presents as an asymptomatic, solitary, variably pigmented, firm to hard nodule – the color may vary from light brown to brown-black (**Figure 9.2a**). Sometimes, the center may be pale.
- When the skin is lightly squeezed from the sides of the lesion, a "dimple" or Fitzpatrick sign appears, owing to tethering to the skin (**Figure 9.2b**). The lesion moves freely over subcutaneous tissue.
- Hemosiderotic dermatofibroma presents as a blue or blue-red colored nodule.
- DD: Malignant melanoma, blue nevus, Spitz nevus.

## Blue nevus

- This is also known as benign mesenchymal melanoma, blue neuronevus, chromatophoroma, melanofibroma, Tieche-Jadassohn nevus, and dermal melanocytoma.
- The etiology is unclear; it is believed to originate from latent dermal melanocytes, gestational remnants of melanocyte migration.

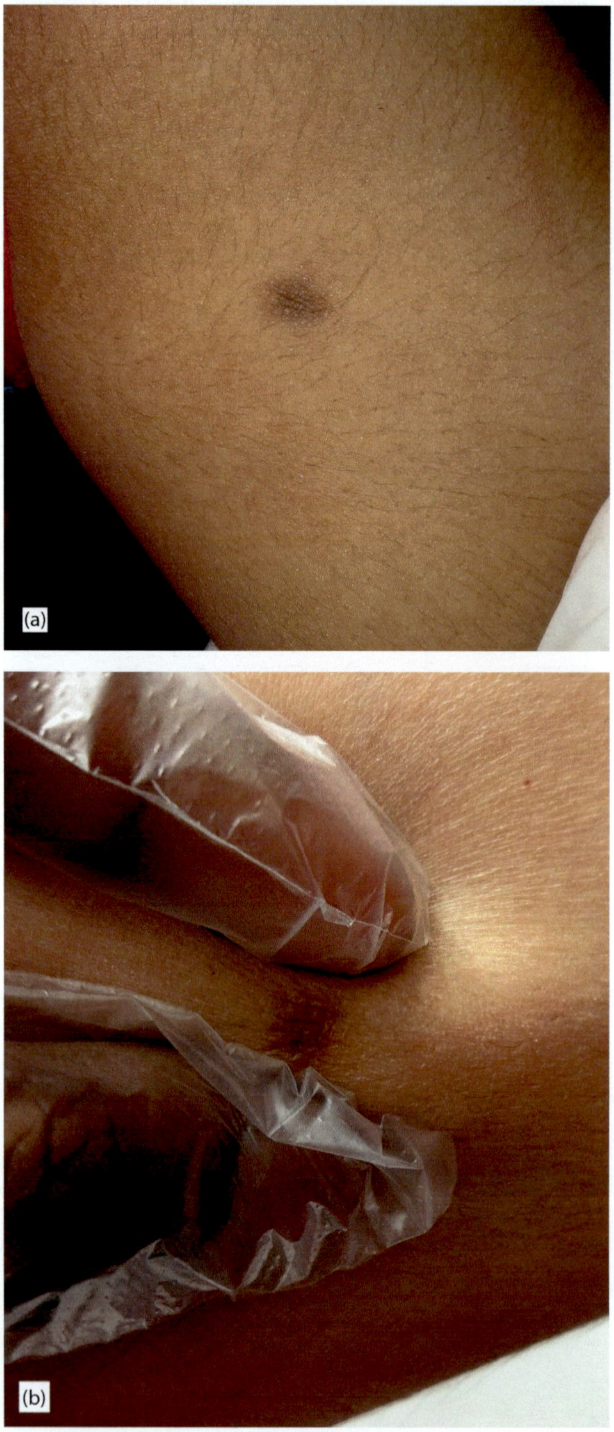


Figure 9.2 **(a)** Solitary, brown nodule on arm in dermatofibroma. **(b)** Pressing the nodule from both sides demonstrated central dimple known as Fitzpatrick sign. (*Continued*)

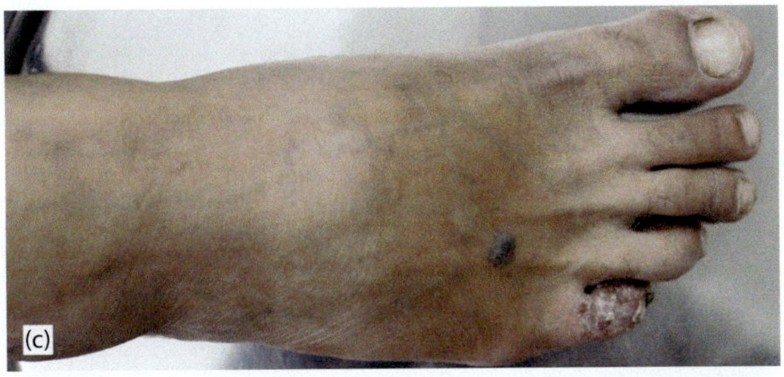

Figure 9.2 (*Continued*) **(c)** Pigmented nodule of blue nevus. (a – Courtesy: Dr. Piyush Kumar, Katihar, India; b – Courtesy: Dr. Deverashetti Srinivas, Nizamabad, India; c – Courtesy: Dr. Balkrishna Nikam, Krishna Institute of Medical Sciences, Deemed University, Karad, India.)

- It is common in children and shows female predilection.
- It presents as a solitary asymptomatic, blue-black, dome-shaped nodule of diameter < 1–2 cm. The lesion can appear anywhere on the body (**Figure 9.2c**).
- The blue color is due to the "Tyndall effect": a scattering of blue light as dermal pigment absorbs the longer visible light wavelengths.
- DD: Malignant melanoma, pigmented dermatofibroma, metastasis, thrombosed plantar wart, or a tattooing effect.

## Pilomatricoma

- Also known as calcifying epithelioma of Malherbe, pilomatricoma is an asymptomatic slow-growing benign cutaneous tumor, differentiating towards the hair matrix of the hair follicle.
- It occurs on the head and neck region in over 50% of cases.
- It is clinically characterized by a deep-seated, firm, non-tender subcutaneous mass adherent to the skin but not fixed to the underlying tissue; blue-red discoloration of overlying skin is characteristic (**Figure 9.3a,b**).
- A pathognomonic sign is that the stretching of the skin over the tumor shows the "tent sign" with multiple facets and angles.
- DD: Inclusion cyst, dermoid cyst.

## Glomus tumor

- Glomus tumors are rare but benign tumors originating from glomus bodies and are mostly seen over the fingertips.
- Subungual glomus tumors are frequently observed in middle-aged women as oval, bluish, or reddish tumors visible through the nail plate (**Figure 9.4**).
- They are also reported to be associated with a history of trauma in the affected area and neurofibromatosis.
- The classic triad symptoms of glomus tumors are pinpoint pain, severe pain, and cold hypersensitivity.
- DD: Neuroma.

## Osler nodes

- Osler nodes are painful, red, raised lesions found on the hands and feet.

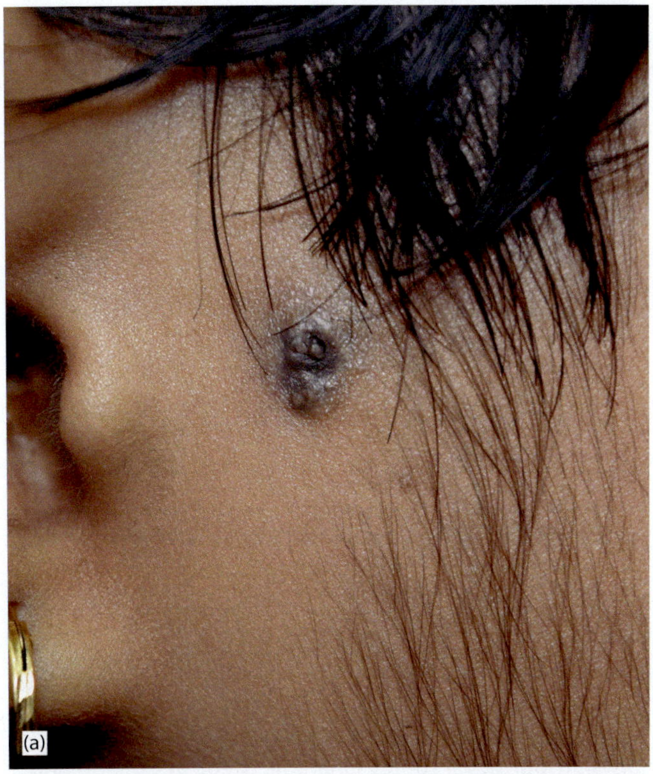

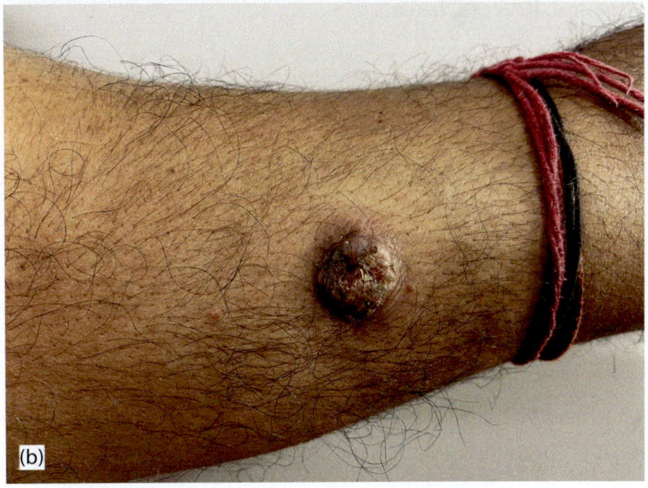

Figure 9.3 **(a)** Subcutaneous nodule of pilomatricoma. The surface changes are secondary to electrocautery done earlier. **(b)** Pilomatricoma presenting as erythematous nodule with crusted surface. (a – Courtesy: Dr. Piyush Kumar, Katihar, India; b – Courtesy: Dr. Esther Nimisha, Jamshedpur, India.)

- They are associated with various conditions, including infective endocarditis, and are brought about by immune complex deposition.
- They occur mainly after the fourth decade of life and more common in males.
- Common sites are fingers, toes, palms, and soles.
- Osler nodes are red-purple, marginally raised, tender lumps, regularly with a pale focus. Pain usually appears 24 hours before lesions.

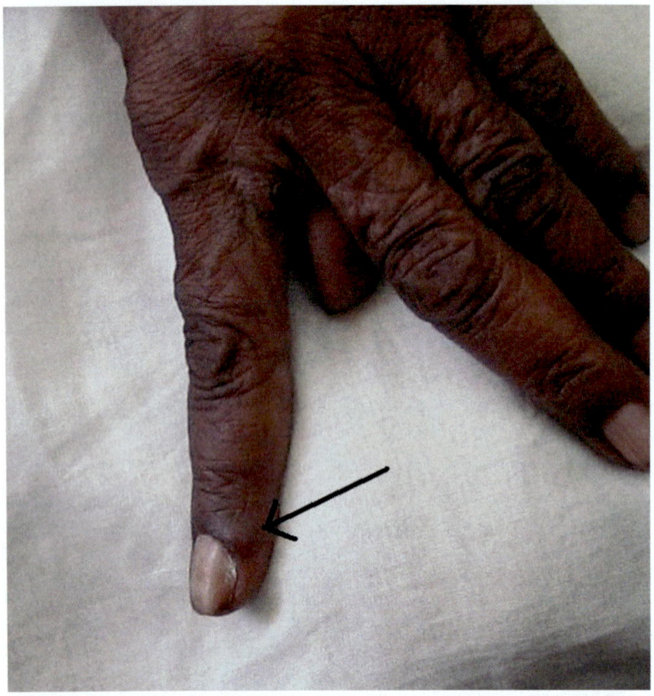

Figure 9.4 Skin-colored, painful nodule (arrow) of glomus tumor. (Courtesy: Prof RC Gharami, Medical College and Hospital, Kolkata, India.)

- They can occur any time on the fingers or toes in endocarditis (generally subacute) and last from hours to a few days.
- Osler nodes are also found in systemic lupus erythematosus, marantic endocarditis, disseminated gonococcal infection, and distal to infected arterial catheter.
- DD: Janeway lesions, cutaneous vasculitis, meningococcemia, gonococcemia, disseminated intravascular coagulation, thrombocytopenia, cholesterol embolization.

## Nodulocystic acne

- It is characterized by development of inflammatory nodules that sometimes soften and become fluctuant (pseudo cysts). They may further evolve into abscesses, or sinus tracts, covered by hemorrhagic crusts (**Figure 9.5**).
- These lesions carry high potential for scarring.

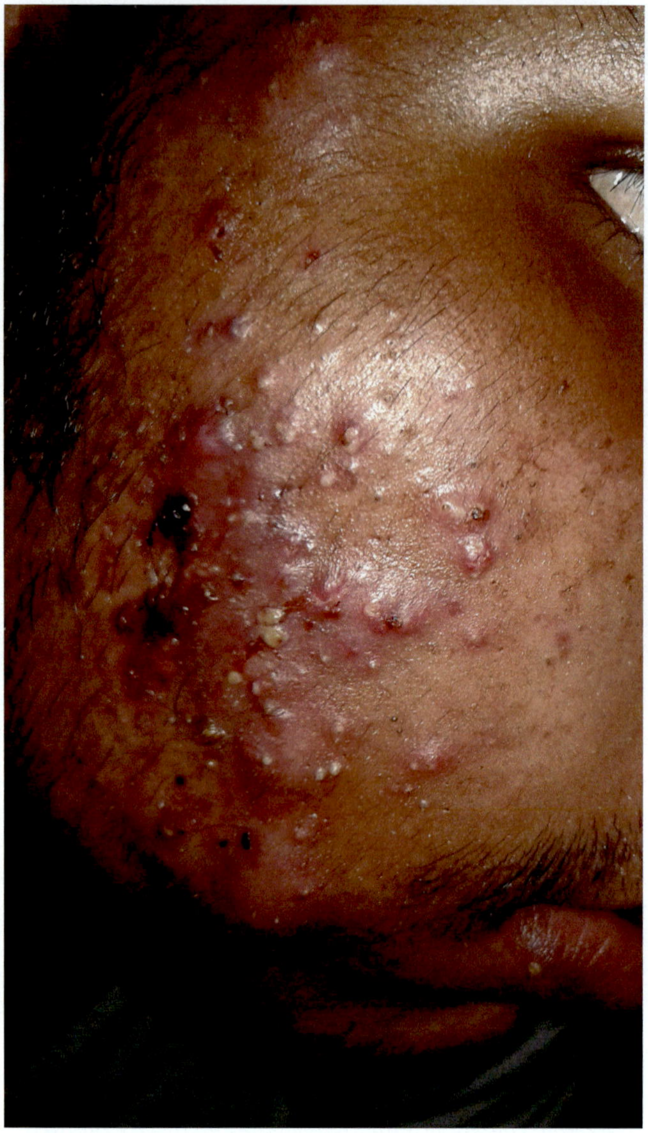

Figure 9.5 Pustules mixed with inflammatory nodules on cheek in nodulocystic acne. (Courtesy: Dr. Piyush Kumar, Katihar, India.)

## Sporotrichosis (rose gardener's disease)

- Sporotrichosis is a subcutaneous fungal infection of the skin presenting after a thorn injury caused by the fungus *Sporothrix schenckii*. The fungus is commonly found on decaying vegetation, rose bushes, twigs, hay, sphagnum moss, and mulch-rich soil.
- It can occur in any age group but is more common in male adults.
- Acral, trauma-prone sites such as fingers, hand, forearm, etc., are commonly affected.
- Cutaneous sporotrichosis can present in three forms: 1) fixed cutaneous 2) lymphocutaneous 3) disseminated.[6]
    - Fixed cutaneous sporotrichosis: The lesions are asymptomatic, erythematous, papules, papulopustules, nodules, or verrucous plaques and occasionally non-healing ulcers or small abscesses. Facial involvement is common, but it can also occur on fingers, arms, or hands.
    - Lymphocutaneous sporotrichosis: A noduloulcerative lesion (sporotrichotic chancre) at the inoculation site and a string of similar nodules along the proximal lymphatic, with or without transient satellite adenopathy, characterizes this form (**Figure 9.6**). These secondary lesions appearing along lymphatic have varied morphology of erythematous papules, nodules, or plaques, having smooth or warty surface, and may soften and ulcerate discharging seropurulent material.
    - Disseminated sporotrichosis: This affects people with immunodeficiency, and symptoms depend on the body part affected. Joint pain, headache, and seizures are common symptoms.

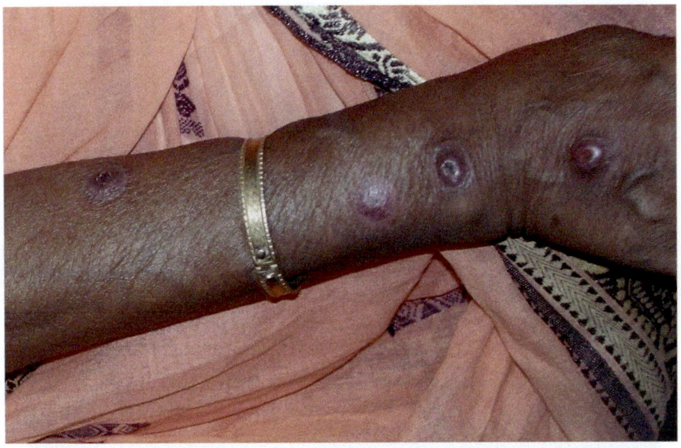

Figure 9.6 Multiple, erythematous, firm nodules with crusted surface in lymphocutaneous sporotrichosis. (Courtesy: Dr. Piyush Kumar, Katihar, India.)

- DD: Cutaneous leishmaniasis, lupus vulgaris, furunculosis.

### Chondrodermatitis nodularis helicis

- Also known as Winkler's disease, nodular chondrodermatitis, ear pressure sores, chondrodermatitis nodularis chronica helicis, and weathering nodules.
- It is seen in association with age and outdoor activities leading to "weathering" of the ear due to chronic UV exposure or cold damage.
- It is common in middle aged men but can occur in any age group and in females.
- The site of affection is the helix or antihelix of the ear.
- It presents as a single or multiple, ovoid or round painful nodule with raised, rolled edges and an ulcer or a crust in its center, seen unilaterally on the helix or antihelix of the pinna.
- On palpation it is firm and usually fixed to the auricular cartilage.
- DD: Warts, actinic keratosis, keratoacanthoma, basal cell carcinoma.

### Hidradenitis suppurativa

- Hidradenitis suppurativa (acne inversa, Verneuil's disease) is a chronic inflammatory condition affecting the skin region bearing apocrine glands.
- It is characterized by inflamed or non-inflamed, deep-seated nodules that may progress to discharging/non-discharging sinus tracts (**Figure 9.7**).
- Commonly affected sites include the axillary, inguinal, and anogenital regions.

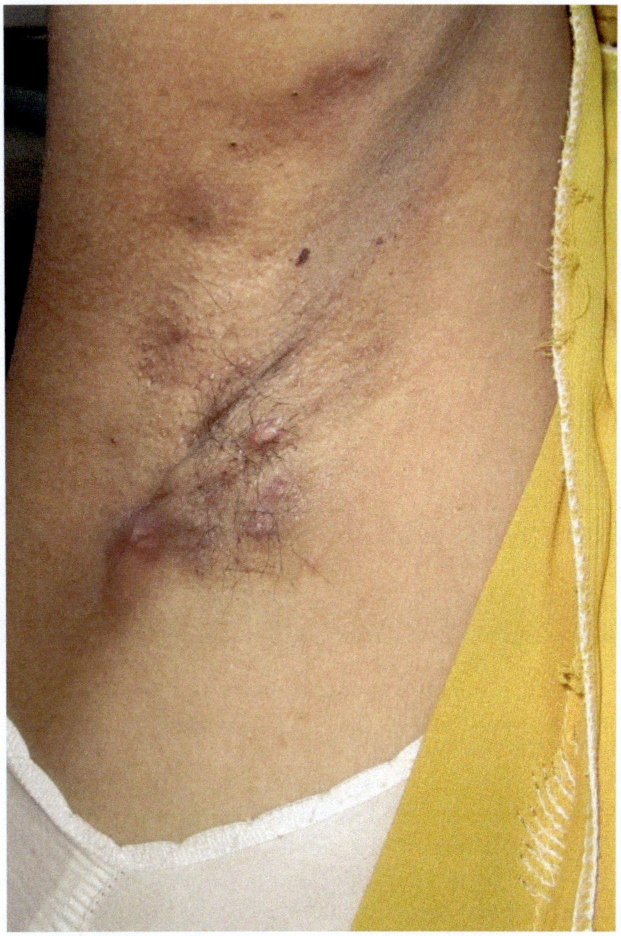

Figure 9.7 Inflammatory nodules and discharging sinuses in axilla in hidradenitis suppurativa. (Courtesy: Dr. Piyush Kumar, Katihar, India.)

### Furuncle (boils)

- Furunculosis (singular: furuncle) is a bacterial infection of the hair follicle and the perifollicular soft tissue caused by *Staphylococcus aureus*.
- It can affect any age group. Risk factors include diabetes, immunodeficiency, poor nutrition and hygiene, and disruption in the epidermal barrier.
- It leads to abscess formation with accumulation of pus and necrotic tissue.
- Commonly affected sites are hair-bearing areas, mainly thighs, buttocks, armpits, shoulders, infra-mammary area, face and neck.
- It starts as a hard, red, painful follicular nodule usually about half an inch in size. Over the next few days, the lesion becomes softer, larger, and more painful. Soon a pocket of pus forms on the top of the boil (**Figure 9.8**).
- In cases of severe infection the surrounding skin turns red, swollen, painful, and warm.
- DD: Folliculitis, carbuncle, hidradenitis suppurativa.

### Leiomyoma

- It is a rare, benign, smooth-muscle tumor originating from the arrector pili muscle.
- It is more commonly seen in female adults.
- It is commonly seen on the extremities, trunk, genitals, and nipples.
- The different subtypes of cutaneous leiomyomas are angioleiomyoma, piloleiomyoma, and genital leiomyoma.
- Lesions may be single or multiple nodules seen in a bunch, linear, dermatomal, or scattered distribution.

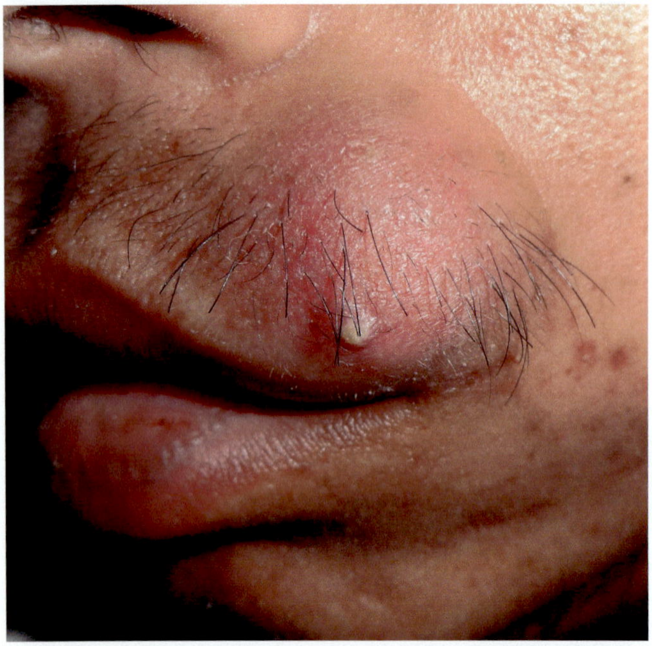

Figure 9.8 Furuncle seen as erythematous nodule topped by a pustule. (Courtesy Dr. Niharika Ranjan Lal, ESIPGIMSR, Kolkata, India.)

The nodules can be skin-colored, pink, red, or brown and vary in size from 2 mm to 20 mm (**Figure 9.9a,b**).

- The presenting complaint is sharp, shooting or aching pain that may occur spontaneously or be associated with pressure, cold temperatures, strong emotion, or light touch.
- Genital leiomyoma are asymptomatic, solitary nodules found on the scrotum, penis, and vulva or on the nipple-areola complex.
- Angioleiomyoma presents as a firm, often painful, subcutaneous nodule on the lower extremity and is most commonly seen in females.
- DD: Keloid, blue rubber bleb nevus, angiolipoma, neuromas, glomus tumors, neurilemmoma, endometrioma, granular cell tumor, eccrine spiradenoma, dermatofibroma.

## Erythema nodosum (subacute migratory panniculitis of Vilanova and Pinol)

- Erythema nodosum (EN) is a non-specific type IV delayed-hypersensitivity cutaneous reaction to various antigens. It may occur in association with several systemic diseases or drug therapies, or it may be idiopathic.
- It is more common in the 25- to 40-year age group and in females.
- Classically, extensor surfaces of lower legs (shins, ankles, or knees) are affected.
- It is clinically characterized by red nodules of different sizes seen on the front and sides of the legs and knees. The thighs, external parts of the arms, face, and neck are less frequently involved, and the size of the lesions there is smaller.
- The nodules are bright-red, hot, painful, and slightly raised above the surrounding skin when they first appear. As the disease progresses they become purple then fade through the color changes of a bruise (**Figure 9.10a–c**).

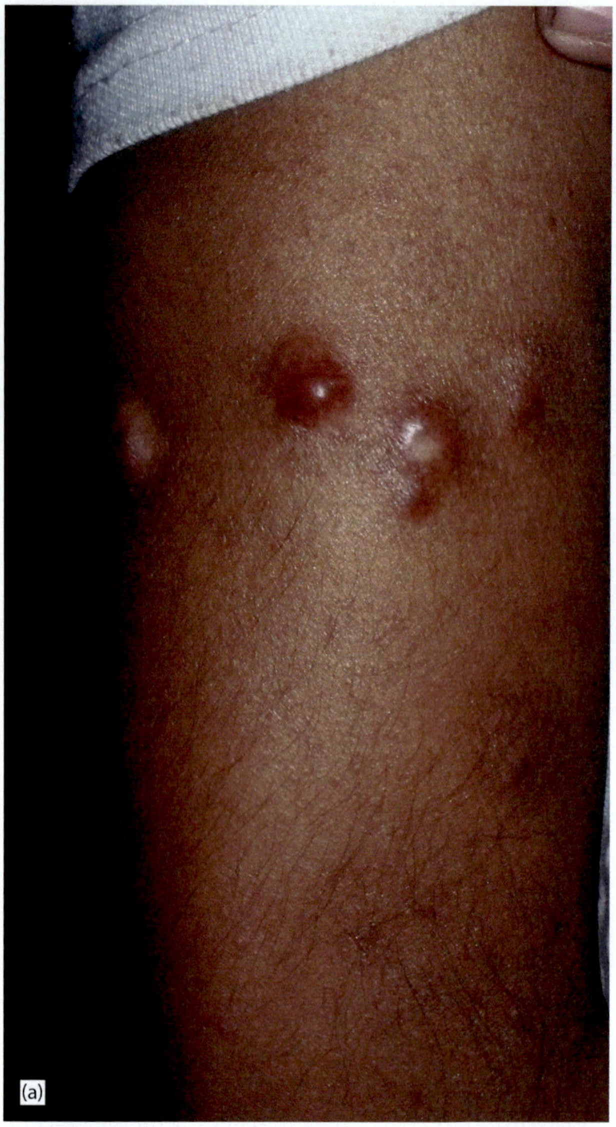


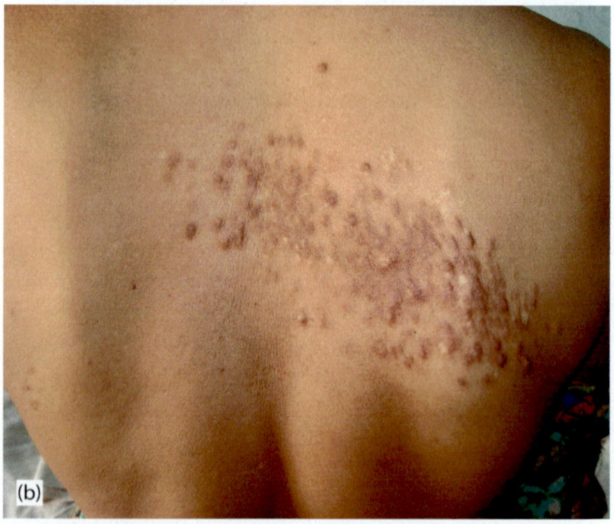


Figure 9.9 **(a)** Grouped erythematous nodules in leiomyoma. **(b)** Zosteriform nodules of leiomyoma. (a – Courtesy: Dr. Piyush Kumar, Katihar, India; b – Courtesy: Dr. Santoshdev Rathod, Smt. NHL Municipal Medical College, SCL General Hospital, Ahmedabad, India.)

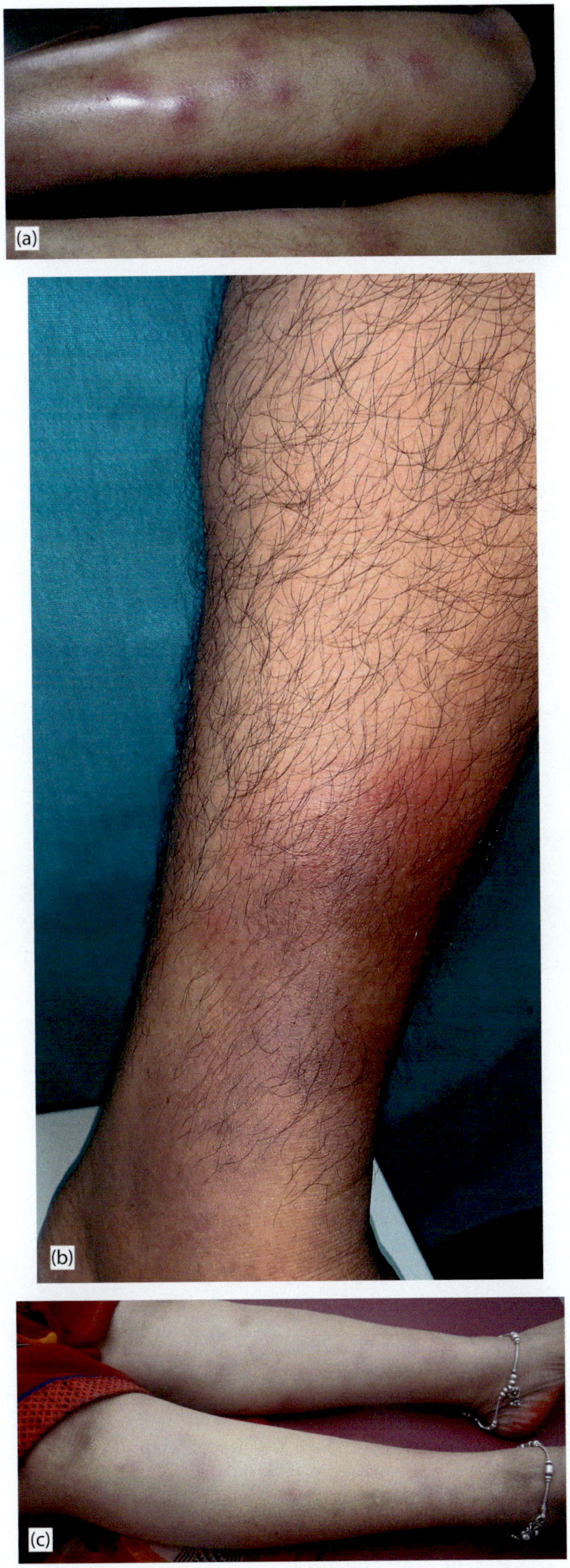


Figure 9.10 **(a)** Erythematous, subcutaneous nodules bilaterally symmetrically distributed on shins in erythema nodosum. **(b)** Erythema nodosum presenting as large nodule with erythematous surface. **(c)** Multiple bilateral erythematous nodules of erythema nodosum. (a–c – Courtesy: Dr. Piyush Kumar, Katihar, India.)

- They continue to erupt in crops for about 10 days. The "bruising" color change starts in the second week, becomes most prominent in the third week, then regresses at any time from the end of the third week to the sixth week.
- Constitutional symptoms include fever, general body ache, and malaise and arthralgias.
- DD: Acute urticaria, erythema induratum (nodular vasculitis), familial Mediterranean fever, insect bites, sarcoidosis, superficial thrombophlebitis, thrombophlebitis, erysipelas.

## Erythema nodosum leprosum (ENL)

- It is the cutaneous manifestation of type 2 lepra reaction characterized by the presence of multiple inflammatory cutaneous nodules and systemic symptoms such as fever, malaise, arthritis, iritis, neuritis, and lymphadenitis.
- More common in 25 to 40 year age group but can occur at any age; it is more common in females.
- Common sites include the face and extensor surfaces of arms and legs.
- It presents as multiple red, firm, painful, blanchable, delicate, cutaneous and subcutaneous nodules or plaques distributed bilaterally and symmetrically. They occur in crops, with lesions found on the face and outer surface of limbs, rarely on the trunk (**Figure 9.11**).

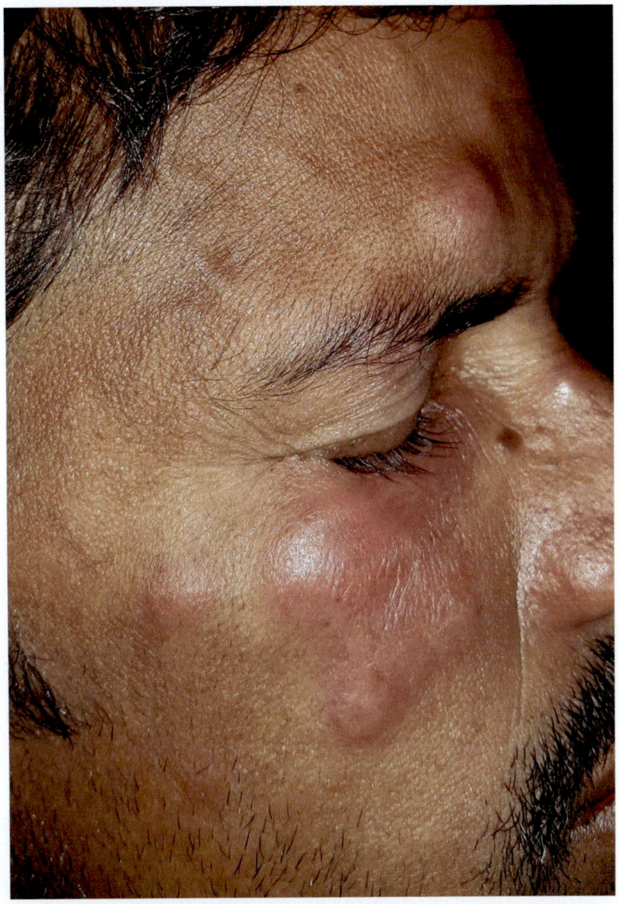

Figure 9.11 Erythematous, shiny subcutaneous nodules and plaque on face in erythema nodosum leprosum. (Courtesy: Dr. Niharika Ranjan Lal, ESIPGIMSR, Kolkata, India.)

- At times they can ulcerate or suppurate – erythema nodosum necroticans (ulcerative ENL).
- These nodule crops are transient, resolving in several days. After regression they leave behind bluish/brownish marks followed by brownish hue in the skin.
- Fever, generalized malaise, pain, conjunctivitis and other constitutional symptoms are also seen.
- DD: Erythema nodosum, erythema induratum (nodular vasculitis), Sweet syndrome, sarcoidosis.

### Localized Sweet's syndrome (SS)

- Also known as acute febrile neutrophilic dermatosis and neutrophilic dermatosis of dorsal hands (NDDH).
- It is an inflammatory condition associated with many systemic diseases.
- Localized SS is an uncommon variant, and there has been a special interest in describing its occurrence on the hands as neutrophilic dermatosis of dorsal hands (NDDH).
- It is mostly seen in middle-aged woman between 30 and 50 years but can also occur in the elderly and in children.
- Commonly affected sites are the forearms, hands, fingers, and palms.
- It presents as erythematous to purplish plaques and nodules that heal without scarring. Fever often precedes the occurrence of nodules (**Figure 9.12**).
- Constitutional symptoms, such as fever, malaise, and arthralgias, can be seen.
- DD: Cellulitis, atypical mycobacterial infection, atypical pyoderma gangrenosum, bullous erythema multiforme.

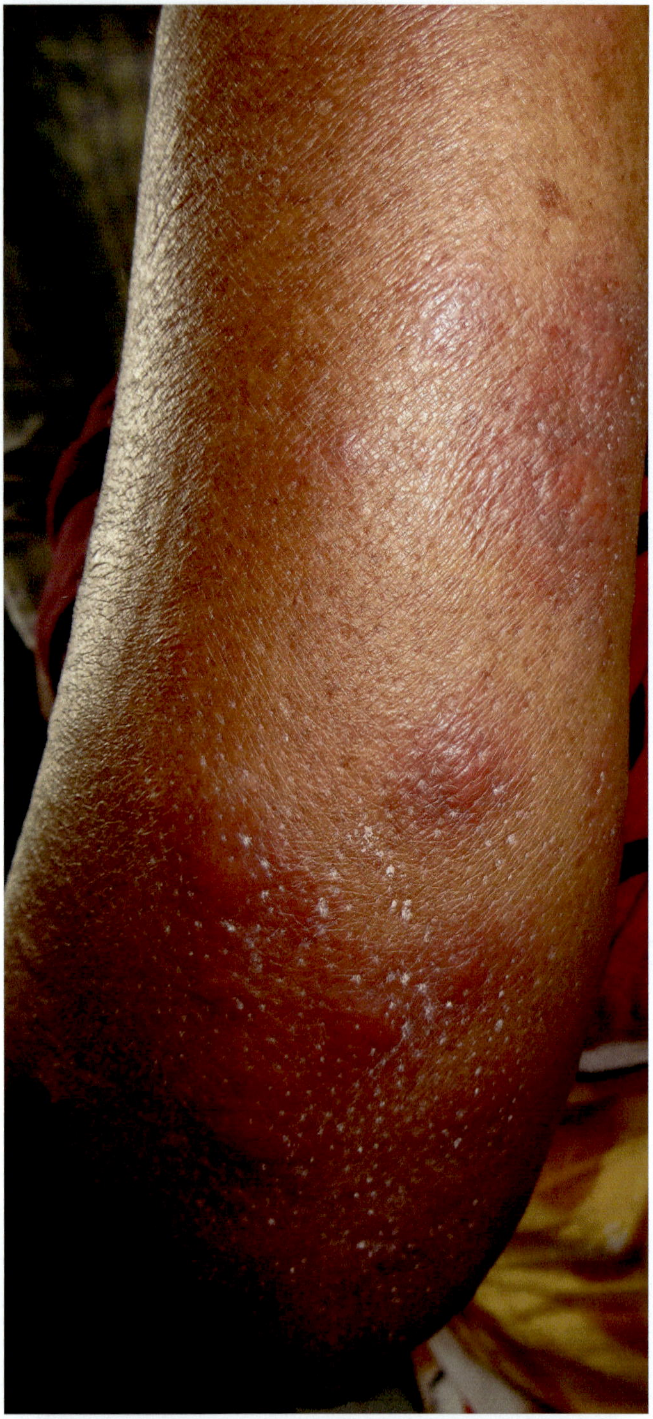

Figure 9.12 Erythematous, shiny, edematous-looking nodules on forearm in localized Sweet syndrome. (Courtesy: Dr. Niharika Ranjan Lal, ESIPGIMSR, Kolkata, India.)

### Leukaemia cutis

- Leukaemia cutis is the penetration of neoplastic leukocytes or their antecedents into the epidermis, the dermis, or the subcutis, bringing about clinically recognizable cutaneous lesions.
- It can occur in any age group but is more common in children and has a male predilection.
- It can occur anywhere on the body.
- It presents as solitary or numerous violaceous to red-dark papules, plaques, or nodules. Nodules may develop central ulceration (**Figure 9.13a**).
- Atypical presentations include indurated plaques, hemorrhagic plaques, perifollicular acneiform papules, macules, ulcers, bullae, and purpuric patches.
- DD: Sarcoidosis, drug eruptions, cutaneous B-cell lymphoma **(Figure 9.13b)**, large-cell lymphoma **(Figure 9.13c)**, cutaneous pseudolymphoma, erythema nodosum, pseudolymphoma.

### Pyogenic granuloma (PG)

- Also known as lobular capillary hemangioma, pyogenic granuloma is a benign vascular tumor that occurs on the skin and mucous membranes; occasionally it can be found subcutaneously or intravascularly.
- It can arise spontaneously in sites of injury or within capillary malformations.
- It has also been associated with certain medications, such as oral contraceptives, retinoids, gefitinib, capecitabine, and afatinib.
- Clinical features include small or large, smooth or lobulated, reddish exophytic vascular nodules that can grow rapidly. Larger lesions become lobulated and sometimes develop into mushroom-like, pediculated tumors.

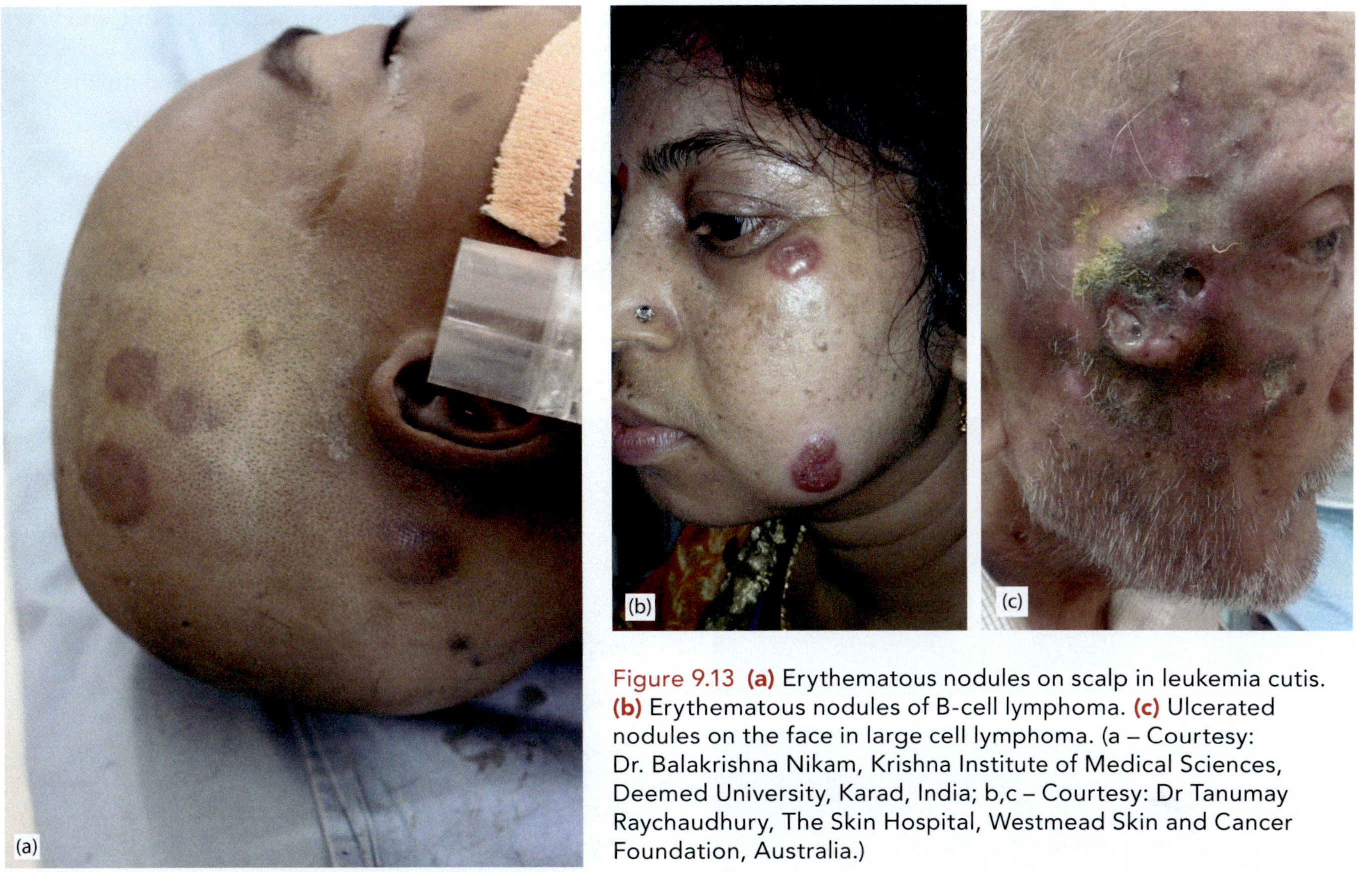


Figure 9.13 **(a)** Erythematous nodules on scalp in leukemia cutis. **(b)** Erythematous nodules of B-cell lymphoma. **(c)** Ulcerated nodules on the face in large cell lymphoma. (a – Courtesy: Dr. Balakrishna Nikam, Krishna Institute of Medical Sciences, Deemed University, Karad, India; b,c – Courtesy: Dr Tanumay Raychaudhury, The Skin Hospital, Westmead Skin and Cancer Foundation, Australia.)

- Common sites are the hands, lower lips and gingiva (**Figure 9.14a,b**).
- PGs have a tendency to bleed profusely.
- DD: Kaposiform hemangioendothelioma, infantile hemangioma, vascular malformations, and Kaposi sarcoma.

## Prurigo nodularis

- Prurigo nodularis is an intensely pruritic, chronic skin condition characterized by localized or generalized hyperkeratotic papules and nodules, typically in a symmetrical distribution.

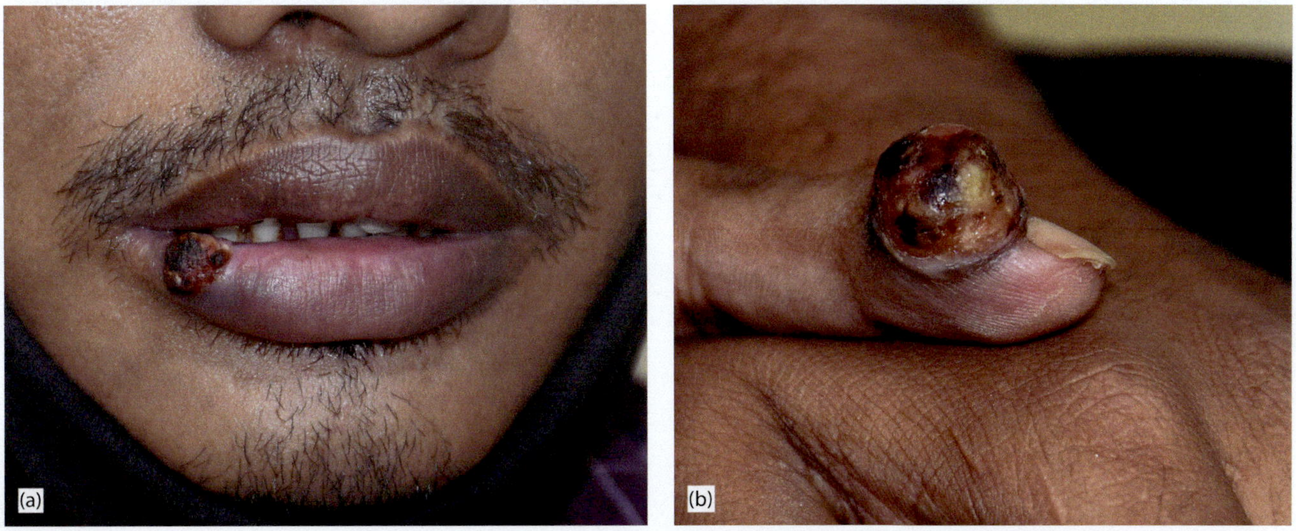


Figure 9.14 **(a)** Lobular capillary hemangioma (pyogenic granuloma) seen as erythematous nodule covered by hemorrhagic crust on the lip. **(b)** Lobular capillary hemangioma on the index finger. (a – Courtesy: Dr. Piyush Kumar, Katihar, India; b – Courtesy: Dr. PC Das and Dr. Piyush Kumar, Katihar, India.)

- They arise in the setting of chronic prurigo and the induction of an uncontrollable itch–scratch cycle.
- They may be associated with underlying dermatoses such as scabies, stasis dermatitis, allergic contact dermatitis, lichen planus, and bullous pemphigoid, and certain internal diseases such as chronic renal failure, diabetes mellitus, cholestatic jaundice. In addition, anxiety disorders, depression, and tactile hallucinations can also lead to chronic pruritus and thereby to prurigo nodularis as well.
- Lesions are distributed in areas accessible to chronic scratching and are often found in a symmetrical distribution over the extensor surfaces, trunk, and lower extremities (**Figure 9.15a–d**).
- Repeated scratching can lead to excoriation, further lichenification, or crusting, often resulting in a hyperpigmented border.
- DD: Kyrle's disease, acquired perforating disorders.

## Nodular scabies

- Nodular scabies is a well-known clinical variant of scabies, characterized by pruritic nodule that persists even after the specific treatment of scabies (**Figure 9.16**).

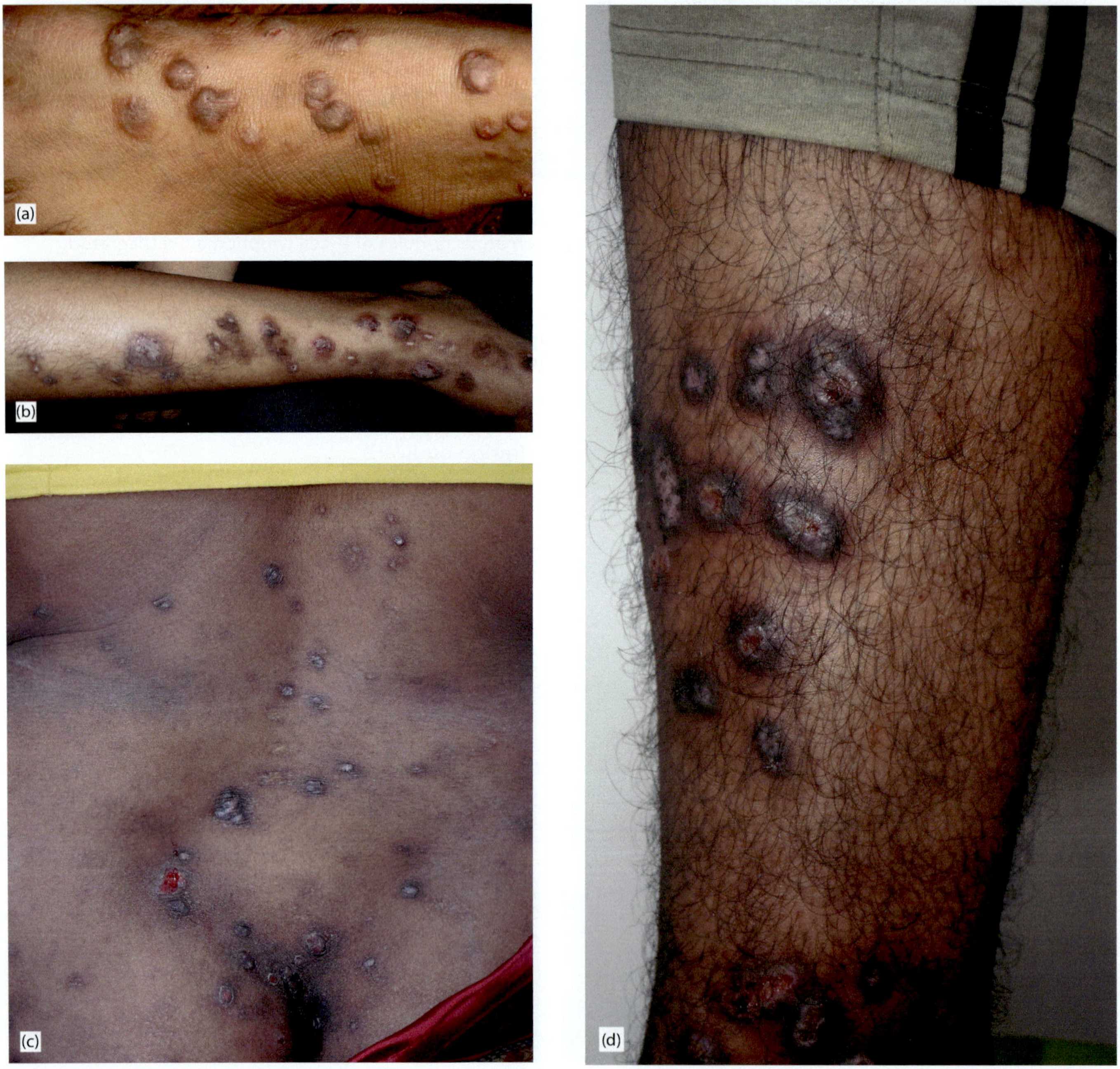


Figure 9.15 **(a)** Hyperpigmented nodules on the dorsum of the foot in prurigo nodularis. **(b)** Hyperpigmented nodules with excoriated top and hemorrhagic crust in prurigo nodularis. **(c)** Excoriated papules and nodules of prurigo nodularis on the lower back. **(d)** Prurigo nodularis presenting as pigmented nodules with eroded tops. (a–d – Courtesy: Dr. Piyush Kumar, Katihar, India.)

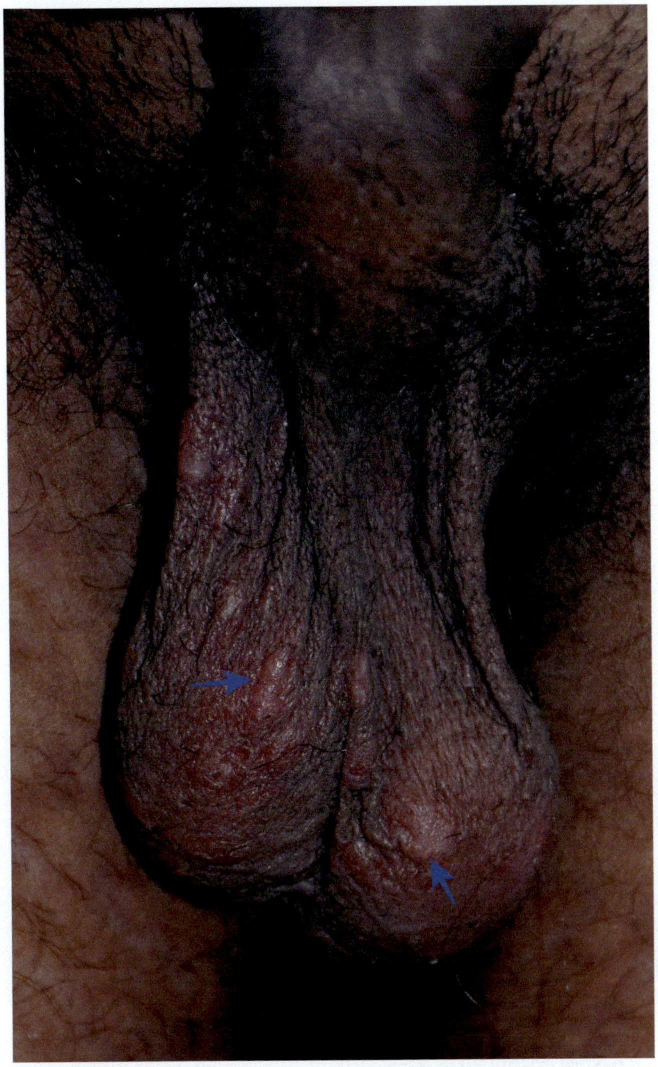

Figure 9.16 Erythematous, shiny papules and nodules on scrotum in nodular scabies. (Courtesy: Dr. Piyush Kumar, Katihar, India.)

- It probably represents the hypersensitivity reaction to retained mite parts or antigens. Genital skin and scrotal skin are the most common sites for such lesions.
- It can also occur in the axilla and over the breast.

## Wells syndrome (Eosinophilic cellulitis)[7]

- Wells syndrome is an uncommon eosinophilic disorder affecting the skin. Affected individuals develop a skin rash that is preceded by a tingling, itching, or burning sensation.
- It can occur in any age group, but is more common in adults; males are commonly affected.
- It is commonly seen on the arms, legs, trunk, etc.
- Initially, it presents as burning or pruritus, as well as localized or diffuse cutaneous erythematous plaques. These lesions are mildly tender, with patients subsequently developing cutaneous edema. In addition to erythema, papules, nodules, blisters, or bullae may occur.
- The second stage is characterized by a progressive involution of the lesions, which occurs over a period of two to eight weeks and can result in morphea-like residual skin atrophy and hyperpigmentation.
- Patients may complain of asthma, joint pain, fever, or fatigue.
- DD: Allergic contact dermatitis, urticaria, insect bites, erysipelas, bacterial cellulitis, Churg-Strauss syndrome.

## Acroangiodermatitis

- Also known as acroangiodermatitis of Mali-Kuiper, pseudo-Kaposi sarcoma, gravitational purpura, stasis purpura.
- Acroangiodermatitis is a reactive angiodysplasia of cutaneous veins related with venous inadequacy or with vascular pathologies, for example, Klippel-Trenaunay syndrome or stump dermatosis in amputees.
- It starts as violaceous macules and patches that progressively form into papules, nodules, or indurated plaques, often bilateral; it is normally situated on the lower edematous extremities.
- Adults are more commonly affected; the condition is more common in males.
- The usual sites of affection are dorsal feet and the extensor surface of lower extremities.
- It presents as confluent, violaceous or dark-colored coalescing papules or nodules covering vast regions of the distal legs. Ulceration and draining may be noted (**Figure 9.17**).
- Bilateral lesions are usually seen in venous inadequacy, while unilateral lesions suggest a basic vascular abnormality.
- DD: Kaposi sarcoma, pigmented purpuric dermatosis, vasculitis, stasis dermatitis.

## Scrofuloderma

- It is a manifestation of endogenous tuberculosis that can present in an isolated form or coexist with pulmonary and disseminated forms of tuberculosis.
- The clinical picture is characterized by the presence of subcutaneous, painless, slow-growing nodules that

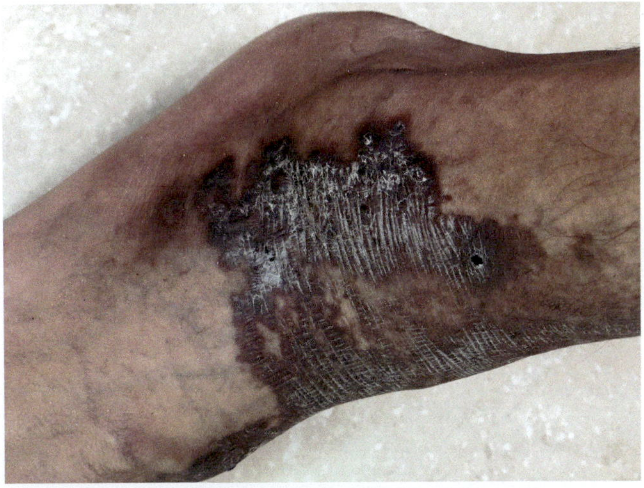

Figure 9.17 Pigmented scaly plaque studded with a few violaceous nodules in acroangiodermatitis of Mali. (Courtesy: Dr. Sunil Kumar Gupta, AIIMS, Gorakhpur, India.)

evolve to ulcers and fistulous tracts with drainage of serous, purulent, or caseous content.

- The evolution is insidious and can evolve with persistent purulent discharge, chronic ulcers, atrophic sequelae, or spontaneous cure.
- Cervical lymph nodes are the most frequently compromised, but there may be involvement of the axillary, inguinal, and pre- and post-auricular, submandibular, epitrochlear, and occipital lymph nodes (**Figure 9.18a,b**).

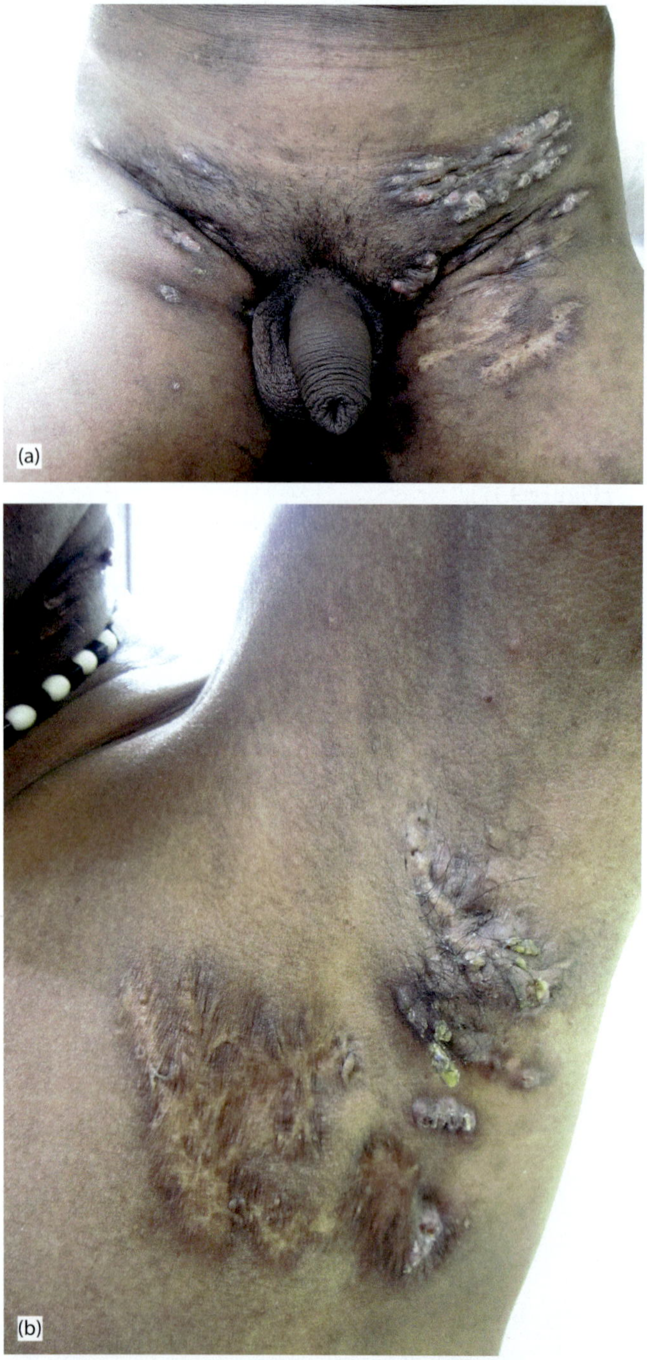


Figure 9.18 **(a)** Scrofuloderma of inguinal region seen as nodules and discharging sinuses. **(b)** Scrofuloderma of axillary region. (a–b – Courtesy: Dr. Panchami Debbarman, Mumbai, India.)

- DD: Bacterial abscesses, hidradenitis suppurativa, atypical mycobacteriosis, sporotrichosis, gummatous syphilis, and actinomycosis.

## Atypical mycobacteria infection

- Atypical mycobacteria are also known as non-tuberculous mycobacteria (NTM), environmental mycobacteria, and mycobacteria other than tuberculosis (MOTT). They are small rod-shaped bacilli, and the disease is caused due to environmental exposure.
- It can occur at any age group but is more common in male adults.
- The usual sites of affection are exposed parts of the body.
- The morphology of the lesion varies depending upon the causative organism.
  - *Mycobacterium marinum* causes fish tank granuloma or swimming pool granuloma. The lesion presents as single papule, nodule, or pustule that breaks open to form ulcers, crusty sores, or abscesses on the elbows, knees, knuckles, or fingers.
  - *Mycobacterium ulcerans* causes buruli ulcer (Bairnsdale ulcer). The lesion starts as a single, painless, pruritic nodule that ulcerates.
  - *M. fortuitum* complex (*Mycobacterium fortuitum, M.chelonae, and M. abscessus*) infection leads to a subcutaneous nodule, non-healing ulcer, abscess, or cellulitis (**Figure 9.19**).
- Constitutional symptoms, such as fever, lymphadenopathy, weight loss, easy fatigability, shortness of breath, chronic diarrhea, and recurrent abdominal pain, may be seen in some cases.
- DD: Bacterial adenitis, lymphoma.

## Nodular vasculitis (erythema induratum of Bazin)

- Erythema induratum of Bazin is a chronic, nodular eruption considered to be a manifestation of tuberculin

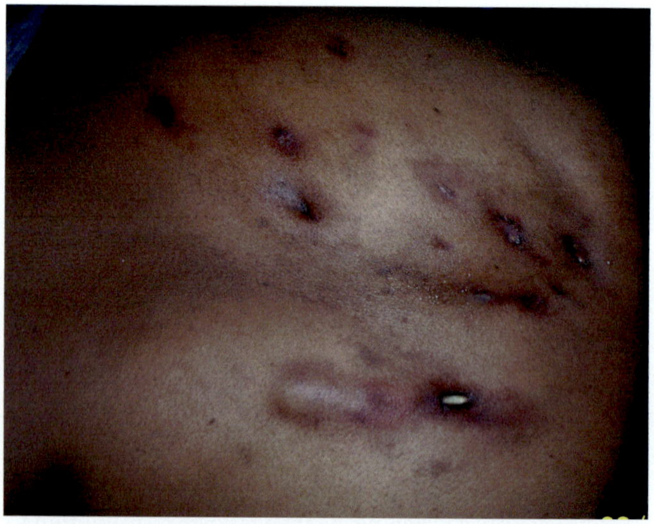

Figure 9.19 Subcutaneous nodules, sinuses, and puckered scars on the back due to *M. fortuitum* complex infection. (Courtesy: Dr. Piyush Kumar, Katihar, India.)

hypersensitivity. Pulmonary and lymph node tuberculosis are the most frequent types of underlying tuberculosis. Other than tuberculosis, associated conditions include *Nocardia* and *Pseudomonas* infection.

- It is commonly seen in females of 20 to 30 years of age.
- The lower legs are the most commonly involved site. Rarely, thighs, and arms may be involved.
- It presents as multiple unilateral or bilateral, erythematous, tender nodules of varying size. Lesions appear in crops and preferentially involve posterior and lateral parts of lower legs. They may ulcerate and heal over in several weeks, with scarring and pigmentation (**Figure 9.20**).
- DD: Erythema nodosum leprosum, erythema nodosum, cold panniculitis, subcutaneous panniculitic T-cell lymphoma.

## Cutaneous polyarteritis nodosa

- Cutaneous polyarteritis nodosa (CPAN) is an uncommon and rare form of cutaneous vasculitis. It involves small and medium-sized arteries of the dermis and subcutaneous tissue.
- Infections (streptococcal, parvovirus B19, mycobacterium, hepatitis viruses B and C)

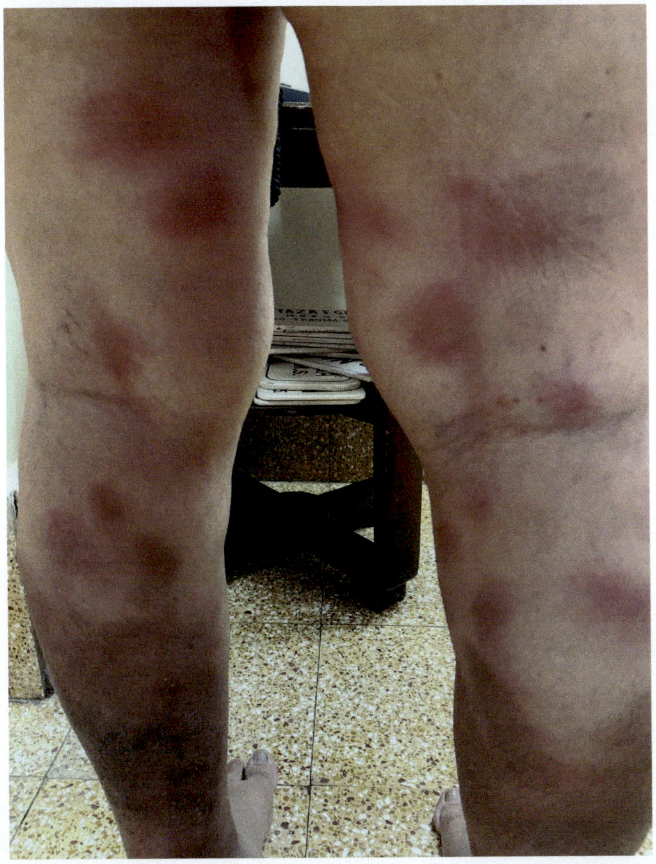

Figure 9.20 Erythematous nodules localized to posterior legs in erythema induratum. (Courtesy: Dr. Swetha Jain, Mumbai, India.)

and connective-tissue diseases (systemic lupus erythematosus, rheumatoid arthritis) may be associated with CPAN.

- It is clinically characterized by tender, erythematous, subcutaneous nodules usually 0.5–3 cm in diameter), mostly on the lower extremities; they may disappear spontaneously or undergo ulceration.
- Other features include livedo reticularis, petechiae, purpura, cutaneous necrosis, and auto amputations.
- Other extracutaneous manifestations include arthralgia, myalgia, constitutional symptoms (such as fever and malaise), and peripheral neuropathy (mononeuropathy and mononeuritis multiplex).
- DD: Erythema nodosum, subcutaneous granuloma annulare, nodular vasculitis.

## Orf

- Orf is also known as ecthyma contagiosum, contagious pustular dermatitis, scabby mouth, and sore mouth.
- It is caused by a large DNA parapox virus contracted by humans from sheep and goats.
- Can occur in any age group but is more common in adult males.
- The lesion usually affects fingers, hands, forearms, or face.
- After an incubation period of three to five days, a small, red, itchy, or painful nodule appears. Lesions may be multiple.
- The lesion is usually firm, red or blue in color, and varies from 2–5 cm in diameter. Over the period of three to six weeks the condition progresses to a vesicle or pustule that gets crusted.
- Constitutional symptoms such as fever and lymphadenopathy may be present.
- DD: cowpox, milker's nodule, anthrax, herpetic whitlow.

## Milker's nodule

- This is also known as milkmaid blisters, paravaccinia, and pseudocowpox.
- It is caused by a double-stranded DNA virus of the genus *Parapoxvirus* in people whose occupation involves close contact with dairy cattle.
- It is commonly seen in adolescents and adults and is more common in males.
- Fingers, hands, or forearms are the most commonly affected sites.
- After an incubation period of 5 to 14 days, lesions of milker's nodules develop as 0.5–1.5 cm, single, pruritic or painful, firm, red or purplish red, mobile dome-shaped papules or nodules. They may evolve to develop targetoid appearance. Focal ulceration or crusting may happen.
- They have a grayish covering in the target stage and a verrucous surface in the papillomatous stage.

- Other variants may incorporate vesicles, flaky patches, or erosions. Local lymphadenopathy, fever, diarrhea, or abdominal cramping might be present.
- DD: Orf, pyogenic granuloma, anthrax, erythema multiforme, staphylococcal abscess.

## Keloid

- A keloid is an abnormal proliferation of scar tissue that forms at the site of a cutaneous injury (e.g., on the site of a surgical incision or trauma); it grows beyond the original margins of the scar and does not regress.
- It is usually seen between 10 to 30 years of age with a slight female preponderance. People with pigmented skin and Asians show a greater tendency to develop keloids.
- It can affect any part of the body but is mainly seen on the chest, shoulders, earlobes, and cheeks.
- It is usually asymptomatic but may be tender, painful, or pruritic. It presents as a localized raised lumpy or ridged area that is flesh-colored, pink, or red with claw-like projections (**Figure 9.21**).
- Keloids tend to be larger than the original wound itself. They may take weeks or months to develop fully.
- DD: Hypertrophic scar, dermatofibroma, lobomycosis.

## Giant molluscum contagiosum

- It is a viral infection caused by molluscipox viruses 1–4, communicated via direct and indirect cutaneous contact, auto-inoculation, and in adults via sexual contact.
- Clusters of cases are seen in swimming pools, play fields, school compounds, and overcrowded houses.

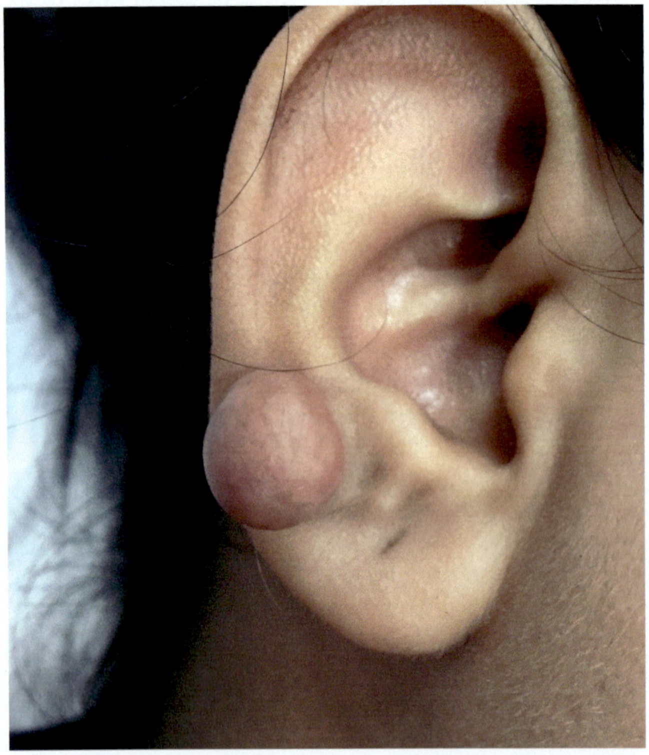

Figure 9.21 Flesh-colored, shiny nodule in earlobe keloid.

- There is no specific predilection; palms and soles are spared.
- It clinically presents as clusters of whitish-pink, small, dome-shaped, umbilicated papules, that may coalesce and/or progress to form giant molluscum (>10 mm) (**Figure 9.22a,b**).
- It may develop eczematous reaction – "eczema molluscatum" – in atopic children.
- DD: Calcinosis cutis, tuberous xanthoma, gouty tophi.

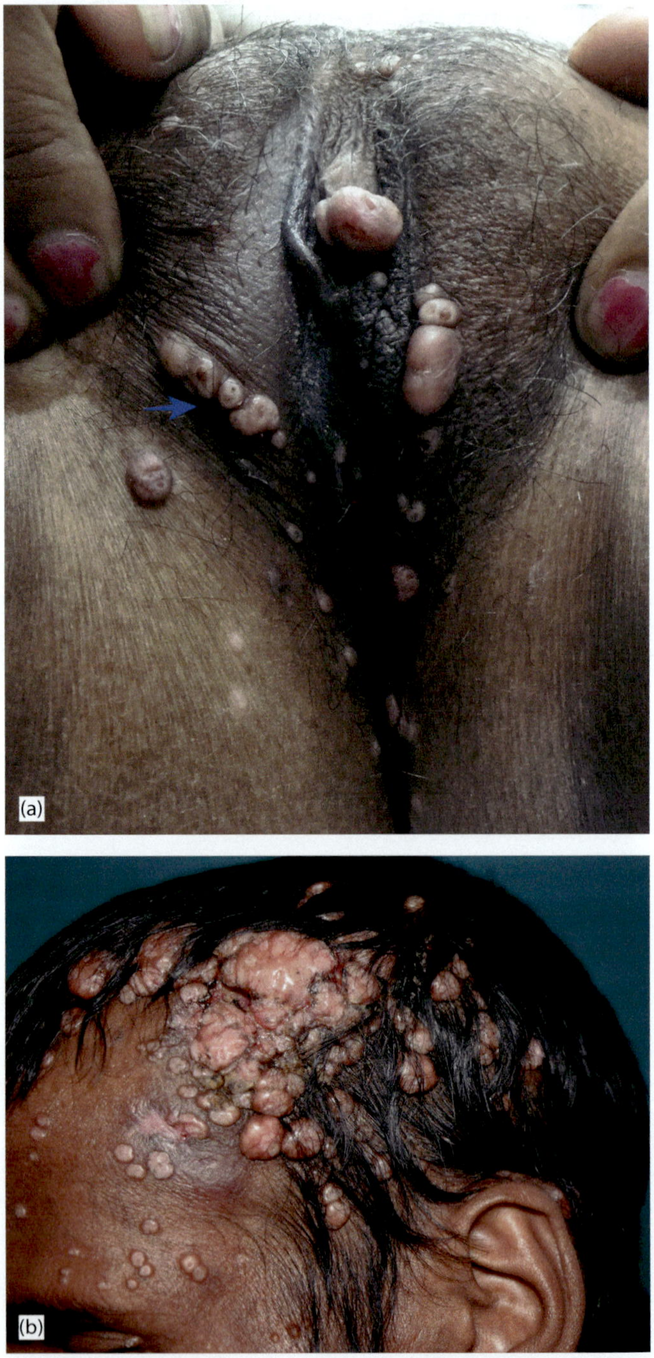

Figure 9.22 **(a)** Erythematous nodules with central umbilication seen in giant molluscum. **(b)** Giant molluscum contagiosum in a seropositive male. (Courtesy: Dr. Piyush Kumar, Katihar, India.)

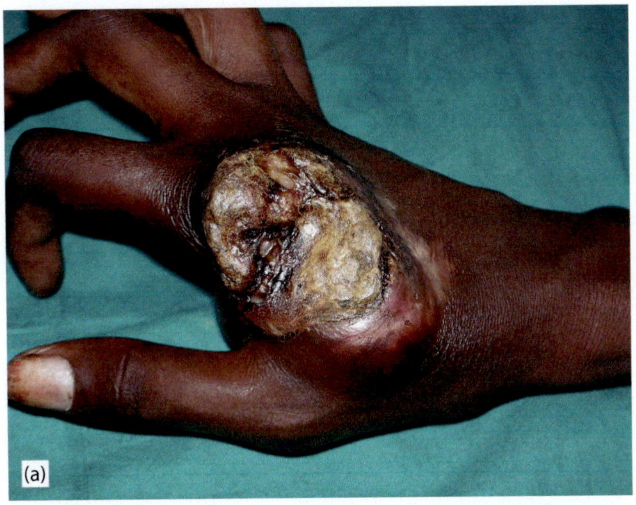


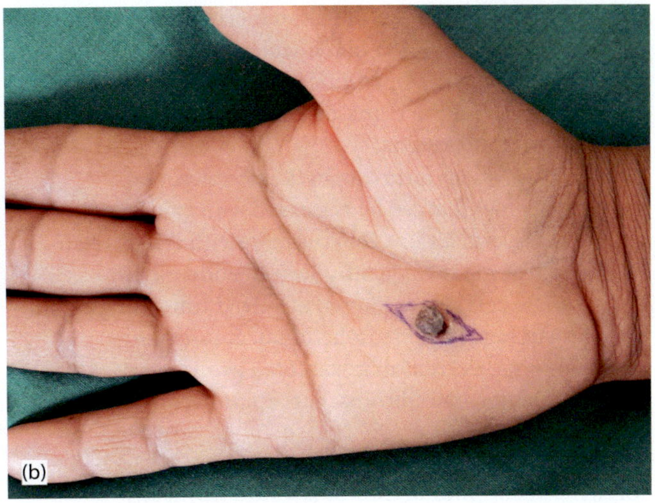


Figure 9.23 **(a)** Amelanotic melanoma presenting as erythematous noduloulcerative lesion covered by crust and eschar. **(b)** Poroma presenting as crusted nodule on the palm. (a – Courtesy: Dr. Piyush Kumar, Katihar, India; b – Courtesy: Dr. Balakrishna Nikam, Krishna Institute of Medical Sciences, Deemed University, Karad, India.)

## Amelanotic melanoma

- Cutaneous amelanotic melanoma (AM) is an amelanotic or a hypomelanotic subtype of cutaneous melanoma that shows no or little pigment on macroscopic inspection or dermoscopic evaluation or lacks melanin pigmentation on histological examination.
- There are three main clinical forms of AM: (a) erythematous macule with epidermal changes on sun-exposed skin, (b) skin-colored dermal plaque without epidermal changes, and (c) papulonodular form.
- The papulonodular form accounts for 58% cases of AM and may present as an ulcerated nodule or a vascular lesion (**Figure 9.23a**).
- Despite the absence of melanin, AMs can be skin-colored, red, pink, or erythematous, among which red AMs account for nearly 70% of AM.
- It often occurs in acral sites, with the highest incidence of 20–28%.
- DD: Pyogenic granuloma, hemangioma.

## Clear cell acanthoma

- It is a rare, benign tumor of unknown etiology.
- Most commonly located on the lower extremities, clear cell acanthomas can also appear on the trunk, forearm, face, and inguinal area, and a few cases of nipple and areola lesions have been reported.
- Lesions are usually solitary; however, there are reports of rare cases of multiple disseminated clear cell acanthomas. These tumors clinically present in middle-aged to elderly individuals.
- Clinically it presents as a solitary red or red-brown, dome-shaped papule or nodule. A peripheral, wafer-like scale (collarette) is classically described in a majority of lesions but may not always be present. The surface may also have a crusted or moist appearance and may bleed with minor trauma.
- DD: Pyogenic granuloma, benign lichenoid keratosis, inflamed seborrhoeic keratosis, eccrine poroma, basal cell carcinoma, squamous cell carcinoma, amelanotic melanoma, and psoriasis.

## Eccrine poroma

- Eccrine poroma is a benign adnexal neoplasm originating from eccrine epithelial cells that show tubular (generally distal ductal) differentiation.
- It commonly presents in fourth to sixth decade of life.
- It usually occurs on palms and soles.
- It presents as asymptomatic or painful, slow-growing, or stable nodular lesions. Clinically, the lesion is noted as solitary skin-colored or pink papule, plaque, or nodule less than 2 cm in diameter. The surface may be ulcerated and sometimes pigmented (**Figure 9.23b**).
- Some patients may develop multiple poromas (poromatosis) simultaneously.
- DD: Granuloma pyogenicum, cutaneous squamous cell carcinoma, melanoma.

## Kaposi sarcoma

- Kaposi sarcoma (KS) is the second most common tumor in HIV patients with CD4 counts less than 200 cells/mm3 and is an AIDs-defining illness.
- Types of KS:
  - Classic type: occurs primarily in patients over 50 years old of Eastern European and Mediterranean descent. These patients are at greater risk for secondary malignancies.
  - Endemic type: unusual predilection for the pediatric population and mirrors HHV-8 seropositivity.
  - AIDS related: second most common tumor in HIV patients with CD4 counts less than 200 cells/mm3 and is an AIDs-defining illness.
  - Iatrogenic: seen in transplant recipients.

- Clinically all forms of KS are characterized by multiple pigmented, painless, non-blanchable, pale-pink to vivid-purple macules or papules.
- Larger plaques on the trunk often follow the skin creases as oblong lesions.
- Occasionally, lesions form exophytic, ulcerated, and bleeding nodules that can be associated with painful edema.
- Oral and visceral lesions are common with AIDS-related KS; lymphedema is frequently seen in endemic KS.
- DD: Spindle cell hemangioma, acquired tufted angioma, kaposiform hemangioendothelioma, cutaneous angiosarcoma, dermatofibrosarcoma protuberans, aneurysmal dermatofibroma, acroangiodermatitis.

## Merkel cell tumor

- Merkel cell carcinoma (MCC) is a rare, clinically aggressive cutaneous neuroendocrine neoplasm with a high mortality rate.
- Clinically it presents as painless subcutaneous mass with a cystic, nodular, or plaque-like appearance.
- Lesions can vastly range in color, most often presenting as red/pink, blue/violaceous, or skin-colored.
- They can exhibit overlying telangiectasia or a shiny surface, and may be confused with basal cell carcinoma.
- Lesions occur in head and neck region in more than 50% cases and have a slighter greater predilection for sun-exposed areas.
- DD: Epidermoid cyst, lipoma, dermatofibroma, amelanotic melanoma, basal cell carcinoma, squamous cell carcinoma, lymphoma, sarcoma.

## Cylindroma

- Cylindromas are benign adnexal tumors showing an eccrine and apocrine differentiation. Solitary cylindroma affects middle-aged and elderly people. Multiple cylindromas are inherited and highly associated with Brooke-Spiegler syndrome.
- Clinically lesions are firm, rubbery nodules with red, pink, or sometimes blue stain that range in size from a few millimeters to several centimeters (**Figure 9.24a**).
- The most frequent location for the solitary form is the head and neck. The multiple form usually occurs on the head and neck followed by the trunk and the extremities and the pubic area. When multiple lesions cover the scalp, the neoplasm is referred to as "turban tumors."
- They are usually painless, but pain or paraesthesia may occur due to nerve compression.
- DD: Trichoepithelioma, spiradenoma, angiolymphoid hyperplasia with eosinophilia (**Figure 9.24b**).

## Granuloma faciale (Lever type)

- Granuloma faciale is an uncommon and benign skin disease portrayed by chronic leukocytoclastic vasculitis with a neutrophilic predominance.
- It is mostly seen in the third to fifth decade of life, with a male predilection.
- It classically affects the face (nose, preauricular area, cheeks, forehead, helix of the ear).
- A typical lesion is an asymptomatic solitary, erythematous nodule, in the case of the Lever subtype. It may also present as multiple soft-brown to red papules, nodules, or plaques.
- The lesions are smooth surfaced with prominent follicular orifices and telangiectasia.
- DD: Erythema elevatum diutinum, sarcoidosis, cutaneous lymphomas, lymphocytoma cutis, discoid

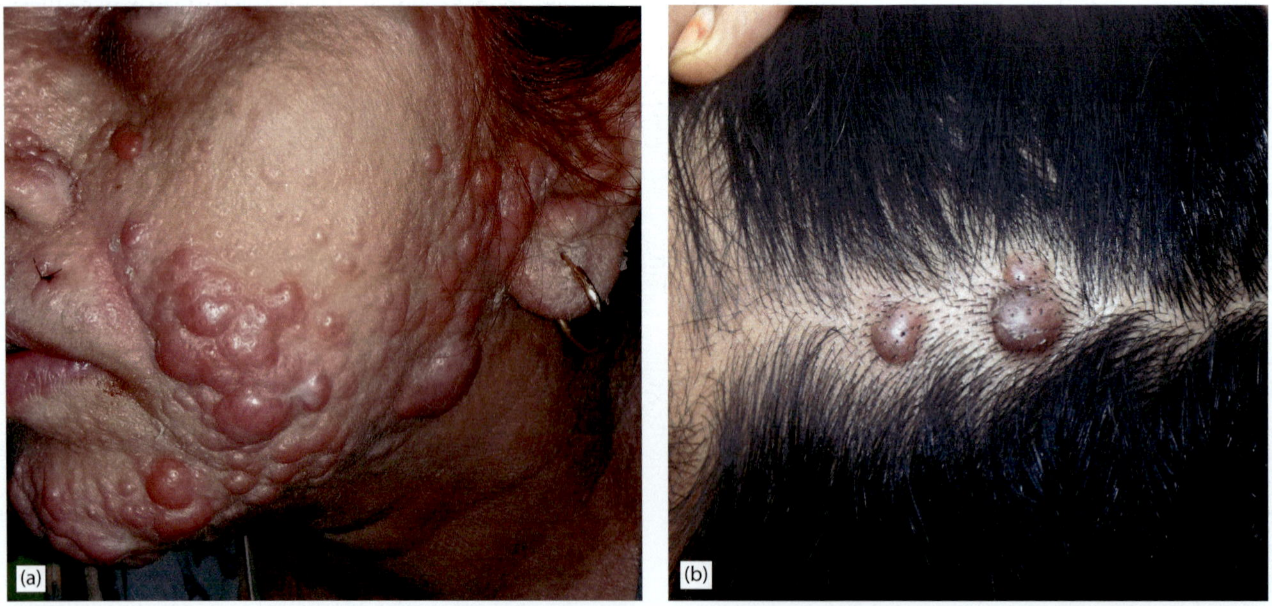


Figure 9.24 **(a)** Multiple erythematous nodules of cylindroma in a case of Brooke-Spiegler syndrome. **(b)** Multiple grouped erythematous nodules of angiolymphoid hyperplasia with eosinophilia. (a – Courtesy: Dr. Hiral Shah, Baroda Medical College, Vadodara, India; b – Courtesy: Dr Piyush Kumar, Katihar, India.)

lupus, basal cell carcinoma, lymphocytic infiltrate of Jessner, fixed drug eruption, lupus vulgaris, and fungal and mycobacterial infections.

## Spitz nevi

- Spitz nevi is also known as epithelioid and spindle-cell nevus, benign juvenile melanoma, and Spitz's juvenile melanoma.
- A spitz nevus is slow- or fast-growing tumor that may arise de novo or within a melanocytic nevi. The exact etiology of growth remains unknown.
- It occurs mainly before the second decade of life; females are more commonly affected.
- Commonly affected sites include face, neck, legs, or oral cavity.
- The most typical lesion is single dome-shaped, red or pigmented papule or nodule (**Figure 9.25a,b**).
- The color may vary from pink to orange-red to pigmented. Pigmented spitz moles have an irregular border and are black, blue, or dark tan.
- DD: Melanoma, Reed nevus, vascular tumors, basal cell carcinoma, juvenile xanthogranuloma, pyogenic granuloma (lobular capillary hemangioma), melanocytic nevi, non-genital warts.

## Cutaneous leishmaniasis

- Leishmaniasis is a parasitic disease with multiple clinical forms and is transmitted by sand flies infected with the protozoa *Leishmania*. The clinical manifestation of the infection depends on the species causing infection and the host's immune response.
- It can occur at any age group but is more common in adults.
- It is more common in males.
- Usually affected sites are exposed areas of the body, mainly the face and extremities.
- Skin lesions develop at the site of inoculation and start as single or multiple small red papules. The lesion gradually enlarges in size and may develop central ulceration. The ulcer is typically painless and may exude pus or may be dry with a crusted scab. The lesions may heal over several months with atrophic scarring (**Figure 9.26a,b**).

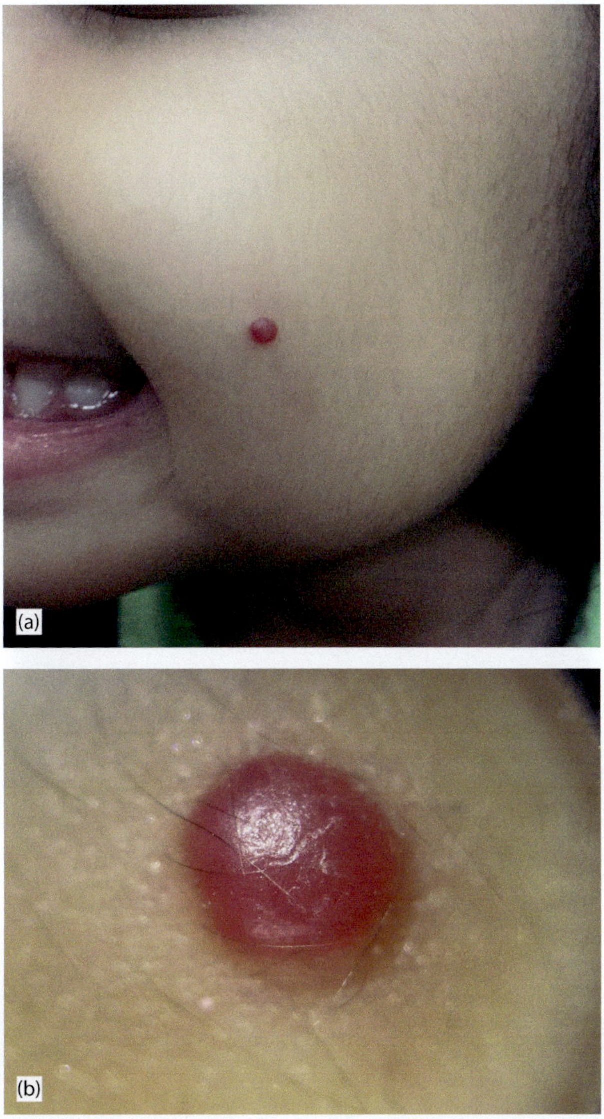

Figure 9.25 **(a)** Spitz nevus. **(b)** Close-up view of spitz nevus.

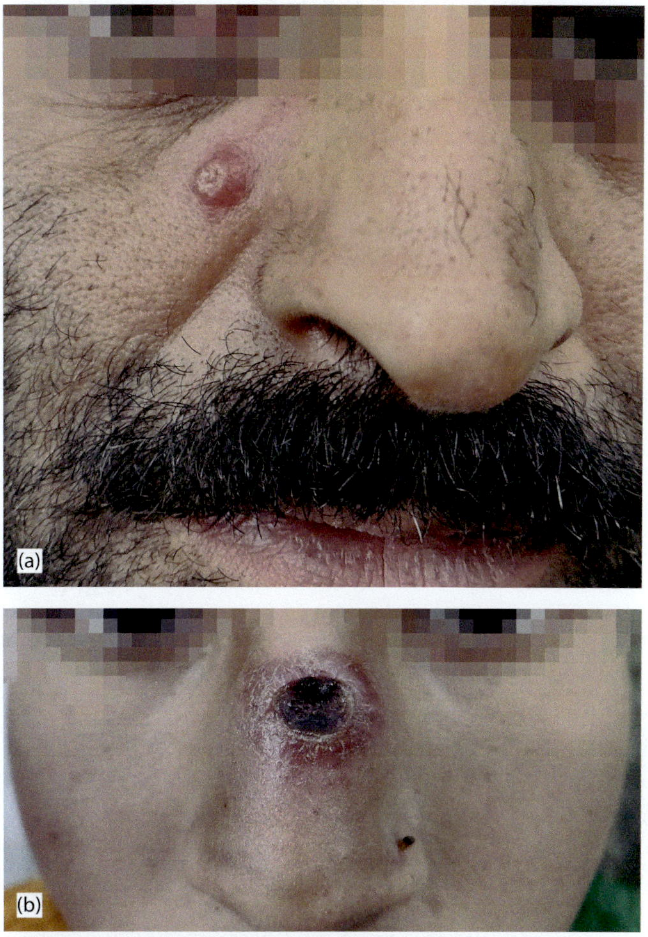

Figure 9.26 **(a)** Cutaneous leishmaniasis presenting as erythematous nodule with central crust on the face. **(b)** Cutaneous leishmaniasis seen as erythematous noduloulcerative lesion on the nose. The surface is notable for eschar. (a,b – Courtesy: Dr. Ennakshee, Government Medical College, Jammu, India.)

- Sporotrichosis spread and chronic disease can occur.
- Mucocutaneous lesions are painful and present after resolution or treatment of primary lesions. They generally affect the mucous membranes of the eyes and genital tracts and may cause extensive disfigurement.
- DD: Chromoblastomycosis, sporotrichosis, Wegener's granulomatosis, lymphomas.

## Schwannoma

- Schwannomas or neurilemmoma are benign encapsulated tumors of nerve sheath origin.
- Although they commonly occur as solitary lesions (90%), they can be associated with several central neurological tumors (usually meningiomas, 5%), neurofibromatosis type 2 (3%), or appear as multiple lesions (schwannomatosis, 2%).
- Clinically, cutaneous schwannomas (CS) usually range in size from 0.25–3.00 cm and generally occur in the head and neck region.
- CS are generally asymptomatic; however, when pain is present, it is usually associated with compression the adjacent structures of nerve and the paraesthesia restricted on the tumor site or radiating along nerve of origin.
- They most often occurs in the fourth and fifth decades of life, without significant evidence of sex predilection.
- DD: Pilomatricoma, epithelial cysts, lipoma, desmoid tumor, and rheumatoid nodule.

## Juvenile xanthogranuloma (JXG)

- JXG is a member of the non-Langerhans cell group of histiocytic proliferative disorders and is a relatively uncommon benign cutaneous fibrohistiocytic lesion.
- JXG is a disease of the young child. Median age of onset is two years, but lesions may be present at birth. Male preponderance is seen.
- Clinically it starts as reddish-yellow macules/papules, which may enlarge and evolve into yellow-brown patches/plaques or nodules with surface telangiectasia. The consistency is generally firm and rubbery. Giant JXG, defined as a lesion greater than 2 cm in diameter, has been reported (**Figure 9.27**).

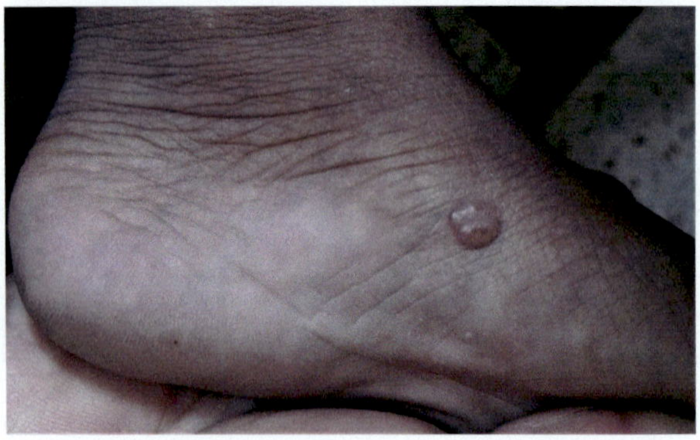

Figure 9.27 Yellow-orange firm nodule of juvenile xanthogranuloma on the foot. (Courtesy: Dr. Anup Kumar Tiwary, Consultant Dermatologist, Yashoda Hospital and Research Center, Ghaziabad, India.)

- Although the head, neck, and trunk are the most common sites for JXG, it can appear anywhere on the body, including the groin, scrotum, penis, clitoris, eyelids, toenails, palms, soles, and lips.
- Extracutaneous involvement is usually restricted to the eye, specifically the iris, but may also occur in bone, lung, and liver.
- DD: Dermatofibroma, Langerhans cell histiocytosis, mastocytosis, Spitz nevus, xanthomas.

## Necrobiotic xanthogranuloma

- Necrobiotic xanthogranuloma, a non-Langerhans histiocytosis, is a subset of inflammatory form of normolipemic xanthoma.
- The age of onset ranges from 17 to 85 years, without any sex predilection.
- The periorbital region is the most frequent site of involvement, followed by the trunk, face, and extremities.
- The most frequent skin lesion is an indurated papule, nodule or plaque. The color varies from violaceous to red-orange, often with a yellowish hue (**Figure 9.28**).

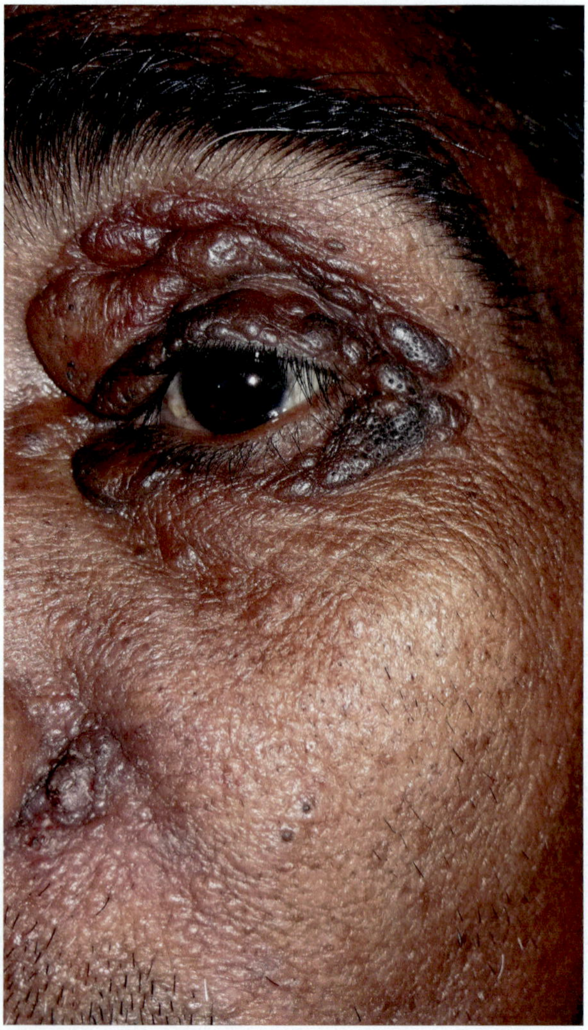

Figure 9.28 Yellow-orange and brownish nodules of necrobiotic xanthogranuloma. (Courtesy: Dr. Hiral Shah, Baroda Medical College, Vadodara, India.)

- There is a characteristic absence of generalized lymphadenopathy.
- Ophthalmic features of necrobiotic xanthogranuloma include eyelid lesions, orbital masses, conjunctival involvement, keratitis and scleritis, episcleritis or anterior uveitis.
- Other systemic findings include hepatosplenomegaly, arthralgia/arthritis, hypertension, generalized sensorineural polyneuropathy, cardiomyopathy, and pulmonary fibrosis.
- DD: Diffuse normolipemic plane xanthoma, granuloma annulare, necrobiosis lipoidica, juvenile xanthogranuloma, and deep xanthomas.

## Chondroid syringoma

- Chondroid syringoma is a benign, skin appendageal tumor.
- It is also known as mixed tumor of the skin as it contains epithelial and mesenchymal stromal components.
- Is usually occurs in middle-aged males.
- The lesions are typically located in the head and neck region.
- They are slow-growing, subcutaneous or dermal nodules. Rarely, rapid growth, ulceration, and necrosis may be noted.
- The malignant form occurs predominantly in females, has no age-related predilection, and is observed more commonly on the extremities.
- DD: Epidermal cyst, pilar cyst, calcifying epithelioma, solitary trichoepithelioma.

## Steatocystoma multiplex[8]

- Steatocystoma multiplex (SCM) is a rare, hamartomatous disorder of the pilosebaceous unit characterized by sebum-containing cysts in the dermis.
- Clinically, it manifests as skin-colored to yellowish, soft or firm, cystic or dome-shaped papules or nodules (**Figure 9.29**).
- The lesions are usually devoid of a central punctum, and yellowish, cheesy, semisolid or oily secretion can be expressed through the same.
- Areas of involvement include the trunk, neck, groin, scalp, and proximal extremities. However, uncommon sites, including face, glutei, breasts, or flexures, may be affected.
- DD: Epidermoid cysts, neurofibromatosis, lipomatosis.

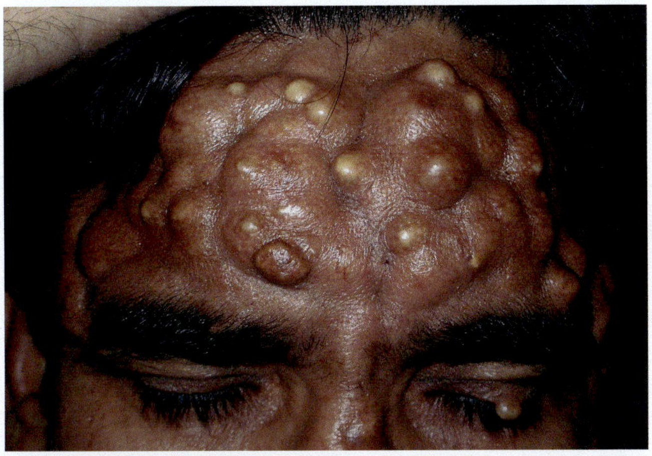

Figure 9.29 Multiple, skin-colored to yellowish nodules in steatocystoma multiplex. (Courtesy: Dr. Piyush Kumar, Katihar, India.)

## Xanthoma (tendinous, tuberous, eruptive, normolipemic)

- Xanthomas are a common manifestation of lipid metabolism disorders.
- These may occur in persons of any age.
- Tuberous xanthoma are the nodules that are frequently localized to extensor surface of elbows, knees, knuckles, and gluteal region (**Figure 9.30**).
- Tendinous xanthoma are firm subcutaneous nodules found in facia, ligaments, and Achilles tendon or extensor tendons of the hands, knees, and elbows.
- DD: Nodular amyloidosis, erythema elevatum diutinum, histoid leprosy.

## Tophus (podagra)

- It is a disorder of hyperuricemia; elevated uric acid levels lead to precipitation of monosodium urate (MSU) crystals in skin, soft tissue, joints, and kidneys.
- It is considered a lifestyle disease; risk factors include high protein and alcohol intake and metabolic syndrome.
- Usually occurs in the fourth sixth decade of life, males commonly more affected than females.
- Acral involvement is most common in distal to proximal joints.

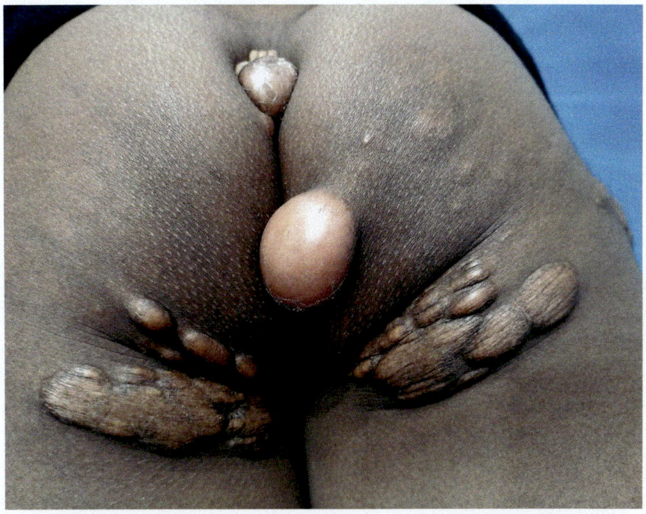

Figure 9.30 Tuberous xanthomas seen as shiny, yellow nodules and plaques on the gluteal region. (Courtesy Dr. Deverashetti Srinivas, Nizamabad, India.)

- Cutaneous lesions are known as tophi and are characterized as firm, skin-colored papules and nodules (**Figure 9.31a,b**).
- Gout nodulosis is a rare presentation of the disease in which multiple nodular tophi develops in the absence of gouty arthritis (**Figure 9.31c**).[9]
- A clinical variant is miliarial gout.
- Joint involvement may present in an acute manner, with excruciating pain and swelling in one joint, commonly the great toe (podagra), and acute episode usually lasts for 7 to 14 days. Multiple episodes result in joint destruction and mutilation.
- DD: Calcinosis cutis, tuberous xanthoma, giant molluscum.

## Dilated pore of Winer

- Dilated pore of Winer results from an obstruction of the follicle ostium in a process similar to that of inflammatory cystic acne.
- Most cases of dilated pore of Winer are diagnosed in individuals older than 40 years.
- A male preponderance is seen.
- A dilated pore of Winer usually appears as a solitary large comedone on the face, predominantly on the upper lip, cheek, or forehead. The lesion can also be found on the trunk, most commonly the back. A rare incidence involving the external ear canal has also been reported.
- The skin surrounding the pore appears to be unchanged, with no inflammation or induration.
- DD: Epidermal inclusion cyst, Favre-Racouchot syndrome, trichilemmal cyst (pilar cyst), trichoepithelioma.

## Tertiary syphilis (gumma)

- Gummas are the characteristic lesions of tertiary syphilis and occur three to ten years after primary infection.
- The condition is more common in males.
- Commonly involved sites are thighs, buttocks, shoulders, forehead, and scalp.

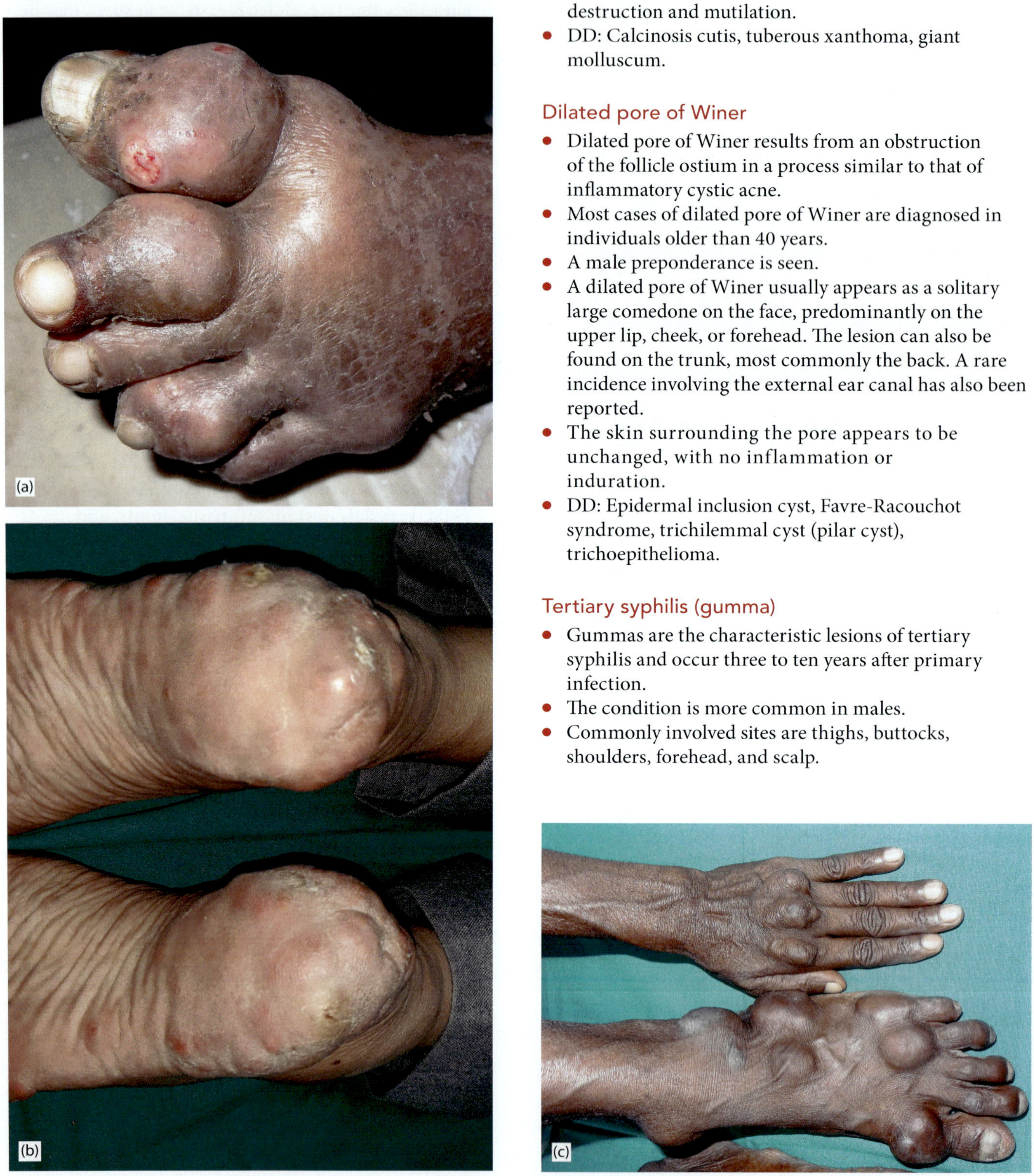


Figure 9.31 **(a)** Multiple tophi on the toes in a patient of gout. **(b)** Bilateral nodules of tophi on the planatar aspect of the feet. **(c)** Multiple tophi on the hand and foot in a case of gout nodulosis. (a,c – Courtesy Dr. Piyush Kumar, Katihar, India; b – Courtesy: Dr Hiral Shah, Baroda Medical College, Vadodara, India.)

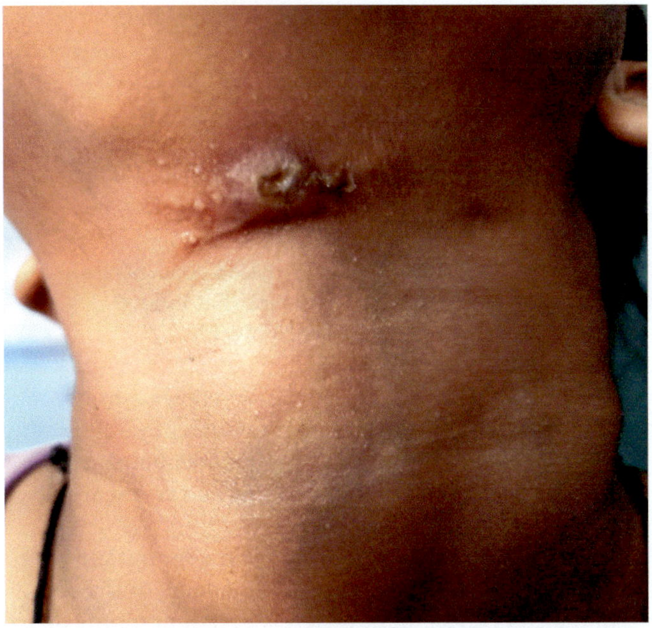

Figure 9.32 Erythematous nodule with crusted surface in tertiary syphilis (gumma). (Courtesy: Dr. Hiral Shah, Baroda Medical College, Vadodara, India.)

- The gumma appear as cutaneous plaques or nodules of irregular shape and outline and are often single lesions on the arms, back, and face. The size of lesions may vary from 2–10 cm (**Figure 9.32**).
- Gummas are usually painless even when they ulcerate. Their central necrotic tissue may turn into a slimy, stringy mass, and it is this that gives rise to the name "gumma." Multiple gummas tend to coalesce, the bridges of skin between them gradually undergoing necrosis. They have a tendency for peripheral healing with tissue-paper scarring.
- Gummas that start in bone or muscle also tend to ulcerate the skin; this form is difficult to differentiate from a nodular syphilide.
- DD: Sarcoidosis, xanthogranulomas, xanthomata.

## Nevus lipomatosus

- Also known as nevus lipomatosus cutaneous superficialis, it is an uncommon benign hamartomatous skin lesion defined by the presence of aggregates of mature adipose tissue among the collagen bundles of the dermis.
- It is more common in children and young adults (first two decade of life); a male preponderance is seen.
- The gluteal region, upper posterior thigh, and lumbar back are most commonly affected.
- Two clinical types are distinguished: the classical type and the solitary type.[10]
    - The classical type, Hoffman and Zurhelle type, consists of multiple soft, non-tender, pedunculated, cerebriform, yellowish or skin-colored papules or nodules in unilateral, band-like, linear, or zosteriform distribution (**Figure 9.33**).
    - The solitary form usually occurs after the age of 20 and presents with a single nodular lesion with no particular predilection sites.
- DD: Nevus sebaceous, skin tags, neurofibroma, lymphangioma, hemangioma, and focal dermal hypoplasia (Goltz syndrome).

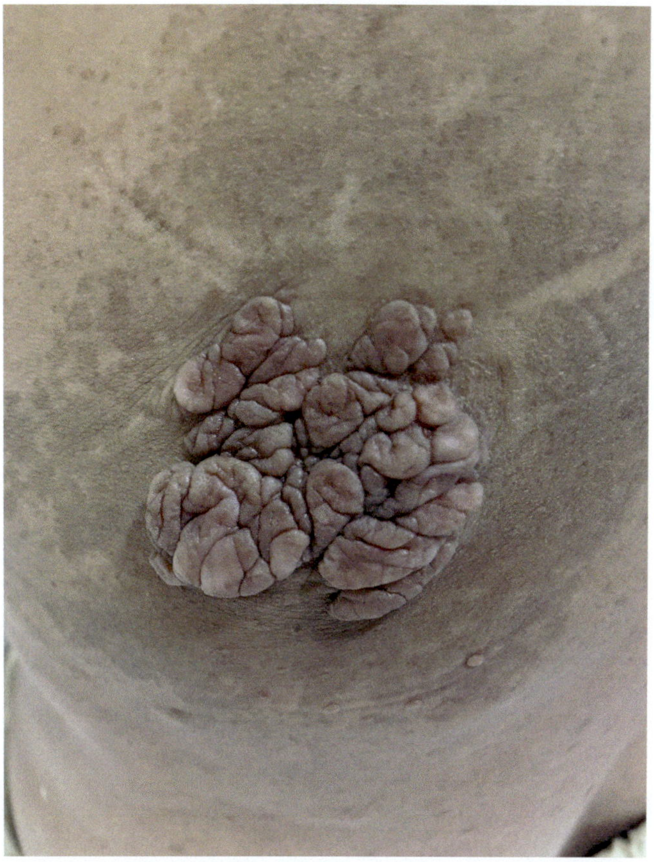

Figure 9.33 Skin-colored, smooth-surfaced, cerebriform nodule of nevus lipomatosus.

## Melanocytic nevus

- Melanocytic nevi are a localized proliferation of nests of nevus cells (melanocytes).
- Most cases are sporadic, but familial occurrence is not uncommon. It may also appear in patients receiving chemotherapeutic agents (BRAF-inhibitor drugs).
- Most frequently seen in the Caucasian race and fair-skinned people, global incidence is 1–1.5%.
- It is classified into
    - Congenital – small, medium, giant
    - Acquired – junctional, intradermal, compound
    - Special types dermal melanocytosis – speckled (lentiginous), nevus of Ota/Hori, café-au-lait macules, Mongolian spots, hairy nevi, halo nevus, perinevoid dermatitis (Meyerson's phenomenon)

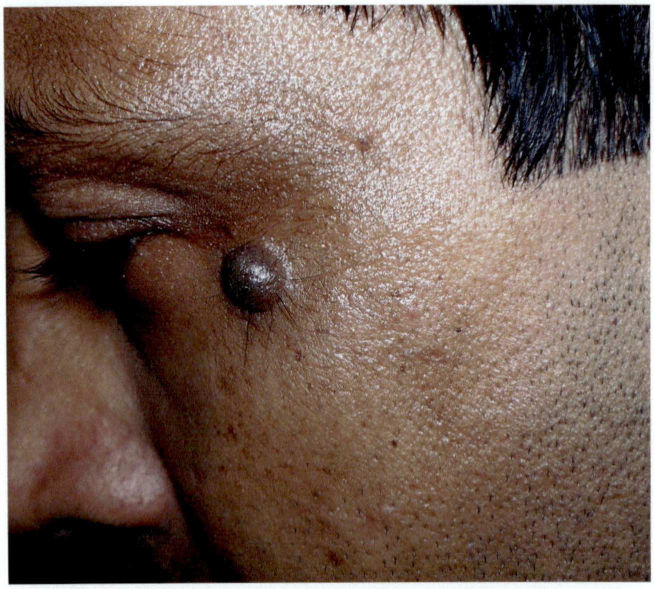

Figure 9.34 Brownish, dome-shaped nodule bearing hair on the face in compound nevus. (Courtesy: Dr. Piyush Kumar, Katihar, India.)

- Melanocytic nevi may present as solitary or multiple pigmented nodules to plaques. The color of the lesion varies and gives clues to the type of nevi – skin-colored (intradermal), dark-brown to black (compound) (**Figure 9.34**), black (congenital), and blue (deep dermal). The surface may show hairs.
- Color of the nevus becomes darker with progression in the Fitzpatrick skin type.
- DD: Mastocytoma, melanoma, verruca plana, acrochordons.

## Mastocytoma

- A mastocytoma is a tumor of mast cells, which are derived from myeloid stem cells and located in connective tissues, predominantly in the skin and mucosal linings.
- *C-kit* gene mutation causes increased concentration of growth factors and interleukins that induce proliferation of mast cells is responsible.
- This usually affects children.
- Lesions are noted as single or a few yellowish-brown pigmented macules, papules, or nodules of variable size. The lesions are generally non-tender but can be associated with intermittent itching and erythema (**Figure 9.35a,b**).
- Rubbing or stroking the lesion can degranulate the mast cells and cause itching, and edema of the skin, known as Darier sign, which is pathognomonic of the disease.
- The blistering and bullous presentation is common in children less than three years of age and can also be present in diffuse and severe forms of the disease.
- The diffuse disease presents with thickened, leathery skin without individual lesions.
- DD: Melanocytic nevus, melanoma, dermatofibroma, insect-bite reaction.

## Nodular melanoma

- Nodular melanoma is a common subtype of melanoma and shows aggressive vertical growth phase from the early stage.

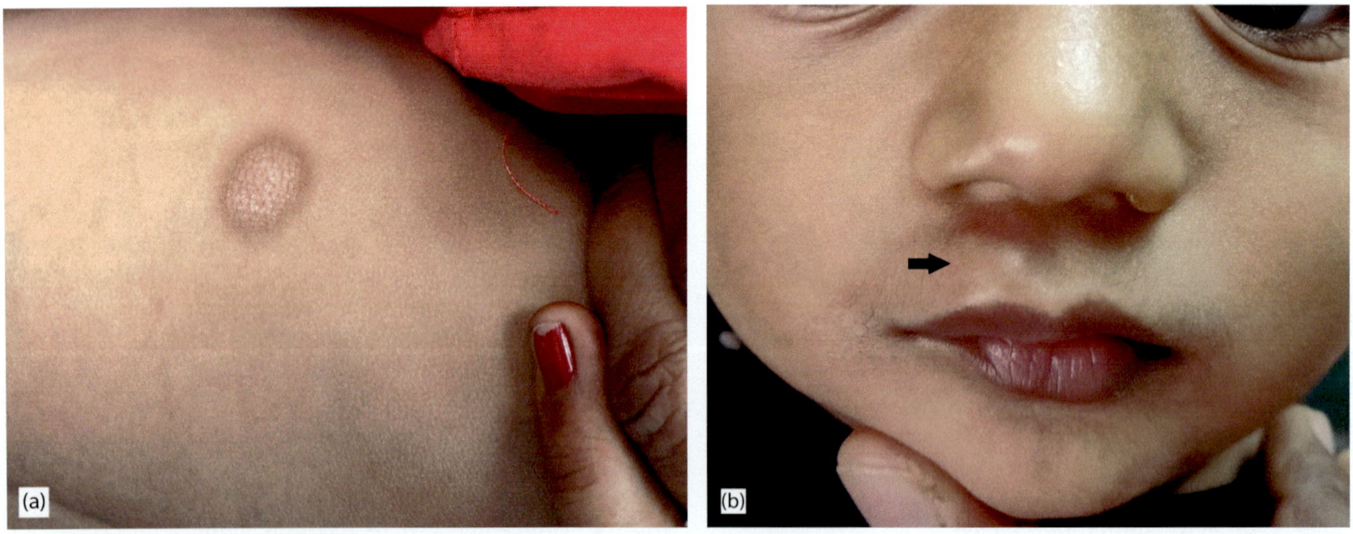


Figure 9.35 **(a)** Solitary nodule of mastocytoma on the leg. **(b)** Flesh-colored nodule of mastocytoma on the upper lip (arrow) of a child. (a – Courtesy: Dr. Sunil Kumar Gupta, AIIMS, Gorakhpur, India; b – Courtesy: Dr. Mandeep Bhukar, Rohtak, India.)

- It can appear de novo in normal-appearing skin or in existing melanoma of other types or dysplastic nevi.
- It is more commonly seen in fair-skinned individuals and is common in elderly men.
- It presents as a solitary rapidly progressing, dome-shaped nodule of black or variegated color (black, red, etc.). The surface shows variable ulceration, bleeding, crusting, or warty surface (**Figure 9.36a**).
- Regional lymph nodes and cutaneous metastases may occur (**Figure 9.36b**). The prognosis is poor.
- In amelanotic melanoma up to one-third of nodular melanomas may not be pigmented and appear red or skin-colored. They carry an even worse prognosis.

### Dermatofibrosarcoma protuberans[11]

- Dermatofibrosarcoma protuberans (DFSP) is a rare soft-tissue tumor that involves the dermis, subcutaneous fat, and, in rare cases, muscle and fascia.
- It typically presents as a slow-growing, firm plaque on the trunk of young adults.

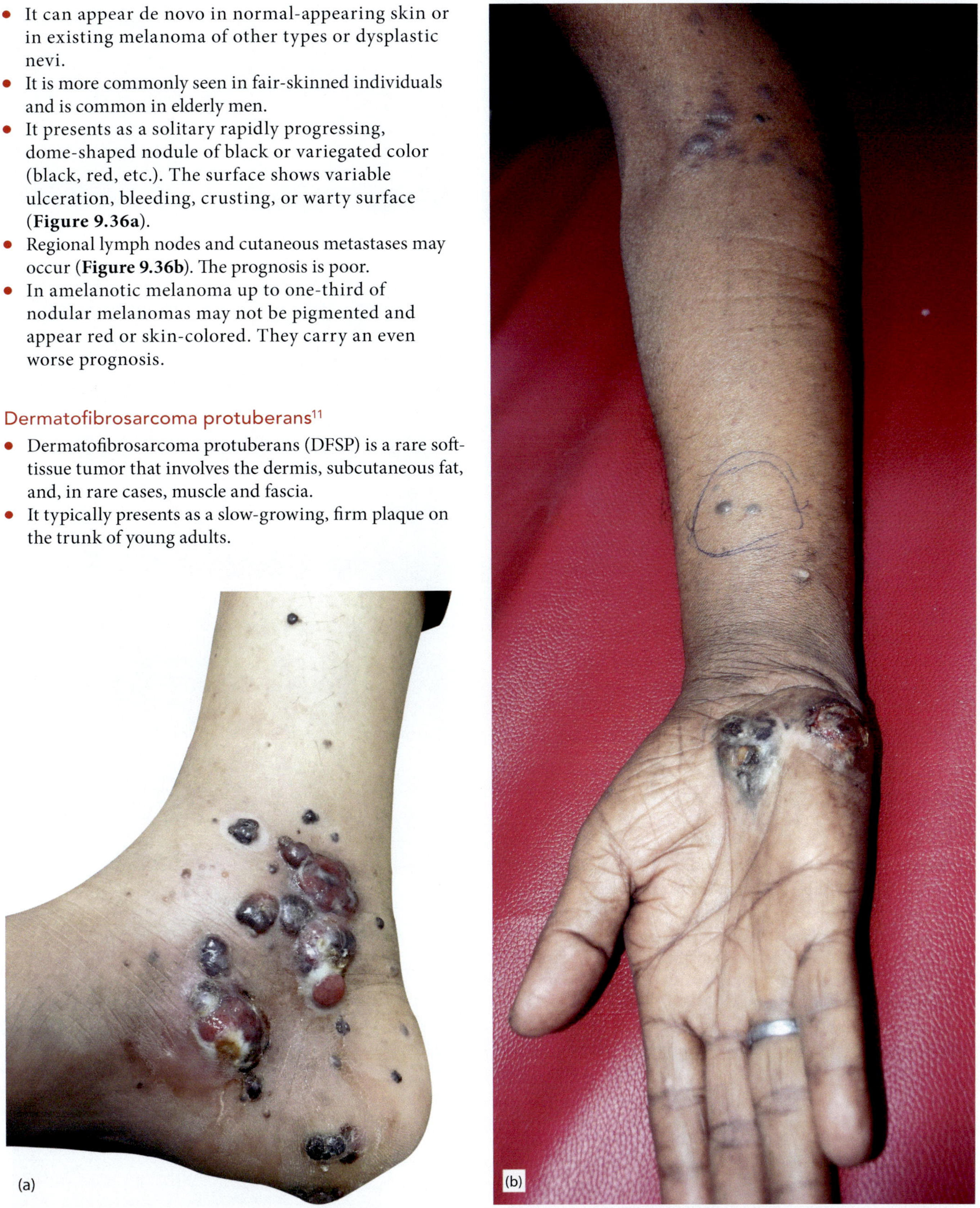


Figure 9.36 **(a)** Erythematous noduloulcerative lesions and multiple black nodules in a case of nodular melanoma with cutaneous metastasis. **(b)** Ulcerated, pigmented nodule of malignant melanoma on the palm, with pigmented nodules of metastatic lesions on the forearm and arm. (Courtesy: Dr. PC Das and Dr. Piyush Kumar, Katihar, India.)

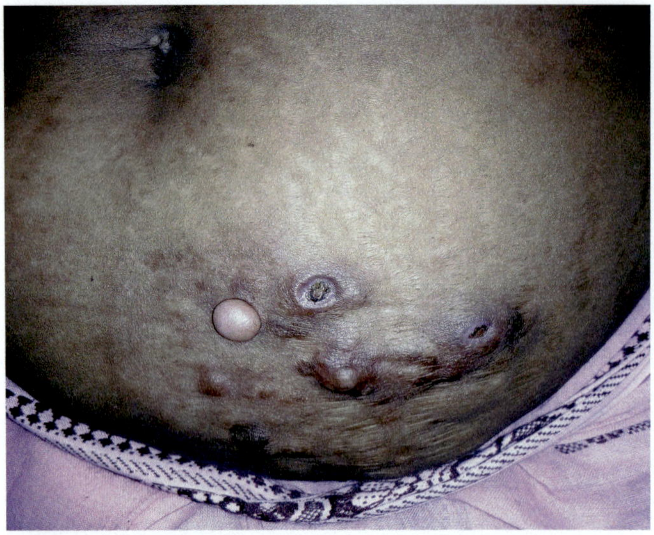

Figure 9.37 Dermatofibrosarcoma protuberans presenting as subcutaneous nodule with flesh-colored and pigmented nodules on its surface. (Courtesy: Dr. Piyush Kumar, Katihar, India.)

- It is clinically characterized by asymptomatic, skin-colored to red-brown indurated plaque which eventually develops multiple raised violaceus to red-brown nodules (**Figure 9.37**).
- As they grow larger, some can ulcerate and become painful. The majority of DFSPs occur on the trunk (50%), followed by the extremities (35%), and then head and neck (15%).
- DD: Cutaneous melanoma, dermatofibroma.

## Mycetoma

- Mycetoma is caused by fungi as well as filamentous bacteria. Lesions are more common on the feet, shins, and hands.
- The earliest clinical manifestation is a hard painless nodule that spreads slowly to produce papules and sinuses that discharge fluid containing granules onto the skin surface (**Figure 9.38a,b**).
- The original site of infection is distorted by local tissue swelling, formation of chronic sinuses, and late bone involvement.
- DD: Bacterial osteomyelitis, tuberculous osteomyelitis, hidradenitis suppurativa, Kaposi sarcoma, and cutaneous tuberculosis.

## Phaeohyphomycosis

- Phaeohyphomycosis is caused by dark-walled (dematiaceous) fungi. These fungi are found in all climates, although they are more common in tropical climates. Immunosuppressed patients with HIV infection or AIDS, transplant recipients, and diabetic patients are more susceptible.
- In subcutaneous phaeohyphomycosis following local trauma or inoculation with foreign material, patients

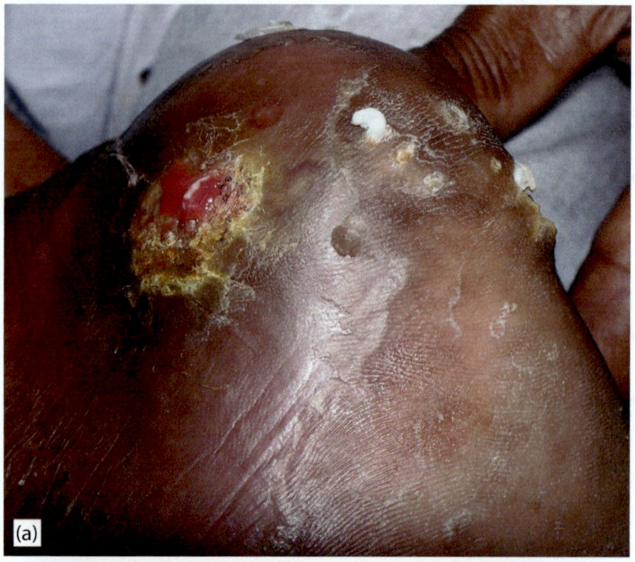

(a)

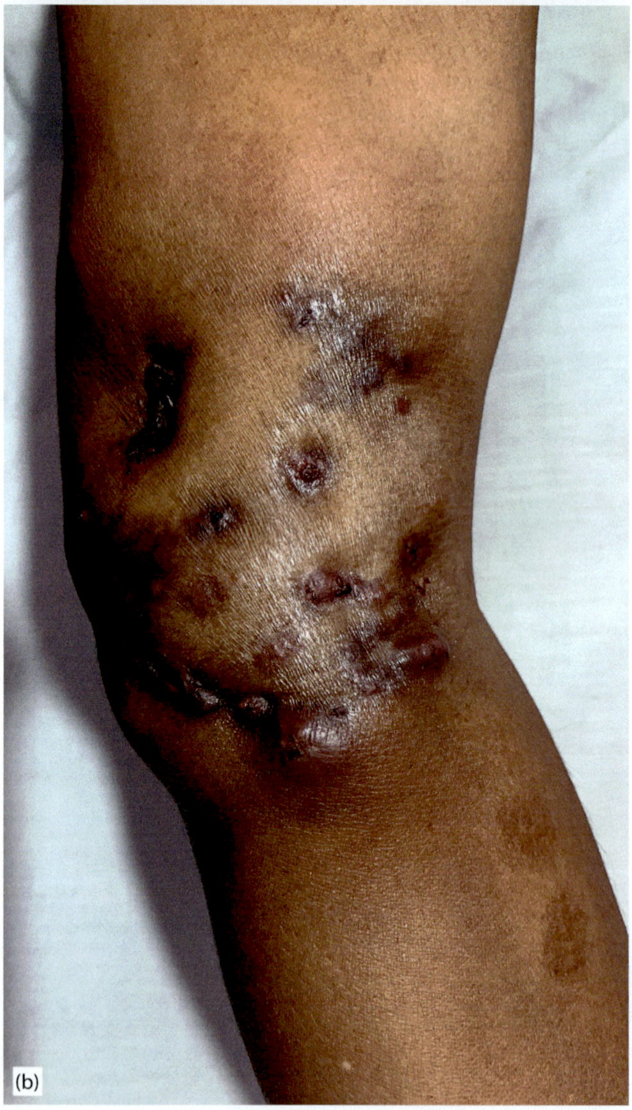

(b)

Figure 9.38 **(a)** Nodule and discharging sinuses on the heel in mycetoma. **(b)** Localized swelling and discharging nodules in actinomycetoma. (a – Courtesy: Dr. Piyush Kumar, Katihar, India; b – Courtesy: Dr Rajeev Ranjan, Ara, India.)

develop a slow-growing solitary lesion (generally a cyst or a nodule, or possibly a plaque or abscess) normally located on the extremities.

- DD: Lipoma, epidermal or synovial cysts, fibromas, foreign body cysts, and bacterial abscesses.

## Histoplasmosis

- This is a chronic granulomatous disease caused by the dimorphic fungus *Histoplasma capsulatum*.
- Skin lesions are not specific and are characterized by their polymorphism, ranging from papules, plaques with or without crusts, pustules, and nodules to mucosal ulcers, erosions, and lesions resembling molluscum contagiosum.
- The most commonly affected sites are the face, trunk, extremities, oral, perianal and genital mucosa. Oropharyngeal ulcers present as painful nodules on the tongue, gums, and larynx.

## Cryptococcosis

- It is an opportunistic fungal infection caused by *Cryptococcus neoformans*.
- Skin lesions are frequently a sentinel for disseminated disease; however, primary cutaneous lesions do occur in immunocompetent persons. The primary cutaneous lesion may be a papule, maculopapular lesion with an ulcerated center or a violaceous nodular lesion. Often there is a discharging sinus that connects to the underlying deep abscess or the underlying bone.

## Neurofibroma

- Neurofibromas are the most prevalent benign peripheral nerve sheath tumor.
- They are comprised of Schwann cells, fibroblasts, perineural cells, and mast cells in a variably myxoid background.
- Patients are often asymptomatic; however, irritation, mild pruritus, pain, or paresthesia, can occur; the most common chief complaint is cosmetic appearance.
- Often appearing as a soft, skin-colored papule or small subcutaneous nodule, they arise from endoneurium and the connective tissues of peripheral nerve sheaths (**Figure 9.39**).
- A characteristic "buttonhole sign" where, on palpation, the lesion retracts into the subcutis and reappears on the release of pressure, is seen.
- Localized neurofibromas can occur anywhere on the body, with a predilection for the trunk, head/neck, and extremities.
- Neurofibromas may appear without any known cause or may be associated with neurofibromatosis.
- DD: Acrochordons, leiomyoma, schwannoma.

## Macro acrochordon

- This is also known as fibroepithelial polyp, skin tag, soft fibroma, and giant acrochordon.

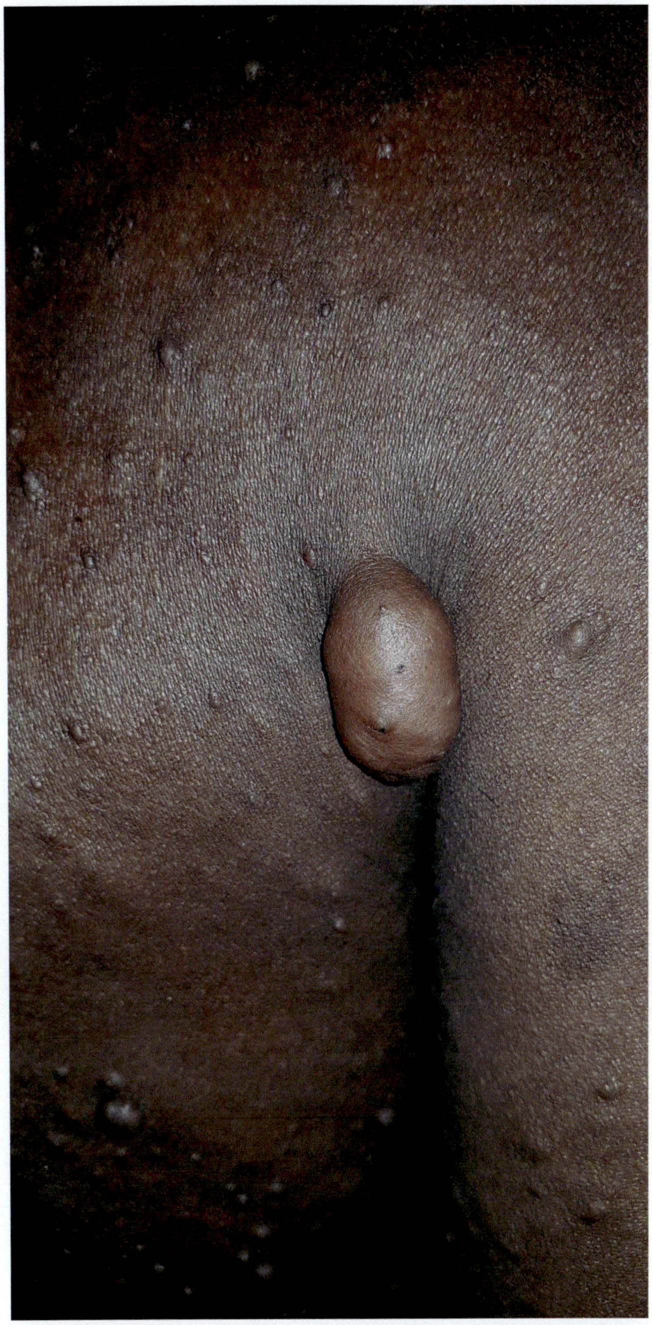

Figure 9.39 Nodule of neurofibroma in a patient of neurofibromatosis type 1. (Courtesy: Dr. PC Das, Katihar, India.)

- Frequent irritation seems to be an important causative factor, especially in persons who are obese. Hormone imbalances may facilitate the development of acrochordons (e.g., high levels of estrogen and progesterone during pregnancy, high levels of growth hormone in acromegaly). Epidermal growth factor (EGF) and alpha tissue growth factor (TGF) have also been implicated in the development of these lesions.
- The onset of acrochordon increases in frequency up through the fifth decade. As many as 59% of persons may have acrochordons by the time they are age 70.

- Commonly, lesions are found on the groin, upper thigh, and back.
- It presents as large, pedunculated, bag-like, soft fibromas (**Figure 9.40a,b**).
- It can cause considerable discomfort for patients when located in the axilla and genital regions.
- DD: Neurofibromatosis Type 1, genital warts, melanocytic nevi, premalignant fibroepithelial tumor (Pinkus tumor), seborrheic keratosis.

## Rheumatoid nodules[12]

- Classic rheumatoid nodules occur in approximately 20% to 25% of patients with seropositive rheumatoid arthritis (RA) and are the most common extra-articular manifestation of RA.

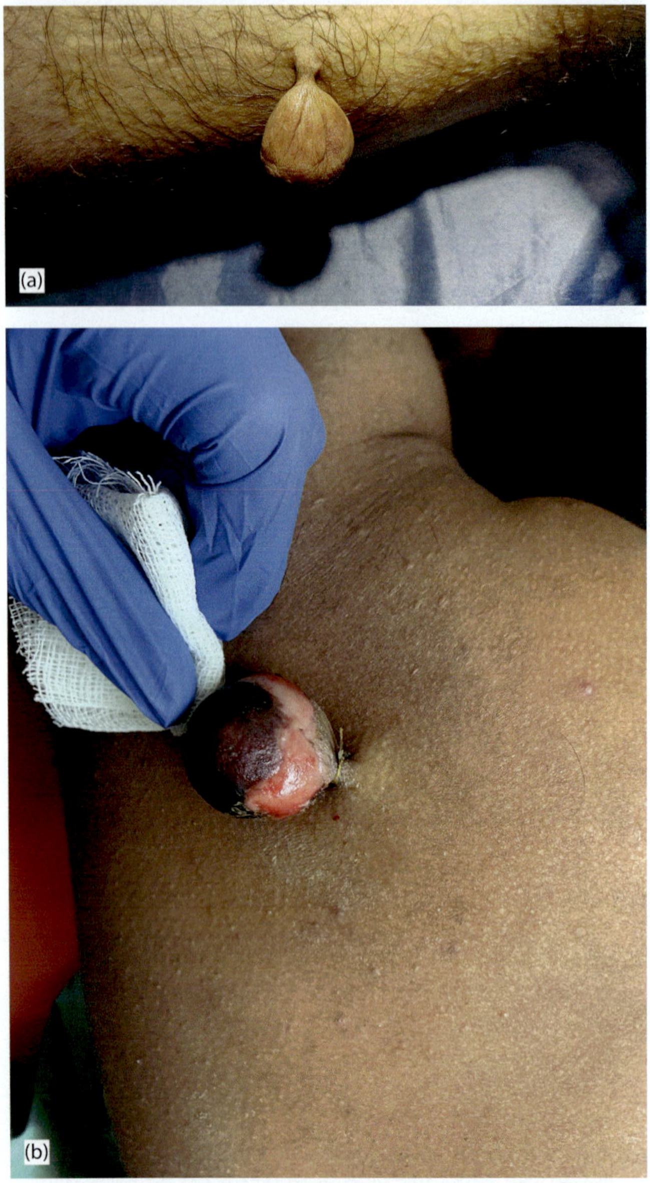

Figure 9.40 **(a)** Skin-colored, soft, pedunculated nodule seen in macro acrochordon. **(b)** Giant acrochordon showing surface necrosis due to a thread tied around its peduncle. (Courtesy: Dr. Piyush Kumar, Katihar, India.)

- Nodules are skin-colored, can be solitary or multiple, and their size ranges from 2 mm to more than 5 cm in diameter.
- They are firm, non-tender, and movable within the subcutaneous tissue; however, they could also be attached to underlying structures such as the periosteum, tendons, or bursae.
- Most rheumatoid nodules are found on areas prone to mild repetitive trauma, such as bony prominences, extensor surfaces, or adjacent to joints.
- They have a predilection for the elbows and fingers.
- They are most frequently found on extensor surfaces of the proximal forearm, metacarpophalangeal, and proximal interphalangeal joints, occiput, back, and heel.
- DD: gouty tophi, subcutaneous granuloma annulare, tumoral calcinosis, fibromas, xanthomas, subcutaneous sarcoidosis.

## Sebaceous hyperplasia

- Sebaceous hyperplasia is a benign dermatosis characterized by asymptomatic solitary or multiple lesions on the face, with a predilection for the forehead.
- Lesions are common in middle-aged persons and occur rarely in early adult life.
- Clinically they are characterized by single or multiple yellow papules or skin nodules, usually 0.2–0.3 cm in diameter with a central area of umbilication.
- DD: Basal cell carcinoma, sebaceous adenoma.

## Lipoma

- It is usually seen in people between 25 and 50 years of age.
- It is more common in males.
- The trunk and upper limbs are the common sites but it can occur on other parts of the body too.
- It is clinically characterized by soft, fluctuant, freely mobile nodules with normal-appearing overlying skin (**Figure 9.41a–c**).
- A characteristic "slippage sign" may be elicited by gently sliding the fingers off the edge of the tumor. The tumor will be felt to slip out from under, as opposed to a sebaceous cyst or an abscess that is tethered by surrounding induration. The overlying skin is typically normal.
- DD: Epidermoid cyst, abscess, liposarcomas.

## Subcutaneous granuloma annulare

- Subcutaneous granuloma annulare (SGA) is a rare type of granuloma annulare (GA), a benign granulomatous inflammatory disease that usually involves the skin or deeper tissues.
- Etiology is unknown; it may be associated with systemic diseases such as diabetes, rheumatoid arthritis, and malignancy.
- It is most frequently seen in children and young adults; males are more commonly affected.

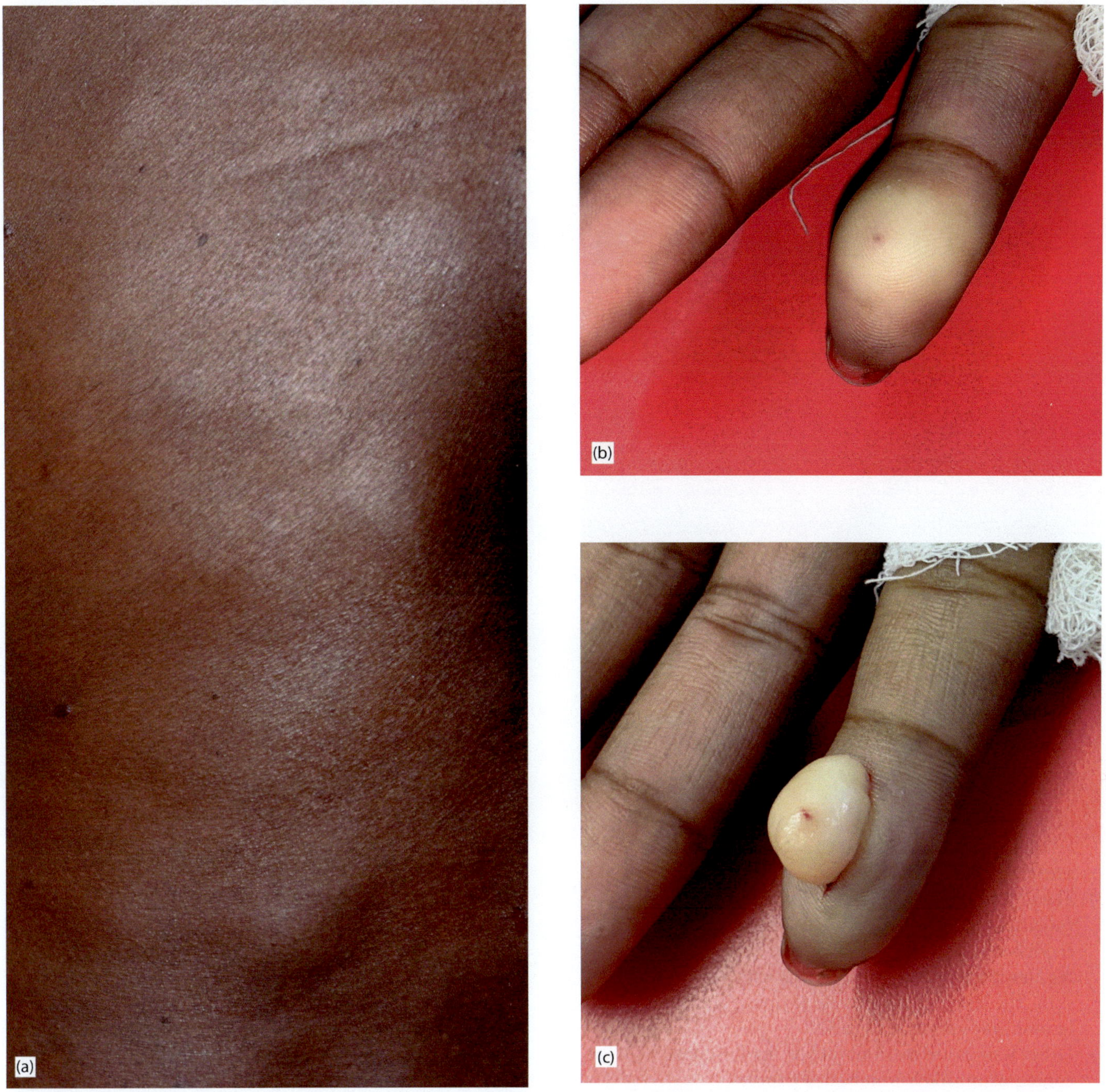


Figure 9.41 **(a)** Subcutaneous nodules of lipoma on the back. **(b)** Lipoma causing pale colored swelling of the pulp of index finger. **(c)** Intraoperative visualization of lipoma. (a–c – Courtesy: Dr. Piyush Kumar, Katihar, India.)

- It is most commonly located on the anterior aspects of the lower legs, hands, head, and gluteal region.
- It is clinically characterized by subcutaneous nodules with no inflammatory appearance at the skin surface (**Figure 9.42**).
- In rare cases, subcutaneous granuloma annulare may extend, involving deeper soft tissues, and produce a destructive arthritis and limb deformity.
- The lesions described in children under the names pseudo rheumatoid nodules and benign rheumatoid nodules are currently considered within the spectrum of subcutaneous granuloma annulare.
- DD: Rheumatoid nodule, necrobiosis lipoidica, epithelioid sarcoma.

## Histoid leprosy[13]

- Also known as histoid Hansen's disease, histoid nodules, mycobacterium leprae histiocytoma (cutis), and leprous histiocytoma.
- Histoid leprosy is considered to be a variant of lepromatous leprosy caused by *Mycobacterium leprae.*

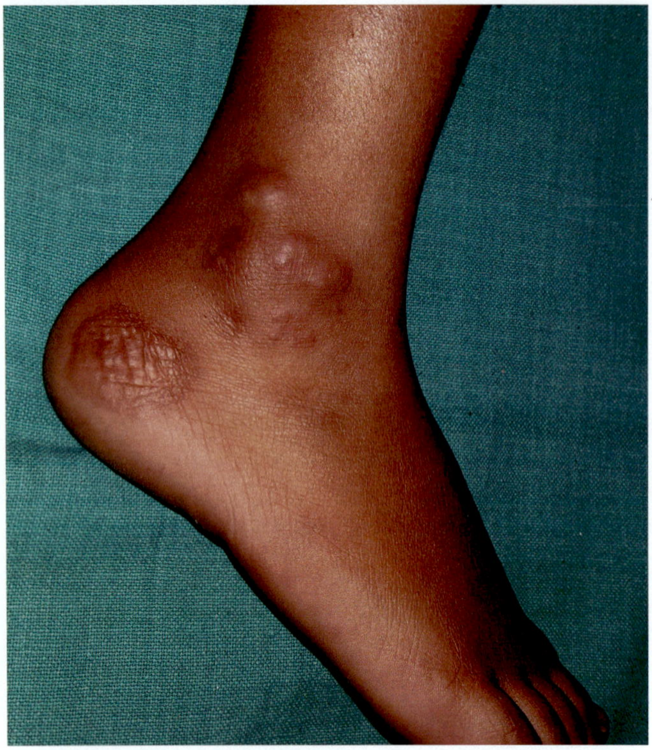

Figure 9.42 Multiple grouped, skin-colored nodules and plaques in subcutaneous granuloma annulare. (Courtesy: Dr. Shahid Hassan, Purnea, India.)

- It may be seen in all ages (most commonly 20–39 years) with male preponderance.
- The lesions are located on the back, buttocks, face, extremities, or over bony prominences. Oral mucosal lesions are rarely seen; palms, sole, and nasal mucosa are not affected commonly.
- The nodules of histoid leprosy may be soft to firm; superficially placed, deeply fixed, or subcutaneous; reddish or skin-colored; and dome-shaped, oval, or regular in contour, with overlying shiny or stretched skin. The lesions may ulcerate at times. The number of lesions may vary from 3 to 50.
- Other lesions are neurofibroid or "molluscum-contagiosum-like" umbilicated papules.
- DD: Lepromatous nodules, ENL, Von Recklinghausen's disease/NF-1, molluscum contagiosum, keloids, post kala-azar dermal leishmaniasis.

## Cutaneous calcinosis (calcinosis cutis)

- It may be iatrogenic, idiopathic, metastatic (increased calcium and phosphate as in renal failure, milk-alkali syndrome, calciphylaxis), or dystrophic (calcification occurs in damaged tissue as in collagen vascular disease, infections, trauma, chronic acne, panniculitis) in origin.
- It is more common in young adults; but the occurrence may vary with type of calcification.
- Acral involvement is common – distal phalanges, tips, etc.; it may be distributed over other areas as well.
- It is clinically characterized by solitary to multiple asymptomatic, flesh-colored to yellow or whitish, hard

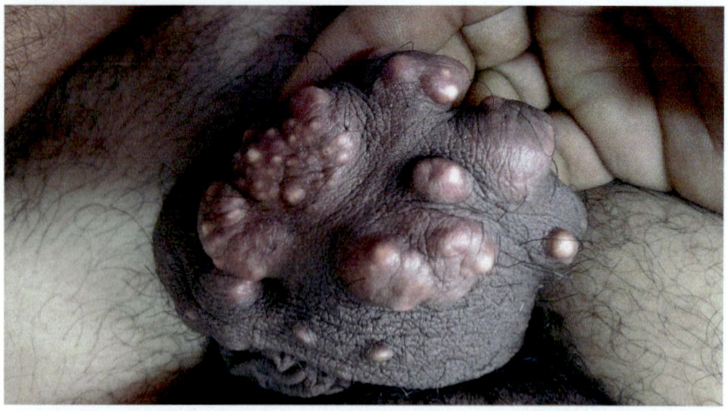

Figure 9.43 Skin-colored and white, shiny nodules on scrotum in scrotal calcinosis. (Courtesy: Dr. Anup Kumar Tiwary, Consultant Dermatologist, Yashoda Hospital and Research Center, Ghaziabad, India.)

nodules (**Figure 9.43**). The lesions may become tender and ulcerate spontaneously to reveal a chalky white discharge, rich in calcium carbonate/phosphate.
- DD: Tophus, mycetoma, giant molluscum, osteoma cutis.

## Osteoma cutis

- Osteoma cutis or cutaneous ossification is a rare and benign dermatological disease characterized by bone formation in the dermis or subcutaneous tissue.
- Primary osteoma cutis (without any pre-existing lesion) can occur in isolation or in association with metabolic syndrome. Secondary osteoma cutis is associated with cutaneous inflammatory processes, scars, dysembryoplasia, or neoplasia.
- The most common site is the face in females and the scalp in males. Other sites of involvement include the breasts, buttocks, and extremities.
- Clinical features can range from asymptomatic single to multiple lesions. They range in size from 0.1–5.0 cm. These lesions may present as papules, plaques, nodules, or as miliary lesions. On palpation, they are hard and can sometimes be responsible for skin discoloration that becomes white or yellowish **(Figure 9.44)**.
- In rare cases, the overlying epidermis may be ulcerated with the release of bony spicules known as perforating osteoma cutis.
- DD: Pilomatricoma, osteochondroma, ossified hair follicle, cutaneous calcinosis.

## Furuncular myiasis

- This is also known as blowfly strike and fly-blown maggot infestation.
- Myiasis is a skin disease caused by the larvae (maggots) of the fly *Dermatobia hominis* and *Cordylobia anthropophaga*.
- It can occur in any age group, and appears more in males.
- Predisposing factors include poor socioeconomic status, poor hygiene, advanced or very young age, psychiatric illness, alcoholism, diabetes, peripheral vascular disease, and physical disabilities.
- Exposed sites most commonly include the fingers, hands, forearms or face, but it can occur anywhere.

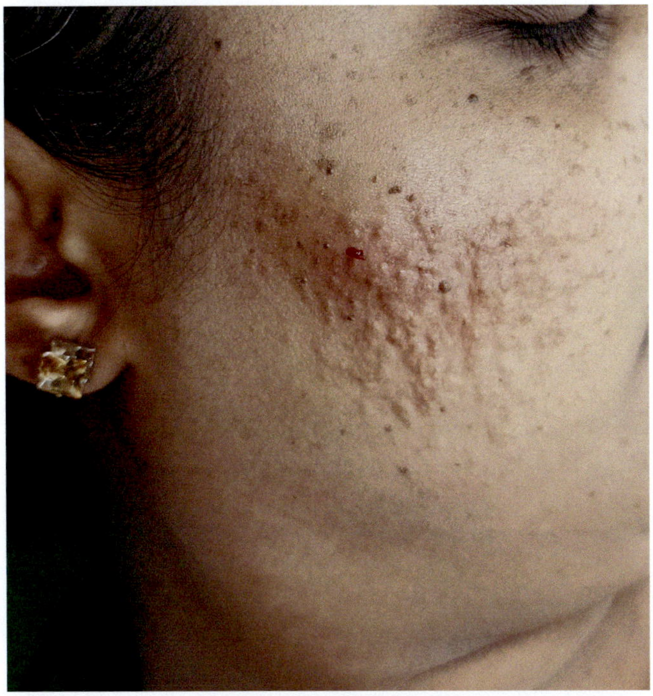

Figure 9.44 Secondary osteoma cutis presenting as hard papulonodules on the face. (Courtesy: Dr Ganesh Avhad, Mumbai, India.)

- The typical lesion presents as an itchy, painful erythematous papule or a nodule with a central punctum. A serosanguinous or purulent discharge from the punctum and end of the larvae is visible.
- The pain associated is sharp and stabbing, with sensation of movement.
- At times it heals, leaving behind slight hyperpigmentation and scarring.
- DD: Furunculosis, cellulitis, abscess, insect-bite reaction, cutaneous larva migrans, leishmaniasis.

## Nodular amyloidosis

- The cause of nodular localized cutaneous amyloidosis is not known, although the amyloid protein is derived from a localized infiltrate of plasma cells.
- It is more common in the fifth to sixth decade and equally seen in males and females.
- It clinically presents as firm nodules on the face, scalp, extremities, trunk, and genitalia; however, acral areas are preferentially involved. Nodules vary from a few millimeters to a few centimeters and may coalesce to form larger plaques. Nodules appear pink to brown or red. Underlying epidermal atrophy has been described.
- Disseminated cases have been described.
- DD: Colloid milium, cutaneous pseudolymphoma, leiomyoma.

## Sarcoidosis

- Sarcoidosis is a multisystem granulomatous disease of unknown etiology.
- It occurs more frequently between ages 20 and 40. There is a second peak of incidence around the age of 60. It is less common in the elderly and rare in children.
- Males are more commonly affected.
- Lesions mostly occur on the face, scalp, back, buttocks and extremities.
- It usually presents as multiple round or oval, infiltrated reddish-brown plaques. They are larger than 10 mm in diameter, tend to be thicker and more indurated and persistent, and are sometimes mammillated.
- Plaques can adopt an annular appearance by means of peripheral extension and central clearing, especially on the forehead and neck. Plaques can simulate lupus vulgaris, necrobiosis lipoidica, morphea, leprosy, leishmaniasis, discoid lupus erythematosus, and granuloma annulare.
- Plaques can be associated with nodular dermal lesions. They can be located on the face, scalp, back, buttocks, and extremities **(Figure 9.45)**.
- An unusual manifestation of sarcoidosis, known as Darier-Roussy sarcoidosis, is characterized by insidious, multiple, firm, asymptomatic to slightly tender, mobile, round to oval, skin-colored nodules. Commonly, they involve the extremities, but the trunk and face can also be affected.

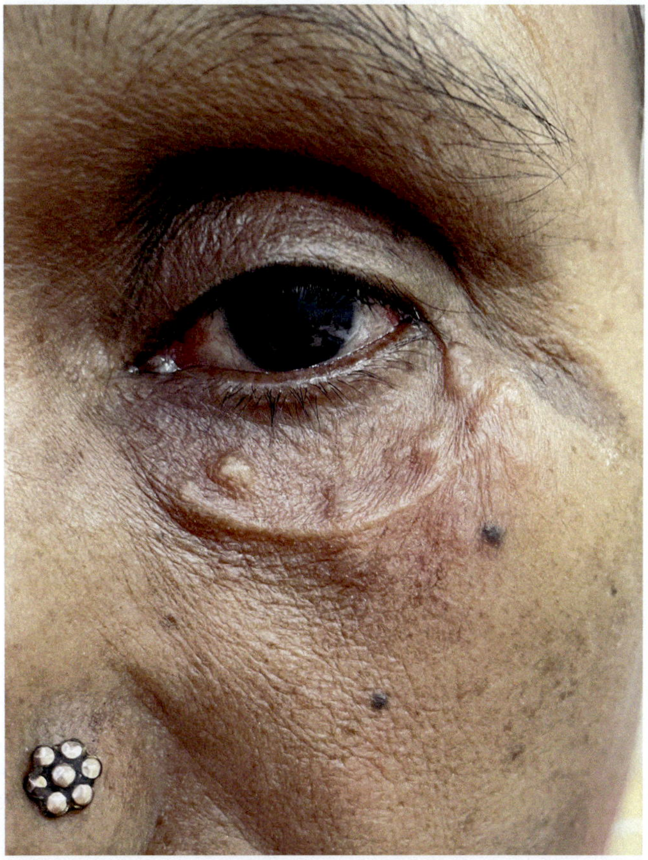

Figure 9.45 Scar sarcoidosis in an elderly lady presenting as dermal nodule with surface mamillations. (Courtesy: Soumyajit Roychoudhury, Berhampore, India.)

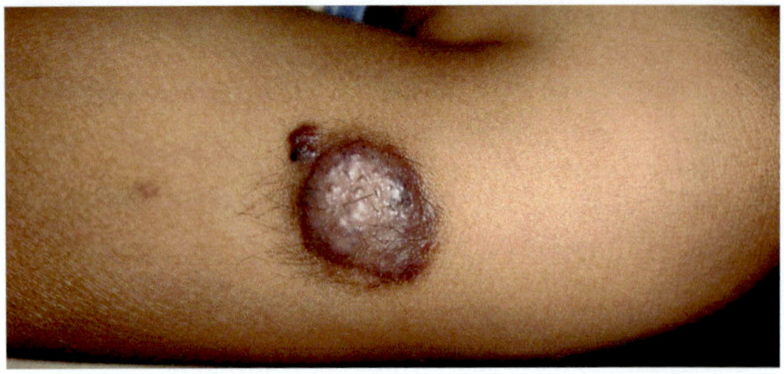

Figure 9.46 Red-brown nodule of eccrine angiomatous hamartoma presenting with pain and hyperhidrosis. Lesional hypertrichosis is appreciable. (Courtesy: Soumyajit Roychoudhury, Berhampore, India.)

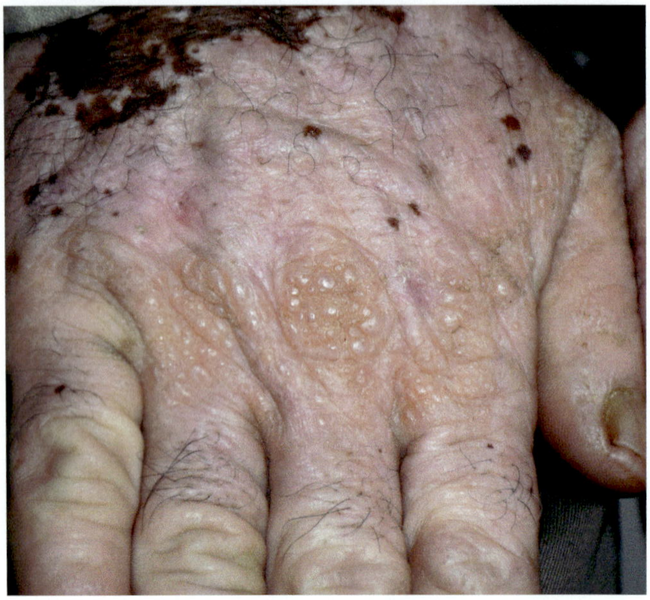

Figure 9.47 Shiny, confluent, smooth-surfaced, pearly papules and nodules of colloid milia. (Courtesy: Dr. Piyush Kumar, Katihar, India.)

- DD: Deep mycoses, cutaneous metastases of visceral neoplasms and melanoma, epidermoid cysts, lipomas, rheumatoid nodules, and erythema induratum.

## Additional images – Figures 9.46, 9.47, and 9.48

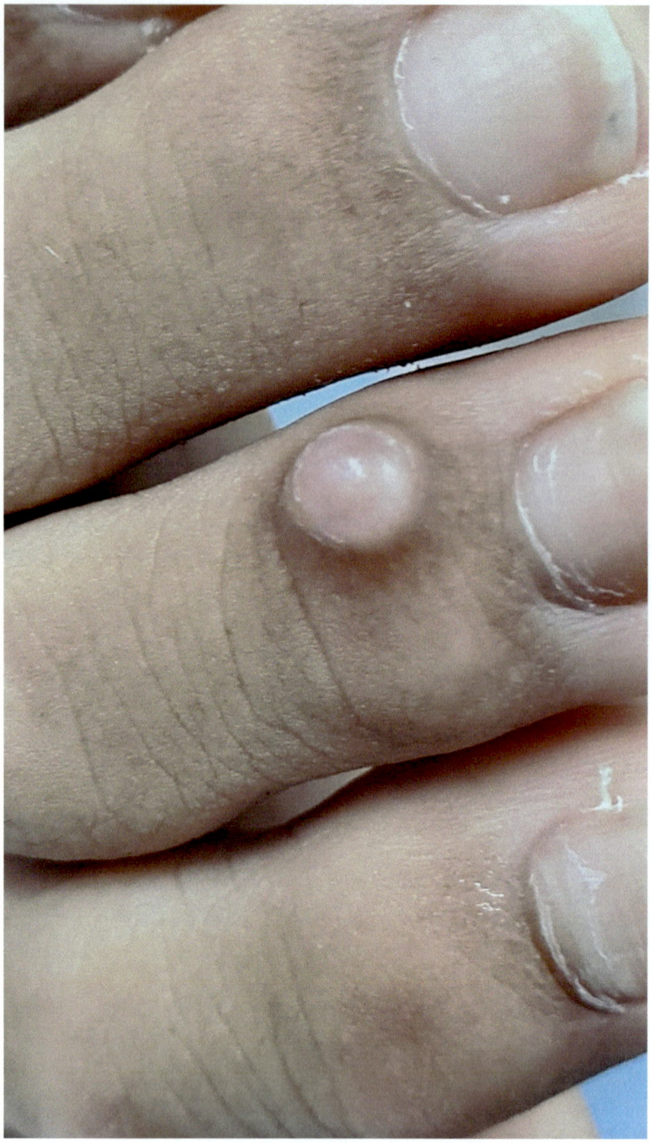

Figure 9.48 Superficial acral fibromyxoma presenting as slow-growing, smooth-surfaced, shiny nodule in the periungual area. (Courtesy: Dr. Tanumay Raychaudhury, Skin and Cancer Foundation, The University of Sydney, Australia.)

## REFERENCES


1. Fitzpatrick JE, High WA, Kyle WL. Urgent Care Dermatology: Symptom-Based Diagnosis. 1st ed. Philadelphia: Elsevier; 2018. Chapter 15. Subcutaneous Diseases. P. 253–268.
2. Lipsker D. Clinical Examination and Differential Diagnosis of Skin Lesions. 1st edition. France: Springer-Verlag; 2013. Chapter 4. Palpable and Solid Lesions. P. 19–28.
3. Higgins JC, Maher MH, Douglas MS. Diagnosing common benign skin tumors.Am Fam Physician 2015;92(7):601–607.
4. Nguyen T, Zuniga R. Skin conditions: Benign nodular skin lesions. FP Essent 2013;407:24–30.
5. Cohen BA. Pediatric Dermatology. 4th ed. Oxford: Saunders Elsevier; 2013. Chapter 5. Nodules and Tumors. P. 126–147.
6. Mahajan VK. Sporotrichosis: An overview and therapeutic options. Dermatol Res Pract 2014;2014:272376.
7. Sinno H, Lacroix JP, Lee J, et al. Diagnosis and management of eosinophilic cellulitis (Wells' syndrome): A case series and literature review. Can J Plast Surg 2012;20(2):91–97.
8. Sharma A, Agrawal S, Dhurat R, Shukla D, Vishwanath T. An unusual case of facial steatocystoma multiplex: A clinicopathologic and dermoscopic report. Dermatopathology (Basel) 2018;5(2):58–63.
9. Kumar P, Das A, Savant SS, Mandal RK, Hassan S. Gout nodulosis: Report of a rare case and brief review. Dermatol Online J 2015;21(1):13030/qt7x98t2jt.
10. Pujani M, Choudhury M, Garg T, Madan NK. Nevus lipomatosus superficialis: A rare cutaneous hamartoma. Indian Dermatol Online J 2014;5:109–110.
11. Das A, Kumar P. Dermatofibrosarcoma protuberans. J Pak Assoc Dermatol 2016;26(2):166–170.
12. García-Patos V. Rheumatoid nodule. Semin Cutan Med Surg 2007;26(2):100–107.
13. Gupta SK. Histoid leprosy: Review of the literature. Int J Dermatol 2015;54(11):1283–1288.

E7

# Nodules: Generalized

SWETALINA PRADHAN, KANANBALA SAHU


## ABSTRACT

Generalized or multiple nodules are the primary lesions in various skin conditions. The characteristic morphology, distribution, and duration of these lesions help in diagnosing a variety of diseases such as infective and neoplastic conditions. This chapter will provide a basic idea in diagnosing skin diseases that present with multiple/generalized nodules.


The text of this chapter is available online at https://routledgetextbooks.com/textbooks/9781032399669/

DOI: 10.1201/9781351054225-18

E8

# Tumors

PC DAS

## ABSTRACT

The term tumor refers to solid elevated skin lesions of more than two centimeters diameter. Papules, nodules, and tumors are skin lesion morphologies usually considered together because they belong to the same type, the difference being that of size only. The same dermatosis may give rise to all three morphologies in the same patient at a particular time in the course of disease progression. In this chapter, the word "tumor" is used in reference to skin lesion morphology rather than neoplasia, which it is often used to mean.

The text of this chapter is available online at https://routledgetextbooks.com/textbooks/9781032399669/



DOI: 10.1201/9781351054225-19

# 10

# Vesicobullous lesions: Localized

NIHARIKA RANJAN LAL

## INTRODUCTION

Vesicles and/or bullae may be the primary morphological manifestation of many skin disorders of localized or systemic pathology. These conditions traditionally come under the purview of vesiculobullous disorders. Approach to vesicobullous disorders may be discussed in more than one ways- etiology wise (genetic, autoimmune, infective etc.), presenting age groups (adults or children), course of the disease (short duration or recurrent and chronic), etc. In this book, author attempts to discuss vesicobullous diseases based on the extent of involvement. In this chapter, blistering diseases expressing on limited skin area of the body are considered. It is important to remember that systemic pathology may present on localized area of the skin initially, so one should keep them in mind when dealing with localized vesicobullous conditions. The clinical approach to diagnose vesicobullous conditions usually involving the limited area of skin has been depicted in **Figure 10.1** and the salient features of conditions are described below.[1–4]

### Pompholyx/dyshidrosiform eczema

- The cause of this condition is unknown; it is usually associated with atopy, contact allergy, psychological stress, hot climate, and palmoplantar hyperhidrosis.
- Clinical features include deep-seated vesicles (sago-like) on the lateral aspect of fingers (**Figure 10.2a,b**) and on palms and soles (**Figure 10.2c**).
- It is extremely pruritic.
- DD: Acute palmoplantar dermatitis, id reaction.

### Epidermolysis bullosa (EB)

- This is an inherited mechanobullous disorder.
- The cause is mutations of genes coding for components of the basement membrane zone.
- There is skin fragility and blister formation on minor trauma/friction.
- There are four types: EB simplex, junctional, dystrophic, Kindler syndrome.
- Electron microscopy, immunofluorescence mapping help in diagnosis.
- Acral blisters heal without scarring; there is mild or no mucosal involvement seen in localized EB simplex (**Figure 10.3a,b**).
- There are herpetiform blisters and mucosal and nail involvement in EBS-DM (Dowling-Meara type).
- In junctional EB, Herlitz type, there is non-healing granulation tissue on areas of non-healing and dystrophic teeth and nails.
- Blisters/erosion with abdominal distension and non-bilious vomiting/and or ureteral and renal abnormalities occur with JEB with pyloric atresia.
- Dystrophic EB is the most severe form and may result in pseudosyndactyly (thin membranous scarring joining two adjacent digits, also called mitten hand deformity) (**Figure 10.3c,d**).
- Lesions in EB heal with varying scarring, milia, and nail loss, most noticeable in dystrophic EB.
- DD: Epidermolysis bullosa acquisita (manifests in adulthood).

### Erythema multiforme

- Infections (*Herpes simplex virus, Mycoplasma*) and drugs are the most important causes.
- Target/iris lesions with three concentric zones develop from inside out: a central dusky area covered with a blister, middle edematous zone, peripheral erythematous (**Figure 10.4a–c**).
- Lesions heal over weeks with hyperpigmentation.
- Mucosal blisters easily rupture into erosions.
- Lesions are usually symmetrical and acral.
- DD: Fixed drug reaction; secondary syphilis; hand, foot, and mouth disease.

DOI: 10.1201/9781351054225-20

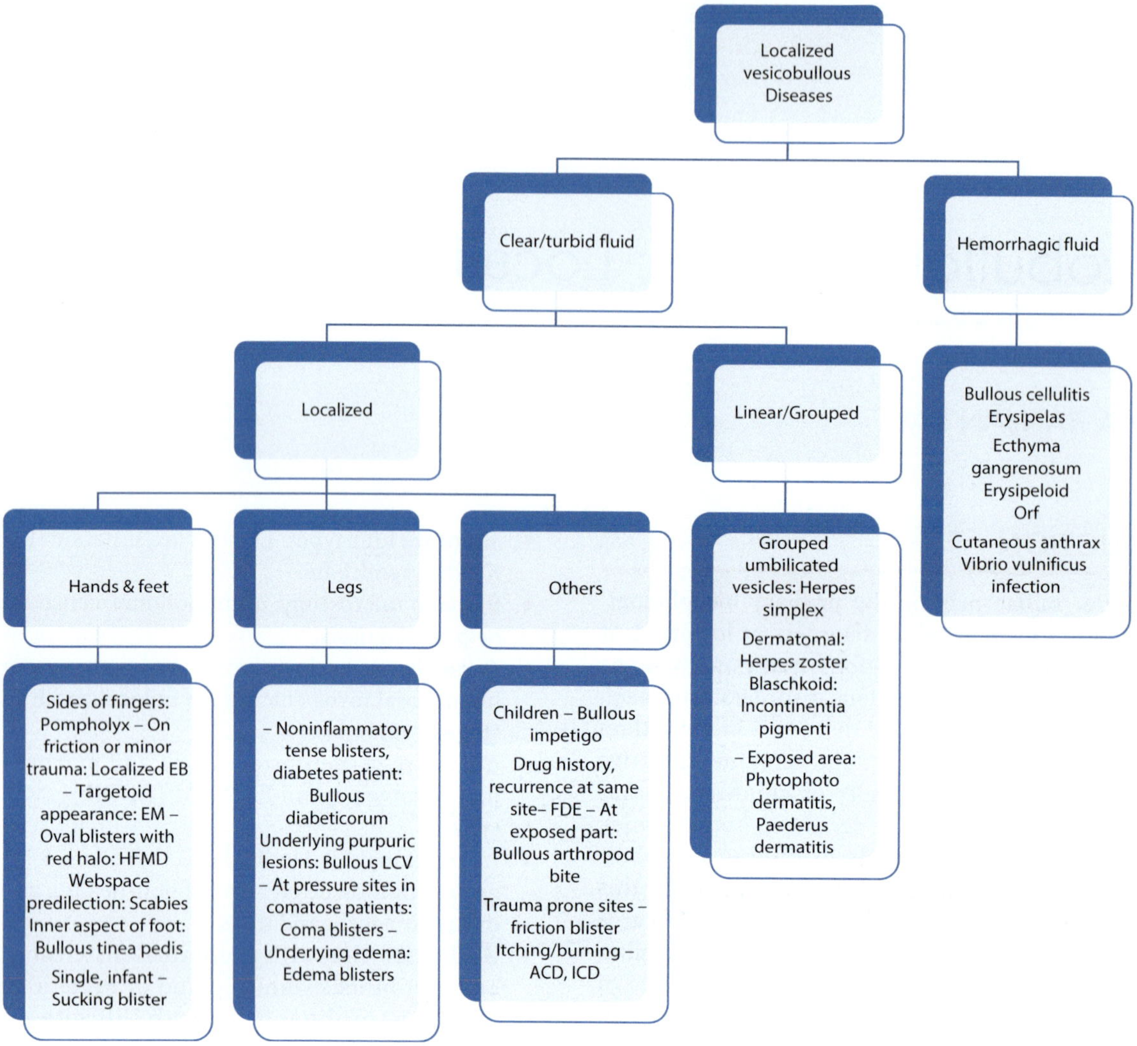


Figure 10.1 Clinical approach to localized vesicobullous diseases (LCV: leukocytoclastic vasculitis, FDE: fixed drug eruption, ACD: allergic contact dermatitis, ICD: irritant contact dermatitis).

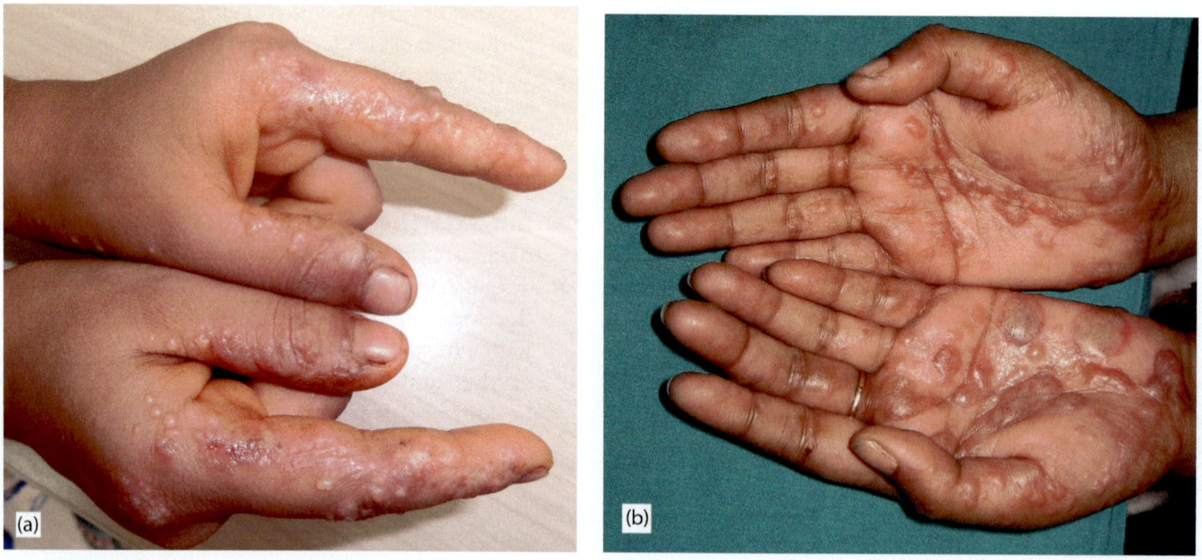


Figure 10.2 **(a)** Deep-seated vesicles on the lateral aspect of fingers in pompholyx. **(b)** Pompholyx over palm. (*Continued*)

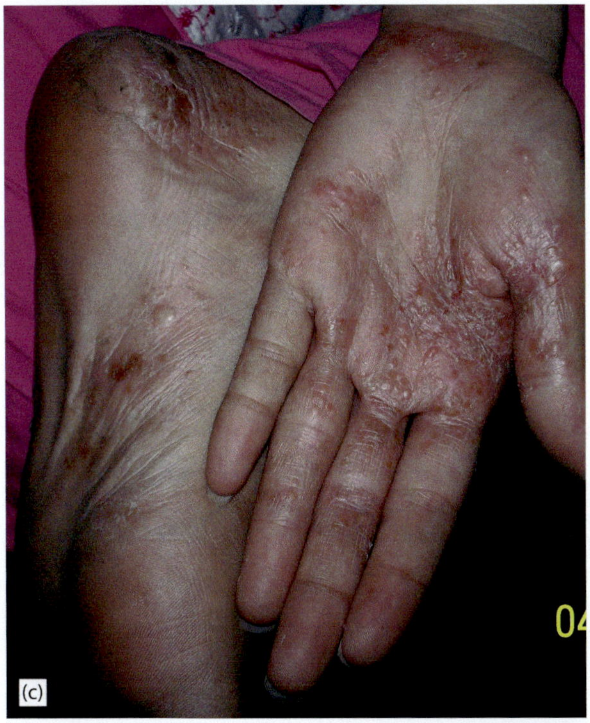

Figure 10.2 (*Continued*) **(c)** Pompholyx affecting the palm and foot. (b,c – Courtesy: Dr. Piyush Kumar, Katihar, India.)

## Hand, foot, and mouth disease

- With this condition, blisters occur on the hands and feet, and sometimes buttocks (**Figure 10.5a–c**).
- Typically, blisters are oval shaped and have an erythematous halo (**Figure 10.5d**).
- Sometimes, they can be more widespread.
- They may have oral aphthae-like ulcers.
- It is associated with a low-grade fever, sore throat, and loss of appetite.
- Usually occurs in children <5 years of age.
- DD: Acropustulosis of infancy, scabies.

## Bullous scabies

- Bulla in scabies is rare.
- They may form because of secondary bacterial infection or autoantibody-mediated or id reaction.

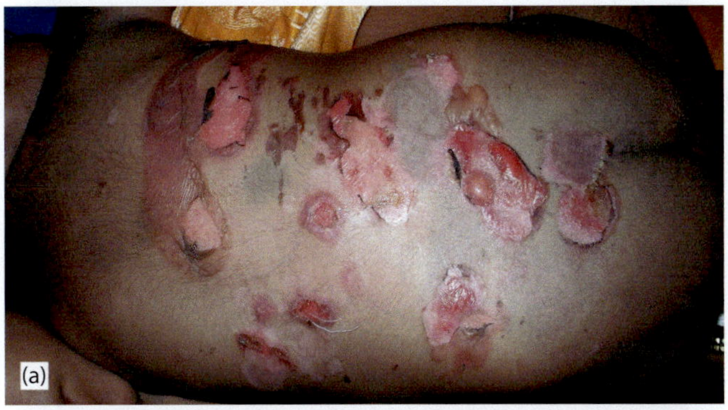

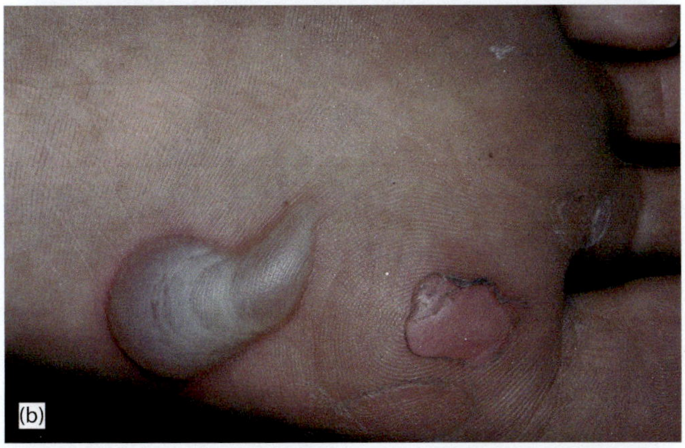

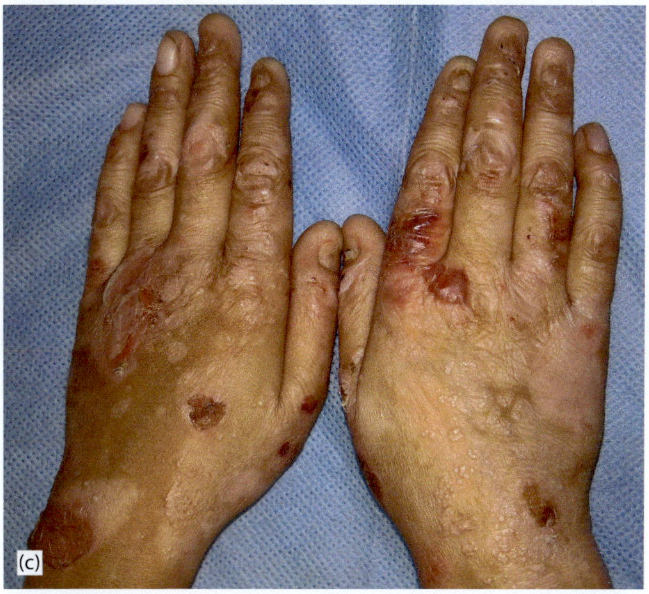

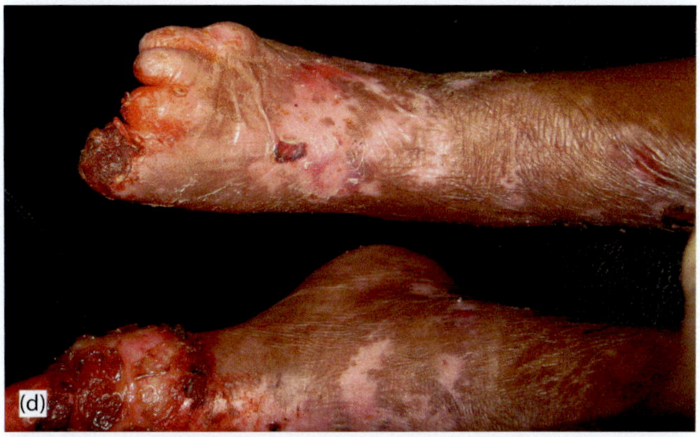

Figure 10.3 **(a)** Flaccid blisters and erosions on the back in epidermolysis bullosa simplex. **(b)** Blister on the sole in epidermolysis bullosa simplex. **(c)** Blister and scars on the dorsa of both hands in dystrophic epidermolysis bullosa. **(d)** Dystrophic epidermolysis bulla resulting in atrophic scarring, pigmentary loss, and loss of nails. Crusted erosions are noted over digits. (a,b,d – Courtesy: Dr. Piyush Kumar, Katihar, India; c – Courtesy: Dr. Vishal Gupta, AIIMS, New Delhi.)

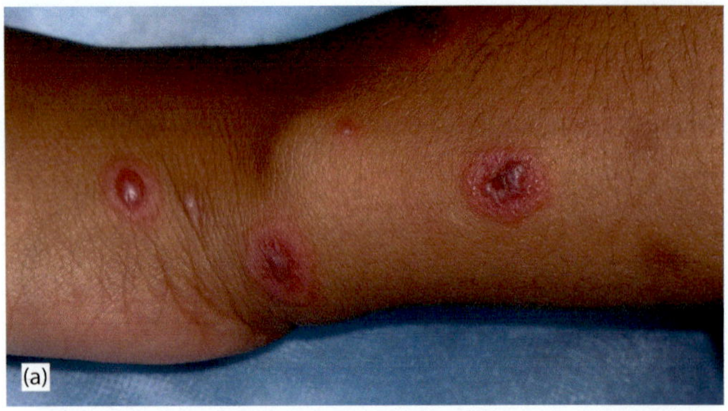

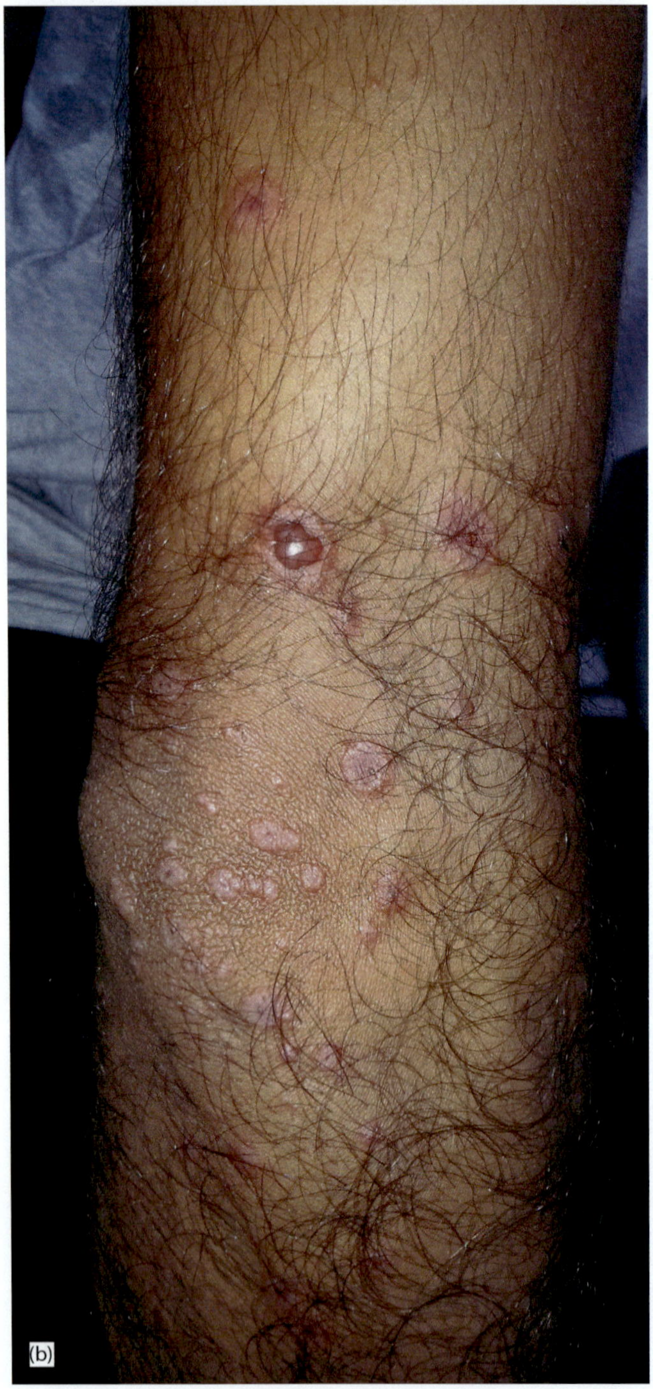

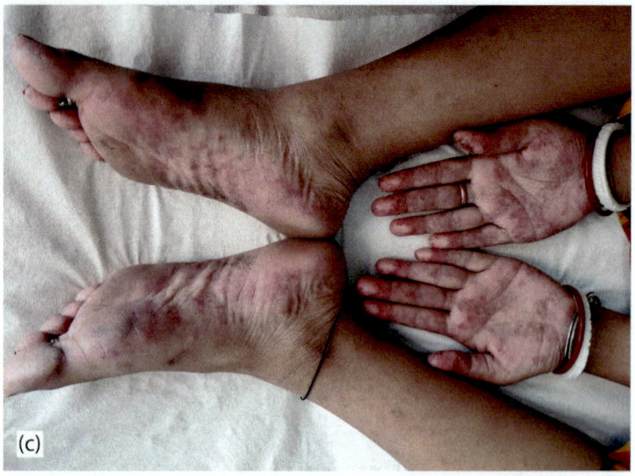

Figure 10.4 **(a)** Erythema multiforme with three concentric zones visible. **(b)** Erythema multiforme with target lesions on upper extremity. **(c)** Erythema multiforme lesions on palms and soles. (a – Courtesy: Dr. Vishal Gupta, AIIMS, New Delhi, India; b – Courtesy: Dr. Piyush Kumar, Katihar, India.)

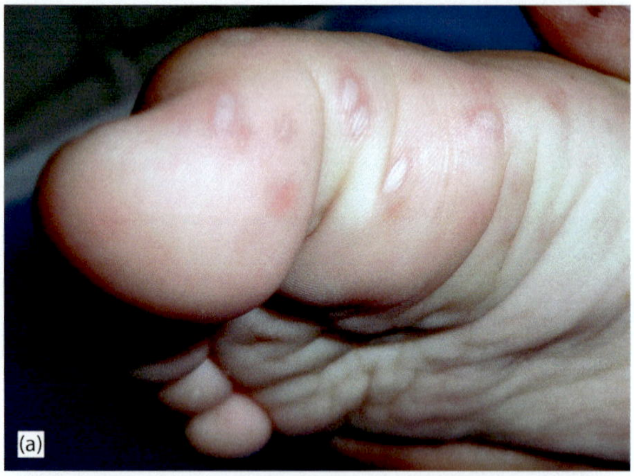

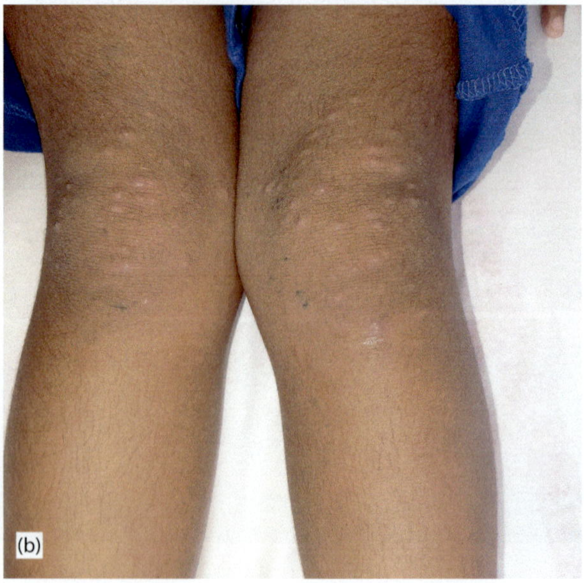

Figure 10.5 **(a)** Oval vesicle surrounded by erythema on the sole in hand, foot, and mouth disease. **(b)** Hand, foot, and mouth disease with blisters on knees. (*Continued*)

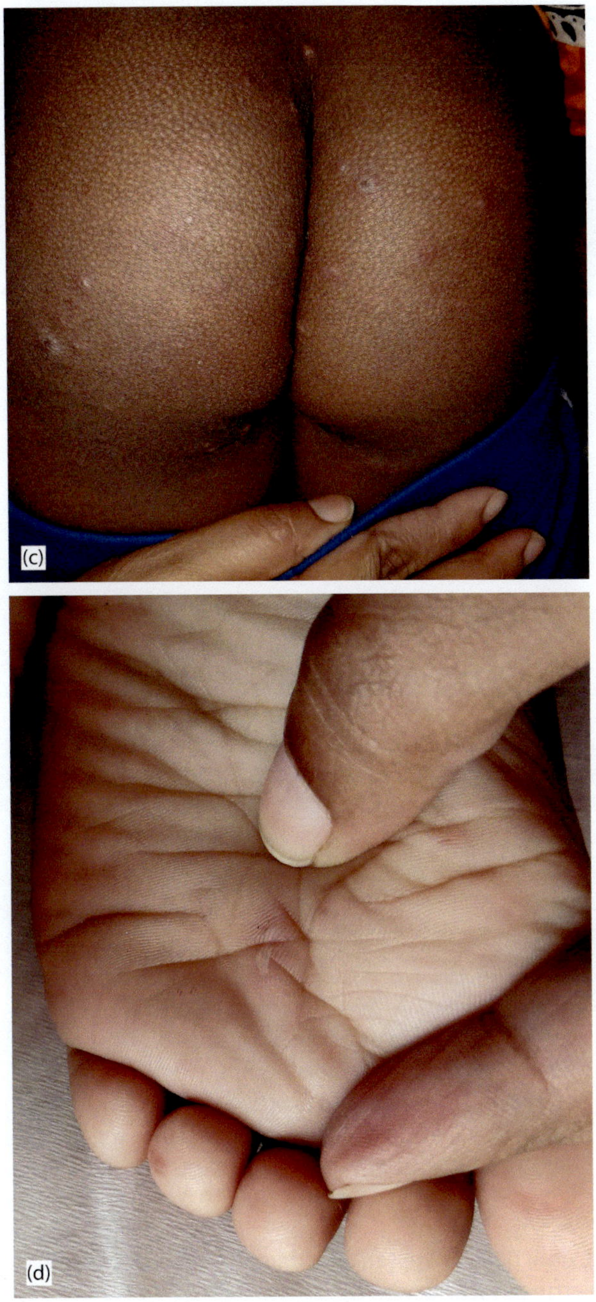


Figure 10.5 (*Continued*) **(c)** Vesicles on buttocks in hand, foot, and mouth disease. **(d)** Characteristic oblong vesicle on sole in hand, foot, and mouth disease. (a – Courtesy: Dr. Vishal Gupta, AIIMS, New Delhi, India.)

- Tense/flaccid bullae appear on a scabies-prone site with/without classic lesion of scabies (**Figure 10.6**).
- They are associated with excoriated papules elsewhere (circle of Hebra) and may burrow.
- DD: Bullous pemphigoid (more on extremities, no response to anti scabietic treatment).

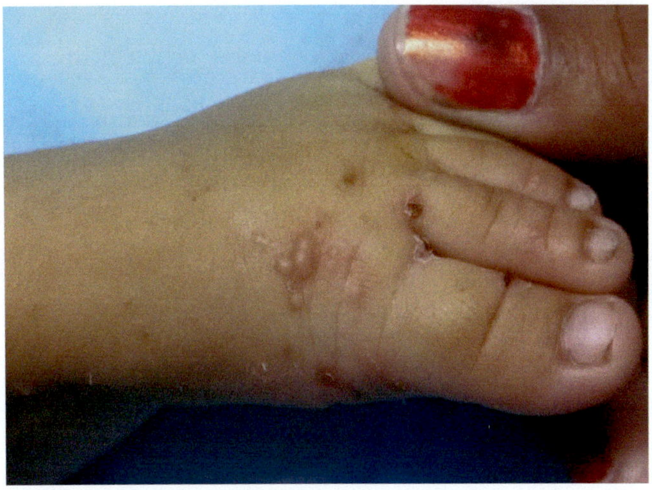

Figure 10.6 A patient with scabies having vesicles and excoriations on the dorsum of the foot. (Courtesy: Dr. Vishal Gupta, AIIMS, New Delhi, India.)

## Vesicobullous tinea pedis

- Vesicobullous tinea pedis is a dermatophyte infection of the soles of the feet and interdigital spaces.
- The most common cause is *Trichophyton rubrum*.
- Clinical features include painful/pruritic vesicobullous lesions on the instep and adjacent plantar surfaces of the feet (**Figure 10.7a,b**).
- It may be associated with "id reaction."
- DD: Pompholyx, allergic contact dermatitis, bullous impetigo.

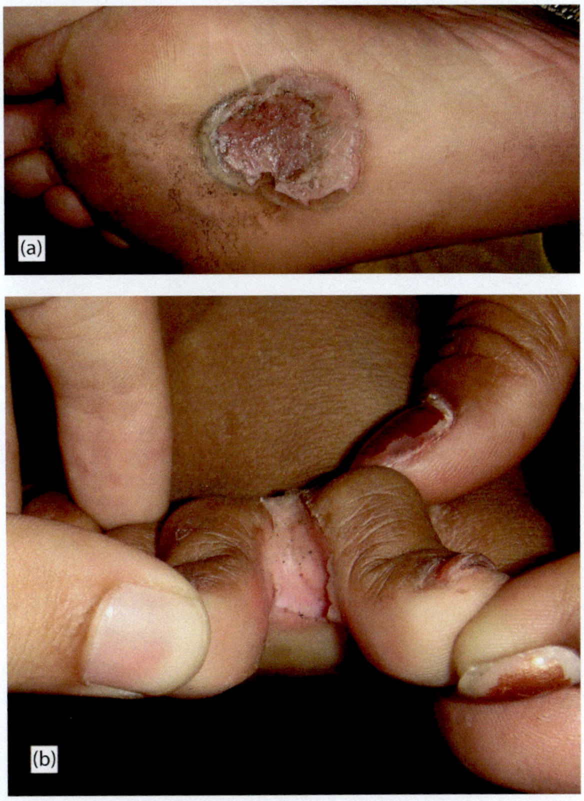


Figure 10.7 **(a)** Plantar surface showing bullous tinea with deroofed lesion and moist floor. **(b)** Same patient with interdigital tinea lesion. (a,b – Courtesy: Dr. Piyush Kumar, Katihar, India.)

## Sucking blister

- A sucking blister is caused by intense suction by the intrauterine fetus.
- It consists of flaccid, serous, blisters of 5–20 mm surrounded by normal skin (**Figure 10.8**).
- The location is the radial border of the forearm, wrist, hand, dorsal part of the thumb and forefinger.
- It is diagnosed as a congenital blister in typical site with good general condition.
- DD: Blistering distal dactylitis.

## Diabetic bulla/bullous diabeticorum

- The cause is spontaneous, non-inflammatory blistering in a diabetes setting.
- Clinical features include asymptomatic, large, asymmetrical tense bulla, usually on acral sites (**Figure 10.9a,b**).
- Signs of inflammation are typically absent.
- DD: Friction bulla, bullous fixed drug eruption, bullous pemphigoid.

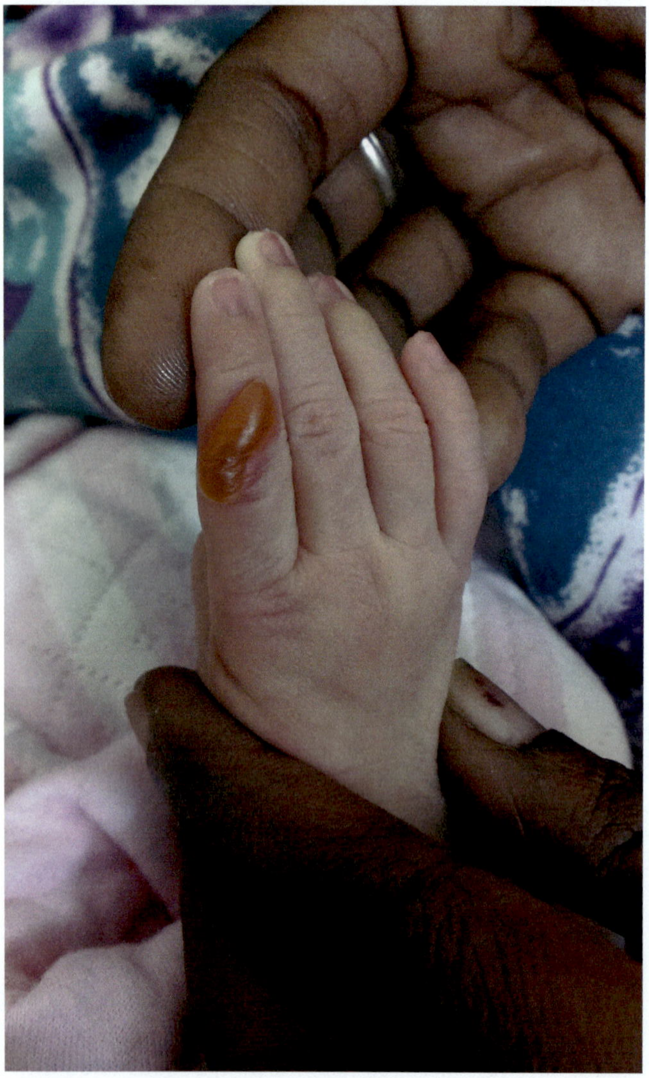

Figure 10.8 Oval flaccid, ducking blister. (Courtesy: Dr. Tanumay Raychaudhury, Sydney, Australia.)

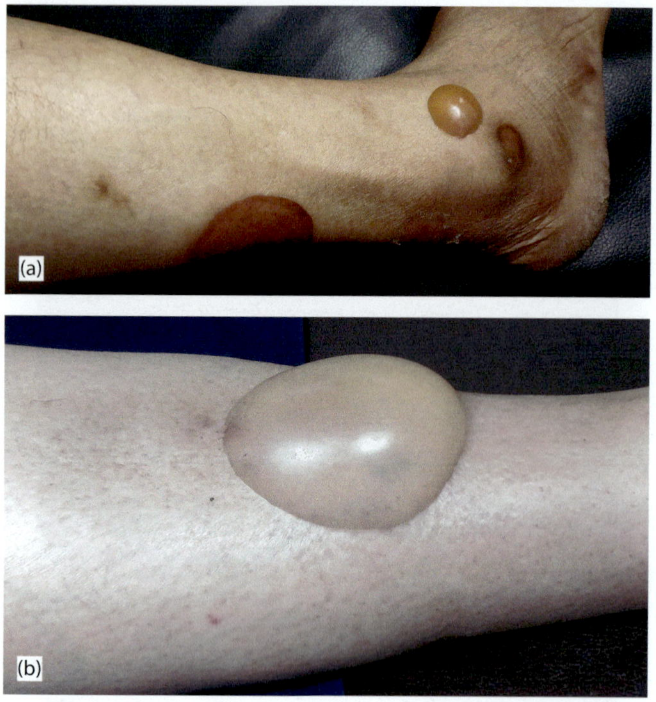

Figure 10.9 **(a)** Non-inflammatory bulla on the leg in diabetic patient. **(b)** Large diabetic bulla. (a – Courtesy: Dr. Anil Patki, Pune, India; b – Courtesy: Dr. Ganesh Avhad, Mumbai, India.)

## Bullous leukocytoclastic vasculitis

- This presents with blisters overlying purpuric macules and papules and with necrotic or hemorrhagic blisters (**Figure 10.10**).
- Bulla formation occurs due to necrosis of the skin overlying areas of small vessel vasculitis.
- Common locations are the lower extremities.
- Bullae appear in crops and may be associated with constitutional features such as fever, malaise, and joint pain.
- DD: Erythema multiforme, septic emboli.

## Coma blister

- Coma blisters are self-limiting blisters occurring in the setting of loss of consciousness (within 48–72 hours).
- Risk factors include neurological diseases, immobilization, metabolic conditions, substance poisoning, and drug overdoses primarily involving barbiturates, opiates, benzodiazepine, alcohol, and other neuropsychiatric medications.
- Blisters develop as a result of tissue hypoxia, ischemia, and local pressure effects.
- Clinical features include tense blisters on erythematous base, usually on pressure-dependent sites such as the fingers, forearms, malleoli, heels, buttocks, medial aspect of the knees, and other bony prominences.
- DD: Bullous cellulitis, friction blister.

## Blistering distal dactylitis

- Blistering distal dactylitis is a localized infection of the anterior pad of the distal phalanx of the digits.

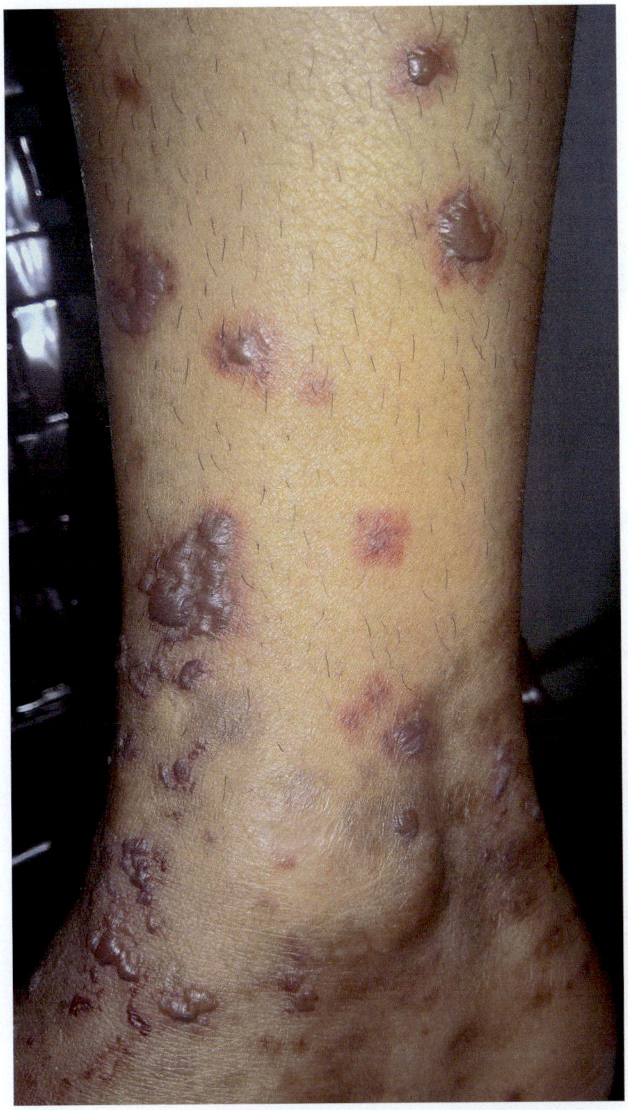

Figure 10.10 Necrotic blisters over purpuric papules in leukocytoclastic vasculitis. (Courtesy: Dr. Vishal Gupta, AIIMS, New Delhi, India.)

- Less common locations of infection include the proximal or lateral nail folds, palmar or dorsal hand, toes, and feet.
- Children are most commonly affected, but cases in adults are occasionally reported as well.
- The most common etiologic pathogen is group A beta-hemolytic *Streptococci* and, rarely, *Staphylococcus aureus*. Multiple bullae tend to occur more commonly with *S. aureus* infection.
- Autoinoculation of the digits from nose picking is proposed to play a role in causing blistering distal dactylitis.
- They present as tense, tender, oval bullae that are filled with thin, seropurulent fluid. These bullae eventually progress to bullae with central erosions or simple erosions with adherent layers of skin.
- DD: Herpetic whitlow, epidermolysis bullosa, bullous impetigo, friction blisters.

## Bullous impetigo

- This condition consists of flaccid transparent or pus-filled bullae, usually in neonates or children (**Figure 10.11a,b**).
- It is not associated with systemic symptoms.
- Common sites are the face, trunk, perineum, and extremities.
- Sometimes, it can have an annular arrangement of blisters with a central honey-colored crust (impetigo circinata) (**Figure 10.11c,d**); it can resemble chronic bullous disease of childhood (periorificial location) and vesicular/pustular tinea infection.
- DD: Neonatal candidiasis, erythema toxicum neonatorum, miliaria pustulosa.

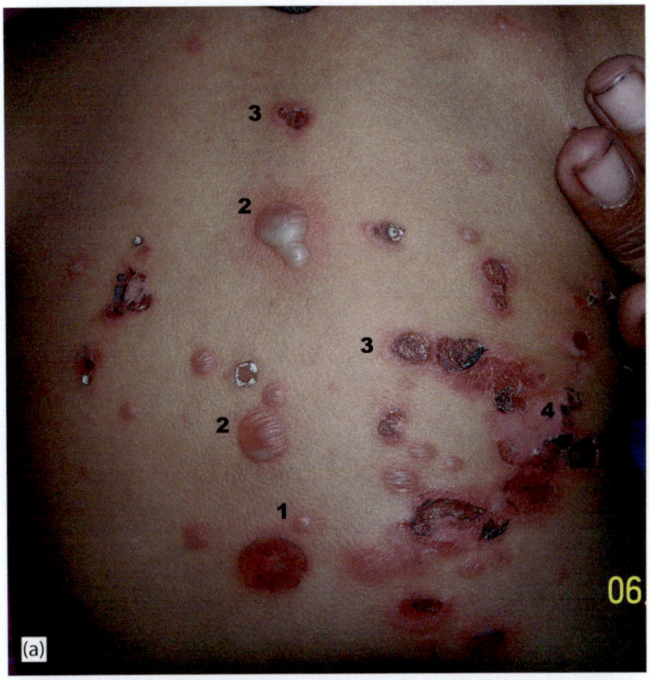


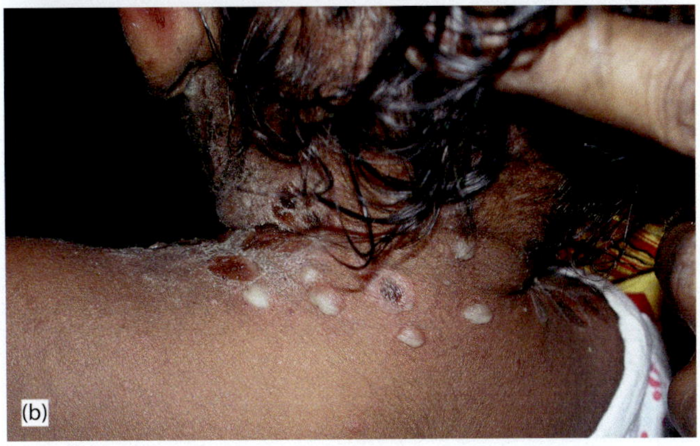


Figure 10.11 **(a)** Bullous impetigo – the lesion starts as a vesicle over an erythematous skin (1) and enlarges to form flaccid blisters with pus in their bottom part (2). Soon blisters rupture to leave erosions covered with crust (3) and ultimately heal with epithelization (4). **(b)** Bullous impetigo over neck. (*Continued*)

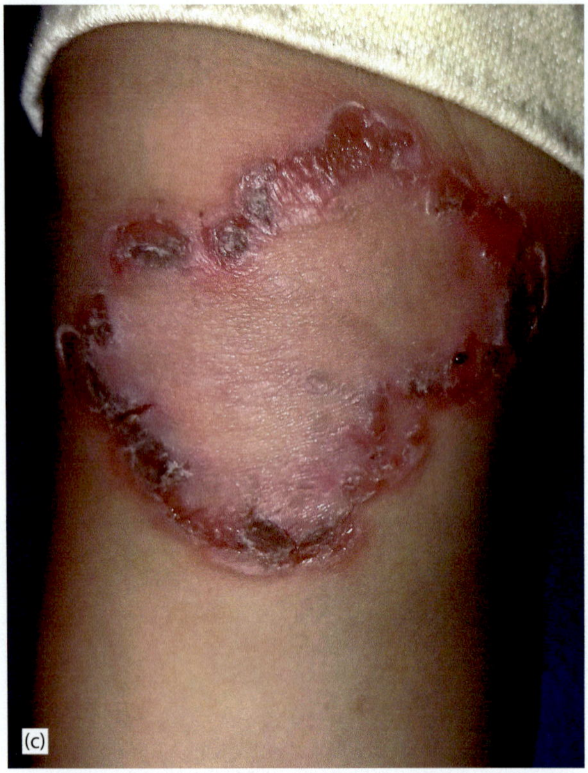

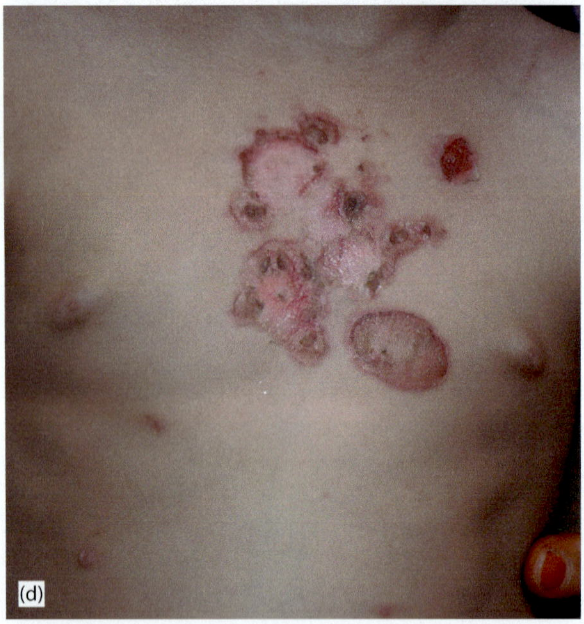

Figure 10.11 (*Continued*) **(c)** Honey-colored annular crust in impetigo circinata. **(d)** Annular lesions of impetigo circinata. (a,b,d – Courtesy: Dr. Piyush Kumar, Katihar, India; c – Courtesy: Dr. Vishal Gupta, AIIMS, New Delhi, India.)

## Bullous fixed drug eruption

- Bullae occur over the central area of dusky erythematous or violaceous round-to-oval macules and plaques (**Figure 10.12a–c**).
- It is associated with pain and a burning sensation.
- Common locations are lips, genitals, and acral sites.
- They heal with significant post-inflammatory hyperpigmentation.

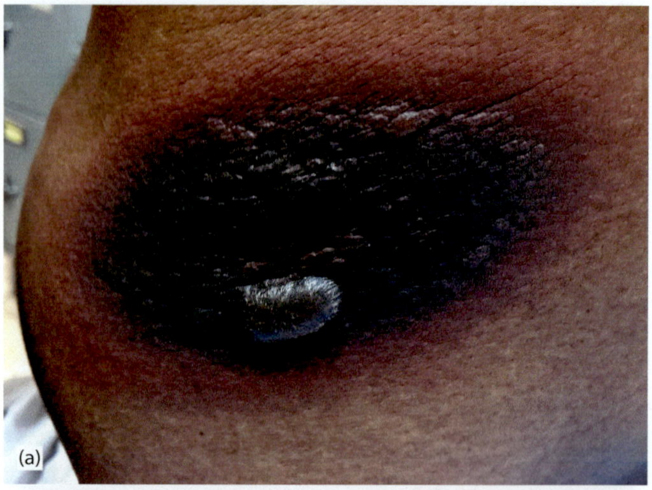

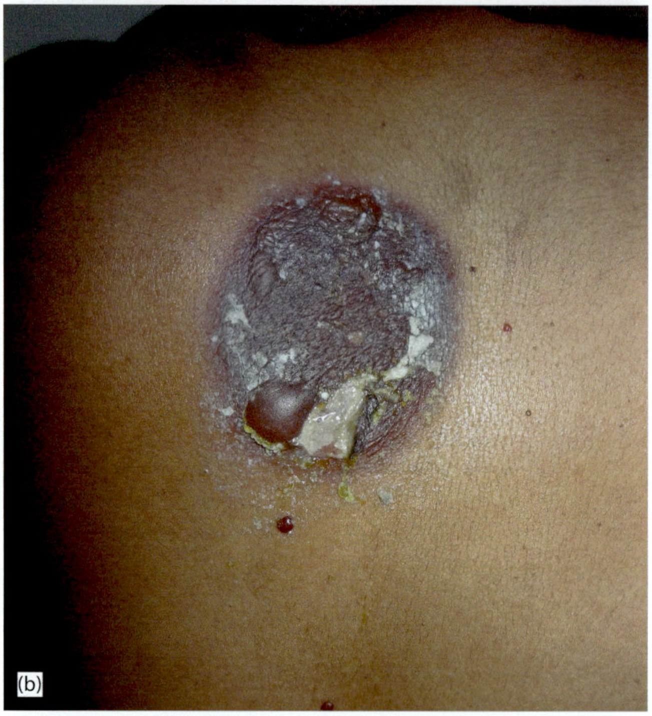

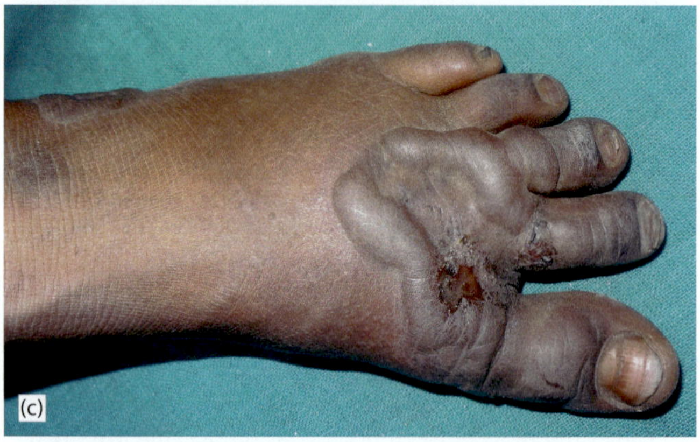

Figure 10.12 **(a)** Bullous fixed drug reaction. Hyperpigmented, oval patch surrounded by erythematous border with vesiculation. **(b)** Bulla over round, erythematous area of skin. **(c)** Bullous fixed drug eruption over the dorsum of the foot. (a – Courtesy: Dr. Vishal Gupta, AIIMS, New Delhi, India; b,c – Courtesy: Dr. Piyush Kumar, Katihar, India.)

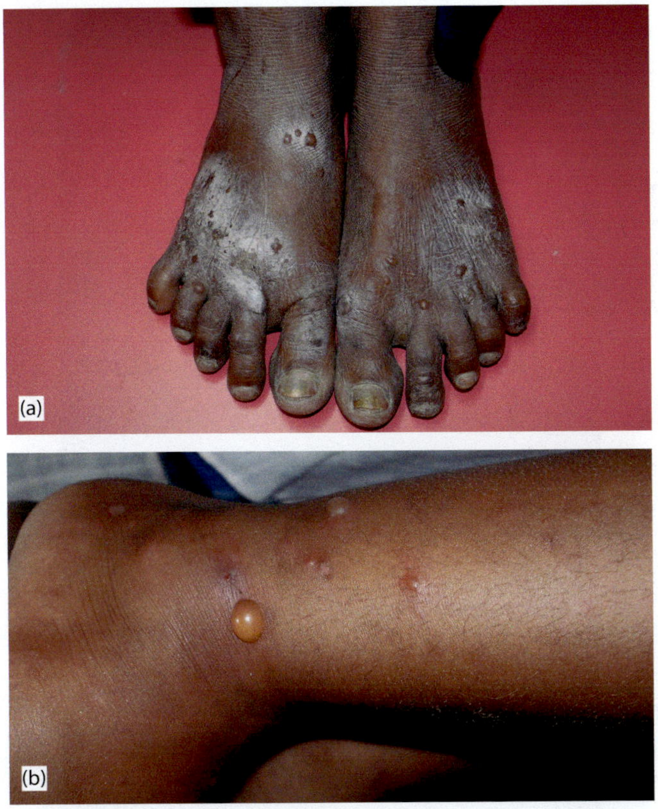

Figure 10.13 **(a)** Tense blisters on the dorsa of both feet due to insect bites. **(b)** Tense blisters of insect bite reaction in a child. (a,b – Courtesy: Dr. Piyush Kumar, Katihar, India.)

- Recurrence at the same site with subsequent implicated drug exposure is typical.

## Bullous insect-bite reaction

- Bullous lesions in reaction to insect bites are common with mosquitoes and bedbugs (**Figure 10.13a,b**).
- Skeeter syndrome is a mosquito saliva-induced large local inflammatory reaction clinically resembling cellulitis.
- Bedbug bites are known as cimicosis.
- Common sites are the arms, shoulders, and legs.

## Friction blister

- Friction blisters result from pressure/shear forces, causing delamination at the level of the stratum spinosum.
- Risk factors include outdoor pursuits (hiking, marathon races).
- The most common sites are the foot and areas with thick stratum corneum.
- Clinical features include distinct bulla on trauma site (**Figure 10.14a–c**).
- DD: Acquired/hereditary epidermolysis bullosa (other trauma-prone areas also involved).

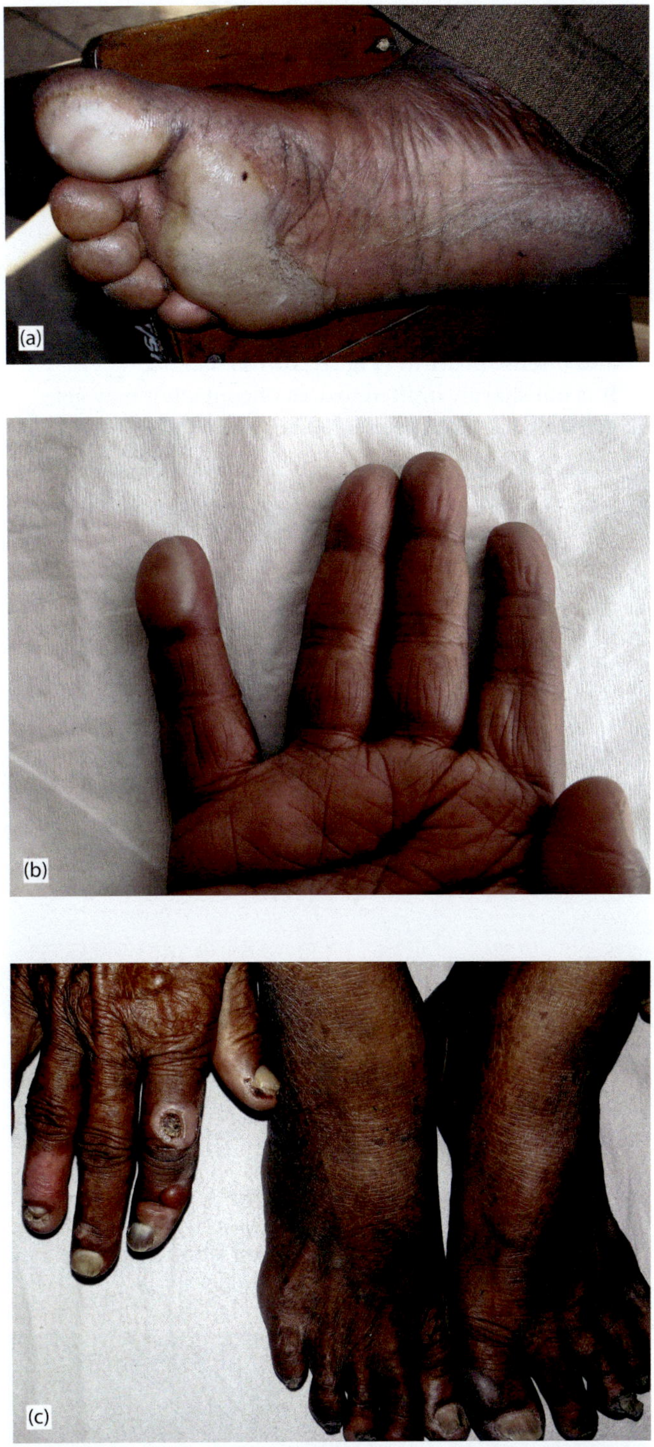

Figure 10.14 **(a)** Friction blisters on the pressure areas of the foot in leprosy. **(b)** Thermal damage resulting in blister on anesthetic hand in borderline tuberculoid leprosy. **(c)** Friction blisters on hand and feet in leprosy. (a – Courtesy: Dr. Piyush Kumar, Katihar, India.)

## Thermal burns

- Burn blisters are a common wound finding for health care providers treating burn patients in burn centers, emergency rooms, and other medical facilities.
- They are unique in that they incorporate several zones of tissue damage due to differences in heat transfer.
- In the inflammatory phase, blisters can occur as a physiological response to burn damage if the epidermis is separated from the underlying dermis.
- Deep partial-thickness blisters are thick-walled and contain white skin; sensation is either impaired or intact.

- Superficial partial-thickness blisters contain weeping skin and are typically thin-walled, with intact sensation (**Figure 10.15a–c**).

## Allergic contact dermatitis

- This is delayed hypersensitivity reaction of skin to contact with foreign substances; on re-exposure, sensitized T cells initiate an inflammatory cascade.
- Causative allergens include nickel, fragrances, neomycin, parabens.
- Clinical features are erythema, edema, vesicles, oozing, and intense pruritus (**Figure 10.16a–c**).
- It is not sharply limited to area of contact; it may get generalized on subsequent exposures.

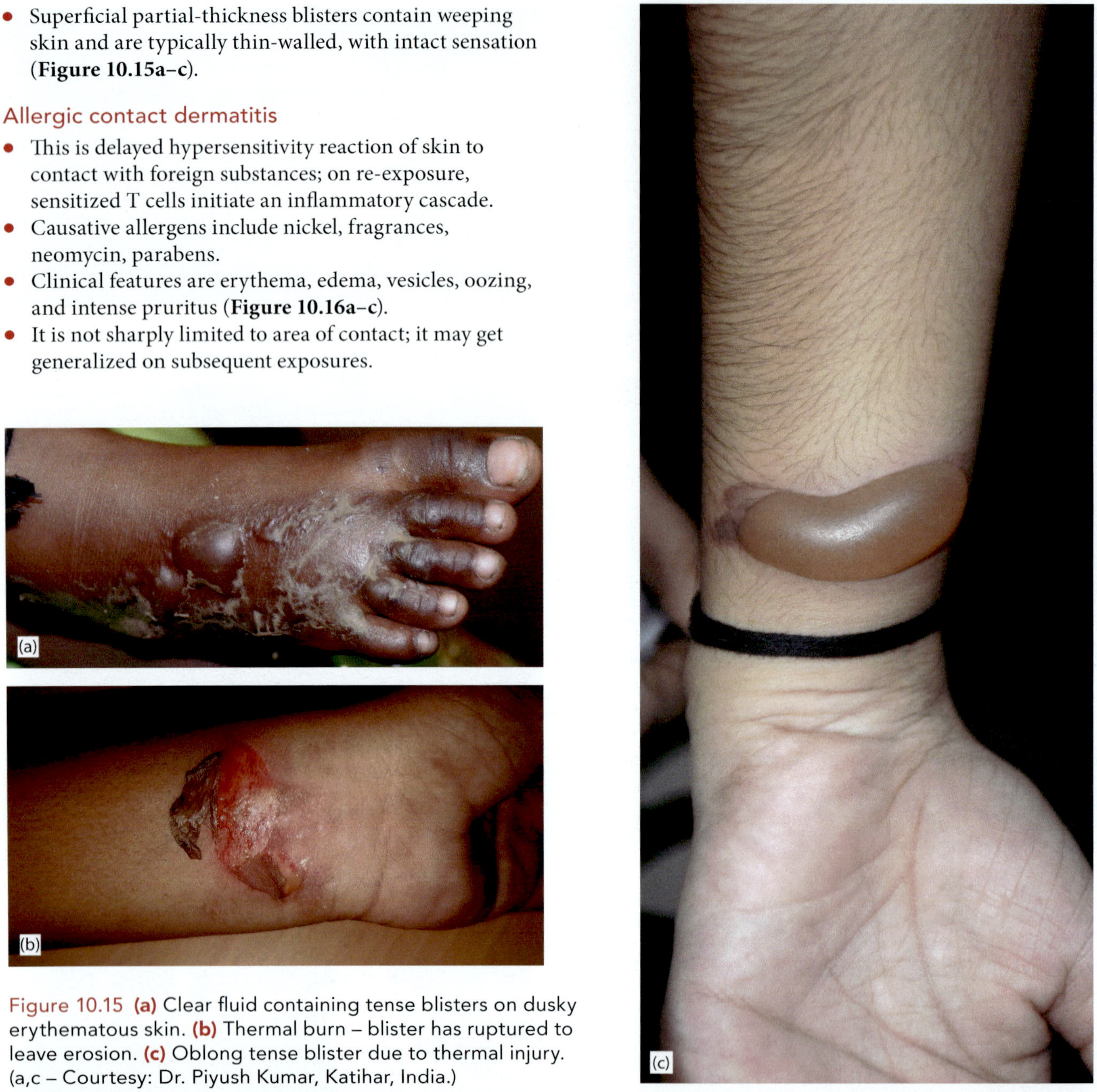

Figure 10.15 **(a)** Clear fluid containing tense blisters on dusky erythematous skin. **(b)** Thermal burn – blister has ruptured to leave erosion. **(c)** Oblong tense blister due to thermal injury. (a,c – Courtesy: Dr. Piyush Kumar, Katihar, India.)

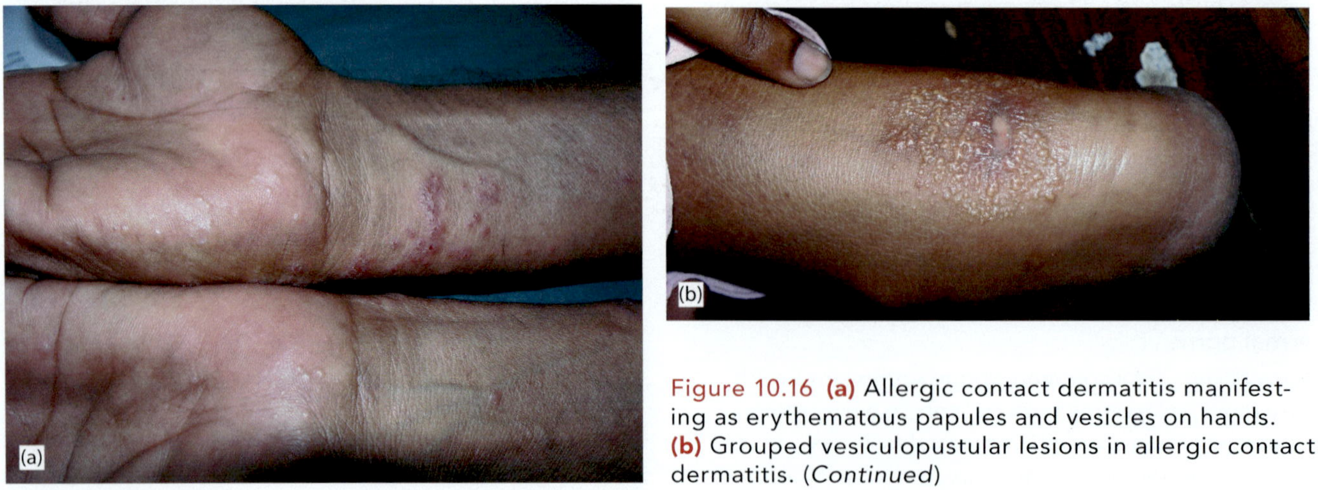

Figure 10.16 **(a)** Allergic contact dermatitis manifesting as erythematous papules and vesicles on hands. **(b)** Grouped vesiculopustular lesions in allergic contact dermatitis. (*Continued*)

- DD: Pompholyx, nummular dermatitis, irritant contact dermatitis.

### Acute irritant contact dermatitis (ICD)

- This is a result of inflammatory and cytotoxic effects caused by exposure to various irritant stimuli, which activate the innate immune system.
- Irritants induce skin barrier disruption and direct cellular damage.
- Symptoms include burning, pain, stinging, pruritus, and soreness.
- Signs are erythema, edema, oozing/exudation, bullae, and erosions (**Figure 10.17a–c**).

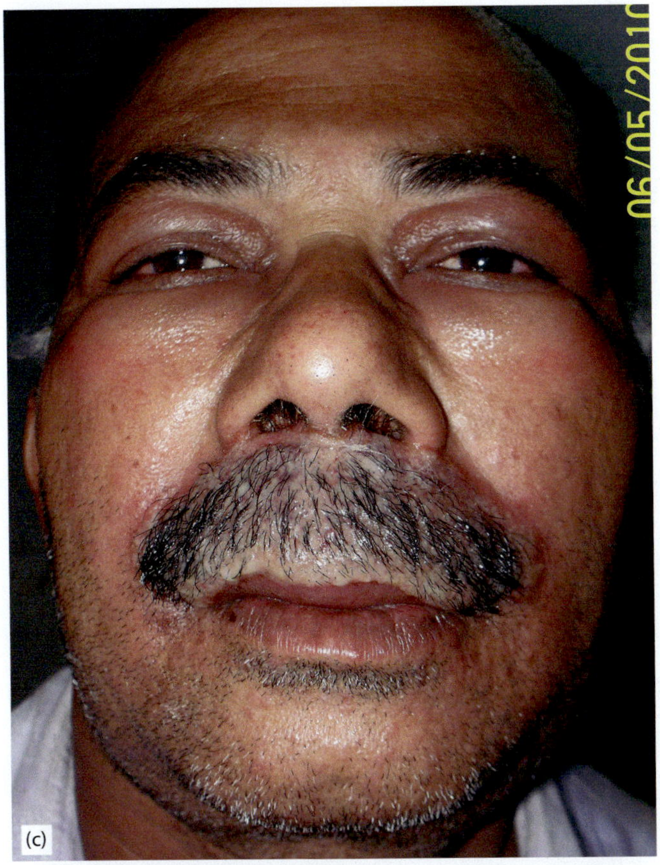


Figure 10.16 (*Continued*) **(c)** Severe allergic contact dermatitis to hair dye manifesting as blisters over eyelids, facial edema and erythema, and oozing. (a–c – Courtesy: Dr. Piyush Kumar, Katihar, India.)

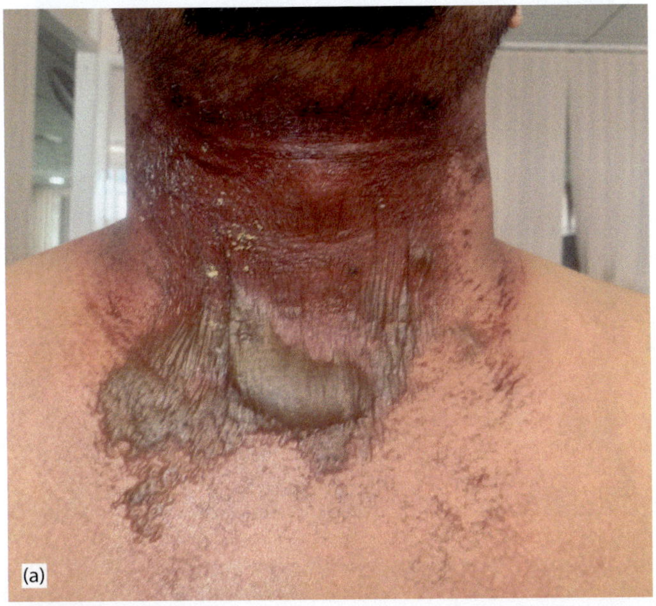


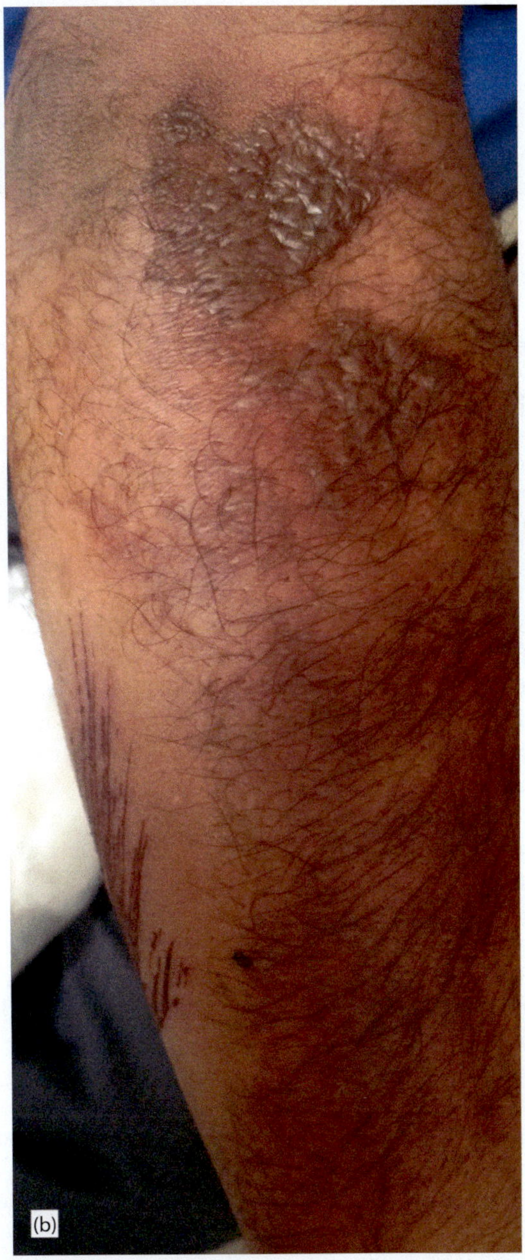


Figure 10.17 **(a)** Flaccid blister and dusky erythematous skin in irritant contact dermatitis to an antiseptic solution containing chlorhexidine gluconate and cetrimide among others. **(b)** Patient applied an antiseptic solution (containing chlorhexidine gluconate and cetrimide among others) over abrasions and developed irritant contact dermatitis. (*Continued*)

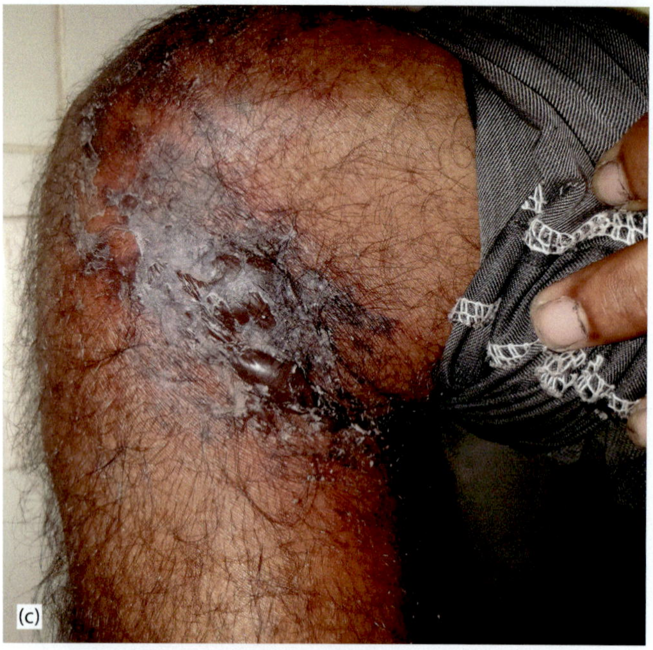

Figure 10.17 (*Continued*) **(c)** Irritant contact dermatitis over medial aspect of knee.

- The severity of the condition and hence, clinical feature depends on the nature, concentration, duration of contact with the irritant chemical, pre-existing skin conditions, mechanical, thermal, or climatic effects.

## Herpes simplex

- This is caused by herpes simplex virus (HSV) types 1 and 2.
- HSV-1 affects above the waist while HSV-2 causes infections below the waist; overlap may occur.
- Infection may be primary or following reactivation.
- HSV-1 mostly causes orolabial infections; it may infect other cutaneous sites also (herpetic whitlow, herpes gladiatorum).
- Grouped vesico-ulcerative lesions occur the on erythematous base palate, gingiva, tongue, lips, and perioral area (**Figure 10.18a–c**).
- Pharyngitis, fever, tender cervical lymphadenopathy may be present.
- HSV2 lesions are seen on the labia majora, minora, cervix, vagina, and mons pubis in females and on the penile shaft in males.
- Perianal lesions may occur, depending on sexual practice.
- Pain, dysuria, fever, tender inguinal lymphadenopathy may be present.
- DD: Paederus dermatitis, bullous fixed drug eruption, aphthous ulcer.

## Herpes zoster (HZ)

- Herpes zoster is caused by reactivation of a latent varicella zoster virus infection.

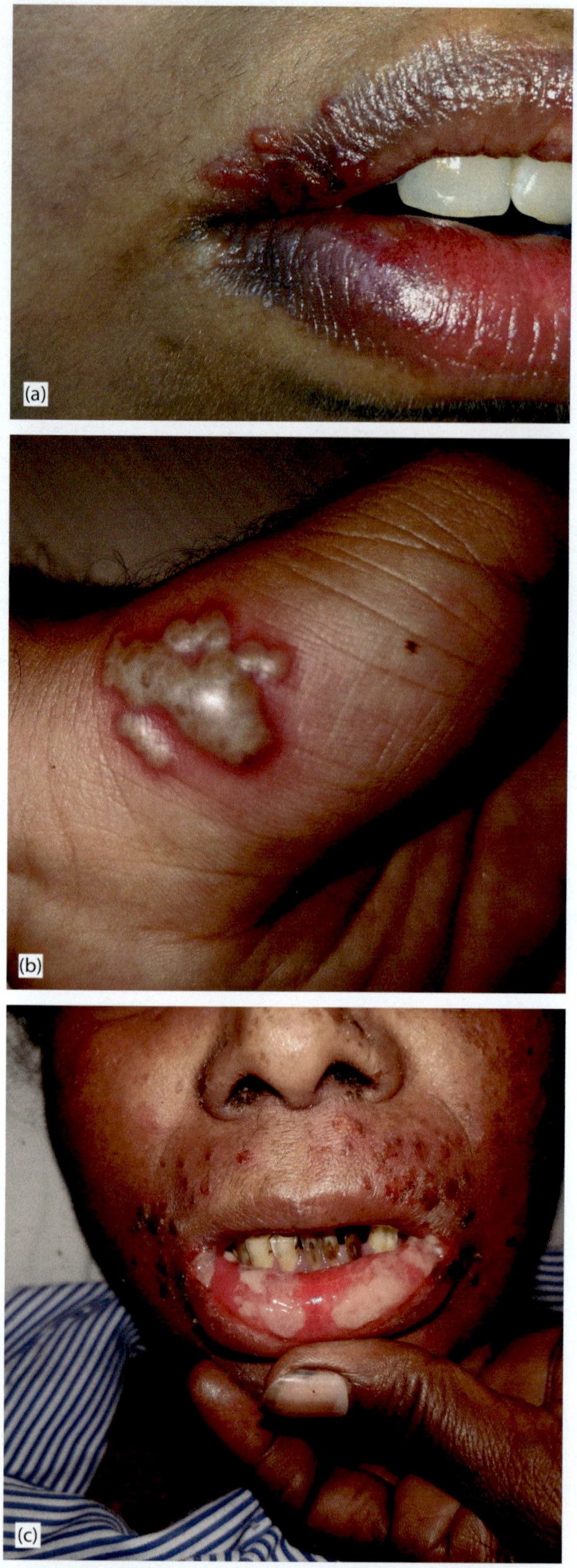

Figure 10.18 **(a)** Herpes labialis. Grouped vesicles on an inflammatory base. **(b)** Multiloculated blisters in herpes simplex on hand. **(c)** Herpes simplex with gingivostomatitis. Oral blisters rupture rapidly, leaving erosions covered with whitish slough. (a – Courtesy: Dr. Vishal Gupta, AIIMS, New Delhi.)

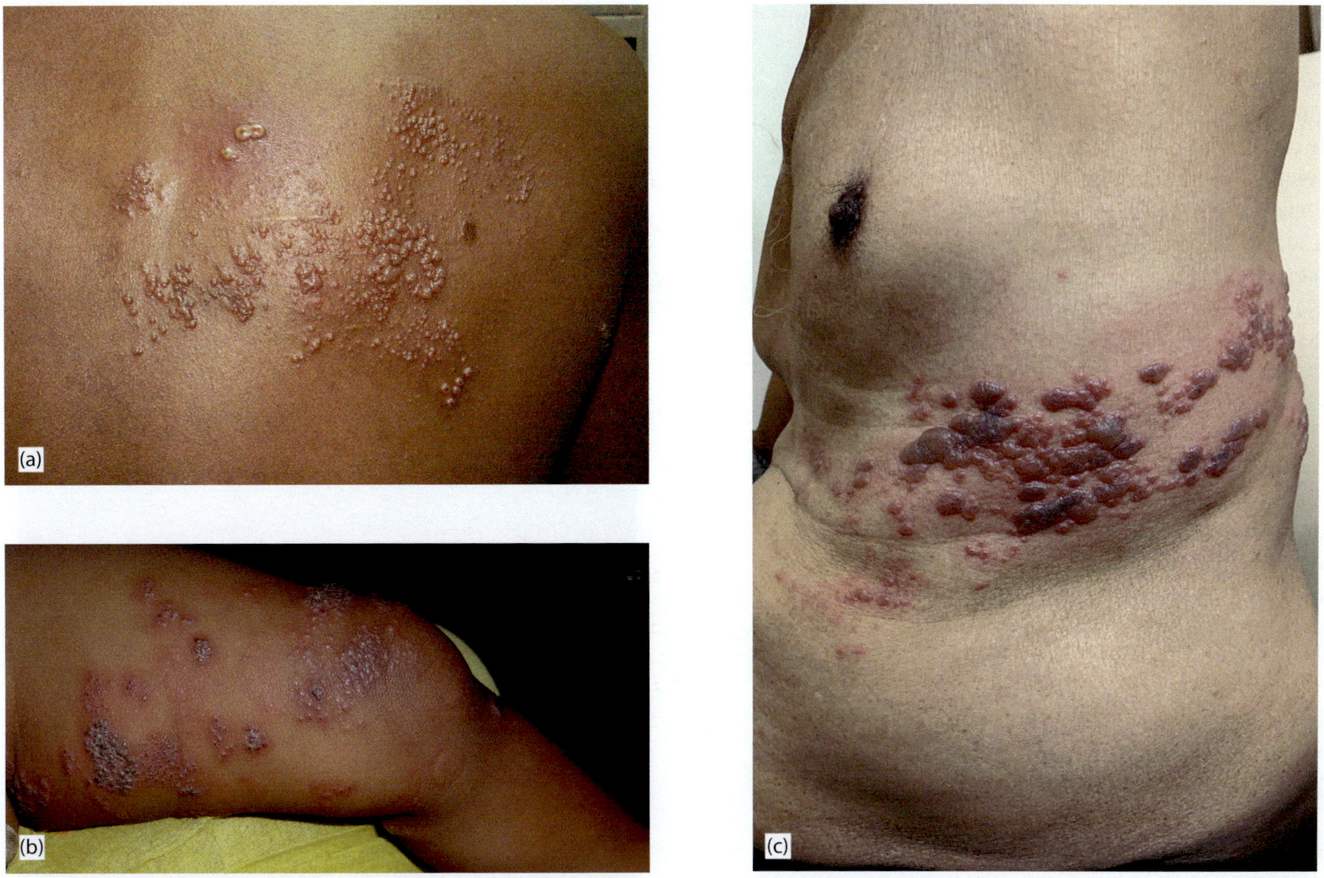


Figure 10.19 **(a)** Herpes zoster presenting as multiple groups of blisters on an inflammatory base along T3–T4 dermatome. **(b)** Herpes zoster along L2–L3 dermatome in an infant. **(c)** Bullae in herpes zoster. (a – Courtesy: Dr. Vishal Gupta, AIIMS, New Delhi; c – Courtesy: Dr. Piyush Kumar, Katihar, India.)

- Prodromal symptoms that herald HZ include pruritus, dysesthesia, and pain along the distribution of the involved dermatome.
- The rash consists of grouped vesicles on a red base in a unilateral, dermatomal distribution (**Figure 10.19a–c**).
- Most commonly affected area is the thoracic dermatome.
- Herpes zoster ophthalmicus may cause keratitis, scarring, and vision loss.
- DD: ICD, herpes simplex.

## Incontinentia pigmenti

- Incontinentia pigmenti (IP), a rare X-linked dominant genodermatosis, is a multisystem, ectodermal and mesodermal disorder accompanied by dermatologic, dental and ocular features. In a minority of cases, neurologic deficits may occur.
- Pathogenesis is mutation of the NEMO gene.
- Stage 1 (vesicular stage) is present at birth or within the first two weeks in 90% of patients; it is characterized by a rash of erythematous blisters, often appearing along the lines of Blaschko (**Figure 10.20**).
- Stage 1 is short lived and may be completed in utero. It is followed by stage 2 (verrucous stage), stage 3 (hyperpigmented stage), and stage 4 (atrophic/hypopigmented stage).
- Stage 2 occurs in about 70% of patients. Eruption of hyperkeratotic verrucous papules and plaques develop over the healing blisters.

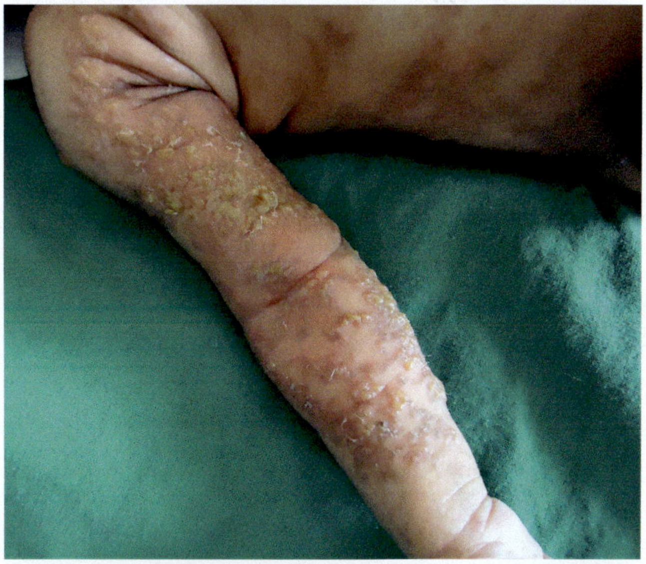

Figure 10.20 Vesicles and crusted erosions along Blaschko's lines in incontinentia pigmenti. (Courtesy: Dr. Sweta Rambhia, Mumbai, India.)

- Stage 3 is seen in 98% of patients as pigmentation (blue-gray or slate to brown) in streaks or whorls.
- Stage 4 is observed in adolescence and persists into adulthood.
- Involvement of appendageal structures may result in vertex alopecia, ridged, pitted, or dystrophic nails.
- Dental abnormalities include delayed dentition, partial anodontia, conical or peg-shaped teeth, or absence of teeth.
- Neurologic manifestations include seizures, mental retardation, developmental delays, spastic paralysis, ataxia, and motor dysfunction.
- Ocular abnormalities include strabismus, cataracts, optic atrophy, retinal dysfunction, uveitis, nystagmus, and blindness.
- Occasionally there may be skeletal and structural anomalies, such as somatic asymmetry, skull deformities, spina bifida, dwarfism, syndactyly, extra ribs, primary pulmonary hypertension, and cardiopulmonary failure.

## Lymphangioma circumscriptum

- Lymphangioma circumscriptum (LC) is a benign lymphatic malformation characterized by dilation of lymphatic vessels in the skin and subcutaneous tissue. These abnormal lymphatic malformations do not communicate to the normal lymphatics.
- The exact cause is unknown. It may be congenital or acquired due to damage of lymphatic vessels from various etiologies.
- However, various growth factors, such as vascular endothelial growth factor-C (VEGF-C) and VEGF-D and their receptors on the lymphatic endothelial cells, may have a role in the mechanism.
- It is commonly found in the chest, mouth, axilla, and tongue.
- It is characterized by translucent, pink-red vesicle bundles with thin membranes, sometimes filled with blood; the vesicles have clear edges and can be scattered or in groups; hyperkeratosis may give rise to a warty appearance (**Figure 10.21a,b**).
- DD: Lymphangiectasia, hemangioma, verruca, molluscum contagiosum, angiokeratoma, and lymphangioendothelioma.

## Paederus dermatitis

- Paederus dermatitis is an irritant dermatitis caused by pederin, a toxin produced by the rove beetle (*Paederus*).
- The hemolymph of the *Paederus* beetle contains this pederin, which is released when crushing the insect onto the skin by the reflex of brushing away the insect.
- Symptoms typically begin between 24 and 48 hours after contact with the insect, the most common being itching and burning or smarting sensation.
- Lesions evolve through an initial erythematous phase followed by vesiculation and subsequent crusting and desquamation.

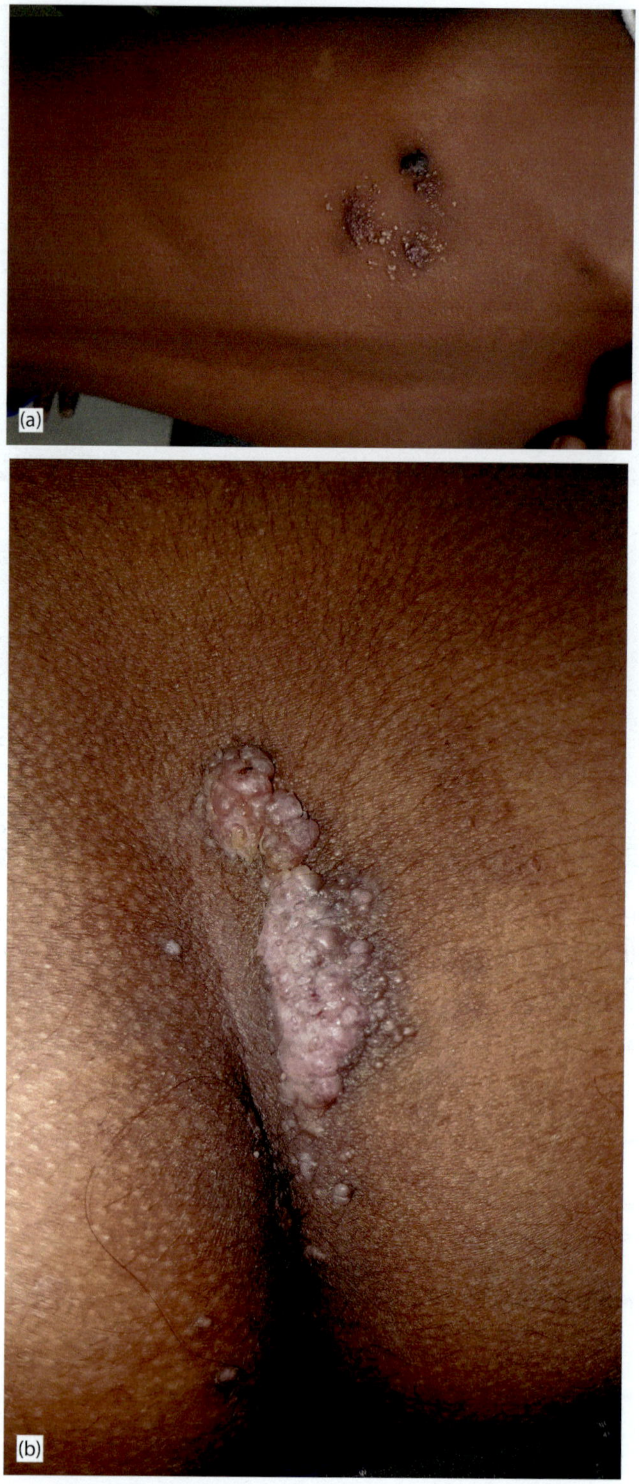


Figure 10.21 **(a)** Lymphangioma circumscriptum presenting as grouped translucent, pink vesicles on the trunk. **(b)** Lymphangioma circumscriptum over the gluteal area. (a – Courtesy: Dr. Piyush Kumar, Katihar, India.)

- Morphological patterns include linear dermatitis (**Figure 10.22a**), kissing lesions (**Figure 10.22b**), localized pustules (**Figure 10.22c**), and, rarely, extensive skin involvement with systemic manifestations such as fever, neuralgia, arthralgia.

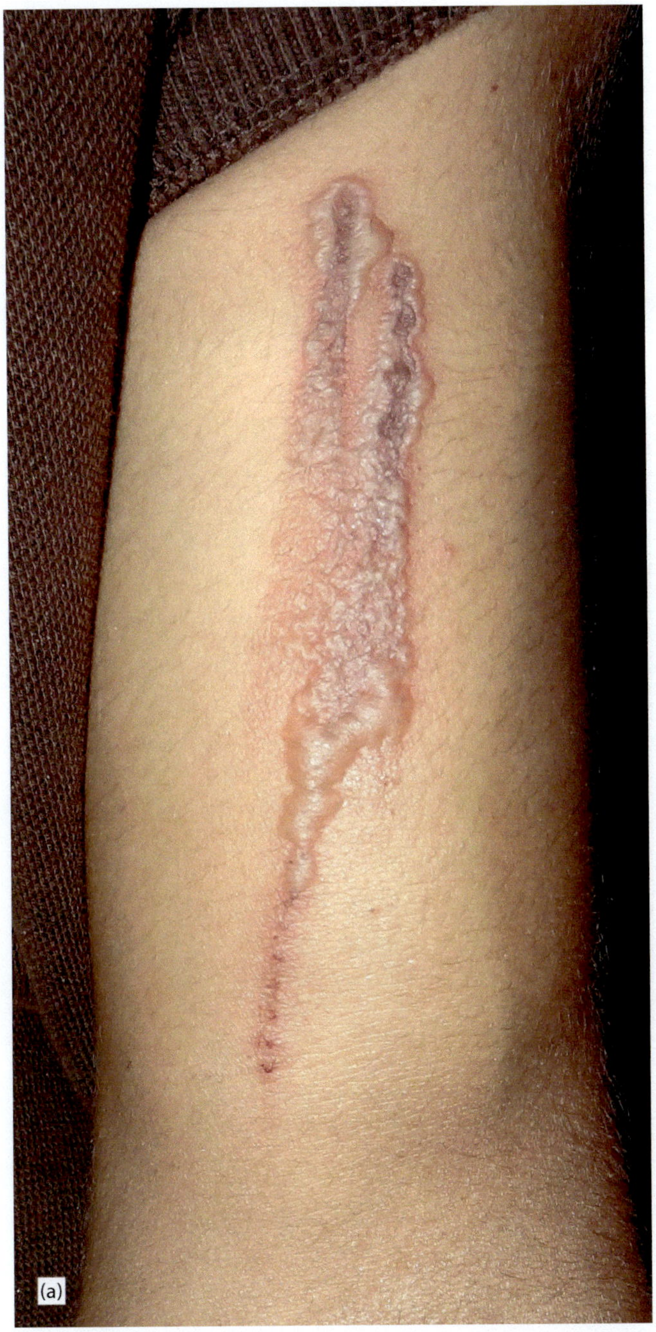

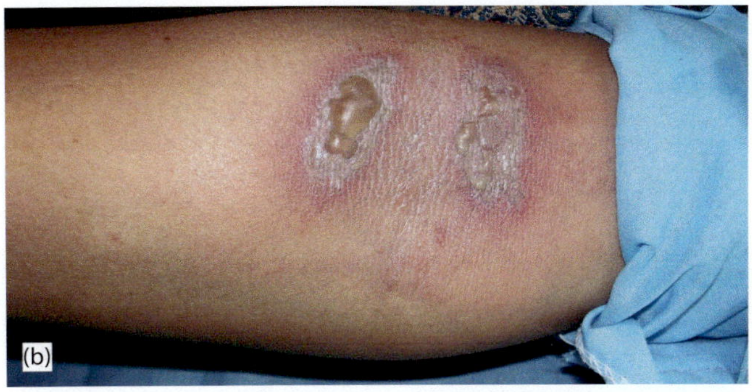

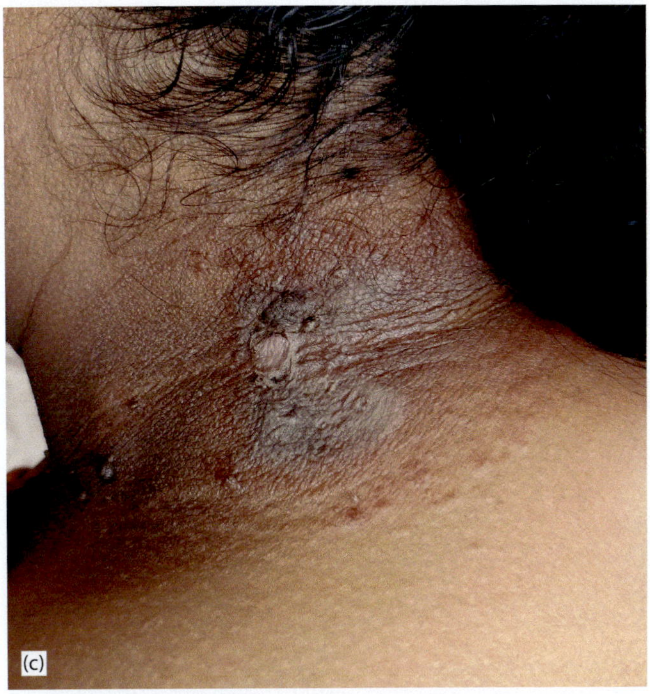

Figure 10.22 **(a)** Paederus dermatitis as vesicopustular lesions on erythematous base, arranged in a linear fashion on the arm. **(b)** "Kissing lesions" in paederus dermatitis – blisters on an erythematous base. **(c)** Irritant contact dermatitis with necrotic skin surrounded by erythema. The epidermal damage is maximum in the center of the lesion. (b – Courtesy: Dr. PC Das, Katihar, India.)

- Moderately severe cases with significant vesiculation may dry out and exfoliate with hyperpigmentation that may last up to a month. Cutaneous necrosis may occur occasionally.
- DD: Herpes zoster, herpes simplex, irritant contact dermatitis, blister beetle dermatitis.

## Bullous cellulitis

- Cellulitis is a bacterial infection of the skin, presenting with poorly demarcated erythema, edema, warmth, and tenderness.
- Portals of entry include toe web-space infections and venous ulcers.
- Streptococcus pyogenes is the most common.
- Clinical features include acute, spreading, poorly demarcated area of erythema, blister formation, and peau d'orange appearance of skin; fever may be present (**Figure 10.23a**).
- DD: Erysipelas (presence of sharp border) (**Figure 10.23b**), necrotizing fasciitis (rapidly spreading, very painful), Sweet syndrome.

## Erysipelas

- Erysipelas is a streptococcal infection involving the upper dermis and extending into the superficial cutaneous lymphatics.

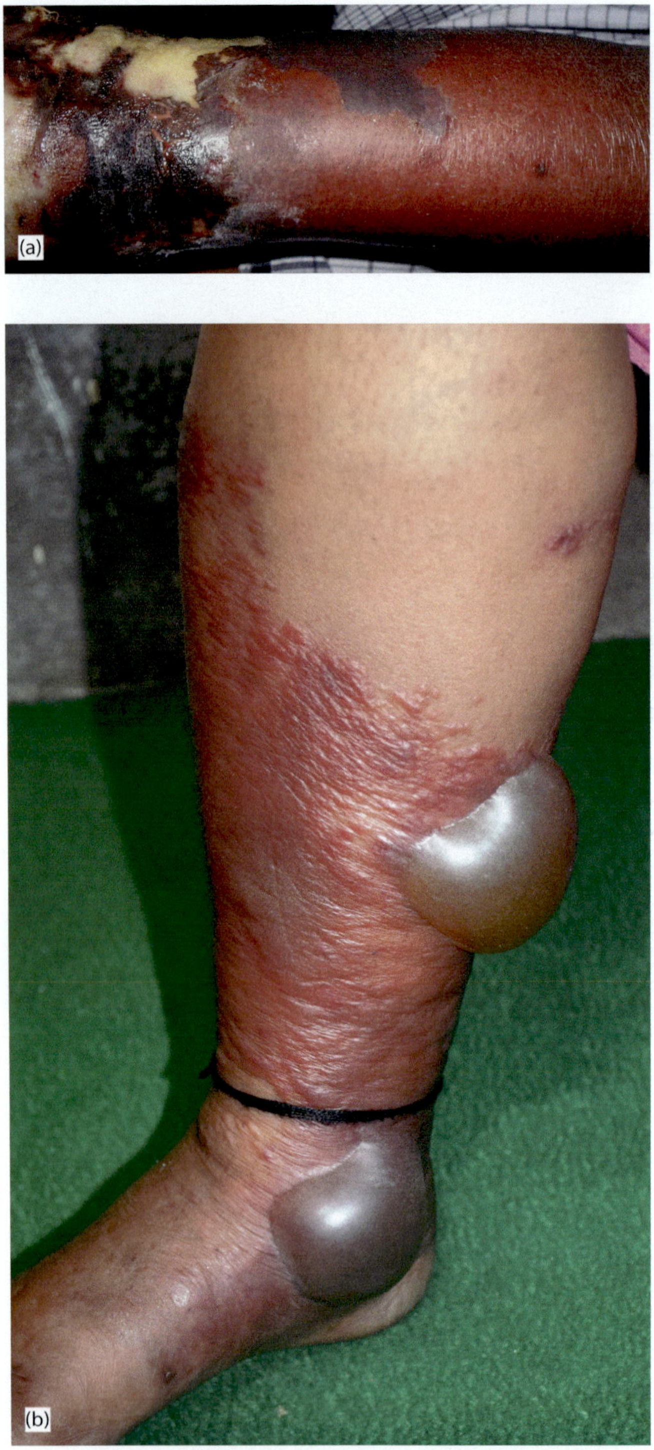


Figure 10.23 **(a)** Swelling, erythema, and erosion in bullous cellulitis. **(b)** Well-defined, erythematous, edematous plaque of erysipelas with tense bullae on its surface. (b – Courtesy: Dr. Piyush Kumar, Katihar, India.)

- Risk factors include lymphatic obstruction, immunosuppression, venous insufficiency, dermatophyte infection.
- Clinical features include high fever, chills, and malaise.
- The cutaneous finding will show fiery red, indurated, shiny plaque with a sharp raised border; lower limbs are involved in 80% of cases (**Figure 10.24a–c**).
- DD: Cellulitis, allergic contact dermatitis, erysipeloid.

## Ecthyma gangrenosum

- This is a condition caused by *Pseudomonas aeruginosa.*
- Risk factors include immunosuppression with severe neutropenia.

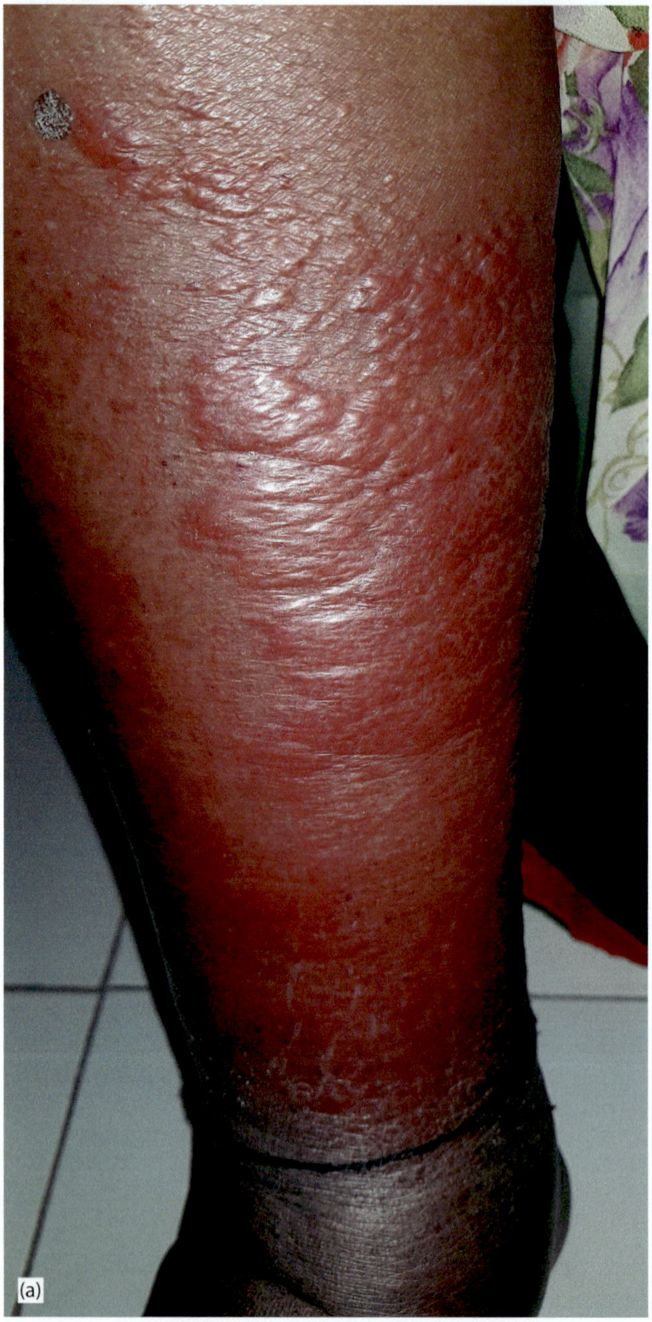


Figure 10.24 **(a)** Well-defined, erythematous, indurated lesion with surface vesiculation in erysipelas. (*Continued*)

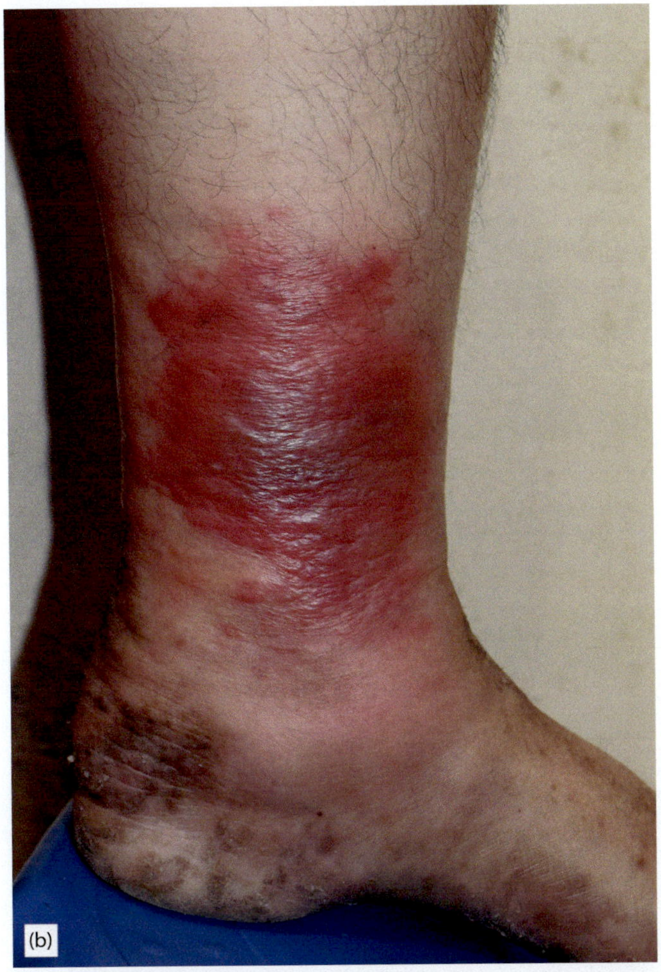


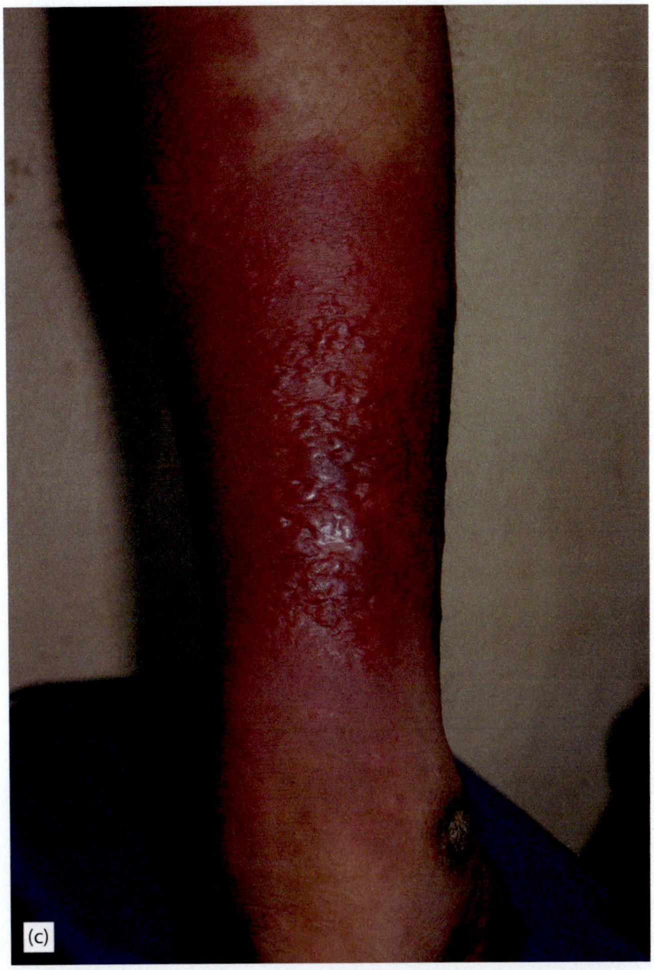


Figure 10.24 (*Continued*) **(b)** Well-defined, erythematous, edematous plaque with surface vesiculation in erysipelas. **(c)** Erysipelas with surface vesiculation. (a – Courtesy: Dr. PC Das, Katihar, India; b,c – Courtesy: Dr. Piyush Kumar, Katihar, India.)

- Erythematous/purpuric macules appear on the skin.
- They evolve into hemorrhagic vesicles and blisters and rupture to form necrotic ulcers with black eschar over extremities and anogenital regions.
- DD: Cutaneous anthrax.

## Erysipeloid

- Erysipeloid is caused by gram positive bacilli *Erysiplothrix rhusiopathiae.*
- It occurs through traumatic inoculation in fishermen/ meat handlers.
- Clinically it manifests as a violaceous to erythematous area of non-suppurative cellulitis.
- Hemorrhagic vesicles may appear.
- DD: Erysipelas, cellulitis, FDE.

## Cutaneous anthrax

- This is caused by occupational exposure to gram positive bacilli *Bacillus anthracis.*
- It affects exposed body parts after contact with infected animals/their hides or carcasses.
- A purpuric macule evolves into a vesicle surrounded by non-pitting edema (**Figure 10.25**).
- The vesicle ruptures into a hemorrhagic ulcer with black eschar.
- DD: Ecthyma gangrenosum, cellulitis, spider bite.

## Vibrio vulnificus infection

- This is caused be gram negative anaerobic bacteria.
- Risk factors include diabetes and chronic liver disease.
- There is often a history of exposure to warm sea water and raw or undercooked seafood consumption.
- Erythematous macules progress to vesicles and hemorrhagic bullae.
- Necrotizing fasciitis may ensue.
- Other features include fever, chills, nausea, vomiting, diarrhea, abdominal cramps, and hypotension.

## Orf

- Orf is an infection caused by *Parapoxvirus* and mainly affects goats and sheep.

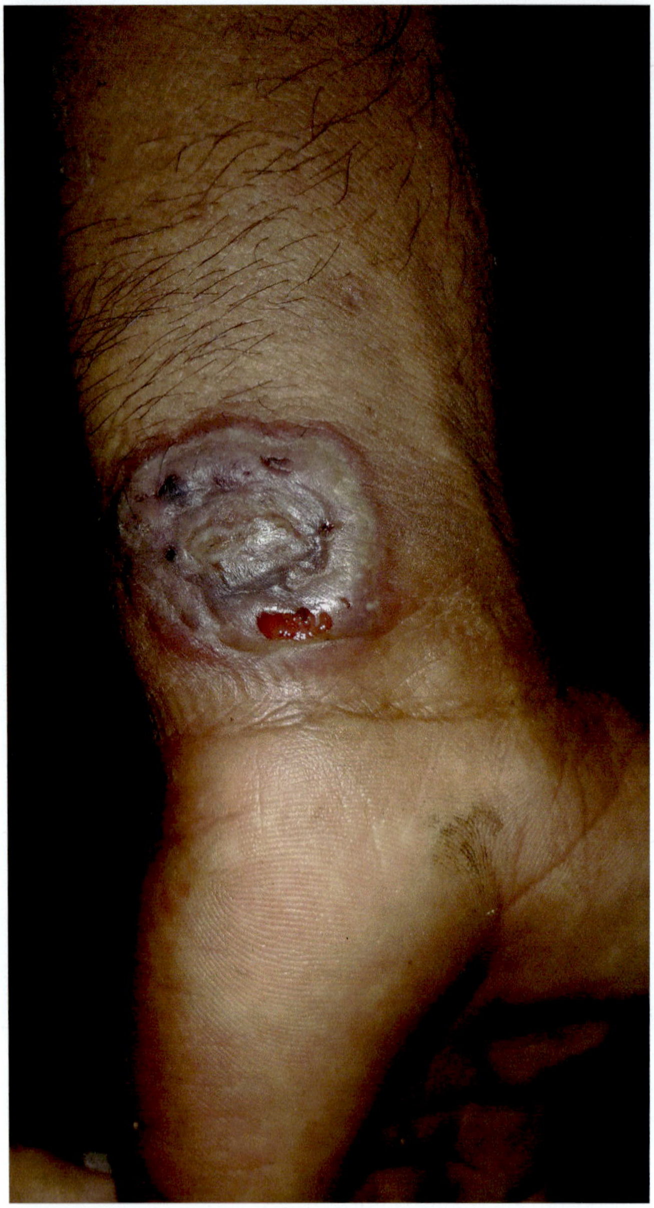

Figure 10.25 Cutaneous anthrax presenting as vesicopustular lesion on an erythematous, edematous base. (Courtesy: Dr. Rajesh Kumar Mandal, North Bengal Medical College, Darjeeling, India.)

- Humans get infected by direct inoculation through cuts or abrasions while handling animals, carcasses, or contaminated equipment.
- A lesion appears three to seven days after contact with an infected animal and evolves slowly over the course of four to eight weeks.
- It starts as a firm red painful papule that expands into a broad, thickened 1- to 3-cm lesion.
- The center of the lesion is red and is surrounded by a white, raised ring with erythematous periphery. The crusting occurs and resolves by three to six weeks, with little to no scarring (**Figure 10.26a,b**).
- DD: Cutaneous anthrax, pyoderma gangrenosum, and herpetic whitlow.

## Hidrocystoma

- Also known as cystadenomas, sudoriferous cysts, and Moll's gland cysts, hidrocystomas are benign cystic tumors derived from either the eccrine or apocrine sweat gland.
- The difference between eccrine hidrocystoma (EH) and apocrine hidrocystoma (AH) can be tabulated as in **Table 10.1**.

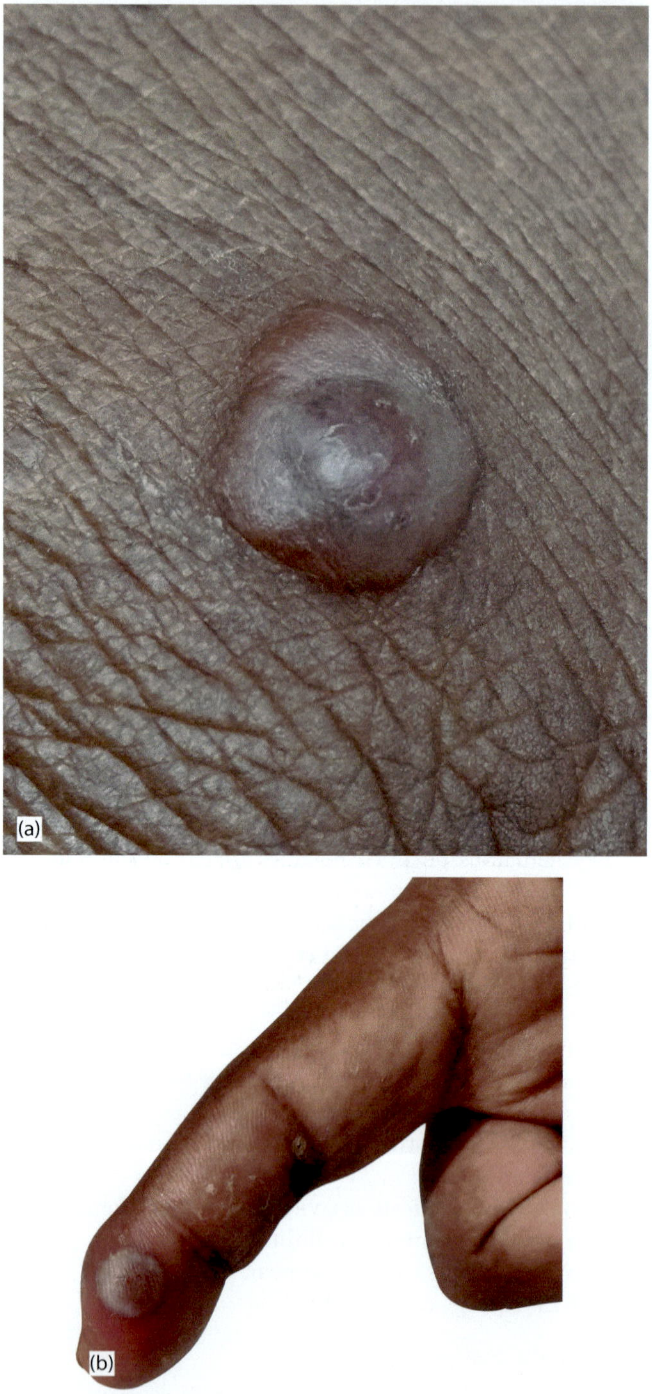


Figure 10.26 **(a)** Blister of orf. **(b)** Vesicopustular lesion of orf on the finger. (a – Courtesy: Dr. Deverashetti Srinivas, Nizamabad, India; b – Courtesy: Dr. Shahid Hassan, Purnea, India.)

Table 10.1 Differences between eccrine hidrocystoma (EH) and apocrine hidrocystoma (AH)

| | Eccrine hidrocystoma | Apocrine hidrocystoma |
|---|---|---|
| **Appearance** | Skin-colored to bluish vesiculopapular lesions (**Figure 10.27a**) | Translucent or semi-transparent, round, skin-colored or bluish vesicles, cystic lesions that contain a watery fluid (**Figure 10.27b**) |
| **Cause** | Obstruction of the eccrine sweat gland, which causes retention of secretions and the appearance of a dilated cystic structure | An adenoma of the coil structure of the apocrine sweat gland |
| **Age** | Usually middle age | Middle age |
| **Sex** | More in women | No sex predilection |
| **Site** | Periorbital area, sparing lid margin | Near lid margin<br>Other sites: penis, axilla, and perianal regions |
| **Number** | Robinson type: solitary<br>Smith and Chernosky type: smaller and multiple | Usually solitary |
| **Effect of temperature** | Become larger on sun exposure | No change |

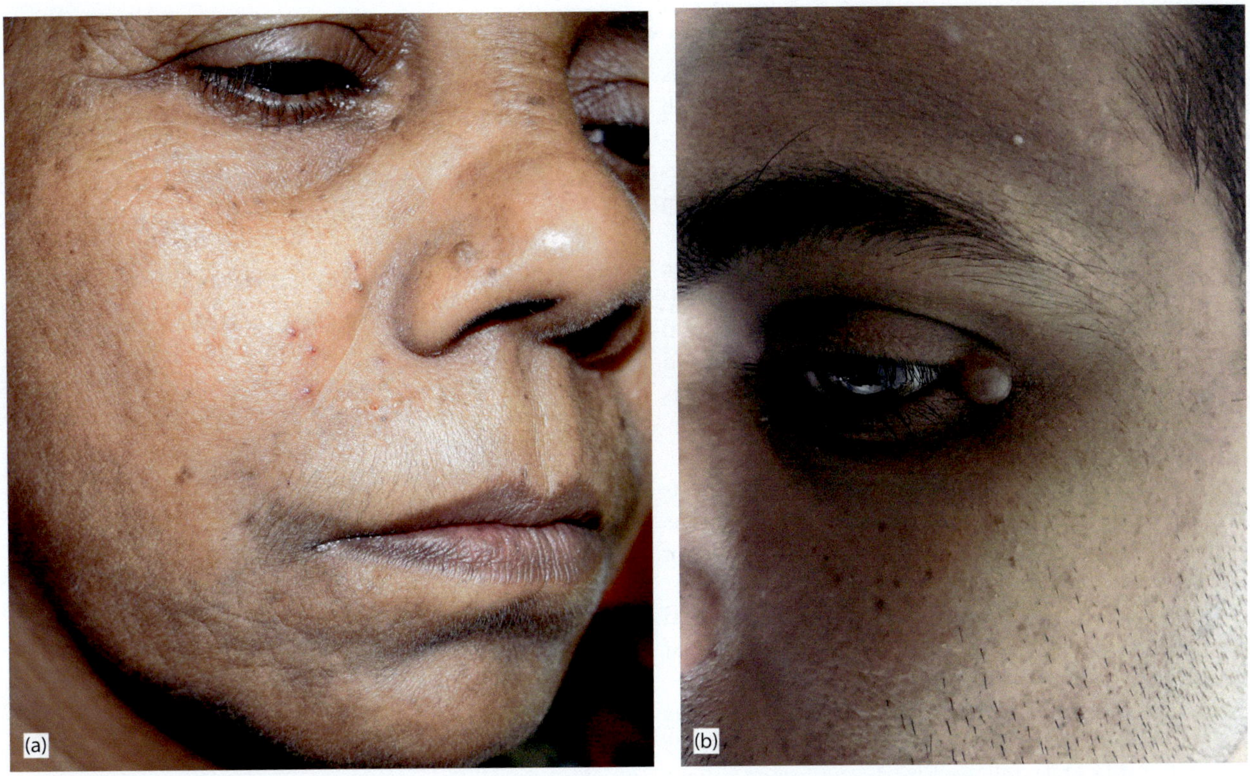


Figure 10.27 **(a)** Tiny, translucent lesions of eccrine hidrocystoma. **(b)** Apocrine hidrocystoma presenting as solitary translucent cyst over lateral canthus. (a – Courtesy: Dr. Piyush Kumar, Katihar, India; b – Courtesy: Dr. Abhishek De, Calcutta National Medical College and Hospital, Kolkata, India.)

- Multiple eyelid AHs are associated with Schöpf-Schulz-Passarge and Goltz-Gorlin syndrome.
- DD: Syringoma, trichoepithelioma, and multiple basal cell carcinomas.

## REFERENCES

1. Hill SF, Murrell DF. Differential diagnosis of vesiculobullous lesions. In, Hoeger P, Kinsler V, Yan A, editors. Harper's Textbook of Pediatric Dermatology. 4th edition. New Jersey: Wiley-Blackwell, 2020. P. 859–867.
2. Hull C, Zone JJ. Approach to the patient with cutaneous blisters. In, Stratman E, Ofori AO, editors. https://www.uptodate.com/contents/approach-to-the-patient-with-cutaneous-blisters
3. Wick MR. Bullous, pseudobullous, & pustular dermatoses. Semin Diagn Pathol 2017;34(3):250–260.
4. Yeh SW, Ahmed B, Sami N, Razzaque Ahmed A. Blistering disorders: diagnosis and treatment. Dermatol Ther 2003;16(3):214–223.

# 11

# Vesicobullous lesions: Generalized

RITI BHATIA AND VISHAL GUPTA

## INTRODUCTION

Vesiculobullous diseases are a distinct group of mucocutaneous disorders characterized by the formation of vesicles or bullae. A wide variety of conditions may present with generalized vesicles and bullae and include viral and bacterial diseases, autoimmune diseases, and genetic diseases among others. A detailed history and clinical examination in most of the cases help us to arrive at a list of clinical differentials. However, a clinician must closely examine the nature of vesicles/bullae (tense, fragile) along with distribution and arrangement (annular, discrete). One should keep in mind that vesicles and bullae, especially flaccid ones, may get ruptured easily, leaving erosions and crusts only, and vesicobullous lesions may not be observed during clinical examination. Examination of surrounding skin (urticarial plaques in pemphigoid gestationis and bullous pemphigoid; lichenoid papules in bullous lichen planus and lichen planus pemphigoides) and demonstration of clinical signs like Nikolsky sign, Asboe-Hansen sign, etc., provide important clues to the diagnosis. However, clinical diagnosis has a somewhat limited role in the diagnosis of autoimmune vesicobullous diseases; biopsy and immunofluorescence studies are conclusive. This chapter discusses the clinical approach to generalized vesicobullous diseases (**Figure 11.1**, **Table 11.1**), followed by discussion on salient features of these conditions.[1–7]

### Miliaria crystallina

- Miliaria crystallina is a self-limiting eccrine gland disorder due to blockage of sweat glands, presenting as fluid-filled vesicles that easily break.
- It is seen mostly in regions with high degrees of heat and humidity as in tropical regions, and is characterized by high-grade fever, hypernatremia, and neutropenia.
- Tiny 1- to 2-mm fragile clear vesicles present on a non-inflammatory base (**Figure 11.2a,b**).
- Common sites are the face, neck, flexures.
- It is usually seen in neonates but can also occur in adults with fever.
- DD: Erythema toxicum neonatorum, bullous impetigo.

### Grover's disease

- This is also known as transient acantholytic dermatosis.
- It usually occurs in middle-aged and elderly people.
- It is characterized by discrete pruritic, papular, or papulo-vesicular eruptions favoring the trunk.
- Eruptions may persist in some patients and the term "papular acantholytic dermatosis" is a preferred term to describe this entity.
- DD: Hailey-Hailey disease, Darier disease.

### Pemphigus vulgaris

- Pemphigus vulgaris is an autoimmune blistering disease due to formation of autoantibodies against desmosomal proteins, desmoglein 1 and 3.
- Clinical features include flaccid blisters that easily rupture to form erosions (**Figure 11.3a,b**), initially beginning from the head and neck and gradually extending to the trunk and flexural area; generalized involvement may occur in severe cases. The erosions

Table 11.1 Vesicobullous lesions in neonates*

| Systemic features | Diseases |
|---|---|
| Absent | • No inflammation – miliaria crystallina<br>• Generalized erythema – epidermolytic ichthyosis<br>• Trauma prone sites – epidermolysis bullosa<br>• Blaschkoid distribution – incontinentia pigmenti<br>• Colored urine – congenital porphyria |
| Present | • Diffuse erythema, Nikolsky sign positive – staphylococcal scalded skin syndrome<br>• Lesional erythema – varicella<br>• Hemorrhagic bullae, petechiae, scaly plaques – Congenital syphilis |

*Entities having prominent vesiculo-pustular lesions are not included here.



DOI: 10.1201/9781351054225-21

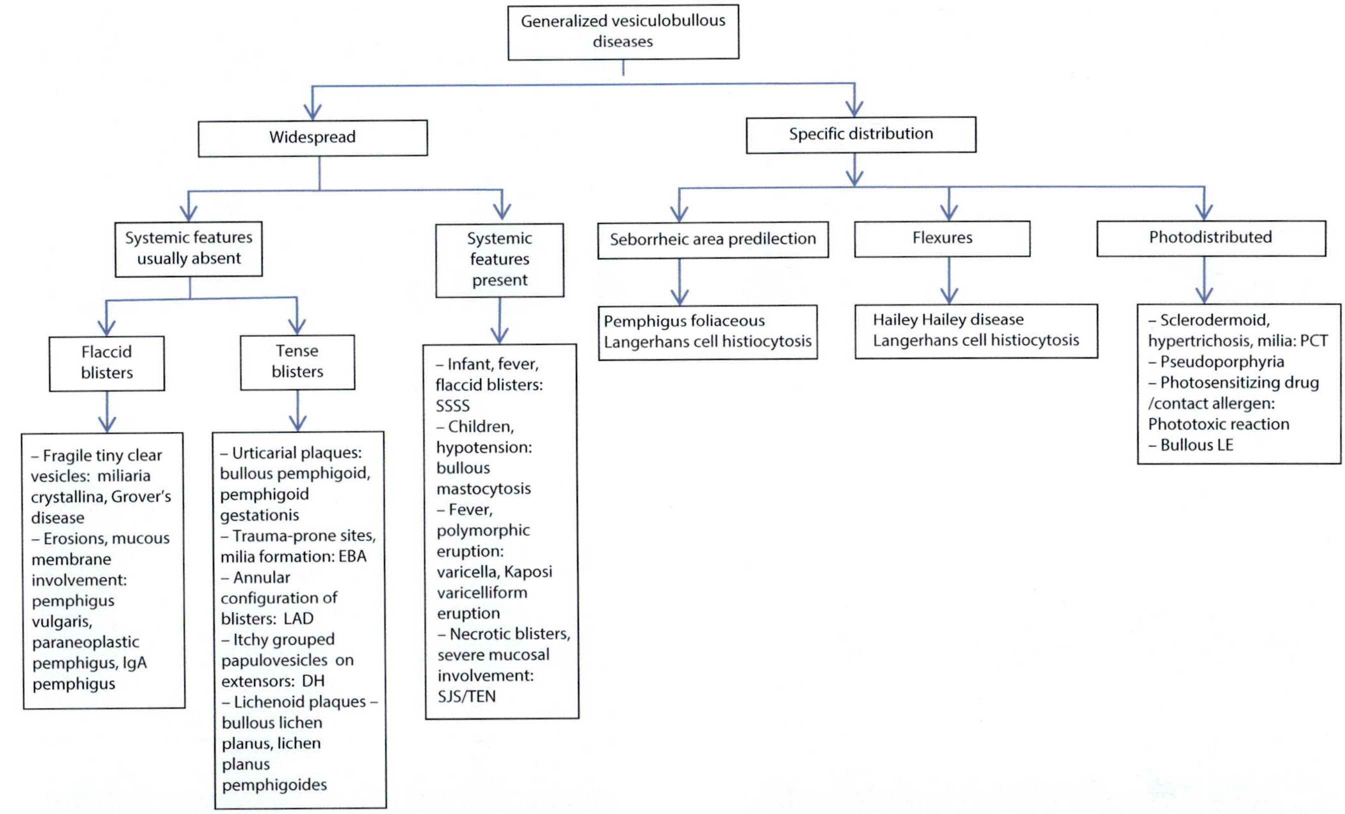


Figure 11.1 Clinical approach to generalized blisters in children and adults. (EBA – Epidermolysis bullosa acquisita, LAD – linear IgA dermatosis, DH – dermatitis herpetiformis, SJS – Stevens Johnson syndrome, TEN – toxic epidermal necrolysis, SSSS – Staphylococcal scalded skin syndrome, PCT – porphyria cutanea tarda).

show a tendency to spread much beyond the size of bullae.

- Bullae may contain a clear or turbid fluid; sometimes turbid fluid may settle in the dependent portion of blister ("hypopyon sign") (**Figure 11.3c**).
- It shows a positive Nikolsky sign (**Figure 11.3d**).
- Mucosal involvement is common: painful oral erosions on the buccal mucosa, tongue, and gingiva;

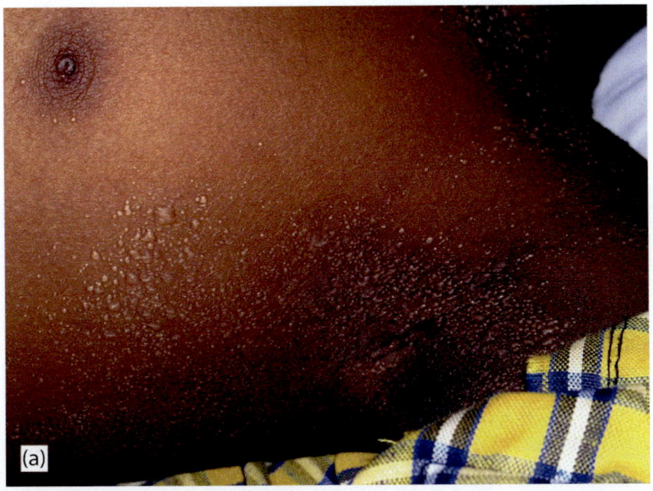

Figure 11.2 **(a)** Tiny, clear vesicles in miliaria crystallina. **(b)** Close-up of lesions of miliaria crystallina. (Courtesy: Dr. Ganesh Avhad, Mumbai, India.)

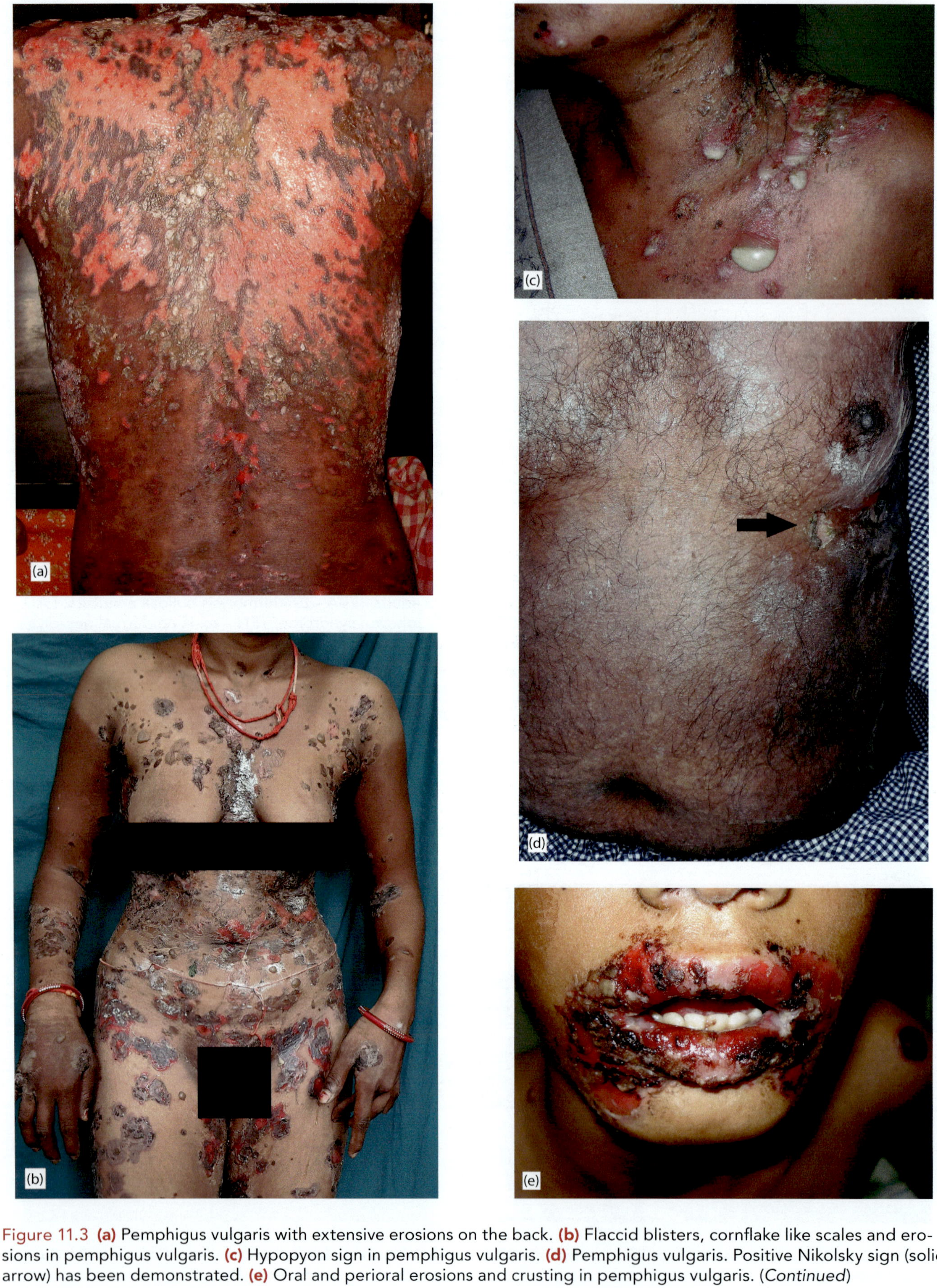


Figure 11.3 **(a)** Pemphigus vulgaris with extensive erosions on the back. **(b)** Flaccid blisters, cornflake like scales and erosions in pemphigus vulgaris. **(c)** Hypopyon sign in pemphigus vulgaris. **(d)** Pemphigus vulgaris. Positive Nikolsky sign (solid arrow) has been demonstrated. **(e)** Oral and perioral erosions and crusting in pemphigus vulgaris. (*Continued*)

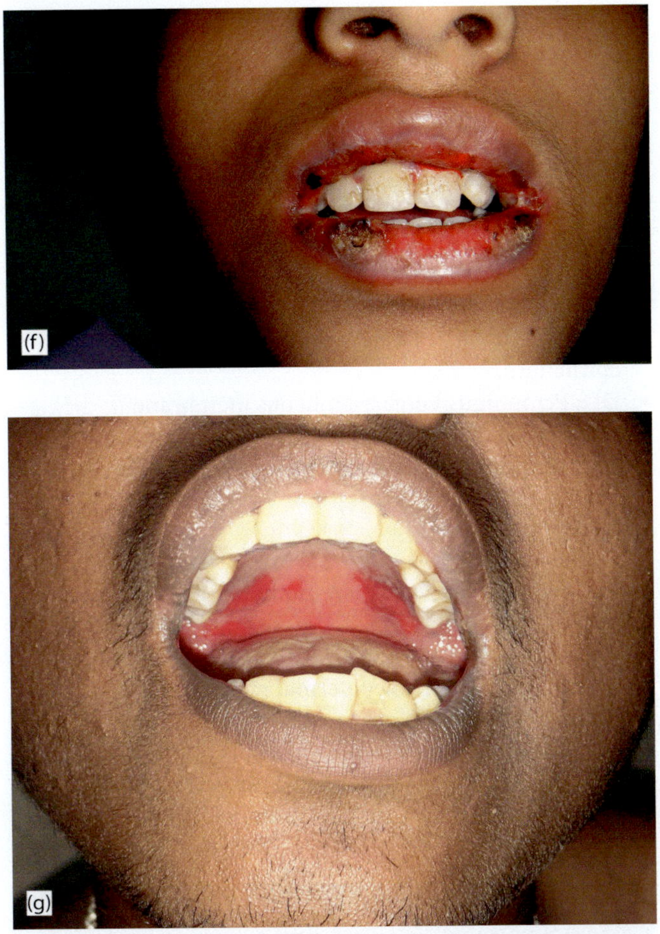

Figure 11.3 (*Continued*) **(f)** Crusted erosions on lip in pemphigus vulgaris. **(g)** Erosions on the hard palate. (a,c,f,g – Courtesy: Dr. Piyush Kumar, Katihar, India b – Courtesy: Dr. Hiral Shah, Baroda Medical College, Vadodara, India.)

genital erosions; oral ulcers with irregular margins (**Figure 11.3e–g**).

- The disease is progressive if untreated; death may occur from sepsis.
- DD: Pemphigus foliaceus (scaly crusted erosions seen more commonly than intact blisters, lacks mucosal involvement), linear IgA pemphigus (annular arrangement), bullous pemphigoid (tense blisters).

## Paraneoplastic pemphigus

- Paraneoplastic pemphigus (PNP) is a rare and often fatal autoimmune blistering disease accompanied by both benign and malignant neoplasms. Skin lesions are thought to be caused by an autoimmune response generated by antibodies to tumor antigens that cross-react with epithelial antigens; autoantibodies are directed against both desmosomal and hemidesmosomal antigens.
- The most frequently reported associated malignancies are lymphomatoid and hematologic (e.g., B-cell lymphoma, chronic lymphocytic leukemia, Castleman disease, Waldenstrom macroglobulinemia, and thymoma – with or without myasthenia gravis).
- Clinically, PNP may manifest in following forms:
    a. Pemphigus-like: superficial vesicles, flaccid vesicles, erosions, crust, and erythema (**Figure 11.4a**).
    b. Bullous pemphigoid-like: scaly erythematous papules, which may or may not be associated with stretched vesicles.

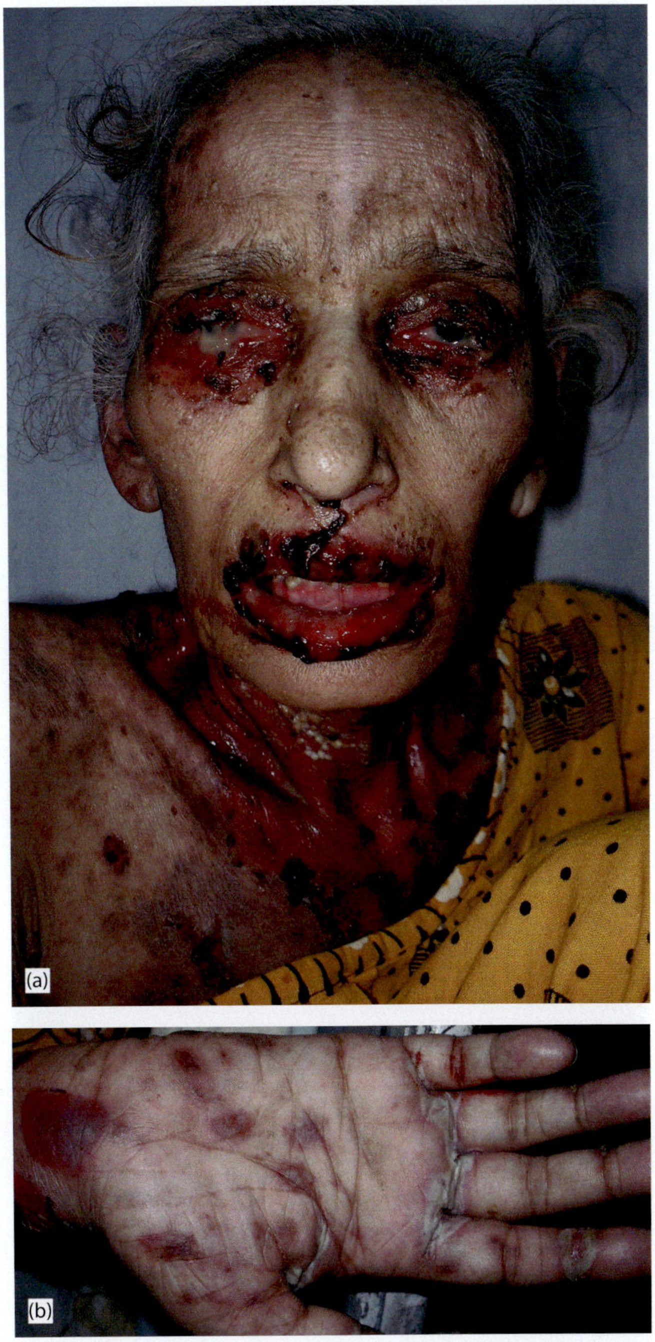

Figure 11.4 **(a)** Pemphigus vulgaris-like cutaneous and mucosal erosions in paraneoplastic pemphigus. **(b)** Hemorrhagic blisters and erythema multiforme-like lesions on the palm in paraneoplastic pemphigus. (*Continued*)

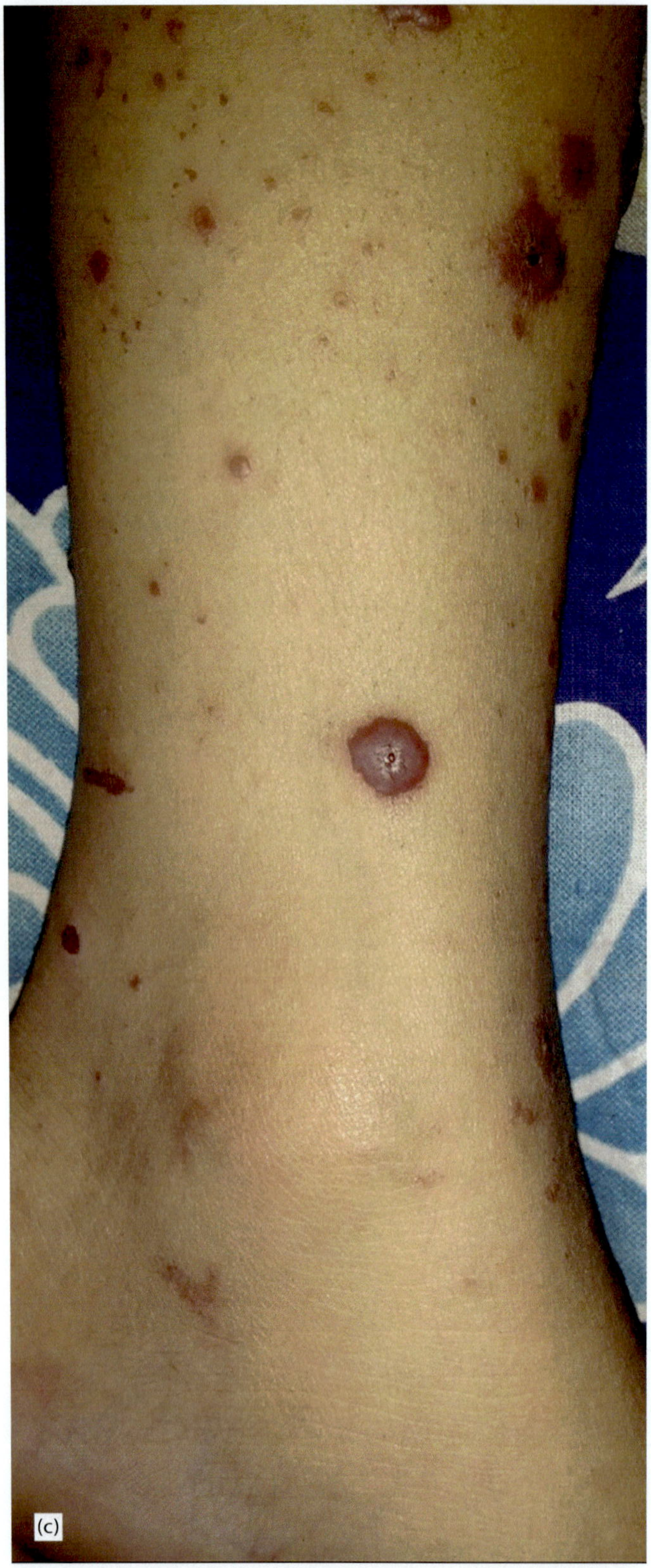


Figure 11.4 (*Continued*) **(c)** Erythema multiforme-like lesions in paraneoplastic pemphigus. (a,b – Courtesy: Dr. Piyush Kumar, Katihar, India; c – Courtesy: Dr. Rajesh Kumar Mandal, North Bengal Medical College and Hospital, India.)

  c. Erythema multiforme-like: polymorphic alterations, mainly erythematous peeling pellets with erosions and sometimes even with hard-to-heal ulcerations (**Figure 11.4b,c**).
  d. Graft-versus-host disease: disseminated dusky-red scaly papules.
  e. Lichen planus-like: small flat scaly papules and intense mucous membrane involvement.
- PNP may involve not only the buccal mucosa but also the mucous membranes of the esophagus, stomach, duodenum, and intestines and also the pulmonary epithelium.
- DD: Pemphigus vulgaris, mucous membrane pemphigoid, erythema multiforme, Stevens-Johnson syndrome, lichen planus, graft-versus-host disease, and herpes simplex virus infection.

## IgA Pemphigus

- IgA pemphigus is common in middle-aged and elderly people.
- There are two types: subcorneal pustular dermatosis (SCPD)-like and intraepidermal neutrophilic type.
- Patients with both types present with flaccid vesiculopustules on erythematous or normal skin (**Figure 11.5a**).
- Pustules tend to coalesce to form an annular or circinate pattern, with crusts in the central area

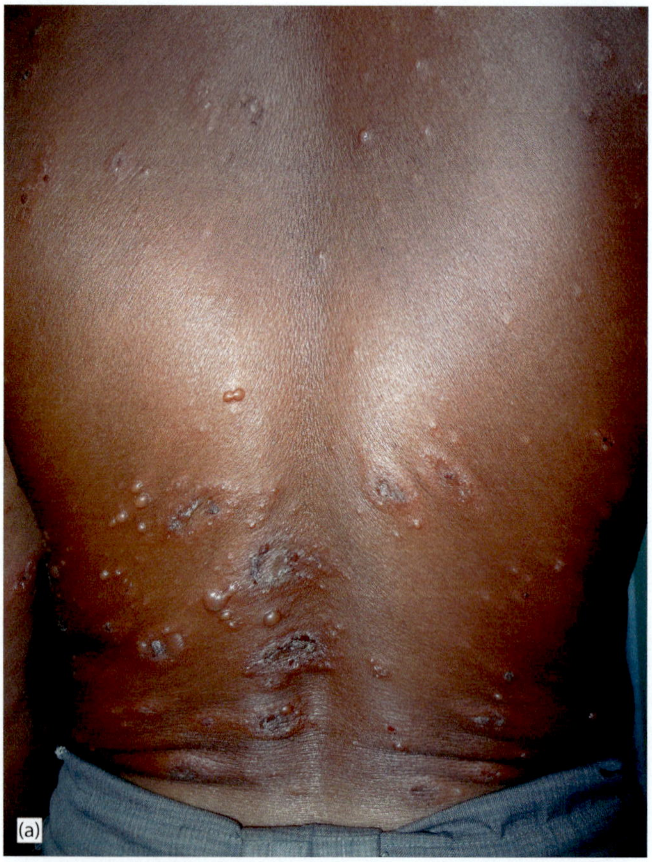


Figure 11.5 **(a)** Vesicles arranged in circinate pattern in IgA pemphigus. (*Continued*)

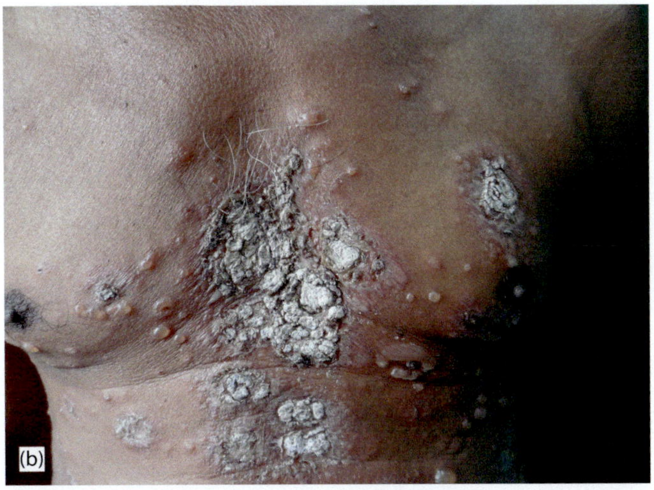


Figure 11.5 (*Continued*) **(b)** IgA pemphigus. (a,b – Courtesy: Dr. Niharika Ranjan Lal. ESIPGIMSR, Kolkata, India.)

(**Figure 11.5b**). It more frequently involves the trunk, intertriginous areas, and flexor aspects of the limbs.
- Mucous membranes are almost never affected.
- DD: Pemphigus vulgaris, bullous pemphigoid, generalized pustular psoriasis (in case of SCPD).

## Bullous pemphigoid

- Bullous pemphigoid is an autoimmune blistering disease characterized by blisters, usually observed in elderly patients.
- It is caused by autoantibodies against BPAg1 and 2.
- Clinical features include the following
  - Non-bullous phase: Mild to severe pruritus alone or associated with urticarial plaques (**Figure 11.6a,b**), eczematous papules/plaques (**Figure 11.6c**).
  - Bullous phase: Blisters are tense with straw-colored fluid (**Figure 11.6d,e**); they can also be hemorrhagic (**Figure 11.6f,g**); the Nikolsky sign is negative. Bullae persist for a longer time compared to those in pemphigus vulgaris, and subsequent erosions do not extend much beyond the size of bullae.
- Eruptions typically heal with hypopigmentation and follicular repigmentation (**Figure 11.6h**), usually with no scarring or milia formation.
- Common locations include the extremities (lower and upper) and the trunk.
- It may also have mucosal involvement.
- DD: Other subepidermal immunobullous disorders such as epidermolysis bullosa acquisita, linear IgA bullous dermatosis, anti-p200 pemphigoid.

## Pemphigoid gestationis

- Pemphigoid gestationis or gestational pemphigoid is a rare pregnancy-associated autoimmune skin disorder that is immunologically and clinically similar to the pemphigoid group of autoimmune blistering skin disorders.

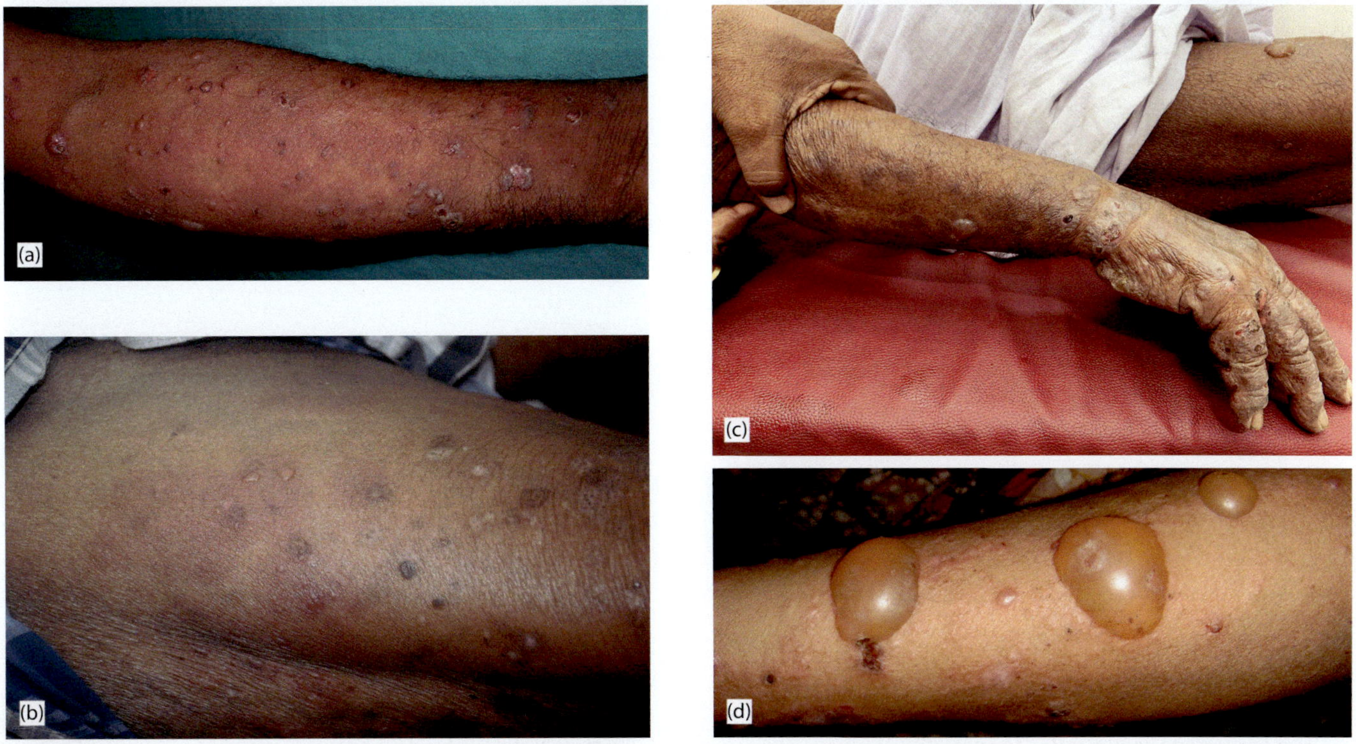


Figure 11.6 **(a)** Urticarial plaque with few vesicles in bullous pemphigoid. **(b)** Urticarial lesion with tense bulla in bullous pemphigoid in an elderly. **(c)** Eczematous plaque with tense bulla in bullous pemphigoid. **(d)** Tense bullae in bullous pemphigoid. (*Continued*)

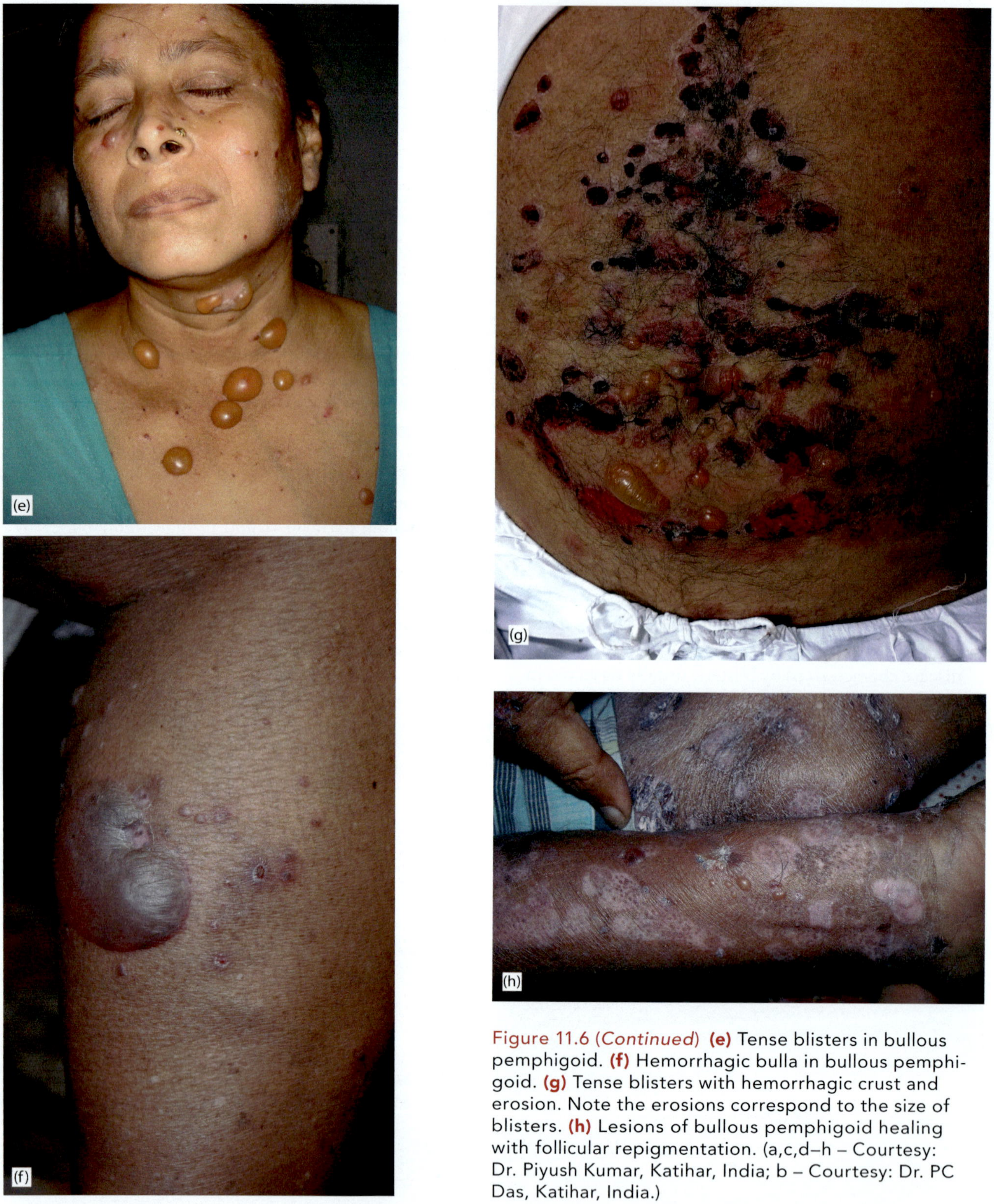


Figure 11.6 (*Continued*) **(e)** Tense blisters in bullous pemphigoid. **(f)** Hemorrhagic bulla in bullous pemphigoid. **(g)** Tense blisters with hemorrhagic crust and erosion. Note the erosions correspond to the size of blisters. **(h)** Lesions of bullous pemphigoid healing with follicular repigmentation. (a,c,d–h – Courtesy: Dr. Piyush Kumar, Katihar, India; b – Courtesy: Dr. PC Das, Katihar, India.)

- It mainly affects multiparous women in their second or third trimester of pregnancy.
- The pathogenesis is similar to that of bullous pemphigoid, caused by autoantibodies directed against two hemidesmosomal proteins, BP180 and BP230, within the dermoepidermal junction, resulting in the formation of bullae and skin erosions.
- PG initially presents with intense pruritus, progressing to polymorphic skin lesions, which are usually urticarial papules and annular plaques.
- It is followed by vesicles and finally large tense bullae on an erythematous background.
- It typically develops on the abdomen, characteristically involving the umbilical region.

- In 90% of the cases, it later spreads to the rest of the abdomen, involving the thighs palms, and soles.
- The mucous membranes and face are usually spared.
- DD: Urticaria, scabies, contact dermatitis, atopic eruption of pregnancy, polymorphic eruption of pregnancy, intrahepatic cholestasis of pregnancy.

## Epidermolysis bullosa acquisita (EBA)

- This is an autoimmune, acquired subepidermal blistering disease.
- It is caused by autoantibodies to collagen VII.
- Clinical features include the following
  - Non-inflammatory type: skin fragility and blistering over trauma-prone areas, healing with scarring, milia formation, dystrophic nails (**Figure 11.7a–c**).
  - Inflammatory type: widespread, tense vesicles and bullae not localized to trauma-prone sites and generally healing with minimal scarring and milia formation. It resembles other chronic bullous disorders.
- DD: Bullous pemphigoid (generalized blister, preceded with itching,), dystrophic epidermolysis bullosa, cicatricial pemphigoid.

## Linear IgA dermatosis/chronic bullous disease of childhood

- Linear IgA dermatosis is a rare autoimmune blistering disease with two clinical forms: childhood type (chronic bullous disease of childhood) and adult type

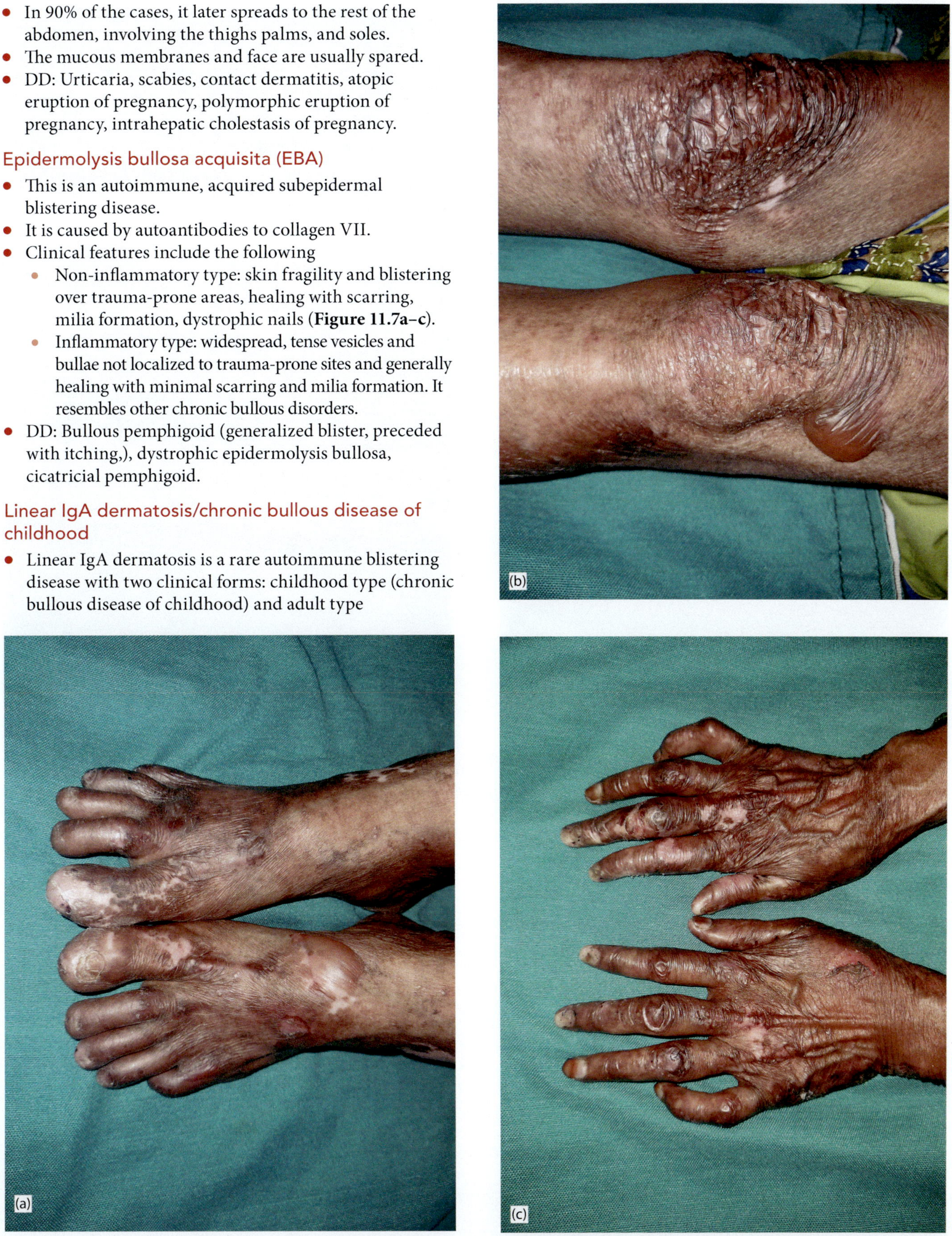

Figure 11.7 **(a)** Tense blisters, scarring, milia, and anonychia in epidermolysis bullosa acquisita. **(b)** Tense blisters and scarring of the skin over knee in EBA. **(c)** Extensive scarring of the skin over hands and anonychia in EBA. *(Continued)*

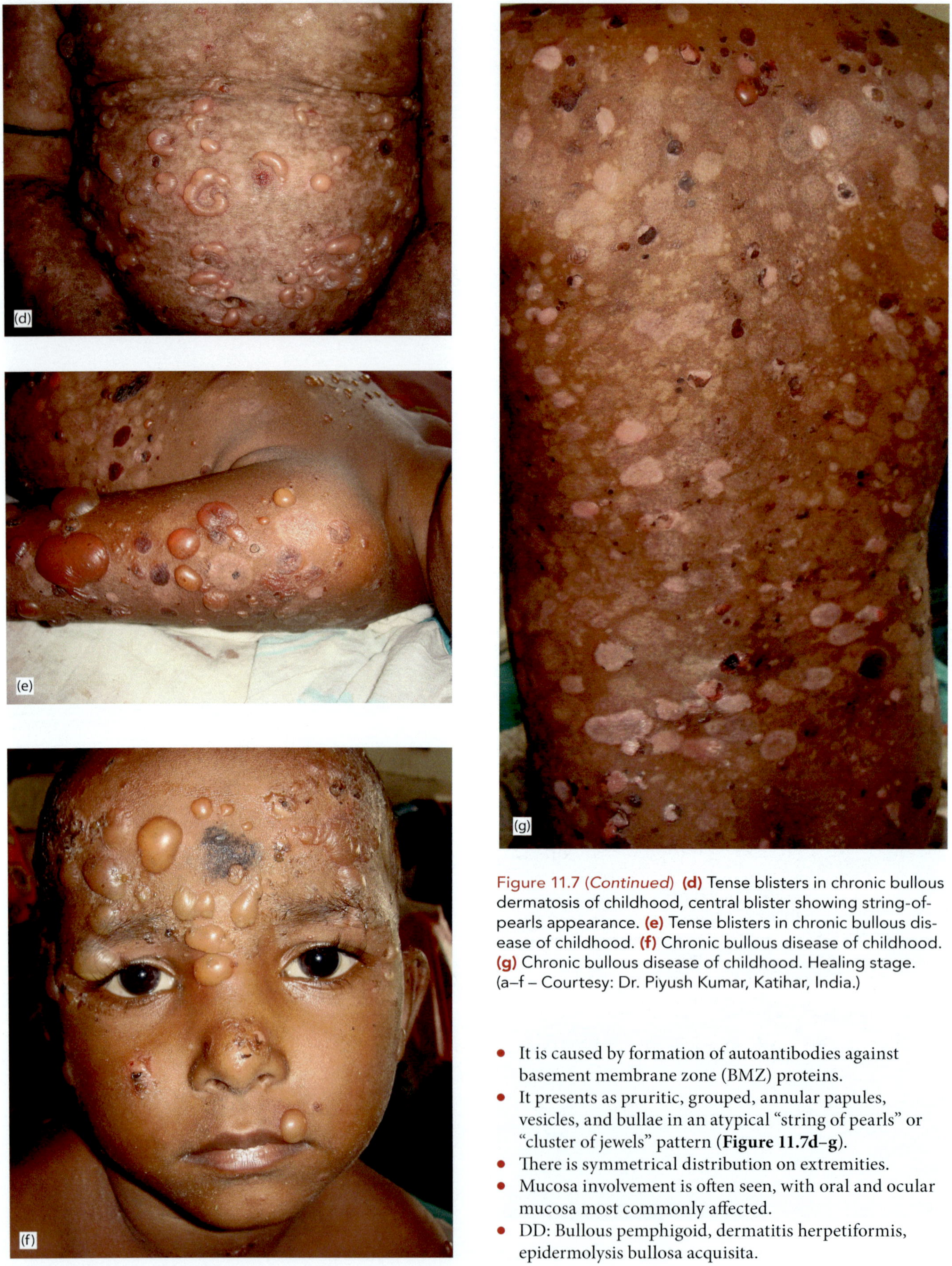

Figure 11.7 (*Continued*) **(d)** Tense blisters in chronic bullous dermatosis of childhood, central blister showing string-of-pearls appearance. **(e)** Tense blisters in chronic bullous disease of childhood. **(f)** Chronic bullous disease of childhood. **(g)** Chronic bullous disease of childhood. Healing stage. (a–f – Courtesy: Dr. Piyush Kumar, Katihar, India.)

- It is caused by formation of autoantibodies against basement membrane zone (BMZ) proteins.
- It presents as pruritic, grouped, annular papules, vesicles, and bullae in an atypical "string of pearls" or "cluster of jewels" pattern (**Figure 11.7d–g**).
- There is symmetrical distribution on extremities.
- Mucosa involvement is often seen, with oral and ocular mucosa most commonly affected.
- DD: Bullous pemphigoid, dermatitis herpetiformis, epidermolysis bullosa acquisita.

## Dermatitis herpetiformis

- Dermatitis herpetiformis presents with intensely pruritic and grouped vesicobullous lesions and urticarial plaques (**Figure 11.8a**).
- It is commonly found on extensor surfaces (elbows, knees, buttocks, shoulders, sacral areas) (**Figure 11.8b**).
- Gluten sensitive enteropathy is seen in most of the patients.

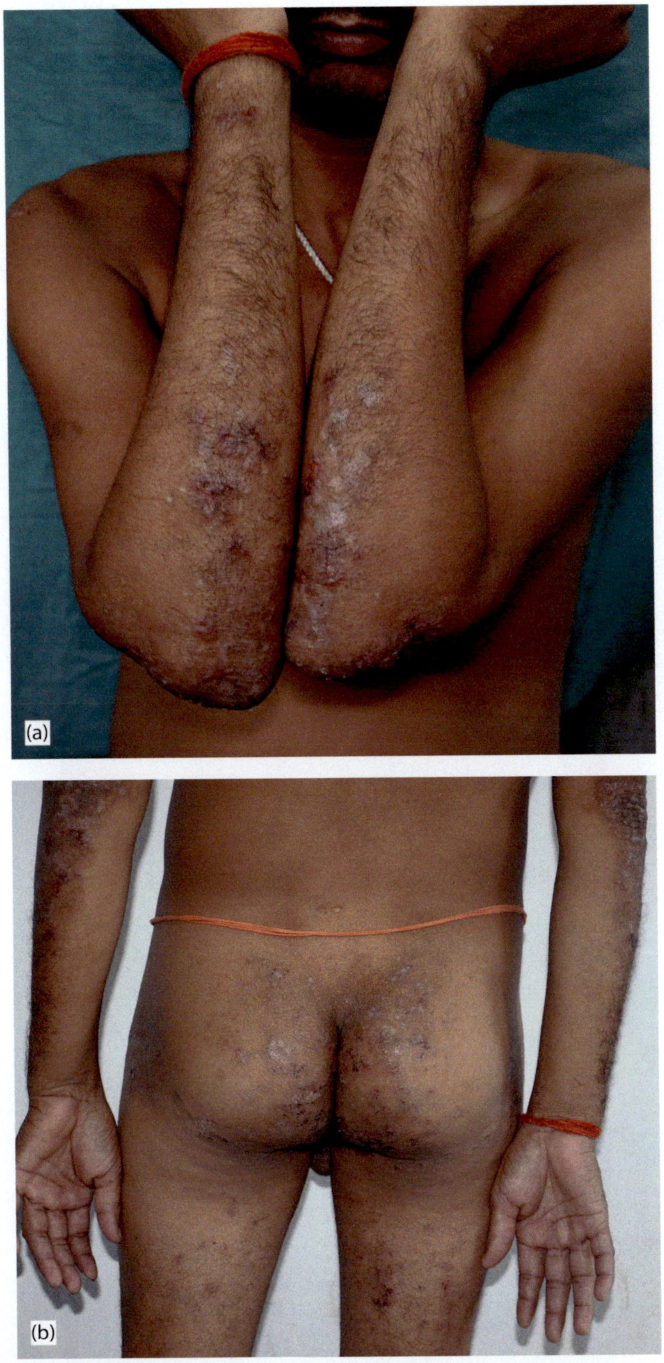


Figure 11.8 **(a)** Excoriated papulovesicles symmetrically distributed on elbow extensors in dermatitis herpetiformis. **(b)** Excoriated grouped papulovesicles on sacral area in dermatitis herpetiformis. (a,b – Courtesy: Dr. Piyush Kumar, Katihar, India.)

- Diagnosis is neutrophilic microabscess and IgA deposits on dermal papillary tips.
- DD: Scabies, id reaction.

## Bullous lichen planus

- Bullous lichen planus (BLP) is an uncommon variant of lichen planus (LP) and results from severe inflammation at the dermoepidermal junction (DEJ), causing a split at the DEJ.
- It is clinically characterized by vesicular and/or bullous lesions developing on pre-existing LP lesions or on perilesional skin (**Figure 11.9**).
- There are two variants of BLP: familial and non-familial.
- Familial variant is more common, occurs at an earlier age with longer duration of disease, more extensive eruptions, and increased tendency to involve nails as compared to non-familial variants. Pathogenesis of familial variants may be attributable to genetic factors.
- Lower extremities are most commonly affected. Nail involvement is characterized by hemorrhagic crusty lesions resulting in exposure of nail bed and nail atrophy
- DD: Lichen planus pemphigoides.

## Lichen planus pemphigoides

- Lichen planus pemphigoides (LPP) is a rare disease usually affecting adults; patients of lichen planus develop autoantibodies against BPAg2 and BPAg1.
- The cause is mostly idiopathic, drugs: ACE inhibitors, PUVA therapy, anti-tuberculosis medications, hepatitis B.
- In LPP, two discrete primary skin lesions occur: lichenoid papules/plaques and tense blisters.

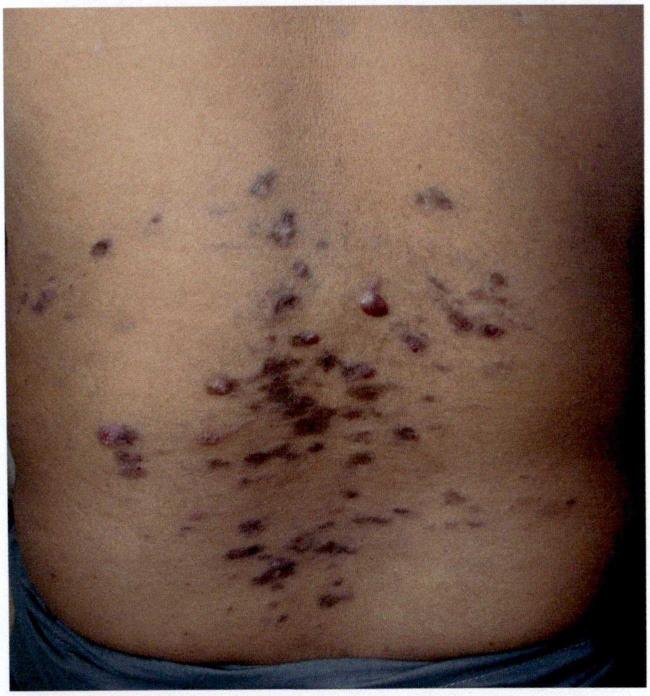

Figure 11.9 Bullae over violaceous papules and plaques in bullous lichen planus. (Courtesy: Dr. Piyush Kumar, Katihar, India.)

- Lichenoid eruptions consist of pruritic violaceous polygonal papules and plaques with a shiny surface.
- Blisters and erosions typically appear after the development of the lichenoid skin changes and classically on previously unaffected skin (**Figure 11.10a**).
- Acral areas are preferred.

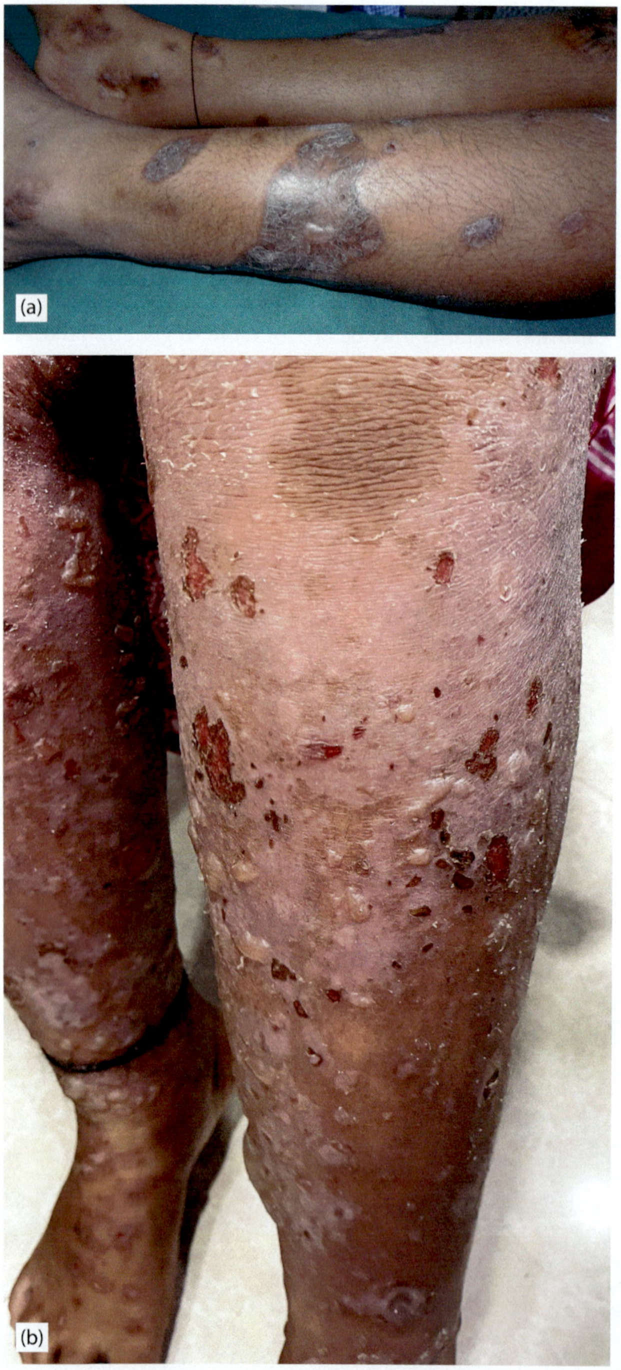

Figure 11.10 **(a)** Lichen planus pemphigoides with tense bulla. The patient has developed lesions preferentially over atrophic scars, an illustration of Ruocco's immuno-compromised district. **(b)** Bullous lichen planus with tense bullae over lichenoid patch and plaques. (a – Courtesy: Dr. Piyush Kumar, Katihar, India; b – Courtesy: Dr Soumyajit Roychoudhury, Berhampore, India.)

- Mucosa and nail involvement may occur at times.
- DD: Bullous lichen planus (blisters limited to LP lesions and perilesional skin) (**Figure 11.10b**), bullous pemphigoid (over urticarial plaques).

## Staphylococcal scalded skin syndrome

- Staphylococcal scalded skin (SSSS) syndrome presents with superficial flaccid bullae that peel off, resulting in sheets of desquamation, and generalized erythema along with facial edema; skin tenderness is present (**Figure 11.11a,b**).

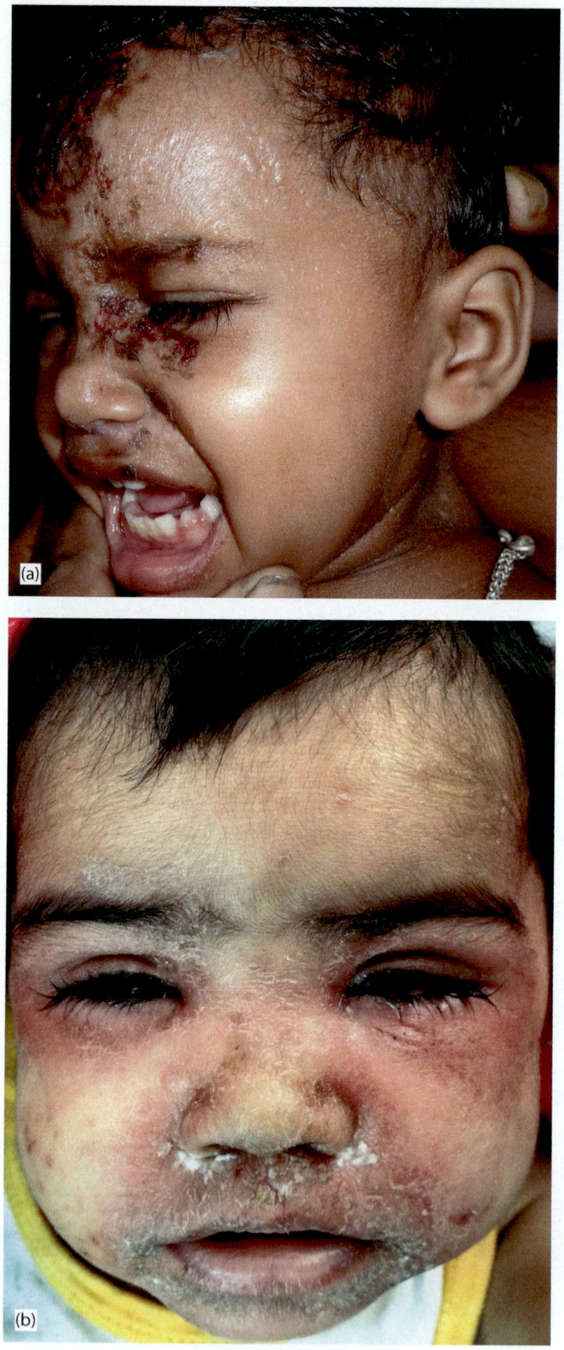

Figure 11.11 **(a)** Superficial flaccid bulla with peeling and erosion in staphylococcal scalded skin syndrome. **(b)** Facial edema with scaling in staphylococcal scalded skin syndrome. (*Continued*)

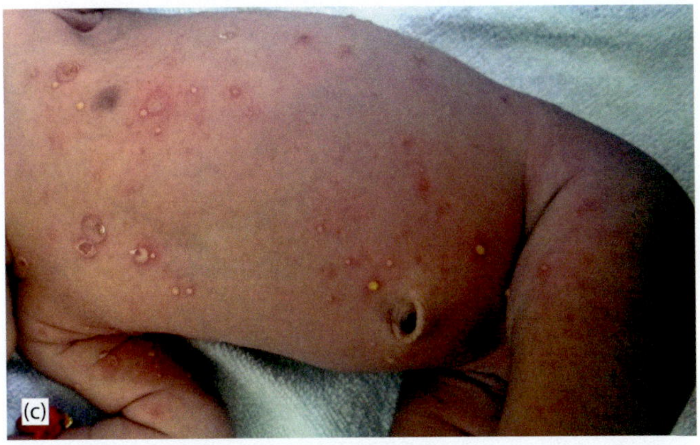

Figure 11.11 (*Continued*) **(c)** Extensive flaccid blisters on the trunk in bullous impetigo.

- The Nikolsky sign is positive.
- There is no mucosal involvement.
- It is associated with fever, malaise, and irritability.
- SSSS is usually seen in infants and children; adults with renal dysfunction are also at risk.
- Healing occurs within 10 to 14 days without any residual changes.
- Common sites start from the perioral area and perineum, followed by generalized involvement.
- Search for the primary site of staphylococcal infection, such as ears, throat, conjunctiva, and umbilicus.
- DD: Viral exanthem, drug reactions, Kawasaki disease, extensive bullous impetigo **(Figure 11.11c)**, toxic epidermal necrolysis (areas of skin necrosis, severe mucosal involvement).

## Diffuse cutaneous mastocytosis

- Mastocytosis is a rare, heterogeneous group of hematopoietic disorders characterized by an abnormal increase and accumulation of mast cells in one or more organ systems.
- Diffuse cutaneous mastocytosis, the rarest and the most severe form, presents with erythroderma, hemorrhagic blisters, and in some cases extensive bullous lesions.
- Onset is commonly seen in first two years of life.
- Lesions are triggered by sudden changes in temperature, irritability, fever, and teething.
- Systemic symptoms include itching, flushing, diarrhea, vomiting, hypotension. and even anaphylactic shock.
- Two clinical variants of diffuse mastocytosis are recognized. The first variant is the "initial bullous presentation," which presents as diffuse erythema, with generalized blistering, and appears early in life. The second variant is the "infiltrative small vesicular type," which presents with limited vesicular blistering and starts with slowly progressive, diffusely distributed yellow–orange infiltrates that evolve into nodular lesions.
- DD: Infections (viral, bacterial, or mycotic infections), genetic diseases (epidermolysis bullosa, epidermolytic hyperkeratosis, incontinentia pigmenti), autoimmune bullous diseases.

## Varicella

- In varicella there are generalized eruption of lesions in varying stages of evolution: papules, papulovesicles, vesicles, pustules, and crusted lesions, (**Figure 11.12a–c**).
- Vesicles with surrounding erythematous halo (characteristic "dew drops on rose petal" appearance) are characteristic. Vesicles may have an umbilicated appearance (**Figure 11.12d,e**).

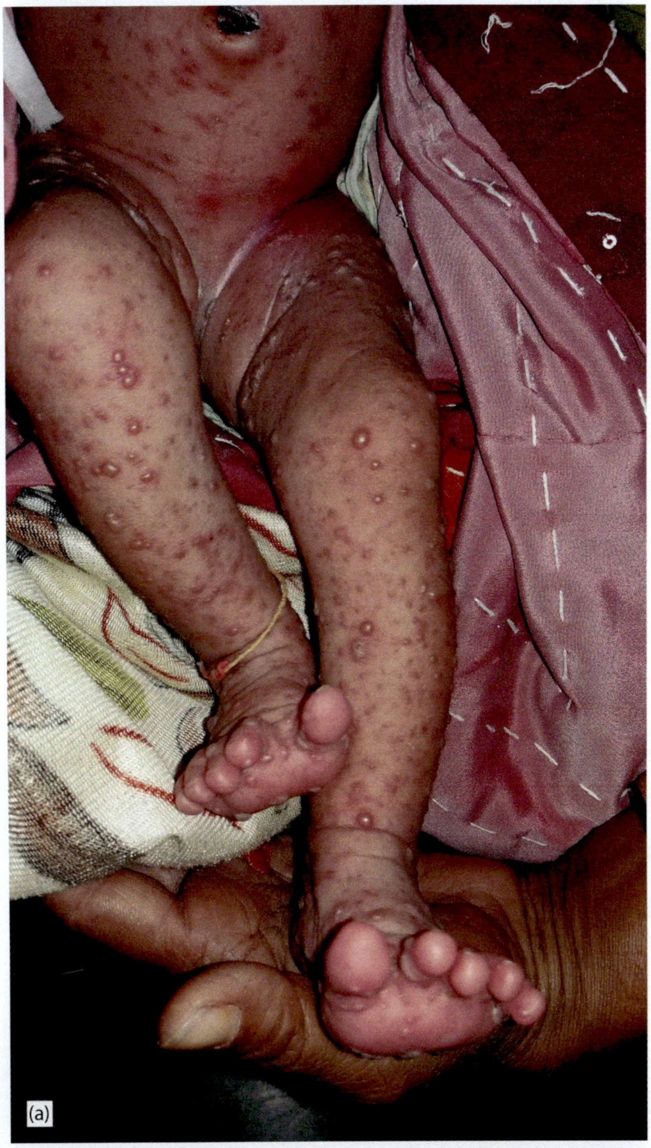

Figure 11.12 **(a)** Neonatal varicella. (*Continued*)

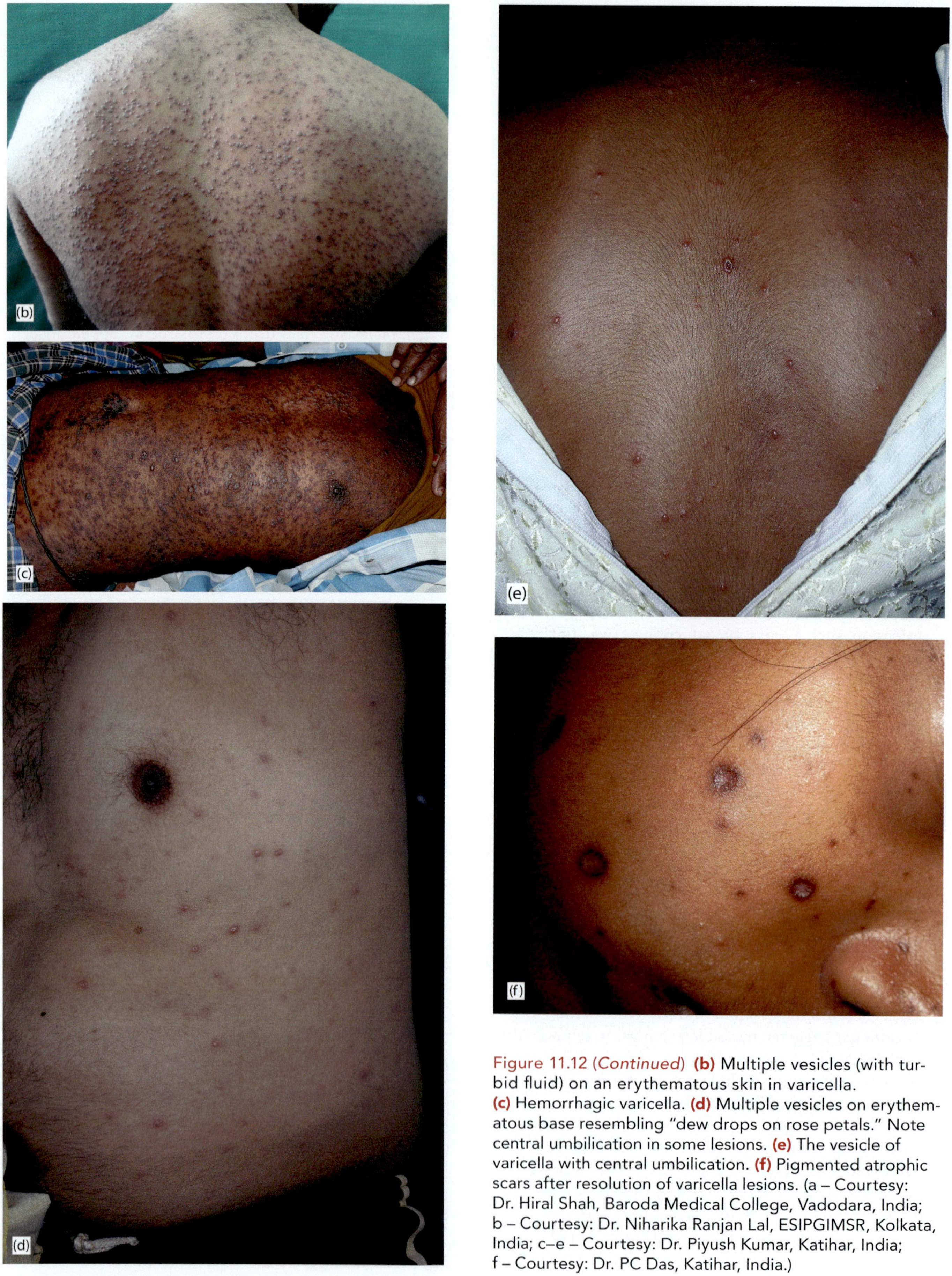


Figure 11.12 (*Continued*) **(b)** Multiple vesicles (with turbid fluid) on an erythematous skin in varicella. **(c)** Hemorrhagic varicella. **(d)** Multiple vesicles on erythematous base resembling "dew drops on rose petals." Note central umbilication in some lesions. **(e)** The vesicle of varicella with central umbilication. **(f)** Pigmented atrophic scars after resolution of varicella lesions. (a – Courtesy: Dr. Hiral Shah, Baroda Medical College, Vadodara, India; b – Courtesy: Dr. Niharika Ranjan Lal, ESIPGIMSR, Kolkata, India; c–e – Courtesy: Dr. Piyush Kumar, Katihar, India; f – Courtesy: Dr. PC Das, Katihar, India.)

- Lesions heal with variable atrophy and pigmentation (**Figure 11.12f**).
- It is associated with constitutional features such as fever, sore throat, and malaise.
- DD: Pityriasis lichenoides et varioliformis acuta, pustular pyoderma gangrenosum, papulovesicular pityriasis rosea, disseminated herpes zoster.

## Kaposi varicelliform eruption

- Kaposi varicelliform eruption (KVE), also known as eczema herpeticum, is a rare and potentially fatal viral infection.
- It is caused mainly by the herpes simplex virus (HSV), predominantly type I. Other viruses, such as coxsackie A 16, vaccinia, and varicella zoster have also been implicated in its pathogenesis.
- It is characterized by widespread clusters of umbilicated vesicopustules and eroded vesicles, alternating with punched-out ulcers covered by hemorrhagic crusts usually located over the head, neck, and trunk (**Figure 11.13**).
- KVE usually develops in patients with existing chronic dermatoses, especially atopic dermatitis; it has also been reported in association with psoriasis, pityriasis rubra pilaris, Darier, Grover's, and Hailey-Hailey diseases, and contact dermatitis (both irritant and allergic), among others.
- The lesions are painful and often associated with fever, malaise, and regional lymphadenopathy.
- DD: Chickenpox, impetigo, contact dermatitis.

## Stevens-Johnson syndrome/toxic epidermal necrolysis

- This presents with dusky erythematous or purpuric macules with a tendency to coalesce (**Figure 11.14a,b**); skin tenderness is present.
- There is rapid progression, with vesicles, bullae, skin necrosis, and epidermal sloughing in a few days (**Figure 11.14c,d**).
- It is usually accompanied by constitutional features.
- There is severe mucosal involvement: ocular, oral and genital mucosa are involved in almost all cases (**Figure 11.14e**).
- DD: Extensive bullous fixed drug eruption, erythema multiforme, acute cutaneous systemic

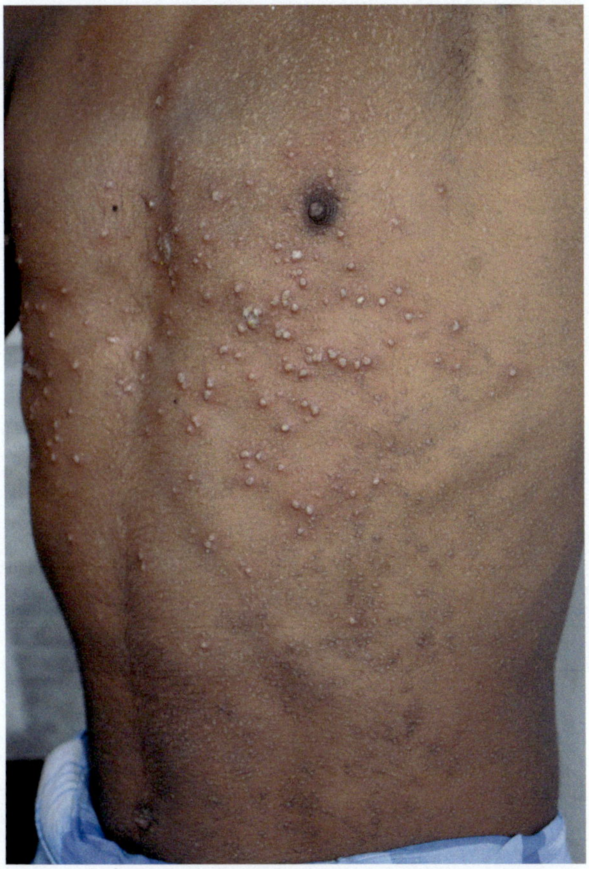

Figure 11.13 Kaposi varicelliform eruption seen as vesicles and pustules in a patient with pre-existing Darier disease. (Courtesy: Dr. Piyush Kumar, Katihar, India.)

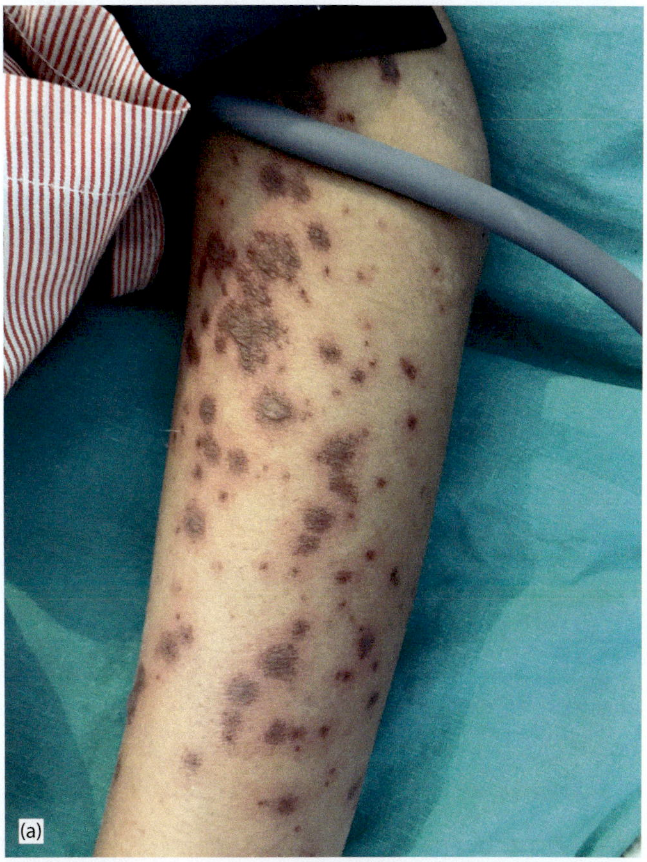


Figure 11.14 **(a)** Dusky, erythematous macules and bullous in a patient of Stevens-Johnson syndrome. (*Continued*)

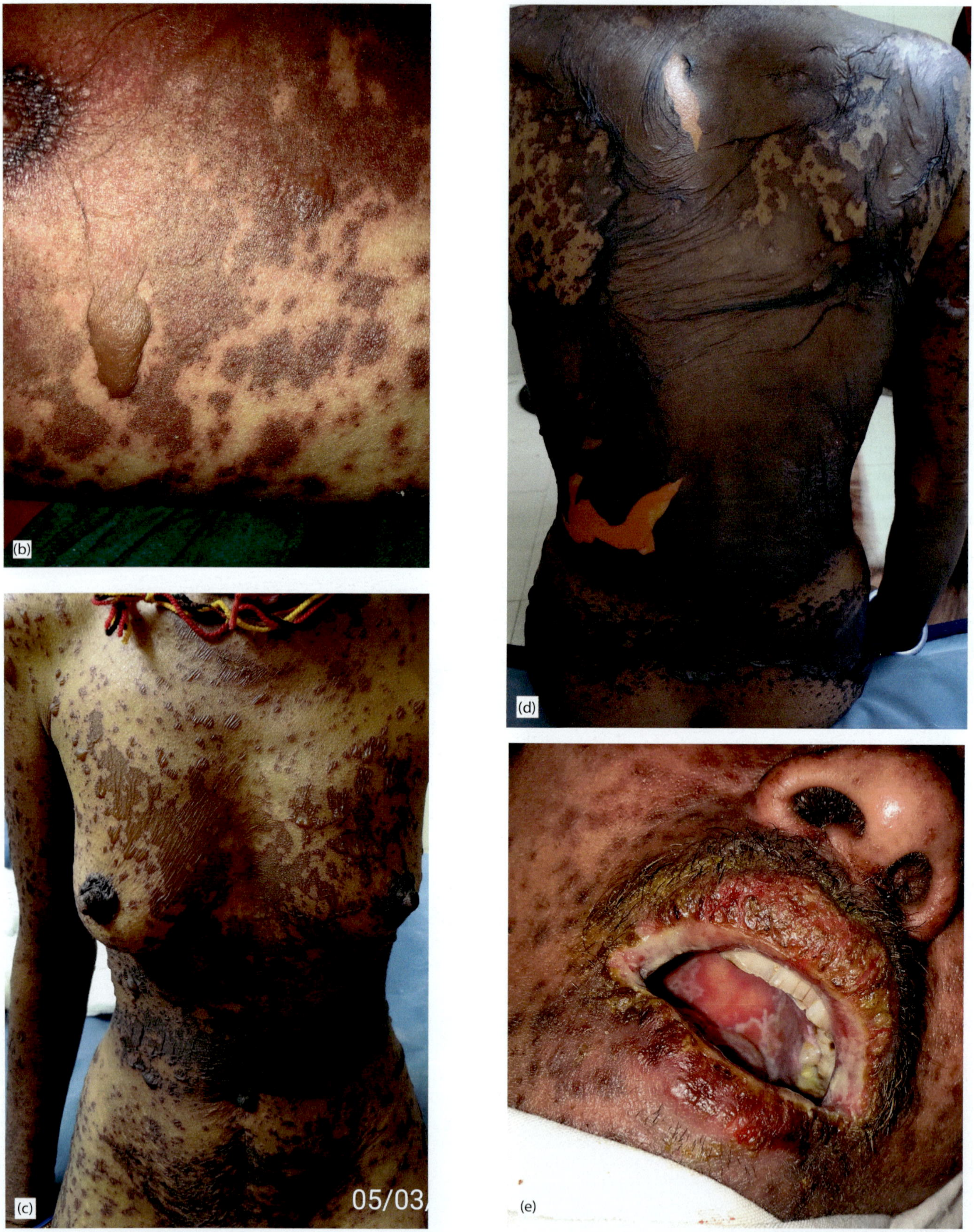


Figure 11.14 (*Continued*) **(b)** Confluent lesions in Stevens-Johnson syndrome. **(c)** Blisters with skin peeling in toxic epidermal necrolysis. **(d)** Extensive epidermal sloughing in toxic epidermal necrolysis. **(e)** Severe erosive mucositis in Stevens-Johnson syndrome. (a,b – Courtesy: Dr. Bhushan Madke, Jawaharlal Nehru Medical College, Datta Meghe Institute of Medical Sciences, India; c–e – Courtesy: Dr. Hiral Shah, Baroda Medical College, Vadodara, India.)

lupus erythematosus (acute syndrome of apoptotic pan-epidermolysis), paraneoplastic pemphigus.

## Pemphigus foliaceus

- Pemphigus foliaceus presents with flaccid, superficial vesicles, and bulla, mostly in seborrheic distribution (**Figure 11.15a**).
- There is prominent scaling and crusting (**Figure 11.15b,c**) but no tendency of lesions to spread (**Figure 11.15d**).
- Mucosas are usually spared.
- The Nikolsky sign is positive.
- DD: Bullous impetigo, pemphigus vulgaris, lupus erythematosus.

## Langerhans cell histiocytosis

- It clinically presents with papules, vesicles, crusts, and petechiae over seborrheic and intertriginous areas.
- Patients may have fever, anemia, thrombocytopenia, pulmonary infiltrates, hepatosplenomegaly, and enlargement of lymph nodes.
- DD: Seborrheic dermatitis, acrodermatitis enteropathica.

## Hailey-Hailey disease

- Also known as familial benign chronic pemphigus, Hailey-Hailey disease is an autosomal dominant genodermatosis.
- Dysregulation of intracellular calcium homeostasis leads to impaired desmosome function and suprabasilar acantholysis of the epidermis.
- Clinically, it is characterized by intertriginous vesicles, erosions, and weeping, fissured plaques; it is complicated by pain, secondary infection, and malodor (**Figure 11.16a–d**). Sometimes, in chronic cases, patients may develop verrucous papules and plaques (**Figure 11.16e**).
- Sometimes lesions may appear on the scalp, antecubital or popliteal fossa, and trunk.
- Conjunctiva, mucosa, and vulva involvement is rarely seen.
- Friction, heat, and sweating tend to exacerbate the disease
- DD: Grover's disease, pemphigus vegetans.

## Porphyria cutanea tarda

- Porphyria cutanea tarda (PCT) is a metabolic disorder caused by reduction and inhibition of hepatic uroporphyrinogen decarboxylase (UROD) enzyme activity.

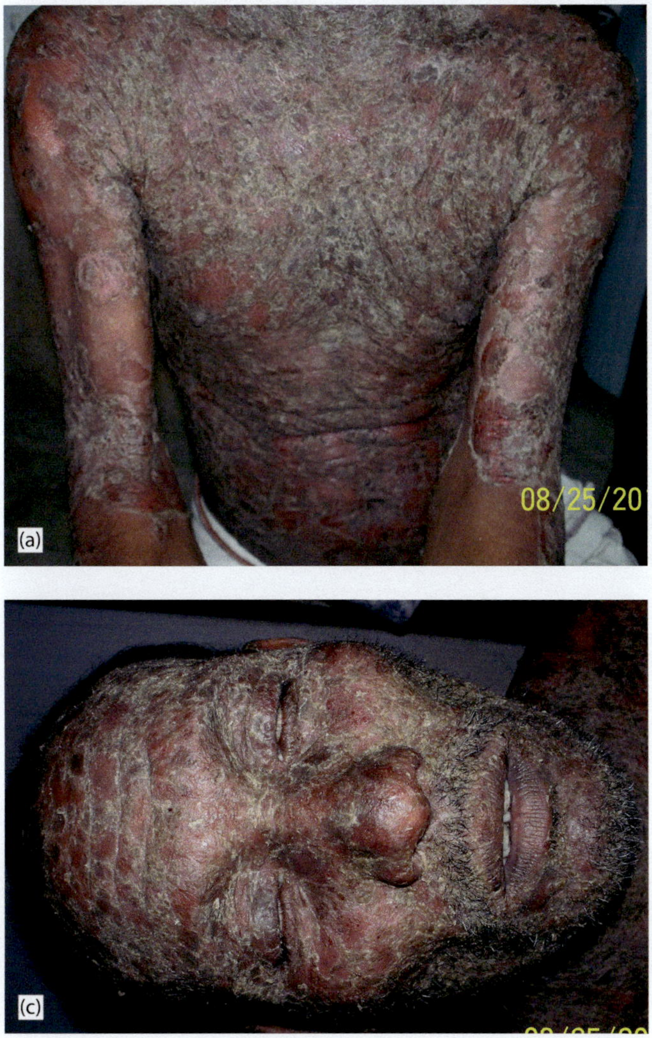


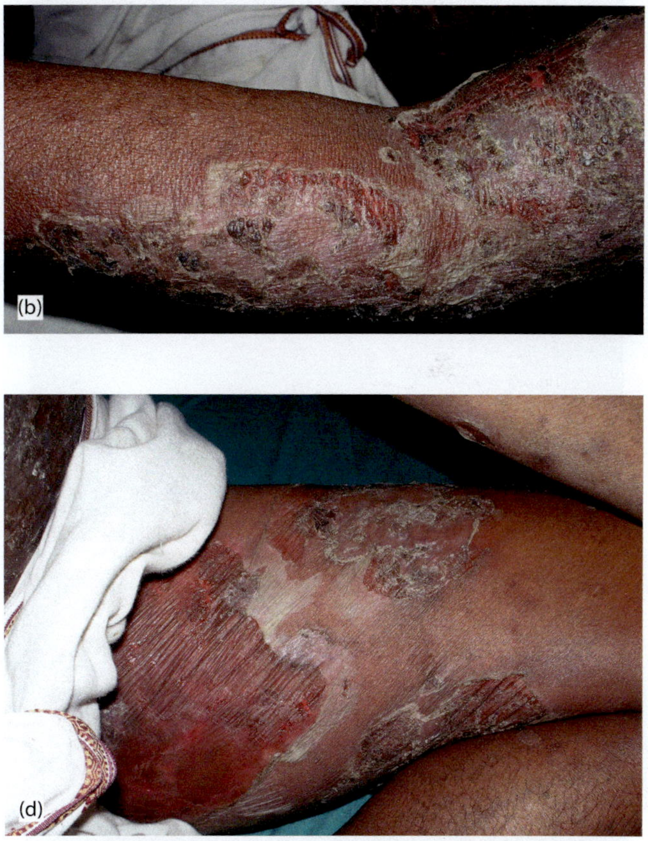


Figure 11.15 **(a)** Crusting and scaling in pemphigus foliaceus in seborrheic distribution. **(b)** Predominant crusted and scaly lesions in pemphigus foliaceus. **(c)** Pemphigus foliaceus. **(d)** Self-limited erosions showing no tendency to spread in pemphigus foliaceous. (a–d – Courtesy: Dr. Piyush Kumar, Katihar, India.)

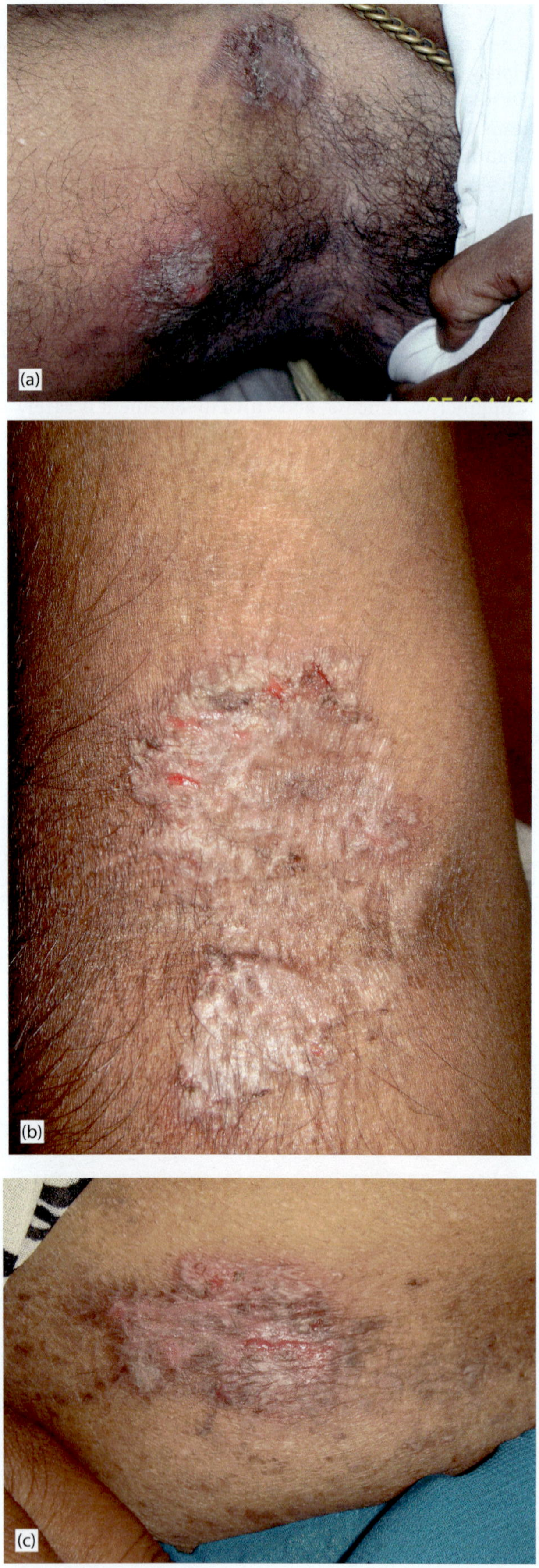


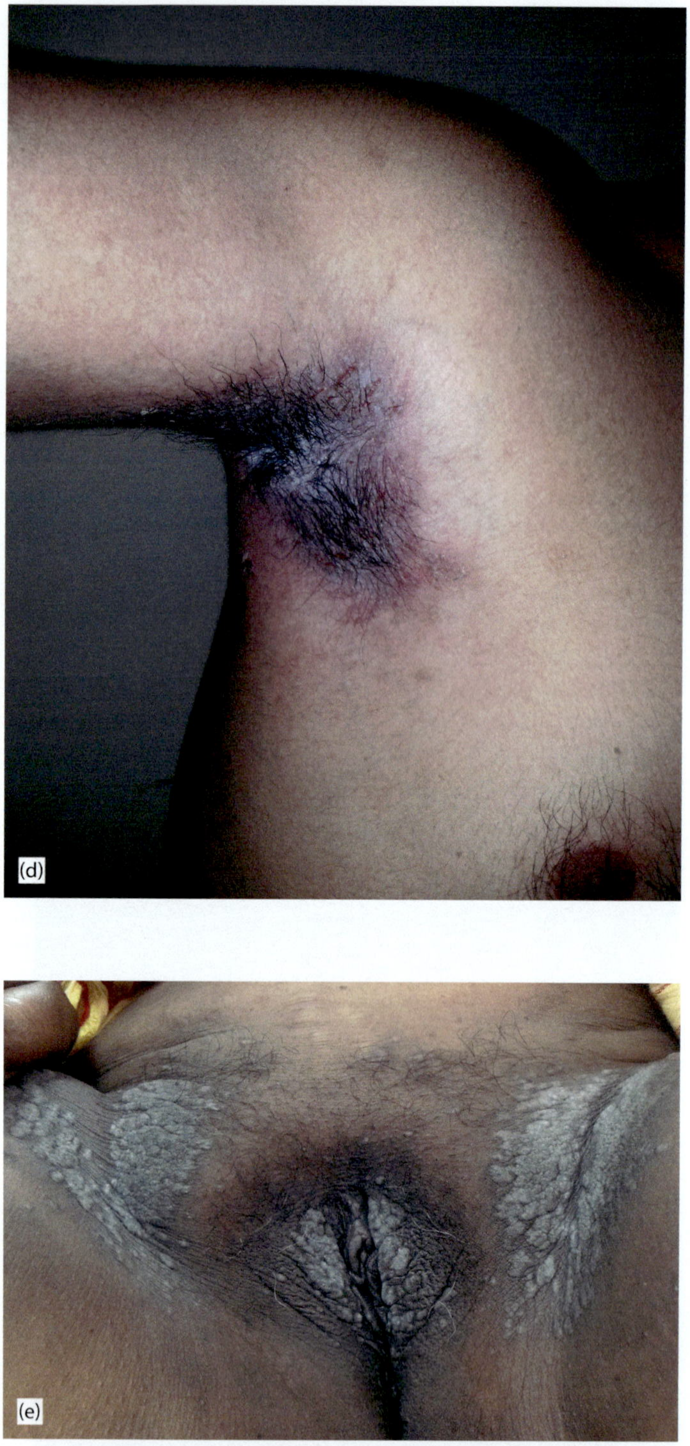


Fig 11.16 **(a)** The groin showing erythema, maceration, vesiculopustular lesions, and fissures in Hailey-Hailey disease. **(b)** Hailey-Hailey disease affecting antecubital fossa. **(c)** The lesion of Hailey-Hailey disease at pressure and friction prone area of the waist. **(d)** Vesicobullous lesions in Hailey-Hailey disease are transient, and patients more commonly present with erythema, fissures, and whitish macerated skin. **(e)** Macerated and verrucous plaques in groin in Hailey-Hailey disease. (a–d – Courtesy: Dr. Piyush Kumar, Katihar, India; e – Courtesy: Dr. Niharika Ranjan Lal, ESIPGIMSR, Kolkata, India.)

- It is characterized by photosensitivity, increased skin fragility, tense blisters and erosions over sun-exposed areas (**Figure 11.17a**).
- Blisters heal with scarring and milia formation (**Figure 11.17b,c**).

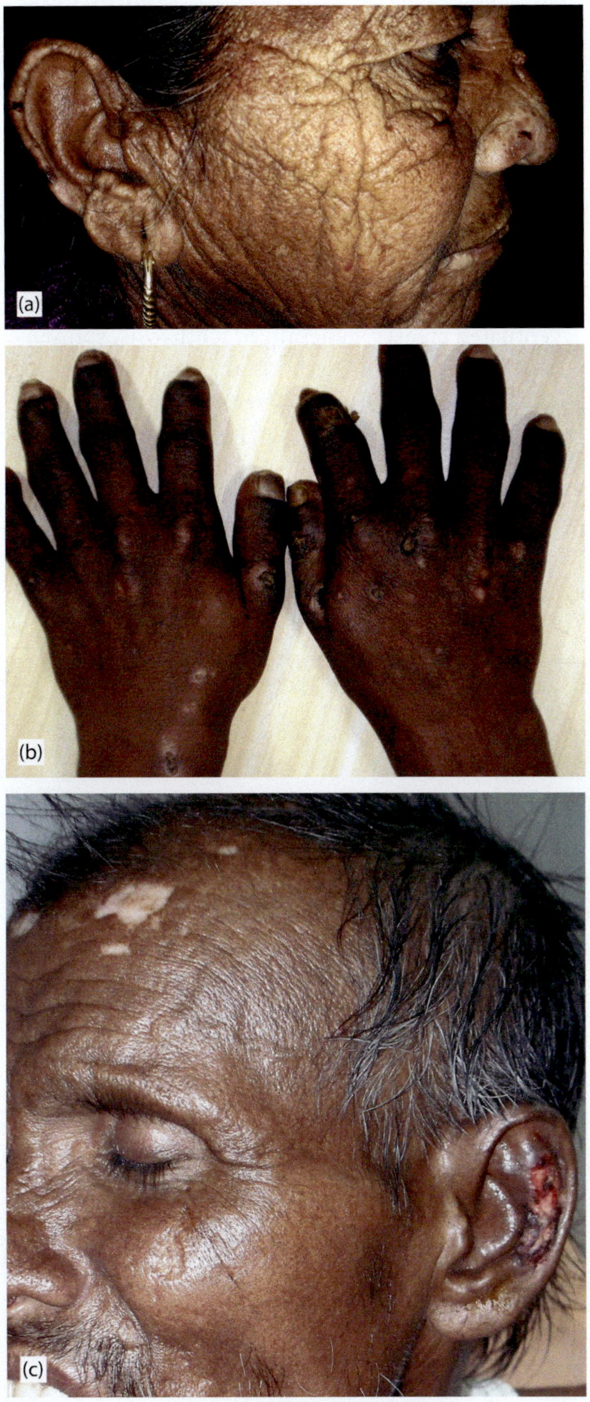


Figure 11.17 **(a)** Crusted vesicles on sun-exposed pinna and nose in porphyria cutanea tarda. **(b)** Blisters healed with scar formation on sun-exposed dorsa of hands in porphyria cutanea tarda. **(c)** Porphyria cutanea tarda. Depigmentation (scalp) and crusted erosion (on pinna). (Courtesy: Dr. Piyush Kumar, Katihar, India.)

- Additional features include hypertrichosis and sclerodermoid features.
- Common sites are sun-exposed areas: the face and dorsum of hands.
- DD: Pseudoporphyria, epidermolysis bullosa acquisita, and phototoxic drug eruption.

### Pseudoporphyria

- Pseudoporphyria is a photosensitive bullous condition resembling porphyria cutanea tarda.
- Risk factors are chronic renal failure, drugs (naproxen), ultraviolet exposure, and genetic predisposition.
- Clinical features include clear fluid filled/hemorrhagic blisters on sun-exposed parts of the body (face, dorsum of hands); it heals with scars and milia formation.
- It resembles PCT clinically and histologically; however, porphyrin levels are normal.
- DD: PCT, EBA (on trauma-prone areas), phototoxic drug reactions.

### Acute phototoxic drug reactions

- These develop in a person exposed to photosensitizing medication in conjunction with sufficient levels of radiant energy.
- They begin within minutes to hours after sun exposure.
- They resemble exaggerated sunburn (**Figure 11.18**).

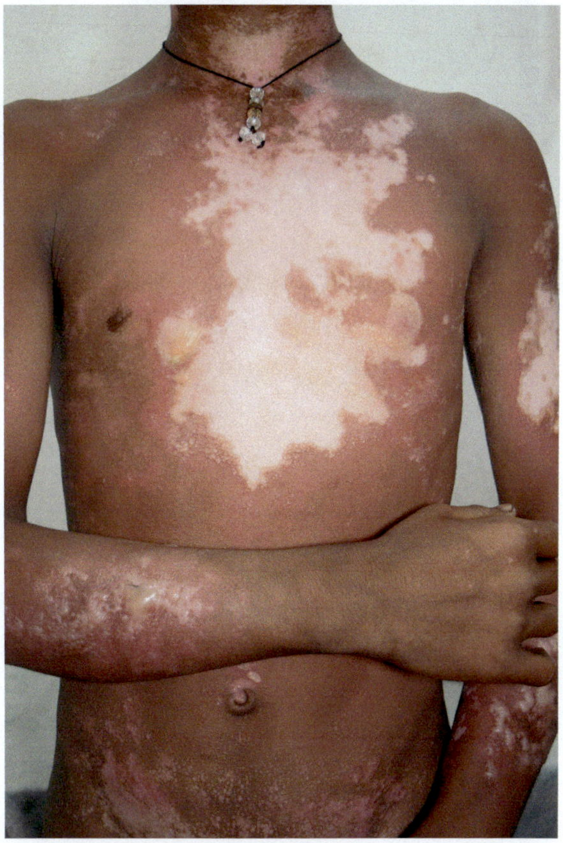

Figure 11.18 Diffuse erythema and vesicobullous lesions of acute phototoxic reaction in a case of vitiligo receiving PUVA therapy. (Courtesy: Dr. Piyush Kumar, Katihar, India.)

- Features include erythema and edema; in severe cases there may be vesicles or bullae, followed by desquamation.
- Common sites include sun-exposed skin areas lithe face, V area of chest, nuchal region, and the dorsum of the hands.
- DD: Photoallergic drug reaction.

## Bullous SLE[8]

- Bullous lesions in SLE may be of three types:
  - Bullous lesions as LE-specific lesions represent severe inflammation, seen in acute cutaneous lupus erythematosus (ACLE) and sometimes subacute cutaneous lupus erythematosus (SCLE); presents like erythema multiforme or toxic epidermal necrolysis.
  - Bullous SLE has autoantibodies against type VII collagen.
  - Rarely, SLE may be seen in association with other autoimmune blistering disorders like pemphigus vulgaris, pemphigus foliaceus, etc.
- Clinical features include blisters on sun-exposed sites; tense blisters form on an erythematous/urticarial base (**Figure 11.19**).
- The face, upper trunk, and proximal extremities are affected.
- Systemic features include fever, weight loss, and arthralgia.
- DD: Pemphigus foliaceus, bullous pemphigoid, bullous fixed drug reaction, vesicobullous lesions of acute LE.

## Epidermolytic ichthyosis (bullous congenital ichthyosiform erythroderma)

- Epidermolytic ichthyosis is an autosomal dominant genetic bullous disease.
- Erythroderma and epidermal blistering are present at birth.
- Blistering diminishes and resolves with age; there is progressive hyperkeratosis.
- Thickened skin, scaling, palmoplantar keratoderma, accentuated creases, generalized ichthyosis, spiny papules, and malodorous body are prominent at advancing age. (**Figure 11.20a–c**).
- Depending upon these clinical grounds, six subtypes of the disease are recognized.
- There is skin fragility, and bouts of blistering are precipitated by fever, skin infections, and friction.
- DD: Epidermolysis bullosa, staphylococcal scalded skin syndrome, bullous pemphigoid.

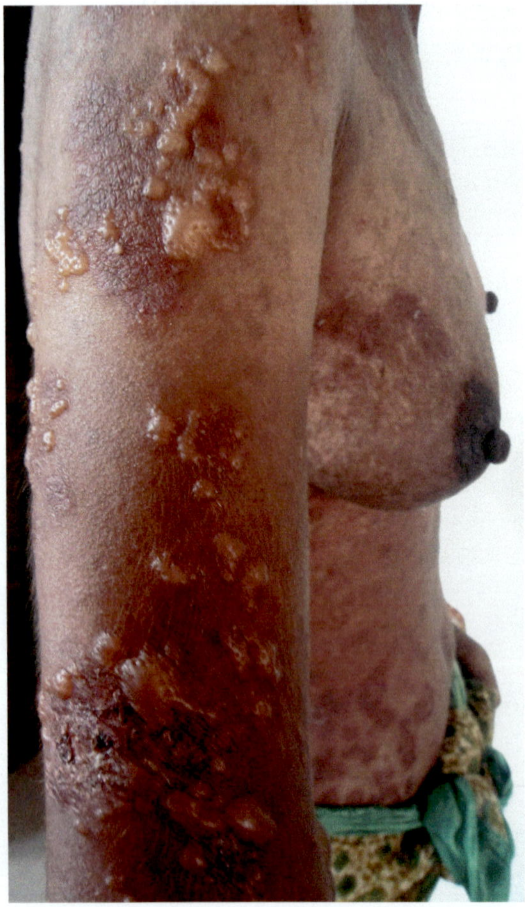

Figure 11.19 Vesicles and bulla over erythematous base in photoexposed distribution in bullous systemic lupus erythematosus. (Courtesy: Dr. Shvetha Jain, Mumbai, India.)

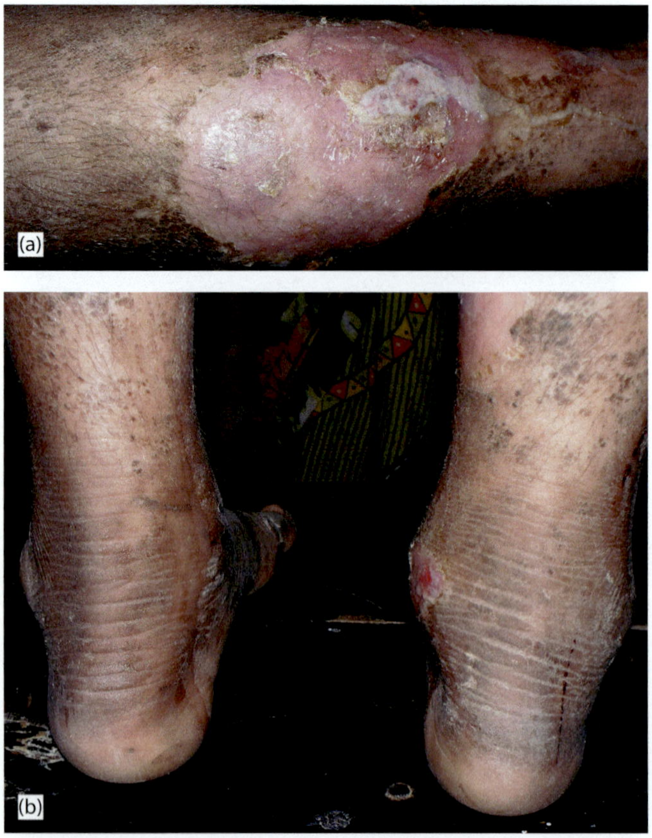

Figure 11.20 **(a)** Superficial erosion and oozing in epidermolytic ichthyosis. **(b)** Parallel ridges of hyperkeratosis mimicking corrugated cardboard on the posterior aspect of the ankle joint. Note a small erosion on the medial aspect of right leg. (*Continued*)

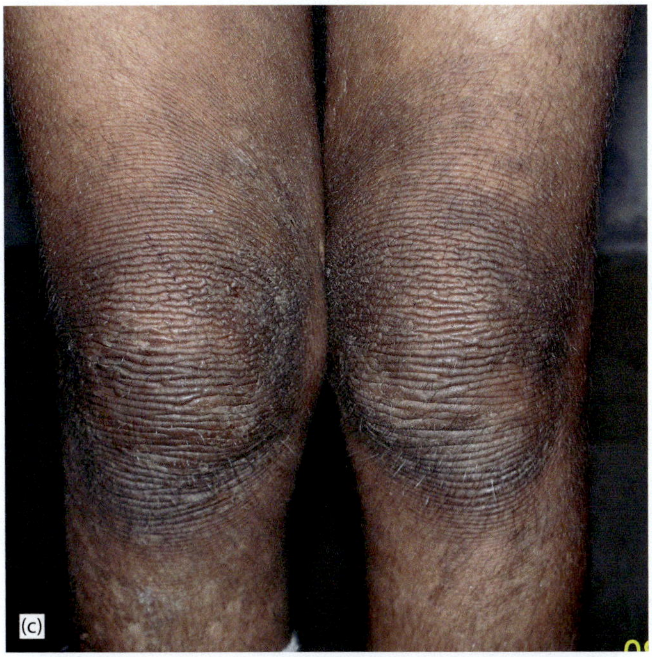


Figure 11.20 (*Continued*) **(c)** Classic "corrugated cardboard" like parallel ridges of hyperkeratosis on the knee joint. (a–c – Courtesy: Dr. Piyush Kumar, Katihar, India.)

## Inherited epidermolysis bullosa

- This presents as tense blisters filled with serous or hemorrhagic fluid on a non-inflammatory base (**Figure 11.21a**).
- Common sites include trauma-prone surfaces: acral sites, elbows, and knees; sometimes it is generalized (**Figure 11.21b–d**).
- Mucosal involvement is variable with laryngeal and esophageal involvement in some cases.
- It heals with atrophic scarring (**Figure 11.21e**) and hyper- or hypopigmentation; there is milia formation in dystrophic forms of epidermolysis bullosa.
- Onset is from birth, in the neonatal period.
- There are variable nail (**Figure 11.21f**) and dental changes, depending on the epidermolysis bullosa subtype (**Figure 11.21g,h**).
- DD: Other skin fragility disorders like porphyria.

## Congenital syphilis

- Congenital syphilis is a multisystem infection caused by *Treponema pallidum* and transmitted to the fetus via the placenta.
- It is asymptomatic at birth; symptoms develop within the first two months of life.
- Early congenital syphilis (first two years of life) usually manifests as characteristic skin lesions, such as vesiculobullous or a macular copper-colored rash on the palms and soles and papular lesions around the nose and mouth and in the diaper area, as well as petechial lesions.
- Other features include rhinitis, bone abnormalities, chorioretinitis, lymphadenopathy, hepatosplenomegaly, and nephrotic syndrome.

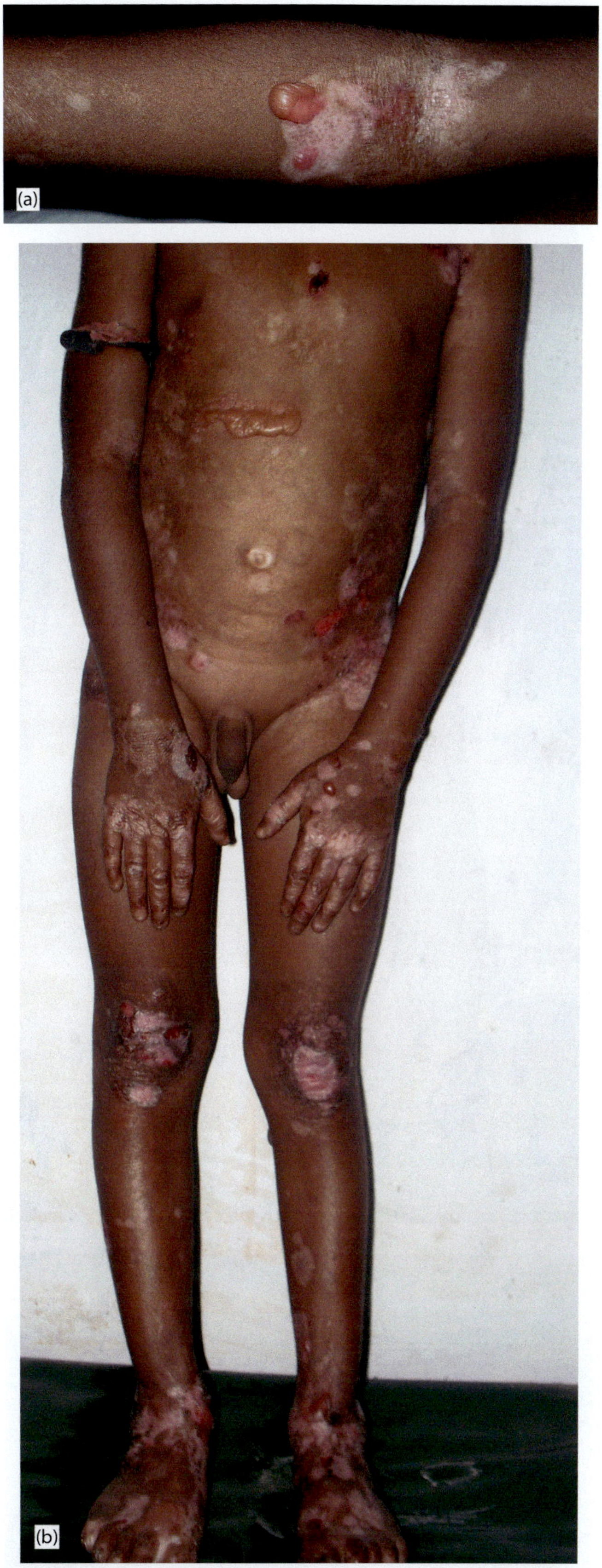


Figure 11.21 **(a)** Blister filled with clear fluid on non-inflammatory base. **(b)** Front view showing blisters, erosions, and scarring on trauma-prone areas in a child with dystrophic epidermolysis bullosa. (*Continued*)

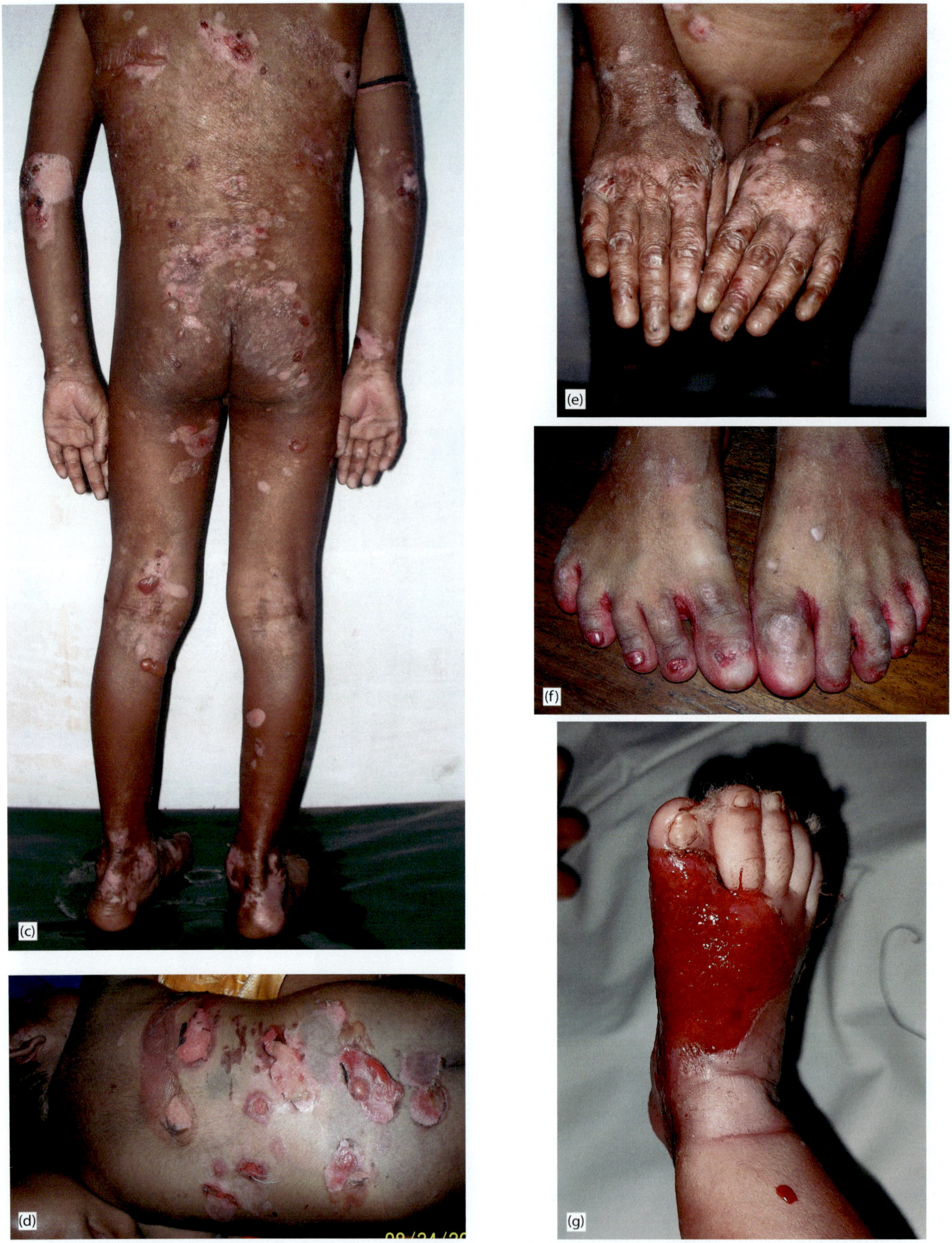


Figure 11.21 (*Continued*) **(c)** Back view of same child. **(d)** Erosions and skin peeling on back of child in epidermolysis bullosa. **(e)** Blisters healed with scarring on hands in dystrophic epidermolysis bullosa. **(f)** Anonychia in a female with dystrophic epidermolysis bullosa. **(g)** Epidermolysis bullosa in a nine-day-old child presenting with erosion with profuse bleeding. (*Continued*)

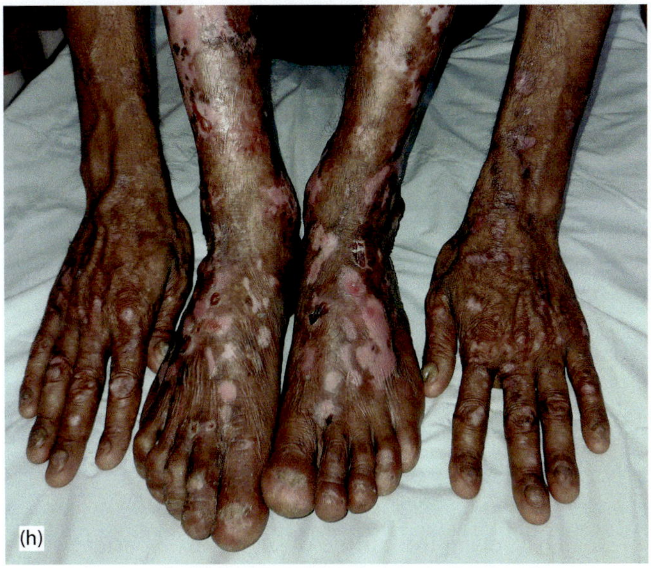


Figure 11.21 (*Continued*) **(h)** Father of the child (Figure 11.21g) has dystrophic epidermolysis bullosa. Note erosions, scarring, and variable degree of nail loss. (a–h – Courtesy: Dr. Piyush Kumar, Katihar, India.)

- Syphilitic pemphigus, a rare bullous variant, most commonly occurs on palms and soles but may be generalized.
- DD: Bullous impetigo, congenital pemphigus, congenital candidiasis.

## REFERENCES


1. Hill SF, Murrell DF. Differential diagnosis of vesiculobullous lesions. In, Hoeger P, Kinsler V, Yan A, editors. Harper's Textbook of Pediatric Dermatology. 4th edition. New Jersey: Wiley-Blackwell, 2020. P. 859–867.
2. Hull C, Zone JJ. Approach to the patient with cutaneous blisters. In, Stratman E, Ofori AO, editors. UpToDate, Waltham, MA.https://www.uptodate.com/contents/approach-to-the-patient-with-cutaneous-blisters. Accessed on 07 April, 2020.
3. van Beek N, Zillikens D, Schmidt E. Diagnosis of autoimmune bullous diseases. J Dtsch Dermatol Ges 2018;16(9):1077–1091.
4. Bogdanov I, Darlenski R, Hristakieva E, Manuelyan K. The rash that presents as a vesiculobullous eruption. Clin Dermatol 2020;38(1):19–34.
5. Jaleel T, Kwak Y, Sami N. Clinical Approach to Diffuse Blisters. Med Clin North Am 2015;99(6):1243–1267, xii.
6. Oberlin KE. Vesiculobullous and Pustular Diseases in Newborns. Cutis 2017;100(4):E18–E21.
7. Zhao CY, Murrell DF. Blistering diseases in neonates. CurrOpinPediatr 2016;28(4):500–506.
8. Ashi, Kumar P. Photosensitivity and Bullous Lesions. In: Rahmani F, Rezaei N, editors. Pediatric Autoimmunity and Transplantation. 1st edition. Cham Switzerland: Springer International Publishing; 2020. P. 337–343.

# 12

# Pustules: Localized

MADHULIKA MHATRE, ASEEM SHARMA, TRUPTI AGARWAL

## INTRODUCTION

Localized pustules can be seen in a variety of infective and inflammatory conditions. Pustular lesions may be seen as exclusive lesions or may occur along with papules (acne vulgaris, rosacea), nodules (nodulocystic acne) or vesicles (pompholyx). Several defining features, including patient's age and general health, distribution of lesions, and duration of lesions aid in making a clinical diagnosis. Follicular localization is usually seen in infective conditions and is another important clinical clue. The clinical approach to the diagnosis of localized pustules has been summarized in **Table 12.1**. Of these listed conditions, a few will be omitted from the detailed discussion owing to the relative rarity of the same.[1–5]

### Folliculitis decalvans

- Folliculitis decalvans is a rare, chronic neutrophilic cicatricial (scarring) alopecia, speculated to be an abnormal response to bacteria, particularly *Staphylococcus aureus*.
- Predisposing factors are trauma and seborrhea.
- It affects young to middle-aged adults.
- Males are affected more than females.
- It affects African Americans more than Caucasians.
- Symptoms include pain, itching, burning sensation, and spontaneous bleeding.
- Clinical morphology is as follows:
    - The initial lesion is an erythematous follicular pustule.
    - It shows livid, bright erythema with yellow-gray scales around follicles associated with follicular hyperkeratosis, erosions. and hemorrhagic crusts (**Figure 12.1**).
    - It progresses to irregularly shaped, atrophic flesh-colored or ivory/white patches of cicatricial alopecia.
    - Tufted folliculitis, with multiple hairs (5 to 20) emerging from a single dilated follicular orifice.
- DD: Dissecting folliculitis of scalp (male patients, boggy confluent nodules), acne keloidalis nuchae (firm papules/nodules over occipital scalp with hypertrophic scarring), erosive pustular dermatosis (elderly women, suppurative, necrotic, erosive papules and plaques), deep fungal infections, bacterial folliculitis (early scarring and lack of ostia).

### Erosive pustular dermatosis of scalp

- This is a chronic inflammatory disease with an unknown cause.
- It is commonly seen in elderly populations and has a female preponderance.
- Risk factors include cutaneous atrophy from any cause, chronic sun exposure, trauma and tissue damage and inflammatory triggers such as HZ, sunburn, hair transplants, topical chemotherapy, cryotherapy, and photodynamic therapy (PDT).
- Patients complain of pain, pruritus, or burning at the site.
- Clinically, it presents as sterile non-follicular pustules, yellow-brown keratotic crusts, and superficial erosions. The surrounding area shows atrophy of affected skin, with scarring alopecia.
- DD: Cicatricial (mucous membrane) pemphigoid, folliculitis decalvans, pemphigus foliaceus, pemphigus vulgaris, Langerhans cell histiocytosis.

### Bacterial folliculitis and impetigo

- Folliculitis is a superficial bacterial infection of the hair follicles with purulent material.
- It primarily affects children but can present in adults as well.
- There is no sex predilection.
- Bacterial folliculitis may occur anywhere on the body, including the face.


DOI: 10.1201/9781351054225-22

Table 12.1 Clinical approach to dermatoses presenting as localized pustules

| Site | Features | Diseases |
|---|---|---|
| Scalp | Children | Tinea capitis*<br>Bacterial folliculitis*<br>Neonatal Langerhans cell histiocytosis |
| | Adult | Folliculitis decalvans*<br>Erosive pustulosis of scalp |
| Face | Children | Impetigo contagiosa and bullous impetigo<br>Neonatal cephalic pustulosis (neonatal acne)*<br>Perioral dermatitis<br>Neonatal Langerhans cell histiocytosis* |
| | Adult | Acne vulgaris*<br>Acneiform eruptions<br>Rosacea (papulopustular)<br>Sycosis barbae*<br>Tinea barbae*<br>Acne keloidalis nuchae*<br>Pseudofolliculitis barbae*<br>Pyoderma faciale |
| | Any age group | Herpes simplex<br>Acute Localized Exanthematous Pustulosis (ALEP) |
| Trunk | Children | Keratosis pilaris* |
| | Adult | Truncal acne*<br>Pityrosporum folliculitis*<br>Gram negative folliculitis*<br>Acneiform eruptions<br>Eosinophilic folliculitis*<br>Subcorneal pustulosis of Sneddon-Wilkinson |
| | Any age group | Miliaria pustulosa |
| Extremities/acral areas | Children | Scabies<br>Infantile acropustulosis<br>Papular urticaria<br>Parakeratosis pustulosa |
| | Adult | Dermatitis cruris pustulosa et atrophicans (DCPA)*<br>Acrodermatitis continua suppurativa of Hallopeau<br>Pustular pyoderma gangrenosum<br>Orf<br>Sporotrichosis |
| Palms and soles | Adult | Contact dermatitis<br>Palmoplantar pustulosis |
| | Any age group | Pompholyx |
| Flexures | Children | Bullous impetigo |
| | Adults | Amicrobial pustulosis of the folds*<br>Hidradenitis suppurativa*<br>Subcorneal pustulosis of Sneddon-Wilkinson |
| | Any age group | Candidiasis*<br>Miliaria pustulosa |
| Anywhere/no site restriction | Any age group | Herpes Zoster<br>Folliculitis*<br>Dermatophyte infection<br>Insect contact dermatitis |

* Follicular pustules

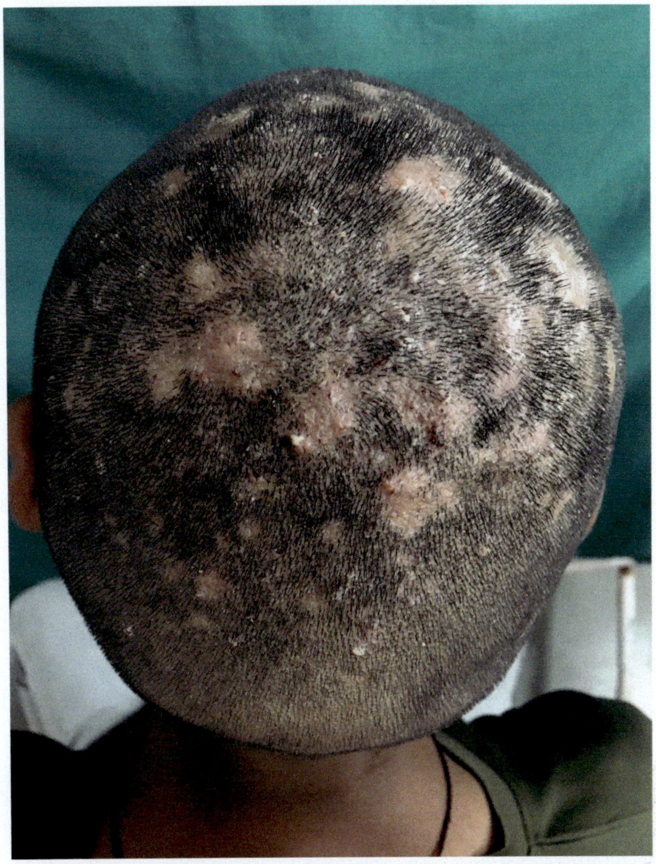

Figure 12.1 Pustules with scaling in folliculitis decalvans. Lesions have healed with scarring. (Courtesy: Dr. Bhushan Madke, Jawaharlal Nehru Medical College, Datta Meghe Institute of Medical Sciences, India.)

- Risk factors include areas of repeated shaving, diabetes mellitus, and immuno-compromised individuals.
- Clinically, folliculitis manifests as clusters of multiple small, raised, pruritic, erythematous lesions less than 5 mm in diameter. Pustules may be present at the centers of the lesions (**Figure 12.2a**). Impetigo occurs most commonly on the face and can present with bullae, honey-colored crusts, erythema, edema, and exudate, commonly in children (**Figure 12.2b,c**).
- DD: Pityrosporum folliculitis, superficial actinic folliculitis, folliculitis following application of epilating agents, folliculitis due to exposure to occupational agents (chemicals, oils) (**Figure 12.2d**), perforating folliculitis (Kyrle's disease).

## Sycosis barbae

- Sycosis barbae is a staphylococcal infection of the entire depth of hair follicle.
- It affects post-adolescents.
- Males are affected more than females.
- The primary site is the beard area.

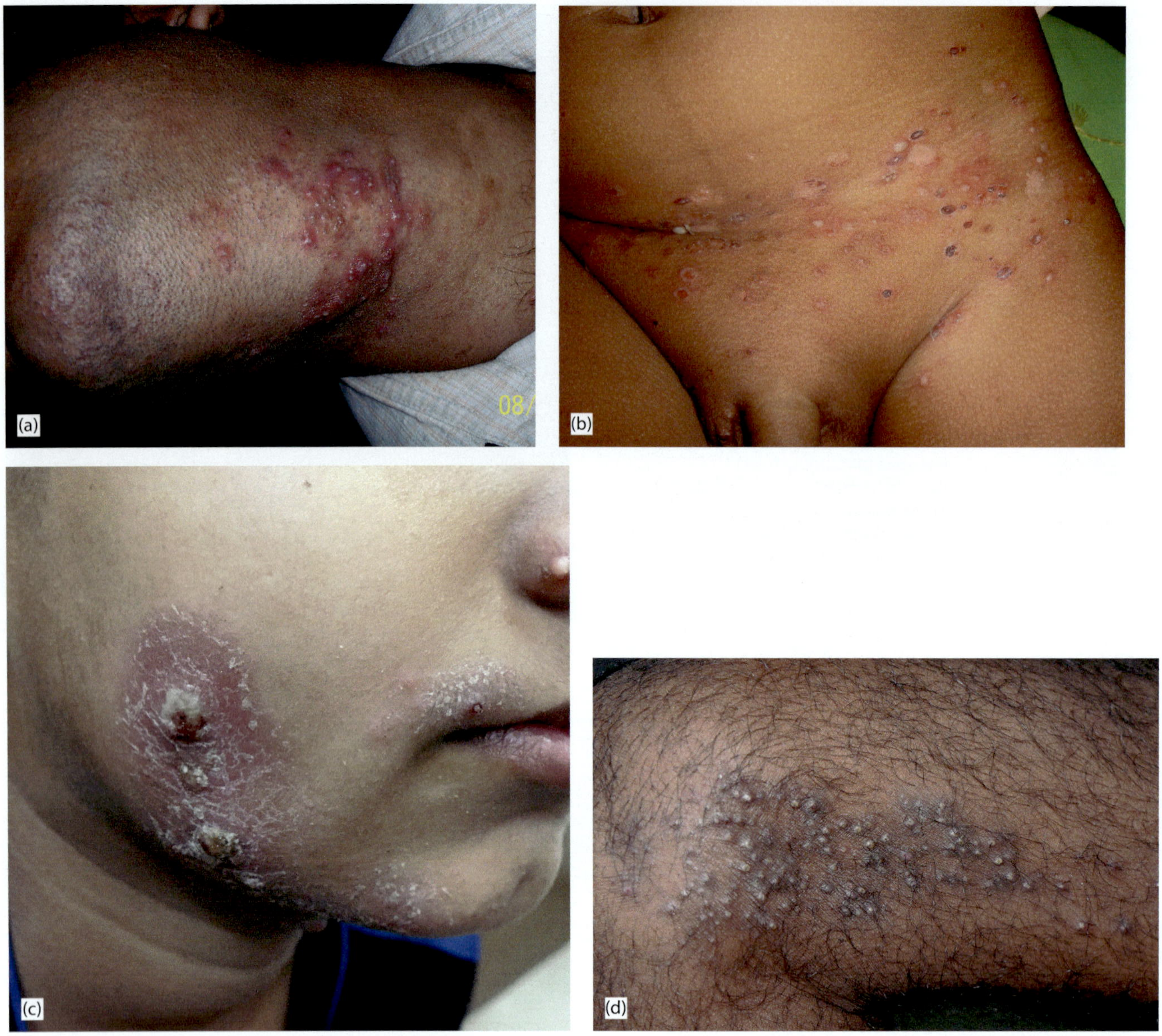


Figure 12.2 **(a)** Closely set pustules pierced by a hair on the erythematous base on neck in bacterial folliculitis. **(b)** Pustules, vesicles, and crusts in a child with bullous impetigo. **(c)** Crusted vesicles and pustules with surrounding erythema in bullous impetigo in a child. **(d)** Follicular pustules due to occlusion by oil. (a,b,d – Courtesy: Dr. Piyush Kumar, Katihar, India.)

- Predisposing factors include seborrhea and indoor work.
- Clinical morphology shows the following:
  - Oedematous erythematous papule or pustule which is folliculo-centric (**Figure 12.3a–c**).
  - Neighboring follicular papules may coalesce to form a plaque studded with pustules resembling a ripe fig; hence the term "sycosis."
  - Lesions are grouped.
  - There is crusting and scaling.
  - The disease runs a chronic relapsing and remitting course and heals with scarring.
- DD: Pseudofolliculitis (typically non-grouped), tinea barbae (typical plaque, may be annular, history of animal contact, relatively asymptomatic or mildly pruritic).

## Tinea barbae

- Three types of dermatophytes account for the majority of infections: epidermophyton, trichophyton, and microsporum.
- The primary site is the beard area.
- It affects adults.
- Dermatophyte infection of the beard area can be superficial and non-inflammatory or deeper and

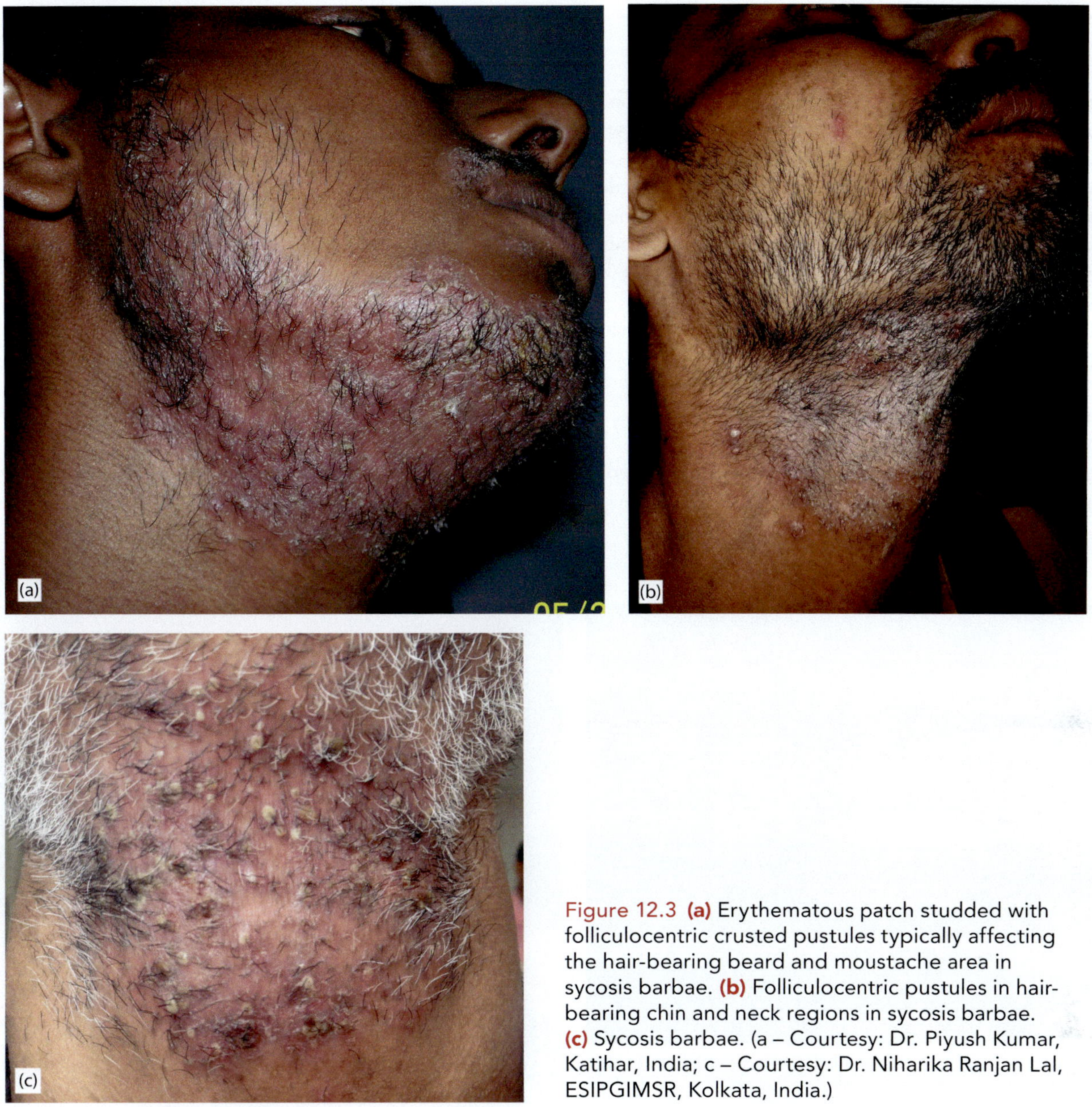


Figure 12.3 **(a)** Erythematous patch studded with folliculocentric crusted pustules typically affecting the hair-bearing beard and moustache area in sycosis barbae. **(b)** Folliculocentric pustules in hair-bearing chin and neck regions in sycosis barbae. **(c)** Sycosis barbae. (a – Courtesy: Dr. Piyush Kumar, Katihar, India; c – Courtesy: Dr. Niharika Ranjan Lal, ESIPGIMSR, Kolkata, India.)

inflammatory (kerion type) and is characterized by scaly, annular plaques with pustules and broken-hairs (**Figure 12.4**) (superficial; most commonly caused by *T. rubrum* or *T. violaceum*) or a deep inflammatory nodule or plaque with pustules and sinus tracts (deep; most commonly by *T. mentagrophytes* or *T. verrucosum*).

- DD: Acne vulgaris, bacterial folliculitis, herpetic sycosis, perioral dermatitis, pseudofolliculitis barbae, sycosis barbae.

## Herpes simplex

- Caused by herpes simplex virus type 1 (HSV-1), this is also known as herpes labialis. It may be a primary or recurrent infection (commonly in immunosuppressed patients).

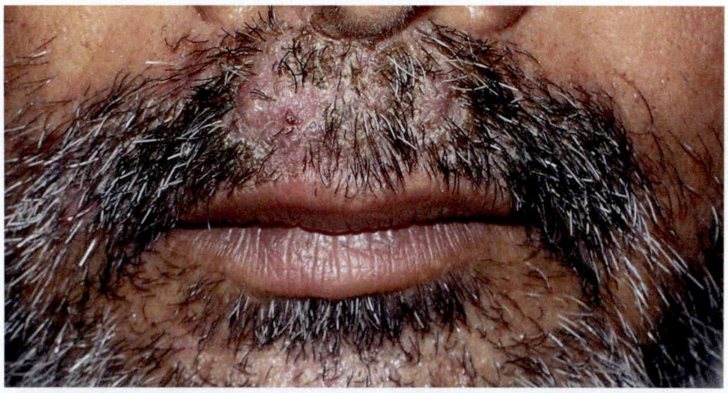

Figure 12.4 Erythematous swelling studded with pustules and loss of hair in the moustache area in tinea barbae. (Courtesy: Dr. Piyush Kumar, Katihar, India.)

- It affects adults and, rarely, children (oropharyngitis more than labialis).
- There is no sex predilection.
- Primary sites are as follows. Labialis: lower vermilion lip margin; Genitalis: labia minora or glans; Whitlow: finger tips.
- Herpes simplex eruptions present as grouped pustules or vesicles on an erythematous base typically on the lower vermilion lip of the face (**Figure 12.5a,b**). They may present similarly in the genital (**Figure 12.5c**) or sacral areas, particularly with recurrent disease. Patients frequently have a history of a prodrome prior to the onset of lesions.
- Precipitating factors include fever, windburn or sunburn, trauma, or stress.
- DD: Aphthous stomatitis, Behçet's disease, bullous pemphigoid, candidiasis, erythema multiforme, fixed drug eruption.

## Neonatal acne/infantile acne

- Also known as acne neonatorum, acne infantum, and neonatal cephalic pustulosis, this is an acneiform eruption that occurs due to the increased sensitivity of the infant's sebaceous glands to maternal hormones during pregnancy.
- It affects newborns or neonates; infantile acne affects infants three to six months of age.
- There is no sex predilection.
- Common sites are the cheeks, chin, and forehead.
- Clinical morphology shows comedones, papules, and pustules and rarely nodules and cysts.
- DD: Folliculitis, perioral dermatitis, milia, miliaria.

## Acne vulgaris

- Acne vulgaris is the most common cutaneous disorder affecting adolescents and young adults.

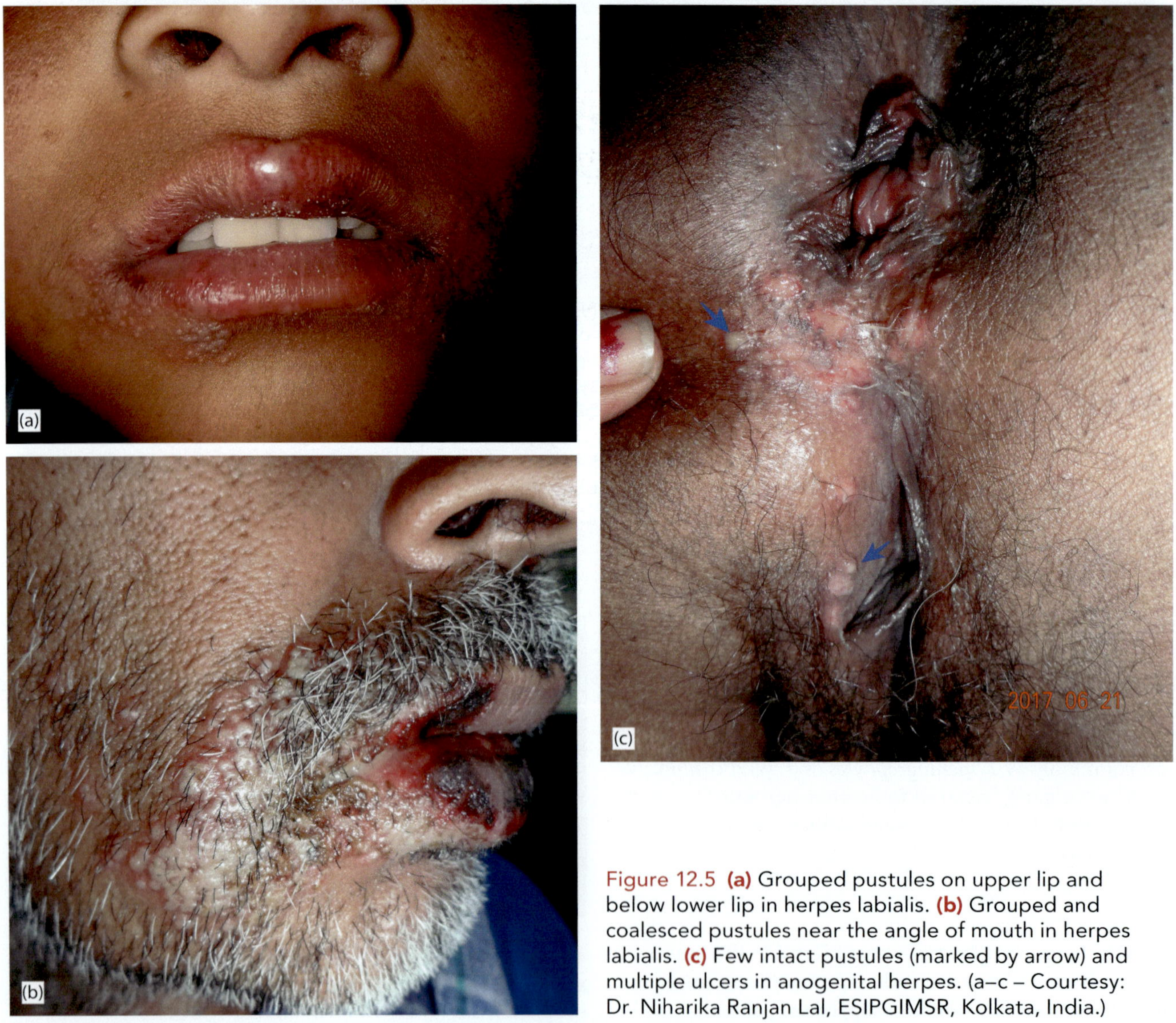


Figure 12.5 **(a)** Grouped pustules on upper lip and below lower lip in herpes labialis. **(b)** Grouped and coalesced pustules near the angle of mouth in herpes labialis. **(c)** Few intact pustules (marked by arrow) and multiple ulcers in anogenital herpes. (a–c – Courtesy: Dr. Niharika Ranjan Lal, ESIPGIMSR, Kolkata, India.)

- Acne vulgaris is a disease of pilosebaceous follicles. Four factors are involved:
  - Follicular hyperkeratinization
  - Increased sebum production
  - *Propionibacterium acnes* (P. acnes) within the follicle
  - Inflammation
- Risk factors include conditions causing androgen excess, use of pomades, family history, stress, use of comedogenic cosmetics.
- It primarily affects adolescent adults but can be seen well into adulthood.
- It affects females more than males.
- The most common sites are areas of the body that have the largest hormonally responsive sebaceous glands, including the face, neck, chest, upper back, and upper arms.
- Clinical picture is typically pleomorphic with pustules along with other characteristic acne lesions including comedones, papules, nodules, postinflammatory hyperpigmentation, and scarring (**Figure 12.6**).
- There may be a history of acne-inducing medication such as glucocorticoids, phenytoin, lithium, isoniazid, epidermal growth factor inhibitors, iodides, bromides, androgens, Vitamins B2, B6, and B12.
- DD: Rosacea (no comedones and presence of telangiectasia), perioral dermatitis (small, grouped erythematous papules sparing vermilion border), pseudofolliculitis barbae and acne keloidalis nuchae (beard and nuchal area affected), folliculitis, steatocystoma multiplex, acneiform eruptions.

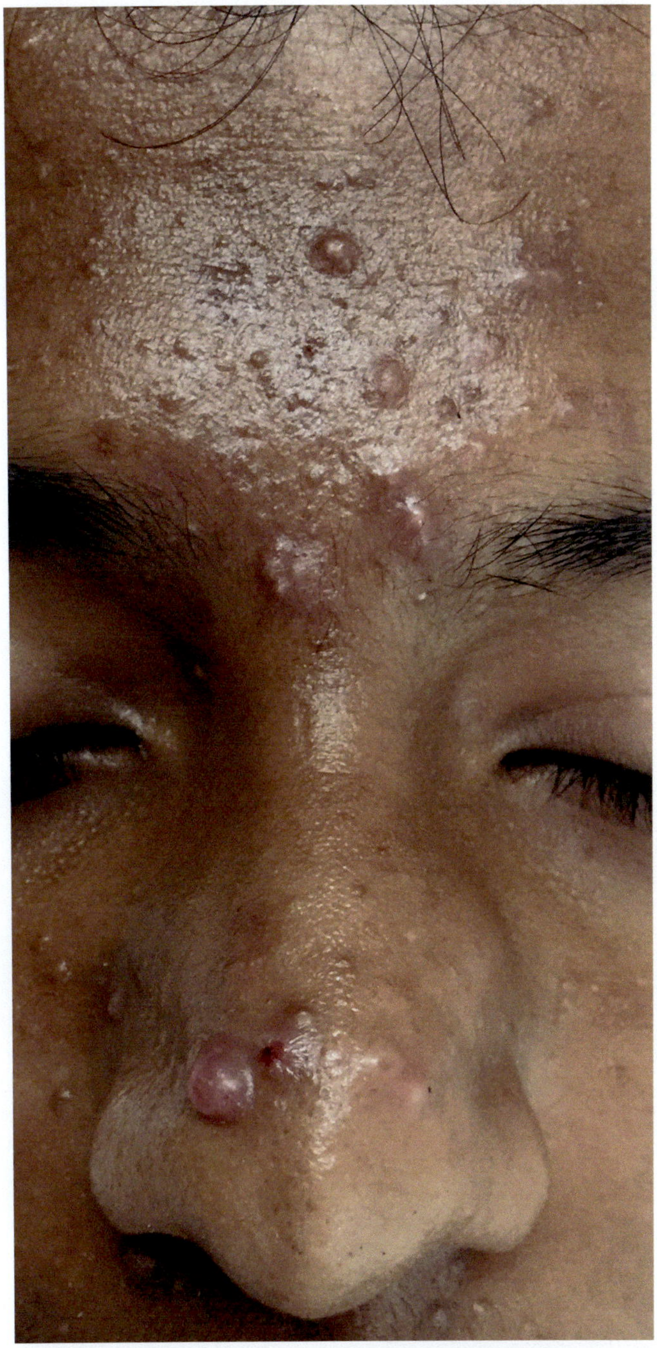

Figure 12.6 Pustules mixed with inflammatory papules over forehead and nose in acne vulgaris.

## Perioral dermatitis (periorificial dermatitis, circumoral dermatitis)

- Deficiencies in skin barrier function and features of atopy have been detected at increased frequency in patients with perioral dermatitis.
- Recent use of topical, nasal, or inhaled corticosteroids may be elicited.
- There is a history of disease flares after topical corticosteroid withdrawal.
- Potential contributors include fluorinated toothpaste, skin moisturizers and cosmetic products, fusobacteria, *Candida albicans*, hormonal fluctuations in women, and oral contraceptive therapy.
- Ages between 16 and 45 constitute the vast majority of cases.
- It affects females more than males.
- The most common site is the perioral region, but a narrow zone around the vermilion border of the lip is usually spared. Less often, the perinasal and periorbital areas are affected.
- It may be asymptomatic or may be accompanied by mild to moderate stinging or burning sensations in the affected areas.
- The skin lesions usually resolve without scarring.
- Clinical morphology shows multiple 1- to 2-mm clustered erythematous papules, papulovesicles, or papulopustules, with or without mild scaling, and sparing of the skin immediately adjacent to the vermilion border of the lip (**Figure 12.7a,b**).
- There may or may not be signs of eczematous dermatitis.
- DD: Rosacea, seborrheic dermatitis, demodex infections, lupus miliaris disseminatus faciei, allergic

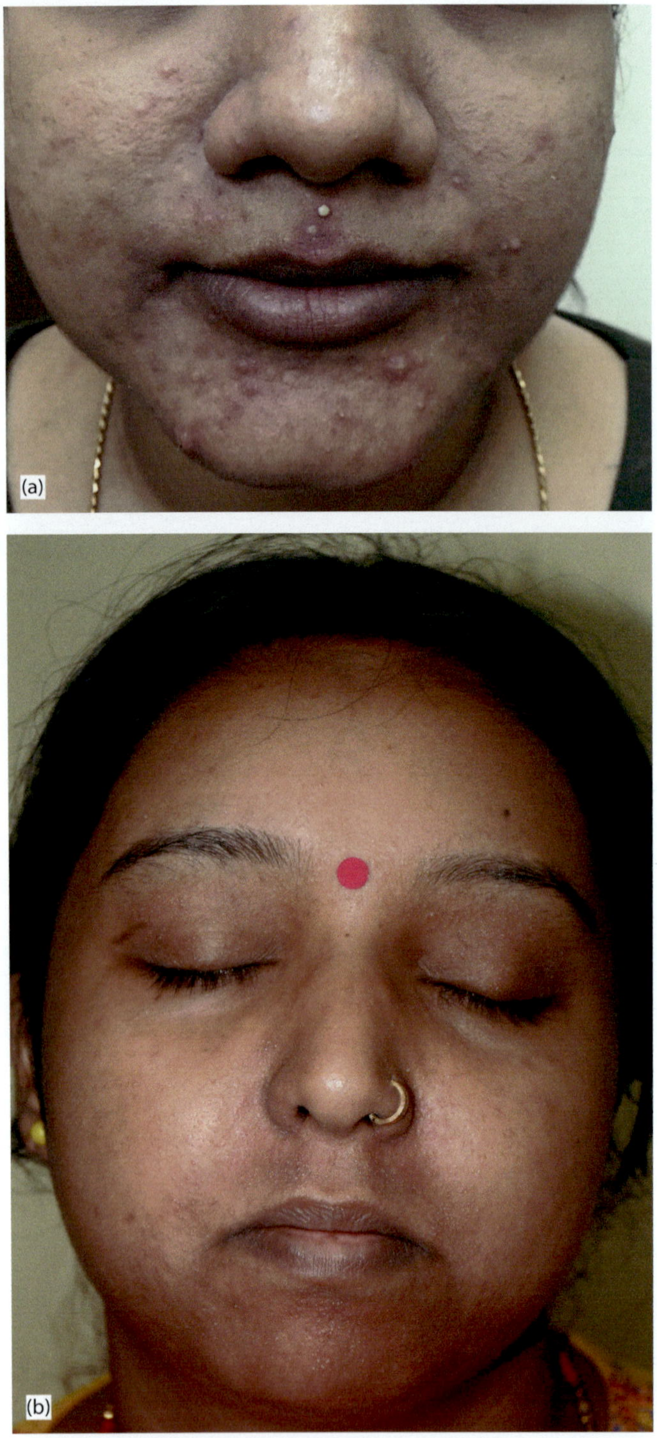


Figure 12.7 **(a)** Perioral pustules in perioral dermatitis. **(b)** Perioral dermatitis presenting as erythema studded with tiny pustules. Note involvement of perioral and periocular area. (a,b – Courtesy: Dr. Piyush Kumar, Katihar, India.)

contact dermatitis (unlike POD, intense pruritus is usually present, scale is often prominent, and lesions fail to improve with antibiotic therapy), impetigo (erosions, vesicles and yellow crusts present; scaling and acne-like papules are uncommon).

## Acne keloidalis nuchae

- Acne keloidalis nuchae is a chronic inflammatory condition.
- It affects post-adolescent young adults.
- It affects males 20 times more than females.
- The most common site is the nape of the neck.
- Risk factors include skin injuries from irritation, occlusion, trauma, friction, and hair-cutting practices.
- Early lesions of acne keloidalis are inflamed papules with marked erythema. Pustules may develop as a result of a sterile, acute inflammatory response to embedded hair or as a manifestation of secondary infection. Papules may be skin-colored, erythematous, or hyperpigmented and coalesce into large plaques and nodules. Secondary infection can lead to pustules and abscess formation in some cases. Over time, continued inflammation leads to pronounced fibrosis and keloid formation. Late stages of presentation include chronic scarring and/or scarring alopecia without active inflammation.
- DD: Bacterial folliculitis (acute condition), dissecting cellulitis, folliculitis decalvans.

## Rosacea (papulopustular type)

- Dysfunction of the innate immune system may contribute to the development of chronic inflammation and vascular abnormalities in rosacea.
- Microorganisms (*Demodex*, *Bacillus olenorium*, and *H. pylori*), ultraviolet radiation, and vascular hyper-reactivity might play a role in pathogenesis.
- A positive family history may be noted.
- Exacerbating factors include exposure to extremes of temperature, sun exposure, hot beverages, spicy foods, alcohol, exercise, irritation from topical products, psychological feelings (especially anger, rage, and embarrassment), and certain drugs such as nicotinic acid and vasodilators.
- It primarily affects adults older than 30.
- It affects females more than males.
- Symptoms include persistent centrofacial redness and pustular eruptions in moderate to severe cases.
- Clinical clues include pustular rosacea found frequently on the central face. Look for telangiectasia, erythema, papules, nodules, thickening of the soft tissue, and sebaceous prominence of the central face. In occasional patients the whole nose may be tender, swollen, and red.
- DD: Acne vulgaris (comedones do not occur in rosacea and inflammation may extend outward well beyond the follicular unit to form plaques),

seborrheic dermatitis (a greasy quality to the scale and involvement of other sites such as the scalp, retroauricular skin, and brow suggest this diagnosis), topical steroid-induced acneiform eruptions (topical corticosteroid use can result in the appearance of monomorphic inflammatory papules and pustules on facial skin; the patient history is valuable for diagnosis), perioral dermatitis (perioral dermatitis presents with numerous small papules with fine scale in the perioral area; sparing of the skin adjacent to the vermillion border of the lip is characteristic), demodicosis (*Demodex* folliculitis) (demodicosis can present with numerous inflammatory papules on the face and is difficult to distinguish from papulopustular rosacea on clinical examination).

## Pityrosporum folliculitis

- *Malassezia (Pityrosporum)* folliculitis (MF) is an acneiform eruption that results from an overgrowth of the *Malassezia* yeast present in the normal cutaneous flora, secondary to occlusion of the follicle or disturbance of normal cutaneous flora. The yeast is primarily found in the infundibulum of the sebaceous glands, as it thrives on the lipid composition of sebum.
- Risk factors include humid environment, tight non-absorbent clothes, excessive sweating, topical or oral antibiotic use, particularly tetracyclines, oral corticosteroid use, immunosuppression.
- It primarily affects adolescents, and affects males more than females.
- It presents as intensely pruritic, 1- to 2-mm, monomorphic follicular papules and pustules. The absence of comedones helps differentiate it from acne (**Figure 12.8**).
- It appears often on the upper back, chest, and shoulders and to a lesser extent on the neck, face (chin and sides of face), or upper arms.
- It may be associated with seborrheic dermatitis or pityriasis versicolor.
- DD: Acne mechanica, acne vulgaris, candidiasis, drug-induced acne, eosinophilic folliculitis, steroid acne, gram-negative folliculitis, *Pseudomonas folliculitis*, rosacea.

## Gram-negative folliculitis

- Gram-negative folliculitis is often seen as a generalized pustular eruption that ranges from mildly symptomatic to being associated with considerable pain and pruritus. This may occur on the face as a sudden pustular flare of acne previously controlled by chronic oral antibiotics.
- Truncal involvement is typically seen in healthy patients after use of recreational hot tubs, with *Pseudomonas aeruginosa* identified as the pathogen on culture.

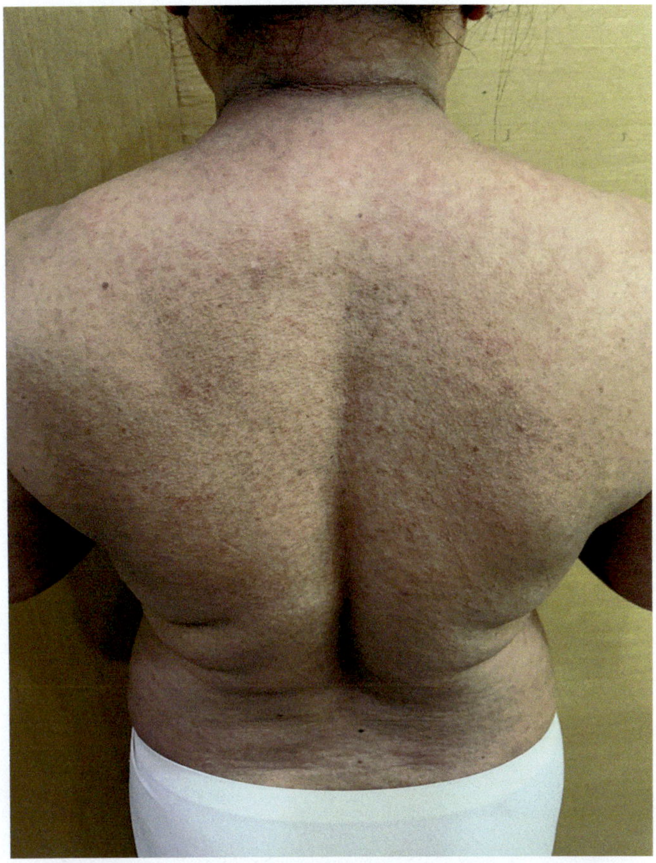

Figure 12.8 Monomorphic papules and pustules on upper back in pityrosporum folliculitis.

- Clinical morphology shows superficial small pustules located in the nasolabial line and on the upper lip and chin, associated with inflammatory papulopustular lesions of the cheeks and perioral region (**Figure 12.9a,b**).
- DD: Acne vulgaris.

## Scabies

- Scabies affects children more than adults.
- There is no sex predilection.
- Risk factors include overcrowding, sharing of linen/clothes/towels.
- There is intense pruritus, more at night; family members may have similar symptoms.
- Clinical morphology shows isolated papules, vesicles, and pustules particularly located in the interdigital web spaces, volar wrists, axillae, breasts, umbilical, and groin areas (**Figure 12.10**).
- DD: Eczema, atopic dermatitis, Langerhans cell histiocytosis, papular urticaria, acropustulosis of infancy, pompholyx.

## Infantile acropustulosis

- Infantile acropustulosis is a chronic, recurrent, self-limited, pruritic, vesicopustular eruption in infants, postulated to be a non-specific hypersensitivity reaction to scabies.

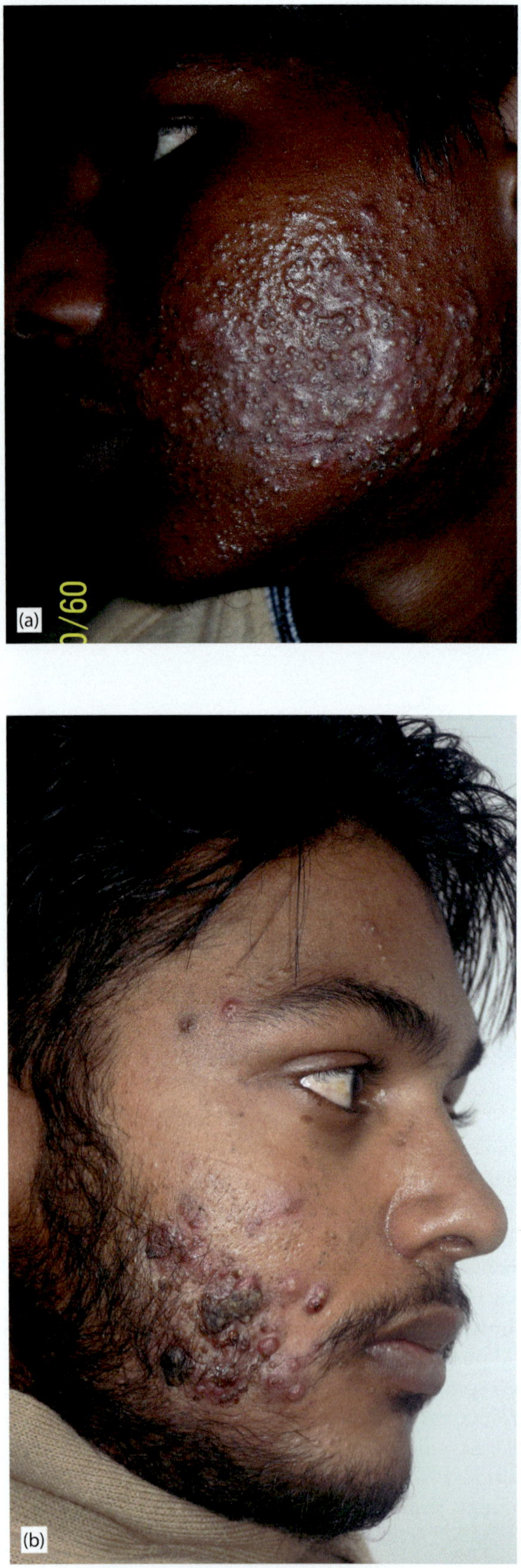


Figure 12.9 **(a)** Pustules in gram negative folliculitis. **(b)** Sudden appearance of erythematous nodules on the cheek in gram negative folliculitis. (a,b – Courtesy: Dr. Piyush Kumar, Katihar, India.)

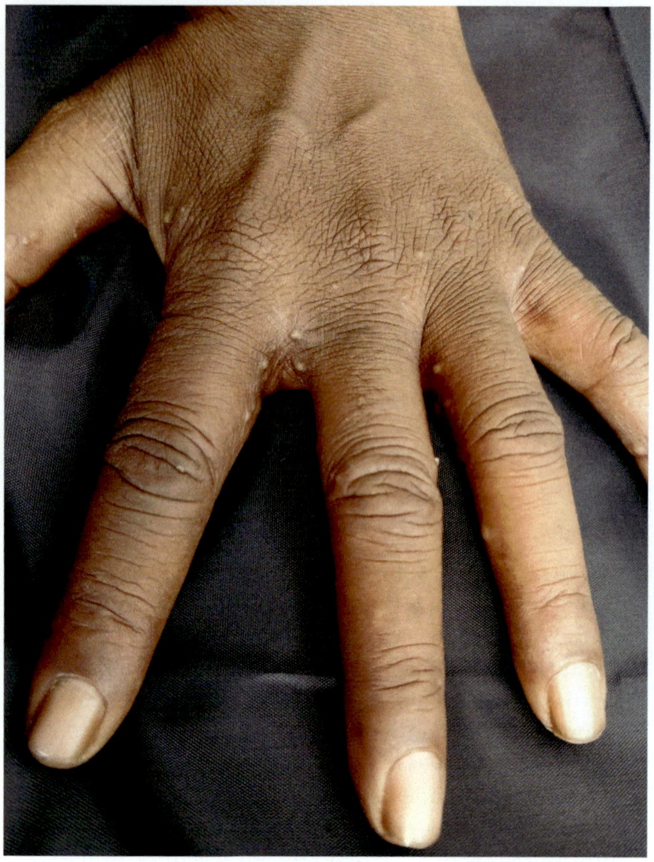

Figure 12.10 Pustules seen in web spaces in scabies. (Courtesy: Dr. Niharika Ranjan Lal, ESIPGIMSR, Kolkata, India.)

- It affects young children during the first two to twelve months of life. Resolution by age three is the norm.
- There is no sex predisposition.
- Symptoms include pruritus and irritability.
- There are recurrent crops of pruritic erythematous macules or papules that progress into vesicles and then pustules.
- Individual bouts may last three to fifteen days and recur in two- to four-week intervals. The attacks occur with progressively diminishing numbers of lesions, and with decreasing frequency, until they cease altogether.
- DD: Dyshidrotic eczema, eosinophilic pustulosis, erythema toxicum neonatorum, fire ant bites, impetigo, Langerhans cell histiocytosis, pustular psoriasis, scabies.

## Parakeratosis pustulosa[6]

- Parakeratosis pustulosa is chronic dermatosis with erythema-squamous lesions with benign clinical course, spontaneous remissions, and improvement with emollients alone in most patients and an obscure etiology.
- It affects children under five years of age.
- It affects females more than males.
- The thumb or middle finger is affected more often than the toes.

Table 12.2 Diagnosis of parakeratosis pustulosa

Major criteria
- Children, particularly young girls <5 years
- Benign course, spontaneous remissions
- Other dermatoses are excluded

Minor Criteria
- Absence of similar disease in family members
- Rare and transient postulation, not extending beyond the initial phase
- Response to topical emollients
- Non-specific histology

- Erythema and scaling of periungual skin are the predominant features, while pustule formation may occur only in the beginning (**Table 12.2**).
- Nail findings include subungual hyperkeratosis and onycholysis with or without nail pitting or ridging.
- DD: Pustular psoriasis (**Table 12.3**), acrodermatitis continua.

## Acrodermatitis continua (pustular acrodermatitis, acrodermatitis continua suppurativa Hallopeau ACH, dermatitis perstans, and dermatitis repens Crocker)

- This is a rare and chronic eruption of sterile painful pustules associated with hyperkeratosis and skin atrophy on the distal fingers and toes.
- It is considered by many to be a localized variant of pustular psoriasis, associated with enhanced polymorphonuclear leukocyte (PMNL) chemotaxis.
- It affects adults 40 to 50 years old.
- Females and males are affected in a ratio of F:M=3:1.
- ACH most often presents at the nail folds of one or two fingers, less frequently on the toes, with small, erythematous pustules that frequently coalesce to form diminutive lakes of pus.
- As individual lesions progress, the affected areas often become hyperkeratotic and scaly as new pustules continue to develop underneath the fissured surface (**Figure 12.11**).
- Over time the skin in these areas may become severely atrophic with shiny erythema.
- Nail involvement includes characteristic pustulation within the nail bed and matrix, leading to onychodystrophy, onychomadesis, onycholysis, or permanent nail loss.

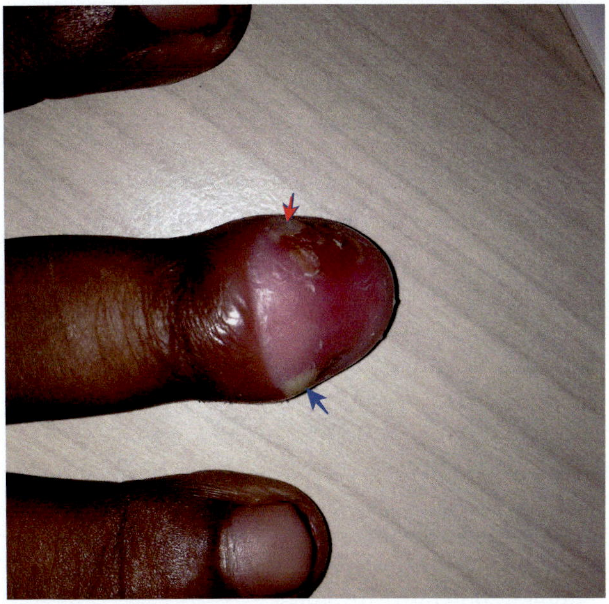

Figure 12.11 Acrodermatitis continua of Hallopeau showing frank pustule (blue arrow), old scaly hyperkeratotic patch (red arrow) with anonychia of affected nail. (Courtesy: Dr. Niharika Ranjan Lal, ESIPGIMSR, Kolkata, India.)

Table 12.3 Clinical differentials of parakeratosis pustulosa

| Features | Parakeratosis pustulosa | Acrodermatitis continua of Hallopeau | Pustular psoriasis of the nails | Nail Psoriasis |
|---|---|---|---|---|
| Age/sex distribution | Young girls | Young females, seldom adult onset | No predilection | No predilection |
| Clinical course | Chronic, benign, painless, recurrent | Aggressive, mutilating, can progress to generalized pustular psoriasis | Aggressive, mutilating | Benign, progressive |
| Spontaneous remissions | Usual | Seldom | None | None |
| Specific Nail changes | Lateral onycholysis, | Distal onycholysis, subungual hyperkeratosis, nail bed pustules, nail dystrophy and loss, distal osteolysis commonly seen | Proximal onycholysis, nail dystrophy owing to nail bed pustules | Proximal onycholysis, subungual hyperkeratosis, pitting, oil-drop, and salmon-patch signs |
| Pustular lesions | Rare/transient | Common (nail bed) | Common (nail bed) | Never |
| Scaling | Sometimes | Tips of digits | Not seen | Periungual |
| Cutaneous lesions | None | None | Lesions of pustular psoriasis | Lesions of plaque psoriasis |
| Histology | Non-specific, mimics eczema | Pustular psoriasis | Pustular psoriasis | Plaque psoriasis |

- Recurrent inflammation may induce sclerosis of underlying soft tissue, muscular atrophy, arthropathy of interphalangeal joints, and osteolysis with resorption of the distal phalanx.
- DD: Pustular psoriasis, palmoplantar pustulosis (does not show propensity for pustules to coalesce, localization over distal extremity, or atrophy and nail loss), acute contact dermatitis (vesicular and not usually pustular, palmoplantar involvement more common, margins are less defined), pustular dyshidrotic eczema, bacterial or viral paronychia, parakeratosis pustulosa (common in children, limited to one finger, resolves spontaneously at puberty).

## Pyoderma gangrenosum (pustular type)

- This inflammatory neutrophilic skin disease is often associated with underlying systemic disorders such as inflammatory bowel disease, arthritis, and lymphoproliferative disorders.
- It affects young to middle-aged adults (40 to 60 years).
- It affects females more than males.
- The eruption may begin as an isolated pustule or scattered lesions on the trunk or extremities. There is surrounding edema and purplish induration, with rapid progression into a large ulcer that heals ultimately with cribriform scars.
- Other types include ulcerative (classic) PG (the most common variant), bullous (atypical) PG, vegetative PG.
- DD: Vasculitis.

## Orf

- Orf is a zoonotic disease caused by a parapox virus and occurring primarily in sheep and goats. It is also known as contagious pustular dermatitis, infectious labial dermatitis, ecthyma contagiosum, thistle disease, and scabby mouth.
- It affects adults more than children.
- It affects males more than females, as it is an occupational hazard.
- Risk factors include occupations like ranchers, veterinarians, butchers, shearers, and shepherds.
- Sites are mainly fingers, hands, and forearms; it rarely appears on the scalp and face.
- It is accompanied by a low-grade fever.
- There may be pruritus.
- Systemic symptoms such as lymphadenopathy, erysipelas-like lesions, and erythema multiforme can occur in up to one-third of cases.
- Clinical morphology shows solitary small, firm, red-to-blue papules then progresses through a series of six stages. The fully developed orf lesion is typically 2–3 cm in diameter, but it may reach 5 cm.
  - Stage 1 (maculopapular or pustular) – A red elevated lesion
  - Stage 2 (targetoid) – A bulla with an iris-like configuration (nodule with a red center, a white middle ring, and a red periphery) (**Figure 12.12a,b**)
  - Stage 3 (acute) – A weeping nodule
  - Stage 4 (regenerative) – A firm nodule covered by a thin crust through which black dots are seen

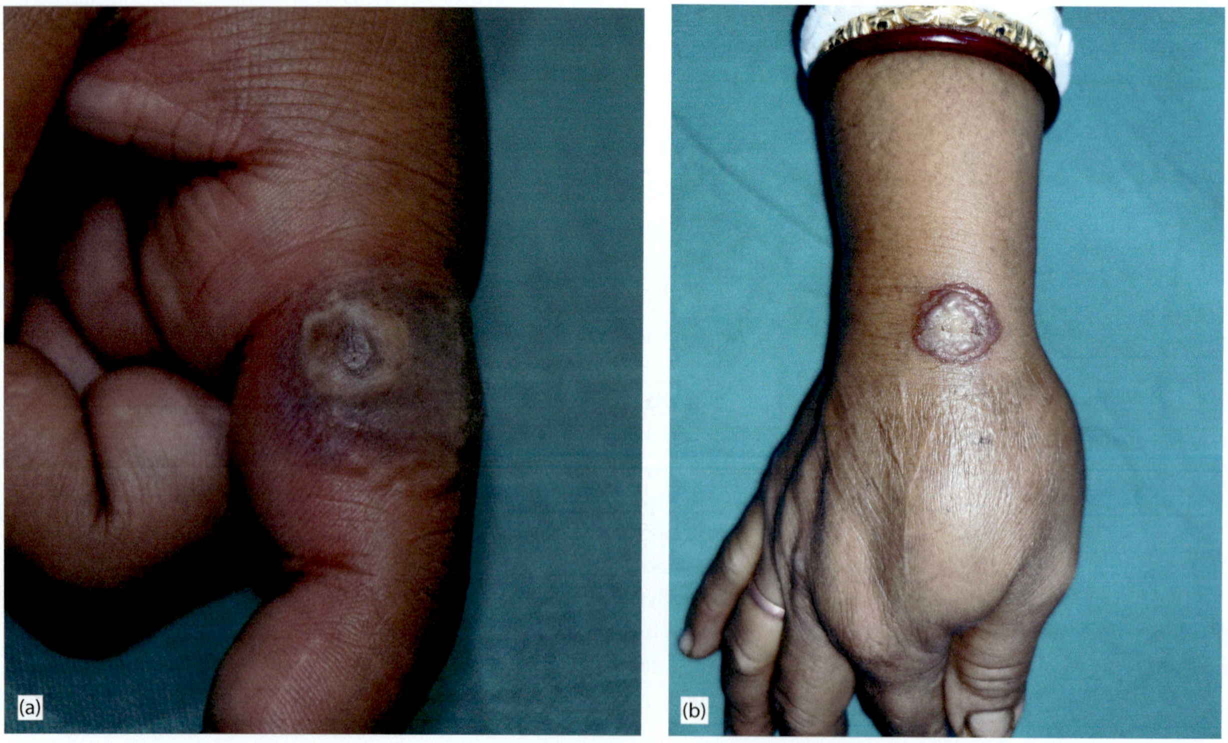


Figure 12.12 **(a)** Pustulonodular lesion of Orf in a young male. Note targetoid appearance. **(b)** Pustular lesion in orf. (a – Courtesy: Dr. Piyush Kumar, Katihar, India; b – Courtesy: Dr. Rajesh Kumar Mandal, North Bengal Medical College, Darjeeling, India.)

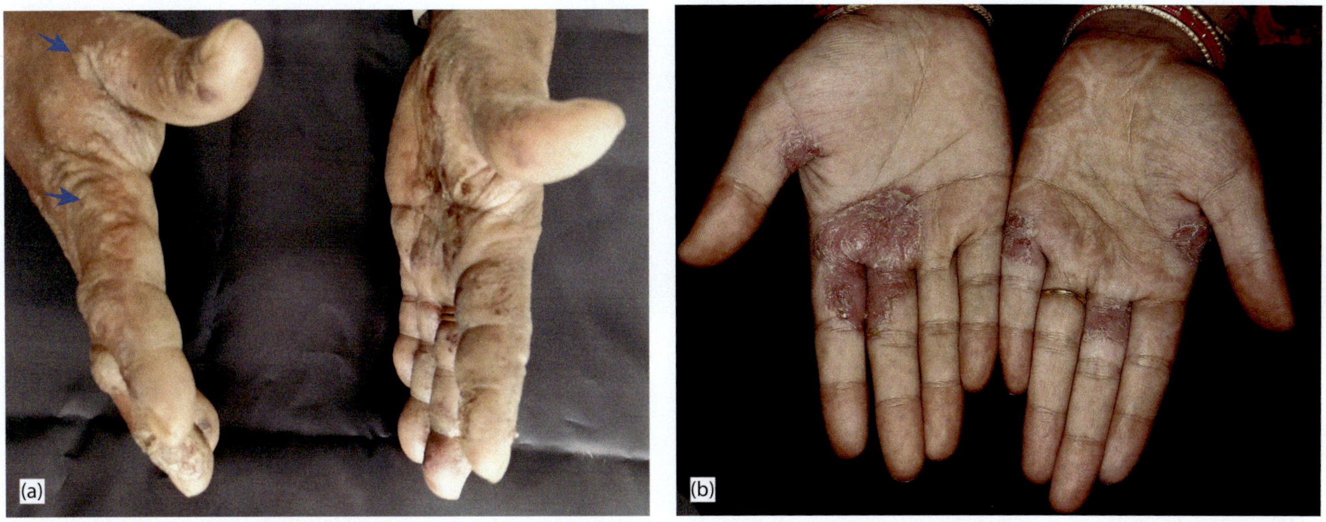

Figure 12.13 **(a)** Pustules (blue arrow), oozing, and scaling on lateral aspect of fingers in pompholyx. **(b)** Pustules and vesicles have eroded to leave erythematous areas with erosions, fissures, and scaling. (a – Courtesy: Dr. Niharika Ranjan Lal, ESIPGIMSR, Kolkata, India; b – Courtesy: Dr. Piyush Kumar, Katihar, India.)

    - Stage 5 (papillomatous) – Small papillomas appearing over the surface
    - Stage 6 (regressive) – A thick dry crust covering the resolving lesion
- DD: Cowpox, pseudocowpox (milker's nodule), furuncle, atypical mycobacteria infections, anthrax.

## Dyshidrotic eczema/pompholyx

- It presents with intensely pruritic, chronic and recurrent, vesicular dermatitis that typically involves the palms and soles and lateral aspects of the fingers (**Figure 12.13a**). Isolated pustules also may occur but rarely are the predominant primary lesions. The vesicles gradually desquamate over one to two weeks, leaving erosions and fissures (**Figure 12.13b**) that slowly resolve.
- DD: Tinea pedis/manuum, contact dermatitis, hand, foot, and mouth disease.

## Palmoplantar pustulosis (PPP)

- It is considered to be a localized form of pustular psoriasis. Psoriasis occurs in 24% of PPP patients.
- It affects people 30 to 50 years of age.
- It affects females more than males.
- Risk factors include tobacco smoking, family history of psoriasis, presence of another autoimmune disorder, and family history of palmoplantar pustulosis.
- Triggers include smoking, infections (especially streptococcal bacterial infections), stress, and medications (steroids).
- It is persistent and painful, leading to a considerable functional impairment.
- Clinical morphology shows sterile pustules and erythematous, scaly skin (**Figure 12.14**).
- DD: Acrodermatitis continua of Hallopeau, allergic contact dermatitis, dyshidrotic eczema, keratoderma blennorrhagicum, secondary syphilis.

## Candidial folliculitis

- This is a follicular infection caused by the yeast *Candida albicans* or other *Candida* species
- Risk factors include immunodeficiency, nutritional deficiencies, endocrine diseases such as dermatomyositis (DM), Cushing's disease, and hypothyroidism.
- It affects the elderly, but may be seen in infants and young adults.

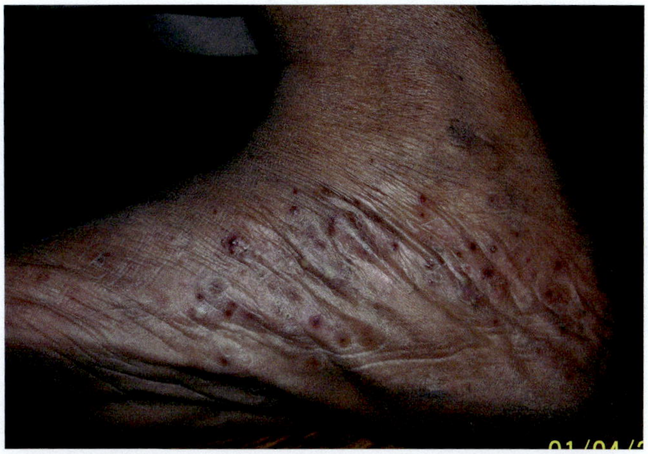

Figure 12.14 Pinpoint sterile pustules with erythema and scaling on lateral aspect of foot in palmoplantar pustulosis. (Courtesy: Dr. Piyush Kumar, Katihar, India.)

- There is no sex predilection.
- It presents as erythema and maceration, with typical satellite pustules and scaling.
- DD: Contact dermatitis, inverse psoriasis.

## Amicrobial pustulosis of the folds (APF)[7]

- This is a recently described neutrophilic dermatosis characterized by relapsing pustular lesions usually occurring in the context of an autoimmune disease.
- It occurs predominantly in cutaneous folds on the scalp and periorificial regions, such as the mouth, external ear canal, and nostrils.
- Affects patients aged 20 to 40 years.
- It affects females more than males.
- Clinical morphology shows folliculo-centric pustules with erythema.
- DD: Extensive folliculitis, pustular psoriasis, subcorneal pustular dermatosis, candidal intertrigo, dermatophyte infections.

## Subcorneal pustular dermatosis (SCPD)

- It is more common in women, with onset usually in their forties.
- It is clinically characterized by recurrent crops of pustules, mainly affecting the intertriginous and flexural areas. The lesions resolve with scaling, but new lesions keep appearing.
- DD: Pustular psoriasis, acute generalized exanthematous pustulosis.

## Hidradenitis suppurativa

- Hidradenitis suppurativa is also known as acne inversa, and in older literature as Verneuil's disease
- The etiology is chronic follicular occlusion.
- The average age of onset is at puberty – second to third decade.
- Females and males are affected in a ratio of F:M=3:1.
- It affects areas of hormonally influenced apocrine sweat glands, including the axillae, mammary, and inguinal regions.
- Risk factors include obesity, hyperandrogenism in females, genetics, infection, and high-glycemic diet.
- Immune factors including cell-mediated immunity is thought to play a role.
- Symptoms include pain and discomfort, purulent discharge, and impaired quality of life.
- Pustules may be evident in early lesions, followed by nodules and discharging abscesses. Follicular rupture and involvement of the apocrine gland occur deeply, resulting over time in extensive scarring and sinus tract formation and chronicity. Multi-headed tombstone comedones are present.
- Complications include fistulae, strictures and contractures, arthropathy, malaise, depression and suicide, lymphatic obstruction, lymphedema of limbs and genitalia, long-term effects of chronic suppuration (anemia, hypoproteinemia and amyloidosis), and squamous cell carcinoma (rarely).
- DD: Follicular pyodermas (superficial, quick-healing, no widespread scarring/induration, no comedones), granuloma inguinale (genital area involved, red ulcers with granulation, easy to bleed), Crohn's disease (perianal and vulval abscesses, fistulae, sinus tracts and "knife-cut" ulcers, previous history of gastrointestinal involvement).

## Herpes zoster

- Herpes zoster is an acute eruption caused by the reactivation of latent varicella-zoster virus and is characterized by painful grouped vesicles and erosions, usually confined to a single dermatome.
- It usually affects adults older than 50.
- There is no sex preponderance.
- The sites affected are dermatomal, rarely multi-dermatomal (if immunocompromised).
- Risk factors include immuno-compromised individuals, old age, stress, and other comorbidities.
- Herpes zoster may present early on as isolated pustules or vesicles with significant discomfort, typically in a dermatomal distribution (**Figure 12.15a,b**).

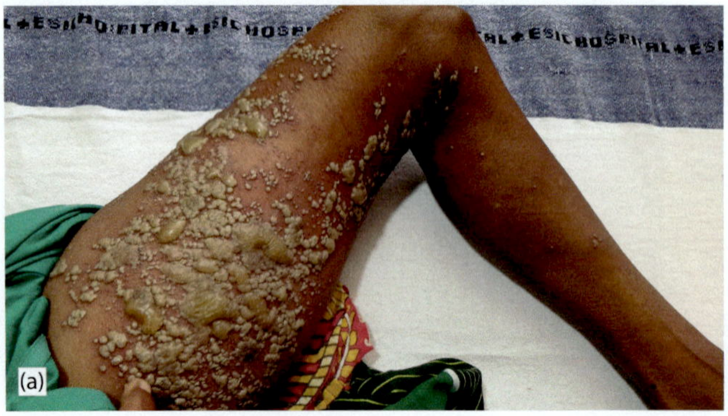

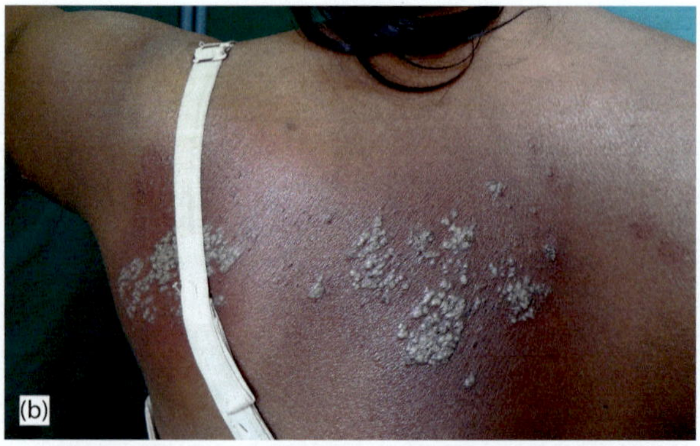

Figure 12.15 **(a)** Grouped pustules coalescing to form large pus-filled bulla along L2–L3 dermatomes in herpes zoster. **(b)** Grouped pustules on erythematous base along T1–T2 dermatome in herpes zoster. (a,b – Courtesy: Dr. Niharika Ranjan Lal, ESIPGIMSR, Kolkata, India.)

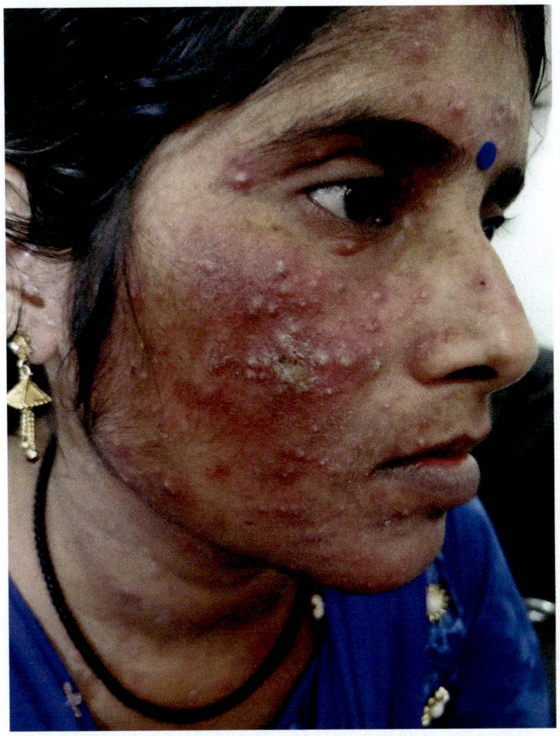

Figure 12.16 Topical steroid abuse on face. Pustules and erythema with hypertrichosis. (Courtesy: Dr. Niharika Ranjan Lal, ESIPGIMSR, Kolkata, India.)

- Symptoms include pain, aching, burning, allodynia, fever, and malaise.
- Common complications include postherpetic neuralgia, bacterial skin infection, and ocular complications, including uveitis and keratitis.
- DD: Zosteriform herpes simplex, cellulitis, erysipelas, folliculitis.

## Chronic glucocorticoid use and abuse

- Chronic topical corticosteroid use can cause pustular lesions on the face and trunk. These lesions are typically asymptomatic.
- It affects young to middle-aged adults.
- It affects females more than males.
- Risk factors include use of whitening creams and over-the-counter medications containing steroids.
- It is generally asymptomatic, but photosensitivity may be present.
- It presents with pleomorphic acneiform lesions, such as papules and pustules, with erythema and mild scaling. Associated dryness, perioral dermatitis, telangiectasia, rosacea-like features, hypopigmentation, and hyperpigmentation may be seen (**Figure 12.16**).
- DD: Acne, rosacea, seborrheic dermatitis, LMDF, demodex folliculitis, contact allergic dermatitis.

## Dermatophyte infections

- Dermatophyte (superficial fungal) infections, such as tinea pedis or corporis, typically occur with papules, plaques, and peripheral scale. Pustules may also be a key primary lesion when follicular units are involved, particularly on the legs, scalp, or forearms.
- Risk factors include occlusive clothing, excessive sweating, immunocompromised, contact with animals, diabetes mellitus.
- Clinical picture depends on the site of affection.
  - Body: Annular erythematous plaques with a border and scaling (**Figure 12.17a,b**).
  - Palms and soles: Diffuse scaling with vesiculo-pustular eruptions occasionally.
  - Scalp: Scaly plaques with follicular pustules (**Figure 12.17c**).
  - Groins: Erythematous annular plaques with maceration.
- Majocchi's granuloma results from dermal invasion and presents with perifollicular papules and pustules.
- DD: Candidiasis, erythema annulare centrifugum, pustular psoriasis, pyoderma.

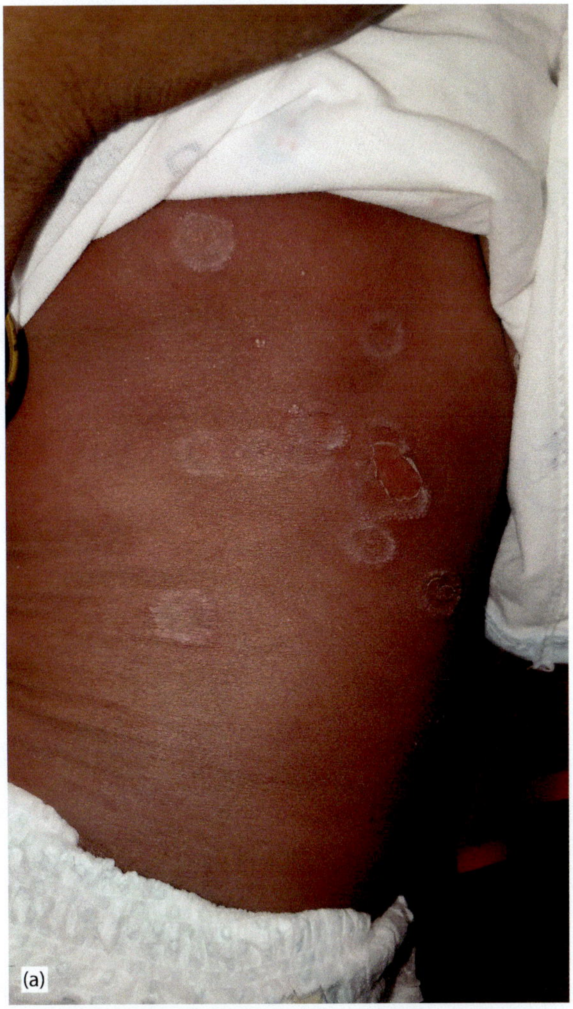


Figure 12.17 **(a)** Annular plaques studded with pustules on the peripheral active margin in tinea corporis in an infant. (*Continued*)

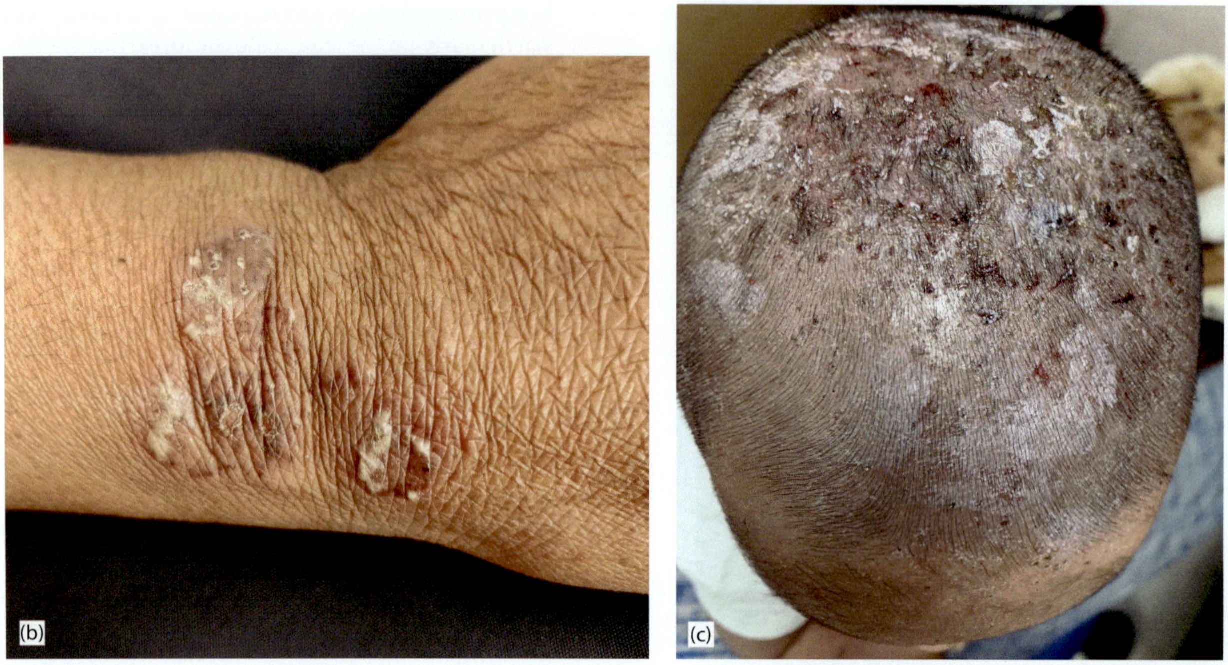

Figure 12.17 *(Continued)* **(b)** Pustules mixed with excoriated papules on active margin in tinea corporis. **(c)** Pustules, crusting, and scales with hair loss over scalp in tinea capitis. (a,b – Courtesy: Dr. Niharika Ranjan Lal, ESIPGIMSR, Kolkata, India.)

## REFERENCES


1. Goldstein BG, Goldstein AO. Approach to the patient with pustular lesions. In: Dellavalle RP, Levy ML, Corona R, editors. UpToDate. 2020. Available from: https://www.uptodate.com/contents/approach-to-the-patient-with-pustular-skin-lesions
2. Mengesha YM, Bennett ML. Pustular skin disorders: Diagnosis and treatment. Am J Clin Dermatol 2002;3(6):389–400.
3. Lipsker D. Clinical Examination and Differential Diagnosis of Skin Lesions. 1st edition. France: Springer-Verlag; 2013. Chapter 29. Pustules. P. 181–182.
4. Fitzpatrick JE, High WA, Kyle WL. Urgent Care Dermatology: Symptom-Based Diagnosis. 1st ed. Philadelphia: Elsevier; 2018. Chapter 12. Pustular Eruptions, Nonfollicular. P. 205–216.
5. Fitzpatrick JE, High WA, Kyle WL. Urgent Care Dermatology: Symptom-Based Diagnosis. 1st ed. Philadelphia: Elsevier; 2018. Chapter 23. Follicular Disorders. P. 375–384.
6. Mahajan VK, Ranjan N. Parakeratosis pustulosa: A diagnostic conundrum. Indian J Paediatr Dermatol 2014;15:12–15.
7. López-Navarro N, Alcaide A, Gallego E, et al. Amicrobial pustulosis of the folds associated with Hashimoto's thyroiditis. Clin Exp Dermatol 2009;34:e561–e563.

# E9

# Pustules: Generalized

ASEEM SHARMA, MADHULIKA MHATRE, TRUPTI AGARWAL

## ABSTRACT

Generalized pustules may evolve from papulo-vesicular lesions or, less commonly, may appear as the primary lesion itself. The latter may be a pointer to serious, life-threatening conditions. This chapter discusses a clinical approach to the diagnosis of various diseases presenting with generalized pustules.

The text of this chapter is available online at https://routledgetextbooks.com/textbooks/9781032399669/

DOI: 10.1201/9781351054225-23

# E10

# Clinical approach to ulcers

SOURABH JAIN

## ABSTRACT

Cutaneous ulcers can develop in a diverse range of pathological processes. The clinical features in these ulcers may not be distinctive in many ulcers, but detailed history and thorough clinical examination can provide clues necessary to arrive at a diagnosis or get a list of differentials. This chapter discusses important features of cutaneous ulcers that can play a role in clinical diagnosis.

The text of this chapter is available online at https://routledgetextbooks.com/textbooks/9781032399669/



DOI: 10.1201/9781351054225-24

13

# Ulcer: Single or few

B SHINY SHULAMITE, CH VENKATA KRISHNA, SRI HARSHA KOLLA, SAI PRASANTH NETI, VIGNASREE A

## INTRODUCTION

Ulcers can be congenital or acquired with various etiologies, such as infective, inflammatory, traumatic, and ischemic. The most common site of skin ulcers is the lower extremities, but they can occur on any body part. Most cutaneous ulcers of the lower extremities are caused by venous insufficiency, arterial insufficiency, or neuropathy (especially of diabetic etiology), and in general such ulcers are not difficult to diagnose. However, many ulcers, especially ulcers associated with or due to systemic inflammatory conditions, may have non-specific clinical findings and are challenging diagnostically. Features that aid in diagnosis include clinical characteristics of the ulcer (as described in Chapter E10), discharge, symptoms, associated systemic features, and co-morbidities. An important pointer to diagnosis is the evolution of ulcer – if there is a presence or absence of primary and secondary lesions over which ulceration has occurred (**Table 13.1**). For example, most infections start with papules/nodules, with secondary ulceration (e.g., cutaneous leishmaniasis, sporotrichosis). Another diagnostic clue is changes in the skin surrounding the ulcer. For example, the presence of purpura and ecchymoses in the background of ulcers is suggestive of necrotizing fasciitis, warfarin necrosis, etc. The clinical approach to the diagnosis of conditions presenting with solitary or few ulcers are outlined in **Table 13.2**, and salient features are discussed below.[1–8]

### Aplasia cutis congenita

- Aplasia cutis congenita (ACC) is a rare, congenital disorder characterized by the focal or widespread absence of skin.
- It usually affects the scalp at midline.

Table 13.1 Evolution of lesions as clinical clue

| Primary/ secondary lesion | Site/ additional clues | Diseases |
|---|---|---|
| Papules/ plaque | Exposed parts | Cutaneous leishmaniasis |
| | Rapid progression into ulcer | Pyoderma gangrenosum |
| | Sun-exposed areas | Basal cell carcinoma, squamous cell carcinoma |
| | On legs; diabetic | Necrobiosis lipoidica diabeticorum |
| Nodule | Over lymph nodes | Scrofuloderma |
| | Lower limbs | Tuberculous gumma |
| | Linear arrangement | Lymphocutaneous sporotrichosis, Nocardiosis |
| | Hand | Fish tank granuloma |
| Vesicles/pustule | Dermatomal | Herpes zoster |
| | Extremity | Cutaneous anthrax |
| Purpura/ ecchymosis | | Calciphylaxis, warfarin necrosis, Nicolau syndrome, vasculitis |
| Erythema and edema | Acral parts | Frostbite, glanders disease |
| | Anywhere | Necrotizing fasciitis |
| Triphasic color change | Acral parts | Raynaud's phenomenon |

DOI: 10.1201/9781351054225-25

Table 13.2 Clinical approach to diagnosis of solitary (or few) ulcers

| Site | Additional clue | Diseases |
|---|---|---|
| Head and neck | Neonates and infants | Aplasia cutis congenita (scalp), ulcerated hemangioma |
| | Children | Scrofuloderma (neck), tubercular chancre (face), noma (face) |
| | Adults | Leishmaniasis, granulomatosis with polyangiitis |
| | Elderly | Basal cell carcinoma, squamous cell carcinoma, herpes zoster, angiosarcoma, temporal arteritis |
| Lower back | Elderly | Decubitus ulcer |
| Abdomen | | Kangri ulcer, warfarin-induced skin necrosis, calciphylaxis |
| Extremities | Children | Tubercular chancre, Ecthyma |
| | Adults | • Anywhere: Nicolau syndrome (history of intramuscular injections), tropical ulcer<br>• Upper extremity: Swimming pool granuloma, sporotrichosis, cutaneous anthrax<br>• Thighs: cholesterol emboli, calciphylaxis, kangri ulcer (inner thighs, history of use of kangri basket)<br>• Lower leg: Livedoid vasculopathy, cryoglobulinemic vasculitis, cutaneous polyarteritis nodosa, venous ulcer (mid-calf), Martorell ulcer<br>• Foot: Trench foot<br>• Distal toes: Thromboangitis obliterans, Raynaud's phenomenon, Frostbite, arterial ulcer (punched out ulcers)<br>• Sole (pressure areas): Neuropathic ulcer |
| | History of exposure to cold | Trench foot, frostbite, Raynaud's phenomenon |
| Genitalia | Single, painless | Syphilis, squamous cell carcinoma (ulcerated tumor) |
| | Single, painful | Trauma, fixed drug eruption |
| | Multiple, painful | Herpes genitalis, chancroid, aphthous ulcer, cutaneous Crohn's disease |
| | Variable, granulation tissue | Donovanosis |
| | Associated with cutaneous blisters and ulcers | Pemphigus vulgaris |
| Anywhere | | Pyoderma gangrenosum, necrotizing fasciitis |

- At birth, 15–30% cases may have superficially eroded to a deeply ulcerated scalp (**Figure 13.1**).
- Large defects of the scalp or scalp defects that involve the underlying skull or dura, with exposure of sagittal sinus, large veins, or brain, may require surgical intervention due to the high risk of infection, hemorrhage, or thrombosis.

## Ulcerated hemangioma

- Ulceration, the most frequent complication of infantile hemangioma (IH), tends to heal poorly and is associated with pain, bleeding, infection, and scarring.
- Ulceration is more common in centrofacial and perineum regions and may be heralded by surfacing of blackish spots or white discoloration (**Figure 13.2**).
- Ulcerated IHs tend to be larger than non-ulcerated ones, and friction, low birth weight, prematurity, and female gender are risk factors associated with ulceration.[9]

## Noma/cancrum oris[10]

- Noma is a rapidly spreading mutilating gangrenous stomatitis caused by normal oral flora that becomes pathogenic during periods of compromised immune status (measles, AIDS, tuberculosis).
- The exact causative organism is not clear, although spirochetes and fusiform bacillus in symbiosis have been considered to be the primary cause of the condition.
- Early features include soreness of the mouth, pronounced halitosis, fetid taste, tenderness of the lip or cheek, cervical lymphadenopathy, a foul-smelling purulent oral discharge, and a blue-black discoloration of the skin in the affected area.
- Without appropriate treatment, the mortality rate is reported to be 70–90%, and surviving patients suffer with functional disturbances and disfigurement.
- DD: Pseudomonas infection, leishmaniasis.

## Tuberculous chancre

- Tuberculous chancre, also known as primary tuberculous inoculation chancre, is a rare form of tuberculosis.
- It develops in individuals not previously sensitized to mycobacterium, occurring most commonly in children, especially those who have not taken the Bacilli Calmette-Guérin (BCG) vaccine.
- It has also been reported in surgical wounds, tattoos and piercing sites, even sexual transmission.

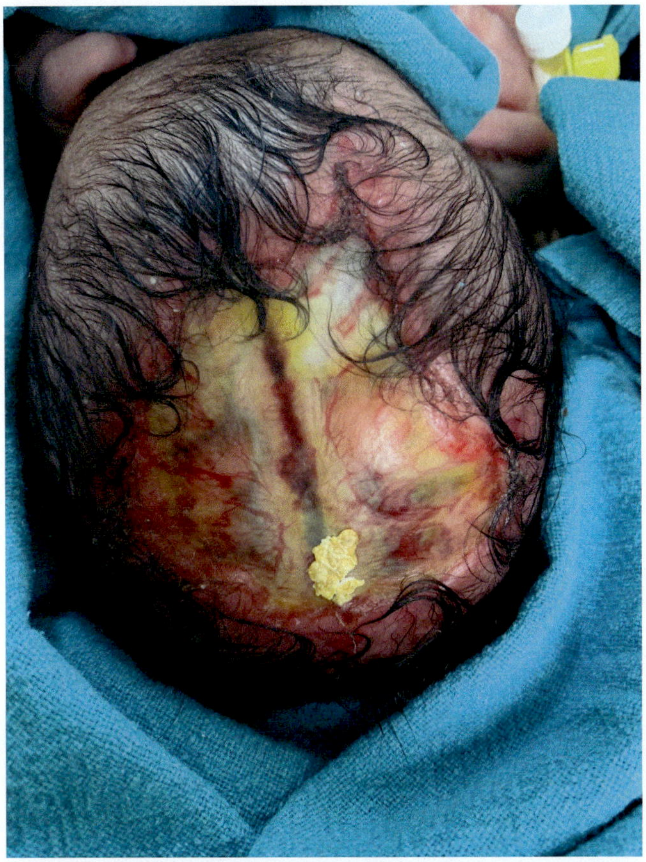

Figure 13.1 Aplasia cutis congenita – large defect in scalp with visible underlying structures. (Courtesy: Dr Rashid Shahid, AIIMS Patna, India.)

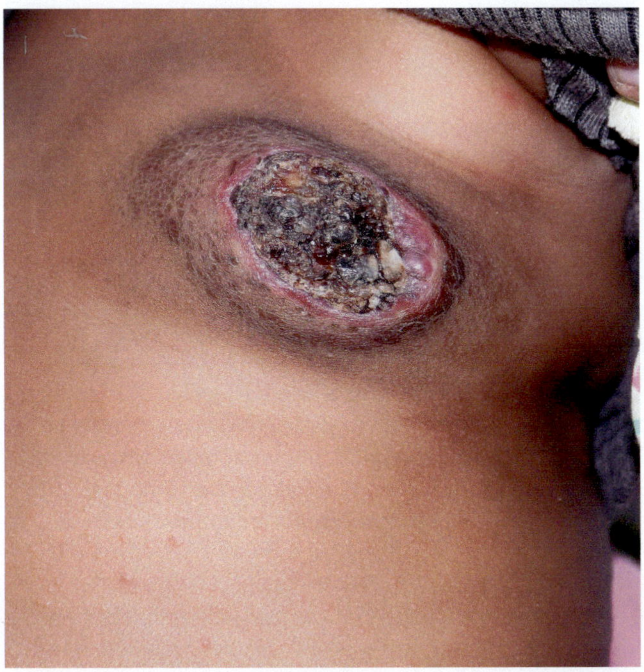

Figure 13.2 Ulcerated infantile hemangioma. (Courtesy: Dr. Piyush Kumar, Katihar, India.)

- It is commonly seen in children, the face and extremities being the most frequently involved sites.
- It is characterized by the appearance at the first site of inoculation, two to four weeks post contact, of a shallow, painless ulcer, with granular base with micro-abscesses or thick crust and undermined borders.[11]
- Painful regional lymphadenopathy is present.
- Spontaneous regression with scarring and regional lymph node calcification may occur, or the patient may develop lupus vulgaris lesions and tuberculosis verrucosa cutis.
- It needs to be differentiated from tubercular gummas.
- DD: Sporotrichosis, leishmaniasis, atypical mycobacteriosis, syphilis, cat scratch disease, and tularemia.

## Tuberculous gumma

- Tuberculous gumma, also known as metastatic tuberculous abscesses, is an unusual form of cutaneous TB.
- It has generally been observed in malnourished children and severely immunosuppressed adults, but its occurrence in immunocompetent individuals is possible.
- It results from hematogenous spread of the mycobacterium from a primary focus during a period of impaired immunity.
- The lesions of tuberculous gumma are typically firm, single or multiple non-tender erythematous nodules.
- Occasionally, the lesions break down and discharge their contents or persist and form ulcers and sinuses (**Figure 13.3a**).
- Limbs are the most frequent site for gummas, especially thighs and buttocks.
- DD: Syphilis gumma, pyoderma gangrenosum, atypical mycobacterial lesions.

## Scrofuloderma[11]

- Scrofuloderma is a common form of cutaneous tuberculosis caused by a lesion in the lymph node, bone, muscle, or tendon that contiguously spreads to the skin.
- Regions most commonly affected include chest, neck, and axillary lymph nodes.
- It begins as painless, subcutaneous nodules, which are called cold abscesses.
- The reddish-blue induration suppurates and breaks down, forming an ulcer with granulation tissue at the base (**Figure 13.3b,c**).
- Sometimes sinuses may develop and communicate directly with areas of deep infection.
- Progression and scarring produce irregular adherent masses, densely fibrous in places and fluctuant or discharging in others.
- DD: Atypical mycobacterial infection, sarcoidosis, blastomycosis, and tertiary syphilis.

## Cutaneous leishmaniasis

- Cutaneous leishmaniasis occurs in the New World and the Old World. Old World disease primarily is caused by *Leishmania tropica* in urban areas and *Leishmania major* in dry desert areas.
- The disease begins as an erythematous papule at the site of the sandfly bite on exposed parts of the body, usually the face.

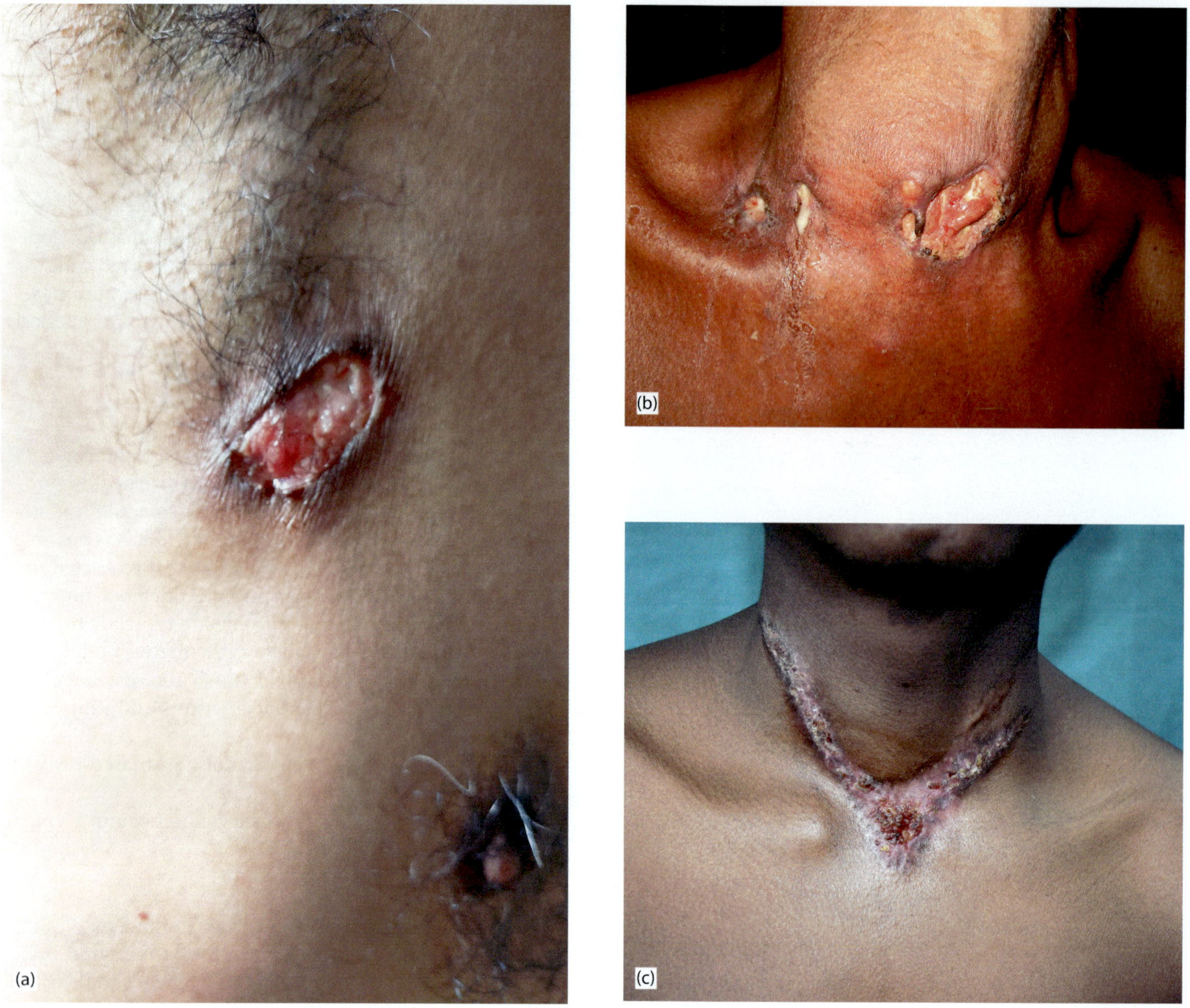

Figure 13.3 **(a)** Tubercular gumma presenting as solitary ulcer with undermined edge and violaceous indurated margin. **(b)** Multiple ulcers with undermined edges and violaceous margin in scrofuloderma. **(c)** Scrofuloderma with lupus vulgaris. (a–c – Courtesy: Dr. Piyush Kumar, Katihar, India.)

- The papule increases in size and becomes a nodule.
- It eventually ulcerates and crusts over. The border is usually raised and distinct (**Figure 13.4**).
- There may be multiple lesions, especially when the patient has encountered a nest of sandflies.
- The ulcer is typically large but painless unless there is secondary bacterial or fungal infection, and it heals with scarring.

## Granulomatosis with polyangiitis

- Initially known as Wegener's granulomatosis, granulomatosis with polyangiitis (GPA) is a necrotizing granulomatous inflammation usually involving the upper and lower respiratory tract and necrotizing vasculitis affecting predominantly small to medium vessels.
- The hallmarks of GPA are systemic necrotizing vasculitis, necrotizing granulomatous inflammation, and necrotizing glomerulonephritis.
- It can involve virtually any organ in the body as generalized disease or as a limited/localized disease.
- Cutaneous vasculitis secondary to GPA can present as papules, nodules, palpable purpura, ulcers resembling pyoderma gangrenosum, or necrotizing lesions leading to gangrene. Cutaneous lesions are found in 50% of patients.
- They are typically located on the lower extremities, but they can also manifest on the face, upper extremities, and the extensor surfaces of the joints. Oral and nasal ulcerations may also occur.
- DD: Pyoderma gangrenosum, mycobacterial infection, deep fungal infections.

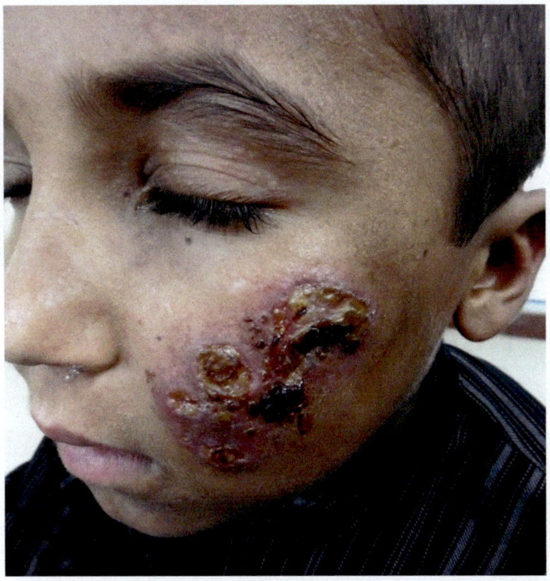

Figure 13.4 Ulcerated plaque covered by crusts in cutaneous leishmaniasis. (Courtesy: Dr. Md Irfan Anwar, Pakistan.)

## Basal cell carcinoma

- Basal cell carcinoma (BCC) typically presents as a shiny, pink or flesh-colored papule or nodule with surface telangiectasia.
- The tumor may enlarge and ulcerate, with rolled waxy borders (**Figure 13.5a,b**).
- The most common sites for nodular BCC are the face, especially the nose, cheeks, forehead, nasolabial folds, and eyelids.
- Patients often give a history of crusting and recurrent bleeding, causing them to seek evaluation.
- Pigmented nodular BCCs are more common in dark-skinned individuals.

## Squamous cell carcinoma[12]

- Cutaneous squamous cell carcinoma (SCC) is a non-melanoma skin cancer that arises from epithelial keratinocytes or their appendages.
- It may arise de novo, as a result of previous exposure to ultraviolet (UV) ionizing radiation or arsenic; within chronic wounds or scars; or from pre-existing lesions, such as actinic keratosis, Bowen's disease (intraepidermal SCC), bowenoid papulosis, or erythroplasia of Queyrat.
- Risk factors include sun exposure, old age, fair skin, and immunosuppression.
- It is locally aggressive and, without treatment, has the potential to metastasize to other parts of the body.
- Most SCCs arise on the sun-damaged skin of the head and neck, with fewer lesions arising on the extremities and occasional tumors occurring on the trunk.
- Early lesions frequently present as red scaly papules.
- Later, lesions may form nodules or firm plaques, either of which can ulcerate (**Figure 13.6a,b**).
- SCC may also present as a non-healing ulcer (**Figure 13.6c–e**).

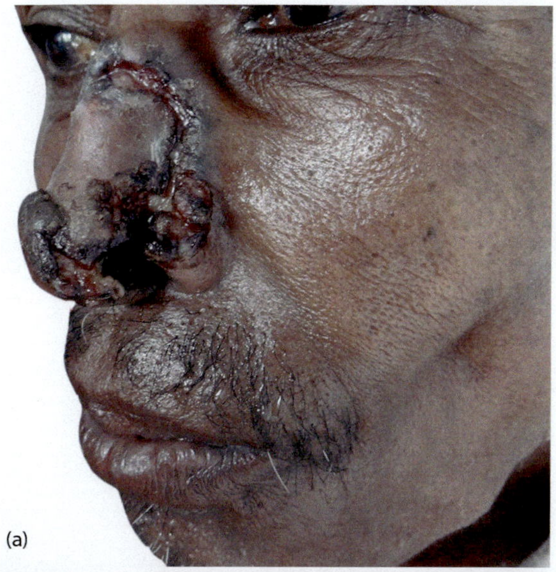


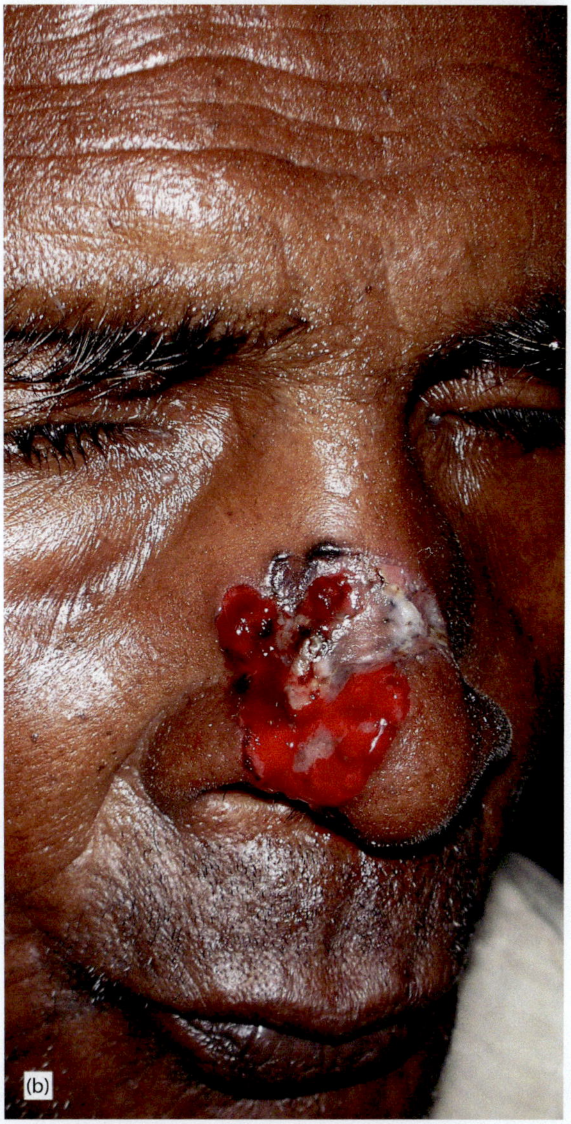


Figure 13.5 **(a)** Basal cell carcinoma causing destruction of left ala nasi and ulceration. **(b)** Ulcerated basal cell carcinoma. (a,b – Courtesy: Dr. Piyush Kumar, Katihar, India.)

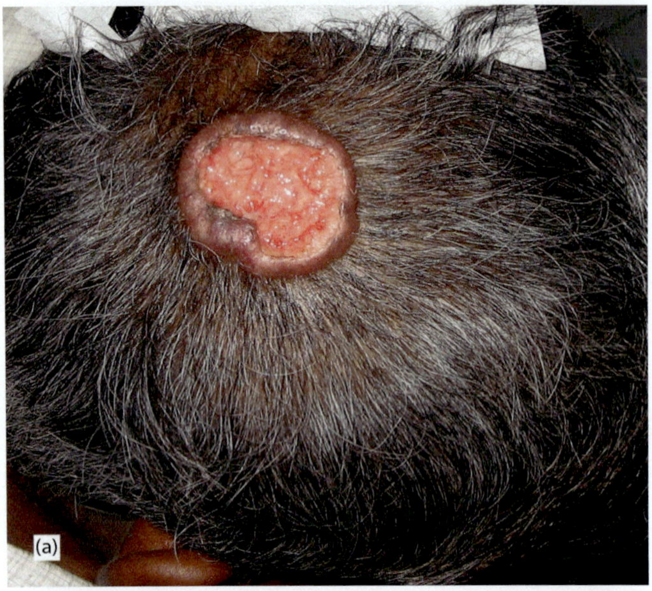


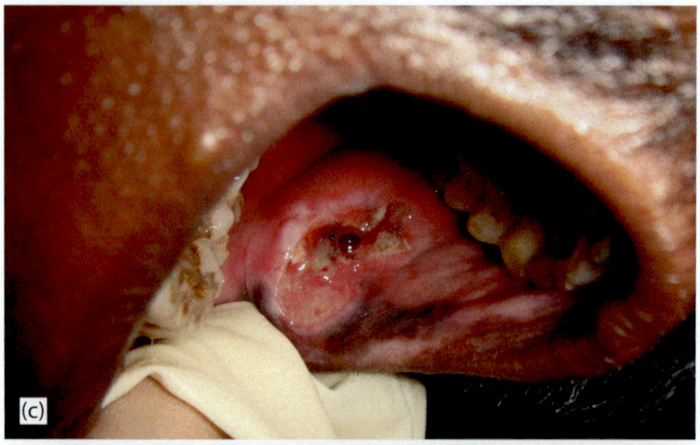


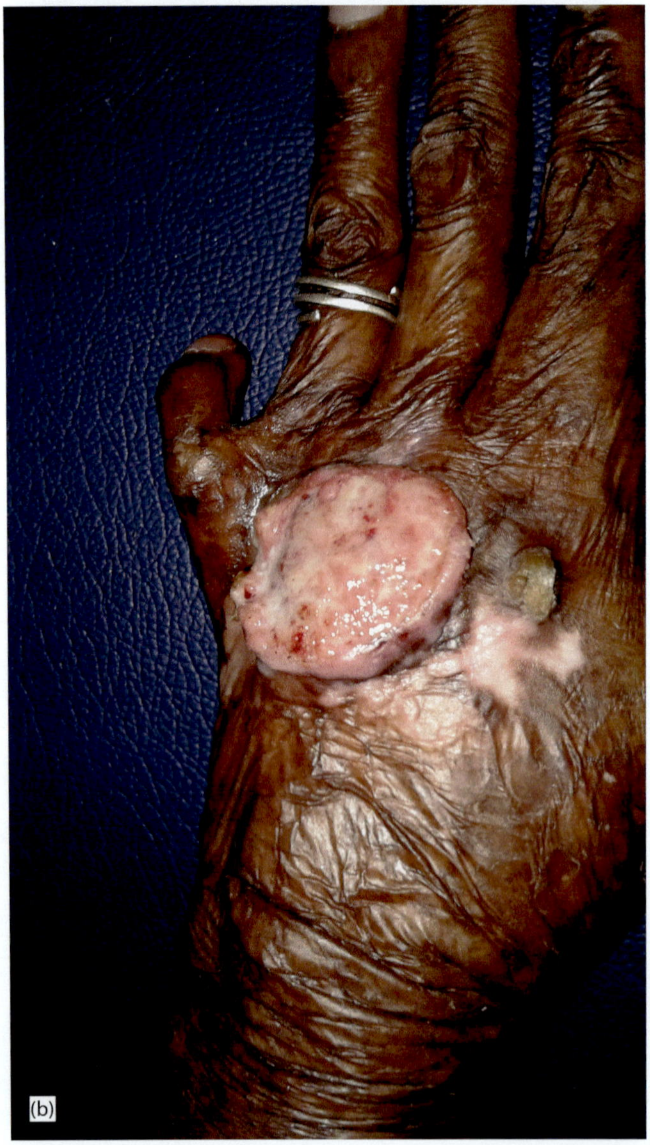


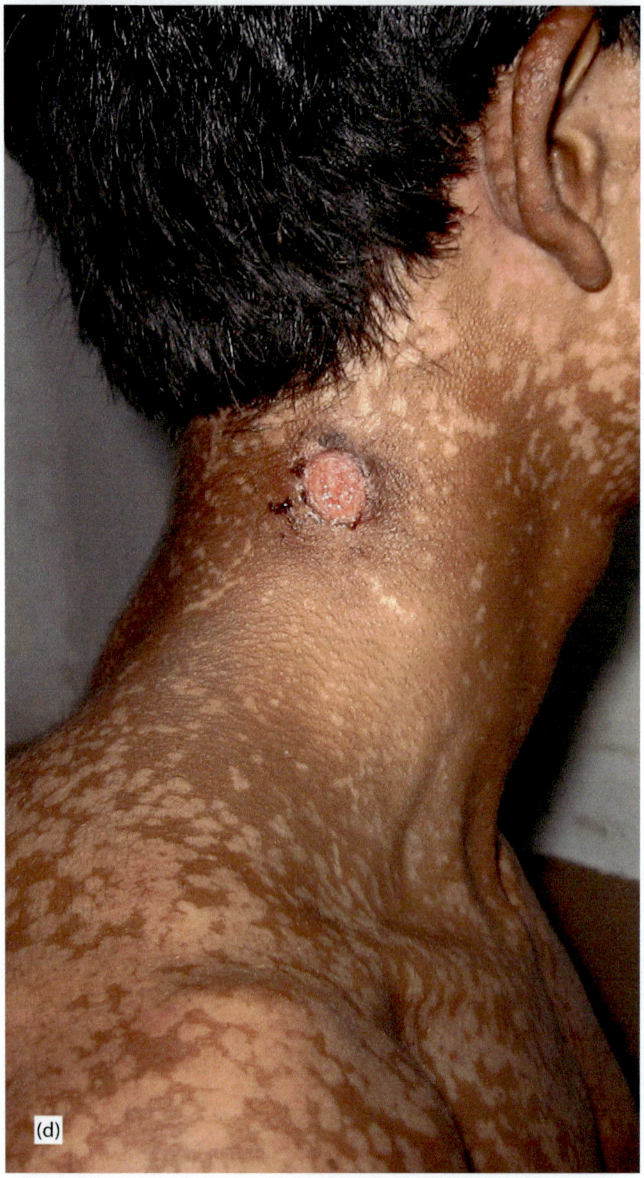


Figure 13.6 **(a)** Ulcerated nodule of squamous cell carcinoma on the scalp. **(b)** Squamous cell carcinoma on the area of previous burn (Marjolin ulcer). **(c)** Squamous cell carcinoma presenting as non-healing ulcer on buccal mucosa. **(d)** Non-healing ulcer of squamous cell carcinoma on the neck in a patient with epidermodysplasia verruciformis. *(Continued)*

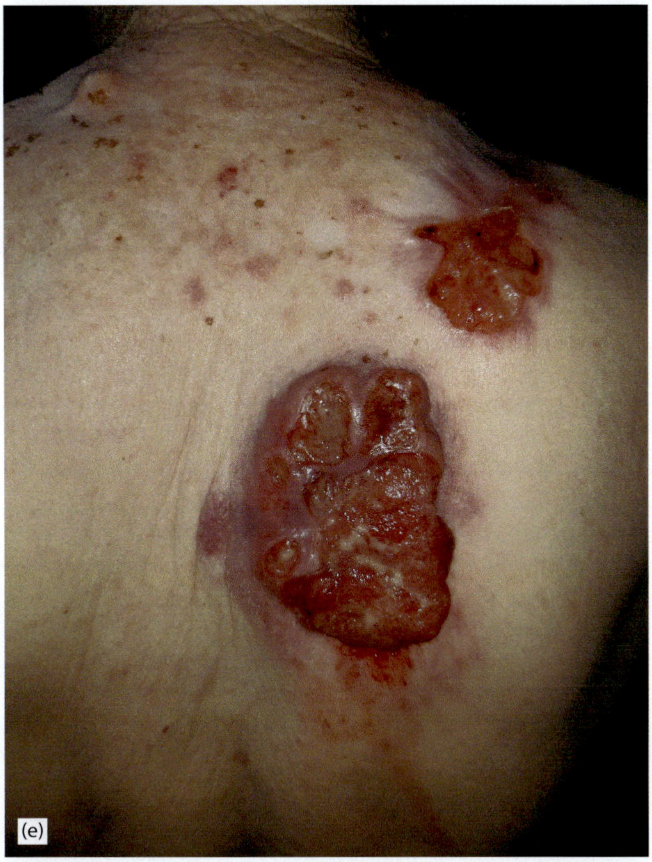


Figure 13.6 *(Continued)* **(e)** Squamous cell carcinoma presenting as non-healing ulcer and large noduloulcerative lesions in a patient with oculocutaneous albinism. (a,b – Courtesy: Dr. PC Das, Katihar, India; c,d – Courtesy: Dr. Piyush Kumar, Katihar, India; e – Courtesy: Dr Hiral Shah, Baroda Medical College, Vadodara, India.)

## Herpes zoster

- Ulcerations in herpes zoster are small and grouped in a linear fashion along a dermatome. They are associated with significant pain and heal with scarring (**Figure 13.7**).

## Temporal arteritis

- Temporal arteritis is a chronic granulomatous vasculitis affecting medium-large cell vessels (external cranial branches of the aorta).
- The incidence of temporal arteritis increases with age, almost exclusively affecting people 50 years of age or older. Women account for 65–75% of patients.
- Typical clinical features include new-onset headache, scalp tenderness, jaw claudication, fever, fatigue, malaise, anorexia, weight loss, and polymyalgia.
- Rarely, patients may present with scalp necrosis.

## Angiosarcoma[13]

- Angiosarcoma is an aggressive, malignant endothelial-cell tumor of lymphatic or vascular origin. It has a high rate of local recurrence and metastasis.

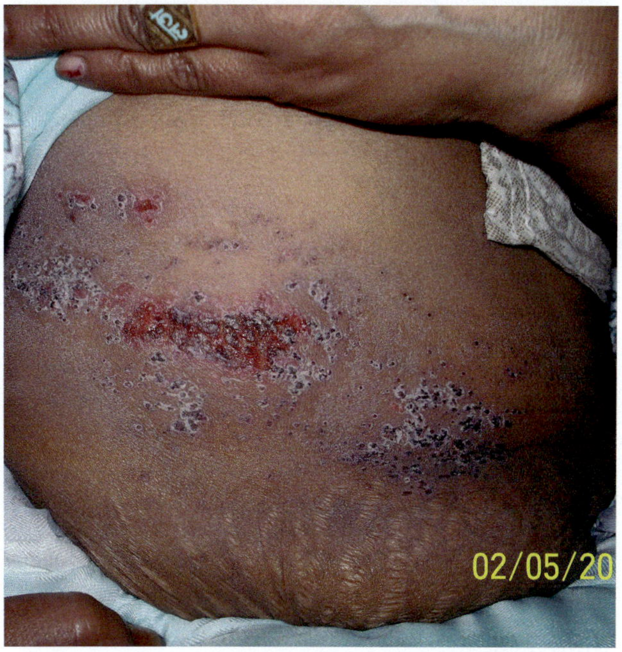


Figure 13.7 Ulcer and crusts in dermatomal distribution in herpes zoster. (Courtesy: Dr. Piyush Kumar, Katihar, India.)

- It is more common in older individuals, with a reported median age between 60 and 71 years; cutaneous angiosarcomas are more prevalent in males.
- The cutaneous form is the most common, accounting for about half of all tumors, with the head and neck being the most frequently involved region. Specifically, the scalp accounts for approximately 50% of all angiosarcoma cases.
- Risk factors include chronic lymphoedema and radiation therapy.
- Patients often present with skin lesions such as an enlarging bruise, a discolored nodule, or persistent ulceration.
- In the early stages, these lesions can be misdiagnosed for benign entities caused by cellulitis, infection, or skin injuries.
- DD: Hemangioblastoma, Kaposi sarcoma, metastatic cancer from an unknown primary site, sinonasal squamous-cell cancer and Merkel cell carcinoma.

## Decubitus ulcer

- Decubitus ulcers, also termed bedsores or pressure ulcers, are skin and soft-tissue injuries that form as a result of constant or prolonged pressure exerted on the skin.
- They occur on bony areas of the body such as the ischium, greater trochanter, sacrum, heel, malleolus (lateral than medial), and occiput.
- Etiology
  - External factors: pressure, friction, shear force, and moisture
  - Internal factors: fever, malnutrition, anemia, and endothelial dysfunction speed up the process of these lesions

- Clinical feature depends on stage of ulcer
  - Stage I describes intact skin with non-blanchable erythema.
  - Stage II pressure ulcers have partial-thickness skin damage with possible blister formation but no subcutaneous tissues visible.
  - Stage III pressure ulcers have full-thickness skin loss with subcutaneous fat exposed but no muscles, bones, or tendons visible.
  - Stage IV pressure ulcers have tissue loss with exposure of muscles, bones, tendons, or vital organs.
- A common hallmark of pressure ulcers is that the area of skin affected typically underrepresents the amount of subcutaneous tissue involved.
- An unstageable pressure ulcer refers to a wound with an undetermined level of tissue injury because the entire base of the wound is covered by slough tissue and/or eschar.[14]

## Kangri ulcer[15]

- This is a squamous cell carcinoma (SCC) that occurs due to keeping lighted coal in a kangri basket (used in remote hilly regions of Kashmir) close to the skin in winter to keep warm.
- The kangri basket, which holds burning coal and dried chinar (*Platanus orientalis*) leaves, is held between the thighs or over the lower abdomen for prolonged periods of 12–18 hours a day.
- Early changes include dyspigmentation, erythema ab igne, induration, and thickening over the medial aspect of upper third of the thighs.
- Malignant transformation is heralded by the development of exophytic growths and ulcers, which often get secondarily infected.

## Calciphylaxis

- Calciphylaxis has been classically described as the sudden development of tender, violaceous, and reticulate lesions that progress to necrotic ulcerations of the lower extremities in patients with renal failure on chronic hemodialysis.
- These ulcers heal poorly and are very painful.
- Areas commonly affected are those with thick adipose tissue, such as the abdomen, breasts, and buttocks.
- Peripheral pulses are preserved, since only the smaller vessels are affected by calciphylaxis.
- There is often an elevated parathyroid (PTH) level (secondary to renal failure), with abnormal calcium and phosphate metabolism.
- Other risk factors include obesity, liver disease, systemic corticosteroid use, and an elevated calcium phosphorus product. In addition, contributing factors are diabetes mellitus, warfarin use, decreased functional protein C and S activity, vitamin D supplementation, and low albumin levels.

## Ecthyma

- Ecthyma is a unique and more invasive form of skin group A Streptococcus infection. In contrast to impetigo, it involves deeper skin tissues, is more painful, and frequently leaves a prominent scar after healing.
- Ecthyma usually arises on the lower extremities of children, persons with diabetes, and neglected elderly patients.
- It begins as a vesicle or pustule overlying an inflamed area of skin that deepens into a dermal ulceration with an overlying crust. The crust of ecthyma lesions is gray-yellow and is thicker and harder than the crust of impetigo. A shallow, punched-out ulceration is apparent when adherent crust is removed. The deep dermal ulcer has a raised and indurated surrounding margin (**Figure 13.8a,b**).
- DD: Ecthyma gangrenosum, pyoderma gangrenosum, insect bite.

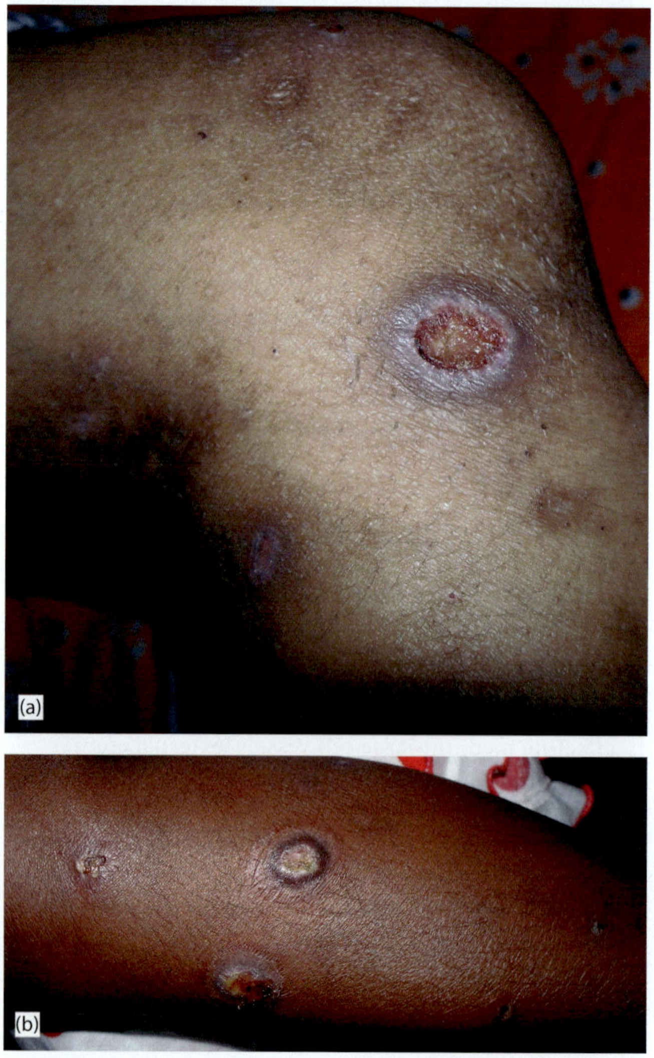


Figure 13.8 **(a)** Ulcer of ecthyma with indurated margin. **(b)** Crusted ulcers in ecthyma. (a,b – Courtesy: Dr. Piyush Kumar, Katihar, India.)

## Swimming pool granuloma

- Also known as fish tank granuloma, this is caused by *M. marinum* infection.
- It is most commonly seen in fishers, oyster workers, swimmers, and aquarium workers, and usually involves the dominant hand.
- The infection starts as a solitary papule or nodule, which grows slowly over several months. Induration and ulceration occur later.
- Sporotrichoid spread and lymphangitis occur subsequently.
- DD: Lupus vulgaris, sporotrichosis.

## Sporotrichosis

- Clinically, sporotrichosis typically manifests as a lymphocutaneous eruption, beginning as a papule or nodule that develops, often within days, at the site of inoculation (**Figure 13.9a**).
- Progressive noduloulcerative lesions following the underlying lymphatics then arise proximally.
- DD: Cutaneous leishmaniasis, nocardiosis.

## Cutaneous anthrax

- Anthrax is a zoonotic disease, and humans are an accidental host. It is caused by *Bacillus anthracis*, a sporulating Gram-positive rod.
- The initial manifestation is of a painless pruritic papule that gradually enlarges over a period of seven to ten days. A serosanguinous discharge may be present.
- Smaller vesicles may be present in the surrounding area, and perilesional edema is characteristic and often disproportionate to the size of the lesion (**Figure 13.9b**).

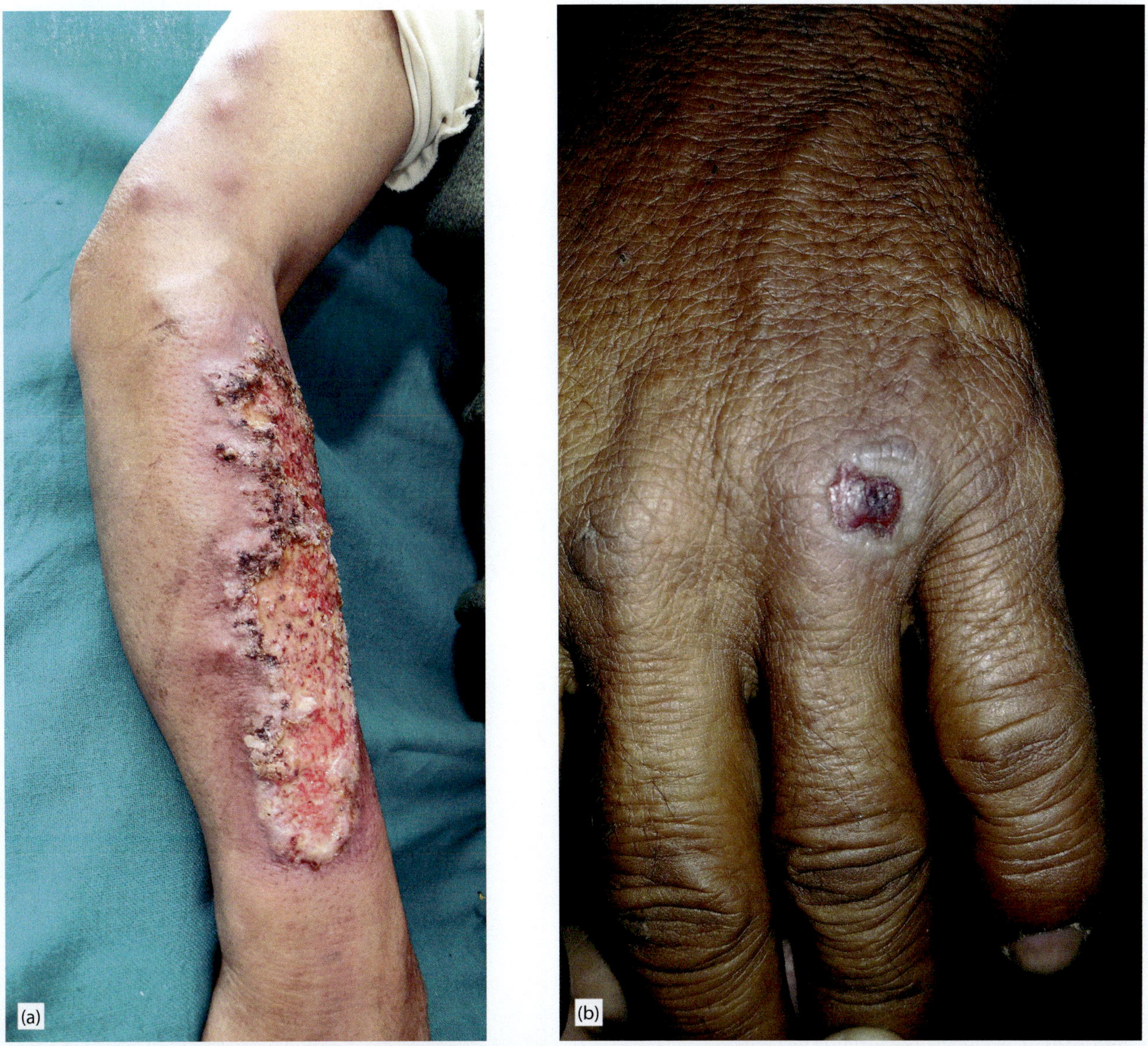


Figure 13.9 **(a)** Ulcerated plaque with erythematous nodules appearing proximally along the lymphatics in a case with ulcerated sporotrichosis. **(b)** Ulcer surrounded by rim of pus in cutaneous anthrax. (a – Courtesy: Dr. Dependra Kumar Timshina, Remedy Clinics, Siliguri, India; b – Courtesy: Dr. Rajesh Kumar Mandal, North Bengal Medical College and Hospital, Darjeeling, India.)

The lesion develops a central depression followed by eschar formation and heals within one to three weeks, with variable scarring.

- More than 90% of the lesions are found on the exposed parts of the body such as the face, neck, hands, and feet.
- DD: Staphylococcal skin abscess, cat scratch disease, tularemia, spider bite, and ecthyma gangrenosum.

## Frostbite

- Frostbite is a freezing, cold thermal injury that occurs when tissues are exposed to temperatures below their freezing point (typically −0.55°C but can occur as high as 2°C) for a sustained period of time.
- It is mainly due to the formation of ice in both intracellular and extracellular compartments.
- It is mostly seen in soldiers, those engaged in winter sports, homeless people, etc.
- Risk increases with alcohol use, smoking, and the presence of peripheral vascular disease.
- In 90% of cases, limbs are affected. It can also affect the face (nose, chin, earlobes, cheeks, and lips), buttocks/perineum (from sitting on metal seats), and penis (joggers and Nordic skiers).
- Classification of severity
    - 1st degree: partial skin freezing present, erythema, edema, hyperemia, but no blisters or necrosis
    - 2nd degree: full thickness freeze, erythema, edema, blistering, black eschar
    - 3rd degree: requires bone amputation
    - 4th degree: major amputation and complicated by systemic effects
- DD: Frostnip, trench foot, pernio.

## Trench foot

- Trench foot is one of three subclasses of immersion foot and is considered a non-freezing cold injury.
- It is often differentiated by the temperature of the exposure and is caused by prolonged exposure to cold but usually not freezing, damp, and sometimes unsanitary conditions.
- Trench foot often begins with a tingling and itching that can progress to numbness.
- In the setting of cold exposure, vascular changes resulting in poor blood flow can result in the feet becoming erythematous or cyanotic.
- The disease has been known to commonly affect the heels or toes but can extend above the foot.
- The skin can appear blotchy, and as the disease progresses, blisters and open sores can occur, which can lead to fungal as well as bacterial infections.
- As the disease continues to advance, skin and tissue may slough off. If the condition is left untreated, gangrene can set in.
- DD: Frostbite, cellulitis.

## Raynaud's phenomenon

- Raynaud's phenomenon is classically described with a triphasic color change of the digits with initial white or pallor (ischemic phase), then blue or cyanosis (deoxygenation phase), followed by red or erythema (reperfusion phase).
- Patients with secondary Raynaud's will describe attacks that are more frequent, painful, often asymmetric and may lead to digital ulcerations.
- These ulcerations can resolve to leave scars or digital pits or may progress to more severe digital necrosis, gangrene, or auto-amputation (**Figure 13.10**).
- Digital ulcerations can become secondarily infected, leading to osteomyelitis, and can require surgical intervention.
- There should be no evidence of tissue gangrene, digital pitting, or tissue injury in primary Raynaud's.
- It is associated with the following:
    - Connective tissue diseases such as scleroderma, lupus, or mixed connective tissue disease.
    - Hematologic causes such as cryoglobulinemia, cryofibrinogenemia, paraproteinemia, or polycythemia.
    - Drug-induced conditions (ergot, methysergide, beta-blockers, bleomycin, cisplatin, clonidine, cocaine, cyclosporine, interferon-alpha, nicotine, and vinblastine).
    - Other vasospastic causes such as pheochromocytoma, carcinoid syndrome, or thyroid disease.

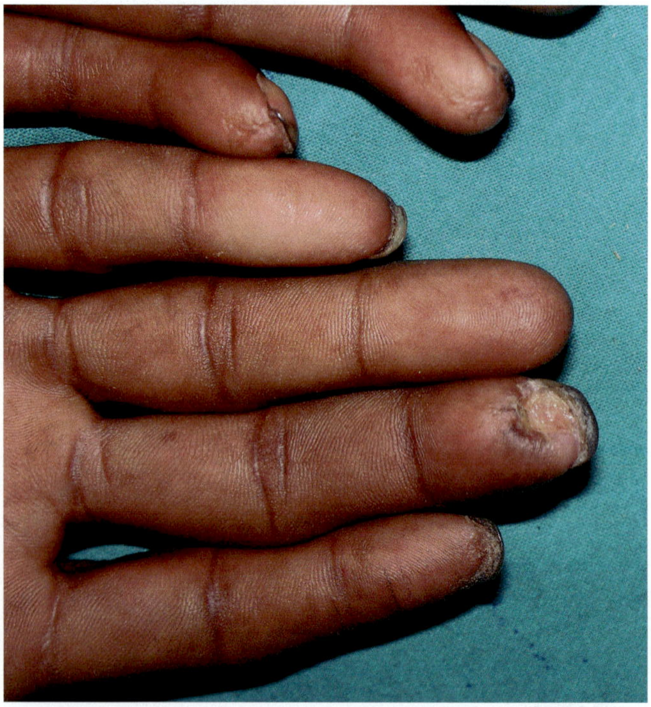

Figure 13.10 Digital ulcer in systemic sclerosis with Raynaud's phenomenon. (Courtesy: Dr. Piyush Kumar, Katihar, India.)

- Numerous structural causes that may include thoracic outlet syndrome, atherosclerosis, brachiocephalic trunk disease as in Takayasu's arteritis, Buerger's disease or thromboangiitis obliterans, or use of vibratory tools such as jackhammers.
- DD: Acrocyanosis, erythromelalgia.

## Necrobiosis lipoidica diabeticorum/necrobiosis lipoidica

- Necrobiosis lipoidica (NL) is characterized by single or multiple asymptomatic red to yellow shiny plaques that gradually enlarge and within which, due to atrophy, dermal blood vessels are readily apparent.
- Ulceration is a complication of NL and commonly develops after trauma to the lesions (**Figure 13.11**).
- Majority of patients have diabetes mellitus, or pre-diabetes.

## Venous ulcer

- Ninety-five per cent of venous ulceration is in the gaiter area of the leg, characteristically around the malleoli.
- Ulceration may be discrete or circumferential. The ulcer bed is often covered with a fibrinous layer mixed with granulation tissue, surrounded by an irregular, gently sloping edge.
- Ulcers occurring above the mid-calf or on the foot are likely to have other origins.
- Lipodermatosclerosis often precedes venous ulceration and is characterized by rigid woody hardness that, at its worst, may result in the leg resembling an "inverted champagne bottle."

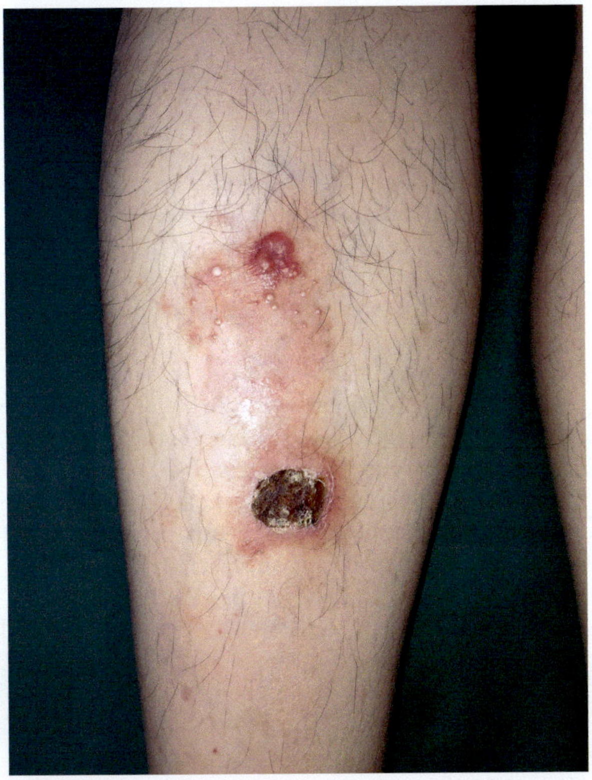

Figure 13.11 Crusted ulcer in necrobiosis lipoidica. (Courtesy: Dr. Sushil S Savant, Mumbai, India.)

- Stasis eczema (erythema, scaling, weeping, and itching) is also common and is distinct from cellulitis. (See Chapter E11.)

## Martorell ulcer

- Martorell ulcer is an uncommon ischemic and extremely painful lesion located in the distal portion of the lower limb, resulting from severe systemic and poorly controlled hypertension. It is common in women between 50 and 70 years of age.
- It is frequently symmetrical and located in the distal third and anterolateral surfaces of the lower limbs.
- Classically, the ulcer has variable depth, necrotic base, and violaceous edges. The presence of satellite lesions and irregular edges are also features that suggest additional cutaneous ischemia.
- Pain in greater intensity than in ulcers of other etiologies, referred to as being disproportionate to the size of the lesion, is the most relevant symptom.
- DD: Venous ulcer, traumatic ulcer, pyoderma gangrenosum.

## Nicolau syndrome

- Nicolau syndrome (embolia cutis medicamentosa) is a rare cutaneous adverse reaction occurring at the site of intramuscular, intra-articular or, rarely, subcutaneous injection of particular drugs.
- Three factors have been proposed to play a final role in the pathogenesis: embolism (of the injected material), angiospasm (secondary to needle prick), and thrombosis. Mechanical pressure exerted by the material placed around the vessel too might play a role.
- The typical clinical presentation is pain around the injection site soon after injection, followed by erythema, livedoid patch, hemorrhagic patch, and finally necrosis of skin, subcutaneous fat, and muscle tissue.

## Tropical ulcer

- Tropical ulcers result from diseases transmitted by mosquitoes and flies in tropical and subtropical countries where the weather is hot and humid.
- Predisposing factors include poor hygiene, low socioeconomic conditions, poor nutrition, poverty, and lack of protection from insect bites.
- Superinfection with *Fusobacterium* species, anaerobic microorganisms (*Bacillus fusiformis*) and spirochetes (*Treponema vincenti*) aggravates these ulcers and delays healing.
- The lesion first appears as a small papule on the lower leg, usually at the site of trauma.
- The ulcer then spreads rapidly, forms a blister, and undergoes necrosis, which is associated with pain, fever, and malaise.
- Within a few weeks the ulcer enlarges to 10–12 cm, and a superficial, necrotic, malodorous, purulent, hemorrhagic black coating develops (**Figure 13.12a,b**).
- After three to four weeks, the edge becomes flatter, and the swelling and pain decrease.
- DD: Buruli ulcer, pyoderma gangrenosum.

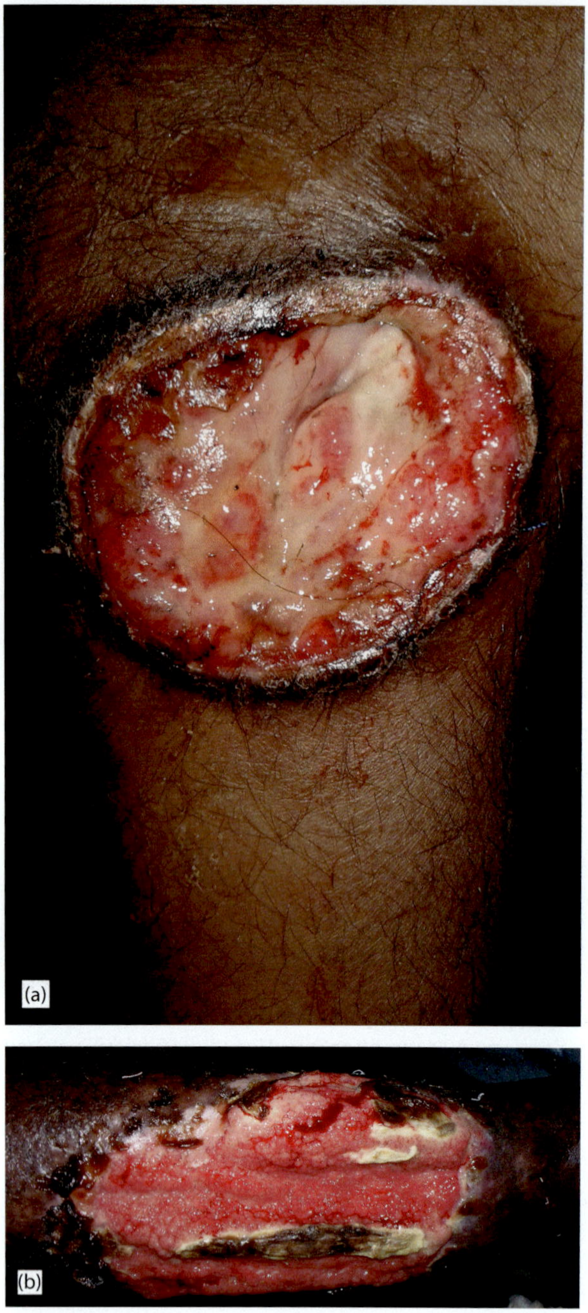


Figure 13.12 **(a)** Tropical ulcer. **(b)** Large tropical ulcer. (a – Courtesy: Dr. PC Das, Katihar, India; b – Courtesy: Dr. Piyush Kumar, Katihar, India.)

## Thromboangiitis obliterans

- Thromboangiitis obliterans (TAO), also known as Buerger's disease, is a progressive, non-atherosclerotic, segmental, inflammatory disease that most often affects small and medium arteries of the upper and lower extremities.
- Risk factors include male gender, and smoking.
- Claudication in the arch of the foot is an early sign and is suggestive of, or even specific to, TAO. This condition is a manifestation of infrapopliteal vessel occlusive disease.
- As the disease progresses, typical calf claudication and eventually ischemic pain at rest and ischemic ulcerations on the toes, feet, or fingers may develop.
- Raynaud's phenomenon is present in greater than 40% of patients with thromboangiitis obliterans.
- Superficial thrombophlebitis differentiates thromboangiitis obliterans from other vasculitides and atherosclerosis.

## Arterial ulcer

- Arterial ulceration typically occurs over the toes, heels, and bony prominences of the foot.
- The ulcer appears "punched out," with well-demarcated edges and a pale, non-granulating, often necrotic base.
- The surrounding skin may exhibit dusky erythema and may be cool to touch, hairless, thin, and brittle, with a shiny texture.
- The toenails thicken and become opaque and may be lost. Gangrene of the extremities may also occur. (See chapter E11.)

## Pyoderma gangrenosum

- Pyoderma gangrenosum (PG) is a reactive non-infectious inflammatory dermatosis falling within the spectrum of the neutrophilic dermatoses and characterized by chronic and recurrent cutaneous ulcers with a necrolytic border.
- It is typically seen in adults, with peak occurrence between the ages of 30 and 50 years and with slight predilection for females.
- Etiology is unknown. Risk factors include female gender, pregnancy, surgery, and a history of underlying disease such as inflammatory bowel disease or hematologic malignancy.
- The lower legs are most frequently affected, although PG can affect any site. The lesion may be precipitated by minor trauma, a phenomenon known as "pathergy."
- Lesions in classical PG, also known as ulcerative PG, present as painful small erythematous or violaceous papules or pustules, which evolve into violaceous ulcers or necrotic plaques.
- One of the hallmark features of classic PG is the presence of an undermined or raised border with a characteristic gun metal gray or violaceous to blue color (**Figure 13.13a–c**). Lesions heal with cribriform scarring.[16]
- DD: Arterial and venous disease, hematological causes (sickle cell disease, cryoglobulinemia, antiphospholipid syndrome), vascular occlusion, vasculitis, infections, calciphylaxis, drug-induced ulceration, primary or metastatic tumors, hypertension (Martorell ulcer) and other inflammatory disorders, including cutaneous Crohn's disease.

## Necrotizing fasciitis[17]

- Necrotizing fasciitis (NF) is a severe, rare, potentially lethal soft-tissue infection that develops in the scrotum and perineum, the abdominal wall, or the extremities.

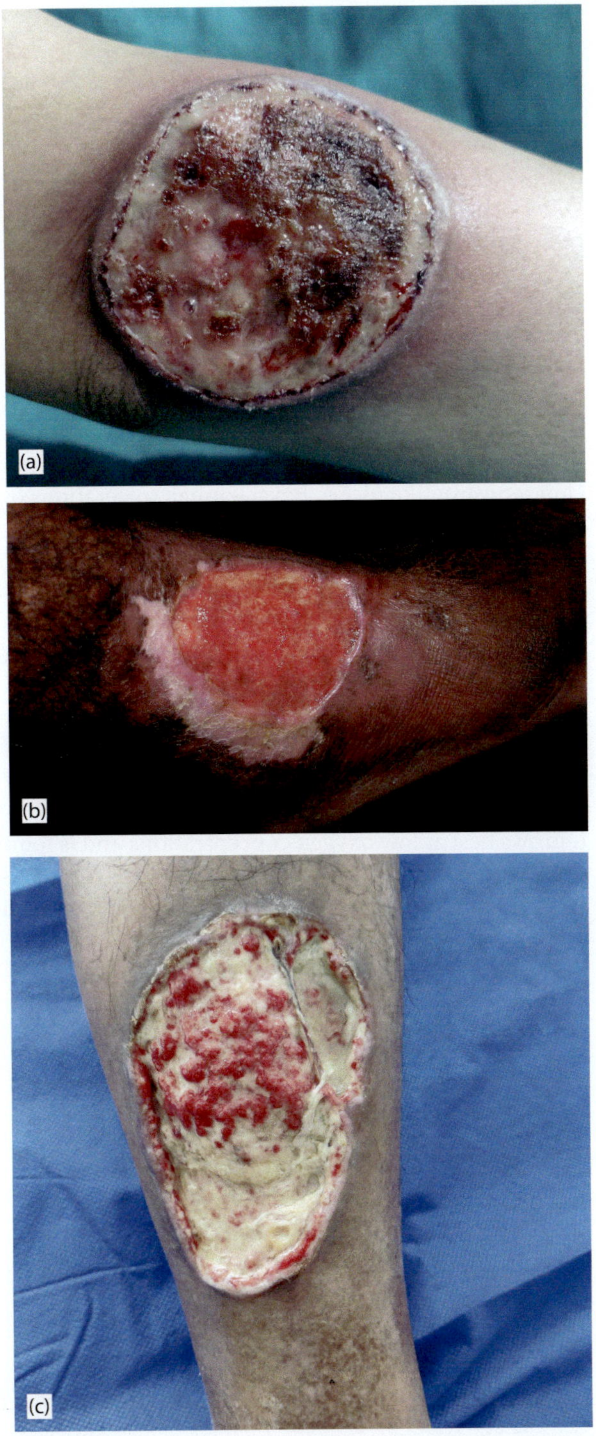


Figure 13.13 **(a)** Ulcer of pyoderma gangrenosum with raised, violaceous margin. **(b)** Pyoderma gangrenosum. **(c)** Pyoderma gangrenosum progresses rapidly and may assume a large size. (a,c – Courtesy Dr. Dependra Kumar Timshina, Remedy Clinics, Siliguri, India; b – Courtesy Dr. Piyush Kumar, Katihar, India.)

- Trauma is the most common identifiable etiology. The majority of patients have a history of minor or major traumas, generally involving external injuries and surgical wounds.
- Responsible pathogens are as follows:
  - Type 1: Polymicrobial (obligate and facultative anaerobes)
  - Type 2: Beta-hemolytic *Streptococcus*
  - Type 3: *Clostridium*, gram negative bacteria, *Aeromonas, Vibrio*
  - Type 4:*Candida, Zygomycetes*
- Risk factors include diabetes mellitus (the most frequent comorbidity). Other common comorbidities include liver cirrhosis, chronic heart failure, obesity, alcohol abuse, immunodeficiency, systemic lupus erythematosus, Addison's disease, pre-existing hypertension, and peripheral vascular disease.
- Patients with NF usually present with the classic triad of symptoms: local pain, swelling, and erythema. Tachycardia (>100 beats/min) and fever are the most common vital sign abnormalities, followed by hypotension (SAP < 100 mmHg) and tachypnea (>20/min).
- However, in the fulminant form of disease, the patient is critically ill, with signs and symptoms of severe septic shock and multiple organ dysfunction syndrome along with extensive necrosis of soft tissue.
- The skin lesion starts with painful edema and erythema. The condition progresses rapidly, and gangrene sets in. The skin becomes dark and ulcerates with eschar formation. The pain subsides after ulceration (**Figure 13.14**).

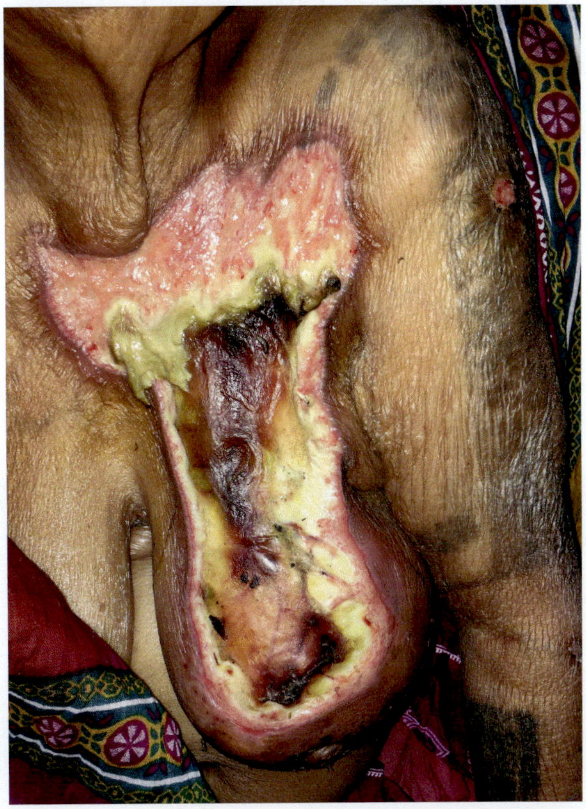

Figure 13.14 Necrotizing fasciitis affecting anterior chest and left breast. (Courtesy: Dr. Piyush Kumar, Katihar, India.)

- Gas formation can lead to crepitus in the overlying skin, indicating anaerobic infection, such as *C. perfringens*.
- Systemic features include hypotension, elevated white blood cell count, metabolic acidosis, coagulopathy, changes in mental status, and weakness.
- DD: Cellulitis.

### Syphilitic gumma

- Cutaneous gummas of tertiary syphilis are dermal or subcutaneous nodules that have a gummy or rubbery consistency.
- They can occur singly or form grouped, annular or serpiginous lesions that have predilection for the scalp, face, chest, legs, and sites of trauma.
- They are painless and frequently ulcerate.

### Ecthyma gangrenosum

- Ecthyma gangrenosum is a rare and invasive cutaneous infection caused by *Pseudomonas aeruginosa* in the majority of cases, typically affecting immunocompromised patients, particularly those with neutropenia.
- The characteristic clinical appearance is red macules that progress to a central area of necrosis surrounded by an erythematous halo (**Figure 13.15**).
- The main sites of ecthyma gangrenosum lesions are the extremities and gluteal or perineal region (57%), although this lesion can spread to other body sites.
- Classically, the pathogen is isolated from the skin lesions as well as from the blood.
- DD: Calciphylaxis, septic emboli, cutaneous anthrax, cutaneous aspergillosis, and pyoderma gangrenosum.

### Warfarin-induced skin necrosis

- Sudden development of paresthesia, edema, petechiae, and ecchymoses progressing to full-thickness necrosis and deep ulcers within three to ten days after the initiation of warfarin therapy should alert the clinician to the possibility of warfarin-induced skin necrosis (WISN).
- WISN has been described in patients on anticoagulation, typically several days after therapy is stopped or on retreatment. It is thought to be the result of a paradoxical hypercoagulable state, possibly due to inhibition of vitamin K–dependent coagulation factors relative to other factors, thus producing a transient imbalance that predisposes to clotting.
- Protein C deficiency, protein S deficiency, and antithrombin III deficiency are considered risk factors in the development of WISN.
- DD: Heparin-induced necrosis associated with heparin-induced thrombocytopenia and thrombosis (HITT).

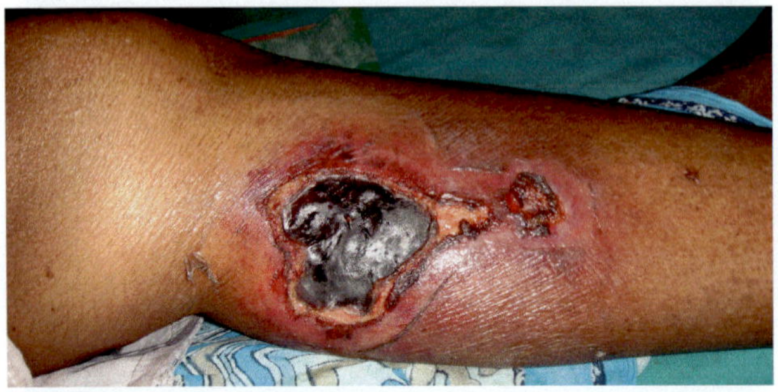

Figure 13.15 Ecthyma gangrenosum with central ulcer and eschar surrounded by erythema. (Courtesy: Dr. Piyush Kumar, Katihar, India.)

### Chemotherapy agents and ulcer[18]

- The antineoplatic agents commonly associated with ulcers are mentioned below.
- Inhibitors of epidermal growth actor receptors (EGFR): Geftinib (pyoderma gangrenosum-like ulcer), Sorafenib.
- Angiogenesis inhibitor: Sorafenib, Sunitinib (pyoderma gangrenosum like ulcer), Bevacizumab (ulcerations over striae distensae).
- BCR-ABL, c-KIT, PDGFR inhibitors: Imatinib (oral ulcers).
- m-TOR inhibitor: Sirolimus (aphthous ulcer).
- Antimetabolites: Methotrexate (dose-dependent ulceration of psoriatic plaques, Mucositis) (**Figure 13.16**).
- Antiproliferative: Hydroxyurea (perimalleolar and pretibial ulcers have been described).

### Buruli ulcer (Bairnsdale ulcer)[19]

- This is caused by *M. ulcerans*.
- It grows best at low oxygen concentrations and is found in muddy or marshy ground.
- It causes necrotizing ulcers in otherwise healthy people.
- The disease begins as indurated nodules that look like insect bites but are painless and cold (not inflamed).
- Within weeks, these lesions grow in diameter and depth, producing edematous plaques with ill-defined borders.

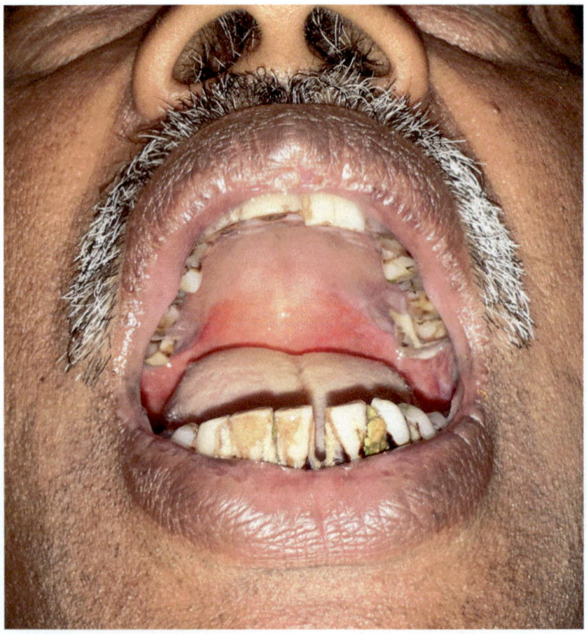

Figure 13.16 Erosive mucositis following methotrexate toxicity. (Courtesy: Dr. Piyush Kumar, Katihar, India.)

- On occasion there is no nodule or plaque and only diffuse swelling.
- Eventually the indurated, necrotic skin sloughs off, creating a painless ulcer with irregular borders and characteristic undermined edges.
- The surrounding skin can show edema and changes in pigmentation.
- Most of the time there is a single lesion; however, small satellite lesions can be present. In many instances the ulcer acquires secondary bacterial infections, giving it a foul smell.
- DD: Pyoderma gangrenosum, metastatic ulcer.

### Tularaemia

- It results from infection with *Francisella tularensis*, a gram-negative bacteria.
- Wild rodents and other small animals are the main reservoir of infection, which is transmitted to humans by bites of ticks, usually of dermacentor species.
- It occurs in all ages and affects males and females equally.
- Clinical features depend on portal of entry, which may be skin, eye, or respiratory and GI tract.
- A red painful and then ulcerated nodule at point of inoculation or tick bite is associated with enlargement and tenderness and later breakdown of regional lymph nodes.
- During the toxemic stage of all forms, cutaneous lesions may develop; a generalized eruption, maculopapular or resembling erythema multiforme, profuse crops of nodules, usually on limbs may occur.
- DD: Tick-borne rickettsial infections.

### Cat scratch disease

- Caused by *Bartonella henselae*, it usually develops after a cat scratch or bite.
- It affects all ages but mostly children and teenagers; it affects both genders.
- The main clinical feature is that three to five days after inoculation a papule may form that progresses through vesicular and blistering stages in two or three days and may ulcerate and often leaves a superficial scar (90% of cases).
- Constitutional symptoms are usually mild, but fever is present in 60% of cases.
- Lymphadenopathy is present in all cases and usually develops within two weeks of the initial papule; it is solitary in 85% of cases but two or three are seen in occasional cases.
- DD: Sporotrichosis, atypical mycobacterial infections.

### Glanders disease

- Also called farcy, Glanders is contacted from affected horses, donkeys, mules, and goats.
- Caused by *Burkholderia mallei*, it is extremely rare nowadays and affects both sexes and any age.
- It is characterized by cellulitis at the site of inoculation, which soon develops into an irregular ulcer with an offensive hemorrhagic purulent discharge.
- Systemic symptoms include headache, malaise, and fever.
- After a few weeks, metastatic lesions begin to appear, which are grouped, dull red papules, pustules or bullae especially over joints and face. These are followed by ulcers that enlarge and coalesce.
- Deep subcutaneous abscesses with multiple sinuses may also occur.
- DD: Melioidosis, pyoderma.

### Myiasis

- Myiasis is an infestation of body tissues by larvae (maggots) of the order Diptera.
- There are three types of cutaneous myiasis: furuncular, traumatic (wound), migratory (creeping).
- Wound myiasis occurs as a complication of war wounds or neglected open wounds (**Figure 13.17**).
    - Risk factors include the following:
        - Wounds with alkaline discharges (attract blow flies)
        - Presence of necrosis
        - Lack of hygiene
        - Low socioeconomic status
        - Extremes of age, mental retardation, diabetes, alcoholism, vascular occlusive disorders
- Furuncular myiasis results from penetration of larva into healthy skin.
    - Caused by *Dermatobia hominis*, and *Cordylobia anthropophaga*.
    - It has a papule/nodule with a central punctum exuding serosanguinous or purulent fluid.
    - The clinical diagnosis rests on visualizing the respiratory spiracle of larva through the punctum or presence of bubbles in the discharge.
    - Pruritus, pain, movement sensation may be present.
    - Vesicular, bullous, pustular, erosive, ulcerative, or ecchymotic lesions are uncommon.

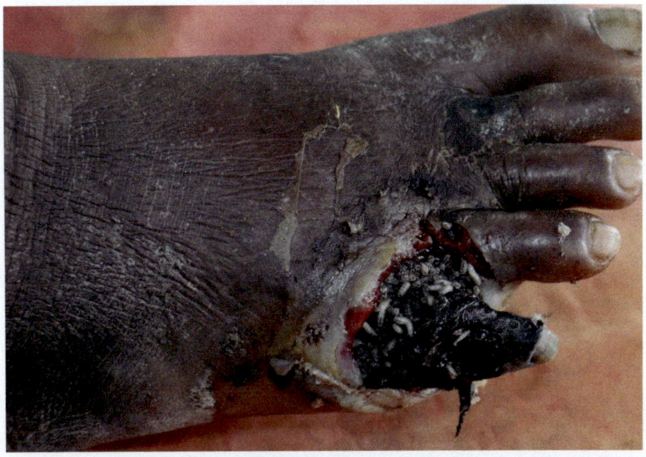

Figure 13.17 Myiasis complicating a traumatic wound in a leprosy patient. (Courtesy: Dr. Piyush Kumar, Katihar, India.)

## Cutaneous Crohn disease

- Cutaneous lesions in Crohn disease could be specific (showing histopathology findings consistent with Crohn disease) or reactive (pyoderma gangrenosum, Sweet syndrome, etc). These cutaneous lesions are often associated with systemic features like abdominal pain, diarrhea, melena, malnutrition and weight loss, fever, and bowel obstruction.
- Specific lesions in Crohn disease may result from direct extension from gastrointestinal Crohn disease or may be metastatic. Cutaneous lesions resulting from direct extension are noted in perianal and orofacial areas.
- Cutaneous lesions developing after direct extension include perianal fissures and fistulae, abscess, and painful ulcers (**Figure 13.18**).
- Metastatic lesions assume the morphology of red/purple plaques and nodules and may ulcerate.

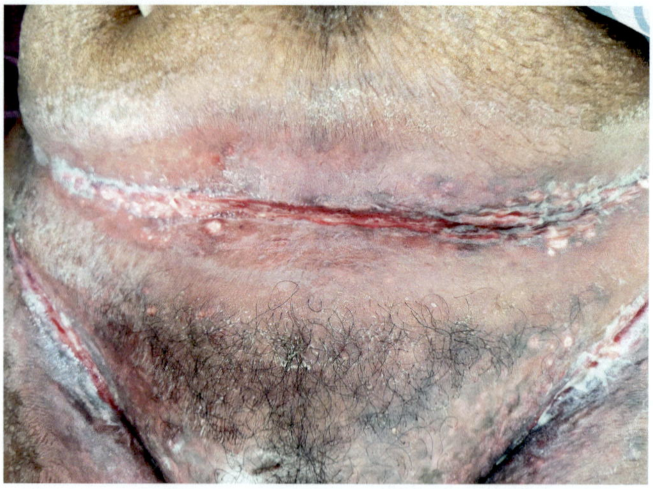

Figure 13.18 Classical "knife cut" ulcers in Crohn disease. (Courtesy: Dr Shekhar Neema, Armed Forces Medical College, Pune, India.)

## Additional images – Figure 13.19a,b

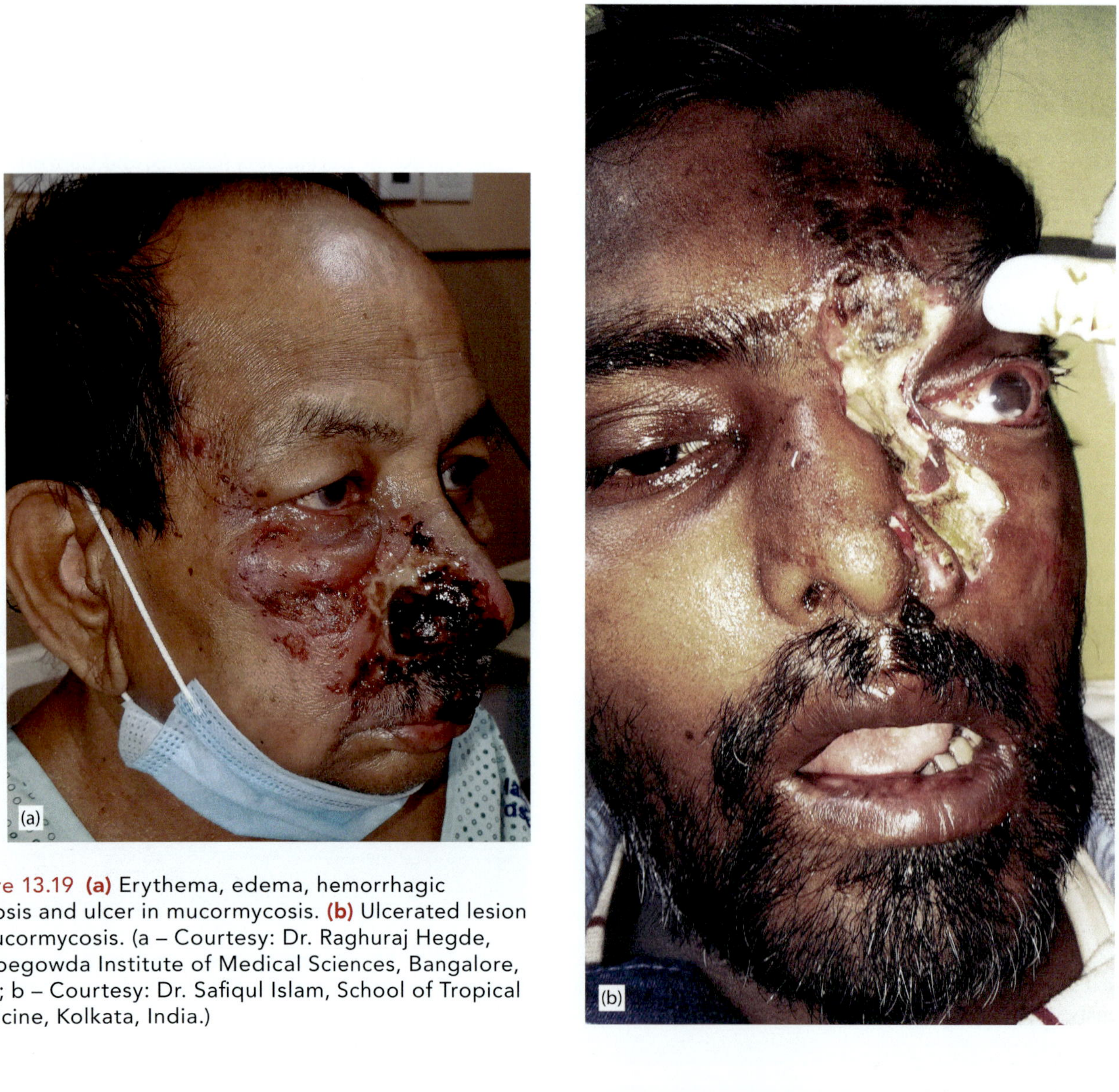


Figure 13.19 **(a)** Erythema, edema, hemorrhagic necrosis and ulcer in mucormycosis. **(b)** Ulcerated lesion in mucormycosis. (a – Courtesy: Dr. Raghuraj Hegde, Kempegowda Institute of Medical Sciences, Bangalore, India; b – Courtesy: Dr. Safiqul Islam, School of Tropical Medicine, Kolkata, India.)

## REFERENCES


1. Lipsker D. Clinical Examination and Differential Diagnosis of Skin Lesions. 1st edition. France: Springer-Verlag; 2013. Chapter 42. Erosions and Ulcerations. P. 219–224.
2. Fitzpatrick JE, High WA, Kyle WL. Urgent Care Dermatology: Symptom-Based Diagnosis. 1st ed. Philadelphia: Elsevier; 2018. Chapter 14. Necrotic and Ulcerative Skin Disorders. P. 231–252.
3. Marks Jr JG, Miller JJ. Lookingbill and Marks' Principles of Dermatology. 6th edition. Philadelphia: Elsevier; 2019. Chapter 19. Ulcers. P. 257–261.
4. Singer AJ, Tassiopoulos A, Kirsner RS. Evaluation and management of lower-extremity ulcers. N Engl J Med 2017;377(16):1559–1567.
5. Roett MA, Mayor MT, Uduhiri KA. Diagnosis and management of genital ulcers. Am Fam Physician 2012;85(3):254–262.
6. Hoffman MD. Atypical ulcers. Dermatol Ther 2013;26(3):222–235.
7. Janowska A, Dini V, Oranges T, Iannone M, Loggini B, Romanelli M. Atypical ulcers: Diagnosis and management. Clin Interv Aging 2019;14:2137–2143.
8. Hoffman MD. Inflammatory ulcers. Clin Dermatol 2007;25(1):131–138.
9. Chang CS, Kang GC. Efficacious healing of ulcerated infantile hemangiomas using topical timolol. Plast Reconstr Surg Glob Open 2016;4(2):e621.
10. Enwonwu CO, Falkler WA Jr, Phillips RS. Noma (cancrum oris). Lancet 2006;368(9530):147–156.
11. Dias MF, Bernardes Filho F, Quaresma MV, Nascimento LV, Nery JA, Azulay DR. Update on cutaneous tuberculosis. An Bras Dermatol 2014;89(6):925–938.
12. Garcia-Zuazaga J, Olbricht SM. Cutaneous squamous cell carcinoma. Adv Dermatol 2008;24:33–57.
13. Gaballah AH, Jensen CT, Palmquist S, Pickhardt PJ, Duran A, Broering G, Elsayes KM. Angiosarcoma: Clinical and imaging features from head to toe. Br J Radiol 2017;90(1075):20170039.
14. Boyko TV, Longaker MT, Yang GP. Review of the current management of pressure ulcers. Adv Wound Care (New Rochelle) 2018;7(2):57–67.
15. Gupta D, Thappa DM. Dermatoses due to Indian cultural practices. Indian J Dermatol 2015;60:3–12.
16. Ahn C, Negus D, Huang W. Pyoderma gangrenosum: A review of pathogenesis and treatment. Expert Rev Clin Immunol 2018;14(3):225–233.
17. Misiakos EP, Bagias G, Patapis P, Sotiropoulos D, Kanavidis P, Machairas A. Current concepts in the management of necrotizing fasciitis. Front Surg 2014;1:36.
18. D'Epiro S, Salvi M, Luzi A, Mattozzi C, Luci C, Macaluso L, Marzocca F, Salvo V, Cantisani C, Paolino G, Calvieri S, Richetta AG. Drug cutaneous side effect: Focus on skin ulceration. Clin Ter 2014;165(4):e323–9.
19. Guarner J. Buruli ulcer: Review of a neglected skin mycobacterial disease. J Clin Microbiol 2018;56(4):e01507–17.

# E11

# Leg ulcers

PIYUSH KUMAR, KOMAL AGARWAL

## ABSTRACT

Lower-limb ulcers are a common presentation in the dermatology department. These ulcers are not only a cause of great concern to the patient but also a diagnostic dilemma to the treating dermatologists. Given the wide array of causes and the often-confusing presentation, the correct diagnosis of leg ulcers is often delayed. In order to address the above issue and for better understanding, this chapter is presented in a lucid form focusing only on the relevant clinical presentations of various ulcers, with due emphasis on the number, shape, site, pain, margin, and associated clinical features, if any.

The text of this chapter is available online at https://routledgetextbooks.com/textbooks/9781032399669/



DOI: 10.1201/9781351054225-26

# E12

# Ulcers: Multiple

PIYUSH KUMAR, RASHMI ROY

## ABSTRACT

Skin ulceration is a major source of morbidity and is often difficult to manage. They can have various etiologies, such as infections, inflammation, and malignancy, among others. Ulcers may be solitary or multiple. Multiple ulcers may indicate an underlying systemic disease, and the physician must know the dermatological as well as systemic signs and symptoms so that early intervention can be made. This chapter discusses the various causes and clinical features of important entities that can present with multiple cutaneous ulcers.

The text of this chapter is available online at https://routledgetextbooks.com/textbooks/9781032399669/

DOI: 10.1201/9781351054225-27

E13

# Scales: Localized

PC DAS

## ABSTRACT

Scale is a secondary skin lesion. Many dermatoses may present with scales at some stage of the disease course, reflecting the ongoing repair and remodeling in the skin. On the other hand, some other dermatoses have scales as the predominant skin lesion. This chapter discusses common conditions presenting with scaling in a localized area.

The text of this chapter is available online at https://routledgetextbooks.com/textbooks/9781032399669/



DOI: 10.1201/9781351054225-28

E14

# Scales: Generalized

AVIJIT MONDAL

## ABSTRACT

Many dermatoses may develop scaling in a generalized distribution during the evolution or resolution of lesions. This chapter, however, focuses on entities that present exclusively or predominantly with generalized scaling.

The text of this chapter is available online at https://routledgetextbooks.com/textbooks/9781032399669/

DOI: 10.1201/9781351054225-29

# E15

# Atrophy

CHIRAG DESAI, RASHID SHAHID

## ABSTRACT

Atrophy of skin, a morphological entity described under secondary skin lesions, is a result of partial or significant loss of epidermis, dermis, subcutis and/or skin appendages leading to overall thinning and loss of elasticity. Apart from primary atrophic conditions, a large number of dermatological diseases and traumatic conditions leave atrophy as sequelae.

The text of this chapter is available online at https://routledgetextbooks.com/textbooks/9781032399669/

 DOI: 10.1201/9781351054225-30

# 14

# Purpura

SANTOSHDEV P RATHOD

## INTRODUCTION

Purpura is extravasation of red blood cells into the skin and/or mucosa and does not blanch on diascopy. Understanding the clinical characteristics of a purpuric lesion (**Box 14.1**) is crucial for generating clinical differentials. Other features that help in clinical diagnosis include age of onset, associated skin lesions, and general status of the patient. Purpuric lesions may be an ominous sign of many life-threatening diseases, including septicemia, vasculitis, purpura fulminans, bleeding disorders, etc., and hence need immediate attention and urgent evaluation by treating physicians. Additionally, purpura in a child (child abuse) or in adults may be a medicolegal concern. This chapter focuses on clinical evaluation of purpuric lesions (outlined in **Table 14.1**), and salient features of different entities are discussed below.[1–6] Additional clinical clues are enumerated in **Table 14.2**.

## PETECHIAE AND ECCHYMOSES

### Idiopathic thrombocytopenic purpura

- Two-thirds of cases occur before 21 years of age.
- There is a strong female preponderance in adults.
- The onset may be gradual or, especially in children, acute.
- Usually the only symptom is a tendency to bleed from gingivae after brushing teeth or into the skin-producing crops of petechiae or larger hemorrhages (**Figure 14.1**).
- The spleen is usually mildly enlarged; gross enlargement should suggest an alternate diagnosis.
- DD: Systemic lupus erythematosus (SLE), drug-induced purpura, disseminated intravascular coagulation, and renal failure.

### Leukemia/bone marrow failure

- Splenomegaly is the major feature.
- Purpura and ecchymoses are among the common cutaneous features.

### Heparin-induced thrombocytopenia

- This can occur in conjunction with heparin-induced skin necrosis.
- This may immediately occur if patient has been sensitized and has received heparin within past 100 days.
- Lesions are most common at subcutaneous injection sites but can occur elsewhere.
- It commonly induces cutaneous findings of simple hemorrhage with ecchymoses and occasionally triggers urticaria or infiltrated plaques.

**BOX 14.1: Clinical characteristics of purpura**

- Based on size
    - Petechiae – flat lesions ≤4 mm, initially bright red and then fading to a rust color.
    - Ecchymosis – flat lesions >5 mm, typically initially red or purple, but color changes to yellow, brown, or green as the lesion ages.
- Based on morphology
    - Palpable purpura – elevated, round or oval, red or purple papules and/or plaques.
    - Retiform purpura – stellate-shaped or branching lesions, with angular or geometric borders. These are usually palpable, but may be non-palpable too.

DOI: 10.1201/9781351054225-31

Table 14.1 Clinical approach to purpura

| Morphology | Features | Diseases |
|---|---|---|
| Petechiae | Prolonged bleeding on trauma | • Acute, mucosal bleeding – immune thrombocytopenia<br>• Rapid onset, meningism, hypotension, shock – acute bacterial sepsis, including invasive meningococcal disease, active hemorrhagic type of disseminated intravascular coagulation (DIC)<br>• Subacute, lethargy, pallor – myelosuppression, non-leukemic bone marrow failure (e.g., myelodysplasia, aplastic anemia, solid tumor infiltration)<br>• Chronic, family history – congenital bleeding disorders including hemophilia and von Willebrand disease<br>• Variable – drug-induced thrombocytopenia |
| | Neurological signs (seizures, hemiplegia, paresthesias) | Thrombotic thrombocytopenic purpura |
| | History of surgery, sepsis, delivery, neoplasm, etc. | Disseminated intravascular coagulation (DIC) |
| | Others | • Lower extremities – pigmented purpuric dermatosis, hypergammaglobulinemic purpura of Waldenstrom<br>• Face and neck – Valsalva-associated petechiae<br>• Superior vena cava area – strangulation<br>• Random – trauma, local pressure |
| Ecchymosis | Onset in elderly | Solar/ senile purpura |
| | Onset in childhood | • Delayed wound healing – genetic disease with collagen/ elastin defects (Ehler–Danlos syndrome, pseudoxanthoma elasticum)<br>• Excessive bleeding – clotting factor deficiency, acquired thrombocytopenia secondary to sepsis or leukemia<br>• Patterned – battered baby syndrome/child abuse |
| | Associated signs | • Macroglossia – systemic amyloidosis<br>• Hemorrhagic bulla, skin necrosis – DIC<br>• Perifollicular petechiae, twisted broken hairs – scurvy<br>• Prolonged bleeding on trauma – liver disease, vitamin K deficiency |
| | Others | Trauma, anticoagulant use |
| Palpable purpura | | • Subacute to chronic course – vasculitis (leukocytoclastic vasculitis, small-vessel vasculitis, small- to medium-vessel vasculitis, ANCA associated vasculitis; see Chapter E48)<br>• Acute, viral illness, coryzal symptoms – papular-purpuric "gloves-and-socks" syndrome |
| Retiform purpura | Systemic inflammation | Medium-vessel vasculitis, ANCA-associated vasculitis, purpura fulminans (DIC) |
| | Without systemic inflammation | • Neurological signs – thrombotic thrombocytopenic purpura<br>• Sick patients – vasoinvasive infections (invasive fungus, pseudomonas, strongyloidiasis, or lucio leprosy)<br>• History of anticoagulant – heparin necrosis, warfarin necrosis<br>• Painful lesions – antiphospholipid antibody syndrome, emboli, calciphylaxis, livedoid vasculopathy |

Table 14.2 Additional clues to clinical diagnosis of purpura

| Clue | Diseases |
|---|---|
| Acute onset | Idiopathic thrombocytopenic purpura, Henoch-Schönlein purpura, medication, trauma, Valsalva-associated petechiae |
| Mucosal bleeding | Platelet disorders, thrombocytopenia, von Willebrand disease |
| Lethargy, fever, bone pain | Leukemia |
| Antecedent infection | Idiopathic thrombocytopenic purpura, Henoch-Schönlein purpura |
| Family history of bleeding | von Willebrand disease, hemophilia |
| Restricted diet/malnutrition | Scurvy or vitamin K deficiency |
| Hepatosplenomegaly | Leukemia |

- Uncommonly, purpuric, tender, sharply demarcated plaques develop at lesional margins. Erythema may sometimes accompany such lesions, and necrosis is frequent.
- DD: Post-transfusion purpura in early stages.

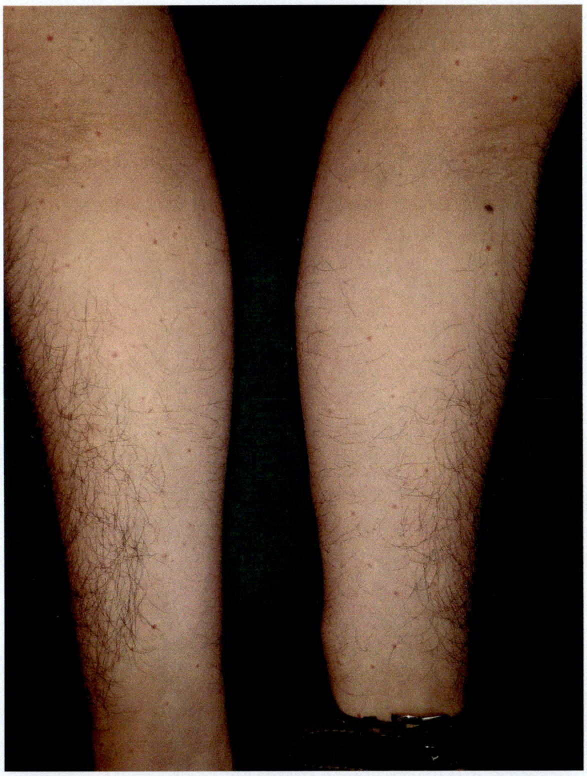

Figure 14.1 Petechiae in idiopathic thrombocytopenic purpura.

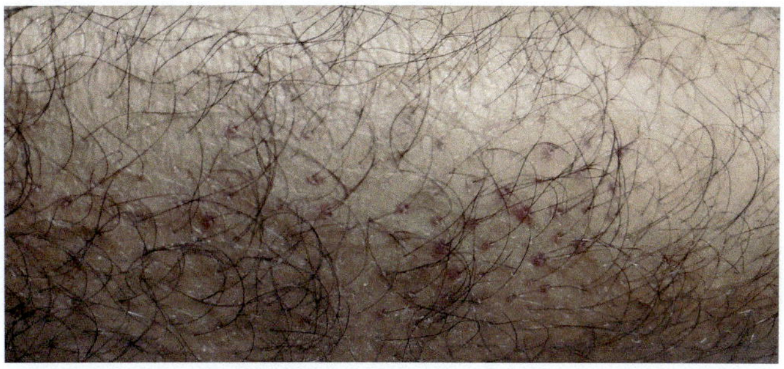

Figure 14.2 Perifollicular petechiae in scurvy. (Courtesy: Dr. Debayan Dasgupta, Berhampore, India.)

## Thrombotic thrombocytopenic purpura (TTP) and hemolytic-uremic syndrome (HUS)

- TTP occurs in adults and HUS in children.
- Purpura is associated with fever, hemolytic anemia and renal and neurological symptoms.
- Childhood HUS is distinguished clinically because it develops one week after diarrhea due to *E. coli* O157:H7.

## Scurvy

- Vitamin C deficiency causes collagen defect.
- Initial skin change is follicular keratosis, with coiled hairs (corkscrew hairs) on the upper arms, buttocks, and lower extremities.
- Later, there is perifollicular hemorrhage with blood pigment discoloration, mainly on the legs (**Figure 14.2**).
- Swollen bleeding gums (spongy bleeding gums), stomatitis, painful joints, and epistaxis occur.

## Actinic purpura

- Actinic purpura presents as purpuric macules on the forearms, hands, face, and neck. They resolve after one to three weeks and may leave residual brown pigmentation (**Figure 14.3a**).
- It occurs most commonly in skin altered by both age and solar radiation but may occur in premature aging syndromes.

## Corticosteroid purpura

- Purpura occurs mainly in the atrophic skin on exposed parts of the hands and forearms or on the legs after minor trauma or spontaneously. It is usually asymptomatic, and purpuras vary in size from a few millimeters to several centimeters, arranged linearly or in geometric shapes.
- The characteristic appearance has non-palpable irregular areas with very little inflammation, which are usually dark purple rather than having the sequential color changes of normal bruises and may persist for several weeks (**Figure 14.3b**).

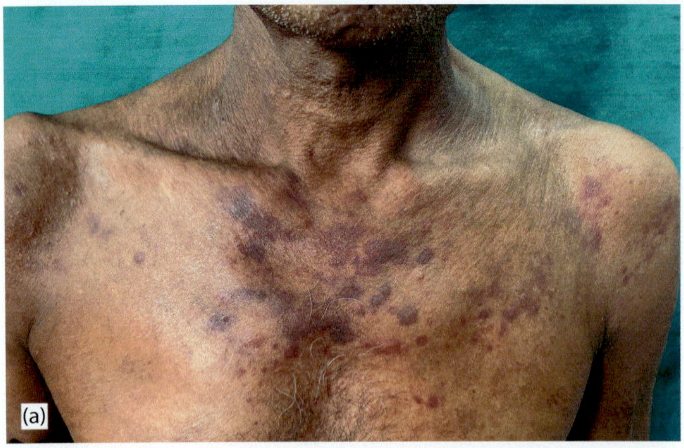

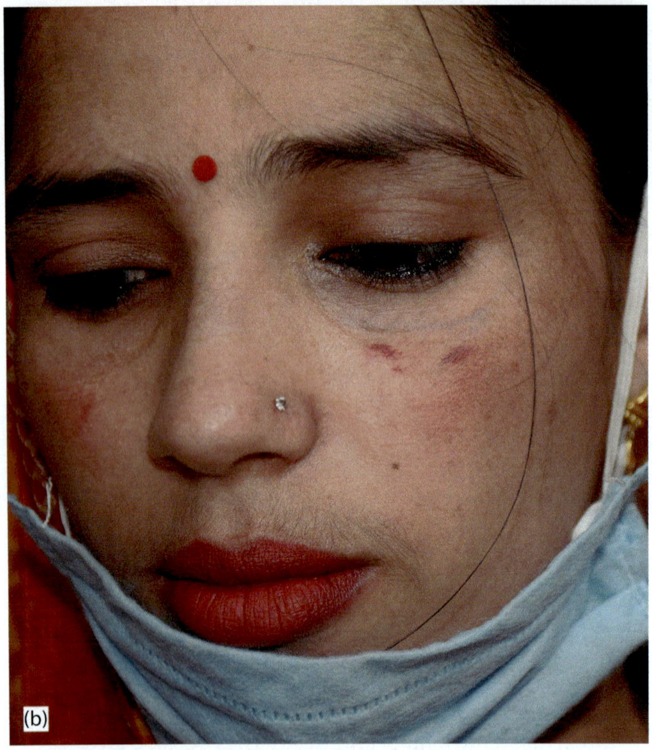

Figure 14.3 **(a)** Ecchymosis in sun-exposed area in a farmer. **(b)** Purpura on the face in a female with long term topical corticosteroid abuse. Note epidermal thinning. (a,b – Courtesy: Dr. Piyush Kumar, Katihar, India.)

## Primary systemic amyloidosis

- Petechiae, purpura, and ecchymoses may occur spontaneously or after normal trauma on normal or clinically involved skin, especially in the body folds (e.g., the eyelids, sides of neck, axillae, umbilicus, oral and anogenital regions). Eyelid purpura after pinching, and periorbital purpura after proctoscopy, coughing, vomiting, or the Valsalva maneuver are characteristic (**Figure 14.4a,b**).
- Purpuric halos may appear around cherry angiomas.

## Hypergammaglobulinemic purpura of Waldenstrom

- Clinically the pattern of purpura is often non-specific, usually consisting of crops of small erythematous macules or palpable purpuric spots on the lower leg, but unusual patterns with reticulate lesions may appear, with itching and burning sensations.
- Prolonged walking, standing, or sitting with legs in dependent positions are obvious provocative factors.

## Valsalva-associated petechiae

- This is the mechanical cause of petechiae.
- Raised pressure leads to a cervico-facial arrangement of purpuric lesions (**Figure 14.4c,d**).

## Coagulation-factor deficiency

- This could be a congenital or acquired deficiency.
- Most commonly encountered are coagulation factor VIII deficiency, coagulation factor IX deficiency, and von Willebrand disease (**Figure 14.5a,b**).
- Onset occurs in neonates and infants.

## Pigmented purpuric dermatoses

- Schamberg's disease
  - This involves a few or many lesions, occurring most frequently on legs, but it may occur anywhere on the body, including the palms.
  - They consist of irregular plaques of orange or brown pigmentation due to hemosiderin, with characteristic "cayenne pepper" spots appearing within and at the edge of old lesions (**Figure 14.6a**).
  - They are usually asymptomatic but may be slightly itchy.
  - Eruption is usually chronic and persists for many years, with slow extension and some clearing of original lesions.
  - DD: Itching purpura.
- Itching Purpura
  - Purpuric lesions usually commence around the ankles and in a few weeks spread to involve the whole legs, sometimes the lower part of the body, and even elsewhere.
  - They are more pronounced at sites of friction with clothing. The lesions consist of erythematous and purpuric macules that may become confluent and often have a characteristic orange color.
  - DD: Carbromal sensitivity, rubber or clothing dermatitis.
- Pigmented purpuric lichenoid dermatosis of Gougerot-Blum
  - The characteristic clinical feature of the dermatosis is the presence of lichenoid papules in association with purpuric lesions similar to those of Schamberg's disease,

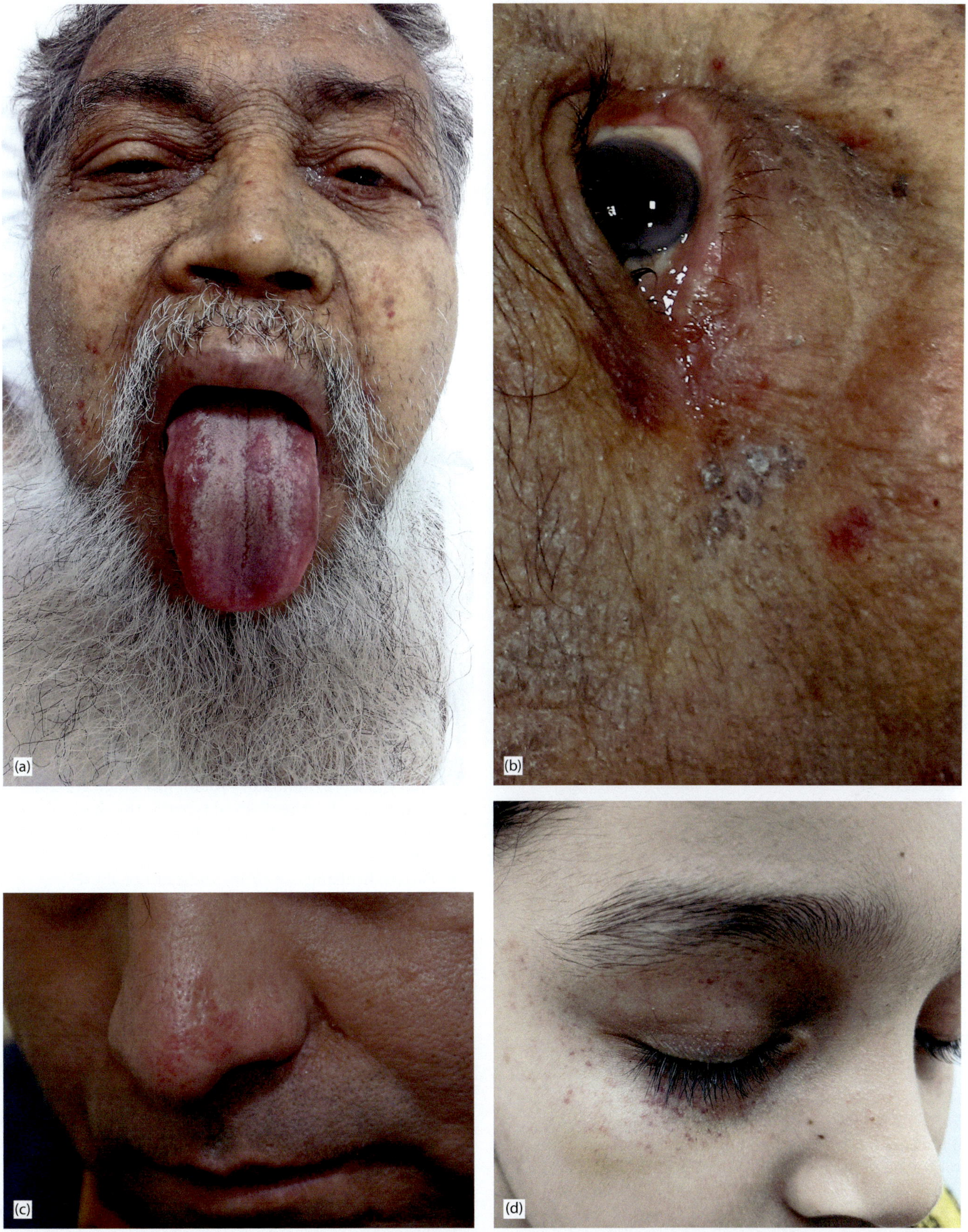


Figure 14.4 **(a)** Primary systemic amyloidosis with facial purpura and macroglossia. **(b)** Periorbital purpura. **(c)** Petechiae over the nose due to Valsalva procedure. **(d)** Periocular petechiae associated with severe coughing. (a,b – Courtesy: Dr. Tanumay Raychaudhury, Skin and Cancer Foundation, The University of Sydney, Australia; c – Courtesy: Dr. Piyush Kumar, Katihar, India; d – Courtesy: Dr Srinivas Devarashetty, Nizamabad, India.)

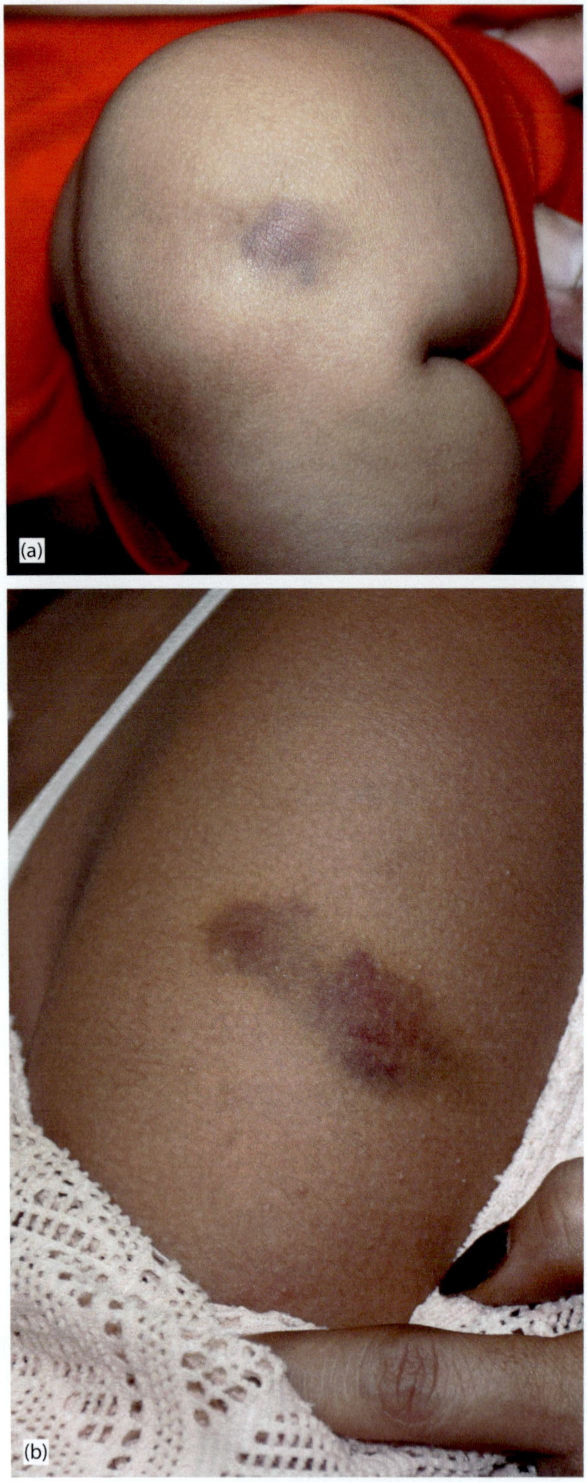


Figure 14.5 **(a)** Purpura in a child with hemophilia. **(b)** Purpura in a girl child with hemophilia. (a,b – Courtesy: Dr. Piyush Kumar, Katihar, India.)

- Lichen aureus
    - This involves a more localized, more intensely purpuric but often asymptomatic eruption that may have rather lichenoid morphology.
    - The lesions are often solitary and may be yellowish, golden, rust-colored or purple (**Figure 14.6b**).
    - They may resemble a bruise, and hence must be distinguished from non-accidental injury in children, but may persist for a few years.
- Purpura annularis telangiectodes
    - Clinical features are distinctive and described in its name. Lesions occur at any site, often in the absence of venous stasis, and may be few in number or very numerous. They consist of small plaques 1–3 cm across that are usually annular from their onset (**Figure 14.6c**).
    - Lesions consist of telangiectases and hemosiderin staining of the skin. They may be purple, yellow, or brown, and may contain "cayenne pepper" spots. Individual lesions persist unchanged for many months or years, or there may be slow centrifugal extension with development of slight central atrophy.

## Battered baby syndrome

- Up to 90% of victims of physical abuse present with skin findings. Although bruising is the most common physical sign of abuse, it is also a frequent finding in any active child. Accidental bruising most commonly occurs over the knees and anterior tibial area.
- Bruising over relatively protected sites such as the upper arms, medial and posterior thighs, hands, trunk, cheeks, ears, neck, genitalia, and buttocks should raise suspicion of abuse, especially if the bruises are extensive and of varying age. Bruising of the genitalia and ears is highly suspicious for abuse.
- Bruises are extremely rare in babies less than six months of age, as they are not yet mobile. Any single soft-tissue injury in a preambulatory infant has a high correlation with abuse. Another helpful factor is the shape of the bruise, which can reflect the shape of the object used to inflict it.
- Pattern bruising is a strong indicator of abuse.

## Vitamin K deficiency

- Vitamin K deficiency bleeding (VKDB) disorder is an uncommon entity that occurs due to inadequate activity of vitamin K-dependent coagulation factors.
- Clinical presentation of late VKDB ranges from life-threatening intracranial hemorrhage to skin bleeds with nodular purpura.
- Though skin bleeding in the form of petechiae, purpura, or ecchymoses may occur in 10–30% of patients, it is a presenting feature in only half of such infants.
- It occurs on the lower extremities, back, chest abdomen, buttocks, upper extremities face, and neck in descending order of frequency.
- These lesions are bluish-violet in color with raised infiltrated purplish centers, and their diameter may vary from 1.5 cm to 7.5 cm. Hematomas may occur at skin puncture sites.

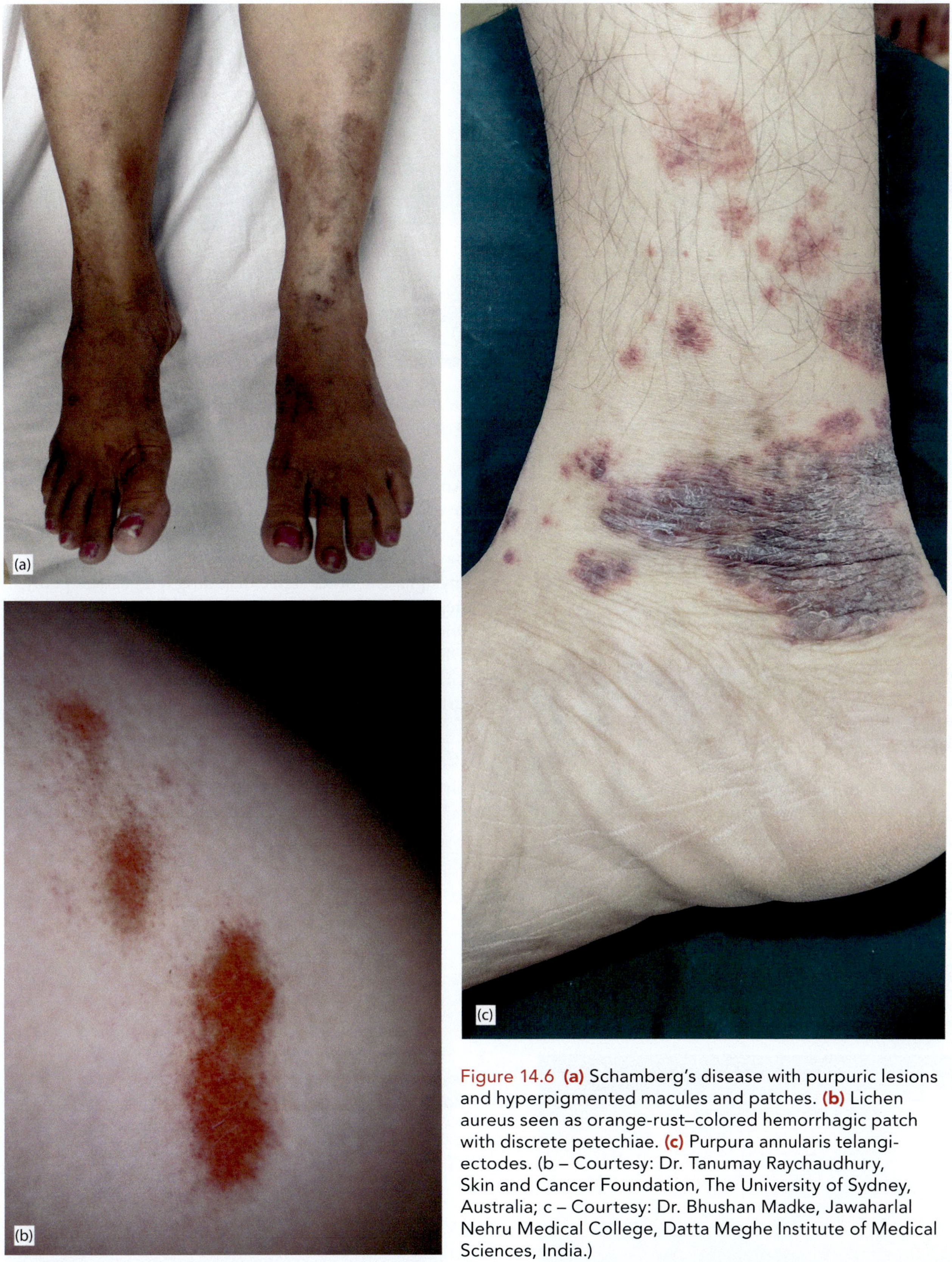


Figure 14.6 **(a)** Schamberg's disease with purpuric lesions and hyperpigmented macules and patches. **(b)** Lichen aureus seen as orange-rust–colored hemorrhagic patch with discrete petechiae. **(c)** Purpura annularis telangiectodes. (b – Courtesy: Dr. Tanumay Raychaudhury, Skin and Cancer Foundation, The University of Sydney, Australia; c – Courtesy: Dr. Bhushan Madke, Jawaharlal Nehru Medical College, Datta Meghe Institute of Medical Sciences, India.)

## PALPABLE PURPURA

### Cutaneous small vessel vasculitis (CSVV)

- CSVV typically presents with palpable purpura ranging in size from 1 mm to several centimeters. It is sometimes macular in early stages but may progress to a wide array of lesions, including urticarial papules, pustules, vesicles, petechiae, or targetoid lesions (**Figure 14.7**).
- The lesions favor dependent sites as well as areas under tight-fitting clothing, reflecting the influence of hydrostatic pressure and stasis on the pathophysiology.
- In general, the lesions are asymptomatic, but they may itch, burn, or sting.
- In differential diagnosis, vasculitis with systemic manifestations must be ruled out.

### Henoch-Schönlein purpura

- At its outset this manifests with the classic findings of purpura, arthralgia, and abdominal pain.
- The cutaneous findings are typically erythematous urticarial papules, which evolve within 24 hours into palpable purpura with hemorrhage. Furthermore, urticaria, vesicles, bullae, and necrotic ulcers may develop.
- Typically involving extensor aspects of the limbs and buttocks in symmetrical fashion, HSP may also affect the trunk and face. It usually fades within five to seven days; however, crops of lesions can recur from a few weeks to several months (**Figure 14.8**).
- DD: Cutaneous small-vessel vasculitis, Wegener's granulomatosis, Churg-Strauss syndrome, microscopic polyangiitis, and other vasculitides.

### Urticarial vasculitis

- Individual lesions (hives) persist for more than 24 hours, often demonstrate purpuric foci, leave post-inflammatory hyperpigmentation, and cause symptoms of burning.

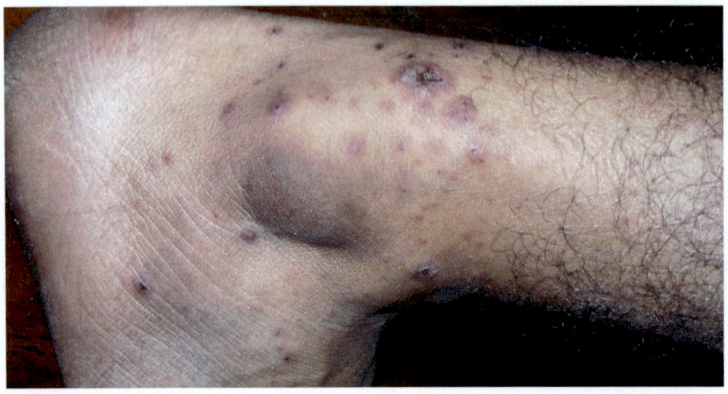

Figure 14.7 Palpable purpura in cutaneous small vessel vasculitis. (Courtesy: Dr. Piyush Kumar, Katihar, India.)

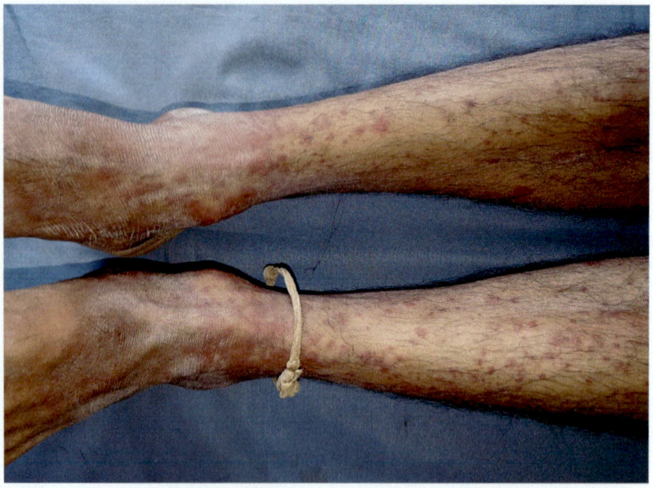

Figure 14.8 Purpuric lesions on the lower limbs in Henoch-Schönlein purpura.

- Angioedema and macular erythema may also occur; livedo reticularis, nodules, and bullae may be evident.
- Patients with the hypocomplemententemic form may have constitutional symptoms such as fever, malaise, myalgia, and other signs, including lymphadenopathy, hepatosplenomegaly, and abdominal pain with or without nausea and or diarrhea.
- DD: Presence of ocular inflammation, angioedema and COPD distinguish it from SLE. Other differentials include urticaria and atypical forms of erythema multiforme.

### ANCA-associated vasculitis

- Granulomatosis with polyangiitis (GPA)
  - The most common cutaneous manifestation of GPA is palpable purpura.
  - Others include tender subcutaneous nodules, papules, vesicles, and petechiae as well as pyoderma gangrenosum-like lesions.
  - Papulonecrotic lesions appear most commonly on the limbs but also occur on the face and scalp.
  - Oral ulcers and "strawberry" gingival hyperplasia are pathognomonic.
  - Saddle nose deformity may result from necrotizing granulomas of the nasal mucosa.
  - DD: Churg-Strauss syndrome.
- Eosinophilic granulomatosis with polyangiitis
  - The first phase, which may continue for years, consists of allergic rhinitis, nasal polyps, asthma, and peripheral blood eosinophilia.
  - The second phase is vasculitis.
  - Palpable purpura and infiltrated nodules (typically located on the scalp or limbs) are the most common skin manifestations.
  - Livedo reticularis, migratory erythema, new onset Raynaud's phenomenon, aseptic pustules or vesicles, and infiltrated papules may also be present.
  - DD: Granulomatosis with polyangiitis (GPA).

### Papular-purpuric "gloves-and-socks" syndrome

- It is considered a reaction pattern to various viral infections and, possibly, bacterial infection and drugs.
- The most established cause is parvovirus B19 infection. Other documented causes include Coxsackie B virus, measles virus, human herpesvirus 6, and drugs (co-trimoxazole).
- Cutaneous lesions start with edema and erythema on the hands and feet in a "gloves-and-socks'" distribution. This is followed by development of painful and/or pruritic, erythematous papular and purpuric lesions in the same distribution. A clinical clue is sharp demarcation of the rash at the wrists and ankles. Rarely, the lesions may progress to vesicles and bullae and ulceration.
- Sometimes other sites, such as the face, trunk, and thighs, may be affected.
- Systemic findings include fever, asthenia, headache, anorexia, and arthralgia.
- Mucosal findings are as follows:
  - Oral mucosa – pharyngeal erythema, erosions, petechiae, and vesiculopustular lesions on the hard and soft palates
  - Genital mucosa – painful edema and erythema
- The condition resolves in a few weeks.

## RETIFORM PURPURA

### Polyarteritis nodosa

- Dermal or subcutaneous nodules are most commonly located on the lower legs near the ankles and may extend proximally to the thighs, buttocks, arms, or hands. These nodules may be tender, which may ulcerate, or more commonly demonstrate livedo reticularis, which may be necrotizing (**Figure 14.9**).

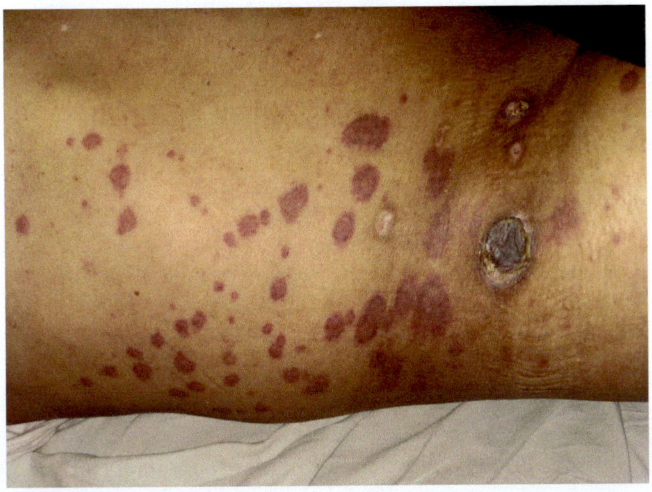

Figure 14.9 Purpuric lesions in polyarteritis nodosa. Note two ulcerated lesions.

- Digital gangrene can ultimately occur.
- In cutaneous polyarteritis nodosa the disease is limited to skin for long periods of time; nodules and ulcers occur, usually on the legs.
- DD: Antiphospholipid antibody syndrome, cholesterol emboli or other factors that can produce non-vasculitic vessel occlusion.

### Purpura fulminans with DIC (septic vasculitis)

- This is usually sepsis-related and presents with disseminated intravascular coagulation (DIC).
- There is widespread cutaneous hemorrhage with sepsis.
- It clinically presents as non-inflammatory (bland) hemorrhage, usually with retiform, stellate or branching configuration, with rapid transition to necrosis and eschar formation (**Figure 14.10a**).
- When patients are on vasopressors, there is an additional component of peripheral gangrene.
- It often affects distal extremities.

### Post-infectious purpura fulminans (PF)

- This is a rapidly progressive disorder.
- It occurs most commonly in the setting of acute severe bacterial or viral infection and as a post infectious syndrome after infections such as primary varicella and scarlet fever.
- It usually occurs seven to ten days after the onset of symptoms of an acute infection.
- Post-infectious PF tends to occur on the lower body, especially thighs, lower legs, and buttocks, and phenomenon such as large-vessel venous thrombosis and systemic microvascular thrombosis and multi-organ failure are uncommon (**Figure 14.10b**).
- Post-infectious PF should be considered strongly if purpura fulminans with extensive necrotic skin lesions with or without DIC develop following nonspecific infection in an otherwise healthy child.

### Lucio phenomenon (LPh)

- It is characterized by the occurrence of painful, red or purpuric macules, of irregular shape, angulated or "stellar," in a patient with diffuse lepromatous leprosy (Lucio-*Latapí* leprosy).
- Lucio phenomenon in lepromatous leprosy or type 2 leprosy reaction is clinically characterized by crops of sharply delineated, purple-red lesions of irregular shape, angulated or "stellar" on the extremities. Lesions are accompanied by a burning sensation and indurations that evolve into necrotic-hemorrhagic lesions.
- Lesions appear on the lower extremities and then spread to the trunk and upper extremities. Patients may present with fever, myalgia, or arthralgia.

### Periumbilical thumbprint parasitic purpura (PTPP)

- It is cutaneous sign of strongyloidiasis seen in the more advanced stages of Strongyloides infection and represents a poor prognostic sign for the patient.

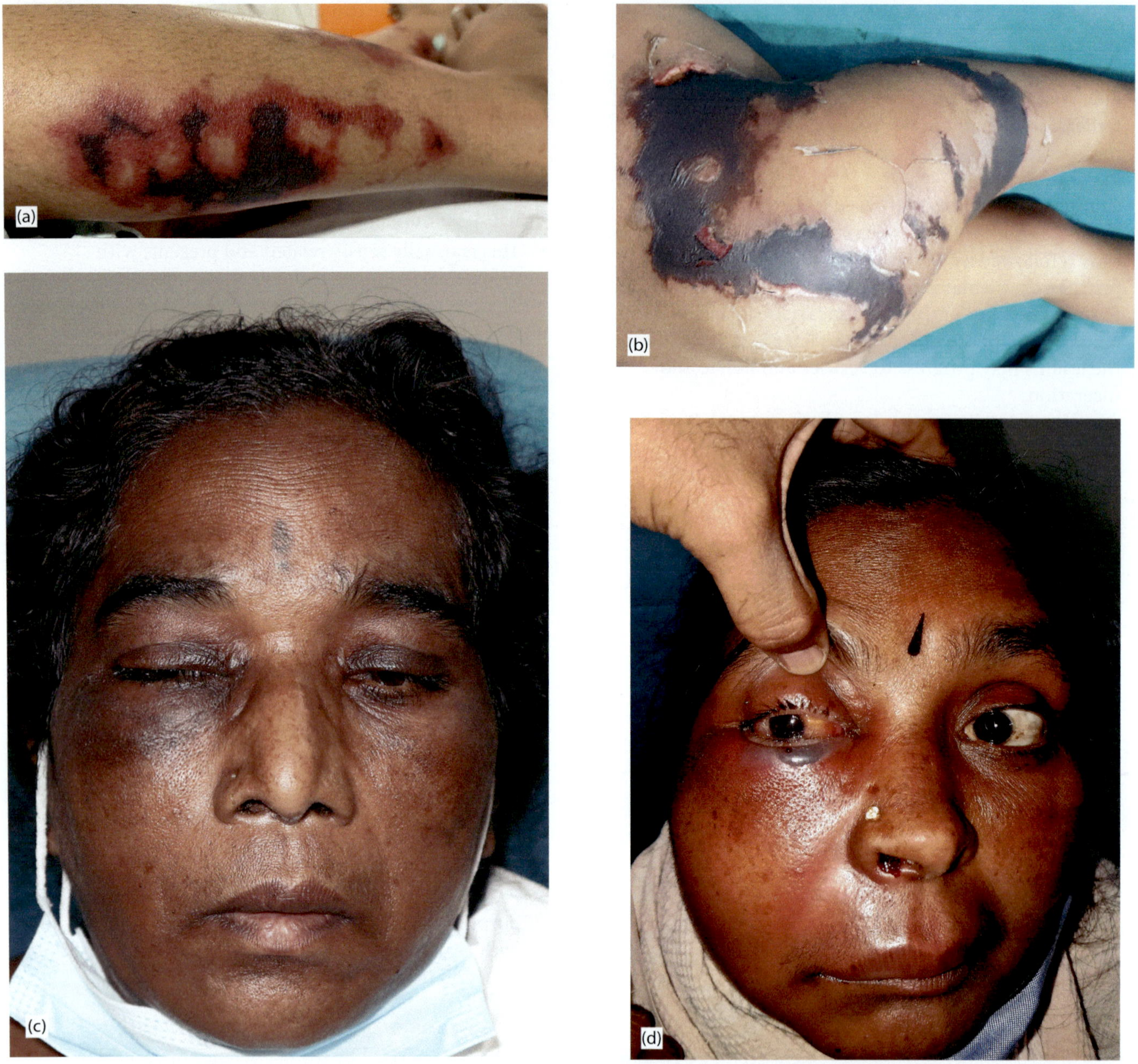


Figure 14.10 **(a)** Stellate purpura in purpura fulminans. **(b)** Purpura and epidermal necrosis in post infectious purpura fulminans. **(c)** Mucormycosis causing periorbital edema with hemorrhagic surface. **(d)** Hemorrhagic bulla in mucormycosis. (a – Courtesy: Dr. Anuradha Priyadarshini, Sri Ramachandra Medical College, Chennai, India; b – Courtesy: Dr. Rajeev Ranjan and Dr. Shalini Sinha, Ara, India; c,d – Courtesy: Dr. Raghuraj Hegde, Kempegowda Institute of Medical Sciences, Bangalore, India.)

- It usually presents as periumbilical purpura that spreads centrifugally throughout the abdomen and groin.
- The purpura is caused by the dermal migration of filariform larvae through vessel walls or the large bowel wall.
- It has been proposed that the periumbilical distribution may result from retrograde venous migration. Additionally, larvae may penetrate into the skin from the abdominal cavity, following migration through the large-bowel wall.

### Angioinvasive fungal infections

- These are acute, rapidly evolving, often fatal infections due to vasculotropic invasive mycoses, such as *Aspergillus* (*flavus, fumigatus, niger*), *Fusarium* (*solani, oxysporum, verticillioides*), and *Zygomycetes* (*Mucor, Rhizopus, Rhizomucor*, and more) (**Figure 14.10c,d**).
- Lesions typically present as tender, rapidly enlarging, bright-red to purple papulonodules that rapidly develop areas of ischemic necrosis, ulcers, and/or hemorrhagic bullae, which may be accompanied by purpura, erythema, warmth, and induration.

### Warfarin necrosis

- Warfarin necrosis typically affects areas of the body with greater adipose tissue, including the breasts, thighs, and buttocks.

### Heparin skin necrosis

- Heparin skin necrosis shows a predilection for sites of subcutaneous heparin or low-molecular-weight heparin (LMWH) injections; if patients are on intravenous (IV) infusions, sites distal to the IV site are more commonly involved.
- It commonly induces cutaneous findings of simple hemorrhage with ecchymoses and occasionally triggers urticaria or infiltrated plaques.
- Purpuric, tender, sharply demarcated plaques develop; retiform extensions that sometimes develop at the lesional margins are characteristic of heparin necrosis.

### Cryoglobulinemia

- Cryoglobulinemia, especially type I, involves colder areas of the body, such as the distal digits and ears.
- Recurrent showers of dependent palpable purpura, sometimes with burning or itching and frequently associated with arthritis or arthralgia, is the classic presentation of mixed (type II and type III) cryoglobulinemia.
- The combination of purpura, asthenia, and arthralgia is termed Meltzer's triad.
- Ulceration, hemorrhagic crusting, or cutaneous infarction is seen in 10–25% of cases.
- Acrocyanosis, Raynaud's phenomenon, urticarial lesions, ulceration, and livedo-reticularis may be present.

### Calciphylaxis

- Calciphylaxis, also known as calcific uremic arteriolopathy, may also produce an occlusion within the vessels, although the most characteristic finding consists of calcification of the media of muscular small- and medium-sized arteries.
- It typically starts as livedo reticularis and progresses to intensely painful, indurated, symmetrical reticulated violaceous plaques with necrosis, usually affecting acral sites as well as fat-rich body areas.

### Cholesterol emboli

- Livedo reticularis of the lower extremities and buttocks is the most common cutaneous manifestation, although the trunk and upper extremities may also be involved.
- The livedoid change may be more pronounced in the standing position and may be missed if only supine examination is performed.
- Cholesterol emboli also result in "blue toe syndrome" and dry gangrene of the digits (**Figure 14.11**).
- Less commonly, petechiae and purpura of the lower extremities are seen with this syndrome.

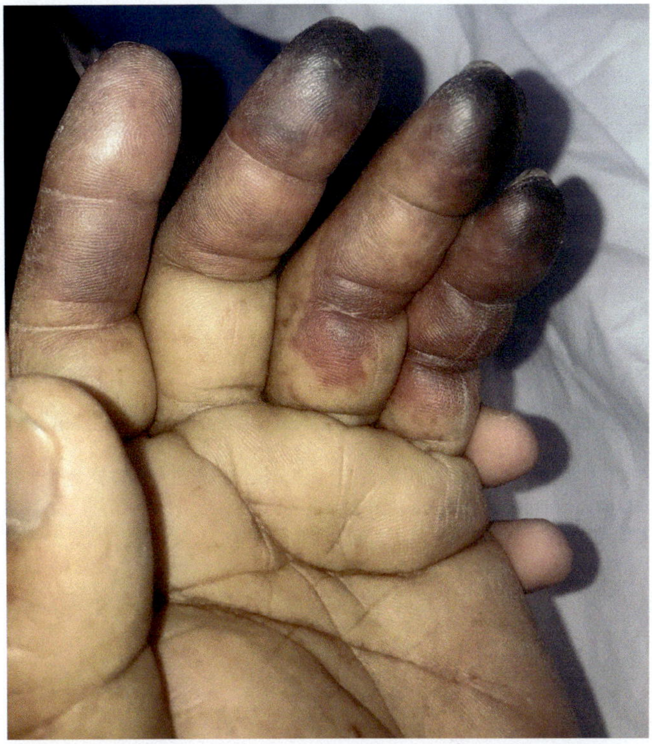

Figure 14.11 Acral purpuric lesions affecting the digits in cholesterol embolization. (Courtesy: Dr. Preema Sinha, Armed Forces Medical Sciences, Pune, India.)

### Anti-phospholipid syndrome (APLS)

- Clinically, APLS presents with a variety of cutaneous findings; retiform purpura, anetoderma, and atrophic blanche are seen, with widespread cutaneous necrosis and multiorgan failure, especially renal and pulmonary.
- APS is characterized by typical clinical manifestations (livedo reticularis, livedo racemosa, livedo vasculitis, thromboembolic phenomena with necrosis and ulceration of the extremities, digital gangrene, purpura, and purpura fulminans) and persistent aPL positivity (at least 12 weeks apart).
- Additionally, Behçet-like lesions, nail-fold ulcers, leg ulcers, cholesterol emboli-like proximal livedo-reticularis with or without distal retiform purpura, acral livedo, degos-like lesions, pyoderma gangrenosum-like lesions, and splinter hemorrhages may be present.

### Livedoid vasculopathy

- It initially manifests as erythematosus or purpuric plaques or papules that are painful and/or pruritic and are most commonly located bilaterally around the ankles (**Figure 14.12**).
- These lesions may ulcerate and then slowly heal over a period of three to four months, forming residual atrophic stellate white scars called atrophie blanche.

### Additional images – Figures 14.13 and 14.14

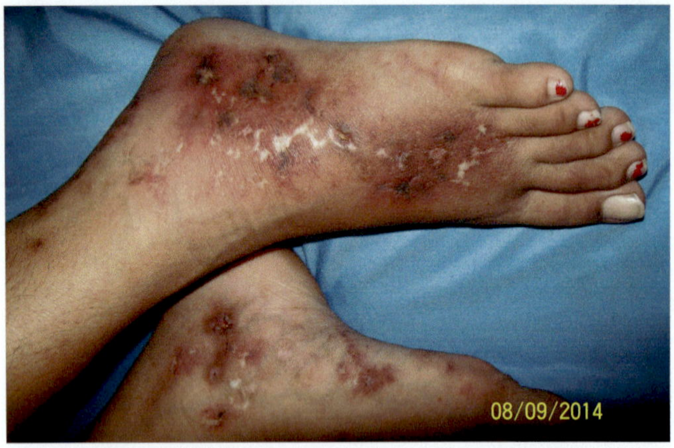


Figure 14.12 Purpuric lesions, ulcers, and atrophie blanche in livedoid vasculopathy.

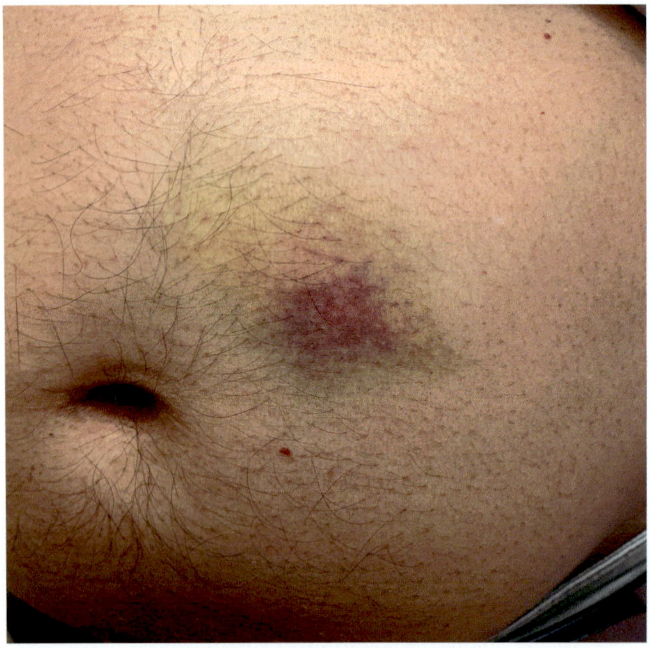

Figure 14.13 Traumatic purpura. Note color changes. (Courtesy: Dr. Piyush Kumar, Katihar, India.)

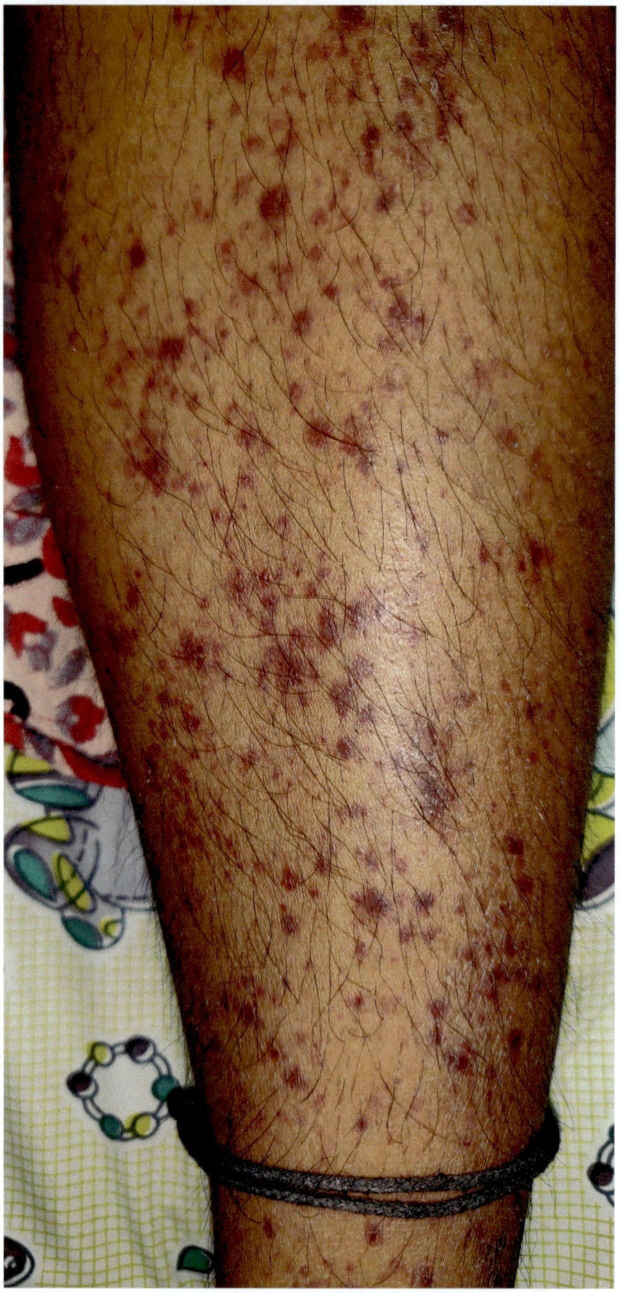

Figure 14.14 Rifampicin-induced thrombocytopenia presenting with purpuric lesions. (Courtesy: Dr. Soumyajit Roychoudhury, Berhampore, India.)

## REFERENCES


1. Arakaki R, Fox L. Updates in the approach to the patient with purpura. Curr Derm Rep 2017: 6;55–62.
2. Piette WW. Purpura: Mechanisms and Differential Diagnosis. In: Bolognia JL, Schaffer JV, Cerroni L, editors. Dermatology. 4th edition. North York: Elsevier Limited; 2018. p. 376–389.
3. Lamadrid-Zertuche AC, Garza-Rodríguez V, Ocampo-Candiani JJ. Pigmented purpura and cutaneous vascular occlusion syndromes. An Bras Dermatol 2018;93(3):397–404.
4. Leung AK, Chan KW. Evaluating the child with purpura. Am Fam Physician 2001;64(3):419–428.
5. Wysong A, Venkatesan P. An approach to the patient with retiform purpura. Dermatol Ther 2011;24(2):151–172.
6. Georgesen C, Fox LP, Harp J. Retiform purpura: A diagnostic approach. J Am Acad Dermatol 2020;82(4):783–796.

E16

# Erythema: Localized

APARAJITA GHOSH, PC DAS

## ABSTRACT

Erythema is an effect on the skin induced by enhanced blood flow. Different physiological and pathological conditions are responsible for the same. Based on the extent of skin involvement, erythema may be localized or generalized, and at the same time it may be a primary event or a coincidental condition. The differentials depend on the pattern and localization of erythema, age of presentation, preceding events, and associated skin lesions.

The text of this chapter is available online at https://routledgetextbooks.com/textbooks/9781032399669/

DOI: 10.1201/9781351054225-32

E17

# Erythema: Generalized

SWETALINA PRADHAN, ARPITA NIBEDITA ROUT

## ABSTRACT

Erythema represents a blanchable red or pink color of skin or mucous membrane. It is caused due to dilation of arteries and veins in the papillary or reticular dermis. Based on the extent of skin involvement, erythema may be localized or generalized, and at the same time it may be a primary event or a condition with prominently associated features such as fever, rash, pustules, crusts, scales, epidermal detachment, and pruritus. This chapter discusses the clinical differentials of generalized erythema.

The text of this chapter is available online at https://routledgetextbooks.com/textbooks/9781032399669/



DOI: 10.1201/9781351054225-33

# E18

# Telangiectasia

SUNIL K KOTHIWALA, KANYA RANI VASHISHT

## ABSTRACT

Telangiectasias are visibly and persistently dilated blood vessels, coursing through the surface of the skin or mucous membrane. They may be localized or widespread in distribution. Telangiectasia in certain disorders may have a site predilection, such as involvement of the photo-exposed areas, upper or lower body half, bulbar conjunctiva, lips, oral mucosa, anterior chest, or proximal nail folds. Segmental and nevoid forms occur as well. Morphologically, localized telangiectasia can be either macular (and further linear, arborized, spider like, punctate, mat-like or diffusely erythematous) or papular. Their color depends on the vessel of origin (capillaries or venules). The presence or absence of atrophy aids in further classification. Etiologically, they may be primary or secondary. In addition, several genodermatoses present with telangiectasia or inherited poikiloderma. While telangiectasia may arise from a multitude of causes, their morphological features, distribution/site predilection, associated cutaneous features, and systemic features as derived from a careful history and examination help in reaching the correct diagnosis. This chapter reviews the possible causes to consider and diagnostic approach in a patient presenting with telangiectasia.

The text of this chapter is available online at https://routledgetextbooks.com/textbooks/9781032399669/

DOI: 10.1201/9781351054225-34

E19

# Cysts and pseudocysts

PC DAS

## ABSTRACT

Cysts may occur in any organ system of the body, and the symptomatology relates to the function subserved by the involved organ. Cutaneous cysts are common lesions that present to dermatologists for cosmetic reasons, mass effect, or secondary changes, such as discharge, inflammation, and infection. Cysts present as superficial or deep swelling morphologically mimicking a papule, nodule, or tumor.

The text of this chapter is available online at https://routledgetextbooks.com/textbooks/9781032399669/



DOI: 10.1201/9781351054225-35

15

# Draining sinuses and fistulas

SUNIL K KOTHIWALA, KANYA RANI VASHISHT

## INTRODUCTION

A sinus tract is an abnormal blind-ended tract that opens onto the skin or into a cavity. A fistula is an abnormal tract connecting the cavities of two internal organs or the cavity of an internal organ with the skin. As sinus and fistula cannot be easily differentiated from each other on cutaneous examination alone, this chapter clubs them together for the purpose of discussing clinical differentials. Etiologically, sinuses and fistulae may be congenital (developmental), traumatic, infective or non-infective. A broad approach considering morphological aspects is outlined in **Table 15.1** and **Figure 15.1**. The salient features of different entities are discussed below.[1–7]

## CONGENITAL OR DEVELOPMENTAL SINUS

Congenital head and neck swellings are usually present at birth but may manifest up to youth. These cystic swellings may be complicated into sinuses and fistulae. They may be facial or cervical in location, and the latter may be either medial or lateral cervical lesions (**Figure 15.2**). The exact position provides important clinical clues as some of the lesions are characteristically midline (e.g., dermoid cyst, dermal spinal tract). Any midline sinus or cystic lesion in a child should be approached with the understanding that deeper connections may be found. Congenital midline cysts should be imaged to exclude deep, especially intracranial connections.

### Dermoid cysts

- These present in an infant as non-tender subcutaneous nodules along an embryonic fusion plane around the eyes or nose. Those on the bridge of the nose often have a sinus tract and a tuft of hairs protruding out, with sebaceous discharge (pathognomonic). It may produce nasal widening with hypertelorism.
- Dermoid cysts can rarely present as sinus or fistula and may have an intracranial extension passing through the foramen cecum, giving rise to meningeal signs and symptoms. Imaging studies are thus advised prior to excision to exclude an intracranial connection.
- DD: Epidermoid cysts are not present at birth; they may occur elsewhere and are not characteristically midline. Nasal gliomas may present as nasal masses.

### Preauricular cysts and pits

- Imperfect fusion of tubercles leads to entrapment of epithelium to form preauricular cysts which connect to the skin via preauricular sinuses.
- Presentations:
    - These usually present as a unilateral asymptomatic cystic nodule or invagination in the preauricular area (just in front of the ascending limb of the helix).
    - Acute infection presents as tenderness and purulent discharge.
    - Chronic infection may result in granulomatous nodule over the opening of sinus.
- DD: First branchial arch sinus, granulomatous nodule may be confused with lupus vulgaris.

### Thyroglossal duct cyst

- During development, the thyroid gland descends from the floor of the pharynx to the anterior neck, forming a tract called thyroglossal duct. Remnants of this duct take the form of fistulae, cysts, or solid masses of ectopic thyroid tissue.
- This is the most common cause of midline swelling of neck in children/young adults.
- It may be located anywhere from the suprasternal notch to the foramen cecum of the dorsal tongue. Hence it may be located either above or below the hyoid. A tract connecting it to the hyoid bone results in characteristic upward movement on swallowing or tongue protrusion.
- Fistulae may form following infection or procedure for the cyst. Intraoral opening may result in unpleasant taste.
- Preoperative neck ultrasonography is the diagnostic tool, whereas postoperative histopathology of the excised cyst and fistula is mandatory to exclude rare occurrence of malignancy.
- DD: Branchial cleft cyst.

DOI: 10.1201/9781351054225-36

Table 15.1 Site predilection of various developmental and acquired sinuses and fistulae

| Onset | Site | Disease | Comment |
|---|---|---|---|
| **Congenital/ Developmental** | Head and neck | Dermoid cyst | Along embryonic closure lines of the head and neck<br>Common sites: around lateral third of the eyebrows, bridge of nose |
| | Face | Preauricular cyst or pit | Small area anterior to the ear |
| | | Lip pit | On lower lip on one or either side of midline |
| | Neck | Thyroglossal cyst | Anterior neck, in close proximity to the hyoid bone |
| | | Branchial cyst or sinus | Along anterior border of sternocleidomastoid, mandibular region (over parotid gland) |
| | | Bronchogenic cyst | Suprasternal notch, pre-sternal area, lower anteromedial aspect of neck |
| ***Acquired*** | Face | Dental sinus | Along mandibular jaw line or submandibular region |
| | | Scrofuloderma | Commonly on the neck or submandibular region |
| | | Actinomycosis | Mandibular region; less commonly chest wall or iliac fossa |
| | | Pyoderma faciale | Cheeks, chin, and/or forehead |
| | | Oral squamous cell carcinoma | Lateral and undersurface of tongue, floor of mouth are common sites |
| | Thorax | Actinomycosis | |
| | Axilla and/or groin | Hidradenitis suppurativa | Axillae (preferential location in women) and perineum (preferential location in men) |
| | | Scrofuloderma | |
| | Inguinal region | Lymphogranuloma venereum | Inguinal region |
| | | Enterocutaneous fistula | Iliac fossa |
| | | Actinomycosis | |
| | Extremities | Milker's sinus | 2nd or 3rd webspace of dominant (usually right) hand |
| | | Botryomycosis | Limbs, perianal area |
| | | Antitrypsin-deficiency panniculitis | Proximal extremities and lower trunk |
| | | Pancreatic panniculitis | Legs |
| | | Mycetoma | Foot |
| | Perianal area | Pilonidal sinus | In or just above the gluteal cleft |
| | | Cutaneous amoebiasis | Perianal region, buttocks |
| | | Malakoplakia of the skin | Perianal and genital area |
| | | Crohn's disease | Genital or perianal area (metastatic cutaneous Crohn's disease); parastomal (non-metastatic cutaneous Crohn's disease) |
| | Variable | Wound myiasis | Pre-existing non-healing wound |
| | | Chronic osteomyelitis | Vertebral bodies, long bones (tibia and femur), foot (in vascular insufficiency/ neuropathy) |
| | | Atypical mycobacterial | Nodules and sinuses, surgical sites infection or follows trauma |
| | | Cutaneous metastasis | |
| | | Others | Trauma, radiotherapy |

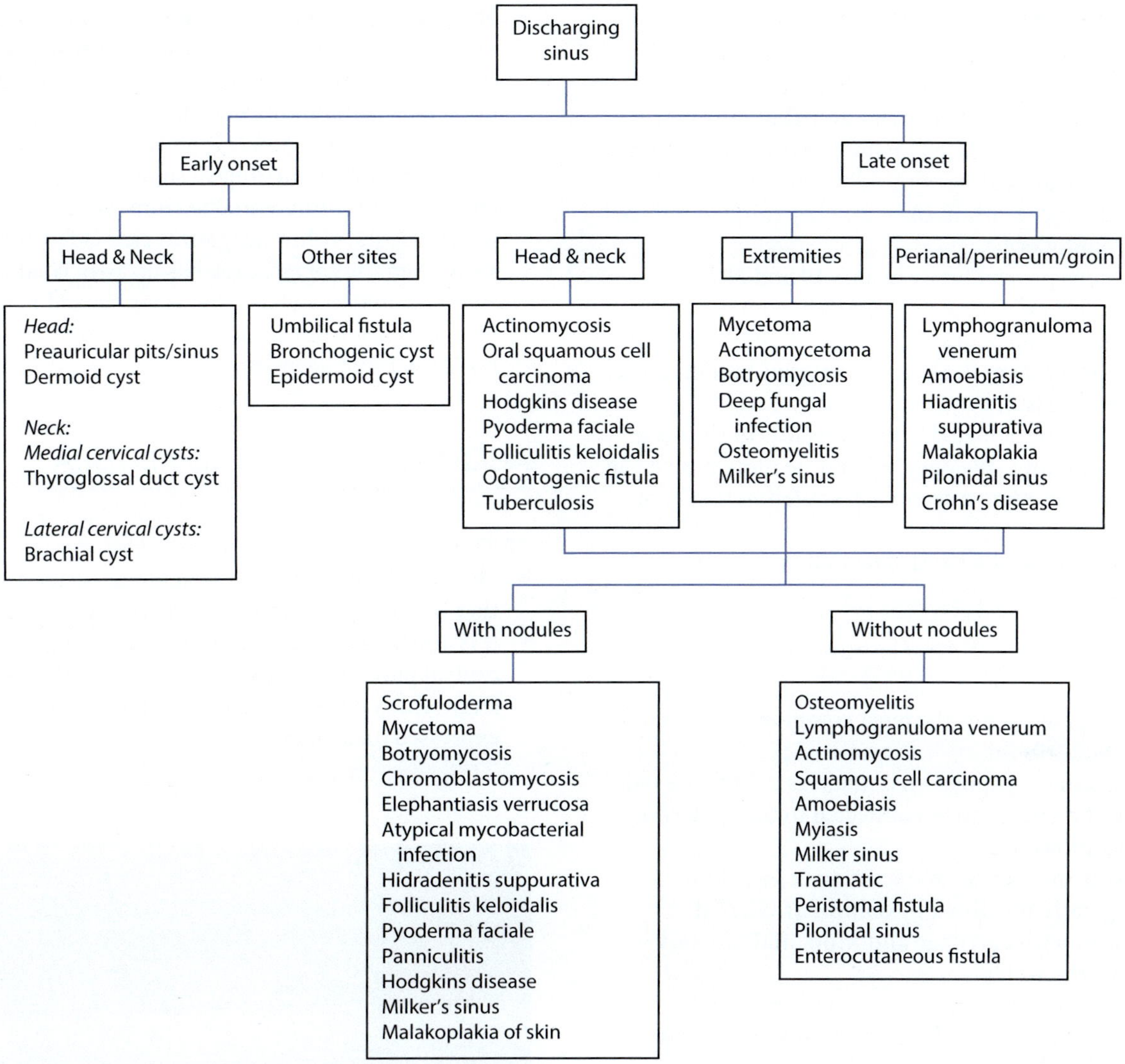


Figure 15.1 Approach to a case of discharging sinus or fistula.

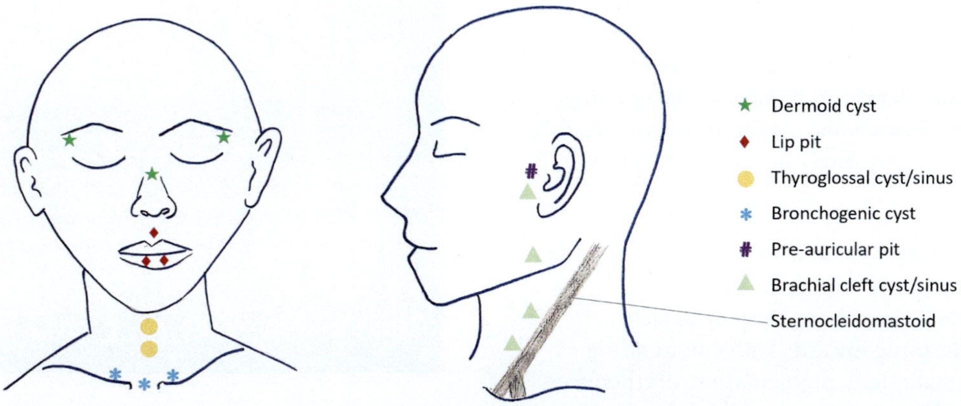


Figure 15.2 Common sites of developmental cysts, sinuses, and fistulae of the head and neck.

### Branchial cleft cyst (lateral cervical cyst)

- Incomplete fusion of branchial arches and their remnant cleft or pouches results in cysts, sinuses, or fistulae. Second branchial arch anomalies are often implicated. Branchial cleft anomalies result in sinus and fistulae communicating with skin (ectoderm), while branchial pouches result in channel opening to internal mucosa (endoderm).
- These lesions present between ages 10 and 30 years, in the preauricular area, mandibular region (over the parotid gland and below the angle of mandible), or the lower third of the neck along the anterior border of the sternocleidomastoid.
- The tract can be palpated, going upwards in the neck from the opening. The opening may be more noticeable because of secretion, infection, granulation tissue, or skin tag.
- DD: Thyroglossal duct cyst, dermoid cyst, cystic hygroma.

### Bronchogenic cysts (subcutaneous bronchogenic cysts)

- A bronchogenic cyst is the most common cystic lesion of the mediastinum.
- It presents in the suprasternal notch as a solitary cystic swelling at birth, at times connected to the epidermis with a fistulous tract.
- The cyst is unilocular and contains clear fluid. Histologically it is lined by columnar ciliated epithelium with cartilage and bronchial mucous glands in the walls.
- The only reported symptoms are swelling and discharge from the sinus. Potential complications are infection and malignant changes.
- DD: Branchial cyst, thyroglossal cyst.

### Umbilical fistula

- Failure of obliteration of the omphalomesenteric duct (vitelline) or urachus (allantois) leads to formation of sinuses, fistulae, cysts or polypoid tumors.
- Urine may be observed at the opening due to a patent urachus duct, while fecal discharge is the result of persistent vitelline duct.
- Intermittent bleeding or mucoid discharge may be present due to development of polyp at the opening.
- An ilio-umbilical fistula may result from laparotomy for Crohn's disease or may rarely occur spontaneously.

### Dermal sinus tract (dermal spinal tract)

- It presents as a congenital midline opening along the spine, most commonly lumbosacral.
- It is usually located just above the gluteal cleft, with the tract heading inwards with surrounding cutaneous stigmata (hair, pigmentation, erythema or inflammation, skin tag, or lipoma). Inability to see the base of the tract by gently separating the skin on either side is another red flag.
- The suspicion of a dermal sinus tract calls for pediatric referral and further imaging. This is because of a possible intradural connection and further chances of infection. Such infants may present with unexplained neurological signs (lower limb weakness, altered bowel/bladder function, meningeal signs).
- DD: It must be differentiated from "coccygeal dimple," which occurs within the gluteal cleft (a few millimeters away from the coccyx top), has no associated cutaneous stigmata, and has a base that is visible and pointed inferiorly towards the coccyx. It is benign and requires no further management.

## ACQUIRED SINUS AND FISTULA

### Epidermoid cyst (infundibular cyst)

- This usually presents as a firm, dome-shaped swelling that is movable over the deeper structures.
- It is attached to the epidermis, and there may be a central punctum (**Figure 15.3**) representing the follicle from which it is derived and from which keratin may be expressed on squeezing.

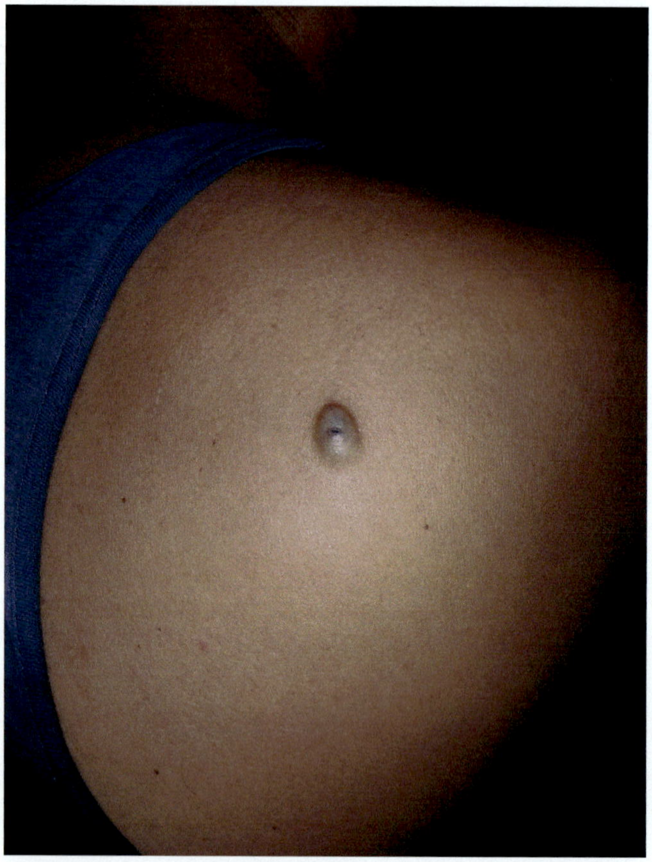

Figure 15.3 Epidermoid cyst with central punctum. Central punctum may be mistaken for a sinus. (Courtesy: Dr. Piyush Kumar, Katihar, India.)

- It may be primary or secondary to traumatically implanted epithelium (thus called "inclusion cyst.")

## Mammary duct fistula

- This typically occurs in a young adult woman who has a history of recurrent abscesses in a breast that has been treated by surgical drainage or has discharged spontaneously.
- There is typically partial inversion of the nipple and a scar or scars at the edge of the areola.

## Milker's sinus

- This is an uncommon foreign body reaction resulting from deep penetration of fragments of cow hair.
- Most lesions involve the second or third web of the right hand, forming tender nodules and discharging sinuses.
- The possible disease courses include disability due to tendon sheath involvement, secondary infections like recurrent cellulitis, or spontaneous cure.

## Dental sinus or fistula (odontogenic fistula)

- It is caused by chronic periapical infection, leading to abnormal tooth canalization, and a periapical abscess that drains externally through the skin.
- It usually consists of one of the mandibular teeth (as maxillary apical abscesses drain internally).
- There is a history of tooth pain. Clinically, either an inflamed abscess or in later stages sprouting granulation tissue around a sinus tract opening may be found along the jaw line or submandibular region (**Figure 15.4a–c**). Palpation may help to course along the sinus tract.
- Dental examination and appropriate radiological evaluation aid in diagnosis.

## Chronic osteomyelitis

- Long-persisting infection of the bone usually follows inadequately treated acute osteomyelitis.
- The most common presentation is persistent discharging of the sinus, with sprouting granulation tissue at its opening (**Figure 15.5**). The sinus tract is adherent to the underlying bone, and the discharge may contain bone chips or spicules. The bone is irregularly thickened, and adjacent joints may be stiff.
- DD: Septic arthritis, gout, sickle cell anemia, mycetoma.

## Scrofuloderma

- This is the most common form of cutaneous tuberculosis seen in children.
- It represents direct extension to the overlying skin from underlying tubercular focus such as lymph node, bone, joint, lacrimal gland, or duct.
- Usually it starts as a bluish-red nodule overlying focus and breaks down to form ulcerations with undermined

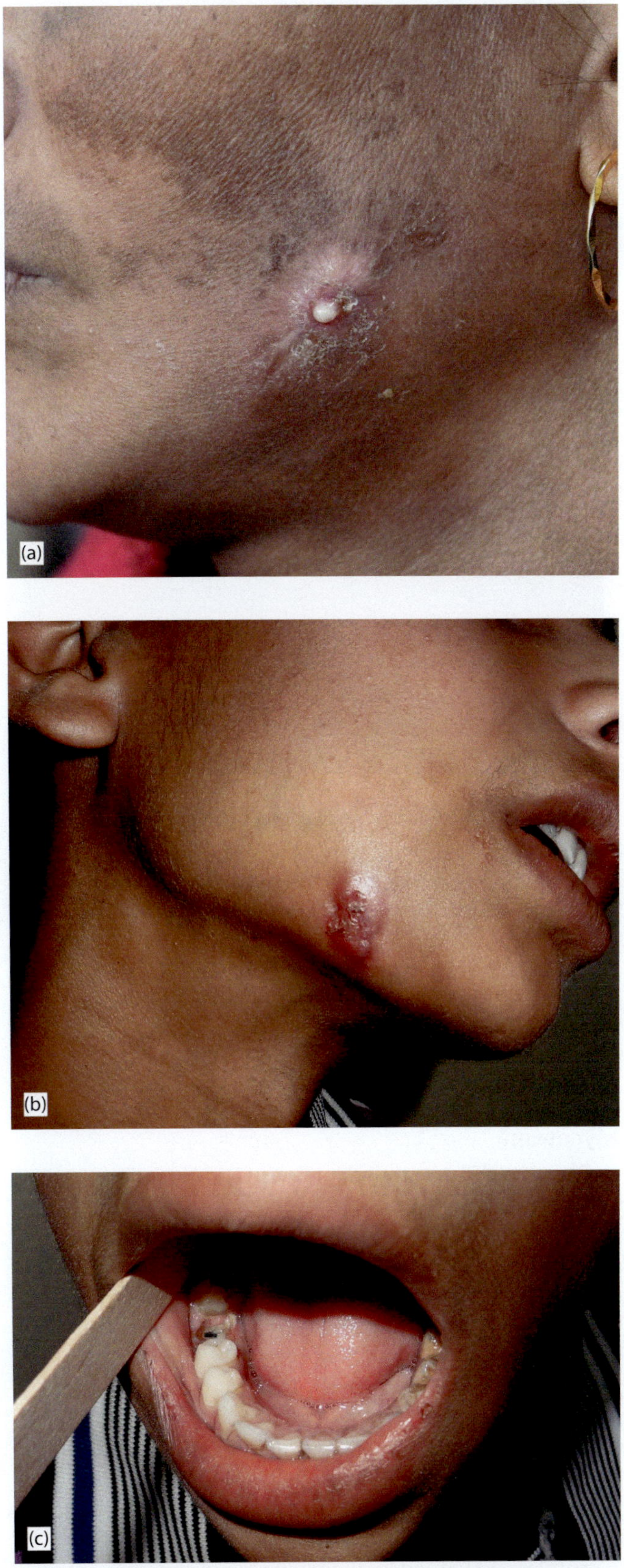


Figure 15.4 **(a)** Dental sinus presenting as erythematous swelling and pus discharge. **(b)** A young boy with dental sinus seen as erythematous crusted swelling in the mandibular region. **(c)** Same boy with dental caries. (a–c – Courtesy: Dr. Piyush Kumar, Katihar, India.)

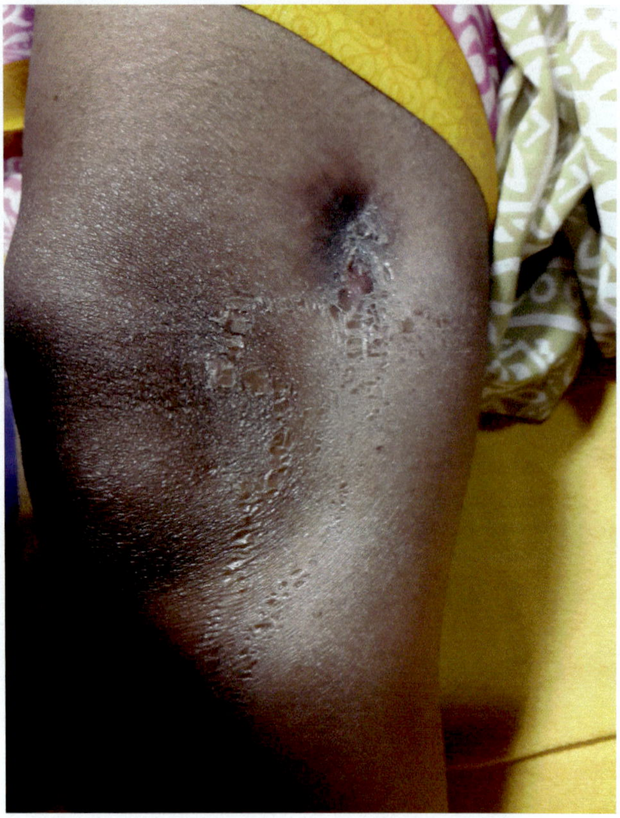

Figure 15.5 Sinus associated with chronic osteomyelitis.

margins (**Figure 15.6a–c**). Numerous discharging sinuses or fistulae intercommunicate beneath involved skin. Sporotrichoid spread has been reported. The most common sites are the neck and submandibular region.

- DD: Lesions caused by environmental (non-tuberculous) mycobacteria, tertiary syphilis, sporotrichosis, actinomycosis, acne conglobata, hidradenitis suppurativa.

## Mycetoma

- This is a chronic granulomatous condition of fungal (more common) or bacterial origin.
- It is characterized by a triad of induration, painless swelling, and multiple sinuses with discharging granules.
- Fungal eumycotic mycetoma is caused by *Madurella mycetomomatis* or *M.grisea* (dark grains) or *Scedosporium, Neotestidina, Acremonium*species (pale grains).
- An inciting factor is penetrating trauma causing subcutaneous implantation of organism.
- The earliest stage is a firm, painless nodule, but with time, papules and pustules appear on the skin surface then break down to form draining sinuses. The whole area becomes indurated and swollen but remains relatively painless. Extension to underlying bones and joints gives rise to periostitis, osteomyelitis, and arthritis. In advanced cases, destruction of bone within an infected area may be almost complete, and gross deformity may result. Usually there are multiple sinus tracts draining purulent or seropurulent discharge; they may remain open for months.

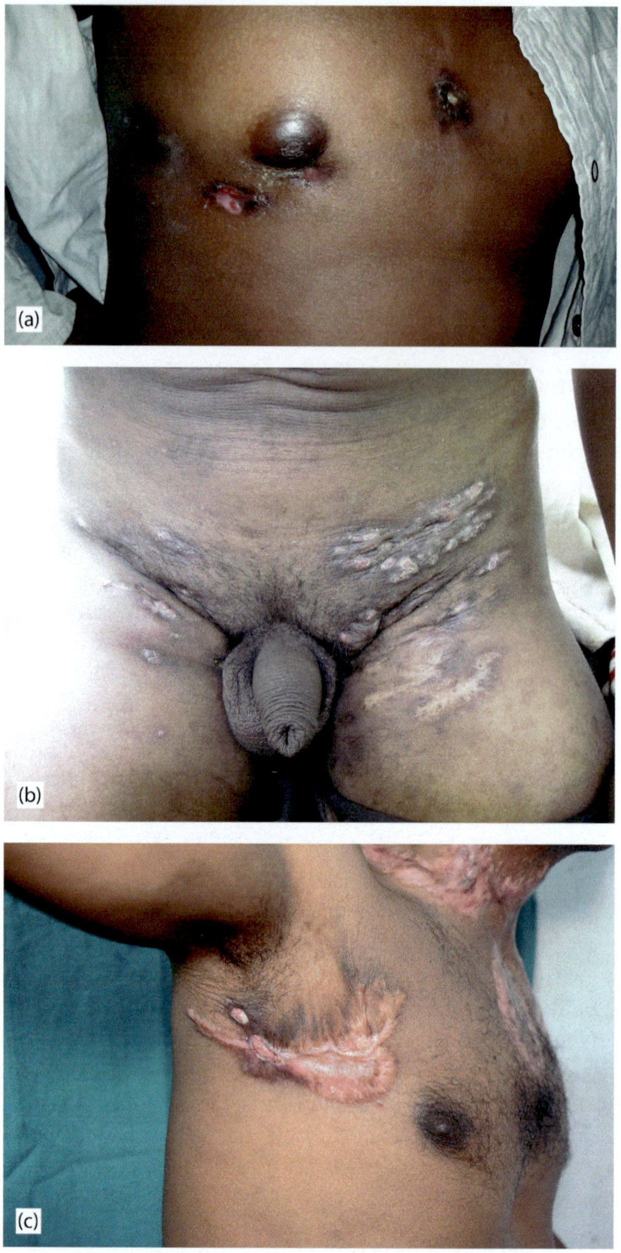

Figure 15.6 **(a)** Scrofuloderma presenting as nodules and discharging sinuses on thorax. **(b)** A young boy with scrofuloderma of inguinal regions. **(c)** Old lesions of scrofuloderma heal with extensive, disfiguring scarring. (b,c – Courtesy: Dr. Piyush Kumar, Katihar, India.)

- Bacterial "Actinomycetoma" can be caused by *Actinomyces* (*A. Israeli* or *A. bovis*) or *Nocardia* species. The swelling is more diffuse without distinct margins, and inflammatory with a more rapid progression and more sinuses (**Figure 15.7a–c**). Bone involvement is faster, producing numerous small cavities.
- Fungal "Eumycetoma" is encapsulated as a well-defined margin. It is less inflammatory with slower progression and fewer sinuses (**Figure 15.7d**). Bone involvement occurs after a longer period of time, forming few but large, clearly defined cavities.

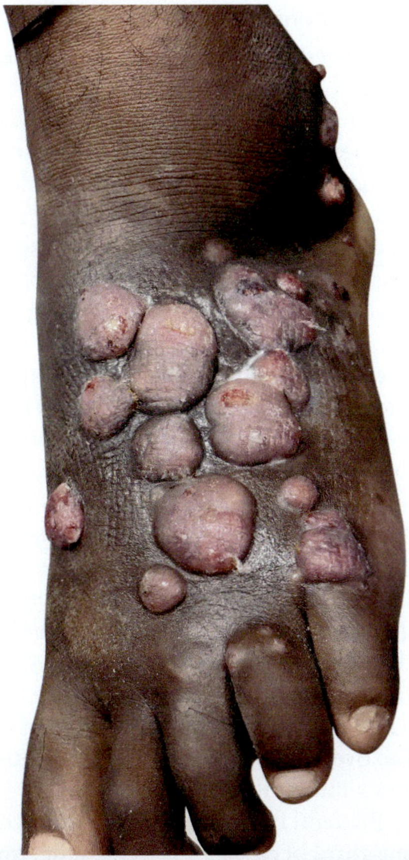

(a)

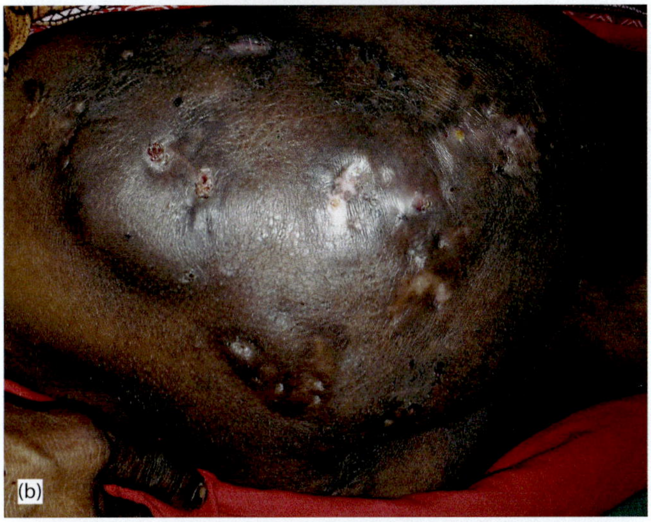

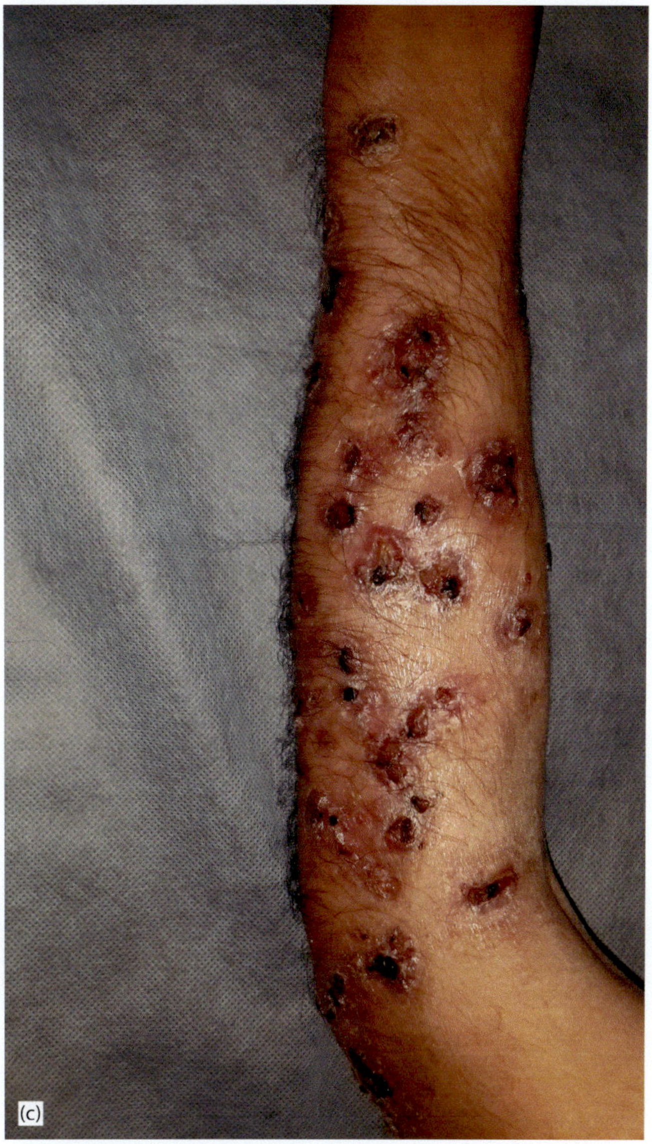

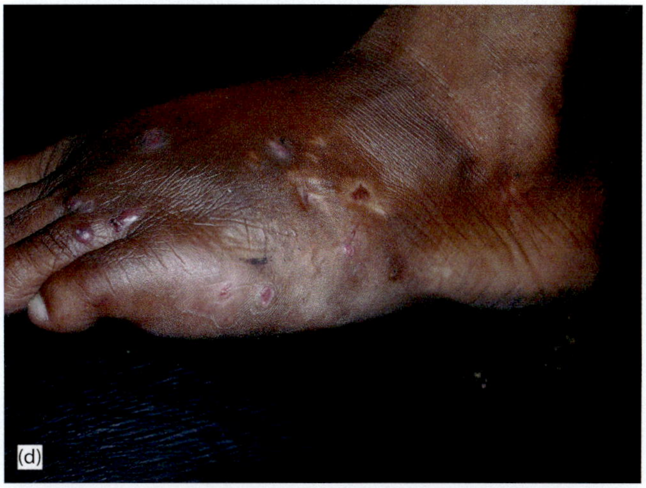

Figure 15.7 **(a)** Unilateral foot swelling with multiple erythematous nodules and sinuses in actinomycetoma. **(b)** Actinomycetoma of the hip region regions. **(c)** Actinomycetoma presenting as multiple discharging sinuses on a background of induration on the forearm. **(d)** A farmer with eumycetoma clinically seen as unilateral foot swelling and multiple discharging sinuses of three years' duration. (a – Courtesy: Dr. Rizwana Barkat, Anugrah Narayan Magadh Medical College & Hospital, India; b – Courtesy: Dr. Piyush Kumar, Katihar, India.)

Table 15.2 Clinical differences between actinomycetoma and eumycetoma

| Features | Actinomycetoma | Eumycetoma |
|---|---|---|
| Progression | Rapid | Slow |
| Inflammation | More | Less |
| Swelling | Deforming, disfiguring | More uniform; contour of the affected part may be maintained |
| Nodules at the sinus openings | Large | Small |
| Granules | White, yellow, red | White, yellow, black |
| Regional lymph node involvement | Common | Uncommon |
| Bone involvement | Early, numerous small cavities | Late, large cavity |

- Eumycetoma may have black granules that show thick septate filaments. Bacterial mycetoma have white/yellow/red granules that, on smear, delineate grains with gram-negative centers and gram-positive radiating, thin hyphae (**Table 15.2**).
- DD: Osteomyelitis, botryomycosis.

## Botryomycosis

- This is a chronic granulomatous bacterial infection, mostly caused by *Staphylococcus aureus* and occasionally *Pseudomonas*.
- The site predilection is limbs more than the perianal area.
- Clinically it presents as multiple subcutaneous nodules, abscesses, ulcers, sinuses, and fistulae discharging yellow granules composed of bacterial masses. Histologically these are coarsely lobulated granules (hence the term "Botryomycosis," referring to groups of granules that resemble grapes).
- Single or multiple abscesses of skin and subcutaneous tissues break down to form serous fluid discharging sinuses that heal in months, leaving behind atrophic scars.
- DD: Actinomycetoma.

## Coccidioidomycosis

- Coccidioidomycosis is caused by *Coccidiodes immitis*, a highly virulent fungus acquired through inhalation.
- Following a flu-like syndrome, lesions may present as
  - Papules, pustules, abscesses, suppurative nodules and discharging sinuses
  - Ulcerations
  - Molluscum contagiosum-like lesions occur in HIV
- Besides pulmonary involvement, systemic involvement includes osteomyelitis and meningitis.

## Lymphogranuloma venereum (LGV)

- This is caused by *Chlamydia trachomatis* (L1, L2, and L3).
- The organism enters through skin breaks or mucous membranes (sexually transmitted) and travels via the lymphatics to multiply within mononuclear phagocytes in regional lymph nodes. Lymphangitis and suppurative lymphadenitis occur. Fistulae and sinus tract formation may ensue. Healing with fibrosis disrupts lymphatic drainage, leading to chronic edema (**Figure 15.8**).
- LGV occurs in three stages:
  - The primary stage, occurring within one month after transmission, is characterized by the appearance of a transient herpetiform ulcer at the inoculation site. It is painless and may go unnoticed, healing rapidly without a scar. DD: Chancroid, granuloma inguinale, herpes genitalis, syphilis.
  - The secondary stage occurs two weeks after the appearance of the primary lesion. It is classically described as the inguinal syndrome, and is characterized by suppurative inguinal lymphadenitis ("Bubo") with matted lymph nodes. The overlying skin becomes violaceous and breaks down into multiple fistulae.

    Bilateral lymph node involvement occurs in one-third of cases. Enlargement of lymph nodes

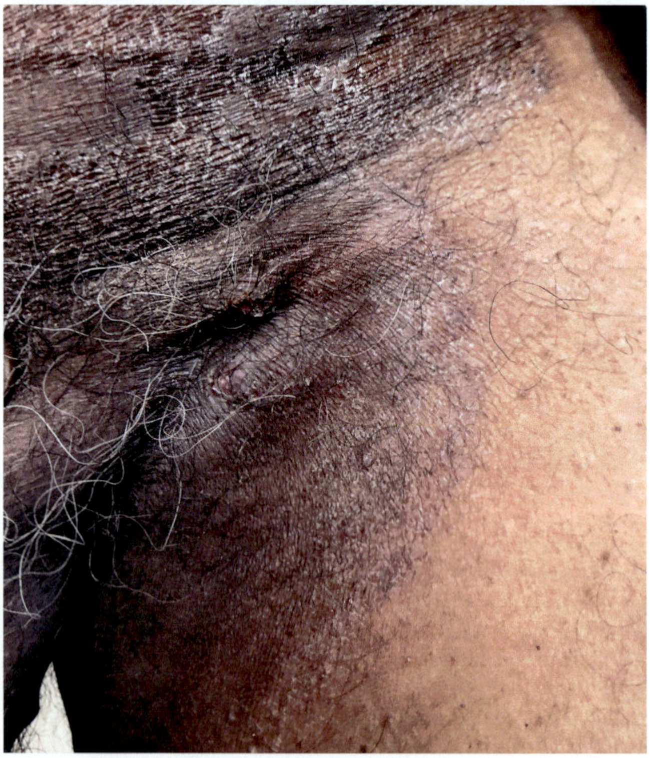

Figure 15.8 Lymphogranuloma venereum with inguinal bubo and sinus. Overlying skin shows scaling of tinea cruris. (Courtesy: Dr. Neethu Mary George, Sri Siddhartha Medical College, Tumkur, India.)

above and below the inguinal ligament (femoral and inguinal lymph nodes) produces the "sign of the groove" in one-third of cases. Constitutional symptoms may be associated. Instead of inguinal bubo, pararectal bubo may also occur. This may present in the rectum as proctitis, with bloody, mucopurulent discharge. DD: Hidradenitis suppurativa, scrofuloderma.
  - The tertiary stage of LGV may occur many years after the initial stages. The manifestations result from fibrosis and lymphatic obstruction. Elephantiasis of the external genitalia causes fistulae and deformity. Esthiomene and saxophone deformity are a result of such involvement of the vulva and penile shaft respectively.

## Actinomycosis

- Actinomycosis is a chronic granulomatous bacterial infection caused by *Actinomyces israelii* and characterized by swelling, discharging sinus, and granules. Histologically there is suppurative granulomatous inflammation.
- These following clinical types haves been described:
  - Cervico-facial ("lumpy jaw"): This is the most common type. Trauma from dental procedures is an inciting factor, with an adjacent tooth or the tonsils being the infective focus. In the early stage it presents as a slow-growing hard swelling that softens and bursts to form multiple erythematous nodules, abscesses, and draining sinuses in the mandibular region (**Figure 15.9**). Discharge contains sulphur granules.
  - Thorax: The lungs and pleura get infected by direct spread from the pharynx or by aspiration. Later a chest-wall nodule appears, which may form discharging sinuses.
  - Iliac fossa: This presents as an abdominal mass with discharging sinuses.
- DD: Blastomycosis, nocardiosis, tuberculosis, odontogenic abscess (dental cyst).

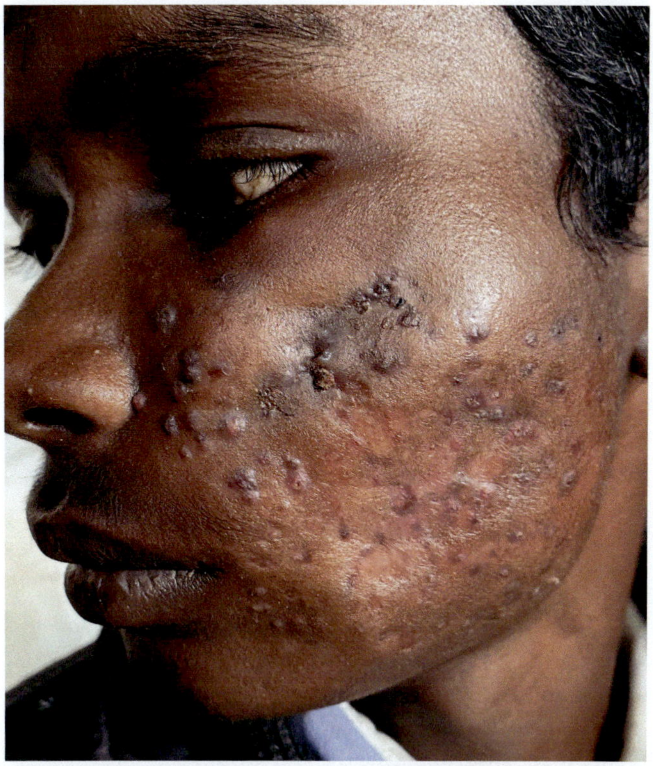

Figure 15.9 Facial actinomycosis presenting as erythematous nodules and sinuses on the cheek. Prior lesions have healed with scarring. (Courtesy: Dr. Rizwana Barkat, Anugrah Narayan Magadh Medical College & Hospital, India.)

## Cutaneous amoebiasis

- **Cutaneous amoebiasis** is caused by *Entamoeba histolytica* transmitted by feco-oral or sexual routes.
- Skin lesions include one or more lesions that appear at the anus or on the buttocks and spread as sloughing, coalescing, and deeply invading ulcers or ulcerated granuloma.
- It is usually seen as a serpiginous painful ulcer with distinct, raised, thickened, often undermined, edges and with an erythematous rim about 2 cm wide, hemopurulent exudate, and necrotic slough. It is associated with regional lymphadenopathy. Pus-discharging sinuses involving the buttocks, perianal/perineal area, and thighs have been described. Vulval lesions in infants with dysentery and penile involvement in homosexual individuals have been reported. A history of dysentery can be a clue in early diagnosis of cutaneous amoebiasis and may be associated with chronic urticaria.
- DD: Tuberculosis verrucosa cutis, syphilis, lymphogranuloma venereum.

## Cutaneous myiasis

- Cutaneous myiasis is an infestation of the skin with larvae (maggots) of a variety of fly species.
- It may present as furuncular, migratory, or wound myiasis.
  - Furuncular myiasis: *Dermatobia hominis*, cordylobia, cuterebra species, *Wohlfahrtia vigil* and *Wohlfahrtia opaca.*
  - Migratory myiasis: Occurs in those who work with horses (*Gasterophilus intestinalis*) or cattle (*Hypoderma bovis*). Presentation is similar to cutaneous larva migrans but the migration is slower and lasts longer for months.
  - Wound myiasis: Caused by *Cochliomyiahominivorax* and infected wounds.
- DD: Insect-bite reaction, cutaneous larva migrans, delusion of parasitosis, abscess, furunculosis.

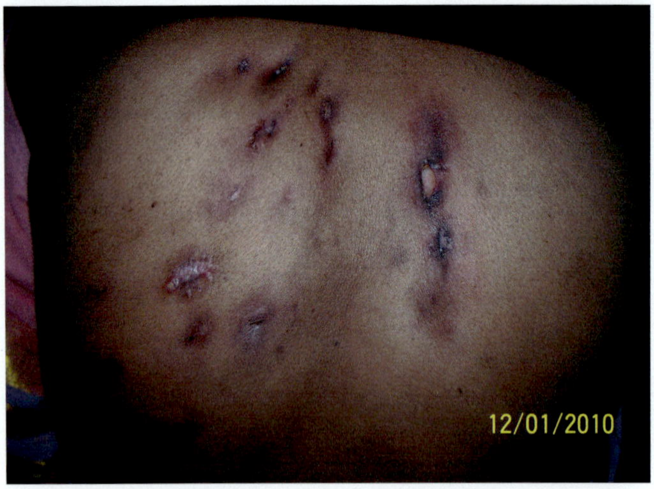


Figure 15.10 Atypical mycobacterial infection presenting as ulcers, sinuses and puckered scarring. (Courtesy: Dr. Piyush Kumar, Katihar, India.)

## Atypical mycobacterial infections

- The atypical mycobacteria *Mycobacterium fortuitum, Mycobacterium abscessus, Mycobacterium chelonae* are together grouped as the "fortuitum complex," atypical mycobacteria that may cause papulopustules, erythematous subcutaneous nodules (most common presentation), ulcers, abscesses, discharging sinuses, or cellulitis. The lesions may at times occur in a sporotrichoid pattern (**Figure 15.10**).
- Trauma, tattoos, and surgery are the major predisposing factors. Resistance to treatment may also be a feature of atypical mycobacterial infection.
- DD: Deep fungal infection, scrofuloderma.

## Hidradenitis suppurativa

- This post-pubertal condition preferentially affects folds that contain both terminal hair and apocrine glands. These include the axillae (preferential location in women) and perineum (preferential location in men). The incidence is higher in women.
- It is characterized by recurrent tender nodules that become fluctuant and suppurate to form sinus tracts. The scarring is extensive. Bridged comedones are a characteristic feature (**Figure 15.11a,b**).
- It forms a tetrad along with conglobate acne, dissecting cellulitis, and pilonidal sinus.
- DD: Actinomycosis, lymphogranuloma venereum, granuloma inguinale, noduloulcerative syphilis.

## Severe acne

- Nodules may extend deeply over a large area, showing little surface involvement. However, if they connect with each other or with deep pustules they may lead to sinus formation as soon as within 24 hours. The lesions are tender, chronic, and treatment-resistant and inevitably result in scarring.

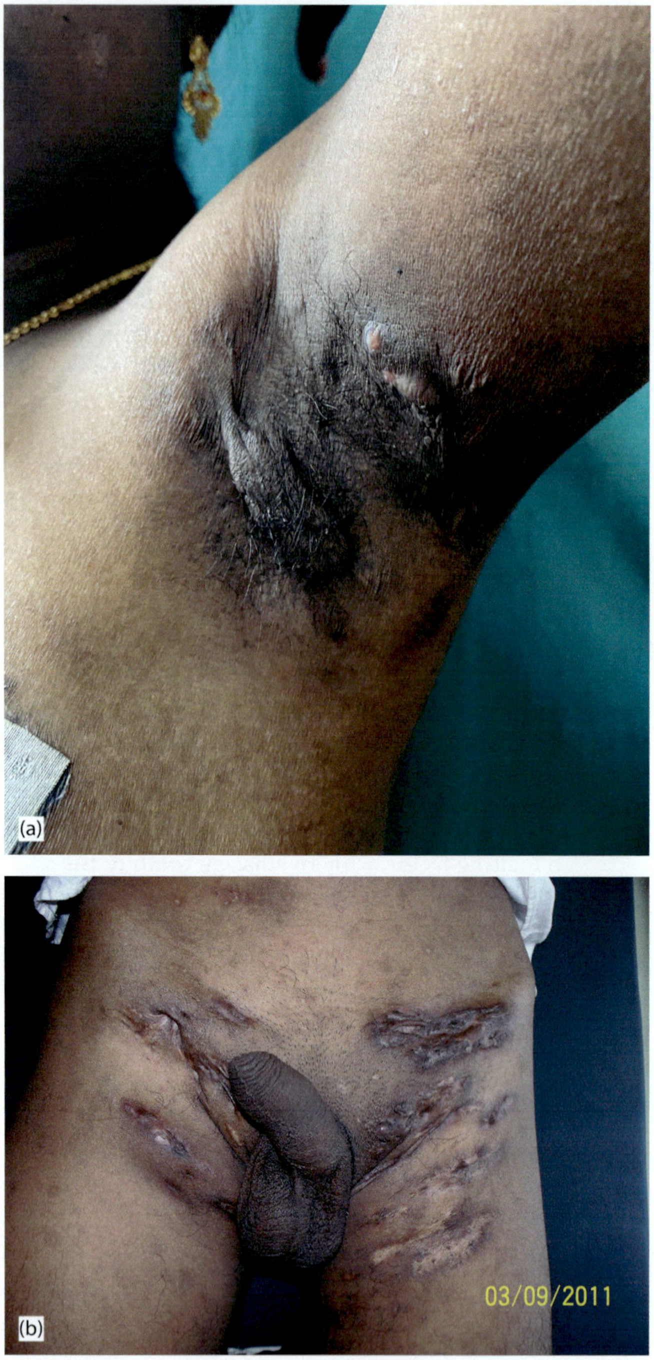


Figure 15.11 **(a)** Hidradenitis suppurativa of the axilla seen as erythematous nodules with sinuses and fluctuant swelling. **(b)** Hidradenitis suppurativa of the inguinal region. (a – Courtesy: Dr. Bhushan Madke, Jawaharlal Nehru Medical College, Datta Meghe Institute of Medical Sciences, India; b – Courtesy: Dr. Piyush Kumar, Katihar, India.)

## Antitrypsin deficiency panniculitis

- This is an inherited deficiency of alpha-1 antitrypsin (a protease inhibitor), producing an ulcerating neutrophilic panniculitis.
- Lesions present as purpuric, tender nodules and plaques on the proximal extremities and lower trunk. The

lesions may become necrotic and break down to form ulcers and sinuses that express an oily brown discharge. The disease course is prolonged, and healing occurs with atrophy and scarring.
- DD: Factitious panniculitis. (antitrypsin deficiency panniculitis has lesions more pronounced than those of trauma); other causes of panniculitis; pyoderma gangrenosum is differentiated by its necrotic, undermined border.

## Malakoplakia of the skin

- It is a rare chronic condition in an immunocompromised host (especially organ transplant recipients) characterized by granulomatous inflammation that is unable to contain a localized bacterial infection (mostly *E. Coli*) effectively. The characteristic macrophages (von Hansemann cells) contain intracytoplasmic Michaelis Gutmann bodies histologically.
- The most common site involved is the genitourinary tract. Skin involvement occurs due to extension from affected internal organ and most commonly affects the perianal and genital area.
- It clinically presents as yellowish-pink soft papules, erythematous indurated nodules, ulcerations, and abscesses with draining sinuses.

## Pancreatic panniculitis

- Pancreatic fat necrosis is a rare complication of pancreatic diseases. All three enzyme categories (lipase, trypsin, and amylase) contribute to the process.
- Clinically it resembles other nodular panniculitis (such as erythema nodosum), with erythematous edematous subcutaneous nodules on the legs more than other areas.
- These lesions may become fluctuant with ulcer or sinus formation, discharging brown oily material representing necrosed adipose tissue.
- DD: Erythema nodosum, erythema induratum, lupus panniculitis, traumatic, alpha-1 antitrypsin deficiency panniculitis.

## Pilonidal sinus

- This arises in or just above the gluteal cleft, where the prerequisites of hair-bearing skin, pressure, and maceration result in chronic inflammation. The pathology initiates when a broken hair follicle penetrates the skin to create a sinus tract filled with cellular debris. Pilonidal sinus may be viewed as a complicated scar with epithelial lined tracts.
- It forms a part of a tetrad along with acne conglobata, dissecting cellulitis of the scalp, and hidradenitis suppurativa.
- Clinically, it is found in teenagers or young adults. It presents as a midline sinus in the sacrococcygeal region (within 5 cm of the gluteal cleft). Chronic, recurrent infection may result in intermittent foul-smelling discharge and pain. Abscess formation may result in more (secondary) tracts that are interconnected and open through multiple sinus openings.
- DD: Perirectal abscess, hidradenitis suppurativa, anal fistula.

## Pyoderma faciale

- Pyoderma faciale is an uncommon eruptive facial disease involving post-adolescent women and resembling severe acne or rosacea.
- It presents as an acute eruption of painful large erythematous coalescing nodules, superficial and deep abscesses, and discharging sinuses, with pronounced background erythema and edema of the cheeks, chin, and/or forehead, and may resolve with scars.
- It differs from acne by the absence of features such as comedones, truncal lesions, and infective organisms on culture.
- It differs from rosacea by the absence of flushing and telangiectatic erythema on the convexities.
- DD: Acne fulminans, severe rosacea, gram negative folliculitis, Sweet syndrome.

## Oral squamous cell carcinoma

- This is the most common malignancy of the oral cavity, seen primarily in middle-aged or elderly men and having a significant association with tobacco and alcohol. The lateral and undersurface of the tongue and floor of the mouth are the common sites. Clinical presentation may range from an irregular exophytic lesion to a painless non-healing ulcer fixed to deeper tissues.
- Untreated disease may destroy oral tissue and extend to the skin on the outer surface of the face to produce a nodular or lobulated growth that appears as a cutaneous discharging sinus.
- DD: Actinomycosis, tuberculosis, nocardiosis, blastomycosis.

## Hodgkin's disease

- There are few reports of abscess presentation of Hodgkin's disease involving liver, lung, chest wall, and brain.
- Suppurative lymphadenitis and discharging sinuses in neck region have also been reported in association with nodular indurated mass in neck.

## Crohn's disease (cutaneous Crohn's disease)

- Cutaneous Crohn's disease presents as lesions that are either metastatic (i.e., distant or non-contiguous with respect to the intestinal disease) or non-metastatic (i.e., contiguous with the intestinal disease). Fistulae may be found in both forms. Histologically all forms uniformly show non-caseating granulomas.
- Metastatic:
  - It presents with genital (labial, scrotal, perianal) or extragenital lesions in the form of dusky erythematous indurated plaques, fissures, ulceration with undermined edges, draining sinuses, fistulae, and scarring.

- Pain usually means that an abscess has formed because of blockage of a fistula.
- Multiple external openings can be encountered all over the buttocks, on the scrotum, and on the thigh; a distinctive sign is the cyanotic hue of the indurated skin.

- Non-metastatic:
    - It involves parastomal fistula associated with ileostomy or colostomy for intestinal Crohn's disease. They are often preceded by abscesses and may be multiple.
    - They signify recurrent disease.

### Enterocutaneous fistula (ECF)

- Most (75%) of ECF are a postoperative complication and the rest are due to other causes (abdominal trauma, cancer, irradiation, inflammatory bowel disease (IBD), ischemic, or infective conditions).
- The ilium is the most common site. It may present with postoperative pain, tenderness, distention, or discharge of enteric contents from the drain site. Peritonitis is a potential complication.
- It can be categorized into low-, moderate-, or high-output fistulae based on the output of enteric contents.

## REFERENCES

1. Rook A, Barker J, Bleiker T, Chalmers R, Creamer D, Griffiths C. Rook's Textbook of Dermatology. 8th edition. Chichester, West Sussex (UK): Wiley Blackwell; 2016.
2. James W, Berger T, Elston D. Andrews' Diseases of the Skin. 11th edition. Philadelphia: Elsevier; 2011, pp. 672–679.
3. Antaya RJ, Schaffer JV. Developmental anomalies. In: Bolognia JL, Schaffer JV, Cerroni L, editors. Dermatology. 4th ed. North York: Elsevier Limited;2018, pp. 1057–1073.
4. Braun-Falco O, Plewig G, Wolff HH, Burgdorf WHC. Cysts and Sinuses. In: Dermatology. Berlin, Heidelberg: Springer; 2000.
5. Foster MT, Moxon CA, Weir E, Sinha A. Dermal sinus tracts. BMJ 2019;366:l5202.
6. Haroun H. Congenital craniofacial and cervical cysts, sinuses and fistulas - A review article.. Sch J Oto 2018;1(1).
7. Goldsmith L, Fitzpatrick T. Fitzpatrick's Dermatology in General Medicine. New York: McGraw-Hill Medical; 2012.

# 16

# Eschar

SUDHIR SINGH

## INTRODUCTION

Eschar is a circumscribed, adherent, hard, black piece of dead tissue (**Figure 16.1a**) that is moist initially, protein rich, and avascular. It implies tissue necrosis, infarction, deep burns, gangrene, or other ulcerating processes. Mostly eschar develops due to some infectious causes, though it may develop due to vasculitis, emboli, etc. It is very important to analyze eschar in a proper context, to reach a definitive diagnosis. For dermatologists, the eschar diagnostic approach and clinical clues to diagnosis are given in **Table 16.1** and **Table 16.2** respectively. The salient features of the diseases are discussed below.[1-5]

### Mucormycosis (zygomycosis)

- Mucormycosis **is** common in diabetes mellitus and immunocompromised patients. Infections in humans are mostly caused by the order *Mucorales* (mucormycosis) and include the genera of *Mucor, Rhizopus, Absidia, Rhizomucor*, and *Cunninghamella*.
- Primary infection can occur by inhalation, by direct inoculation into damaged skin, or by ingestion. Wounds and burn injuries are predisposed to primary cutaneous infection.
- More often it starts with acute onset of pain and swelling on or near the eye or nose.
- The clinicopathologic hallmarks of cutaneous zygomycosis are vascular invasion, ischemic infarction, and necrosis, which result in painful erythematous nodules and plaques that ulcerate rapidly and form central black eschars.
- Rhinocerebral disease is the most common form of the disease and starts as acute sinusitis with fever, nasal congestion, purulent nasal discharge, headache, and sinus pain. Soon it progresses to involve contiguous structures over a course of few days. Tissue necrosis is a prominent feature of the disease and manifests as palatal eschars (**Figure 16.1b**), destruction of the turbinates, perinasal swelling, and cutaneous necrosis with eschar formation and black discharge.
- Cutaneous mucormycosis follows after trauma (including surgical sites) or wounds. The disease starts

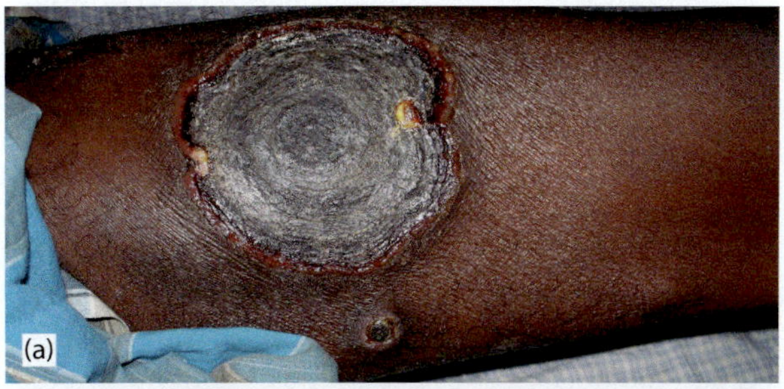

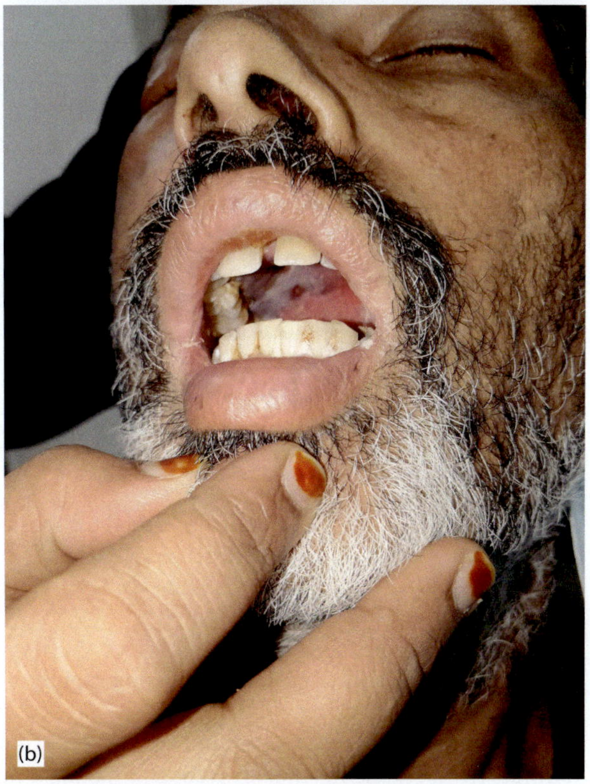

Figure 16.1 **(a)** A well-developed eschar seen as thick, well-circumscribed, hard, dark black area of dead skin. **(b)** Palatal hemorrhage and necrosis in mucormycosis. (a – Courtesy: Dr. Piyush Kumar, Katihar, India; b – Courtesy: Dr. Raghuraj Hegde, Kempegowda Institute of Medical Sciences, Bangalore, India.)

DOI: 10.1201/9781351054225-37

Table 16.1 Clinical approach to diseases presenting with eschar

| General state | Number of lesions | Diseases |
|---|---|---|
| Febrile | Solitary | • Around eye and nose – mucormycosis<br>• Extremities – necrotizing fasciitis<br>• Genital and perineal area – Fournier gangrene<br>• Perineum, groin, axilla, neck – scrub typhus<br>• Hands, fingers, leg, face – anthrax<br>• Extremities – tularemia, rat bite fever, capnocytophaga<br>• Finger, toes, nose – plague |
| | A few | • Anterior nares, nasal bridge, palate – Aspergillosis<br>• Anogenital region, extremities – ecthyma gangrenosum<br>• Toes and feet – cholesterol embolization syndrome<br>• Extremities – purpura fulminans, phaeohyphomycosis, hyalohyphomycosis |
| Afebrile | Solitary | • Extremities – antiphospholipid antibody syndrome<br>• Mastectomy skin flaps/reverse sural artery flaps – flap necrosis<br>• Breast, buttocks, abdomen, thigh – warfarin necrosis<br>• Subcutaneous injection site – heparin necrosis<br>• Extremities snakebite, spider bite (Loxosceles)<br>• Face and extremities – amebic infections |
| | A few | • Abdomen, thigh, and hips – calciphylaxis<br>• Extremities – Lucio's phenomenon<br>• Feet, hand, ears, lips, nose – frostbite<br>• Over sacrum, ischial tuberosity, greater trochanter, heel – decubitus ulcer |

as painful cellulitis-like lesions, progressing rapidly with eschar formation.

- Post-traumatic mucormycosis is an uncommon variant; it differs from cutaneous mucormycosis in having a rare association with diabetes mellitus, mostly localized to the skin, and having a better prognosis.
- It is caused by various species (*Apophysomyces elegans* complex and *Saksenaea vasiformis*).
- A history of trauma following traffic accidents (37%), domestic violence (15.1%), or natural disasters (13.4%) is present.

Table 16.2 Clinical clues to eschar

| General state | Clues to the diagnosis |
|---|---|
| Febrile | • Diabetes mellitus – mucormycosis, necrotizing fasciitis (Fournier gangrene)<br>• Underlying malignant disease, initial lesion hemorrhagic vesicle or pustule – ecthyma gangrenosum<br>• History of travel to endemic areas – scrub typhus, tularemia, plague, anthrax<br>• Sinonasal or pulmonary disease – invasive Aspergillosis<br>• Disease starting as purpura – purpura fulminans<br>• History of trauma or surgical interventions – Fournier gangrene<br>• History of (H/O) Interventional procedures or cardiovascular surgery – cholesterol embolization syndrome<br>• Infiltrated skin lesions – Lucio's phenomenon<br>• Rash with migratory polyarthralgia – rat-bite fever<br>• H/O splenectomy, alcohol-induced liver disease – capnocytophaga<br>• H/O HIV/organ transplant – amebic infections<br>• Immunosuppressed patient – phaeohyphomycosis<br>• Immunocompromised hosts – hyalohyphomycosis |
| Afebrile | • Cardiovascular diseases – arterial insufficiency,<br>• Arterial and venous thrombosis and pregnancy loss – antiphospholipid antibody syndrome<br>• Renal disease – calciphylaxis<br>• Flap surgery – flap necrosis<br>• Involvement of pressure prone areas – decubitus ulcer<br>• On treatment with anticoagulants – warfarin/ heparin necrosis<br>• White/bluish skin with numbness – frostbite<br>• Burn – thermal or chemical burn<br>• Bite – snakebite, Loxosceles bite |

## Necrotizing fasciitis

- It is a life-threatening infection by group *A Streptococcus*, involving soft tissue and fascia.
- It is commonly seen in diabetes, immunosuppressive conditions, chronic alcoholics, and smokers.
- In the early stage, pain (out of proportion to skin involvement), swelling, and erythema develop at the site; these progress rapidly to dusky bullous lesions in one to three days (**Figure 16.2a**).
- DD: Often confused with cellulitis (**Figure 16.2b**) and abscesses; pain out of proportion to erythema tenderness beyond involved area, indistinct margin, and near absence of lymphangitis differentiate early necrotizing fasciitis from other entities.

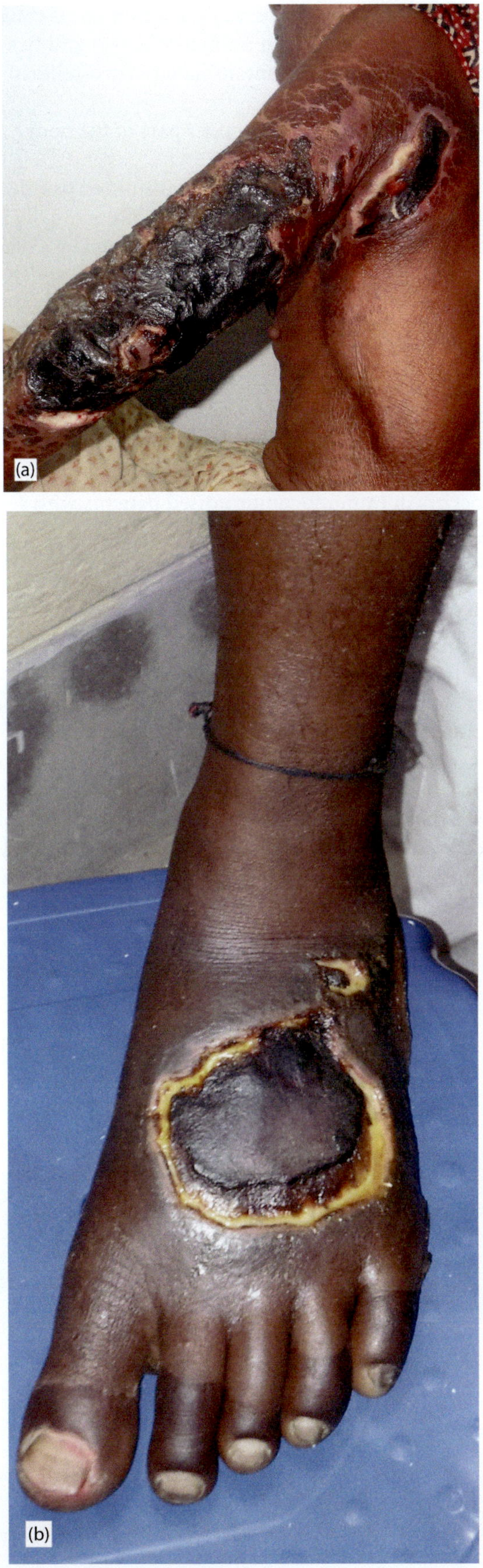

Figure 16.2 **(a)** Necrotizing fasciitis with eschar and ulcer. **(b)** A severe case of cellulitis with eschar. (a,b – Courtesy: Dr. Piyush Kumar, Katihar, India.)

## Fournier gangrene

- It is a type of necrotizing fasciitis affecting genital or perineal skin and soft tissue following trauma or instrumentation.
- It is commonly seen in diabetes patients in the fifth to the sixth decade with a male to female ratio of 10–25:1.
- Cultures commonly show polymicrobial infections by aerobes and anaerobes, which include *Escherichia coli, Staphylococcus aureus, Streptococcal species,* and *Pseudomonas aeruginosa.*
- The scrotum, penile shaft, perineum, and abdomen are involved commonly in men, whereas in women the vulva and perineum are affected (**Figure 16.3**).
- Initially, patients develop pain and swelling, which progress rapidly to tissue ischemia and eschar formation.

## Rickettsia infection[4,6]

- Rickettsiae now include a polyphyletic group of microorganisms in the class proteobacteria, comprising species belonging to the genera *Rickettsia, Orientia, Ehrlichia, Anaplasma*, and *Neorickettsia.*
- Rickettsiae are separated into the spotted fever group and the typhus group based on common genetics, immunologic patterns, and intracellular growth characteristics.
- Spotted fever rickettsiae are injected into the host through the saliva of the feeding tick, whereas typhus group rickettsiae enter through the feces of infected human body lice or fleas.
- There are two major families: the *Ixodidae* (hard ticks) and the *Argasidae* (soft ticks).

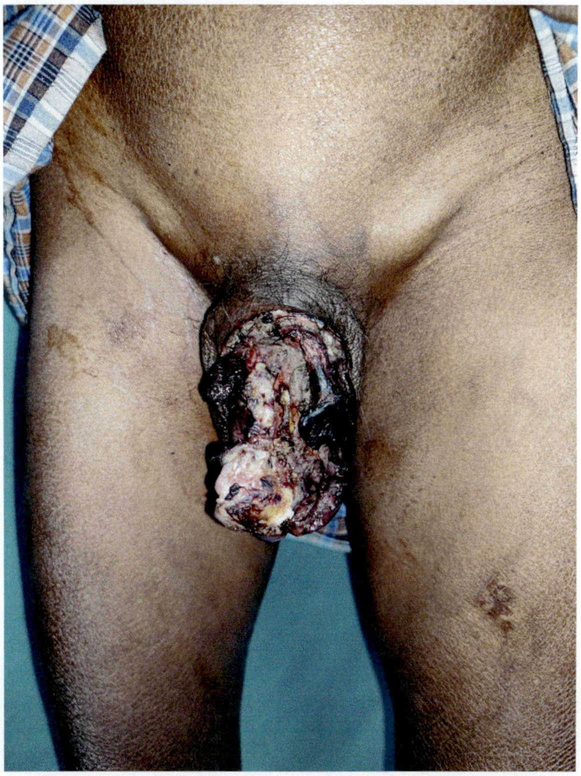

Figure 16.3 Fournier gangrene. (Courtesy: Dr. Rajesh Kumar Mandal, North Bengal Medical College, Darjeeling, India.)

- *Dermacentor* ticks typically attach to the head and neck or the upper trunk. *Ixodes* ticks tend to attach on the trunk, whereas *Amblyomma* ticks prefer the lower extremities.
- Rickettsial diseases of dermatological importance are summarized in **Table 16.3**.

## Tularemia[7]

- Tularemia is caused by *Francisella tularensis*, a gram-negative coccobacillus found in rabbits and rodents and reported mainly in the northern hemisphere.
- The cutaneous form of tularemia in humans is caused by direct contact with an animal reservoir and tick bites or exposure to a contaminated hydro-telluric environment.
- Lesions are located on the upper part of the body (extremities).
- In ulceroglandular tularemia, a painful red papule appears at the inoculation site that evolves rapidly into a necrotic chancreform ulcer often covered by a black eschar. Regional lymph nodes are large and tender.

## Ecthyma gangrenosum[8,9]

- This is most commonly caused by *Pseudomonas aeruginosa* (73%), other bacteria (*Escherichia coli, Aeromonas, Klebsiella pneumoniae, Haemophilus influenzae*), as well as fungi (*Candida, Aspergillus species, Fusarium*).
- It occurs in immunocompromised patients with severe neutropenia, particularly those with an underlying malignant disease.
- It is described in two types: localized (non-septicemic) form, in which lesions are localized at the site of inoculation of the organism into the skin, and classical (bacteremic) form due to hematogenous spread.
- It is most commonly located in the anogenital area or on the extremities.
- Lesions progress rapidly within 12 to 24 hours from erythematous or purpuric macules to hemorrhagic vesicles or bullae, which rupture and become necrotic ulcers with a central black eschar. The surrounding tissue is erythematous and tender (**Figure 16.4a–c**).

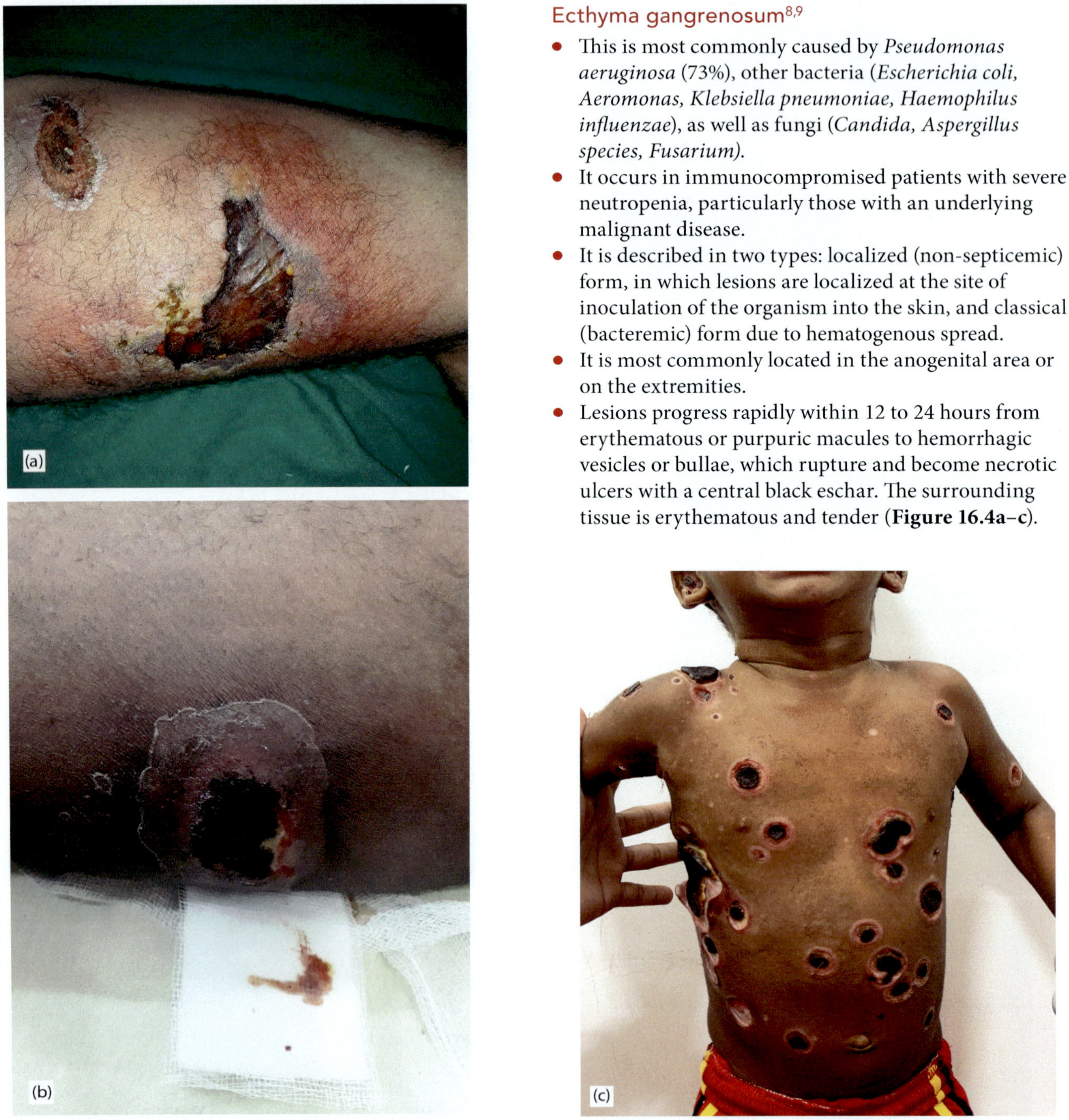


Figure 16.4 **(a)** Ecthyma gangrenosum. Central black eschar with surrounding erythematous tissue. **(b)** Ecthyma gangrenosum. Necrotic ulcers with a central black eschar and erythematous halo. **(c)** Multiple lesions of ecthyma gangrenosum in a child due to sepsis following an episode of varicella. (c – Courtesy: Dr PC Das and Dr Piyush Kumar, Katihar, India.)

Table 16.3 Rickettsial diseases

| Disease | Vector/ reservoir | Incubation period | Clinical features | Systemic features |
|---|---|---|---|---|
| Scrub typhus (*Orientia tsutsugamushi*) (**Figure 16.5a–c**) | Trombiculid mite (*Leptotrombidium deliense*)/ mites and the rodents | 1–2 weeks | Eschar is common in warm, damp areas of the body (perineum, groin, and axilla).<br>An erythematous papule appears within two days of the chigger bite, which ulcerates and forms eschar in 50–70% patients.<br>The regional lymph nodes are enlarged and tender. | High grade fever (40°–40.6°C). Hepatosplenomegaly and relative bradycardia pneumonitis may develop.<br>Deafness and tinnitus occur in about 20%. |
| Rocky Mountain spotted fever RMSF (*Rickettsia rickettsii*) | *Dermacentor variabilis* (dog tick), *Dermacentor andersoni* (wood tick), *Amblyomma americanum* (lone star tick), *Rhipicephalus sanguineus* (brown dog tick)/pet dog | >2–14 days | Males; adults 40–64 years, children <10 years.<br>Rash begins on ankles, wrists, and forehead and spreads centripetally.<br>Erythematous blanching macules and papules 2–4 days after fever onset; and may be hemorrhagic. Originally called "black measles." | Neurologic disease, thrombocytopenia, acute renal failure, hepatitis.<br>The classic triad of fever, rash, and history of tick bite. |
| Mediterranean spotted fever (*Rickettsia conorii*)<br>African tick bite fever ATBF (*R. africae*) | *Rhipicephalus sanguineus* (brown dog tick)<br>*Amblyomma hebraeum and Amblyomma variegatum* tick | 5–7 days | Tache noir, occurring in about 13%–68% as an erythematous, indurated papule with a central necrotic eschar.<br>Rash may be morbilliform or vesicular.<br>Multiple tick bites, multiple eschars (seen in 50% of patients with ATBF) | Mild disease (mainly in children) has a good prognosis.<br>Lymphadenitis; distinguish ATBF from RMSF |
| Rickettsial pox (*Rickettsia akari*) | *Liponyssoides sanguineus* rodent mite/house mouse, *Mus musculus* | 7 days (eschar), 7–24 days (systemic symptoms and rash) | It starts as a painless, erythematous, indurated papule at bite site and evolves into a vesicle, followed by eschar formation.<br>Regional lymphadenopathy is common. | Clinically resembles varicella (chickenpox)<br>Self-limiting |
| Endemic typhus (*Rickettsia typhi; Rickettsia felis*) | *Xenopsylla cheopis* (rat flea), *Ctenocephalides felis* (cat flea) | 1–2 weeks (12 days) | Extremely high fever, 41.1°C (106°F), malaise, headache, rash after 4–5 days<br>Erythematous macules and/or papules involving the trunk more than the extremities.<br>Palms and soles are rarely involved. | Thrombocytopenia, transaminitis, and hyponatremia are common, though usually mild |
| Epidemic typhus (*Rickettsia prowazekii*) | *Pediculus humanus var. corporis* (human body louse), *Neohaematopinus sciuropteri* lice, *Orchopeas howardii* fleas | 1–2 weeks (8 days, average) | Starts as erythematous macules over axillary folds and upper trunk after 4–5 days, which become papular and petechial.<br>Lack of eschar<br>The eruption spreads centrifugally but spares the face, palms, and soles.<br>Predilection for colder months | Acral gangrene, cerebral thrombosis may occur.<br>Brill–Zinsser disease (BZD) can occur in survivors who may suffer recrudescent of the previous infection |

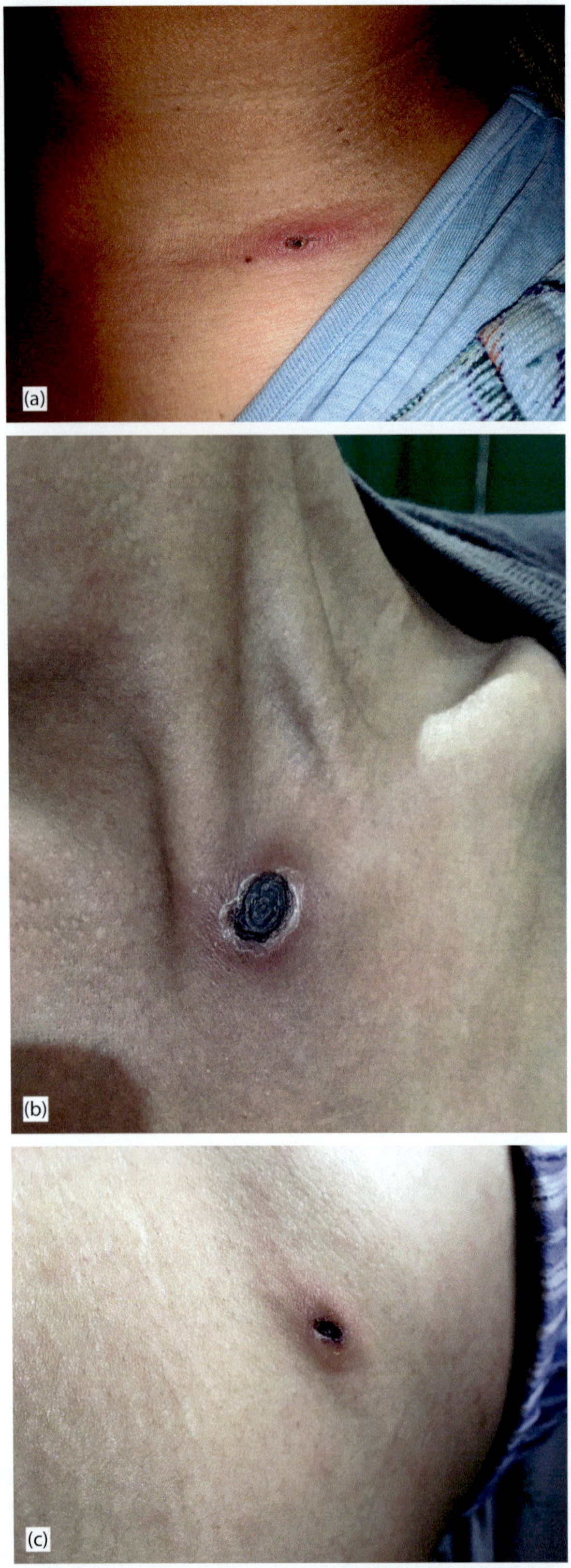


Figure 16.5 **(a)** Scrub typhus with erythematous plaque with central eschar. **(b)** Well-developed eschar in scrub typhus. **(c)** Scrub typhus. (a – Courtesy: Dr. Kalyan Ghosh, Darjeeling, India; b – Courtesy: Dr. Kilangwabang Pongener, Nagaland, India; c – Courtesy: Dr. Kilangwabang Pongener, Nagaland, India.)

- DD: Noma caused by *Fusobacterium,* which occurs in young debilitated infants; septic emboli due to organisms such as *E. coli, Aeromonas hydrophila, Burkholderia cepacia, Candida, Fusarium, Aspergillus,* and other saprophytic fungi.

## Anthrax

- Anthrax is caused by *Bacillus anthracis.*
- It can present in four forms: *cutaneous* (95%), *inhalational* (known as woolsorter's disease), *gastrointestinal,* and *injectional* (seen in IV drug use, primarily in heroin addicts).
- Cutaneous anthrax transmission (approximately 95% of cases) is by the introduction of spores via breaks in exposed skin. The sites involved are exposed parts of the hands, legs, and face.
- Incubation period is about three to seven days.
- It presents initially as an anti-inflammatory papule that rapidly develops into a bulla surrounded by intense edema and infiltration within another 24 to 36 hours. It then ruptures spontaneously, and a dark-brown or black eschar is visible, surrounded by vesicles situated on an indurated area (**Figure 16.6**).
- The lesion is painless and non-tender, associated with tender suppurative regional adenitis. Pustules are seldom present.
- DD: Staphylococcal carbuncle (prominent tenderness), brown recluse spider bite.

## Plague[10]

- It is a flea-borne zoonosis caused by *Yersinia pestis,* associated with the term "the Black Death."
- Transmission to humans occurs through the bite of infected fleas.
- In humans, it classically presents with three forms: bubonic (80–85% cases), septicemic, and pneumonic.
- A skin lesion may develop at the site of the bite in 25% cases, especially over fingers, toes, or the nose, and often go unnoticed. The patient may develop a pustule, vesicle, papule, or an eschar.
- Within a few days, painful regional lymphadenopathy develops, involving single or multiple nodes. Most commonly inguinal nodes, followed by axillary or cervical nodes, are involved.

## Aspergillosis

- Invasive infection with Aspergillus is classically seen during acute periods of neutropenia in hematopoietic stem cell transplant patients, certain hematologic malignancies, GVHD, cytomegalovirus infection, and solid-organ transplant patients.
- *A. fumigatus* is the most common cause of disseminated infections, although emerging strains of *A. flavus, A. niger,* and *A. terreus* are accounting for more disease.
- Cutaneous manifestations of disseminated Aspergillosis occur in only 5%–10% of patients.
- Aspergillosis should be suspected in patients presenting with pneumonia, CNS involvement, and nasal passage

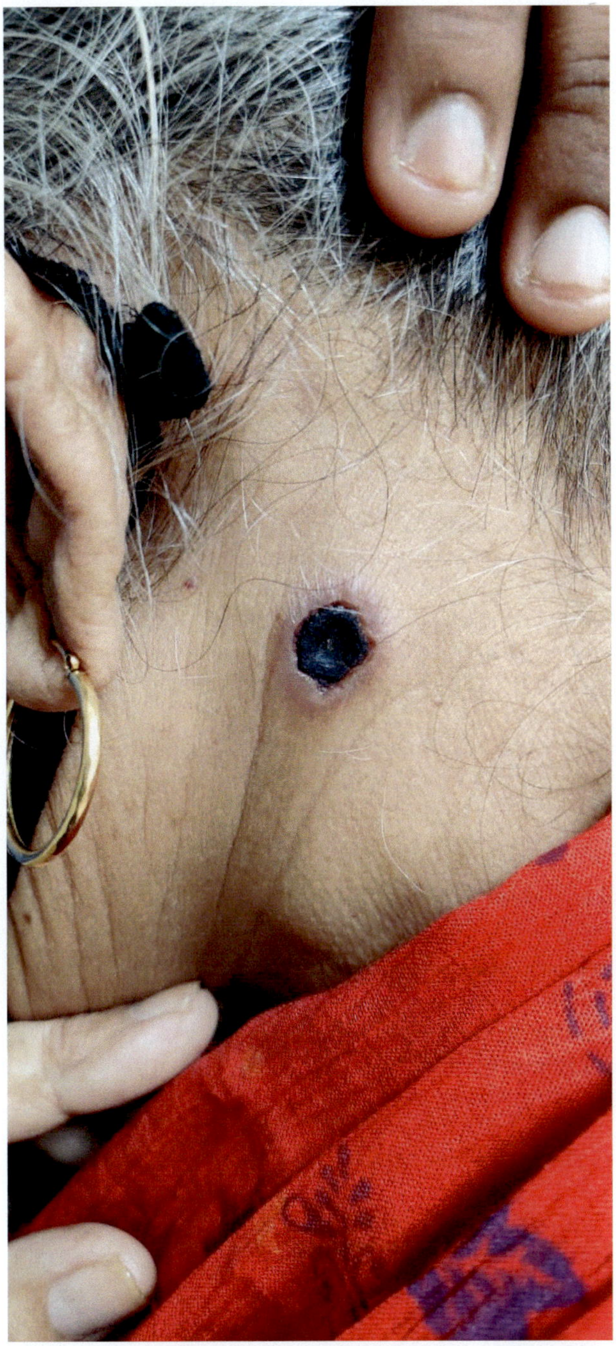

Figure 16.6 Anthrax. Eschar with a rim of induration. (Courtesy: Dr Ajay Rai, Lucknow, India.)

and paranasal sinuses disease that can develop ulcer followed by an eschar.
- Lesions occur in the anterior nares and on the nasal septum, palate, and skin overlying the nasal bridge. Patients with disseminated Aspergillosis often present with unremitting fever despite antibiotic use.
- Lesions begin as single or multiple painful, erythematous papules, nodules, or plaques. They rapidly expand and develop central hemorrhagic vesicles or bullae, then eschar.
- In burn victims, Aspergillus typically colonizes the burn eschar.

## Purpura fulminans

- Purpura fulminans is usually seen in relation to acute sepsis, idiopathic post-infectious form, and in neonates.
- In acute sepsis-associated or secondary purpura fulminans, infection with *Neisseria meningitidis, Staphylococcus aureus,* groups *A* and *B hemolytic streptococci, Streptococcus pneumoniae,* and *Haemophilus influenzae.*
- Postinfectious purpura fulminans can manifest within 10 days of an antecedent illness, most commonly following streptococcal or varicella infections in children.
- Neonatal purpura fulminans are most often seen in association with homozygous protein C deficiency.
- Cutaneous microvascular occlusion in sepsis with DIC presents clinically as ecchymosis, usually with a retiform, stellate, or branching configuration and symmetrical gangrene of extremities. Patients develop non-blanching tender purpura with erythematous halo and indurated borders with rapid transition to necrosis and eschar (**Figure 16.7**).
- DD: Catastrophic antiphospholipid antibody syndrome.

## Cholesterol embolization syndrome

- Also known as blue or purple toe syndrome, this is an entity in which cholesterol crystal or atheroma debris (cholesterol, platelet, and fibrin) embolizes distal arteries.
- It is commonly seen in elderly patients after endovascular procedures (valve replacement or stent placement) but can occur spontaneously.
- Constitutional features, such as fever, anorexia, myalgia and weight loss, may be seen. It commonly affects the kidneys (31.5%), skin (15.5%), and gastrointestinal tract (13.4%).
- The most common skin finding is livedo reticularis; blue or purple toes, ulcers, gangrene, and purpuric lesions are also seen.
- DD: In arterial thromboembolism onset is acute and leads to abrupt organ dysfunction, whereas in

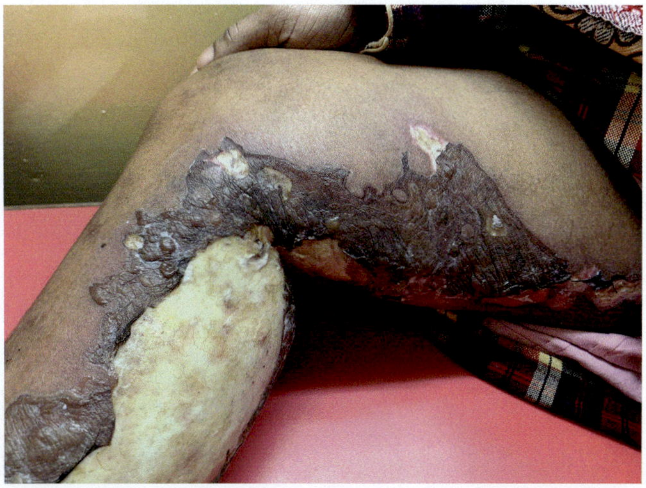

Figure 16.7 Purpura fulminans following disseminated intravascular coagulation (DIC). (Courtesy: Dr. Piyush Kumar, Katihar, India.)

cholesterol embolization syndrome onset is subacute or chronic and causes slow end organ dysfunction. Another distinguishing feature of cholesterol embolization syndrome is that arterial pulsations are palpable as it involves smaller arteries and arterioles.

### Lucio's phenomenon

- Lucio's leprosy (LuLp) is a diffuse form of LL, commonly seen in Mexico and Costa Rica.
- The skin looks waxy and shiny, as there is diffuse infiltration of skin without the previous appearance of discrete lesions.
- Infiltration of the ear lobes and forehead, and loss of eyebrows and sometimes eyelashes give a mask-like appearance known as lepra bonita, or beautiful leprosy. Lucio's phenomenon may be seen in untreated patients.
- It is characterized by multiple, well-defined, irregular purpuric lesions evolving into massive ulcerations, involving the extremities and healing with atrophic scarring (**Figure 16.8a**).
- DD: Antiphospholipid antibody syndrome and necrotic ENL (**Figure 16.8b**). ENL is associated with lymphadenopathy and arthritis. Bacteriological and morphological indices show high positivity in Lucio's phenomenon.

### Arterial insufficiency (ischemic) ulcer

- This is generally seen in hypertensives, smokers, diabetic, and hyperlipidemia patients. In a progressive disease, the diagnosis of thromboangiitis obliterans, or Buerger's disease, should be considered.
- The ratio of the popliteal to brachial pressure is called the ankle-brachial index (ABI); if it is less than 0.75, arterial insufficiency exists; and if it is less than 0.5, the insufficiency is substantial.
- Ischemic ulcers are mostly located on the lateral surface of the ankle or the distal digits.
- The initial red, painful plaque breaks down into a painful superficial ulcer with a surrounding zone of purpuric erythema (**Figure 16.9a,b**).
- Granulation tissue is minimal; little or no infection is present; and a membranous inactive eschar forms over the ulcer.
- Associated findings include decreased or absent pulses, coolness of the extremity, and claudication on exercise.
- DD: Cholesterol emboli.

### Antiphospholipid antibody/lupus anticoagulant syndrome (APLS)

- It is characterized by venous thrombosis, arterial thrombosis, pregnancy loss, or thrombocytopenia in conjunction with the presence of antiphospholipid antibodies.
- It is mostly seen in young to middle-aged patients, with a strong female predominance.
- APLS may occur as a primary or secondary disorder.
- Primary APLS comprises 53% of cases. Secondary antiphospholipid syndrome can be associated with systemic lupus erythematosus, malignancy, lymphoproliferative disorders, infections, drugs, and autoimmune diseases.

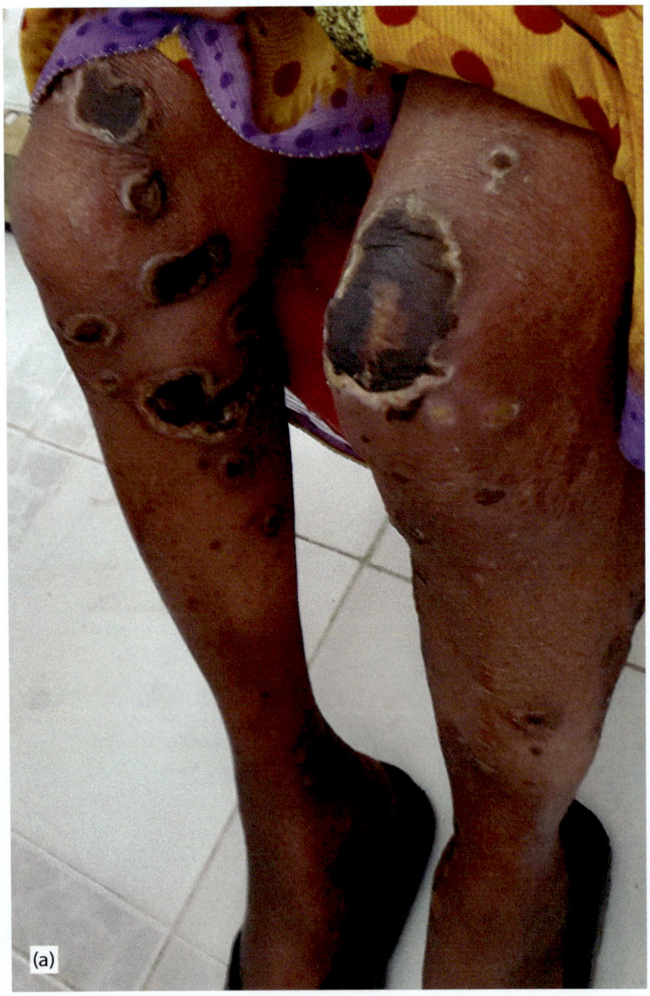


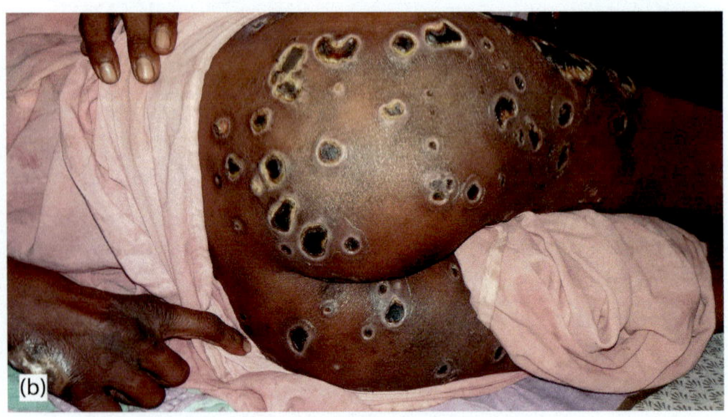


Figure 16.8 **(a)** Lucio's phenomenon. Multiple well-defined round to oval and geographic ulcers covered with eschar. **(b)** Erythema nodosum leprosum necroticans with multiple ulcers covered by eschars. (a – Courtesy: Dr. Vikrant Saoji, Nagpur, India; b – Courtesy: Dr. Hiral Shah, Baroda Medical College, Vadodara, India.)

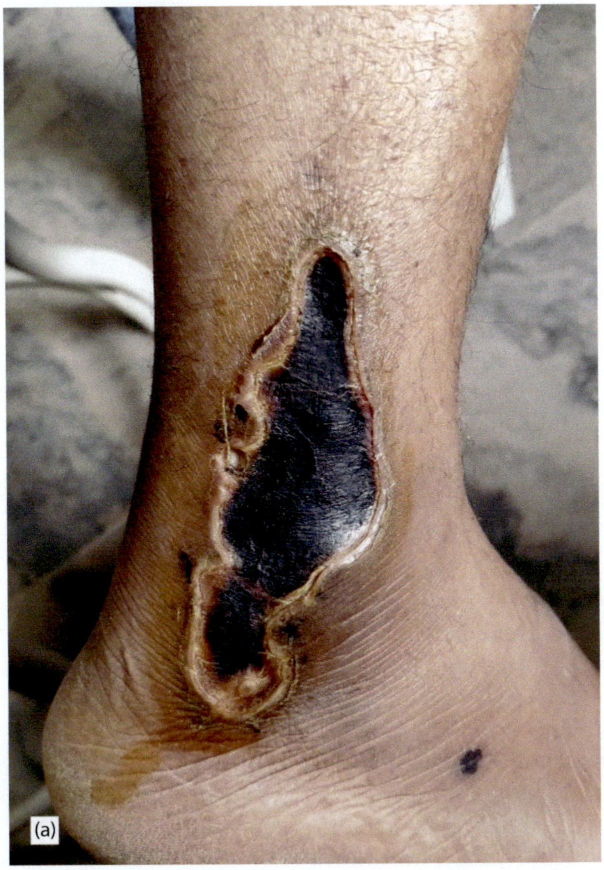

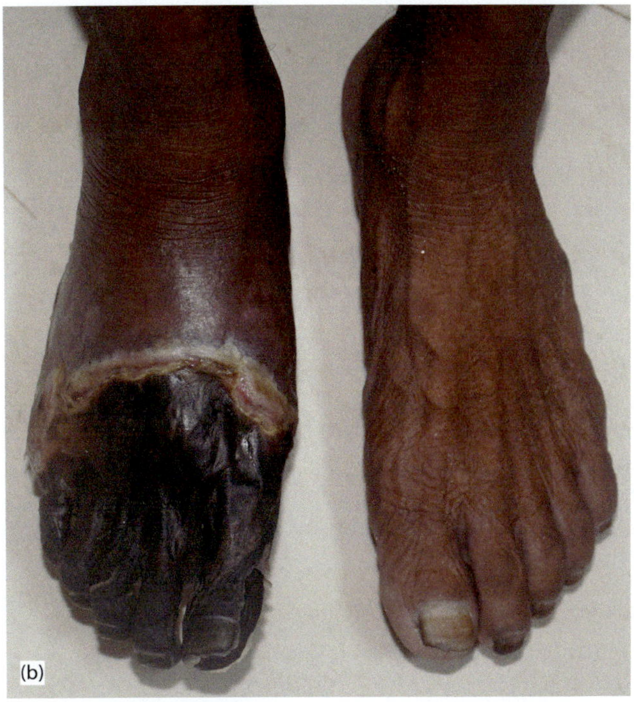

Figure 16.9 **(a)** Arterial insufficiency ulcer. Membranous eschar over the ulcer with a surrounding zone of purpuric erythema. **(b)** Arterial insufficiency ulcer with eschar of distal foot. (a – Courtesy: Dr. Ajay Rai, Lucknow, India; b – Courtesy: Dr. Piyush Kumar, Katihar, India.)

- The most common finding is livedo reticularis found on the extremities; other findings include leg ulcers, pseudovasculitis, digital gangrene, cutaneous necrosis, and splinter hemorrhages.
- Catastrophic APLS is an uncommon variant that presents with widespread cutaneous necrosis and multiorgan failure, especially renal and pulmonary.

## Calciphylaxis/calcific uremic arteriolopathy

- Also known as calciphylaxis, this is a rare but life-threatening cutaneous condition associated with hyperparathyroidism.
- Calciphylaxis is seen in patients of chronic renal failure, secondary hyperparathyroidism, alcoholic liver disease, and occasionally after chemotherapy, even in patients with normal renal function.
- Peak incidence is after the sixth decade, more commonly in females (>80%). Calciphylaxis results from calcium deposition in the walls of small- to medium-sized vessels, resulting in vascular occlusion and skin necrosis.
- Typical sites involved are abdomen, thighs, and hips, but breasts may be involved.
- Patients initially develop violaceous patches that may exhibit a mottled or reticular pattern that become indurated and painful, with eventual ulceration and eschar formation that proceeds to tissue gangrene (**Figure 16.10**).

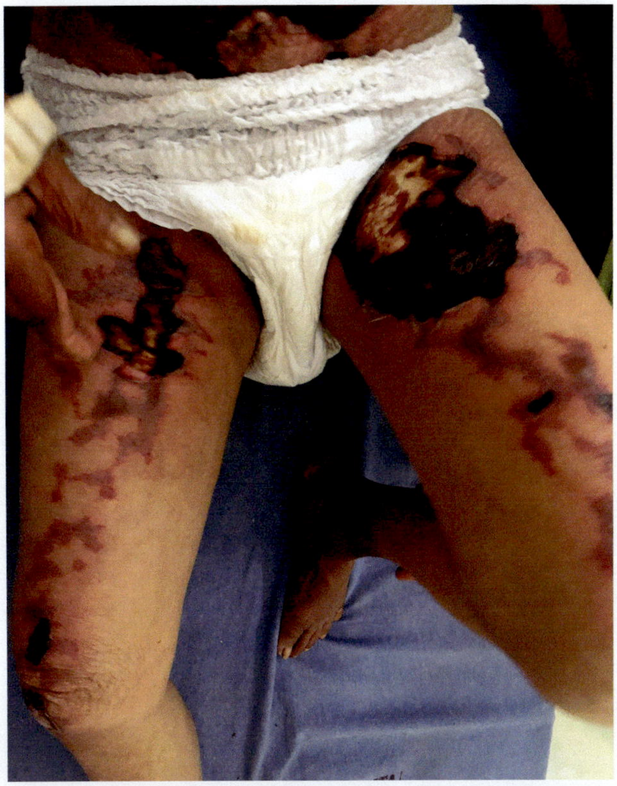

Figure 16.10 Calciphylaxis with reticulate purpura and cutaneous necrosis (eschar). (Courtesy: Dr. Neethu Mary George, Sri Siddhartha Medical College, Tumkur, India.)

- A calcium-phosphate product of greater than 70 mg/dL has often been cited as a risk factor.
- DD: Hyperoxaluria.

## Flap necrosis[11]

- Local flap reconstruction may cause complications related to ischemia, tension, hematologic, or infectious cause.
- The incidence of mastectomy skin flaps ranges from 5%–30%, but in dermatologic surgeries, the incidence of flap necrosis is lower.
- Skin flap viability is influenced by surgical and patient factors (smoking, diabetes, hypertension, and obesity). Compromised skin flap perfusion can lead to necrosis.
- For improving flap survival, minimize tissue undermining and dissection, or use a delayed phenomenon.

## Pressure ulcer (decubitus ulcer)

- Defined as a localized area of necrosis caused by ischemia, this results from compression of soft tissue between a bony prominence and an external surface.
- The predominance is 80% superficial ulcers and 20% deep ulcers. The sacrum is the site of 60% of all sores are over, while the ischial tuberosities, greater trochanter, and heel account for 15%.
- The lesion evolves from blanchable erythema to necrosis of all tissues down to and including bone and joints. When pressure is relieved, sores go through a process of debridement, where necrotic slough forms a hard dry black eschar (**Figure 16.11**, **Table 16.4**).

## Coumadin (coumarin, warfarin) necrosis

- Lesions usually develop within 10 days of starting coumarin therapy in approximately 1 out of 10,000 patients.

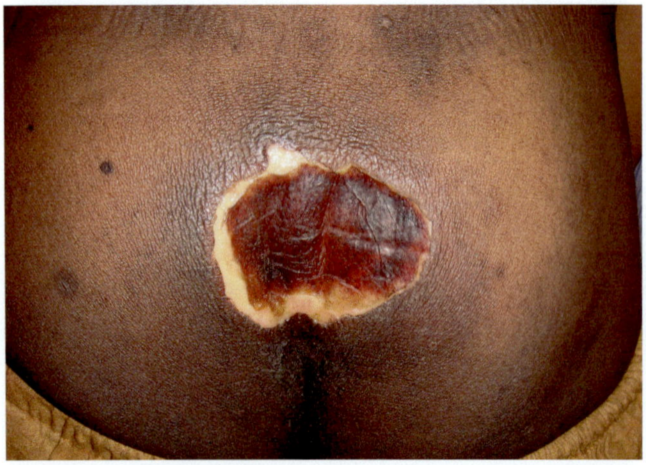

Figure 16.11 Pressure ulcer covered with eschar. (Courtesy: Dr. Piyush Kumar, Katihar, India.)

Table 16.4 European Pressure Ulcer Advisory Panel (EPUAP) classification scheme

| Stage I | Non-blanching erythema of intact skin |
|---|---|
| Stage II | Partial-thickness skin loss involving epidermis and/or dermis |
| Stage III | Full-thickness skin loss with necrosis of subcutaneous tissue down to but not through underlying fascia |
| Stage IV | Full-thickness with penetration to fascia, muscle, bone |

- The risk of coumadin necrosis is increased if loading doses (10 mg or more) of warfarin are used and if a second form of anticoagulation such as heparin therapy is not used to cover the initial phase of anticoagulant therapy.
- The peak incidence is between the sixth and seventh decades and has a male:female ratio of 1:4.
- Sites involved are the breasts (**Figure 16.12**), buttocks, abdomen, and thighs, with abundant fat and reduced blood supply.
- Coumadin necrosis usually presents as the sudden onset of pain within affected areas, followed by well-demarcated erythema, progressing to hemorrhage, necrosis, and often hemorrhagic bullae or eschar.
- DD: Although coumadin necrosis may rarely involve acral areas, acral cutaneous purpura in patients on coumarin is more likely to be due to cholesterol embolus – so-called purple (blue) toe syndrome.

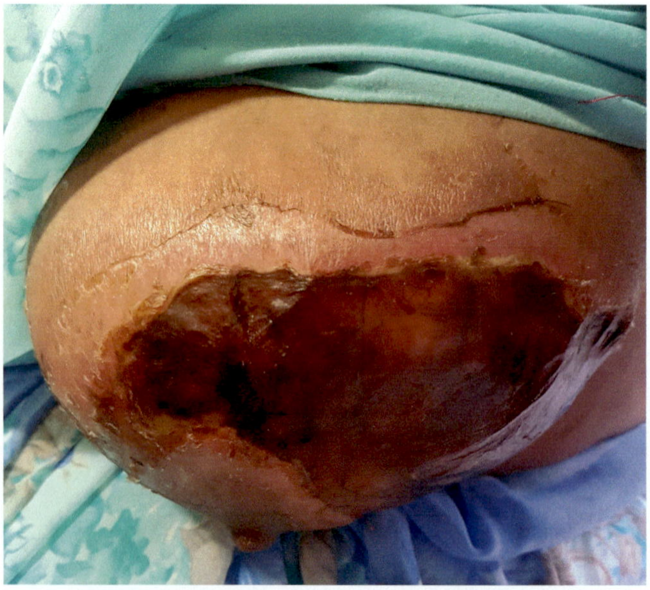

Figure 16.12 Warfarin necrosis with superficial eschar and surrounding erythema. (Courtesy: Dr. Shekhar Neema, Armed Forces Medical College, Pune, India.)

## Heparin necrosis

- Cutaneous heparin necrosis is thought to occur as part of the heparin-induced thrombocytopenia (HIT) syndrome in at least 22% of patients with heparin-induced skin lesions.
- A heparin-dependent antiplatelet antibody is the pathogenic basis of HIT and apparently of heparin-induced skin necrosis. This antibody causes both thrombocytopenia and the aggregation of platelets in vessels, leading to thrombosis (white-clot syndrome).
- Unfractionated heparin is three times more likely to be associated with HIT following orthopedic surgery compared with low molecular-weight heparin.
- Lesions appear around five to seven days after initiation of heparin. Lesions are most common at subcutaneous injection sites but can occur elsewhere.
- Heparin administration commonly induces ecchymoses, purpuric tender, sharply demarcated plaques sometimes with retiform extensions. Erythema may sometimes accompany such lesions, and necrosis is frequent.
- Unlike skin necrosis induced by warfarin, heparin-induced skin necrosis can recur if heparin is restarted, as it is an immune-related condition.

## Burns

- Due to different modalities such as thermal, chemical, electrical, or radiation, burns usually present acutely to clinicians. Burn depth usually is determined by the intensity of the source, duration of contact, and location on the body.
- Heat (and other injury mechanisms) can denature proteins, leading to loss of plasma membrane integrity and cell necrosis (**Figure 16.13**).
- Burns may be classified according to the depth of thermal injury (**Table 16.5**).

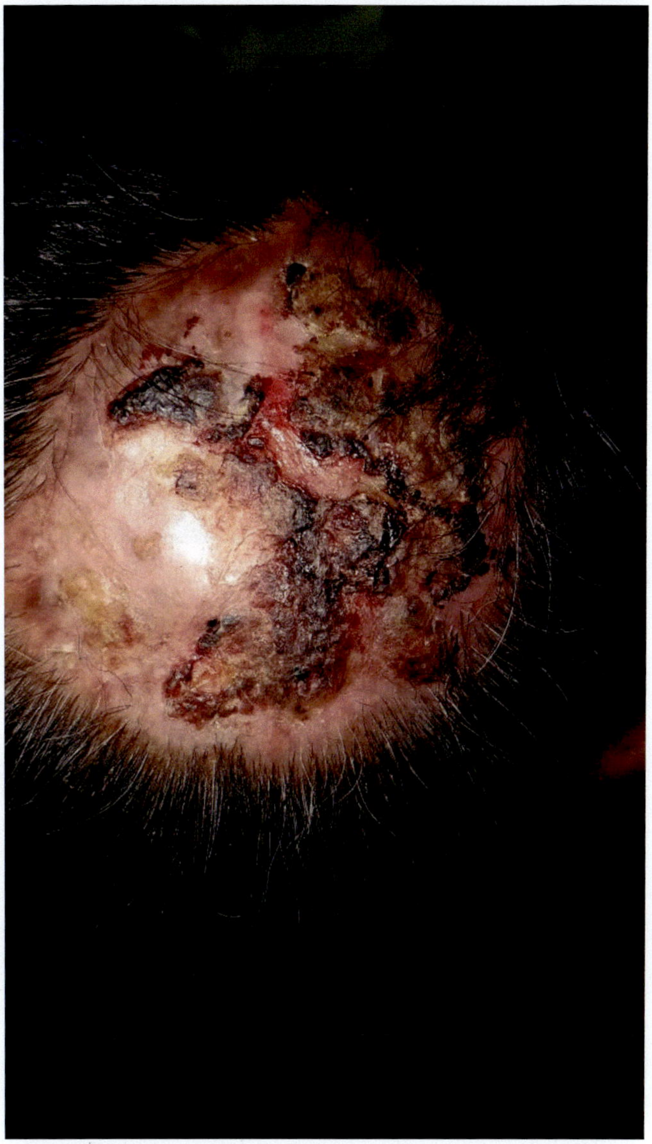

Figure 16.13 Electric burn. Dry, waxy irregular eschar over the scalp. (Courtesy: Dr. Ajay Rai, Lucknow, India.)

## Frostbite[12]

- Tissue damage resulting from exposure to sub-zero degree Celsius temperature is known as frostbite or freezing cold injury.
- Sites prone to develop frostbite are feet, hands, ears, lips, and nose.
- Initially, the skin becomes white and blanched, along with numbness. Later the exposed part becomes dark and purplish.
- Within 4 to 24 hours upon rewarming superficial frostbite develops pale white blisters, while deep frostbite may show hemorrhagic blisters or gangrenous changes.
- Eschar will be evident in 10 to 15 days.

Table 16.5 Classification of burns

| Type | Depth of thermal injury | Sensation | Morphology |
|---|---|---|---|
| Superficial burns (first degree) | Epidermis | Painful | Erythematous, blanch on pressure |
| Partial-thickness burns (second degree) | Epidermis and dermis | Painful | Pink or cherry red, blister, blanch on pressure |
| Full-thickness burns (third degree) | Epidermis, dermis, and subcutaneous tissue | Not painful | Form an eschar, appear dry and leathery, can feel firm and waxy on palpation, and is non-blanching |

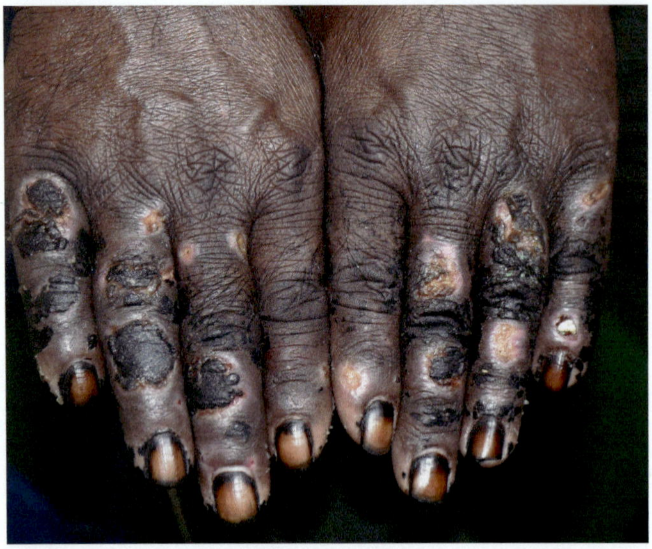

Figure 16.14 Chromic induced ulcers and eschars on the hands. Note pigmentation of the nails. (Courtesy: Dr. Piyush Kumar, Katihar, India.)

## Chemical burns

- It results in irreversible cell damage and necrosis at the site of exposure. There is usually a rapid onset of painful erythema, often within minutes.
- The dead skin turns brown and later black, usually without blistering, and forms a hard eschar (**Figure 16.14**).
- Phenol (carbolic acid) is a protoplasmic poison that produces a white eschar on the surface of the skin. It can penetrate deep into the tissue.
- Most acids (e.g., sulphuric, nitric, hydrochloric, chromic) coagulate skin proteins.
- Some acids can discolor (e.g. nitric acid turns the skin yellow).
- Alkalis (e.g., sodium, calcium, potassium hydroxides; wet concrete; sodium, and potassium cyanides) degrade lipids and penetrate deeper into the skin. The dead skin turns brown and later black, usually without blistering, and forms a hard eschar.

## Snakebite

- Signs and symptoms of snakebite depend upon the species of snake, so identification of snake is essential.
- Venomous snakes belong to three major families, *Elapidae* (cobras, kraits, adders, mambas, coral snakes), *Viperidae* (rattlesnakes, vipers), and *Hydrophiidae* (sea snakes).
- The venom of elapid snakes is highly neurotoxic, and some species, such as *Naja* spp. Cobras, have additional cytotoxicity. Viper venoms are unique for causing bite-site swelling and tissue destruction.
- Local effects, including skin blistering, limb swelling, and tissue necrosis, are caused by vipers. Local blistering can lead to necrosis of full skin thickness, which can get secondarily infected.
- Puncture marks at the wound help in the diagnosis of snakebite.

## Loxosceles[13]

- Bites of the brown recluse spider or fiddle-back spiders (*Loxosceles reclusa*) vary from mild, local reactions to severe ulcerative necrosis, a reaction known as necrotic arachnidism.
- In necrotic cutaneous loxoscelism, systemic symptoms are mild. Within minutes or hours, severe pain develops at the site of the bite, accompanied by erythema, edema, and a central bulla.
- The hallmark – central blue/purple discoloration – develops, surrounded by an ischemic halo and an outer ring of erythema (the “red, white, and blue” sign). The initial wound may progress to become necrotic, and an eschar develops within three or four days. Eventually, deep ulcers develop (**Figure 16.15**).

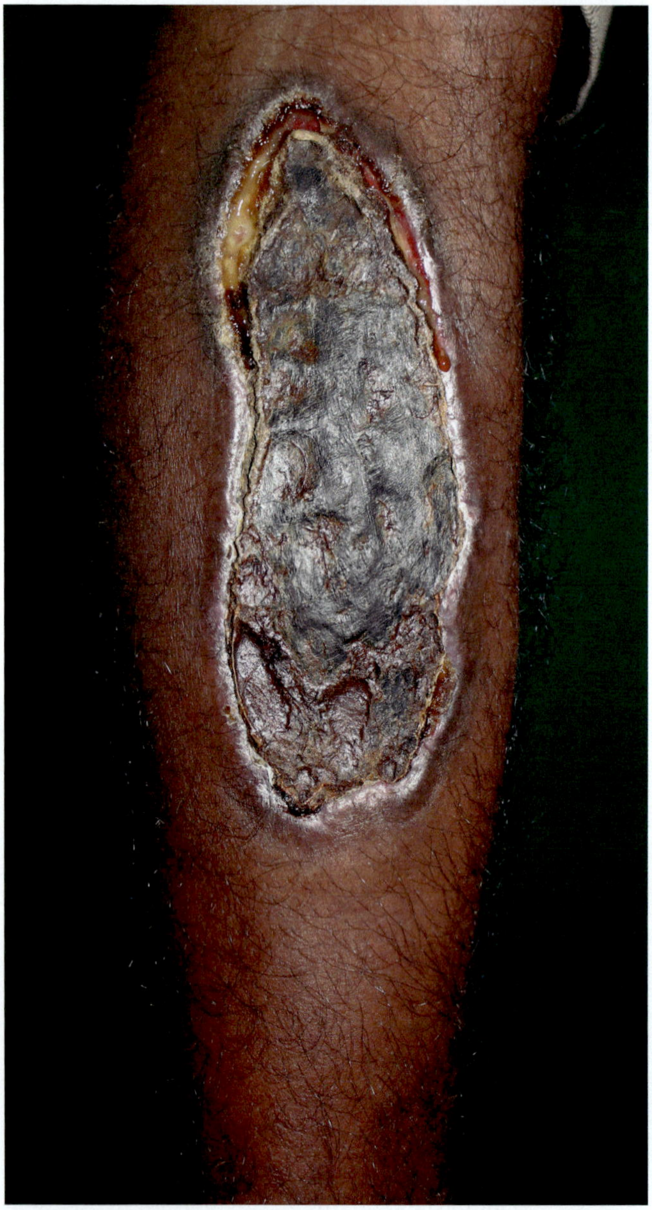

Figure 16.15 Loxosceles with thick adherent eschar. (Courtesy: Dr. Shekhar Neema, Armed Forces Medical College, Pune, India.)

- DD: Pyoderma gangrenosum, erythema migrans of Lyme disease, cutaneous anthrax, and chemical burns.

## Tegenaria

- *Tegenaria agrestis*, the hobo spider or "aggressive house spider," is the predominant cause of necrotic arachnidism.
- The local cutaneous effects are similar to those caused by the brown recluse. Induration and paresthesia of the bite site may develop within 30 minutes.
- Vesicle formation often occurs during the first 36 hours. Eschar formation may follow in severe cases, with necrosis and sloughing of the underlying tissue.

## Amebic infections

- Amebas of the genera *Acanthamoeba, Naegleria,* and *Balamuthia* may also cause skin lesions. Infection is more common in HIV-positive patients and organ transplant patients.
- The extremities (lower more than upper) and the face are commonly involved.
- Lesions present as pink or violaceous nodules that then enlarge, suppurate, and form ulcers with a necrotic eschar.
- DD: Pyoderma gangrenosum.

## Rat-bite fever (sodoku, spirillum minor)

- Caused by a spiral flagellate organism *Streptobacillus moniliformis*, and is transmitted by the bite of a rat. It can be transmitted through food or water contaminated with feces or urine.
- Inflammation and an eschar may form at the wound site within 10 to 12 days, accompanied by fever, malaise, and regional lymphadenopathy. Approximately 75% of patients develop the maculopapular, petechial, or purpuric rash.
- As the infection progresses, 50% of individuals will develop migratory polyarthralgia and myalgia in large and small joints of extremities.

## Capnocytophaga (formerly dysgonic fermenter type 2 [DF2])

- *Capnocytophaga canimorsus* is part of the normal oral flora of healthy dogs and cats.
- Capnocytophaga infections occur following exposure to or bites from dogs.
- Necrotizing eschar at the site of the bite is a characteristic finding. Cellulitis, non-specific macular or maculopapular lesions, erythema multiforme, petechiae, purpura fulminans, and symmetrical peripheral gangrene may be seen.

## Phaeohyphomycosis

- Phaeohyphomycosis is caused by dematiaceous fungi *Exophiala jeanselmei.*
- Subcutaneous disease occurs most frequently as indolent abscesses at the site of minor trauma (so-called "phaeomycotic cyst").
- Systemic phaeohyphomycosis is caused by *Bipolaris spicifera* and *Scedosporium prolificans* in immunocompromised patients.
- Disseminated disease may also begin as a skin infection, although catheter sepsis is a recognized cause of disseminated infection.
- The lesions usually appear as dry, black, leathery eschars with a scalloped, erythematous, edematous border.

## Hyalohyphomycosis

- Hyalohyphomycosis is caused by *Penicillium, Acremonium, Trichoderma, Scedosporium,* and *Paecilomyces.*
- They generally do not cause the disease except in immunocompromised patients. Localized hyalohyphomycosis has also occurred in immunocompetent patients after traumatic implantation.
- There is no classic clinical morphology to the lesions, but keratotic masses, ulcerations, ecthyma gangrenosum-like lesions, erythematous nodules, dark eschars, and disseminated erythema have been described.

## Injuries caused by fire coral and coral cuts

- Coral injuries may be caused by nematocyst stings or lacerations.
- In contrast to the stings of true corals, the sting of the fire coral, *Millepora alcicornis*, is quite painful.
- Within one to several hours a pruritic erythematous papular eruption appears, which in severe cases may become pustular and, in rare cases, may progress to necrosis and eschar formation.
- Lesions heal in 1 to 2 weeks, often with post-inflammatory hyperpigmentation.

## Cowpox

- This is caused by orthopoxvirus after contact with infected cats or cattle.
- Sites involved are usually the hands, arms, or face.
- A lesion evolves from a painful papule within five to seven days at the inoculation site and becomes vesicular and hemorrhagic, which ulcerates within two weeks, and forms crusts with a hard black indurated eschar 1–3 cm in diameter. Healing takes place in four to eight weeks and usually leaves scarring.
- Constitutional symptoms and lymphangitis are common.
- DD: Orf and milker's nodules as well as primary tuberculosis, anthrax. In anthrax, the eschar forms by day six. The amount of surrounding edema and induration is much more marked than in orf. Scarring is common after cowpox.

## Milker's Nodule

- Milker's nodule is caused by the paravaccinia virus (also called pseudocowpox virus) in individuals in close contact with cattle.
- Incubation period for the milker's nodule is four to seven days.

- It commonly occurs on the hands, occasionally on the face.
- Lesions start as red or pruritic macules and then evolve into papules and papulovesicles with a target-like appearance. The lesions then develop into bluish or violaceous tender nodules. Some ulcerate or have a central depression, which results in the formation of eschars with a crust. Lesions heal in four to eight weeks. Lymphangitis is often present. Lymphadenopathy is not common.
- DD: The lesion of anthrax is more hemorrhagic, with rapid progression to an eschar. Tularemia and syphilis are associated with chancres.

## REFERENCES


1. Dunn C, Rosen T. The rash that leads to eschar formation. Clin Dermatol 2019;37(2):99–108. doi:10.1016/j.clindermatol.2018.12.003.
2. Liaqat M, Halpern AV, Green JJ, Heymann WR. The Rickettsioses, Ehrlichioses, and Anaplasmoses. In: Kang S, Amagai M, Bruckner AL, Enk AH, Margolis DJ, McMichael AJ, Orringer JS, editors. Fitzpatrick's Dermatology. 9th edition. New York, NY: McGraw-Hill Education; 2019. P. 3306–3323.
3. Monsel G, Delaunay P, Chosidow O. Arthropods. In: Griffiths CEM, Barker J, Bleiker T, Chalmers R, Creamer D, editors. Rook's Textbook of Dermatology. 9th edition. West Sussex: John Wiley & Sons; 2016. P. 34.1–34.55.
4. Prakash JAJ. Scrub typhus: Risks, diagnostic issues, and management challenges. Res Rep Trop Med 2017 Aug 7;8:73–83.
5. Wysong A, Venkatesan P. An approach to the patient with retiform purpura. Dermatol Ther 2011 Mar–Apr;24(2):151–172.
6. Weerakoon K, Kularatne SA, Rajapakse J, Adikari S, Waduge R. Cutaneous manifestations of spotted fever rickettsial infections in the Central Province of Sri Lanka: A descriptive study. PLoS Negl Trop Dis 2014 Sep 18;8(9):e3179.
7. Maurin M, Gyuranecz M. Tularaemia: Clinical aspects in Europe. Lancet Infect Dis 2016;16(1):113–124. doi:10.1016/S1473-3099(15)00355-2.
8. Vaiman M, Lazarovitch T, Heller L, et al. Ecthyma gangrenosum and ecthyma-like lesions: Review article. Eur J Clin Microbiol Infect Dis 2015;34:633–639.
9. Martínez-Longoria CA, Rosales-Solis GM, Ocampo-Garza J, Guerrero-González GA, Ocampo-Candiani J. Ecthyma gangrenosum: A report of eight cases. An Bras Dermatol 2017;92(5):698–700. doi:10.1590/abd1806-4841.20175580.
10. Dillard RL, Juergens AL. Plague. In: StatPearls. Treasure Island (FL): StatPearls Publishing; August 10, 2020.
11. Robertson SA, Jeevaratnam JA, Agrawal A, Cutress RI. Mastectomy skin flap necrosis: Challenges and solutions. Breast Cancer (Dove Med Press) 2017;9:141–152. Published 2017 Mar 13.
12. Basit H, Wallen TJ, Dudley C. Frostbite. In: StatPearls. Treasure Island (FL): StatPearls Publishing; June 30, 2020.
13. Tibballs J, Winkel KD. Envenomation Syndromes. In: Shaffner DH, Nichols DG, editors. Rogers Textbook of Paediatric Intensive Care. 5th edition. Philadelphia: Wolters Kluwer; 2016. P. 515–540.

17

# Cutaneous horn

SATISH S SAVANT, SUSHIL S SAVANT

## INTRODUCTION

- Cutaneous horn (Cornu cutaneum) is a morphological designation referring to an elongated, densely compacted hyperkeratotic conical projection above the surface of the skin, overlying any of the wide variety of cutaneous lesions and resembling a miniature horn of an animal but differing from it by having a cornified instead of bony core.
- Its peak occurrence is reported in people aged 50 to mid-70s because cutaneous horns with underlying premalignant and malignant lesions are more common in this age group.

Table 17.1 Conditions associated with cutaneous horn

| Condition | Diseases |
|---|---|
| Benign | Verruca vulgaris, seborrheic keratosis, pyogenic granuloma, molluscum contagiosum, fibroma, epidermal cyst, in fundibular cyst, dermatofibroma, angioma, angiokeratoma, benign lichenoid dermatosis, epidermolytic acanthoma, verrucous epidermal nevus, organoid nevus, nevus sebaceous of Jadassohn, sebaceous adenoma, papillary eccrine adenoma, benign epithelial hyperplasia, prurigo nodularis, cutaneous leishmaniasis, discoid lupus inverted follicular keratosis, micaceous pseudoepitheliomatous balanitis, trichilemmoma, trichilemmal cyst. |
| Premalignant | Actinic keratosis, arsenic keratosis, keratoacanthoma, Bowen's disease. |
| Malignant | Squamous cell carcinoma, basal cell carcinoma, sebaceous carcinoma, granular cell tumor, adenocarcinoma, metastatic renal cell carcinoma, Kaposi sarcoma, Paget's disease, malignant melanoma. |

- They are found to be more prevalent in sun-exposed areas, with underlying various benign (61.1%), premalignant (23.2%), and malignant (15.1%) conditions (**Table 17.1**). Clinical importance attached to cutaneous horn is in detection of type of underlying lesions.[1–4]

## CLINICAL FEATURES[1-6]

- Individuals with fair to light-skinned complexions are more susceptible, though it can be seen in all populations.
- They are found more commonly over sun-exposed areas of the body (approximately 30%), such as the scalp, upper face, peri-orbicular, ear, lips, neck, chest, and shoulders. However, they are also found over areas not exposed to sun, such as penis, mucosa of the lower lip, and nasal vestibule.
- Cutaneous horns are well-circumscribed keratinous white, yellow, pink, brown, black (mixtures of various shades) projections situated above the skin surface over the underlying benign premalignant or malignant lesions (**Figures 17.1** to **17.7**).

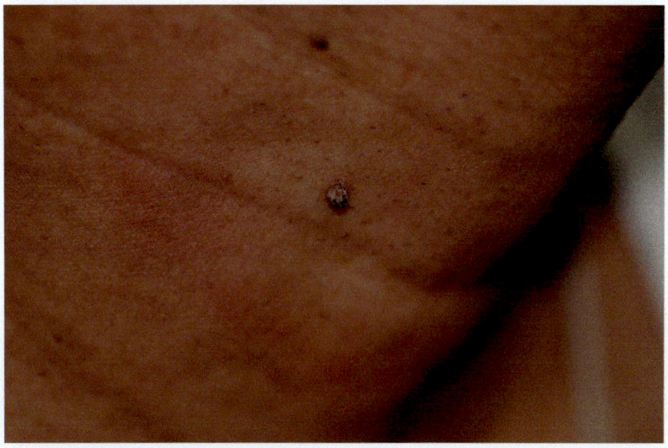

Figure 17.1 Cutaneous horn on the neck.

DOI: 10.1201/9781351054225-38

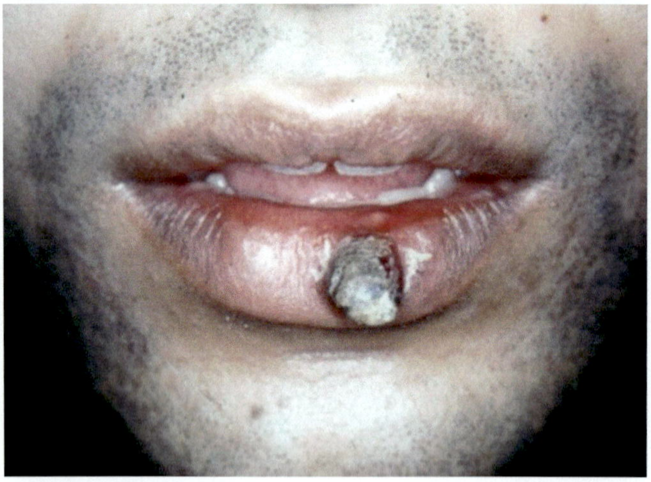

Figure 17.2 Cutaneous horn on lower lip. The underlying lesion in this case was verruca vulgaris.

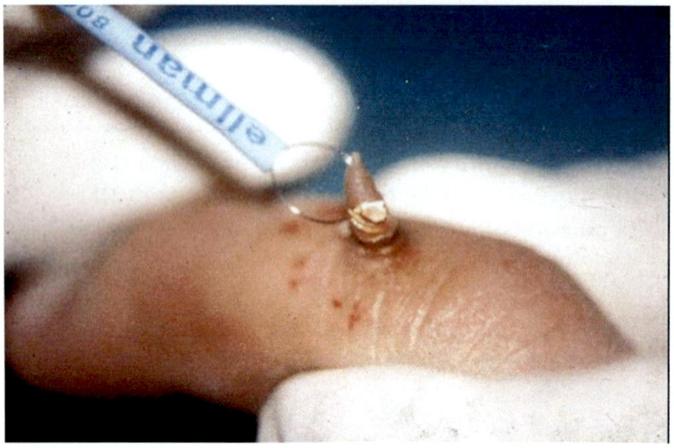


Figure 17.3 Cutaneous horn on the tip of finger.

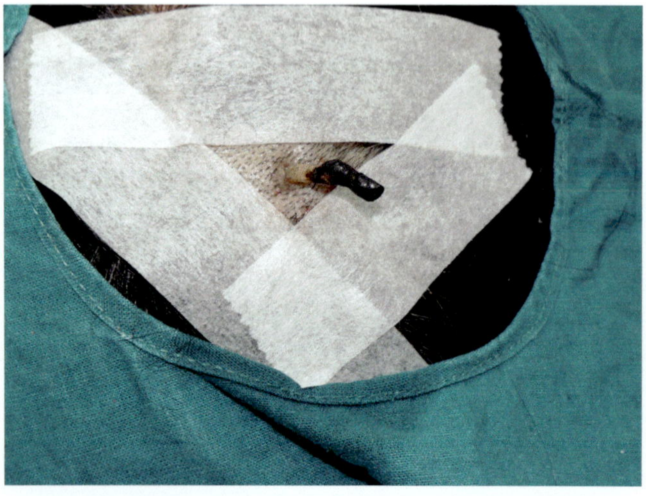

Figure 17.4 Long slender cutaneous horn on the scalp.

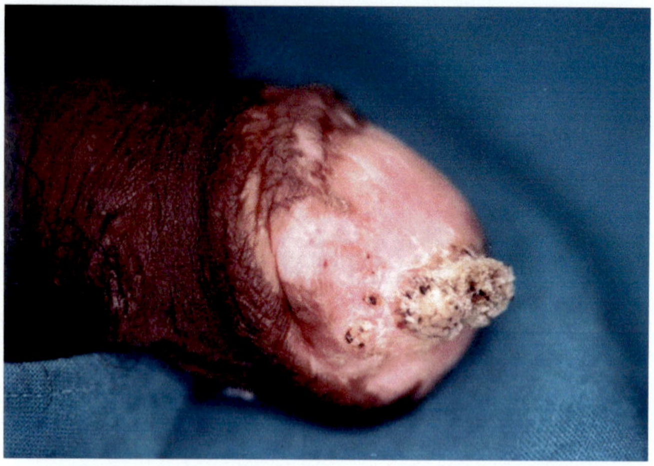

Figure 17.5 Multiple cutaneous horns on the penis in a case of Bowen's disease.

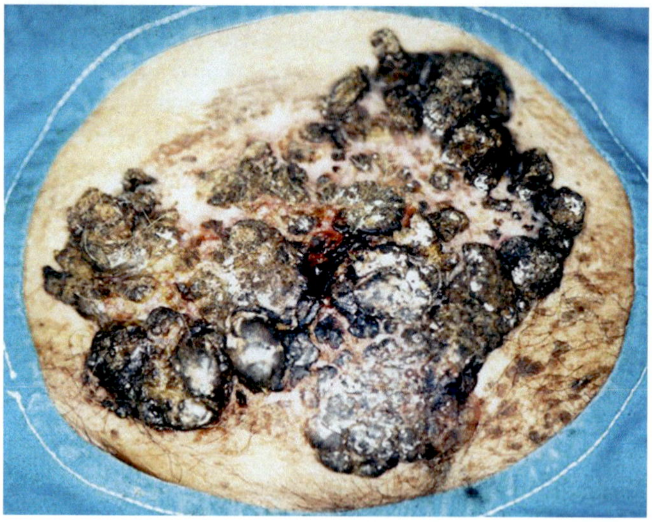

Figure 17.6 Multiple cutaneous horns in a case of Bowen's disease with squamous cell carcinoms (SCC) on the abdomen.

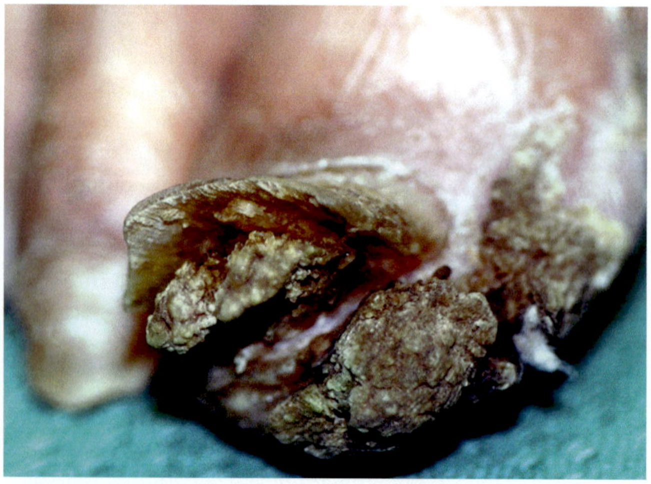

Figure 17.7 Multiple cutaneous horns on the great toe in a case of subungual Bowen's disease.

**BOX 17.1: Risk factors indicating possibility of underlying lesions being malignant**

- Previous history of actinic keratosis or skin cancer
- Male sex
- Fair skin
- Advanced age
- Presence of lesion in sun-exposed area
- Presence of erythema, inflammation, tenderness, infiltration, or indurations at the base
- Large base or larger width to height ratio
- Bleeding
- Giant size
- Increased verrucosity and presence of multiple horns

- They grow slowly over a long period of time (several years) and vary in sizes from a few millimeters to as long as 25 centimeters.
- They are considered giant if they are more than 1 cm. in height.
- They occur in different shapes, such as conical, cylindrical, curved, straight, pointed, and can be corrugated transversely as well as longitudinally.
- They are firm to hard in consistency, with little or no sensation.
- The base of the lesion may be flat, nodular, or crateriform.
- They are usually solitary but can have an associated smaller satellite lesion, or they can also be multiple.
- Cutaneous horns are slow-growing and cause very little physical discomfort unless they are mechanically pulled or when they are present in areas of physical irritation. However, they are cosmetically disfiguring and cause social discomfort for the patient.
- The main clinical importance, as stated earlier, is concern for the lesion underlying it, and hence deep excisional biopsy is indicated to rule out any premalignant or malignant lesion. The clinical diagnosis of underlying lesions is almost impossible; however, certain factors (enlisted in **Box 17.1**) raise suspicion of malignant lesions.

## REFERENCES


1. Fernandes NF, Sinha S, Lambert WC, Schwartz RA. Cutaneous horn: A potentially malignant entity. Acta Dermatovenerol Alp Pannonica Adriat 2009;18(4):189–193.
2. Rush PS, Cockerell CJ. Cutaneous horn. Available from https://emedicine.medscape.com/article/1056568-overview. Accessed on 09.04.2020.
3. Mantese SA, Diogo PM, Rocha A, Berbert AL, Ferreira AK, Ferreira TC. Cutaneous horn: A retrospective histopathological study of 222 cases. An Bras Dermatol 2010;85(2):157–163.
4. Copcu E, Sivrioglu N, Culhaci N. Cutaneous horns: Are these lesions as innocent as they seem to be? World J Surg Oncol 2004;2:18.
5. Sathyanarayana SA, Deutsch GB, Edelman M, Cohen-Kashi KJ. Cutaneous horn: A malignant lesion? A brief review of the literature. Dermatol Surg 2012;38(2):285–287.
6. Pyne J, Sapkota D, Wong JC. Cutaneous horns: Clues to invasive squamous cell carcinoma being present in the horn base. Dermatol Pract Concept. 2013 Apr 30;3(2):3–7.

# SECTION 3

# Regional dermatology

PIYUSH KUMAR, PC DAS

The skin is the largest organ of the human body, and despite its apparent uniform appearance, it has numerous regional variations both structurally and functionally. These variations enable skin to perform the region-specific tasks efficiently. Structural variations include difference in thickness of skin, presence or absence of specialized structures such as mucosa or nails, density of pilosebaceous units and eccrine glands, adipose tissue layer thickness, vascularity, innervation, presence/absence of horny layer, colonization by skin flora, and underlying lymph nodes. One or more of these structural variations make skin a heterogeneous structure composed of many unique topographical regions. For example, thicker skin in palms and soles can handle the trauma more effectively, while thinner skin over eyelids makes it easy for periorbital muscles to lift it; buccal mucosa houses the special receptors for taste, while genital mucosa has dense sensory receptors for sexual pleasures. All these regional variations are also associated with diseases that are localized to the specific regions of the body. Thus, each region is anatomically predisposed to develop a unique set of dermatoses. In addition, the microenvironment of a region may modify the morphology of a particular dermatosis. For example, axillae are constantly warm, occluded, and moist, leading to frequent macerations noted in diseases like Darier disease. Additionally, skin has some specialized structures such as mucosa, hairs, and nails that are affected by some unique dermatoses and may have distinctive presentations of various dermatoses.

Another factor that makes one skin region different from another one is external influences in the form of friction, occlusion, pressure, sun exposure, external trauma, and temperature, to name a few. One of the most common environmental insults is sun exposure, which is localized to sun-exposed areas and can be easily appreciated if one looks at areas that are not generally exposed to sun, such as the post-auricular area, upper eyelid, and so on. Skin folds are special areas that create a special environment (occlusion, moist, warmth) that makes it suitable for growth of certain organisms such as dermatophytes.

Considering anatomical variations and influence of external factors, it becomes obvious that skin has many unique regions that are predisposed to a different set of dermatoses. Recognition of variations in the localization of various dermatoses and awareness of the changes in the morphology of a particular dermatosis in different regions are essential components of skills required for making a clinical diagnosis.

DOI: 10.1201/9781351054225-39

# E20

# Scalp

PC DAS

## ABSTRACT

While most skin disorders affect the scalp skin in a manner the same as elsewhere on the body, a few conditions affect the scalp more frequently than other body sites. Additionally, the frequency and morphology of various dermatoses on scalp may be affected by presence or absence of hairs on the scalp. This chapter discusses the clinical approach to the diagnosis of various dermatoses commonly affecting scalp.

The text of this chapter is available online at https://routledgetextbooks.com/textbooks/9781032399669/

DOI: 10.1201/9781351054225-40

# E21

# Periorbital area

ANUP KUMAR TIWARY

## ABSTRACT

There are various cutaneous diseases that preferentially involve the periorbital region. Some systemic diseases, such as dermatomyositis, lupus, and histiocytosis, may also present with cutaneous changes in this area. To differentiate and make the correct diagnosis, it is imperative to identify the morphology, distribution, and other clinical characteristics of periorbital dermatoses. This chapter briefly describes the clinical approach to the diagnosis of periorbital dermatoses.

The text of this chapter is available online at https://routledgetextbooks.com/textbooks/9781032399669/


DOI: 10.1201/9781351054225-41

# E22

# Ears

DIVYA SACHDEV

## ABSTRACT

Dermatoses of the ear fall under the purview of various medical disciplines such as dermatology, otorhinolaryngology, and general medicine. The ear is anatomically a unique structure as it is composed of elastic cartilage covered by skin and is poorly vascularized. The dermatoses of the external ear may serve as a mirror to various systemic diseases such as Frank's sign for coronary artery disease, bluish discoloration of ear in alkaptonuria, etc. At the same time, there are numerous dermatoses that are specific for the ear, such as juvenile spring eruption, acanthoma fissuratum, etc. Therefore, it is imperative to familiarize ourselves with the various dermatoses that may affect the ear.

The text of this chapter is available online at https://routledgetextbooks.com/textbooks/9781032399669/

DOI: 10.1201/9781351054225-42

E23

# Nose

DIVYA SACHDEV


## ABSTRACT

The nose is affected in a variety of dermatological diseases. Being the most prominent part of mid-face, it is anatomically, physiologically, esthetically, and psychologically important. Any dermatosis affecting the nose has physical as well as grave psycho-social impacts on the health of the patient. Therefore, it is imperative to familiarize ourselves with the various presentations of skin diseases that may affect the nose in order to facilitate early diagnosis and proper management.


The text of this chapter is available online at https://routledgetextbooks.com/textbooks/9781032399669/



DOI: 10.1201/9781351054225-43

# 18

# Oral mucosa

SUNIL KOTHIWALA, KANYA RANI VASHISHT

## INTRODUCTION

The oral cavity is oval shaped and is separated into the oral vestibule and the oral cavity proper. It is bound by the lips anteriorly, the cheeks laterally, the floor of the mouth inferiorly, the oropharynx posteriorly, and the palate superiorly. The epithelium that lines the oral mucosa derives mostly from ectoderm except posterior one-third of the tongue, which derives from endoderm. In contrast to the skin, the oral epithelium exhibits different patterns of keratinization, with higher proliferation rate. The masticatory mucosa (hard palate, gingiva, and alveolar mucosa) has keratinized or parakeratinized (retained nuclei in the stratum corneum) squamous epithelium. The tongue has parakeratinized, non-keratinized, and specialized epithelia (papillae). The buccal mucosa and vestibule have non-keratinized stratified or parakeratinized squamous epithelia, respectively. The supporting connective tissue is of ectomesenchymal origin.

The oral cavity can be affected primarily by disease of mucosa and adjoining structures as well as by systemic diseases. Many dermatological conditions, including genetic, inflammatory, infective and neoplastic disorders, can also occur in oral mucosa with similar clinicopathologic features. Occasionally, the oral cavity can be the only site of a skin disease, as in lichen planus, pemphigus, and mucous membrane pemphigoid. Diagnosing and treating mucosal lesions of the mouth, including the gums, is challenging for most clinicians because of the wide variety of conditions that can present with similar-appearing lesions. This chapter explores both common and uncommon oral pathologies, and it follows conventional classification of lesions. Oral mucosal lesions can be divided based on color of lesion (i.e., white, erythematous, and pigmented) and morphology of lesions, such as ulcerative, verrucous, and lump and swellings (**Tables 18.1** and **18.2**). It emphasizes clinical description of lesions, common sites of pathology, and differential diagnosis. Gingival hyperplasia and cheilitis are described separately.[1-9]

## WHITE LESIONS

White lesions of the oral mucosa are multifactorial group of disorders, the color of which is produced by scattering of the light through an altered epithelial surface (**Figure 18.1**).

The oral mucosa becomes white due to

1. Excess production of keratin intrinsically or from benign keratotic disease (genodermatoses) or dysplasia

Table 18.1 Approach to oral pathologies based on color of lesion

| White lesions | Red lesions | Pigmented lesions |
|---|---|---|
| Leukoplakia | **Hereditary** | Melanotic macule |
| Leukoedema | Vascular malformation | Amalgam tattoo |
| Hairy leukoplakia | Hereditary mucoepithelial dysplasia | Heavy metal deposition |
| Lichen planus | **Acquired** | Drug-induced pigmentation |
| Geographic tongue | Trauma | Smoker's melanosis |
| Hairy tongue | Thermal burn | Freckles and lentigines |
| Candidiasis | Radiation mucositis | Pigmented nevi |
| Fissured tongue | Median rhomboid glossitis | Nevus of Ota |
| Nicotinic stomatitis | Denture-related stomatitis | Melanoma |
| White sponge nevus | Erythroplakia | Melanoacanthoma |
| Dyskeratosis congenital | Plasma cell gingivitis | Addison's disease |
| Pachyonychia congenital | Lupus erythematosus | Peutz-Jeghers syndrome |
| Chemical burn | Anemia | |
| | Thrombocytopenic purpura | |
| | Inflectional mononucleosis | |
| | Reiter's disease | |

DOI: 10.1201/9781351054225-44

Table 18.2 Approach to oral pathology based on morphology of lesions

| Ulcerative lesions | | Verrucous lesions | Lump and swelling |
|---|---|---|---|
| **Prior history of vesicobullous lesions** | **Without history of vesicobullous lesions** | | |
| Herpes simplex | Aphthous ulcer | Papilloma | Angioedema |
| Herpes zoster | Behçet's disease | Verruca vulgaris | Abscess |
| Herpangina | Syphilis | Condyloma accuminatum | Mucocele |
| Hand, foot, and mouth disease | Tuberculosis | Focal epidermal hyperplasia | Ranula |
| Erythema multiforme | Leprosy | Verrucous xanthoma | Fibroma |
| Stevens-Johnson syndrome | Leishmaniasis | Acanthosis nigricans | Pyogenic granuloma |
| Toxic epidermal necrolysis | Eosinophilic ulcer | Darier disease | |
| Pemphigus | Squamous cell carcinoma | | |
| Bullous pemphigoid | | | |
| Cicatracial pemphigoid | | | |
| Pemphigoidgestationis | | | |
| Linear IgA disease | | | |
| Dermatitis herpetiformis | | | |
| Bullous lichen planus | | | |
| Epidermolysis bullosa | | | |
| Epidermolysis bullosa acquisita | | | |

2. Excess production of keratin in response to injury (e.g., friction or biting)
3. Thickening of the epithelium
4. Damage to epithelial cells from direct and identifiable contact injury

## Leukoplakia

- This is defined as a precancerous white patch or plaque firmly attached to the oral mucosa.
- Tobacco, alcohol, chronic local friction, and *Candida albicans* are important predisposing factors.
- Clinically it can be divided into two types: homogeneous (common) and non-homogeneous (**Table 18.3**).
  - The homogeneous type is usually a thin, flat, and uniform white plaque with at least one area that is well demarcated, with or without fissuring (**Figure 18.2a,b**).

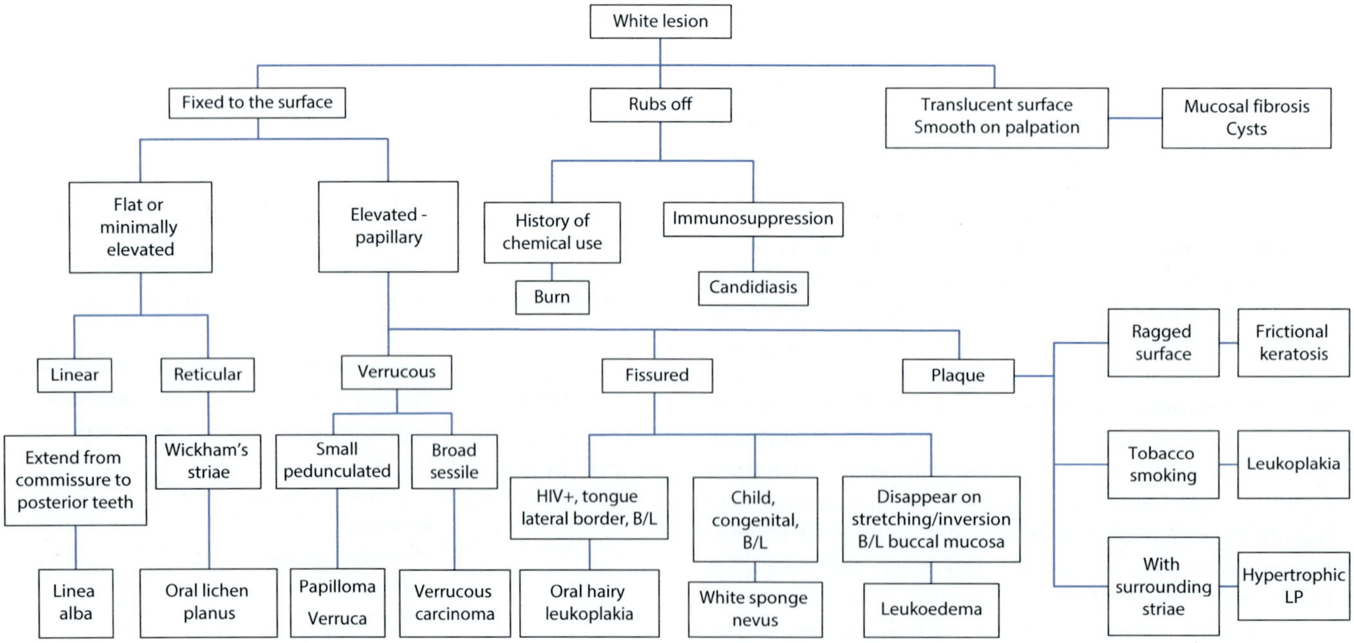


Figure 18.1 Clinical approach to white lesions of the mucosa.

Table 18.3 Main differences between localized leukoplakia and proliferative leukoplakia

| | Localized leukoplakia | Proliferative verrucous leukoplakia |
|---|---|---|
| Epidemiology | Men > Women | Women > Men |
| Association with smoking | Strong | Weak |
| Location | Single site,<br>Ventral tongue and floor of mouth are most common sites | Multifocal<br>Gingiva is most common site |
| Dysplasia or SCC at first biopsy | 40% | <10%, mostly atypical verrucous hyperplasia or KUS |
| Malignant transformation | 3–15% overall, 1–3% per year | 70–100% overall, 10% per year |
| Treatment | Easy to ablate or excise because localized | Difficult to treat because multifocal |

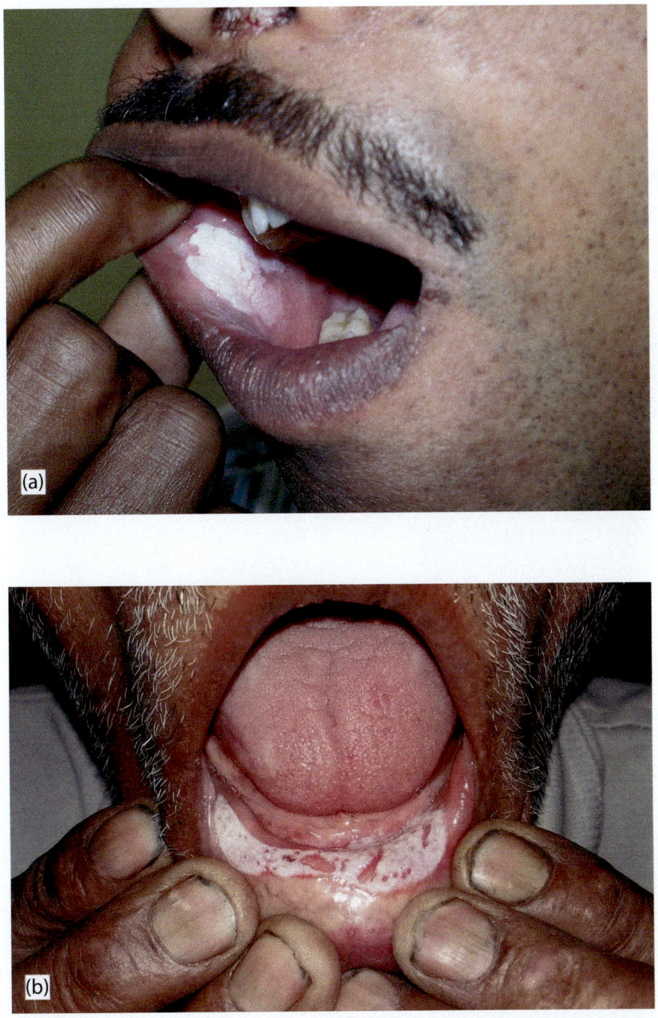

Figure 18.2 **(a)** Well-demarcated localized white plaque on buccal mucosa lip in homogenous leukoplakia. **(b)** Homogenous leukoplakia of the lip. (a – Courtesy: Dr. Piyush Kumar, Katihar, India; b – Courtesy: Dr. Hiral Shah, Baroda Medical College, Vadodara, India.)

    - Non-homogeneous lesions can have the presence of speckled or erythroplakic and nodular or verrucous areas (**Figure 18.3**).
    - Proliferative verrucous leukoplakia presents as irregular, white, exophytic plaque with a papillary surface and characterized by relative progression and spread (**Figure 18.4**).
- The most common sites are the buccal mucosa, tongue, floor of the mouth, gingiva, and lower lip.
- Malignant transformation for localized leukoplakia varies between 3% and 15%. Speckled and verrucous

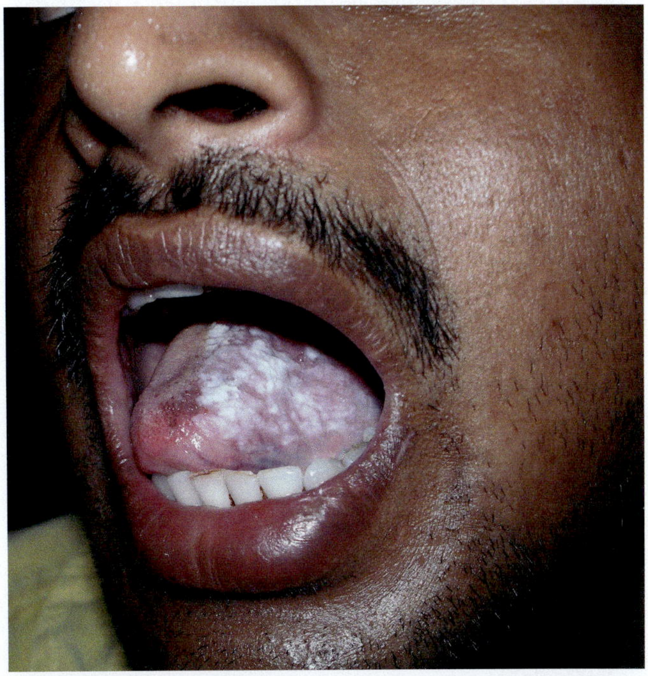

Figure 18.3 Non-homogenous leukoplakia having mild verrucous surface. (Courtesy: Dr. Piyush Kumar, Katihar, India.)

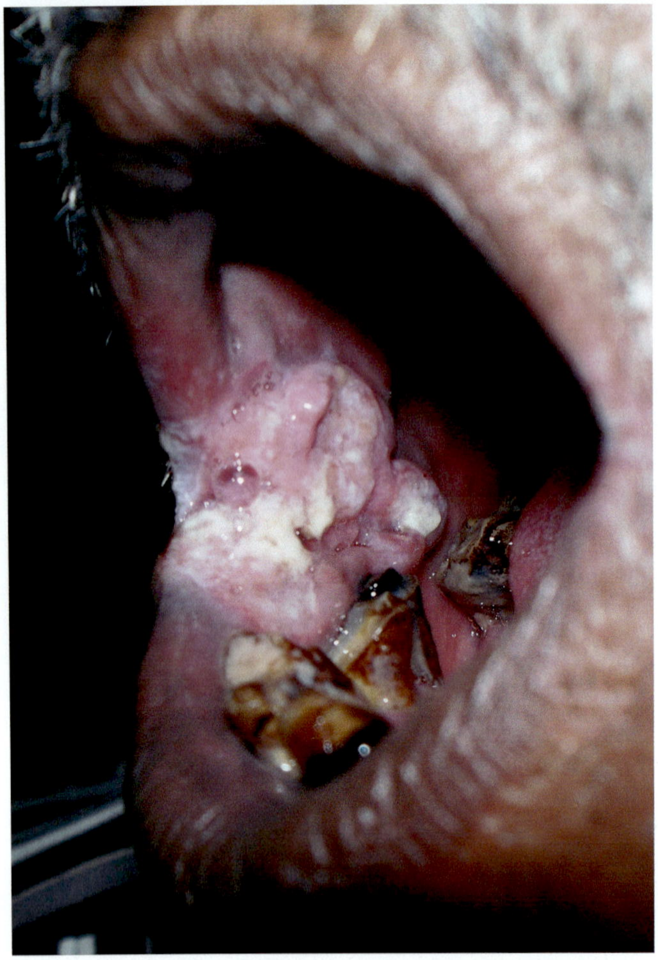

Figure 18.4 Proliferative verrucous leukoplakia. (Courtesy: Dr. Piyush Kumar, Katihar, India.)

leukoplakia have a greater risk for malignant transformation than the homogeneous form.
- DD: Leukoedema, lichen planus, keratosis of unknown significance (KUS), squamous cell carcinoma, in situ and invasive, verruca vulgaris, chronic chewing, chemical burn.

## Leukoedema

- This is a normal anatomical variation. It usually occurs over the buccal mucosa.
- It results from increased thickness of the epithelium and intracellular edema of the prickle-cell layer.
- Clinically, it is characterized by a whitish-gray edematous lesion with a slightly wrinkled surface, which characteristically disappears when the mucosa is averted and stretched.
- DD: Leukoplakia, white sponge nevus, oral hairy leukoplakia.

## Hairy leukoplakia

- Hairy leukoplakia is a non-precancerous lesion, one of the most common and characteristic lesions of human immunodeficiency virus (HIV) infection,
- Epstein–Barr virus seems to play an important role in the pathogenesis.
- It commonly appears bilaterally on the lateral margins of the tongue, and may spread to the dorsum and the ventral surface.
- Clinically it presents as asymptomatic white, elevated plaque with vertically oriented corrugations on surfaces that cannot be rubbed off.
- DD: Geographic tongue, frictional keratosis, pseudo-hairy leukoplakia, hyperplastic candidiasis.

## Lichen planus

- This is a common chronic mucocutaneous disease mediated by CD8+ T cell-mediated autoimmune phenomena.
- Skin involvement in mucosal lichen planus is 40%.
- Mucosal involvement in lichen planus is 40–60%.
- The buccal mucosa, tongue, and gingiva are the sites of predilection.
- Six clinical types have been described.
  - Reticular: white papules that coalesce to form a network of lines (Wickham's striae, **Figure 18.5a–d**)
  - Erosive/ulcerative: well to ill-defined shallow ulcer with overlying fibrin clots (**Figure 18.6a–d**)

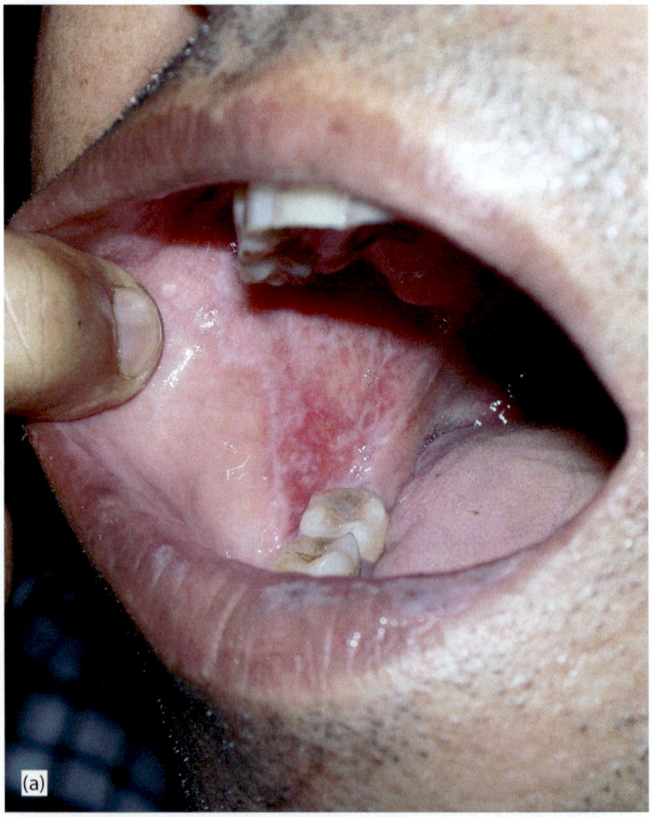


Figure 18.5 **(a)** Reticular lichen planus with Wickham striae on buccal mucosa. *(Continued)*

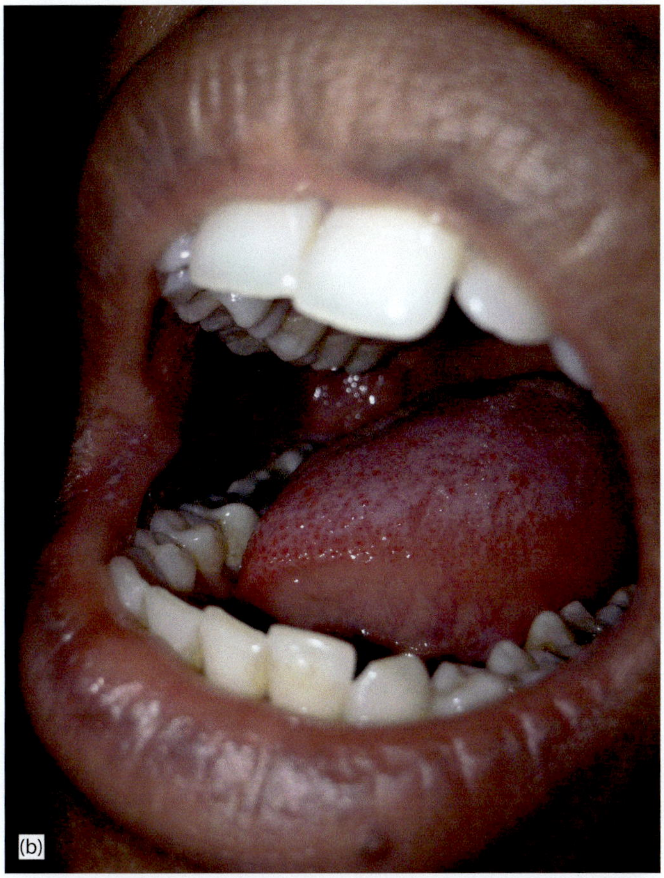


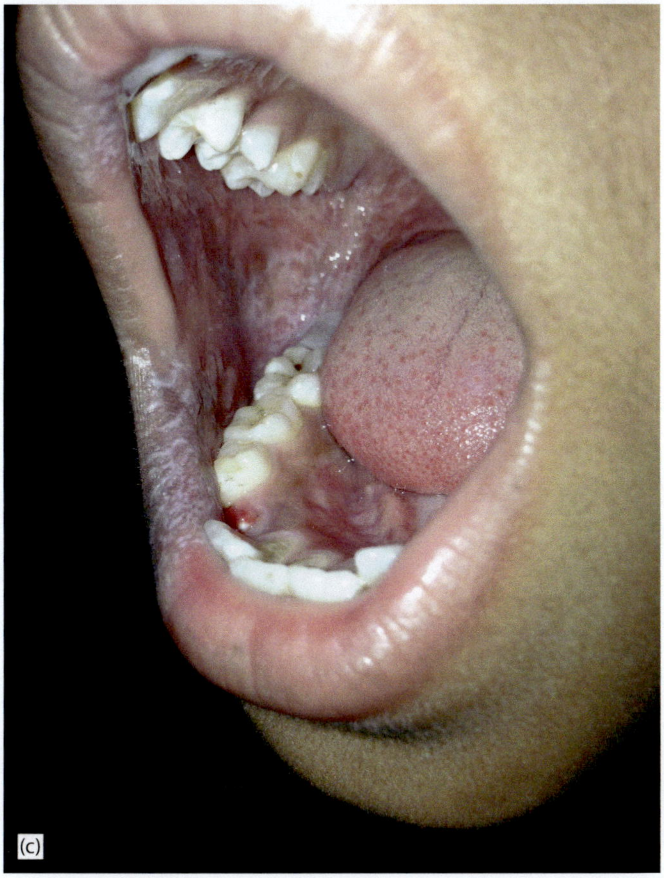


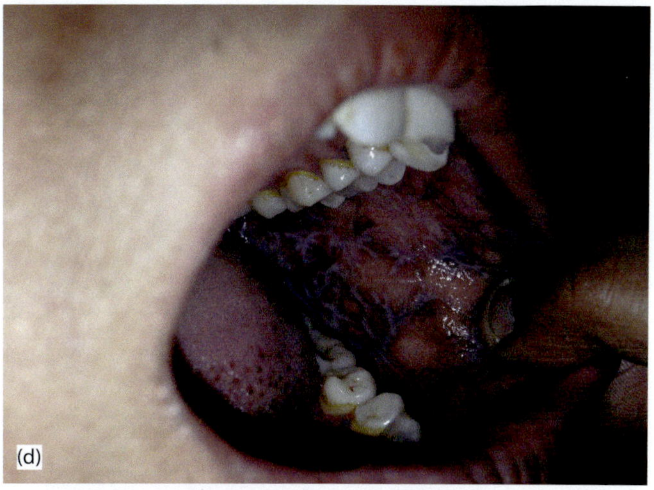


Figure 18.5 (*Continued*) **(b)** Reticular whitish plaque of lichen planus on tongue. **(c)** Reticular oral lichen planus affecting buccal mucosa and lip. **(d)** Reticular lichen planus with pigmentation. (a – Courtesy: Dr. Piyush Kumar, Katihar, India.)

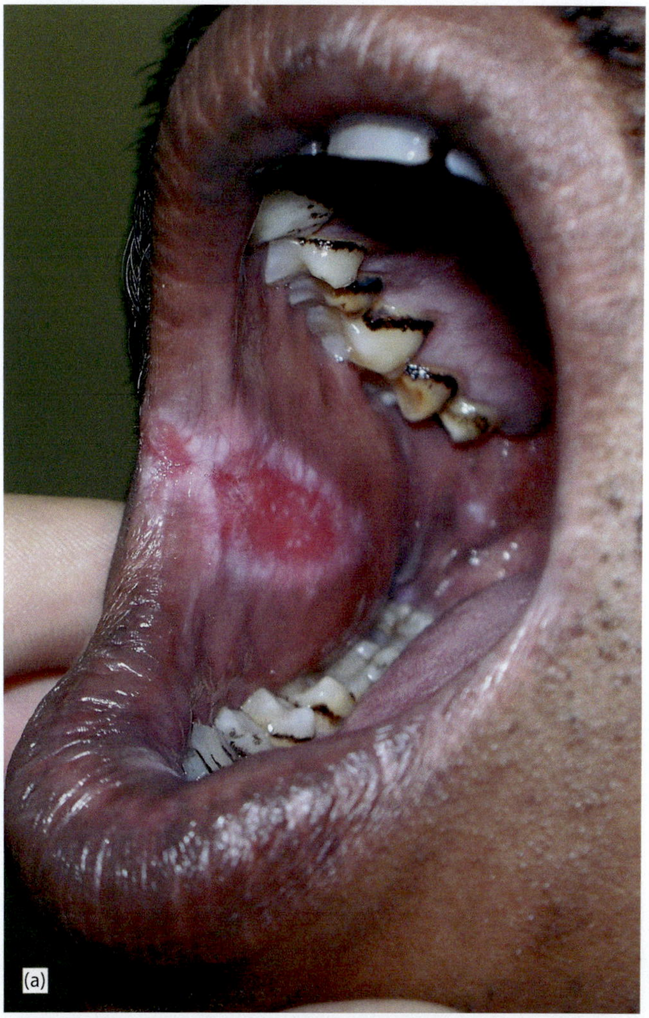


Figure 18.6 **(a)** Erosive lichen planus on buccal mucosa. (*Continued*)

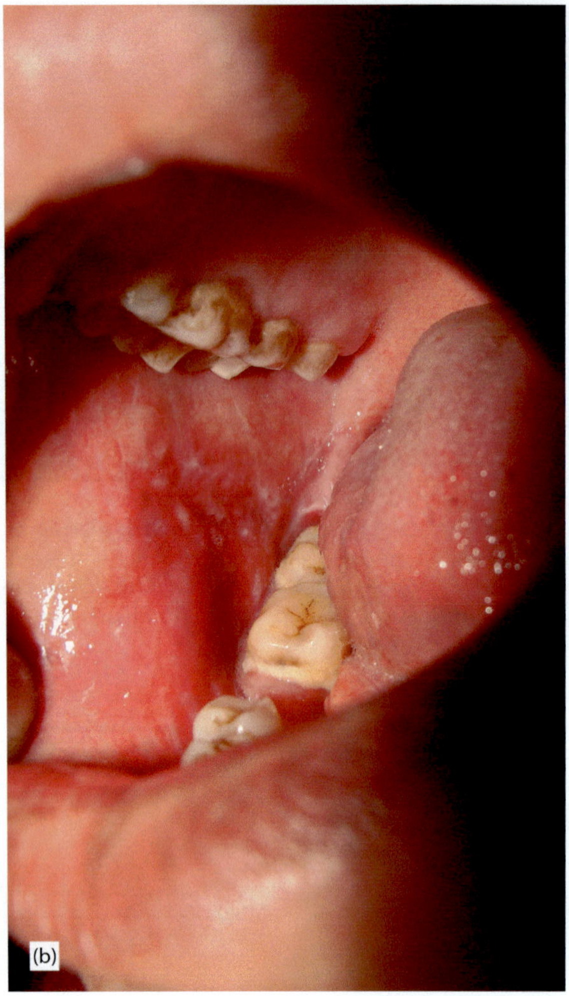


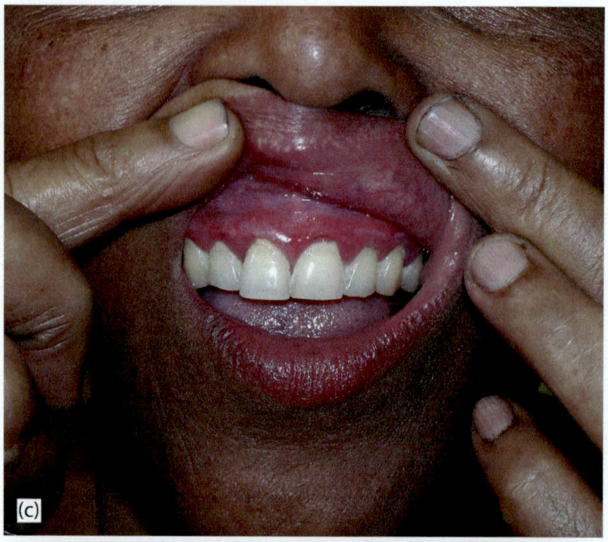


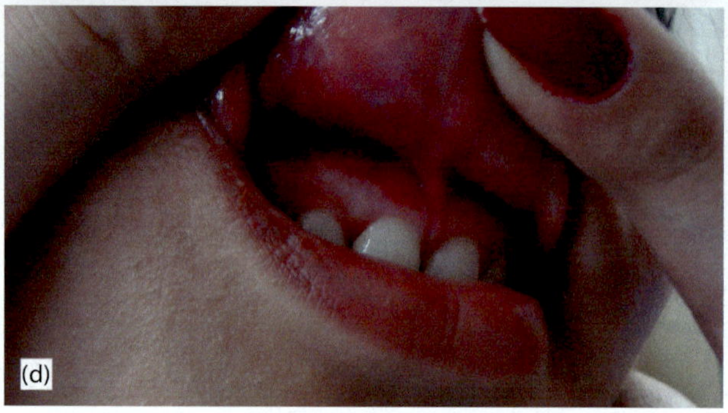


Figure 18.6 (*Continued*) **(b)** Erosive lichen planus on buccal mucosa. **(c,d)** Erosive lichen planus affecting gingiva. (a,c – Courtesy: Dr. Piyush Kumar, Katihar, India.)

- Atrophic: shiny plaques often with Wickham striae in surrounding mucosa (**Figure 18.7**)
- Hypertrophic: leukoplakia with Wickham striae (**Figure 18.8a,b**)
- Bullous: intact blisters that lead to erosive LP after rupture (**Figure 18.9**)
- Pigmented: discrete to coalescing brown patches (**Figure 18.10a,b**)

- The lesions may appear as a mixture of clinical subtypes.
- DD: Lichenoid drug reaction, mucous membrane pemphigoid.

## Geographic tongue

- Geographic tongue is a common benign condition, primarily affecting the tongue and rarely other oral mucosa sites (geographic stomatitis).
- It presents as multiple, irregularly shaped, well-demarcated, red, map-like smooth patches, typically surrounded by a slightly elevated

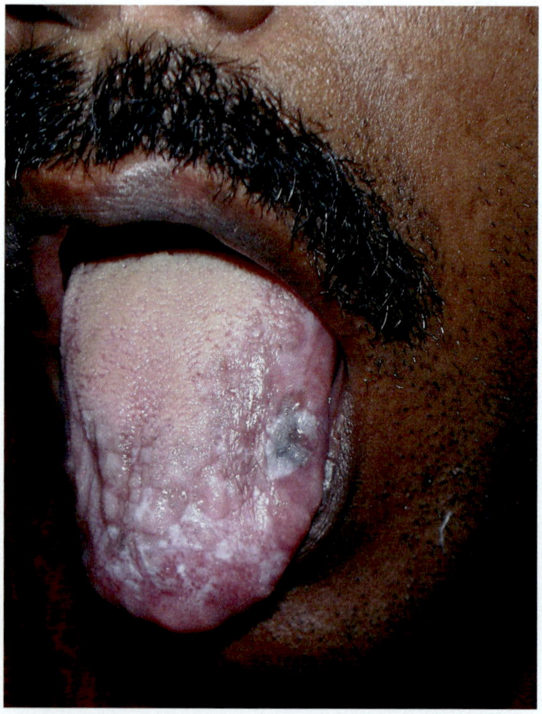

Figure 18.7 Atrophic lichen planus. (Courtesy: Dr. Piyush Kumar, Katihar, India.)

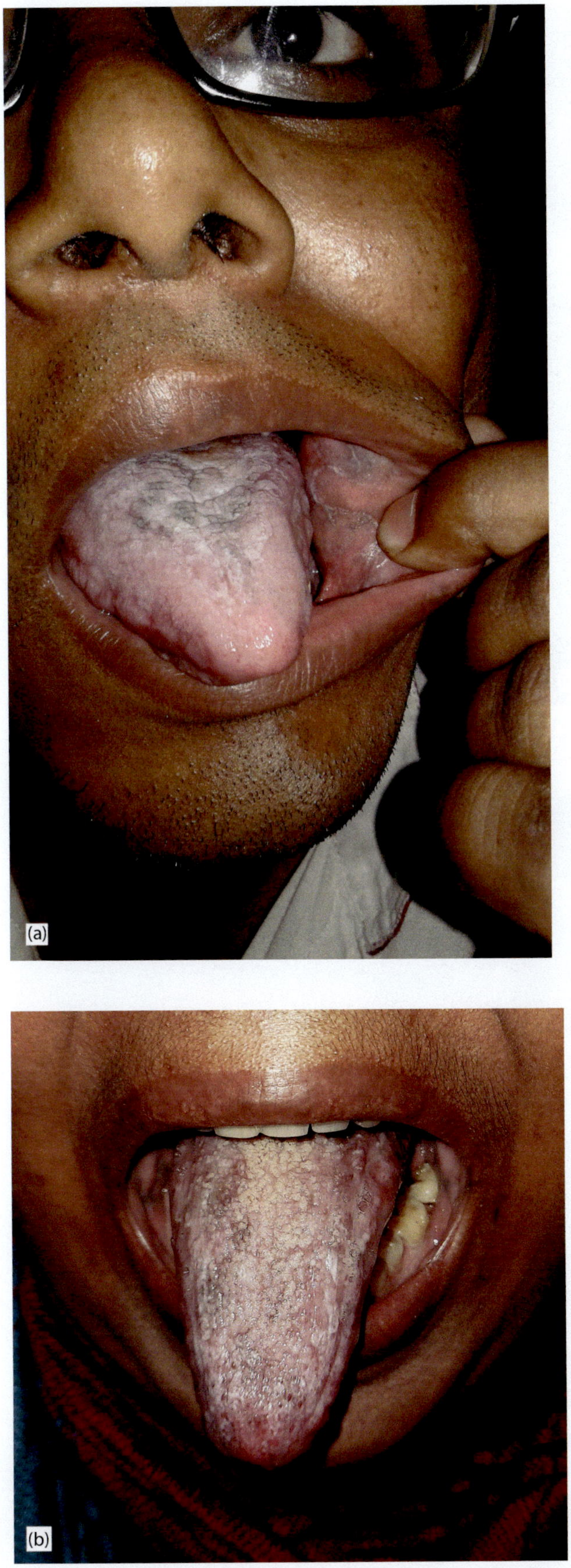

Figure 18.8 **(a,b)** Hypertrophic lichen planus. (Courtesy: Dr. Piyush Kumar, Katihar, India.)

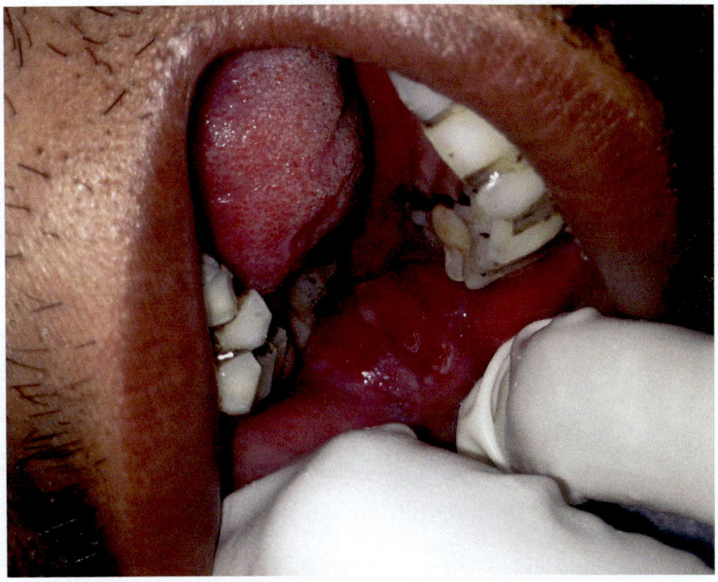

Figure 18.9 Ulcer following bullous lichen planus.

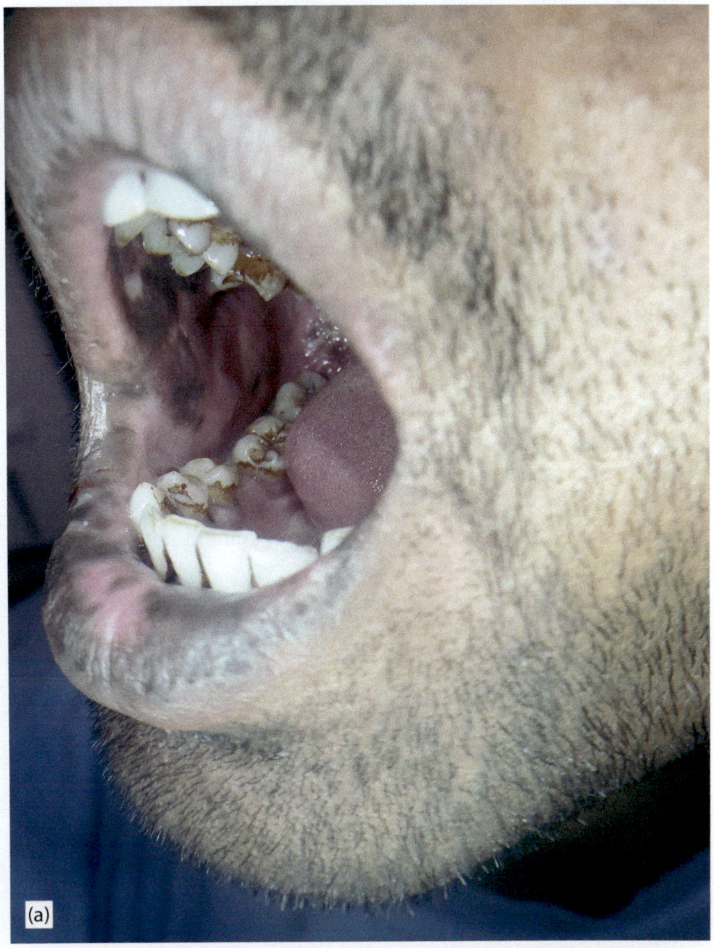

Figure 18.10 **(a)** Multiple dark-brown macules on buccal mucosa and lip. (*Continued*)

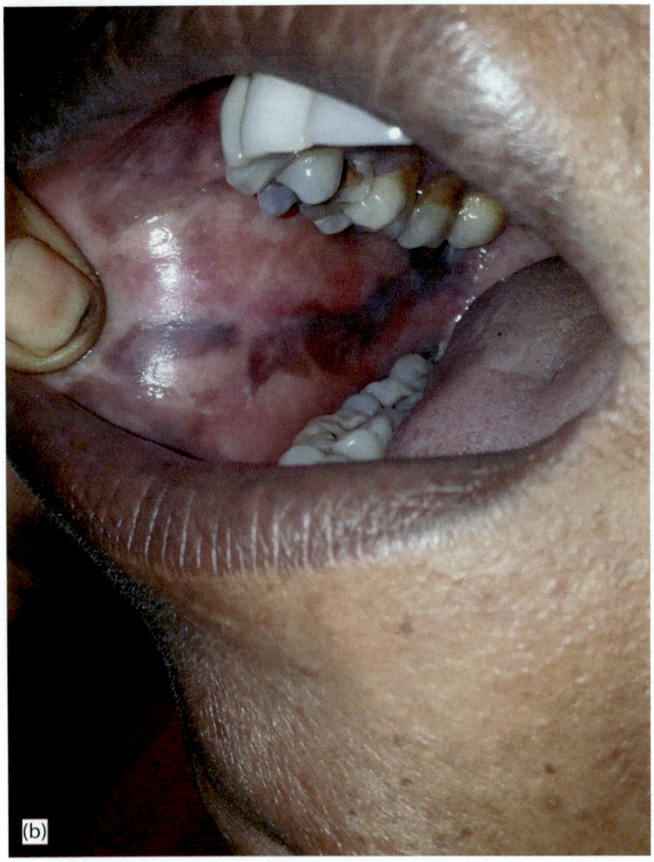

Figure 18.10 (*Continued*) **(b)** Pigmented lichen planus. (a – Courtesy: Dr. Ashutosh Ranjan, Chhapra, India; b – Dr. Hiral Shah, Baroda Medical College, Vadodara, India.)

whitish border on the dorsum of the tongue (**Figure 18.11a,b**).

- It is also known as benign migratory glossitis because the lesions persist for a short time in one area, then disappear completely and reappear in another area. The condition is usually asymptomatic and often coexists with a fissured tongue.
- DD: Chemical burns, fissured tongue, lichen planus, candidiasis.

## Hairy tongue

- This is characterized by a marked accumulation of keratin on the filiform papillae of the tongue, resulting in a hair-like pattern.
- Poor oral hygiene, oxidizing mouthwashes, antibiotics, excessive smoking, radiation therapy, emotional stress, and bacterial and Candida species infections are predisposing factors.
- It is usually asymptomatic and appears as elongation of the filiform papillae on the dorsal surface of

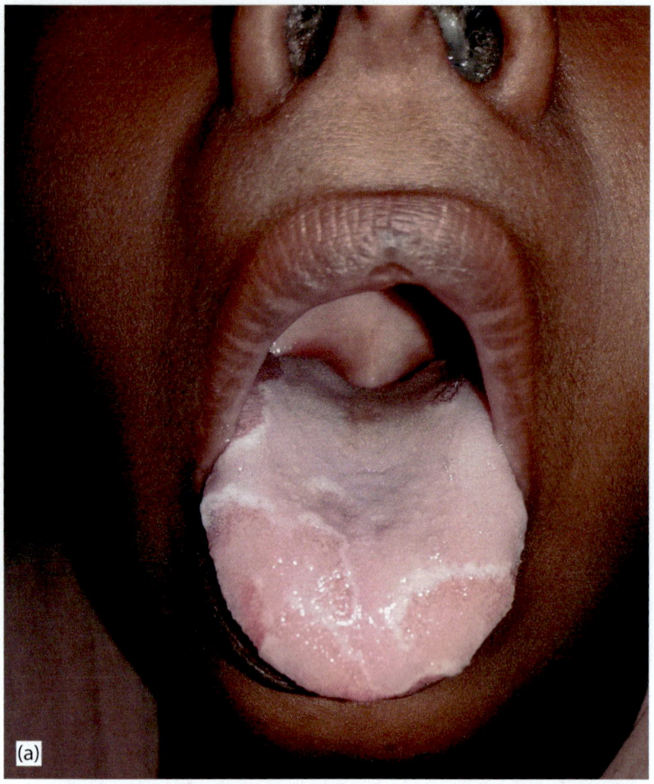

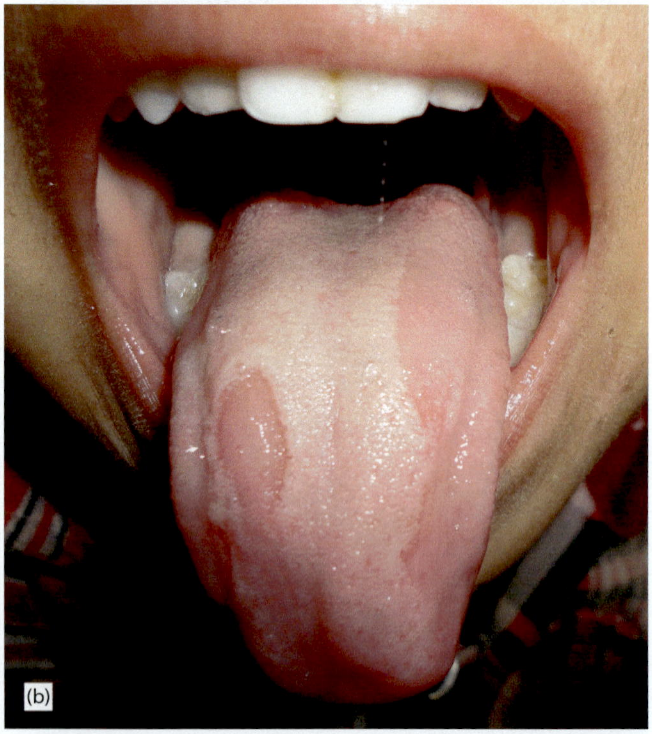

Figure 18.11 **(a)** Geographic tongue presenting with map-like well-demarcated smooth patches surrounded by white borders. **(b)** Geographic tongue. (b – Courtesy: Dr. Piyush Kumar, Katihar, India.)

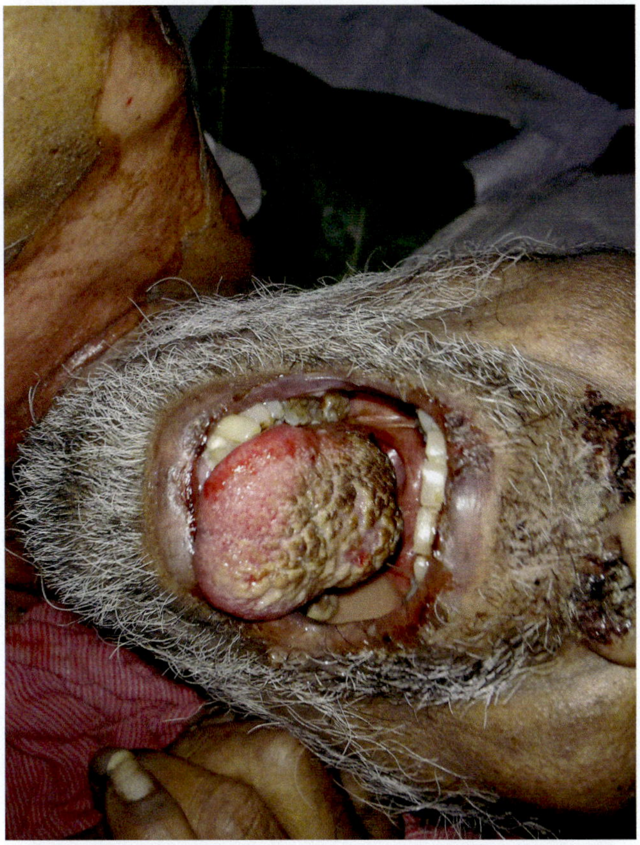

Figure 18.12 Hairy tongue in a patient of paraneoplastic pemphigus. (Courtesy: Dr. Hiral Shah, Baroda Medical College, Vadodara, India.)

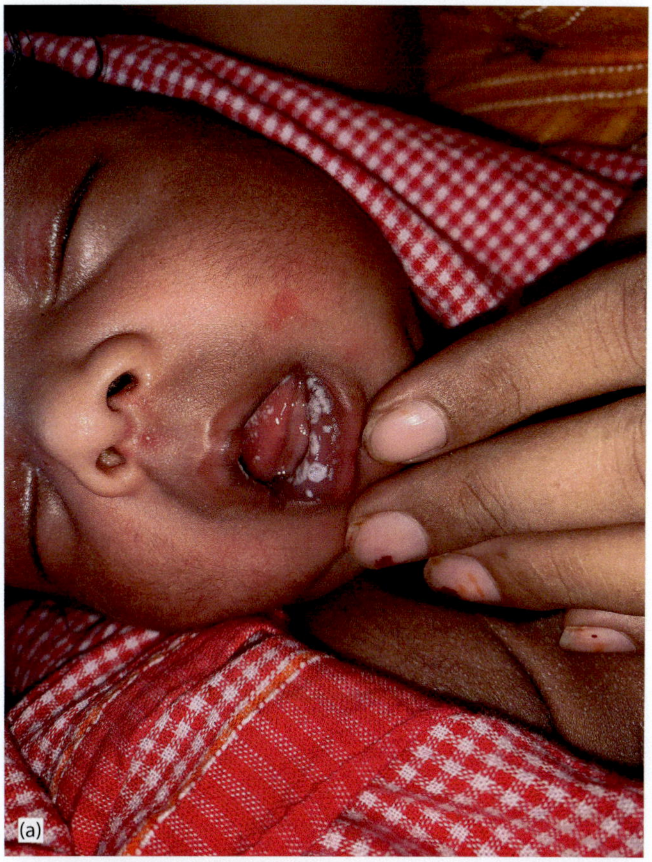

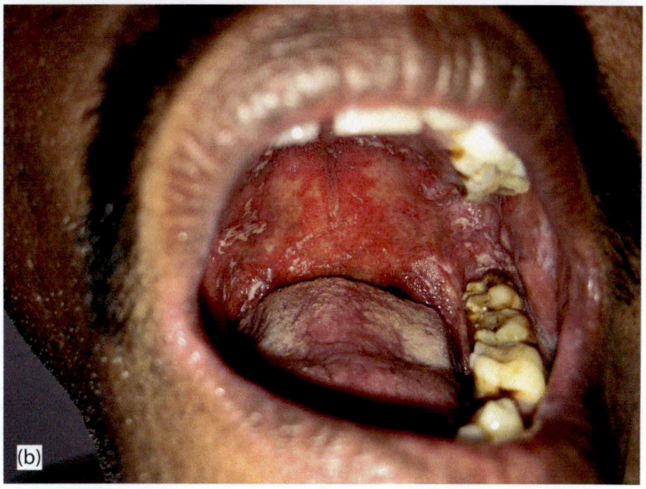

Figure 18.13 Oral candidiasis presenting as **(a)** slightly elevated white plaque on lip mucosa, **(b)** with erythema all over oral cavity in case of oral thrush. (Courtesy: Dr. Piyush Kumar, Katihar, India.)

the tongue, giving a whitish to brown-black color (**Figure 18.12**).

- DD: Amalgam tattoo, drug-induced pigmentation, heavy metal deposits.

## Candidiasis

- This is the most common oral fungal infection.
- It is usually caused by *Candida albicans* and less frequently by other fungal species (*C. glabrata, C. krusei, C. tropicalis, C. parapsilosis*).
- Predisposing factors are local (poor oral hygiene, xerostomia, mucosal damage, dentures, and antibiotic mouthwashes) and systemic (broad-spectrum antibiotics, steroids, immunosuppressive drugs, radiation, HIV infection, hematological malignancies, neutropenia, iron-deficiency anemia, cellular immunodeficiency, endocrine disorders).
- Oral candidiasis is classified as
    - Primary, consisting of lesions exclusively on the oral and perioral area.
        - Pseudomembranous candidiasis is the most common form of the disease and is clinically characterized by creamy-white, slightly elevated, removable spots or plaque (**Figure 18.13a,b**).
        - Nodular candidiasis is a chronic form of the disease; it appears clinically as a white, firm, and raised plaque that usually does not detach from mucosa (**Figure 18.14**).
        - Other subtypes include erythematous, papillary hyperplasia of the palate and candida-associated

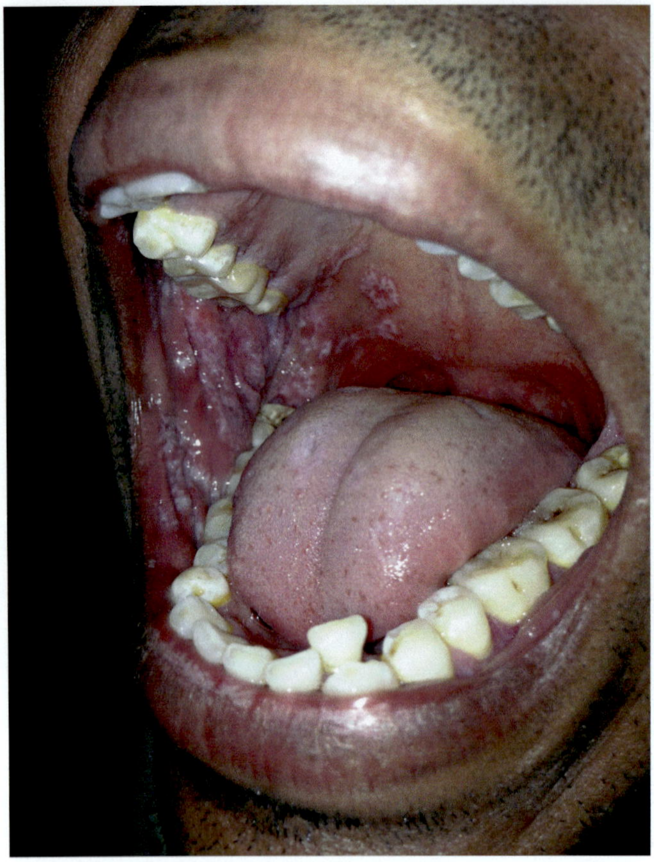

Figure 18.14 Nodular candidiasis presenting as white, raised, non-scrapable plaque on soft palate, oropharynx, and buccal mucosa.

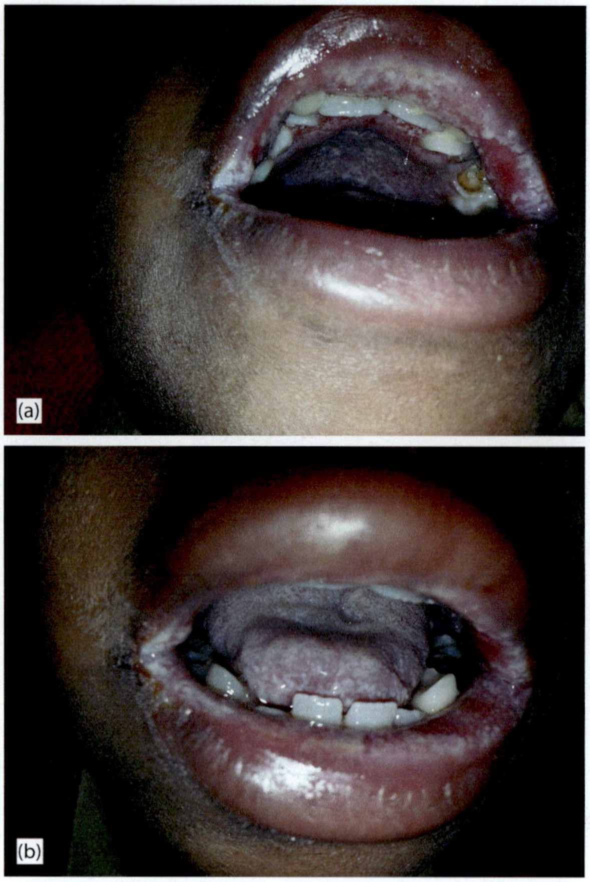

Figure 18.15 **(a,b)** Mucocutaneous candidiasis showing diffuse involvement of oral cavity and angle of mouth. (Courtesy: Dr. Hiral Shah, Baroda Medical College, Vadodara, India.)

lesions (angular cheilitis, median rhomboid glossitis, denture stomatitis).
- Secondary, consisting of oral lesions of mucocutaneous disease.

- Mucocutaneous candidiasis is a heterogeneous and rare group of clinical syndromes, characterized by chronic lesions of the skin, nails, and mucosae, and usually associated with immunological defects. Oral lesions appear as white and usually multiple plaques that cannot be wiped off (**Figure 18.15a,b**).

## Fissured tongue

- This is a benign condition affecting the dorsum of tongue in the form of shallow or deep and prominent groves of variable depth and size. Many times it is associated with a focal whitish coating of tongue (**Figure 18.16**) or geographical tongue (**Figure 18.17**).
- The etiology is not clearly defined, but sometimes it is seen in orofacial granulomatosis, Melkersson-Rosenthal syndrome, Down syndrome, and pustular psoriasis.
- It is usually asymptomatic, but painful or burning sensations develop when food debris get arrested in grooves or it is associated with geographic tongue. The prominence of the condition appears to increase with increasing age.

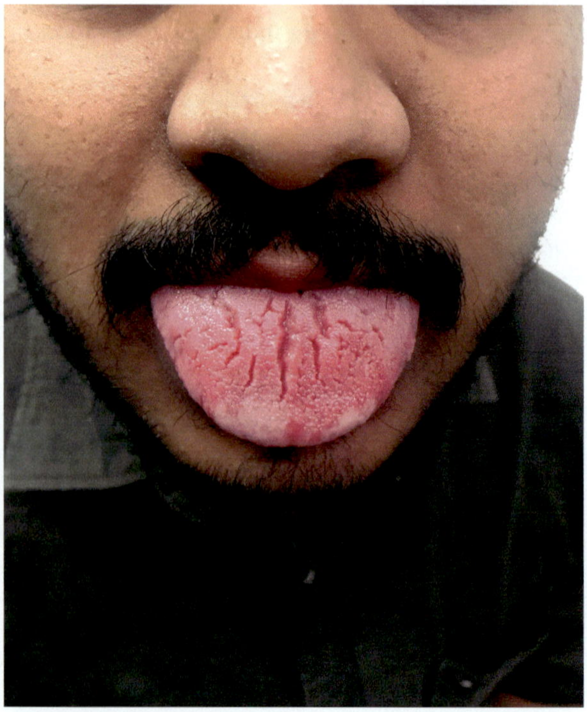

Figure 18.16 Multiple shallow and deep grooves on dorsum of tongue with whitish coating at tip of tongue.

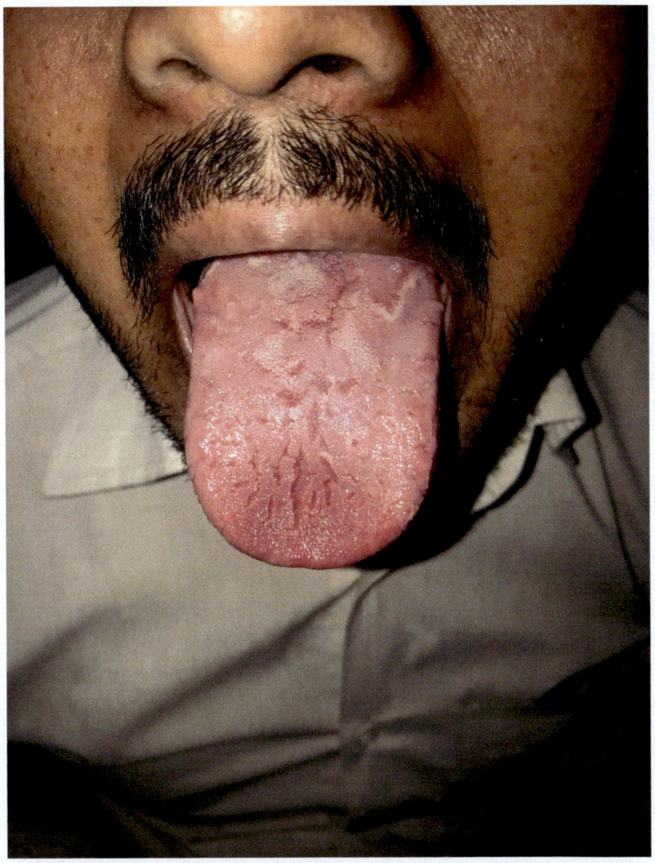

Figure 18.17 Fissured tongue with geographic tongue.

### Nicotinic stomatitis

- Nicotinic stomatitis is a common keratosis associated with heavy pipe and cigar smoking; it exclusively occurs on the hard palate. It is non-premalignant, in contrast to reverse smoker's palate.
- Clinically, it starts with erythema; gradually it becomes wrinkled and diffuse grayish-white in color, with numerous punctate red-centered micronodules that represent the inflamed and dilated orifices of the minor salivary gland ducts.
- DD: Candidiasis, leukoplakia, hairy leukoplakia.

### White sponge nevus

- This is a hereditary dyskeratotic hyperplasia of mucous membrane.
- Autosomal dominant inheritance usually appears in early childhood.
- It presents at symmetrical white, thickened, velvety lesions with multiple furrows and a spongy texture.
- Buccal mucosa and the ventral surface of the tongue are the sites of predilection

### Dyskeratosis congenita

- This is related to autosomal recessive or X-linked inheritance.
- It is characterized by hyperpigmentation, atrophic skin areas, telangiectasia, nail dystrophy, hyperhidrosis, skin and mucosal bullae, blepharitis and ectropion, and anemia.
- The most common oral lesions are leukoplakia, atrophy of papillae, intraoral brown pigmentation, recurrent blisters, taurodont teeth (enlarged pulp chambers and short roots), and dental caries.

### Pachyonychia congenita

- This is an autosomal dominant inheritance
- It is characterized by symmetrical nail thickening, palmoplantar hyperkeratosis, hyperhidrosis, blister formation, follicular keratosis, and oral lesions.
- Oral leukokeratosis presents as thick, painful, white or grayish-white plaques, usually on the tongue and buccal surface in first year of birth. It may interfere with suckling and breastfeeding.

### Chemical burn

- This is injury to the oral mucosa caused by topical application of caustic agents.
- Clinically, the affected mucosa is covered with a white membrane due to necrosis. The necrotic epithelium can easily be scraped off, leaving a red, bleeding surface. The lesions are painful.

# ULCERATIVE LESIONS

## Preceding with vesico-bullous lesion

### Herpes simplex virus infection

- This is a common viral infection usually caused by herpes simplex virus (HSV) type 1 and rarely type 2 (HSV-2).
- The primary infection typically occurs early in life, with viral latency in neural ganglia.
- Reactivation can occur because of several triggers, including immunosuppression, any febrile disease, physical trauma, and stress.
- Clinical presentation and characteristics include the following:
    - Primary herpetic gingivostomatitis:
        - Clinically it starts with erythema and edema with numerous coalescing vesicles that rapidly rupture, leaving painful small, round, shallow ulcers covered by yellow fibrin. New lesions continue to develop during the first three to five days. The ulcers heal in 10 to 14 days. Gingiva may be purple and edematous. Perioral lesions may also present.
        - The primary episode is commonly associated with malaise, anorexia, irritability, fever, and enlarged and tender anterior cervical lymph nodes.

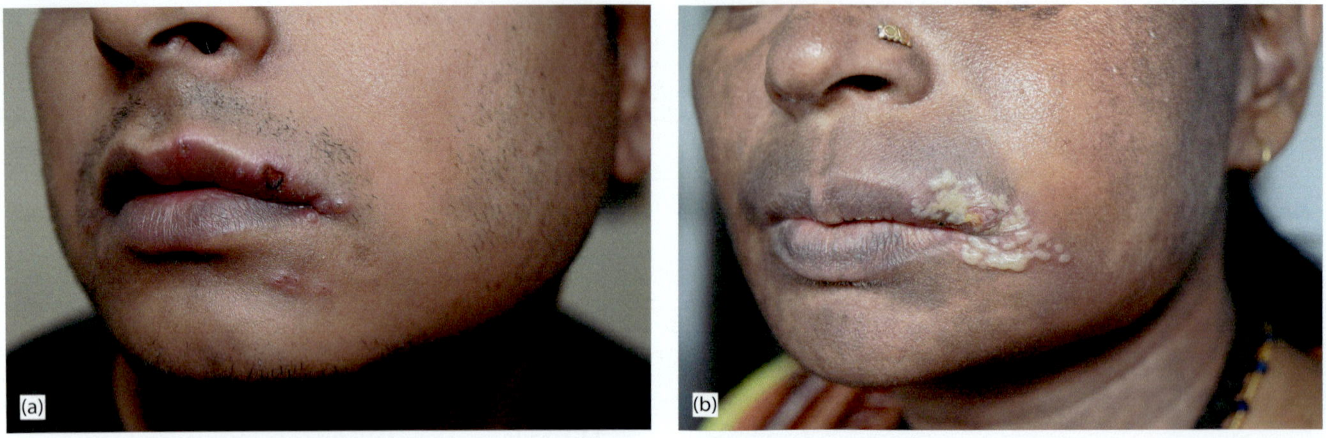


Figure 18.18 **(a)** Multiple grouped vesicles and erosions in herpes labialis. **(b)** Multiple grouped pustules in herpes labialis. (a,b – Courtesy: Dr. Piyush Kumar, Katihar, India.)

- Recurrent herpes labialis:
  - The lesions develop as three to five vesicles at vermilion border of lip and last at least 48 hours (**Figure 18.18a,b**).
  - Lesions may get secondarily infected with staphylococcus or streptococcus (**Figure 18.19**).
- Recurrent intraoral herpes simplex infection:
  - It presents as ulcers with white border and sometimes with dendritic appearance. In immunocompromised individuals, chronic slowly progressive ulcerative or nodular lesions may present.
- DD: Herpetiform aphthous ulcer; herpangina; erythema multiforme; hand, foot, and mouth disease.

## Herpes zoster

- It is an acute self-limiting viral infection caused by varicella zoster characterized by unilateral involvement.
- Oral manifestations are a result of involvement of the second and third branches of the trigeminal nerve. Prodromal symptoms such as pain and tenderness – usually associated with headache, malaise, and fever – may develop two to four days before the appearance of oral or skin lesions consisting of clusters of vesicles and within two or three days evolve into pustules and ulcers, covered by crusts (**Figure 18.20**). The lesions persist for two to three weeks.
- DD: Herpes simplex, erythema multiforme.

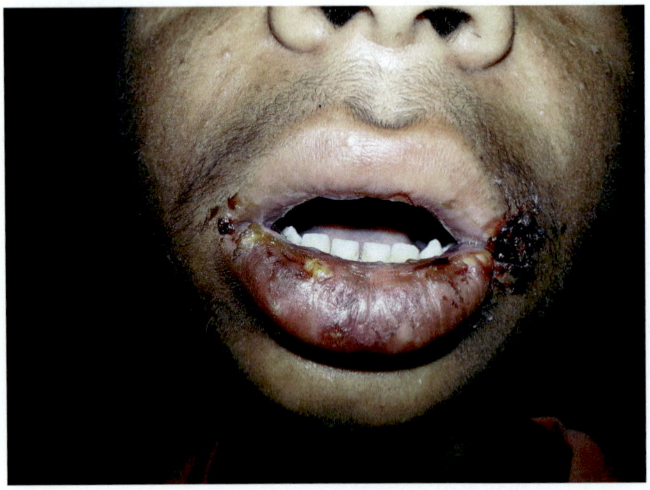

Figure 18.19 Herpes labialis with secondary infection. (Courtesy: Dr. Hiral Shah, Baroda Medical College, Vadodara, India.)

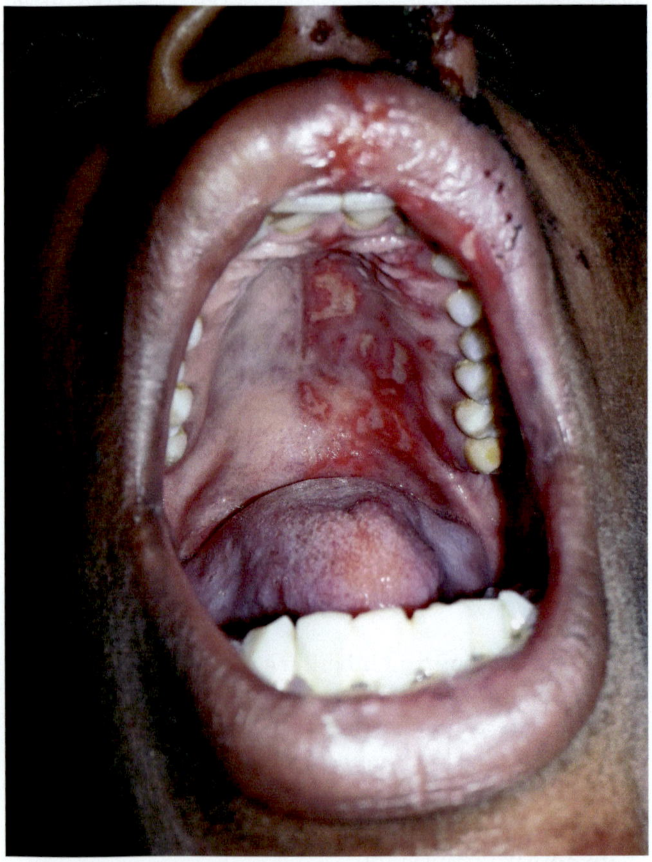

Figure 18.20 Multiple erosions on hard palate and lip in case of herpes zoster. (Courtesy: Dr. Hiral Shah, Baroda Medical College, Vadodara, India.)

## Herpangina

- It is an acute self-limiting viral infection caused by coxsackievirus group A, types 1–6, 8, 10, and 22, frequently affecting children and young adults.
- Oral lesions consist of small, numerous vesicles surrounded by intense erythema that rupture to form painful ulcers that heal within 7 to 10 days. Characteristically, the lesions appear on the soft palate and uvula, tonsillar pillars, and posterior pharyngeal wall.
- Other clinical features are fever, sore throat, dysphagia, headache, and malaise.
- DD: Aphthous stomatitis, drug eruption, hand-foot-mouth disease, primary herpes gingivostomatitis.

## Hand, foot, and mouth disease

- It is an acute self-limiting contagious viral infection caused by coxsackievirus A16.
- It usually affects children and young adults, and often occurs in epidemics.
- Oral manifestations are always present, and are characterized by small vesicles (5 to 30 in number) surrounded by an erythematous halo. Vesicles rapidly rupture to form painful, shallow ulcers (2 to 6 mm in diameter) (**Figure 18.21a–d**).
- The buccal mucosa, tongue, and labial mucosa are the most commonly affected sites.

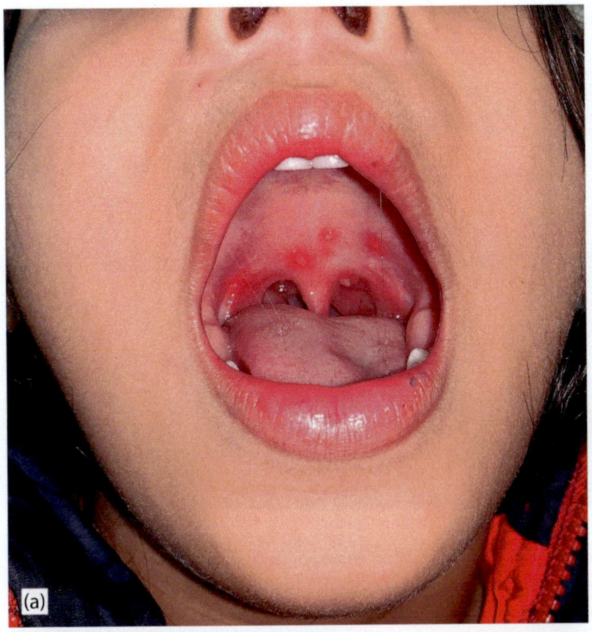


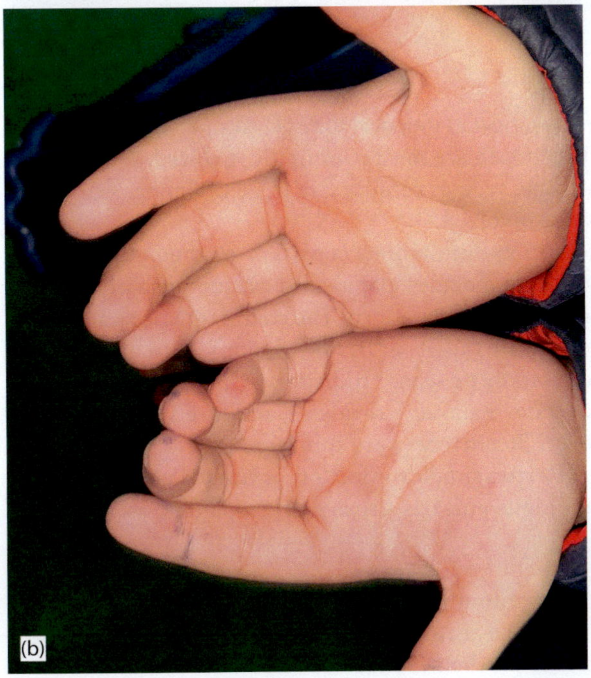


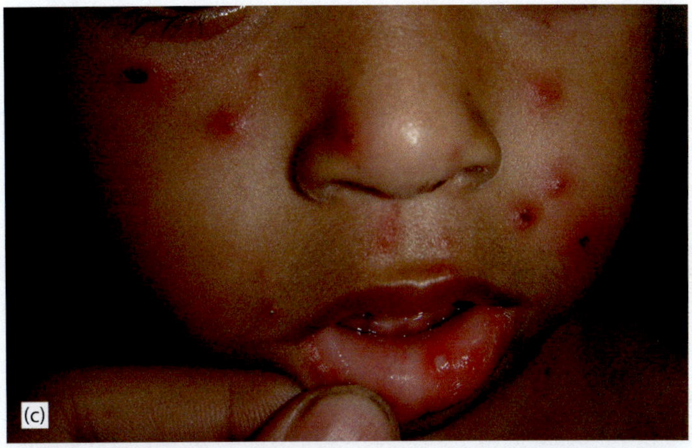


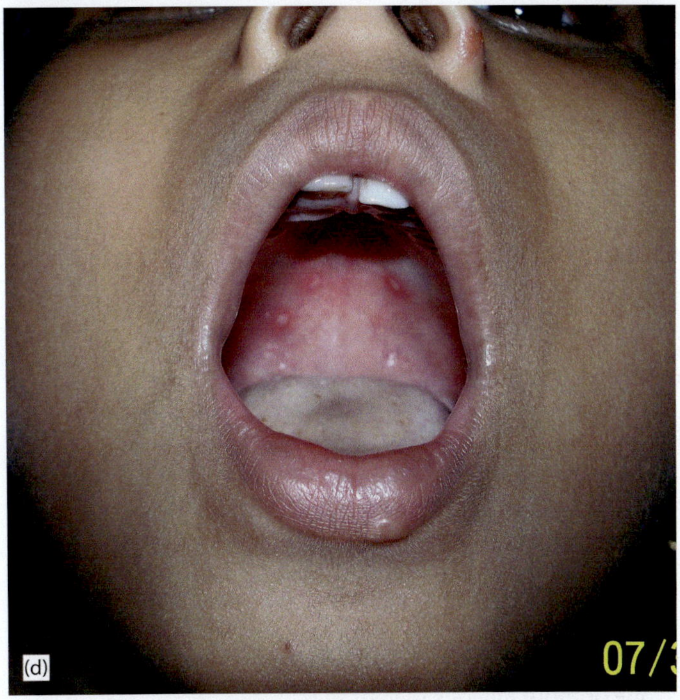


Figure 18.21 **(a)** Shallow ulcer surrounded by erythematous halo on soft palate and uvula. **(b)** Skin lesions on palms. **(c)** Multiple vesicles and ulcers on labial mucosa with skin lesions on face. **(d)** Vesicles and ulcers on palate. (*Continued*)

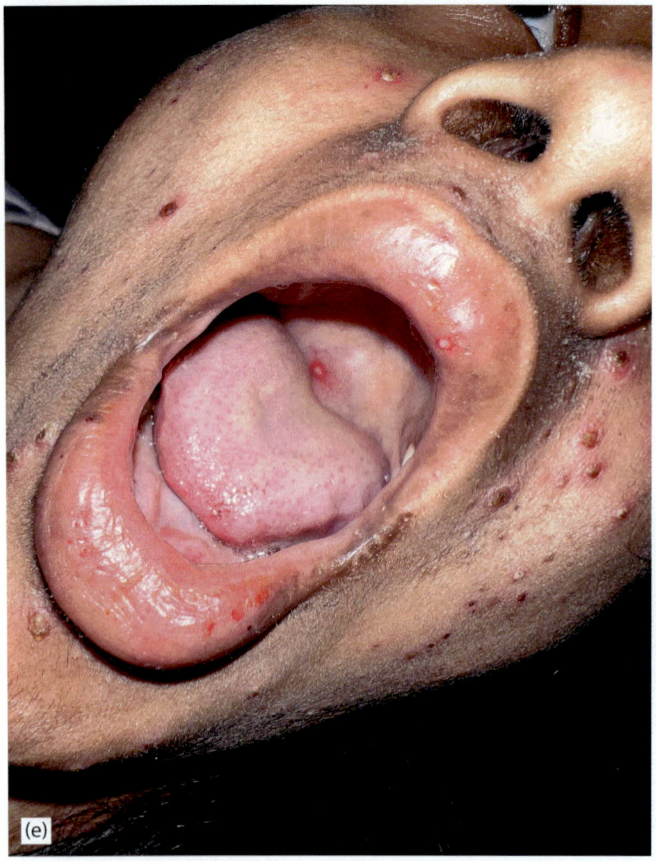


Figure 18.21 (*Continued*) **(e)** Ulcer on the lip and hard palate in varicella. (a–d – Courtesy: Dr. Piyush Kumar, Katihar, India; e – Courtesy: Dr PC Das, Katihar, India.)

- Skin lesions are not constant, and present as small vesicles with a narrow red halo on dorso-lateral surfaces of the fingers and toes, palm, soles, and buttocks.
- The disease lasts five to eight days.
- DD: Aphthous ulcer, herpes simplex, herpangina, varicella (**Figure 18.21e**).

## Erythema multiforme

- It is an acute, self-limiting immune-mediated mucocutaneous disease triggered by an infection such as herpes or *Mycoplasma pneumoniae*, drugs, radiation, or malignancies involving skin and mucosa.
- It may present within a wide spectrum of severity. Erythema multiforme minor represents a localized eruption of typical target-like lesions (predominantly acral) with minimal or no mucosal involvement. Erythema multiforme major is more severe presentation with involvement of up to 10% of body surface area and one or more mucous membranes.
- The oral lesions present as coalescing small vesicles that rupture within two or three days, leaving irregular, painful erosions covered by a necrotic pseudomembrane (**Figure 18.22a,b**).

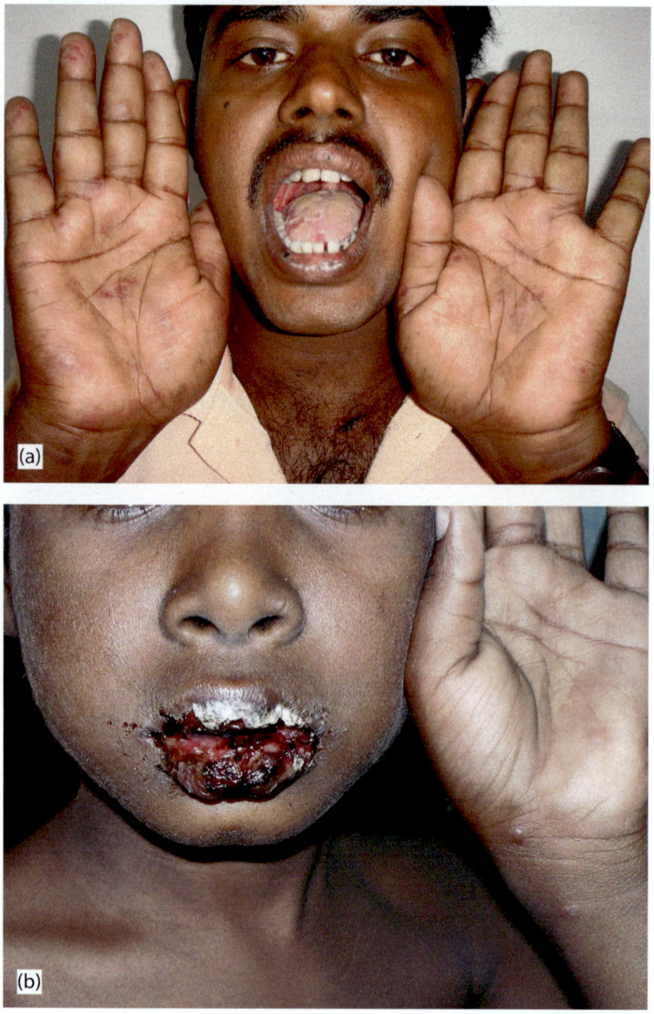


Figure 18.22 **(a)** Irregular erosions on tongue and buccal mucosa with classical targetoid lesions on palm. **(b)** Erosions covered with necrotic pseudomembrane on labial mucosa.

- The lips, buccal mucosa, tongue, soft palate, and floor of the mouth are most commonly involved. Other mucosae, such as conjunctiva or genital mucosa, may also be involved.
- The skin manifestations consist of erythematous, flat, round macules, papules, or plaques, usually in a symmetrical pattern. The characteristic skin patterns are target- or iris-like lesions. Skin bullae may occasionally be seen. Prodromal symptom, such as headache, malaise, arthralgias, and fever, may also be present. Recurrences are common.
- DD: Herpes simplex infection, aphthous ulcer, pemphigus vulgaris, erosive lichen planus.

## Stevens-Johnson syndrome

- This is predominantly drug induced.
- Oral lesions are always present, and presentation includes erythema, edema, and extensive vesicle

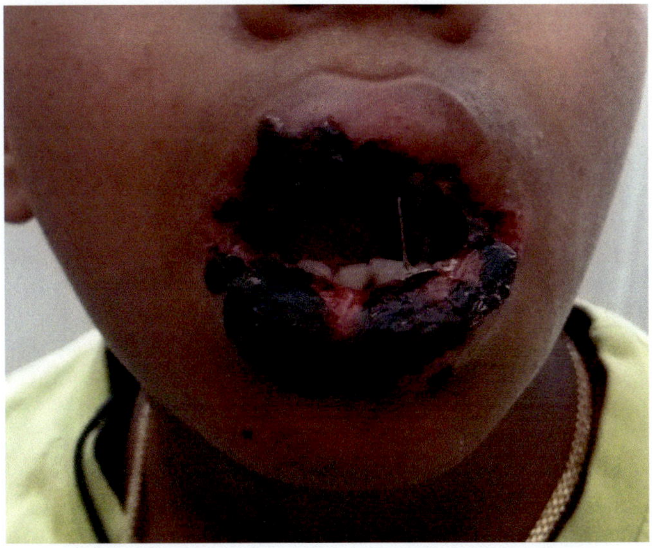

Figure 18.23 Erythema, edema, erosions with severe hemorrhagic crusting on labial mucosa in patient with Steven Johnson syndrome. (Courtesy: Dr. Hiral Shah, Baroda Medical College, Vadodara, India.)

formation, followed by painful erosions covered by grayish-white or hemorrhagic pseudomembrane or necrosis (**Figure 18.23**).
- The primary site is the oral cavity, and it may extend to the pharynx, larynx, and esophagus. The ocular lesions consist of conjunctivitis, uveitis, symblepharon, or even panophthalmitis. The genital lesions are balanitis or vulvovaginitis, and scrotal erosions.
- The skin manifestations may vary from very mild to severe in the form of maculopapular rash, blisters, urticarial plaques, or targetoid lesions with two zones of color. The innermost is vesicular, purpuric, or necrotic surrounded by erythema.
- DD: Erythema multiforme major, Behçet disease, pemphigus, pemphigoid, primary herpes simplex.

## Toxic epidermal necrolysis

- This is a potentially life-threatening condition triggered by drugs (sulfonamides, anticonvulsants and NSAIDs) in genetically sensitive individuals.
- It usually begins with an influenza-like prodrome characterized by low-grade fever, malaise, arthralgias, conjunctival burning sensation, rhinitis, and headache.
- The oral manifestations consist of diffuse erythema, edema followed by vesicles and painful hemorrhagic erosions, primarily on the lips and periorally as well as on the buccal mucosa, tongue, and palate. Hemorrhagic crusting of lips is a common finding. Ocular, genital, and other mucous membrane lesions are common (**Figure 18.24**).
- Skin lesions start with symmetrical morbilliform discrete lesions and gradually coalesce to become flaccid

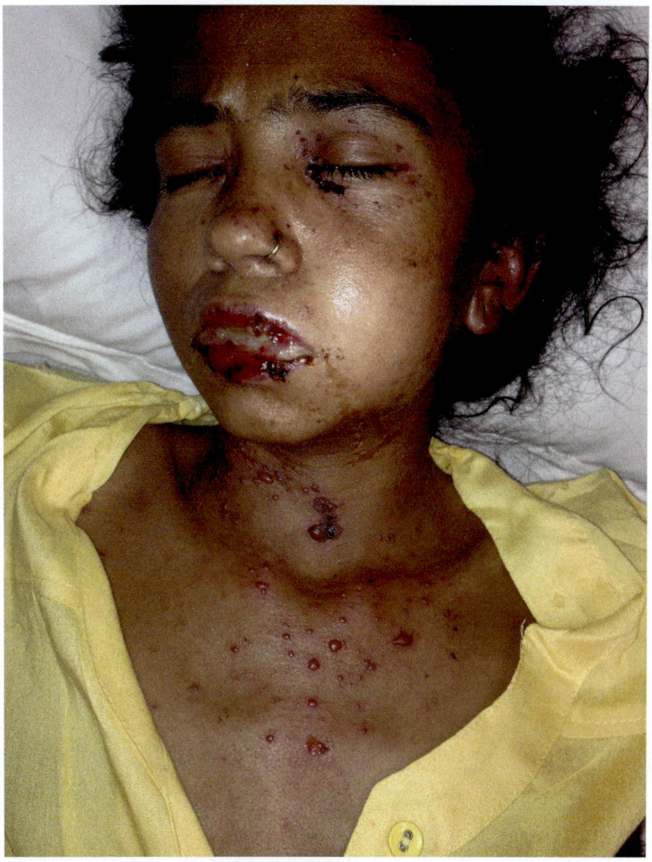

Figure 18.24 Toxic epidermal necrolysis presenting with erythema and edema of labial mucosa with erosions covered with hemorrhagic necrotic pseudomembrane with eye and skin lesions.

bullae. The epidermis sloughs in sheets, leaving a moist, denuded dermis. Nikolsky's sign is positive.
- DD: Stevens-Johnson syndrome, pemphigus vulgaris, severe and extensive burns.

## Pemphigus vulgaris

- Pemphigus vulgaris is a severe chronic bullous autoimmune mucocutaneous disease due to antibodies against antigens Desmoglein 1 and 3.
- Oral lesions are characterized by vesicobullous lesions, which rapidly rupture, leaving painful erosions with a tendency to extend peripherally (**Figure 18.25**).
- The buccal mucosa, labial mucosa, palate, tongue, floor of the mouth, and gingiva are often involved. Lesions may develop over other mucosa.
- The skin lesions present as small vesicles or flaccid bullae on normal skin that rupture quickly, leaving persistent erosions. Nikolsky's sign is positive.
- DD: Cicatricial pemphigoid, bullous pemphigoid, linear IgA disease, epidermolysis bullosa acquisita, toxic epidermal necrolysis.

## Bullous pemphigoid

- This is a chronic autoimmune mucocutaneous bullous disease.

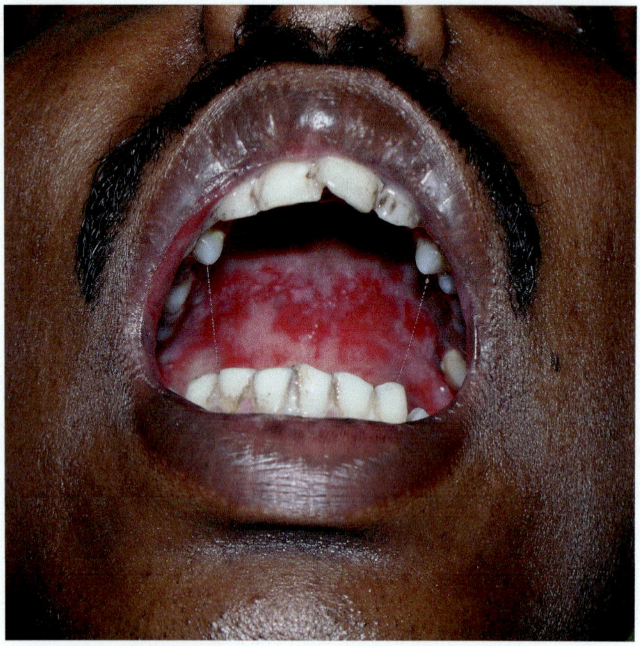

Figure 18.25 Multiple coalescing erosions on soft palate. (Courtesy: Dr. Piyush Kumar, Katihar, India.)

- Bullous pemphigoid antigens (BP180, BP230) are the main target antigens.
- Oral mucosa is affected in about 20–40% of cases, other mucosae may also be affected.
- The oral lesions usually follow cutaneous manifestations and begin as bullae that soon rupture, leaving shallow ulcerations.
- Skin lesions are always present and begin as a non-specific generalized rash followed by large, tense bullae that rupture, leaving denuded areas without a tendency to extend peripherally.
- DD: Pemphigus, cicatricial pemphigoid, linear IgA disease, dermatitis herpetiformis, epidermolysis bullosa acquisita, pemphigoid gestationis.

## Cicatracial pemphigoid

- This is a chronic autoimmune bullous mucocutaneous disease that primarily affects mucous membranes and results in atrophy or scarring.
- Bullous pemphigoid antigen (BP180), laminin 5, integrin B4, and type VII collagen are the main target antigens.
- Oral manifestations are seen in almost all patients, but other mucosae and, rarely, the skin may be involved. The oral lesions often begin on the gingiva as recurrent vesicles or bullae that rupture, leaving large, superficial painful ulcerations that lead to epithelial atrophy or scarring on healing.
- Among other mucosae involvement, ocular lesions consist of conjunctivitis, symblepharon, entropion, trichiasis, dryness, and corneal opacity, frequently leading to blindness.
- DD: Bullous pemphigoid, linear IgA disease, epidermolysis bullosa acquisita, pemphigus, erosive lichen planus, discoid lupus erythematosus.

## Pemphigoid gestationis

- This is a rare autoimmune subepidermal blistering disease occurring in the second or third trimester of pregnancy or in the early postpartum period.
- The target antigen is 180 kD, a hemidesmosomal antigen (BP 180).
- It usually affects the skin, and mucosal lesions occur in less than 20% of cases.
- The oral lesions usually follow the skin lesions and present as multiple, usually hemorrhagic, bullae that rupture quickly, leaving painful ulcerations.
- The buccal mucosa, palate, tongue, and gingiva are the most frequently affected areas.
- The skin manifestations present as urticarial plaques that usually start from periumbilical region and spread peripherally. Lesions progress to form tense vesicobullous lesions and soon rapture, leaving painful ulcerations.
- DD: Bullous pemphigoid, cicatricial pemphigoid, linear IgA disease, dermatitis herpetiformis, epidermolysis bullosa acquisita.

## Linear IgA disease

- Linear IgA disease is a chronic autoimmune subepidermal bullous disease characterized by the linear deposition of IgA along the basement membrane zone.
- Oral lesions occur in about 20–30% of cases, and are characterized by the formation of bullae that soon rupture, leaving superficial, non-specific ulcerations. Other lesions include erythematous patches, desquamative gingivitis, or erosive cheilitis.
- The skin lesions consist of bullae that may be discrete or arranged in a herpetiform pattern described as the "cluster of jewels" sign, or tense vesicles or bullae may be seen at the edge of annular or polycyclic lesions giving appearance of string of pearls.
- DD: Cicatricial pemphigoid, bullous pemphigoid, pemphigus, dermatitis herpetiformis, pemphigoid gestationis.

## Dermatitis herpetiformis

- This is a chronic autoimmune recurrent cutaneous bullous disease associated with gluten sensitive enteropathy.
- The oral mucosa is affected in 5–10% of cases, and oral lesions include erythematous patches, papules, or vesicles. The vesicles appear in a cyclic pattern and rupture rapidly, leaving shallow, painful ulcerations.
- The tongue, buccal mucosa, and palate are more frequently involved.
- Cutaneous lesions are always present and appear as erythematous papules or plaques, with herpetiform vesicles symmetrically distributed over extensors.
- DD: Bullous pemphigoid, cicatricial pemphigoid, linear IgA disease, pemphigus, herpetiform ulcers.

### Epidermolysis bullosa

- This is an inherited mechanobullous disorder characterized by blister formation in response to trauma. The lesions appear at birth or early in infancy.
- Oral manifestations are more common in the junctional and dystrophic forms. Oral lesions present as bullae, usually in areas of friction, that rupture, leaving shallow ulcers and, later, atrophy and scarring.
- Dysplastic teeth may be seen in the severe forms of the disease. Leukoplakia and squamous cell carcinoma may develop on the scars.
- DD: Pemphigus, cicatricial and bullous pemphigoid, linear IgA disease, bullous dermatosis of childhood, epidermolysis bullosa acquisita.

### Epidermolysis bullosa acquisita

- This is a rare, non-inherited, chronic, autoimmune bullous disease involving the skin and mucous membranes.
- The target antigen is type VII collagen.
- Oral lesions occur in more than 50% of cases and present as solitary or multiple bullae and painful erosions involving gingiva and buccal mucosa. Significant scarring and dysfunction may occur.
- Skin lesions present as hemorrhagic bullae and ulcerations, usually at the sites of mechanical irritation. The lesions heal with scarring and milia.
- DD: Cicatricial pemphigoid, bullous pemphigoid, linear IgA disease, pemphigus, genetic epidermolysis bullosa, systemic lupus erythematosus, porphyria cutanea tarda.

## Without preceding with vesicobullous lesions

### Traumatic ulcers

- Cheek bite, facial trauma, dentures, and chemical or thermal burn are common cause of trauma.
- They occur on the tongue, lips, and buccal mucosa.
- They usually appear as a single, painful soft ulcer with a smooth red or whitish-yellow surface and thin erythematous halo (**Figure 18.26**).

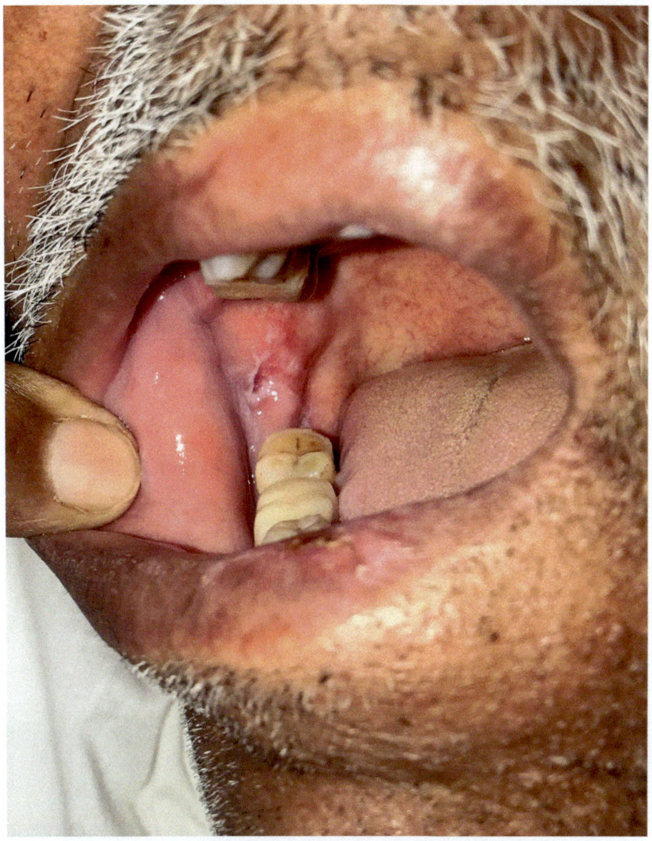

Figure 18.26 Single soft ulcer with red base.

- They heal without scarring within 6 to 10 days, spontaneously or after removal of the cause.
- DD: Carcinoma, aphthous ulcer, infections like tuberculosis, syphilis and mycoses.

### Recurrent aphthous stomatitis

- This is a common disease that affects at least 20% of the population.
- There are three clinical patterns: minor, major, and herpetiform (**Table 18.4**).

Table 18.4 Different clinical patterns of aphthous ulcer

| | Minor aphthous | Major aphthous | Herpetiform aphthous |
|---|---|---|---|
| Prevalence | 80% of RAS | 10% of RAS | 10% of RAS |
| Age | Adolescence | adolescence | Young adult |
| Site | Vestibule, labial, buccal mucosa and floor of mouth | Any site | Any site |
| Number of lesions | 1–6 | 1–6 | 10–100 |
| Size of lesions | 2–4 mm | >10 mm | 1–2 mm |
| Clinical | Painful, round ulcers covered by a whitish-yellow membrane and surrounded by a red halo (**Figure 18.27**) | Larger, last longer deep painful ulcers, recurs more frequently (**Figures 18.28, 18.29**) | Small, painful, shallow ulcers, with a tendency to coalesce into larger irregular ulcers |
| Duration | 7–12 days | 3–6 weeks | 1–2 weeks |
| Evolution | Heal without scarring | May heal with scarring | Heal without scarring |

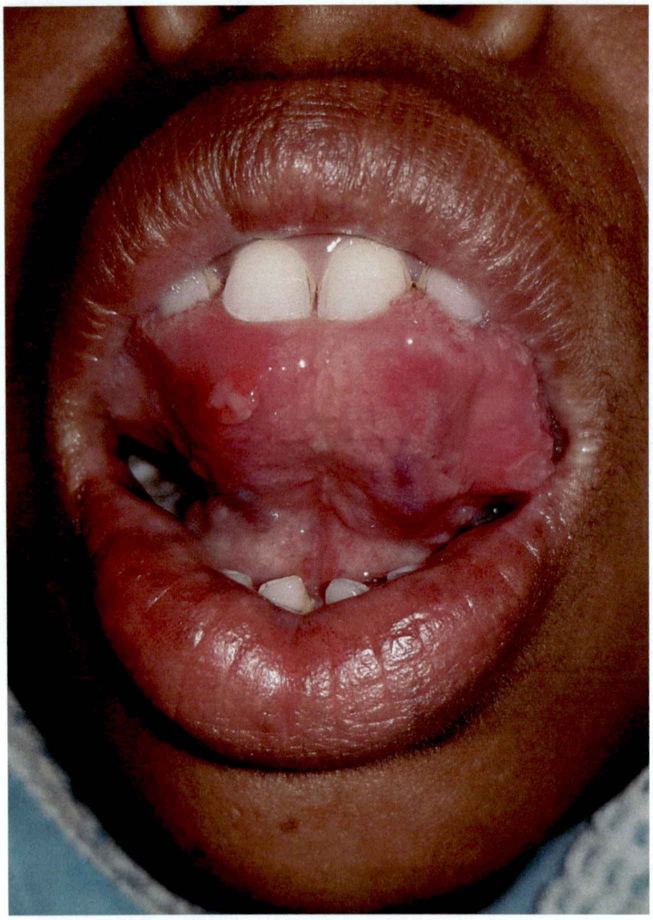

Figure 18.27 Small, shallow ulcer with whitish-yellow membrane on base and surrounded by red halo. (Courtesy: Dr. P C Das, Katihar, India.)

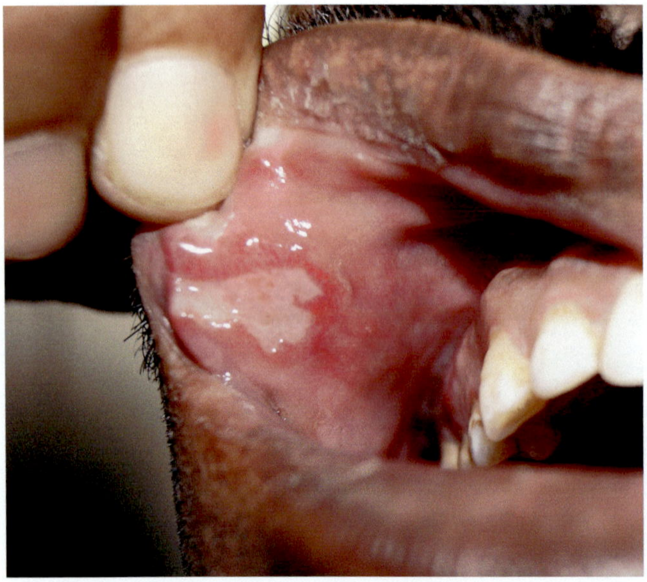

Figure 18.28 Large, deep ulcer on inner aspect of lip.

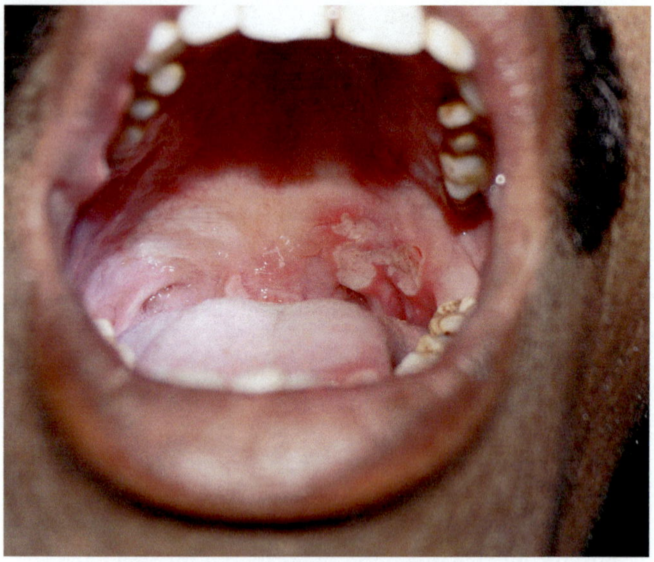

Figure 18.29 Aphthous ulcers seen as multiple ulcers with whitish membrane on palate.

- DD: Herpes simplex, hand-foot-and mouth disease, chancre, Behçet's disease, cyclic neutropenia, erythema multiforme, FAPA syndrome, Sweet syndrome.

## Behçet's disease

- Behçet's disease is a chronic multisystem inflammatory disorder with an association with HLA-Bw51, HLA-B5, HLAB27, and HLA-B12 alleles.
- It is more prevalent in male of 20 to 30 years of age.
- Diagnosis is made on the presence of recurrent aphthous stomatitis (**Figure 18.30**) and two or more of genital ulcers, eye lesions, skin lesions, and pathergy test.
- Major criteria include the following:
  - Recurrent oral ulceration: recurrent aphthous stomatitis, which recurred at least 3 times in a 12-month period
  - Recurrent genital ulceration: aphthous ulceration or scarring
  - Skin lesions: erythema nodosum, papulopustular lesions
  - Neuro-ocular lesions: conjunctivitis, iritis with hypopyon, uveitis, retinal vasculitis, reduced visual acuity. Syndromes resembling disseminated sclerosis, pseudobulbar palsy or neurosyphilis meningoencephalitis
  - Positive pathergy test
- Minor criteria include the following:
  - Arthritis, arthralgia, thrombophlebitis, vein thrombosis, arterial occlusion and aneurysms, pulmonary, renal, and gastrointestinal manifestations

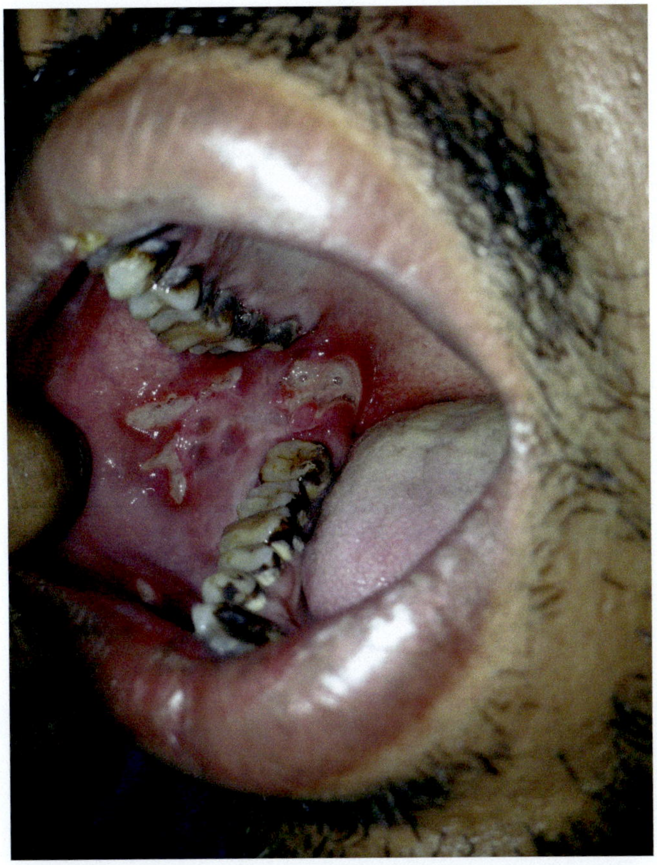

Figure 18.30 Major aphthous ulcers with prominent surrounding erythema on buccal mucosa in case of Behçet's disease.

- DD: Recurrent aphthous stomatitis, Reiter's syndrome, ulcerative colitis, erythema multiforme, Stevens-Johnson syndrome, syphilis, Sweet syndrome.

## Syphilis

- Syphilis is a common sexually transmitted disease caused by *Treponema pallidum*.
- Different types of oral lesions develop in primary, secondary, tertiary, and congenital syphilis.
- Primary: Known as chancre characterized by a painless ulcer with a smooth surface, raised borders, and an indurated base over lip, tongue, and tonsils.
- Secondary: Three types of lesions may present.
  - Mucous patches (painless, shallow, rounded erosions covered with gray macerated scaling)
  - Irregular, serpiginous erosions/ulcers – "snail track ulcers"
  - Condylomata lata (smooth, papillated, or covered with cauliflower-like vegetation)
- Tertiary: A gumma is a soft, painless non-malignant growth mostly occurring on hard palate (**Figure 18.31a**), which eventually ulcerates. Palatal perforation and fistula formation may also happen.
- Congenital: Oral lesions are high-arched palate, short mandible, rhagades, Hutchinson's teeth, and Moon's or mulberry molars.
- DD: Lepromatous leprosy, traumatic ulcer, aphthous ulcer, tuberculosis, herpes simplex, other infective

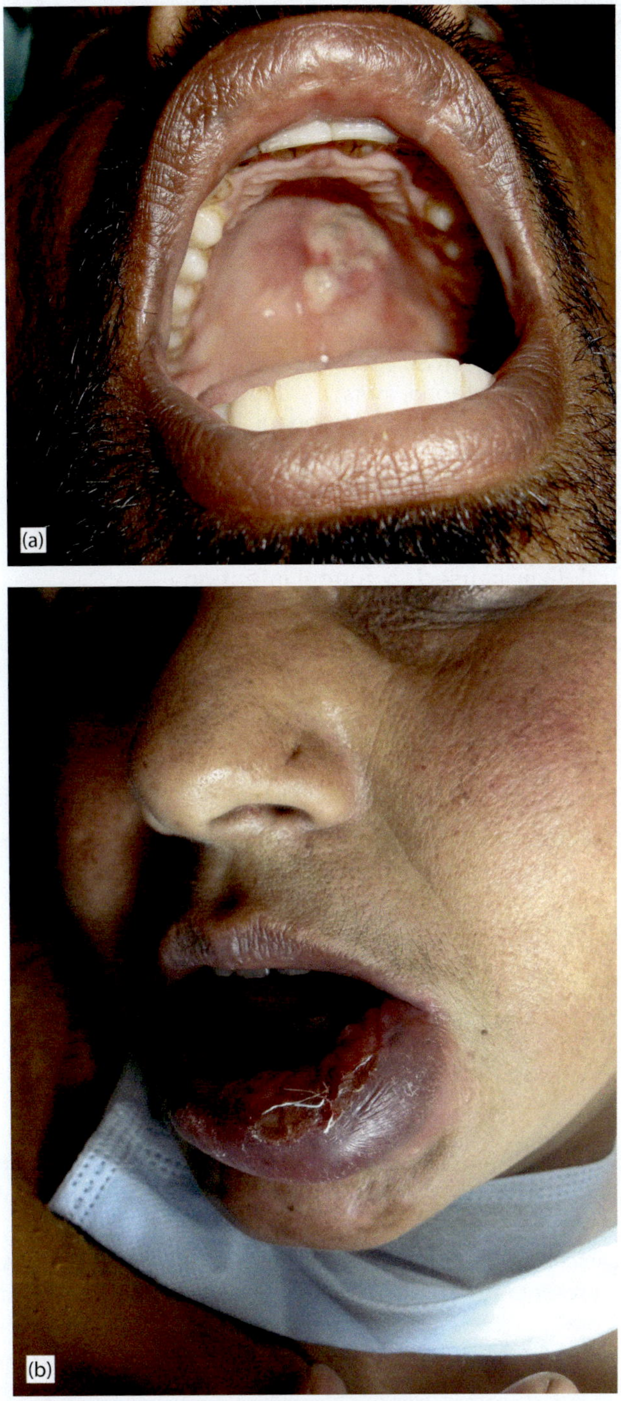

Figure 18.31 **(a)** Gumma lesion presenting as soft painless ulcer on hard palate in tertiary syphilis. **(b)** Erythematous edematous plaque with central ulceration on lip in case of leishmaniasis. (*Continued*)

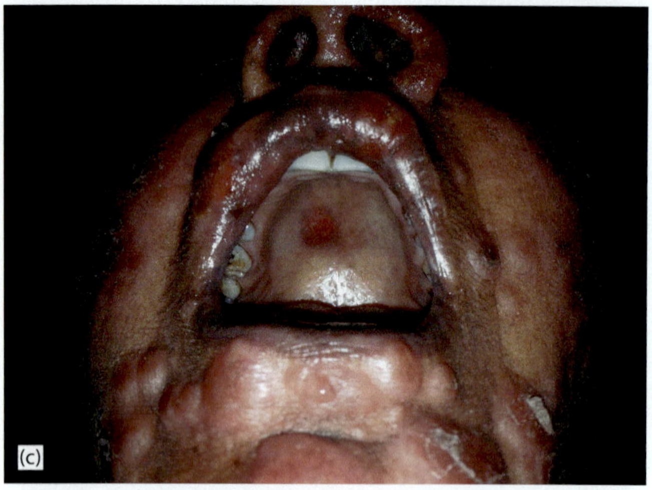

Figure 18.31 (*Continued*) **(c)** Erythematous plaque with ulceration on hard palate and lips, with multiple skin lesions in the case of leprosy. (a – Courtesy: Dr. Santoshdev Rathod, Ahmedabad, India; c – Courtesy: Dr. Hiral Shah, Baroda Medical College, Vadodara, India.)

oral ulcers (**Table 18.5**), infectious mononucleosis, candidiasis, erythema multiforme, lichen planus.

## Oral ulcer caused by fungal infection

- Aspergillosis – palatal necrosis
- Blastomycosis – oral ulcer
- Paracoccidioidomycosis – oral ulcers and lymphadenopathy
- Cryptococcosis – oral ulcers
- Histoplasmosis – nodular lesion or ulcers
- Phycomycosis (mucormycosis, zygomycosis) – palatal ulceration
- Sporotrichosis – oral ulcer rare
- Coccidioidomycosis – oral ulcers rare

## Eosinophilic ulcer

- This is a rare self-limiting benign condition caused by trauma.
- It presents as solitary or multiple painful ulcers with an irregular surface, a raised border, and covered with a whitish-yellow pseudomembrane.
- DD: Major aphthous ulcer, traumatic ulcer.

## Rarer causes of oral ulcer

- Other rarer causes of oral ulceration are summarized in **Table 18.6**.

## Squamous cell carcinoma

- This represents about 90% of oral cancers. It occurs more frequently in men than in women.
- Predisposing factors are tobacco smoke, alcohol, sun exposure, poor oral hygiene, dietary deficiencies, iron deficiency, liver cirrhosis, and infections.
- Common sites are lateral border, the ventral surface of the tongue, lips, and floor of the mouth.

Table 18.5 Other infective causes of oral ulcer

| Infection | Acute necrotizing gingivitis (Noma) | Tuberculosis | Gonorrhea | Leishmaniasis |
|---|---|---|---|---|
| Causative organism | *Fusobacterium nucleatum*, *Prevotella intermedia*, *Borrelia vincentii*, *Streptococcus*, *Staphylococcus* | *Mycobacterium tuberculosis* | *Neisseria gonorrhoeae* | Mucocutaneous- *L. braziliensis*, *L. guyanensis*, *L. panamensis* Post-kala azar dermal leishmaniasis – *L. donovani*, *L. infantum*, *L. tropica*. *L. chagasi* |
| Sites | Buccal mucosa, lips, and the adjacent bone | Dorsum of tongue, lip, buccal mucosa palate | | Tongue, lip, buccal mucosa, palate |
| Clinical presentation – oral manifestations | Necrotizing ulcerative gingivitis, necrotizing ulceration covered with yellow-brown fibrin and debris | Tuberculous ulcer; painless and irregular, thin undermined border, vegetating surface, usually covered by a gray-yellowish exudate | Oral mucosal erythema, edema and ulceration | Central ulceration with surrounding erythematous, edematous plaque (**Figure 18.31b**) |
| Other manifestations | Salivation, halitosis, fever, malaise, and regional lymphadenopathy | Osteomyelitis of the jaws, periapical granuloma, regional lymphadenopathy, and scrofula | | |
| Differentials | Tuberculosis, leukemia | Mycoses, malignancy, syphilis | | Lepromatous leprosy (**Figure 18.31c**) |

Table 18.6 Other causes of oral ulceration

| Causes | Disease | Oral lesions |
|---|---|---|
| Nutritional | Low iron | Aphthous ulcer |
| | Folate, vitamin B12 deficiency | Glossitis |
| | | Angular stomatitis |
| Hematological | Leukopenia | Painful, deep, irregular ulcer covered with whitish membrane with minimum red halo |
| | Agranulocytosis | Multiple necrotic ulcers covered by a grayish-white or dark and dirty pseudomembrane without a red halo. |
| | | Severe necrotizing gingivitis Periodontal destruction |
| | Myelic aplasia | Gingival bleeding, |
| | | petechiae, and ecchymoses. |
| | | Necrotic ulceration |
| | Myelodysplastic syndrome | Persistent and recurrent ulcerations |
| | | Gingival hemorrhage Periodontitis |
| | Leukemia | Ulceration |
| | | Mucosal pallor |
| | | Gingival hemorrhage and swelling |
| | | Petechiae, ecchymoses |
| | | Tooth loosening |
| | Lymphoma | Diffuse painless swelling with or without ulceration on soft palate, tongue, gingiva and tonsillar area. |
| | Wegners granulomatosis | Solitary or multiple oral ulcer with red halo in tongue, palate and buccal mucosa |
| | | Gingival enlargement (strawberry appearance) |
| | | Oral ulceration |
| | Mycosis fungoides | Red or white areas |
| | Pseudolymphoma | Ulcer over palate |
| | Histiocytosis | Gingival swelling |
| | | Periodontal destruction |
| | | Oral ulceration |
| | | Nodular/glandular lesions in labial or buccal mucosa in multicentric reticulohistiocytosis |
| | Hypereosinophilic syndrome | Oral erosion (buccal, gingival or labial mucosa) |
| | Hypoplasminogenemia | Oral ulceration |
| | | Gingival swelling |
| Gastrointestinal | Pyostomatitis vegetans | Deep fissures |
| | | Pustules |
| | | Papillary projections |
| | Crohn's disease | Linear ulcer along buccal sulcus |
| | Orofacial granulomatosis | Thickening and folding of mucosa (cobblestone appearance) |
| | | Mucosal tags |
| | | Lip swelling, angular stomatitis |
| Immune defects | HIV | Recurrent ulceration |
| Vasculitis | Polyarteritis nodosa | Transient submucosal nodule |
| | | Ulceration, hemorrhage |
| | Giant cell arteritis | Ulceration and necrosis of tongue or lip |
| Iatrogenic conditions | Chemotherapy- or radiotherapy-induced mucositis | |
| | Bone marrow transplantation | |
| | Graft-versus-host disease | Atypical diffuse ulcerations Lichenoid lesions |
| | | Oral bleeding, xerostomia, and infections |

- Early lesions appear as a white lesion (**Figure 18.32a**), a red lesion, or both, or even as an exophytic mass (**Figure 18.32b**). However, the most common clinical presentation is erosion or an ulcer (**Figure 18.32c**). Exophytic mass presents as reddish-white colored papillary or verrucous surface with indurated base.
- A chronic lesion is an indurated ulcer with an irregular papillary surface, elevated borders, and a hard base on palpation (**Figure 18.33a–c**).

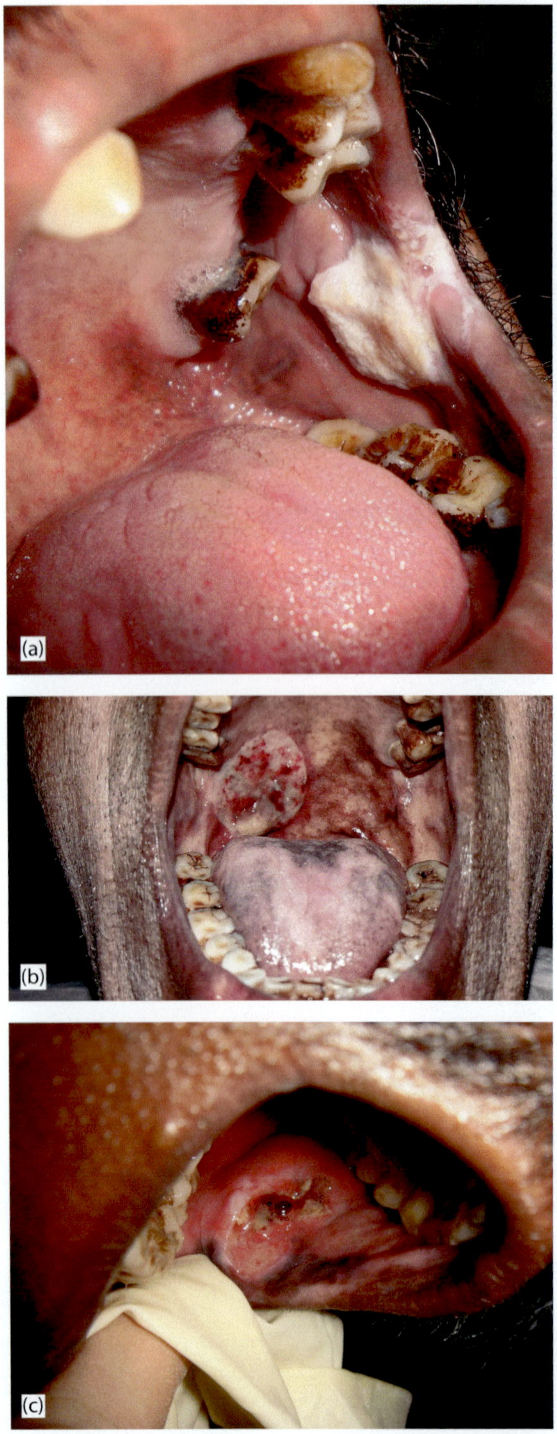


Figure 18.32 Early lesions of squamous cell carcinoma, **(a)** white plaque on buccal mucosa, **(b)** red white exophytic growth on palate, **(c)** ulcer on buccal mucosa (a,c – Courtesy: Dr. Piyush Kumar, Katihar, India; b – Courtesy: Dr. Hiral Shah, Baroda Medical College, Vadodara, India.)

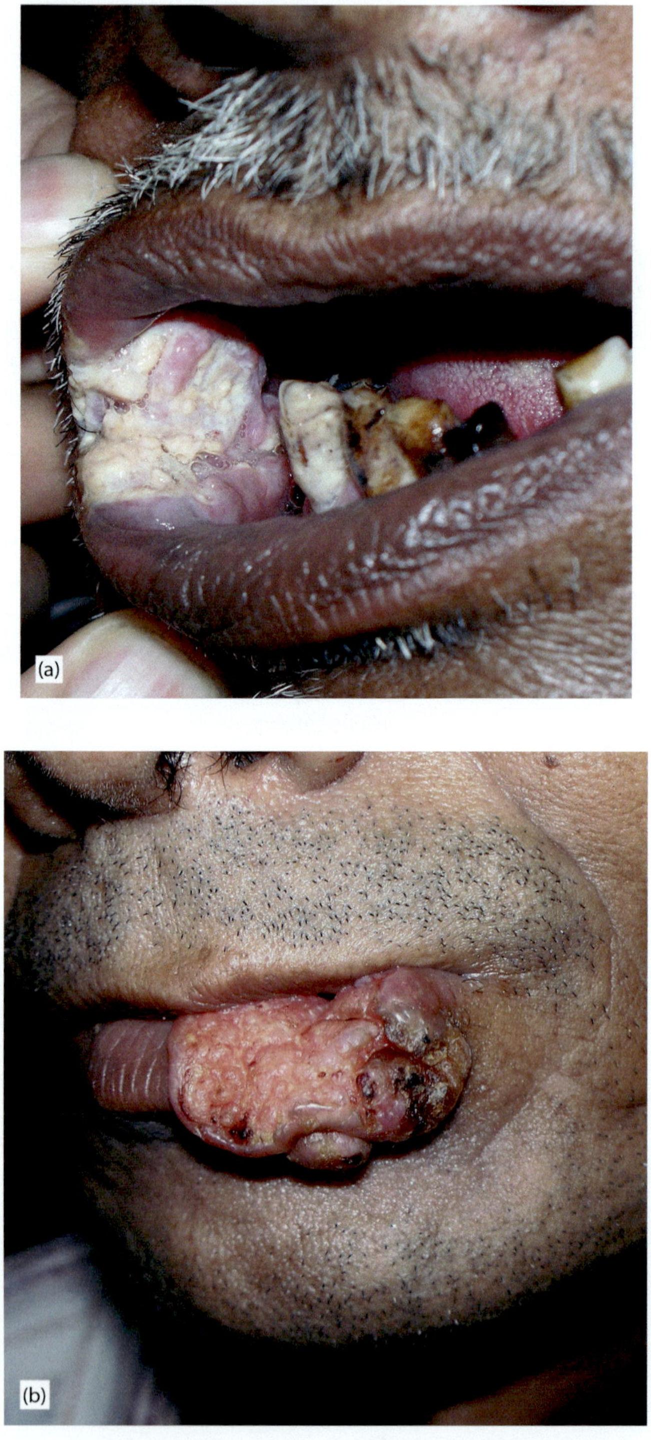


Figure 18.33 Chronic lesion of squamous cell carcinoma in form of **(a)** hard verrucous leukoplakia with ulceration, **(b)** verrucous growth with ulceration. (*Continued*)

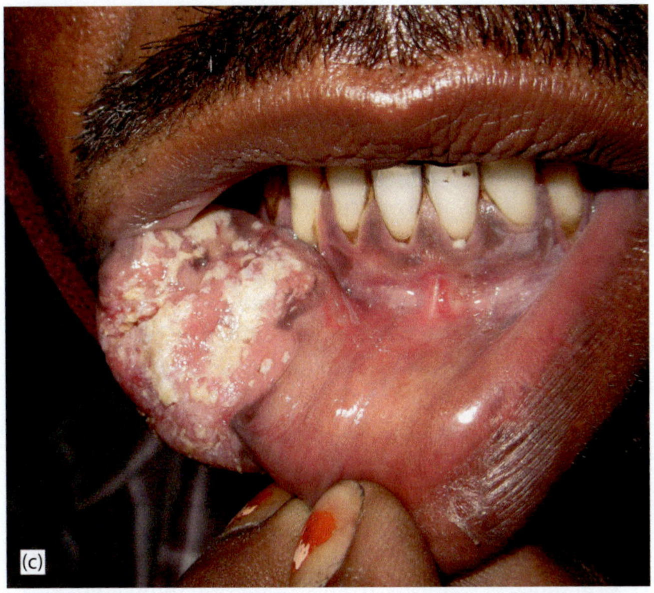


Figure 18.33 (*Continued*) **(c)** Squamous cell carcinoma presenting as hard verrucous leukoplakia with ulceration. (Courtesy: Dr. Hiral Shah, Baroda Medical College, Vadodara, India.)

- There is cervical lymph node enlargement, hard and fixed to tissue.
- DD: Traumatic ulcer, tuberculosis, systemic mycoses, syphilis, eosinophilic ulcer, Wegener granulomatosis.

## PIGMENTED LESIONS

Pigmented lesions represent a variety of clinical entities, ranging from physiologic changes (e.g., racial pigmentation) to manifestations of systemic illnesses (e.g., Addison's disease) and malignant neoplasms (e.g., melanoma and Kaposi sarcoma). Oral pigmentation may be exogenous or endogenous in origin. Exogenous pigmentation is commonly due to foreign-body implantation in the oral mucosa. Endogenous pigments include melanin, hemoglobin, hemosiderin, and carotene (**Figure 18.34a**).

### Melanotic macule

- Most common oral mucosal lesions of melanocytic lesions develop due to functional hyperactivity of regional melanocytes.
- It appears as small, solitary, brown to black, well-demarcated, uniformly pigmented lesions that develop mostly in adult females (**Figure 18.34b**).
- The lower lip, gingiva, and palate are the most common areas.

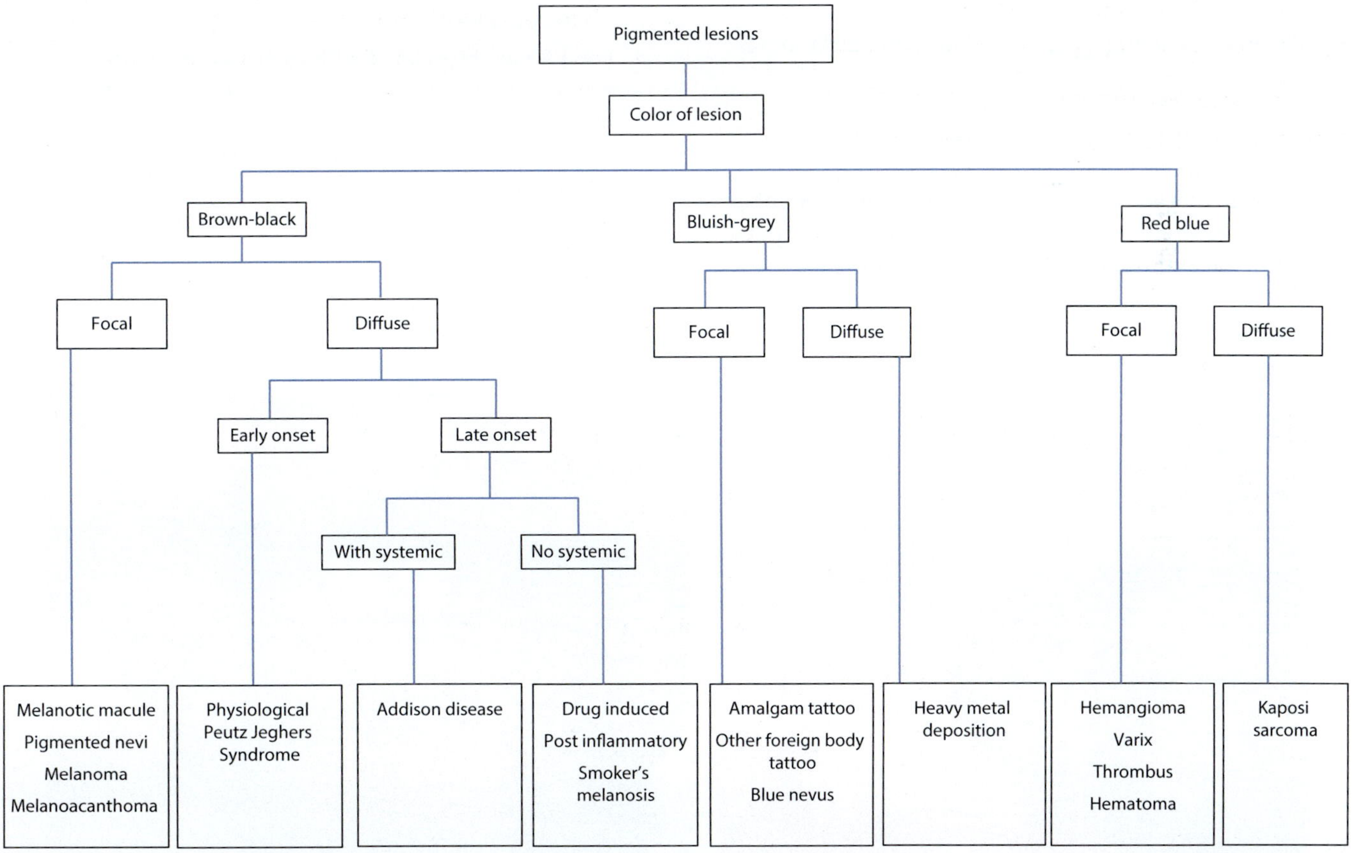


Figure 18.34 **(a)** Clinical approach to pigmented lesions of the mucosa. (*Continued*)

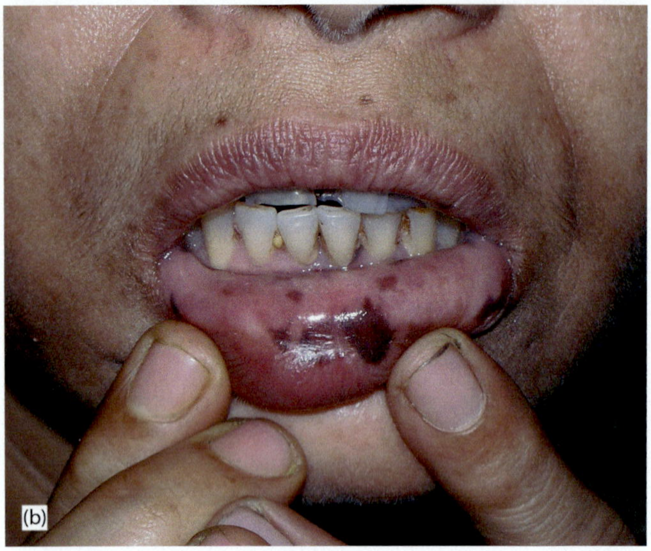


Figure 18.34 (*Continued*) **(b)** Melanotic macule. (b – Courtesy: Dr. Piyush Kumar, Katihar, India.)

## Amalgam tattoo

- This is a common iatrogenic disorder developing due to implantation of dental amalgam into oral mucosa.
- It presents as a well-defined irregular or diffuse flat gray, bluish-black discoloration, usually involving the gingival mucosa of the lower jaw.
- DD: Freckles, lentigo, pigmented nevi and melanoma.

## Heavy-metal deposition

- This is caused by ingestion or exposure to heavy metals (i.e., bismuth, lead, silver, mercury, etc.).
- Exposure to lead or bismuth leads to development of a bluish line along the marginal gingiva or similar spots within the gingival papillae, while diffuse bluish-black discoloration may be seen with exposure to silver (**Figure 18.35a,b**).
- DD: Amalgam tattoo, drug-induced pigmentation.

## Drug-induced pigmentation

- This is a relatively common condition caused by increased melanin production or drug metabolite deposition.
- Most common drugs causing mucosal pigmentation are antimalarials, tranquilizers, minocycline, azidothymidine, ketoconazole, and phenolphthalein.
- It may appear as focal irregular brown or black macules or plaques or diffuse pigmentation (**Figure 18.36**).
- The buccal mucosa, tongue, palate, and gingiva are the most commonly affected sites.
- DD: Heavy-metal deposition, fixed drug eruption.

## Smoker's melanosis

- It is a benign abnormal melanin pigmentation of the oral mucosa resulting from stimulation of melanocytes from tobacco.
- It more commonly occurs in women, and the intensity of pigmentation depends on duration and dose.
- There are multiple brown-pigmented areas, usually located on the anterior labial gingiva of the mandible.
- Pipe smoking may lead to pigmentation of the buccal mucosa and palate.

## Freckles and lentigines

- Freckles are associated with increased melanin production, while lentigines are associated with an increased number of melanocytes.
- They appear as solitary and well-demarcated asymptomatic round brown macules, less than 5 mm in diameter. The vermilion border of the lower lip is the most common site and rarely occurs inside oral cavity.

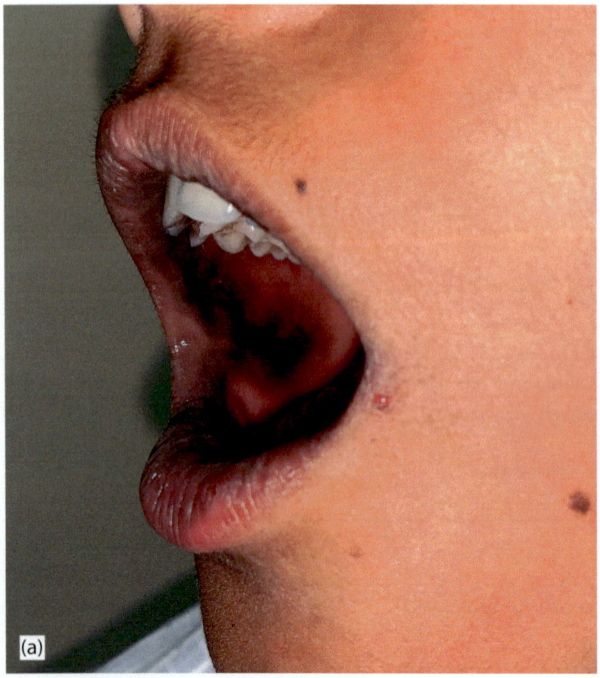


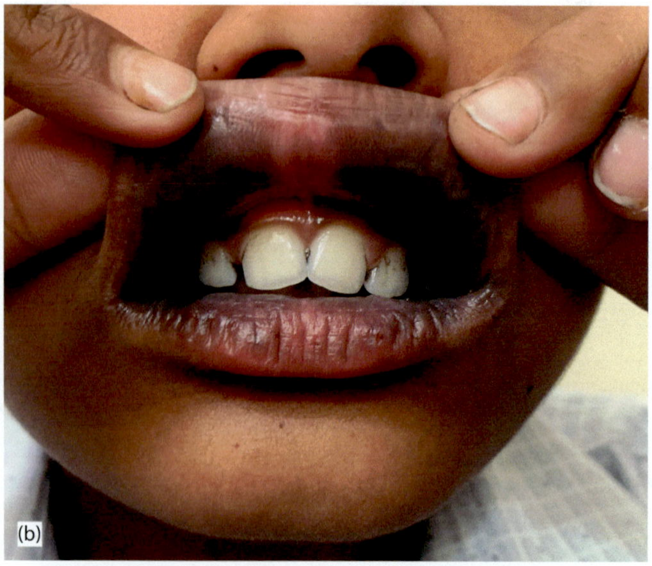


Figure 18.35 **(a,b)** Diffuse bluish-black pigmented macule on lip, buccal mucosa, and gingiva due to exposure to silver. (Courtesy: Dr. Piyush Kumar, Katihar, India.)

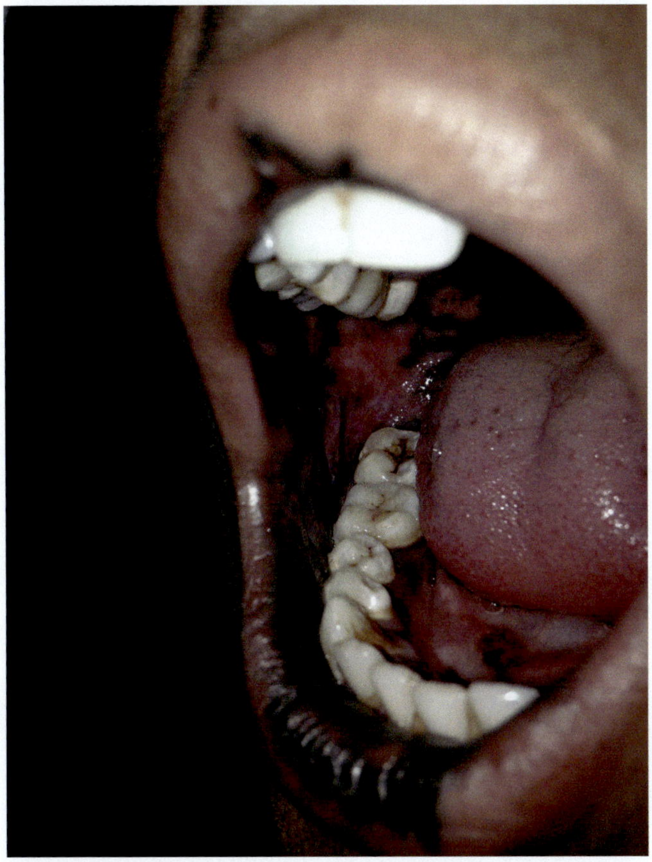

Figure 18.36 Diffuse dark-brown irregular pigmented macules.

## Pigmented nevi

- These involve a benign proliferation of melanocytes and "nevus cells," rare in the oral mucosa.
- Among pigmented nevi, the intramucosal type is the most common in oral cavity, followed by blue nevi. Junctional and compound nevi are rare in oral cavity.
- They present as an asymptomatic small, well-demarcated, solitary, brown or blue, well-circumscribed macule or plaque.
- The hard palate, buccal, labial and gingival mucosa, and lips are the most typical sites.
- Nevus cells tend to be round, ovoid, or spindle-shaped, while the basal layer melanocytes are dendritic in appearance.
- Intramucosal, compound, and junctional nevi likely share a common pathogenesis, while blue nevi cells usually reside deep in the connective tissue, giving the lesion a bluish tint.

## Nevus of Ota

- It is a developmental disorder characterized by hamartomatous presence of the melanocytes; it predominantly involves the skin of the face and eyes, and mucous membrane.
- It usually appears in early childhood and more commonly occurs in females.
- Clinically it presents as multiple mottled black or brown macules of variable size over the face in distribution of the first and second branches of the trigeminal nerve. Ipsilateral sclera may also be involved.
- The oral cavity may have blue-black macules commonly involving the palate and buccal mucosa.

## Melanoma

- Primary oral melanomas are rare and represent less than 1% of total melanomas. The most common sites are the hard palate and maxillary gingiva.
- Clinically, it presents as a well-circumscribed or irregular, black or brown, focally or diffusely pigmented macule, plaque, or nodule that may be ulcerated. Diffuse but contiguous pigmentation is of more concern than diffuse non-contiguous pigmentation.
- Based on clinical and histopathological criteria, oral melanoma is classified into three forms: lentigo maligna melanoma (best prognosis), superficial spreading melanoma (good prognosis), and nodular melanoma (poor prognosis).

## Addison's disease

- Addison's disease is caused by trauma, autoimmune disease, infectious agents, neoplasia, genetic disease, certain medications, and iatrogenic causes.
- Mucocutaneous pigmentation is often one of the earliest clinical manifestations of hypoadrenocorticism.
- It is clinically characterized by diffuse or patchy dark-brown pigmentation, due to melanin production. The buccal mucosa, palate, lips, and gingiva are the most common sites of involvement (**Figure 18.37a,b**).

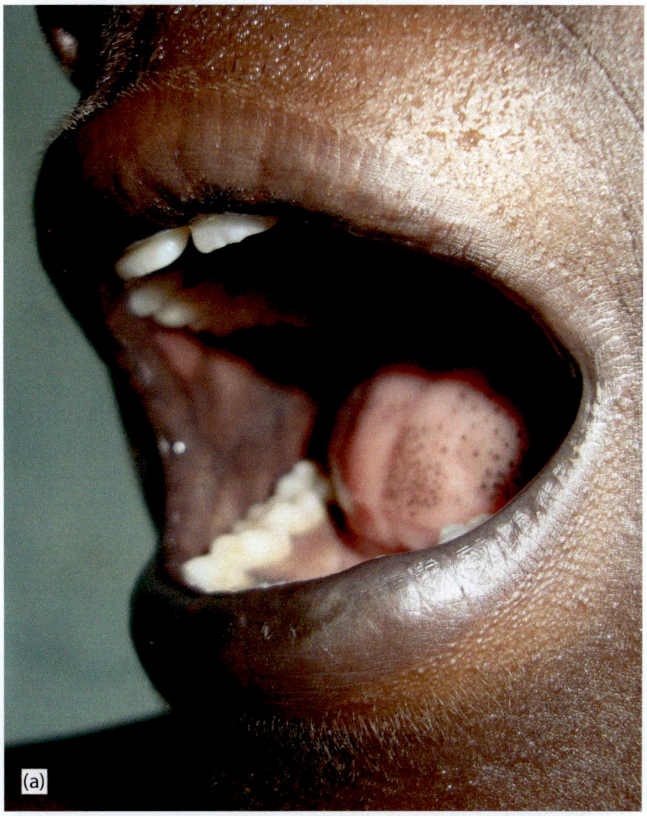


Figure 18.37 **(a)** Diffuse dark-brown pigmentation of buccal mucosa and gingiva. (*Continued*)

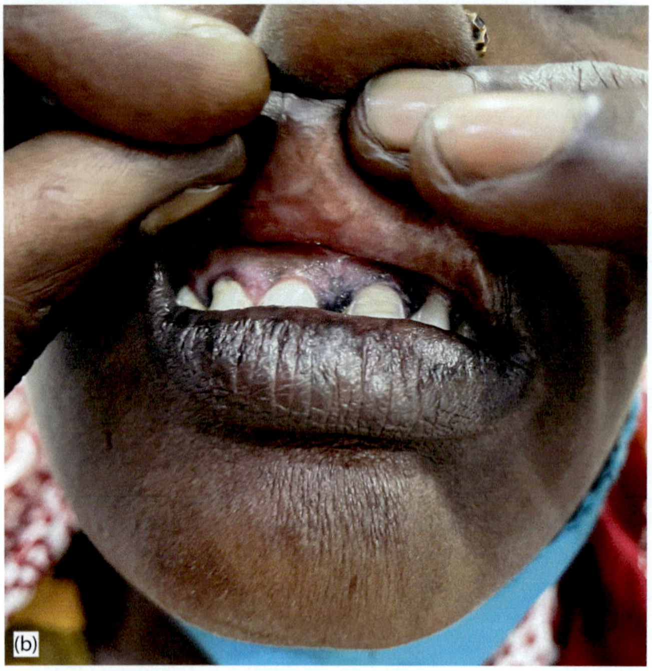

Figure 18.37 (*Continued*) **(b)** Pigmentation of lip and gingiva in Addison's disease. (a – Courtesy: Dr. Santoshdev Rathod, Ahmedabad, India; b – Courtesy: Dr. Soumyajit Roychoudhury, Berhampore, India.)

### Peutz-Jeghers syndrome

- This is a rare genetic disorder of autosomal dominant inheritance, characterized by mucocutaneous pigmentation and intestinal polyposis.
- Oral manifestations are the most important diagnostic findings and consist of oval or round, brown or black macules or spots, 1–10 mm in diameter (**Figure 18.38a,b**).
- The perioral skin, lips, buccal mucosa, and tongue are the most common sites affected.
- The skin lesions consist of numerous, usually perioral, dark spots.
- Intestinal polyps (hamartomas) are constant findings, usually in the jejunum and ileum.

### Melanoacanthoma

- This is a relatively uncommon melanocytic lesion that may cause rapid, diffuse, and dark pigmentation of a large mucosal area.
- It usually presents as an asymptomatic, solitary, ill-defined, rapidly enlarging, macular pigmentation mostly involving buccal mucosa.

# RED LESIONS

## Hereditary disorders

1. Vascular lesions (**Table 18.7**)
2. Hereditary mucoepithelial dysplasia
   - This is an autosomal dominant dyskeratotic epithelial syndrome affecting oral and other mucosae.
   - It occurs on the palate and gingiva.
   - It presents as intraoral erythematous maculo-papular lesions and periorificial red patches.

## Acquired disorders

### Traumatic erythema

- It can present either as an ecchymosis or as a hematoma, which appears as an irregular, flat area with a bright or deep red color.

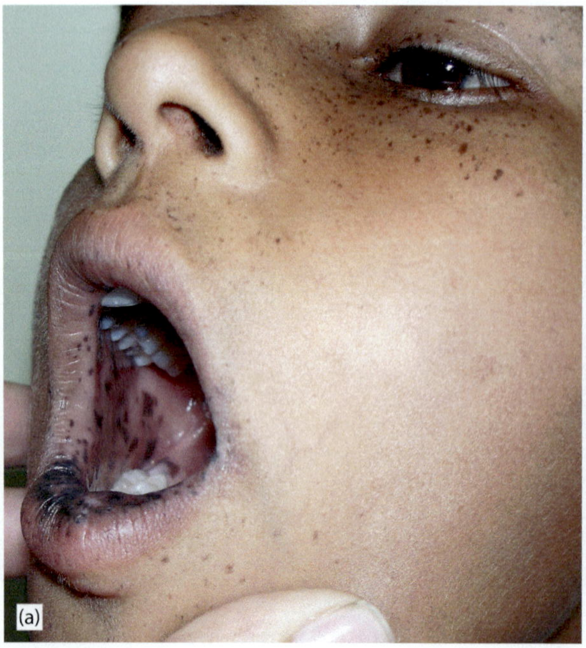

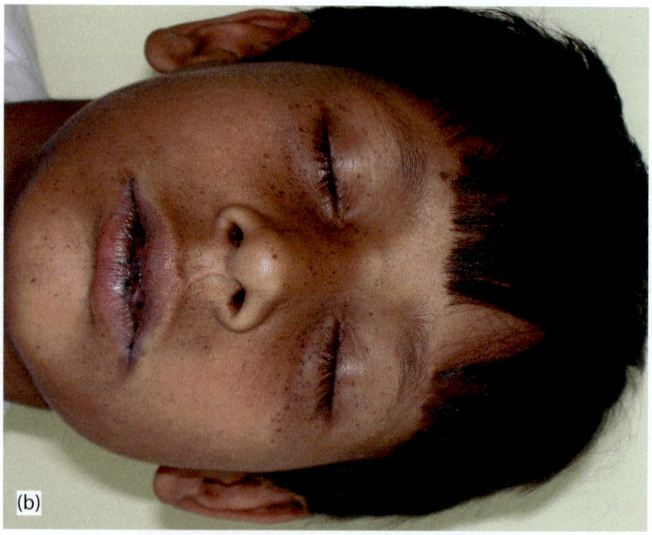

Figure 18.38 **(a)** Multiple dark brown to black macules in oral cavity. **(b)** Pigmented macules on the lip and periorbital area. (Courtesy: Dr. Piyush Kumar, Katihar, India.)

Table 18.7 Vascular causes of erythematous mucosal lesions

| Vascular condition | Type of lesions | Sites |
|---|---|---|
| Vascular malformation (**Figure 18.39a–c**) | Depends on the nature of vessels involved<br>• Capillary malformation: Erythematous patch<br>• Venous malformation: Red- blue papulonodular lesions<br>• Mixed: variable clinical presentation | Anywhere in the buccal cavity |
| Hereditary hemorrhagic telangiectasia syndrome (**Figure 18.39d,e**) | Telangiectasia<br>Hemorrhagic vesicles, nodules, papules, and ulcers | Lip<br>Gingiva, buccal mucosa |
| Sturge-Weber-Krabbe syndrome (**Figure 18.40a,b**) | Slight vascular hyperplasia to Hemangioma | Gingiva |
| Klippel-Trenaunay-Weber syndrome | Hemangioma<br>Macroglossia<br>Maxillary hyperplasia<br>Gingival fibromatosis | Gingiva |
| Blue rubber-bleb nevus syndrome | Soft, compressible and non-tender bluish vascular swelling | Buccal mucosa, retromolar trigone and ventrolateral tongue |
| Maffucci syndrome | Hemangioma | Tongue |

- Common sites include the lips, tongue, and buccal mucosa.
- DD: Other causes of hematoma (i.e., thrombocytopenia, anticoagulant therapy).

## Thermal burn

- It appears as a red, painful erythema that may undergo desquamation, leaving erosions.
- It usually heals spontaneously in about a week.
- DD: Chemical burn, traumatic lesions, herpes simplex.

## Radiation mucositis

- This is an adverse effect of radiation therapy for head and neck tumors.

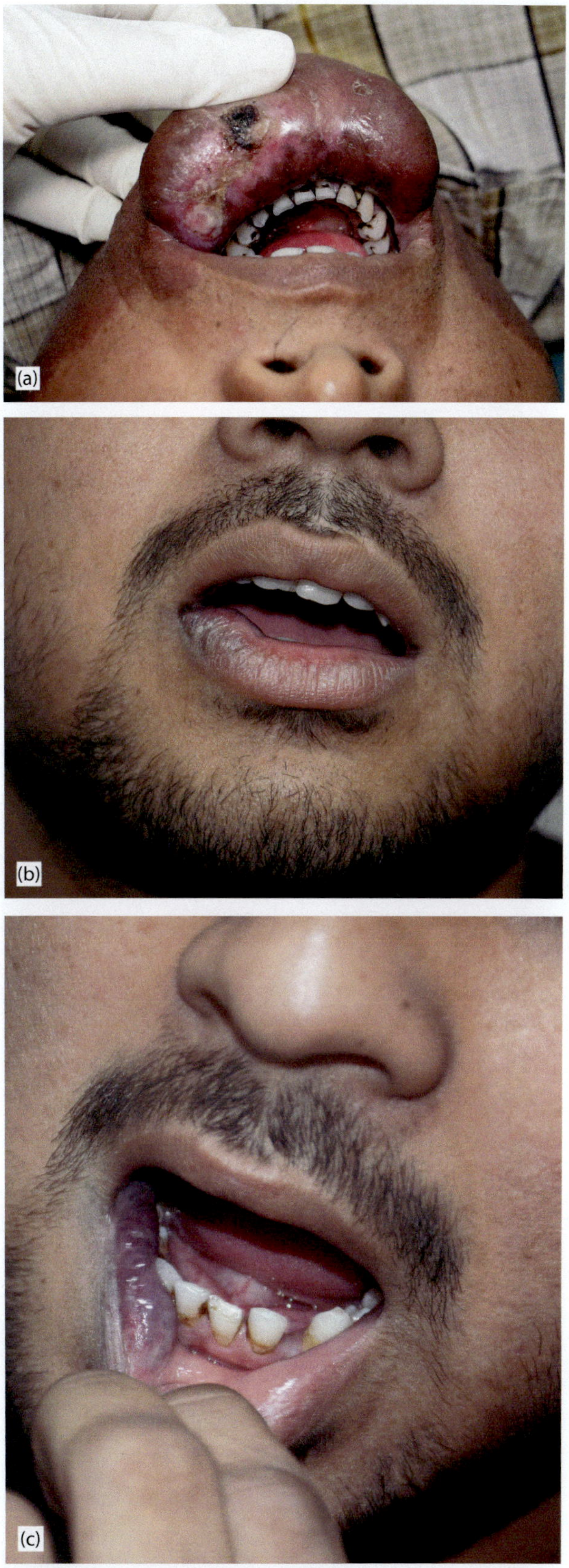


Figure 18.39 **(a)** Diffuse swelling of lower lip in capillary malformation. Note the surface ulceration. **(b)** Soft compressible red-blue focal swelling of the lip in venous malformation. **(c)** Inner aspect of the swelling. Bluish discoloration of dorsum of tongue. (*Continued*)

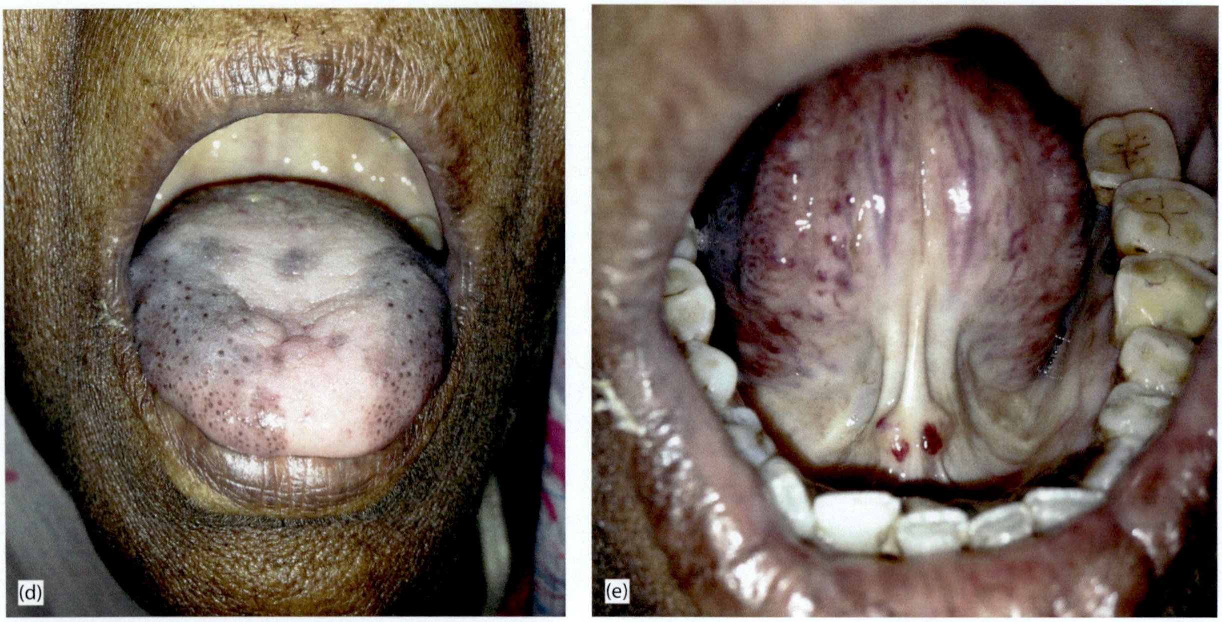


Figure 18.39 (*Continued*) **(d)** Hereditary hemorrhagic telangiectasia syndrome with multiple telangiectatic papules on tongue. **(e)** Telangiectasis on the ventral aspect of tongue in Hereditary hemorrhagic telangiectasia syndrome. (a–c – Courtesy: Dr. Piyush Kumar, Katihar, India.)

- Early lesions in form of erythema and edema usually start at the end of first week of therapy.
- At a later stage it may have erosions and ulcers covered with yellow-white exudate.
- Associated features are dryness of mouth, taste alteration, and burning and pain during mastication, swallowing, and speech.

## Median rhomboid glossitis

- This is a rare condition that may be associated with candidiasis and affect the dorsum of the tongue exclusively.

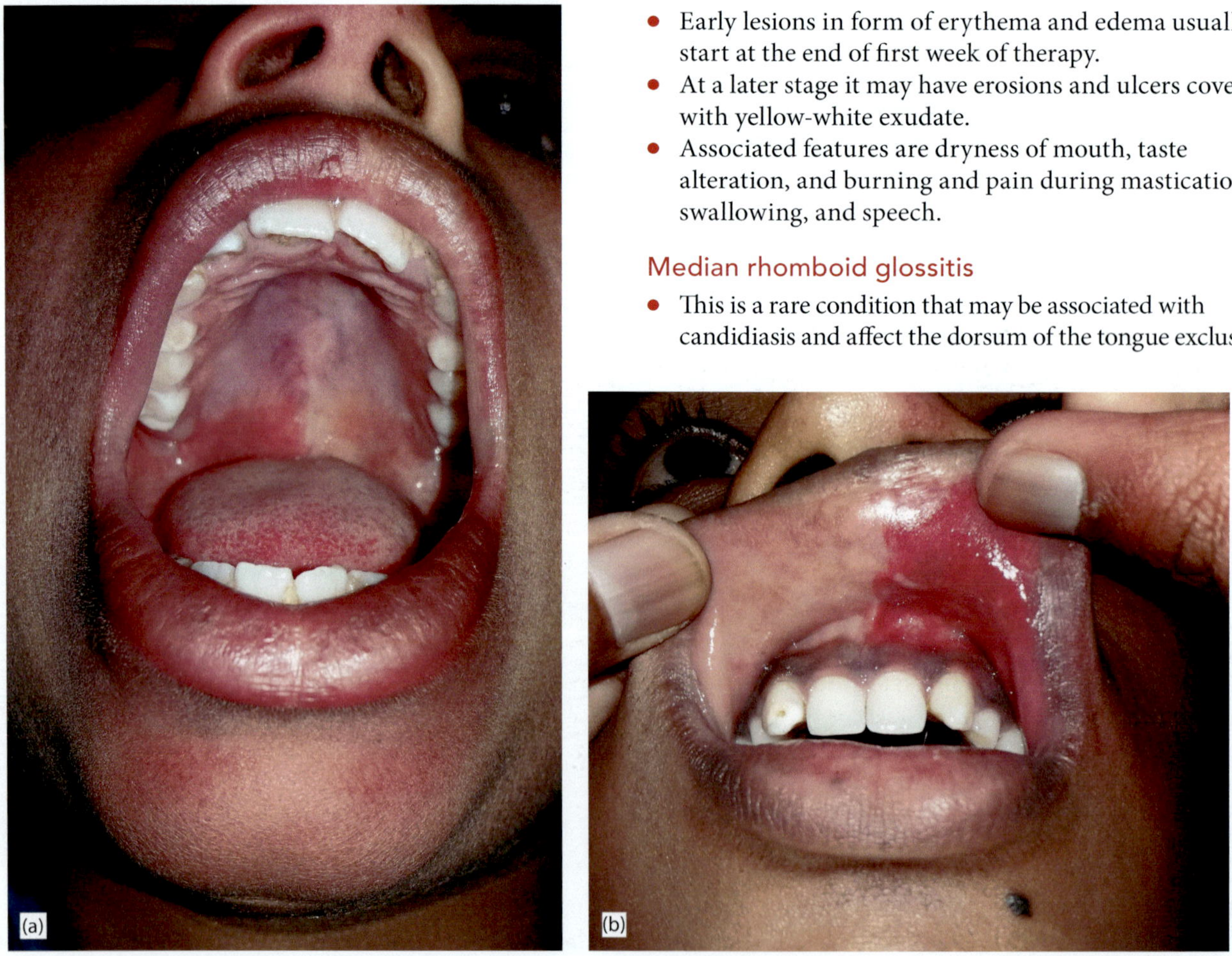


Figure 18.40 **(a)** Unilateral dusky erythematous plaque involving oral cavity, chin, lip, and nose. **(b)** Bright erythematous macule involving the lip in a case of port wine stain. (Courtesy: Dr. Hiral Shah, Baroda Medical College, Vadodara, India.)

- It is typically a rhomboidal-shaped erythematous central lesion anterior to the sulcus terminalis. The surface of lesion may be smooth or lobulated. Sometimes erythematous candidiasis in the palate may coexist.

## Denture-related stomatitis

- It is a common condition consisting of mild inflammation and erythema in patients who wear dentures continuously for long time.
- Caused by mechanical trauma from dentures, it is a tissue response to accumulated microorganisms between dentures and infections with Candida species mainly.
- It is characterized by diffuse chronic erythema and edema, and sometimes petechiae are restricted to denture area and white spots that represent accumulations of candidal hyphae. Mucosa below lower dentures is rarely involved.
- Newton's three clinical types:
  - Type 1: localized mild inflammation or a pinpoint hyperemia
  - Type 2: generalized simple type, more diffuse erythema involving a part of or the entire denture-covered mucosa
  - Type 3: a granular type, inflammatory papillary hyperplasia commonly involving the central part of the hard palate and the alveolar ridge

## Erythroplakia

- It is a premalignant lesion frequently occurring on the glans penis and rarely on the oral mucosa. It occurs more frequently at 50 to 70 years of age.
- It usually involves the floor of the mouth, the ventrum of tongue, or the soft palate.
- It appears as a usually asymptomatic, erythematous, smooth, well-demarcated plaque with velvety surface. On biopsy, 75–90% cases of erythroplasia show severe dysplasia, carcinoma, or carcinoma in situ.
- DD: Erythematous candidiasis, lichen planus, early SCC.

## Plasma cell gingivitis

- This is a unique gingival disorder due to local allergens or chronic infection, characterized histopathologically by chronic inflammatory infiltration of plasma cells.
- It appears as localized or widespread erythematous glossy lesions with edema and frequently accompanied by burning sensation.
- DD: Candidiasis, desquamative gingivitis, erythroplakia.

## Lupus erythematosus

- Oral lesions may develop in 15–25% of cases in discoid lupus erythematosus (DLE) and 30–45% of cases in systemic lupus erythematosus (SLE).
- The oral lesions are characterized by a well-defined central erythematous atrophic area surrounded by a sharp elevated white border with fine irregular perpendicular white paint-brush–like lines. Common sites are the palate and buccal mucosa (**Figure 18.41a–c**).
- Telangiectasia, petechiae, edema, erosions, ill-defined superficial ulcerations, and white hyperkeratotic plaques may be seen.

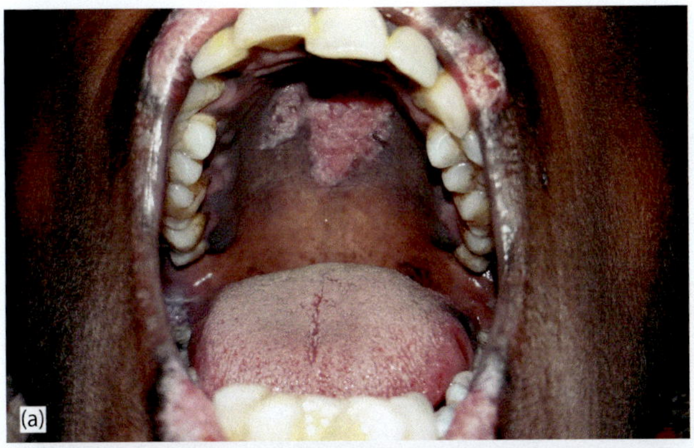
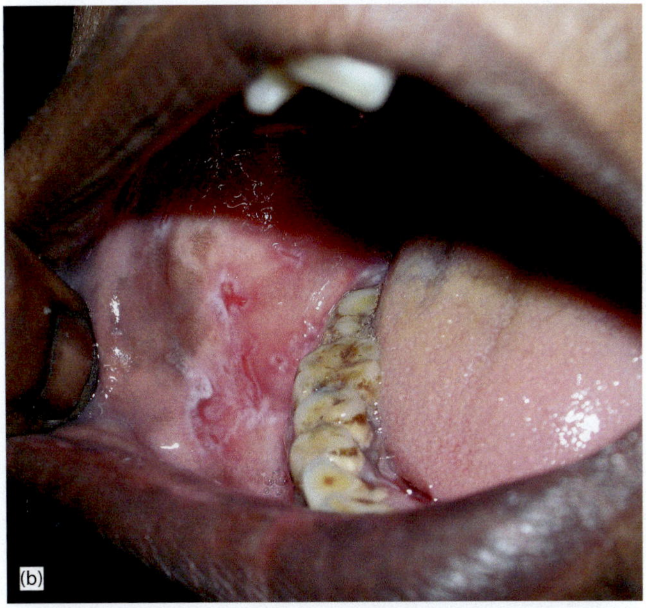
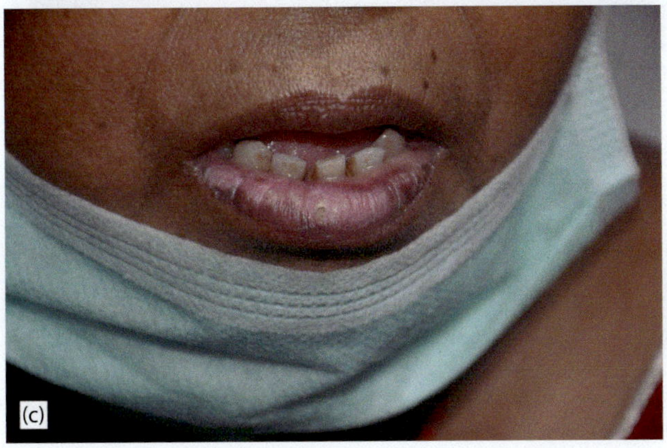

Figure 18.41 **(a)** Central erythematous atrophic plaque with whitish border involving palate and **(b)** small erosions surrounded by whitish border on buccal mucosa. **(c)** Erythematous plaque of discoid lupus erythematosus on the lip. There are some focal verrucous changes. (a – Courtesy: Dr. Hiral Shah, Baroda Medical College, Vadodara, India; c – Courtesy: Dr. Piyush Kumar, Katihar, India.)

- Common symptoms are dryness, soreness, and a burning sensation.
- DD: Lichen planus, speckled leukoplakia, erythroplakia, cicatracial pemphigoid.

## Anemia

- In anemia, pernicious anemia, iron-deficiency anemia, and Plummer-Vinson syndrome usually affect the oral mucosa.
- Iron-deficiency anemia may manifest as atrophic glossitis (flattening of the tongue papillae), mucosal pallor, and angular cheilitis.
- In megaloblastic anemia, painful atrophy of the entire oral mucosa and tongue (glossitis), stomatitis, recurrent aphthous ulcers, and magenta tongue are common features.
- Sickle cell anemia may manifest as orofacial pain, gingival enlargement, buccal mucosa pallor, and alveolar bone changes (step ladder appearance).
- Aplastic anemia presents as oral and facial petechiae, gingival hyperplasia, spontaneous gingival bleeding, hemorrhagic bullae, candidiasis, and herpetic lesions.

## Thrombocytopenic purpura

- This is characterized by hemorrhagic petechiae, ecchymoses, blisters, or even hematomas, usually located on the palate and buccal mucosa (**Figure 18.42a,b**).
- Spontaneous gingival bleeding is a constant early finding.
- DD: Aplastic anemia, leukemias, SJS-TEN.

## Infectious mononucleosis

- It is an acute, self-limited infectious disease caused by Epstein-Barr virus transmitted through saliva transfer; it primarily affects children.
- Prodromal symptoms include anorexia, malaise, headache, fatigue, and fever.
- Oral manifestations consist of palatal petechiae, uvular edema, tonsillar exudate, gingivitis, and rarely ulcers may also appear.
- Other features are maculopapular skin rash, sore generalized lymphadenopathy, hepatosplenomegaly, maculopapular skin rash, and sore throat.
- DD: Leukemia, diphtheria, secondary syphilis, thrombocytopenic purpura.

## Reiter's disease

- It is an uncommon multisystemic disorder involving the genitourinary tract, conjunctiva, and joints.
- The disease is mediated by an immunological mechanism that is triggered by infectious agents in genetically susceptible individuals and predominantly affects young men aged 20 to 30 years.
- Major clinical manifestations are symmetrical arthritis, nongonococcal urethritis, conjunctivitis, balanitis, prostatitis, cervicitis, psoriasiform skin lesions, and palmoplantar keratoderma.
- Oral involvement may occur in 20–40% of the cases and is characterized by erythematous papule or diffuse erythematous areas intermixed with thin whitish dots or lines and painful superficial erosions over buccal mucosa, gingiva palate, and lips.
- The tongue lesions may mimic geographic tongue.
- DD: Behçet's disease, geographic tongue, and SJS-TEN.

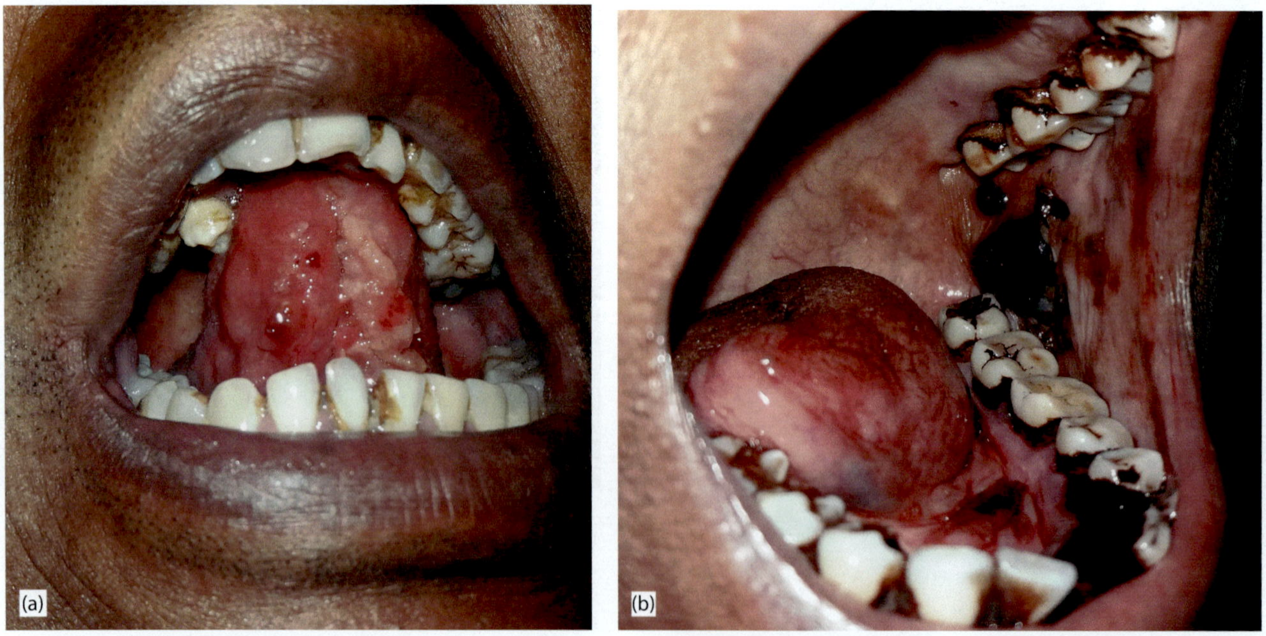


Figure 18.42 **(a)** Multiple hemorrhagic papules on ventral aspect of tongue. **(b)** Large vesicle and bullae on buccal mucosa. (Courtesy: Dr. Hiral Shah, Baroda Medical College, Vadodara, India.)

## VERRUCOUS LESIONS

### Papilloma due to chronic irritation

- Chronic irritation or trauma of mucosa may lead to benign proliferation of stratified squamous epithelium.
- Clinically presents as 0.5- to 1-cm whitish gray, painless, exophytic, well-circumscribed pedunculated lesions with finger like projections giving a rough or cauliflower appearance (**Figure 18.43a,b**).

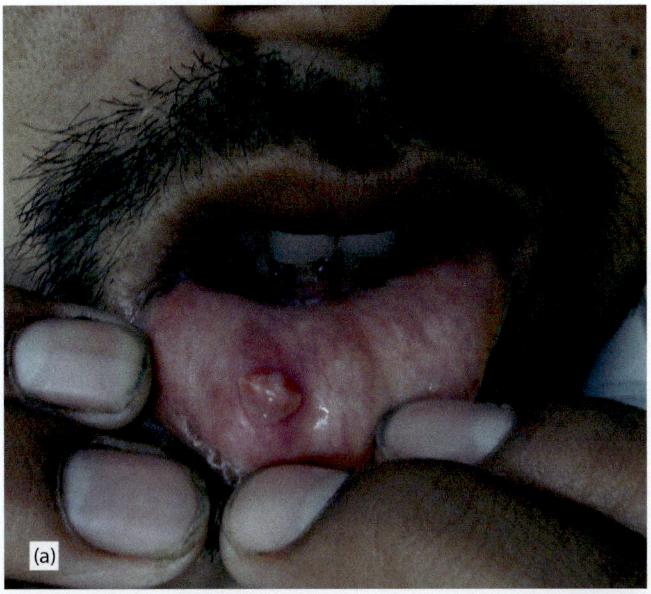


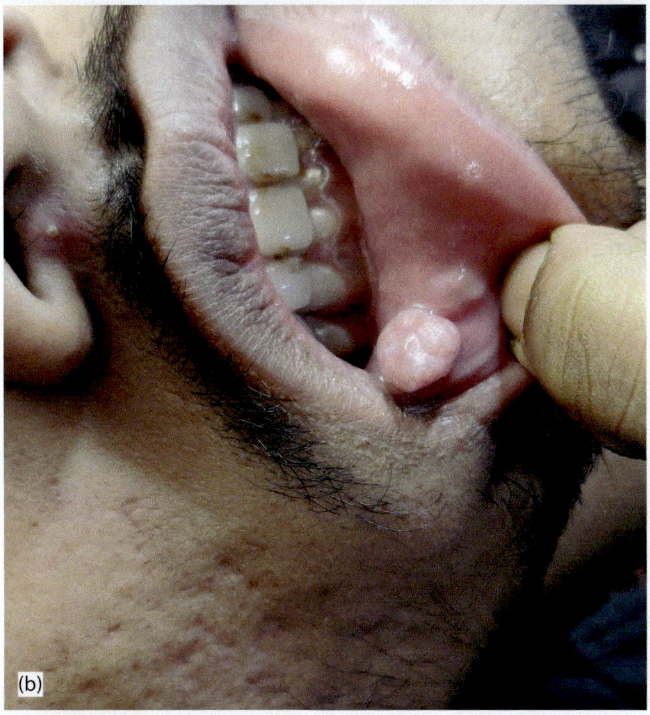


Figure 18.43 **(a)** Repetitive trauma resulting in solitary pinkish-white growth forming a papilloma on labial mucosa. **(b)** Single, sessile, well-defined exophytic cauliflower like growth on labial mucosa. (b – Courtesy: Dr. Shweta Jain, Mumbai, India.)

- Common sites are the ventral tongue, frenulum, and soft palate.
- DD: Verruca vulgaris, verrucous carcinoma, condyloma acuminatum.

### Verruca vulgaris

- An infection caused by human papillomavirus (HPV), it rarely involves oral mucosa and is more common in children.
- Common types of HPV responsible for oral lesions are types 2, 4, and 40.
- The vermilion border and the lip mucosa, keratinized surface of gingiva, commissures, and tongue are common sites.
- Clinically, it appears as a single or multiple painless, white, small, sessile, and well-defined exophytic growth with a cauliflower surface (**Figure 18.44**).
- DD: Papilloma, condyloma acuminatum, focal epithelial hyperplasia.

### Condyloma acuminatum

- Sexually transmitted benign lesions usually involve the anogenital region; they may rarely may occur in oral cavity.
- It is caused by the human papillomavirus types 2, 6, and 11.
- Sites are the labial mucosa, soft palate, and lingual frenum.

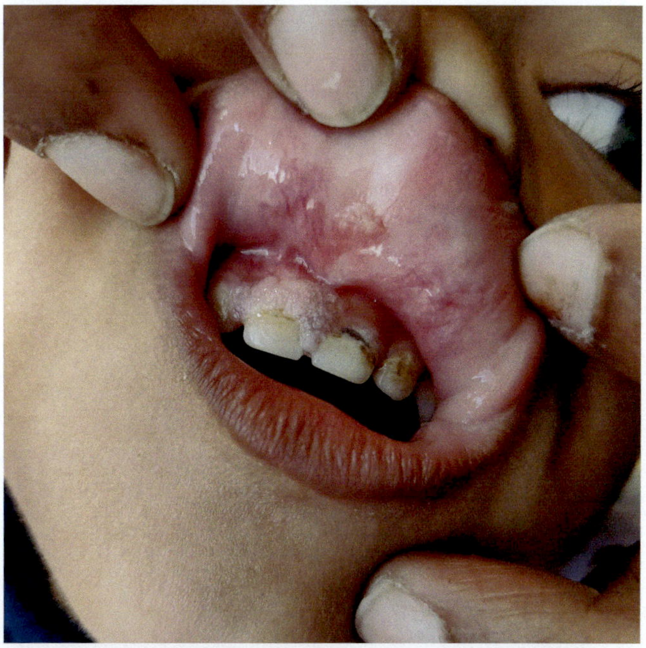

Figure 18.44 Verrucous plaques of verruca vulgaris involving the upper gingiva and adjacent inner surface of upper lip. (Courtesy: Dr. Dependra Kumar Timshina, Remedy Clinic, Siliguri, India.)

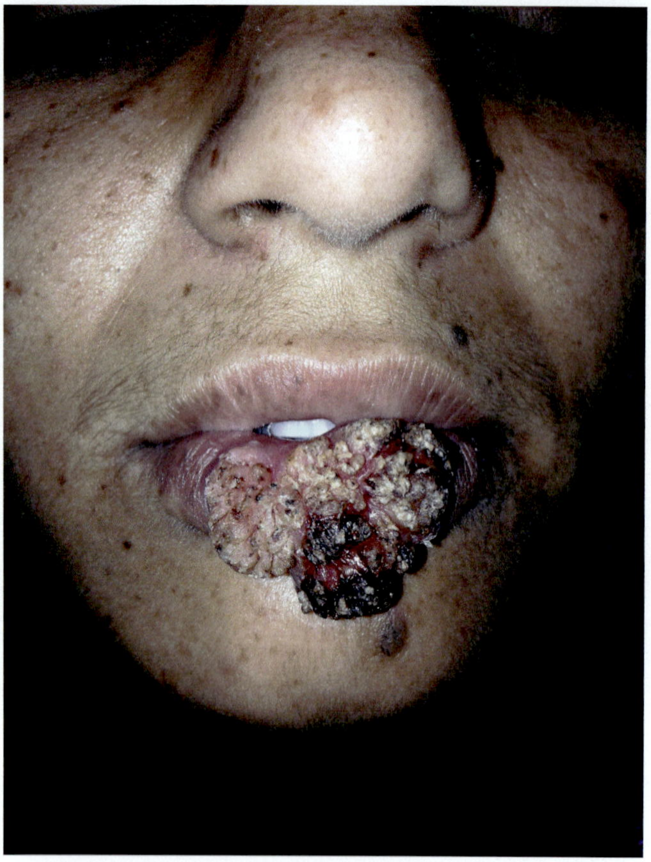

Figure 18.45 Large verrucous growth with marked induration and hemorrhage on lower lip.

- Clinically, lesions are similar to papilloma but larger in size and more clustered, dense, and deeply rooted (**Figure 18.45**).
- DD: Papilloma, verruca vulgaris, focal epithelial hyperplasia, early verrucous carcinoma.

## Focal epithelial hyperplasia (Heck's disease)

- Benign hyperplastic lesions caused by HPV 13 and 32 are increasingly seen in HIV-positive individuals.
- Sites are the buccal, labial, and lingual mucosa.
- Clinically it presents as mucosal-colored multiple soft, smooth, painless, sessile, dome-shaped nodules or plaques 3–10 mm in diameter and lacking papillary surface.
- DD: Condyloma acuminatum, verruca vulgaris, and multiple papillomas.

## Verruciform xanthoma

- Verruciform xanthoma is rare hyperplastic disorder caused by trauma.
- Sites are the gingiva, alveolar ridge, tongue, and palate.
- It presents as a reddish-yellowish, well-demarcated, painless, sessile, slightly elevated lesion. It has a cauliflower-like surface (**Figure 18.46a,b**).
- DD: Papilloma, verruca vulgaris, condyloma acuminatum, verrucous carcinoma.

## Verrucous carcinoma

- It is a slow-growing, well-differentiated low-grade variant of squamous cell carcinoma presenting

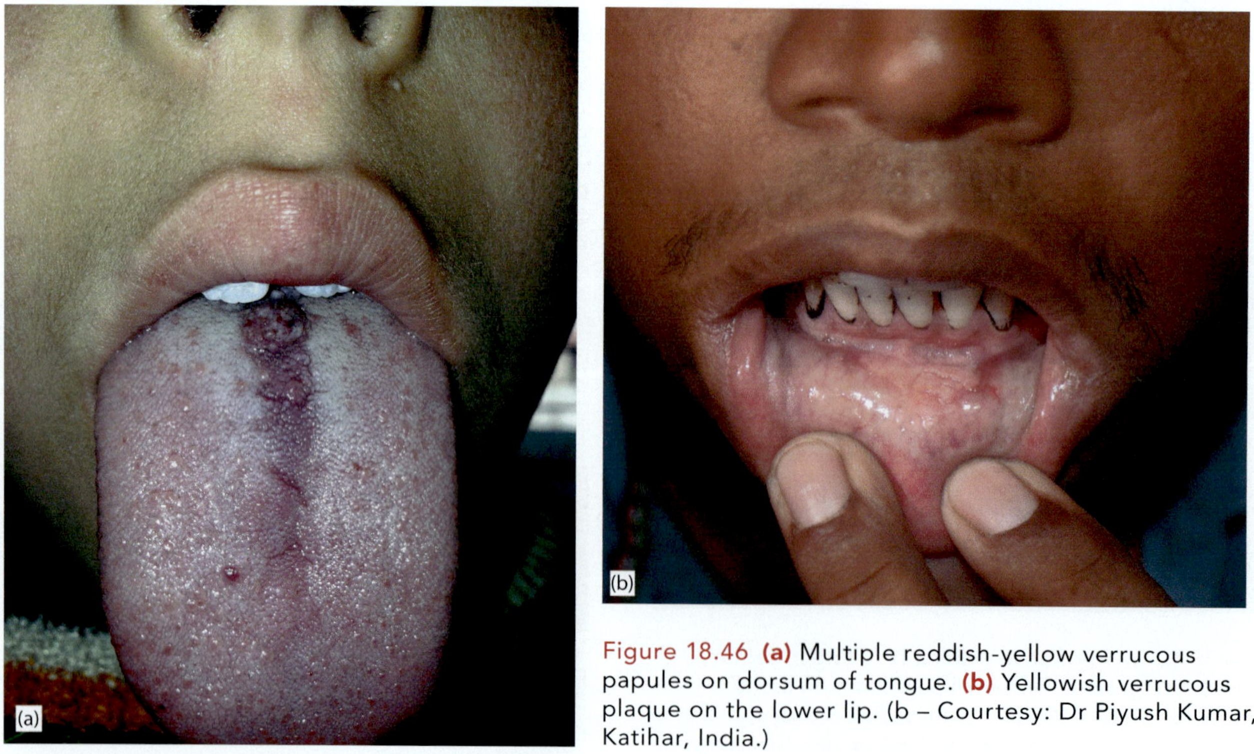


Figure 18.46 **(a)** Multiple reddish-yellow verrucous papules on dorsum of tongue. **(b)** Yellowish verrucous plaque on the lower lip. (b – Courtesy: Dr Piyush Kumar, Katihar, India.)

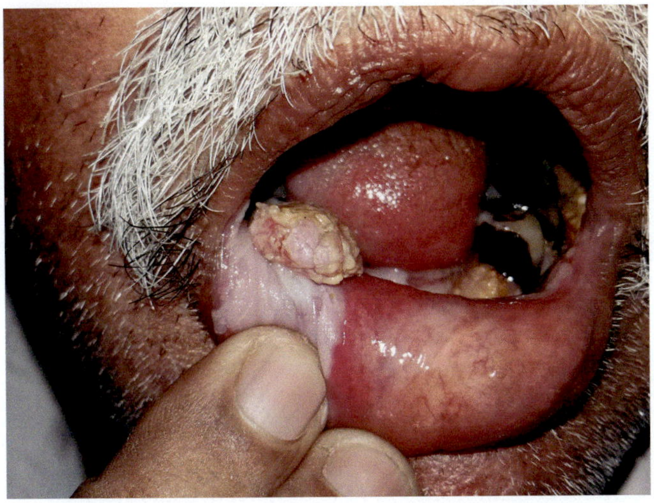

Figure 18.47 Verrucous carcinoma with leukoplakia. (Courtesy: Dr. Hiral Shah, Baroda Medical College, Vadodara, India.)

as an exophytic, whitish mass with a papillary or verruciform surface (**Figure 18.47**).

### Acanthosis nigricans

- Approximately 40% of malignant acanthosis nigricans (AN) show oral lesions.
- Sites are the vermilion border of lips, tongue, and gingiva.
- Clinically it presents as mucosal-colored multiple, small, painless, papillomatous and verrucous lesions. Mild gingival swelling, hypertrophy, and elongation of the filiform papillae (shaggy tongue) have also been reported. Unlike skin lesions, oral AN is rarely pigmented.
- DD: Focal epithelial hyperplasia, multiple papillomas, lipoid proteinosis, multiple verruca vulgaris, pemphigus vegetans.

### Darier disease

- Darier disease is an autosomal dominant inherited dyskeratotic acantholytic disorder.
- Site are the palate, gingiva, buccal mucosa, and tongue.
- Oral lesions occur in 20–40% of cases and appear as small multiple whitish confluent papules, which may become hypertrophic, assuming a cobblestone or papillary pattern (**Figure 18.48**).
- DD: Acanthosis nigricans, papillary hyperplasia of palate.

## LUMPS AND SWELLINGS

### Angioedema

- It can be caused by
  - Allergic angioedema: drugs (local anesthetics, angiotensin converting enzyme inhibitors), exposure to latex or certain food substances.

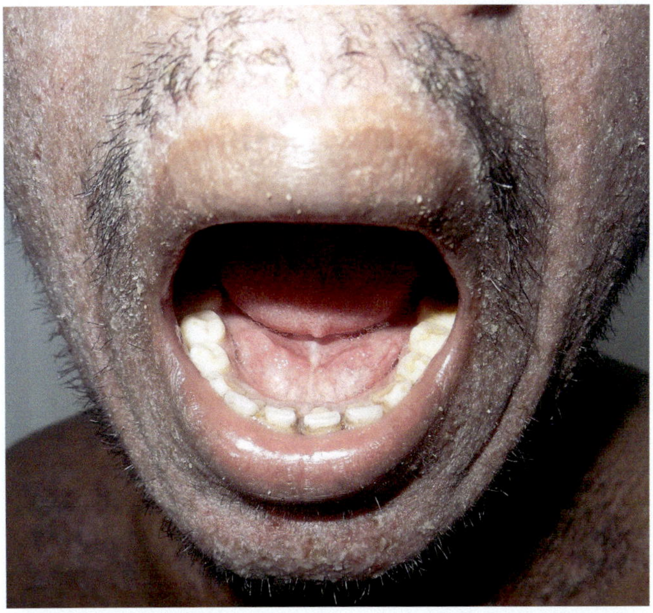

Figure 18.48 Multiple whitish confluent papules on floor of mouth. (Courtesy: Dr. Piyush Kumar, Katihar, India.)

  - C1 esterase inhibitor deficiency:
    - Hereditary – onset occurs in childhood
      - Type I: low levels of functionally normal C1-esterase inhibitor
      - Type II: dysfunctional C1-esterase inhibitor
    - Acquired – usually occurs in adulthood
- The swelling may affect lips, tongue, or other areas.
- It is usually only mild and transient but has potential for obstruction of the airway.

### Abscesses

- These are mostly odontogenic in origin as a consequence of dental caries.
- Rarely they may be the result of trauma, a foreign body, or infections such as actinomycosis, nocardiosis, or botryomycosis.
- They usually discharge in the mouth on buccal gingiva but sometimes discharge palatally, lingually, on the chin or submental region.

### Mucocele (mucous cyst or ranula)

- This is a benign, common, mucus-containing cystic lesion of the minor salivary glands in the oral cavity.
- These lesions are not true cysts, not having an epithelial lining.
- Based on location, they can be superficial (directly under the mucosa), classic (in the upper submucosa), or deep (in the lower corium). Deeper mucoceles are more common.

- Based on histological features, two types of mucoceles are described.
  - Extravasation cysts are pseudo-cysts that result from extravasation of mucous in the peri-glandular connective tissue by a rupture of the salivary duct with a partial epithelial lining (mucous pseudocyst, 92%).
  - Retention cysts surrounded by salivary tissue with an epithelial lining composed of one or two layers of flat or cuboidal epithelial cells (true mucous cyst, 8%).
- It appears as a painless dome-shaped, translucent, whitish-blue smooth-surfaced swelling ranging in size from a few millimeters to centimeters (**Figure 18.49a**). The lesion may become irregular and whitish due to multiple cycles of rupture and healing caused by trauma or puncture.
- Sites are the lower lip, floor of the mouth, cheek, palate, retromolar fossa, and the tongue; the upper lip is usually spared.
- Larger lesions most often affect the floor of the mouth; these are called ranulas because of the similarity to the throat pouch of frogs (**Figure 18.49b**).
- When the mucus accumulates in the deep soft tissues, the presentation is as an enlarging, painless mass assuming the pink coloration of the mucosa.
- The treatment of choice for a deep mucocele and the classic form is surgical excision, which should include the immediate adjacent glandular tissue.

## Fibroma

- It is considered a reactive hyperplastic connective tissue growth rather than a true neoplasm. Accidental biting, other trauma, and irritation are major causative factors.
- It typically presents as an asymptomatic, well-defined, firm, sessile or pedunculated pink papule or nodule with a smooth surface of normal epithelium (**Figure 18.50a**).
- Most common sites are the tongue, buccal mucosa, and lips.
- Angiofibroma is a characteristic lesion of tuberous sclerosis. They are present as discrete to coalescing skin-colored to dark-brown firm papules, nodules, and plaques. Rarely an oral cavity can also be involved, and the gingiva is the most common site. Usually they are located on

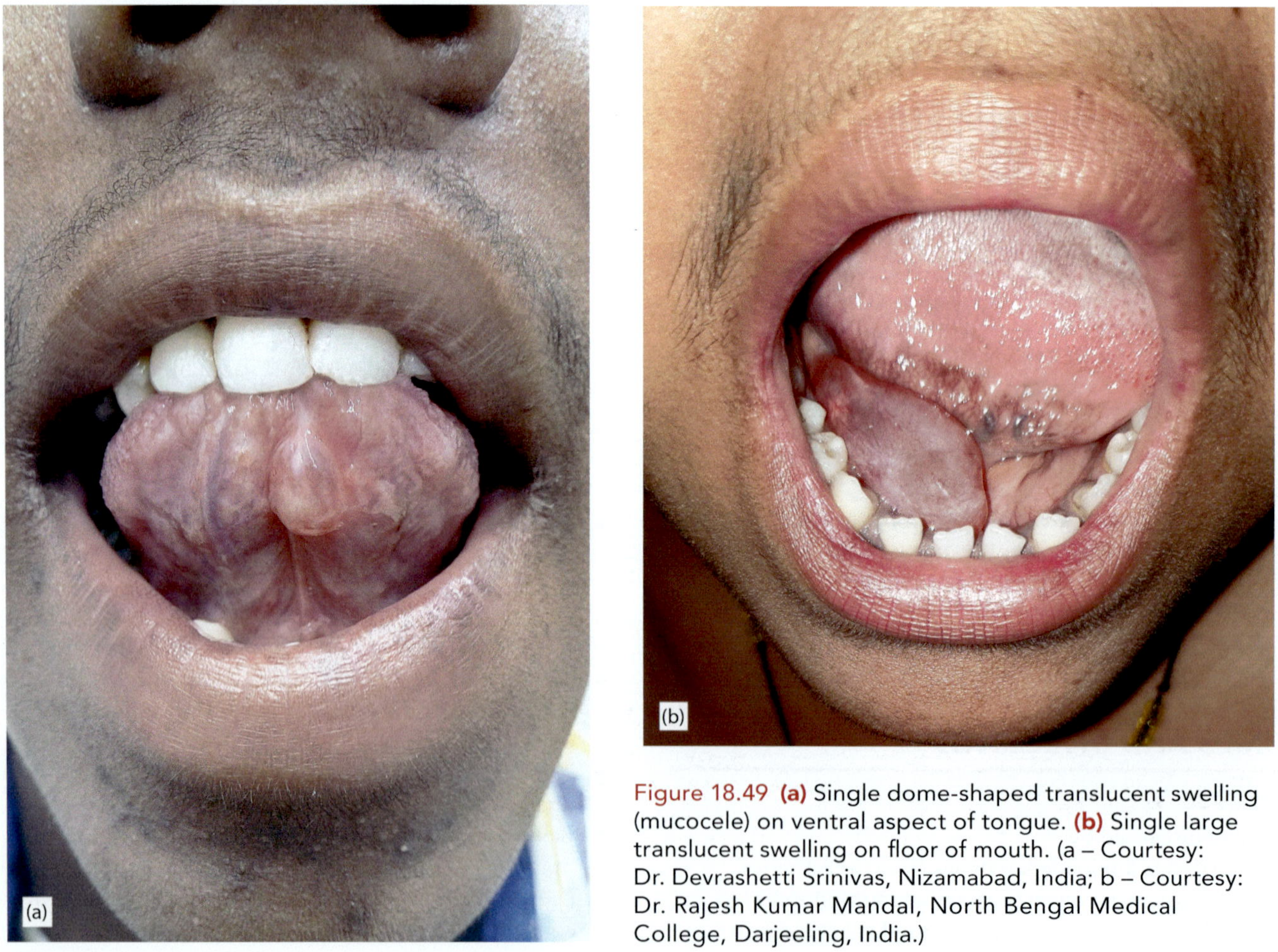


Figure 18.49 **(a)** Single dome-shaped translucent swelling (mucocele) on ventral aspect of tongue. **(b)** Single large translucent swelling on floor of mouth. (a – Courtesy: Dr. Devrashetti Srinivas, Nizamabad, India; b – Courtesy: Dr. Rajesh Kumar Mandal, North Bengal Medical College, Darjeeling, India.)

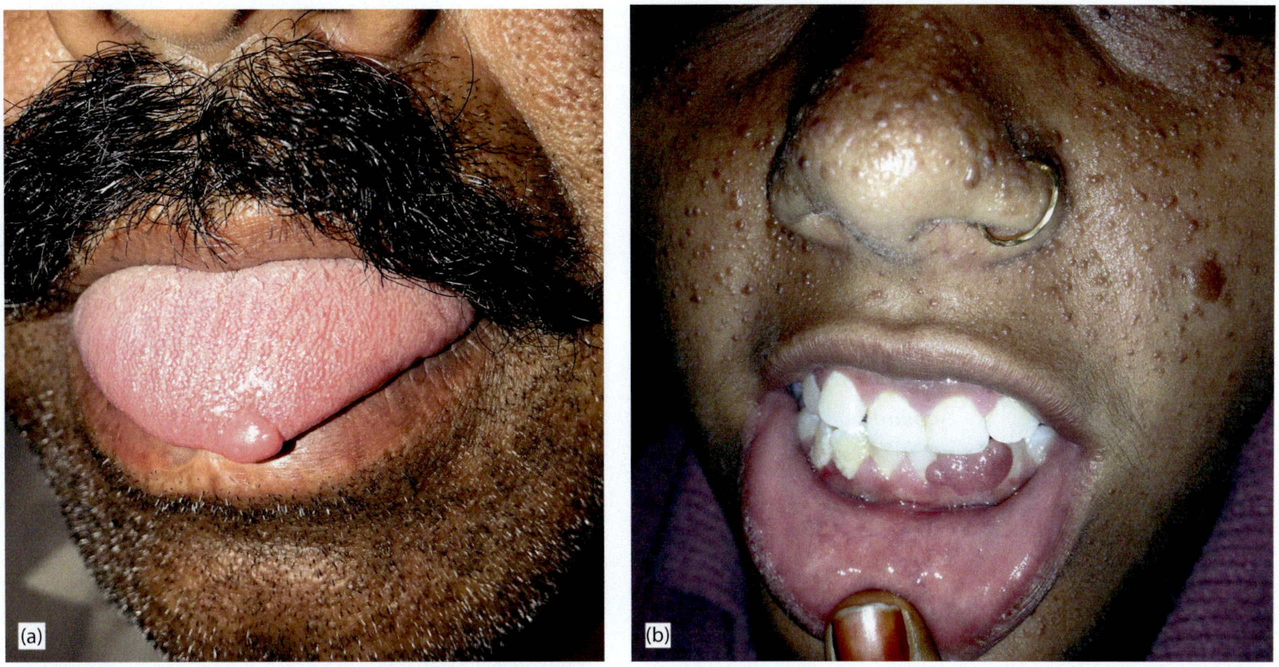

Figure 18.50 **(a)** Well-defined firm papule on tip of tongue. **(b)** Gingival fibroma presenting as erythematous firm nodular plaque with numerous angiofibromas on face in patient tuberous sclerosis.

the face, involving the nose, nasolabial fold, and cheek (**Figure 18.50b**).

## Pyogenic granuloma

- A painless, red, firm, vascular reactive growth presents as a pedunculated or sessile mass with a smooth or lobulated surface. Sometimes it may ulcerate and have a covering of whitish fibrinous membrane. It is soft to the touch and has a tendency to bleed easily.
- The gingiva is the most common site, followed by the tongue, lips, and buccal mucosa (**Figure 18.51a,b**).

## Gingival hyperplasia

It is characterized by overgrowth of submucosal tissue covered with normal epithelium, leading to enlargement of the gingiva (**Table 18.8**). It can present as generalized or localized enlargement.

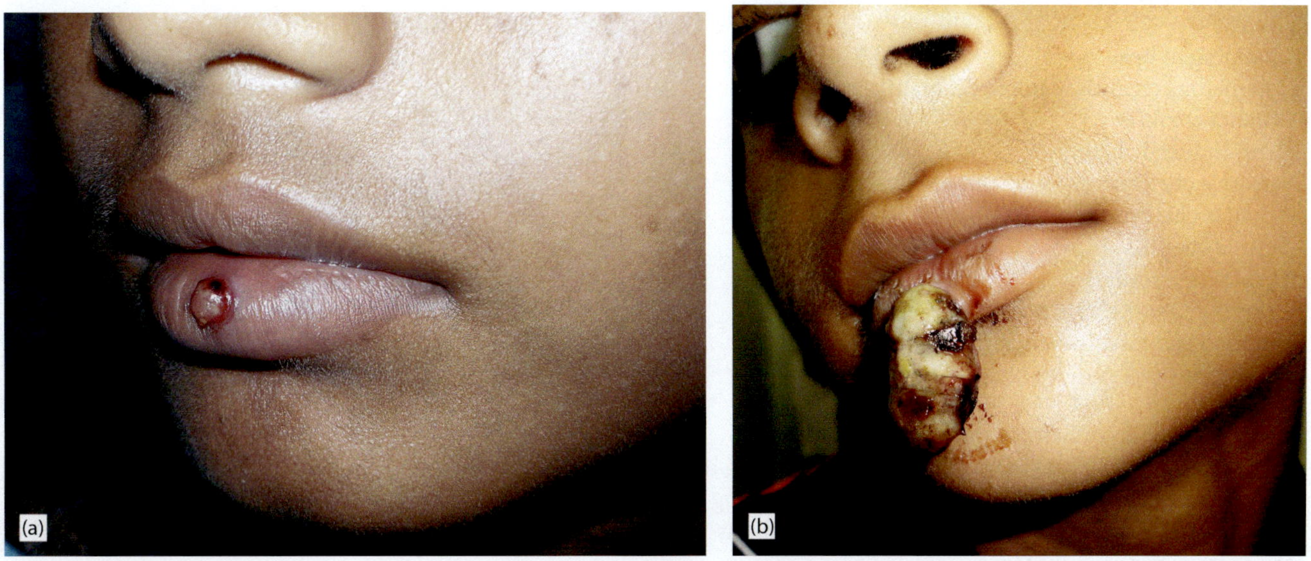

Figure 18.51 **(a)** Pyogenic granuloma seen as friable, eroded erythematous nodule on the lip. **(b)** Large protruding lesion of pyogenic granuloma lip. (a,b – Courtesy: Dr. Piyush Kumar, Katihar, India.)

Table 18.8 Causes of gingival hyperplasia

| Generalized gingival hyperplasia | Localized gingival hyperplasia |
|---|---|
| *Congenital*<br>• Hereditary gingival fibromatosis<br>• Mucopolysaccharidosis<br>• Hypoplasminogenemia<br>*Acquired*<br>• Hyperplastic gingivitis<br>• Mouth-breathing gingivitis<br>• Pregnancy<br>• Puberty<br>• Scurvy<br>• Hematological (leukemia, aplastic anemia, lymphoma)<br>• Drug-induced (phenytoin, calcium channel blockers, cyclosporine, oral contraceptive)<br>• Systemic (Wegener's granulomatosis, primary amyloidosis, sarcoidosis, Crohn's disease, Kaposi sarcoma) | *Congenital*<br>• Fabry syndrome<br>• Cowden syndrome<br>• Tuberous sclerosis<br>• Sturge-Weber angiomatosis<br>• Gingival granular cell tumor<br>*Acquired*<br>• Abscess (periodontal abscess)<br>• Cysts (gingival cyst, eruption cyst)<br>• Pyogenic granuloma<br>• Neoplasms (peripheral giant-cell granuloma, peripheral ossifying fibroma) |

# LIP LESIONS

## Cheilitis

It is an inflammatory condition that may be primary in origin or secondary due to disease of nearby skin and mucosa.

Causes

- Chapping of lips
- Eczematous cheilitis – atopic dermatitis
- Contact cheilitis
- Drug-induced cheilitis
- Infective cheilitis
- Angular cheilitis
- Actinic cheilitis
- Cheilitis glandularis
- Granulomatous cheilitis
- Factitious (exfoliative) cheilitis

### Lip-licking dermatitis

- It is due to chronic cheilitis.
- It is characterized by erythema, scaling, and crusting of the lips and the perioral skin (**Figure 18.52**). Fissuring may also occur in severe cases. A burning sensation is the most common symptom.
- DD: Perioral dermatitis, eczematous cheilitis, contact cheilitis.

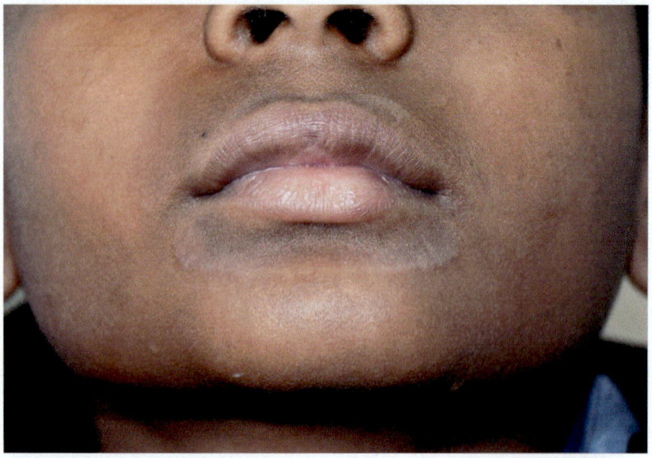

Figure 18.52 Lip-licking dermatitis presenting as scaling and pigmentation around the lips. (Courtesy: Dr. Piyush Kumar, Katihar, India.)

## Contact cheilitis

- Common irritants or allergens include lipsticks, mouthwashes, dental preparations, and food.
- It is confined to the vermilion border of both lips.
- It is characterized by mild edema and erythema, followed by irritation and thick scaling (**Figure 18.53**).

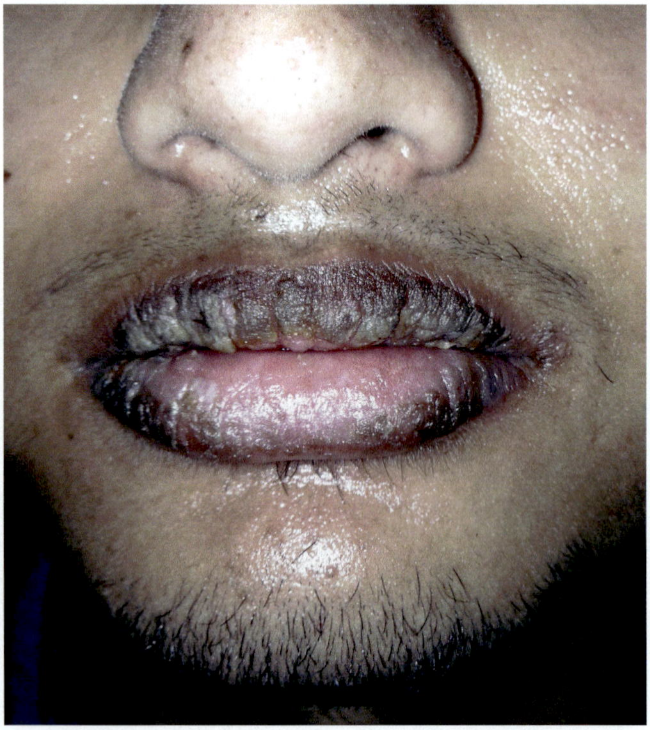

Figure 18.53 Diffuse erythema, edema, and thick scaling on both lips.

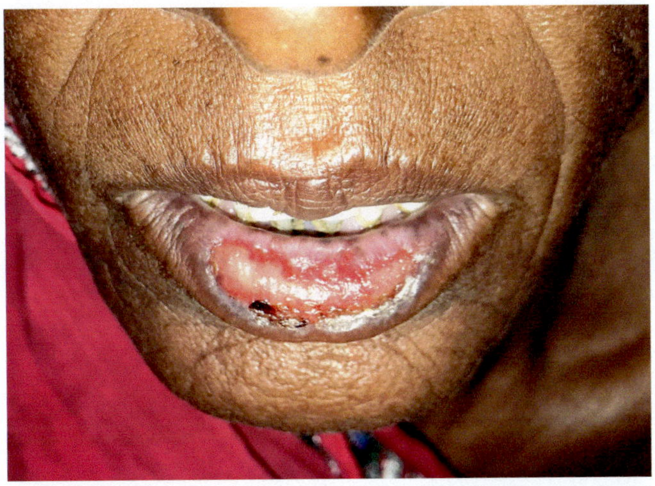

Figure 18.54 Lower lip having central erosion surrounded by erythematous plaque.

## Actinic cheilitis

- Actinic cheilitis is a chronic degenerative disorder of the lower lip due to long sun exposure.
- The premalignant condition usually occurs in people more than 50 years of age.
- It starts as mild erythema, edema with fine scaling and dryness. It slowly progress to thinned, smooth epithelium with mixed whitish-gray and erythematous plaques. Erosions and nodular lesions may also develop (**Figure 18.54**).
- DD: Leukoplakia, lichen planus, lupus erythematosus, early squamous-cell carcinoma, cheilitis due to radiation.

## Angular cheilitis

- It is caused by infections, immune deficiency, nutritional deficiency, or mechanical trauma.
- Characteristic triangular lesions consist of erythema, maceration, and edema at one or both commissures, associated with burning sensation and dryness. In severe cases linear fissures radiating from the angle of mouth to the mucocutaneous border may be present (**Figure 18.55**).

## Exfoliating cheilitis

- This chronic inflammatory disorder more commonly develops in young females with a personality disorder.
- Most of the time it is confined to the vermilion border of lips.
- It is associated with a burning sensation.
- Usually it starts from the middle of the lower lip and spreads to involve the whole of the lower or both lips; it persists in varying severity for months or years and leads to hyperkeratotic thickening, fissuring, and crusting (**Figure 18.56**).

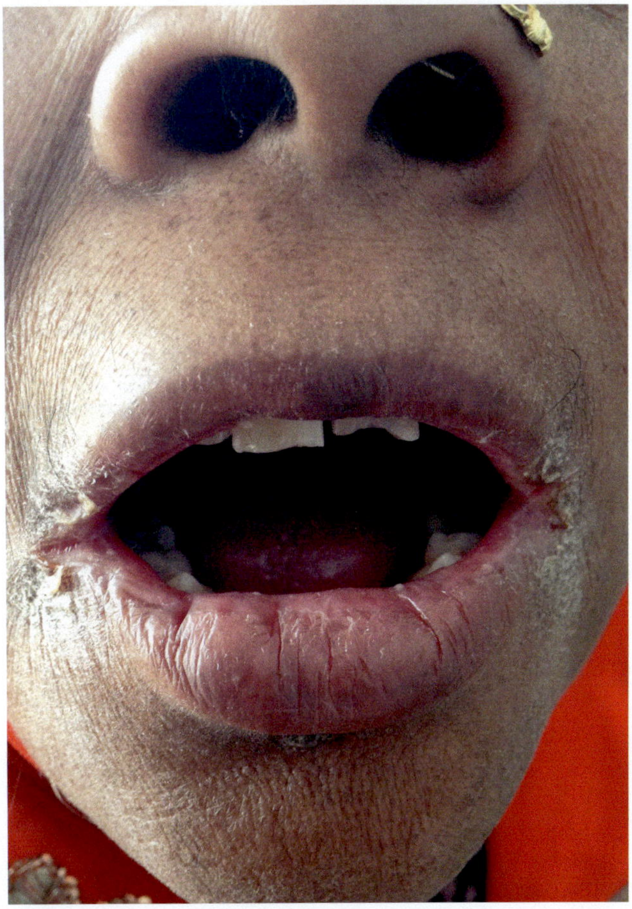

Figure 18.55 Angular cheilitis.

## Cheilitis glandularis

- It is due to inflammation and swelling of the salivary glands of the lips. It may be premalignant in 20–30% of cases.
- It clinically presents as swelling of lower lip, with dilated pinhead-sized orifices of salivary glands.

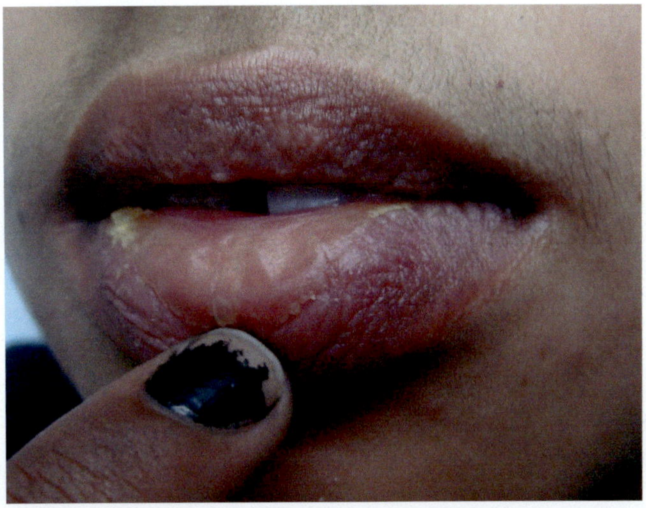

Figure 18.56 Exfoliating cheilitis.

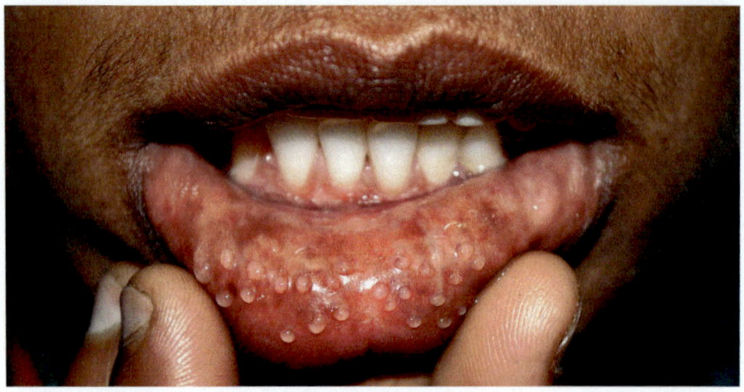

Figure 18.57 Mucous fluid coming out from the orifices in glandular cheilitis. (Courtesy: Dr. Sanjay Khare, MGM Medical College, Indore, India.)

On squeezing them, mucous saliva comes out (**Figure 18.57**).

- Volkmann's cheilitis is a severe and suppurative form in which the lip is tender, enlarged, and covered with crusts and scales covering salivary duct orifices.
- DD: Cheilitis granulomatosa, Melkersson-Rosenthal syndrome, Crohn's disease, sarcoidosis, cystic fibrosis.

### Granulomatous cheilitis

- This is a chronic swelling of the lip due to granulomatous inflammation of unknown cause.
- The granulomatous changes are confined to the lip, and this is generally regarded as a monosymptomatic form of Melkersson-Rosenthal syndrome.
- **Melkersson-Rosenthal syndrome**
  - It appears in a relapsing and remitting course. First episodes may subside in hours or days, but recurrent episodes may persist longer.
  - It is characterized by a sudden diffuse nodular swelling of upper lip, lower lip, or cheek in decreasing order of frequency, labial swelling (75% of cases), facial edema (50% of cases), facial nerve palsy of lower motor neuron type (30%), fissured tongue (20–40%), and regional lymphadenopathy (50% of cases).
- It presents as a painless, persistent, and diffuse swelling of one or both lips. Small vesicles, erosions, and scaling may also occur (**Figure 18.58**).
- DD: Cheilitis glandularis, Crohn's disease, sarcoidosis, cystic fibrosis, lymphangioma, angioneurotic edema.

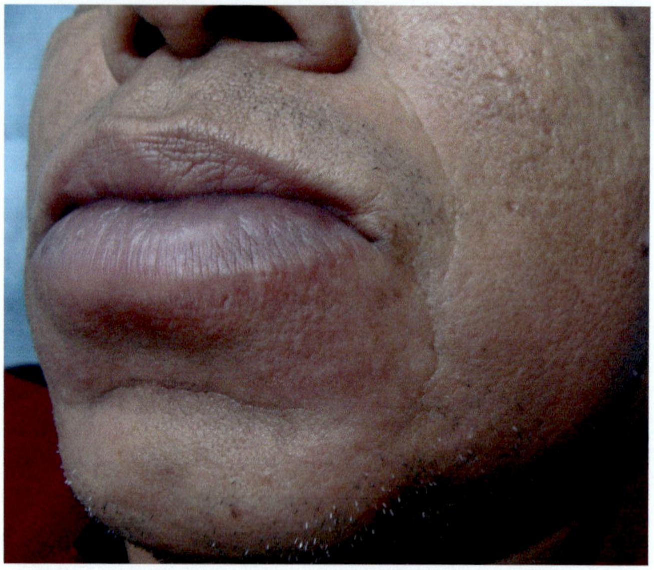

Figure 18.58 Diffuse swelling of lower lip in case of granulomatous cheilitis. (Courtesy: Dr. Hiral Shah, Baroda Medical College, Vadodara, India.)

## REFERENCES


1. Laskaris G. Pocket Atlas of Oral Diseases. 2nd edition. New York: Thieme; 2005.
2. Villa A, Woo SB. Leukoplakia—A Diagnostic and Management Algorithm. J Oral Maxillofac Surg 2017;75:723–734.
3. Maymone MBC, Greer RO, Burdine LK, Dao-Cheng A, Venkatesh S, Sahitya PC et al. Benign oral mucosal lesions: Clinical and pathological findings. J Am Acad Dermatol 2019;81:43–56.
4. Maymone MBC, Greer RO, Kesecker J, Sahitya PC, Burdine LK, Cheng AD et al. Premalignant and malignant oral mucosal lesions: Clinical and pathological findings. J Am Acad Dermatol 2019;81:59–71.
5. Scully C. Dermatoses of the Oral Cavity and Lips. In: Griffiths CEM, Barker J, Bleiker T, Chalmers R, Creamer D, editors. Rook's Textbook of Dermatology. 9th edition. Oxford: Blackwell Science; 2016. pp. 110.1–110.93.
6. Çerman AA, Altuna IK. Oral pigmentation. J Pigment Disorder 2016;3:234.
7. Fitzpatrick SG, Cohen DM, Clark AN. Ulcerated lesions of the oral mucosa: Clinical and histologic review. Head Neck Pathol 2019;13:91–102.
8. McNamara KK, Kalmar JR. Erythematous and vascular oral mucosal lesions: A clinicopathologic review of red entities. Head Neck Pathol 2019;13:4–15.
9. Kauzman A, Pavone M, Blanas N, Bradley G. Pigmented lesions of the oral cavity: Review, differential diagnosis, and case presentations. J Can Dent Assoc 2004;70:682–683.

E24

# Tongue

MEENAZ KHOJA, SABHA MUSHTAQ

## ABSTRACT

The tongue is the most mobile organ of the body and is the special organ for taste. It is also closely linked to the digestive system and speech. The appearance of the tongue gives an assessment or diagnosis of various diseases of regional and systemic importance.

The text of this chapter is available online at https://routledgetextbooks.com/textbooks/9781032399669/

DOI: 10.1201/9781351054225-45

# E25

# Axillae and groins

SHVETHA JAIN

## ABSTRACT

The axillae and groin areas are commonly affected by various dermatoses. Most common lesions involving these areas may be readily identified and easily managed. However, at times there may be diagnostic dilemmas when they are involved secondarily to underlying systemic diseases.

The text of this chapter is available online at https://routledgetextbooks.com/textbooks/9781032399669/



DOI: 10.1201/9781351054225-46

# E26

# Umbilicus and periumbilical region

DIVYA SACHDEV

## ABSTRACT

The umbilicus may be affected in various congenital or acquired malformations, primary cutaneous disease – both localized and generalized – and various systemic conditions. Additionally, benign, malignant, and metastatic tumors may involve the umbilicus, and some of them are unique to this site. This chapter discusses a morphological approach to the diagnosis of various signs and dermatoses involving the umbilical and periumbilical region.

The text of this chapter is available online at https://routledgetextbooks.com/textbooks/9781032399669/

DOI: 10.1201/9781351054225-47

# E27

# Palms and soles

PRERNA, RASHID SHAHID

## ABSTRACT

Palms and soles may be affected by a variety of dermatoses localized to these areas, widespread dermatoses, and systemic diseases. As palms and soles are specialized skin with thicker stratum corneum, various dermatoses may not manifest themselves with typical morphology. Also, mechanical trauma frequently experienced by these sites may alter the morphology, contributing to diagnostic confusion. This chapter discusses the clinical approach to various palmoplantar dermatoses.

The text of this chapter is available online at https://routledgetextbooks.com/textbooks/9781032399669/


DOI: 10.1201/9781351054225-48

19

# Male genitalia

PIYUSH KUMAR, RASHID SHAHID

## INTRODUCTION

Various dermatoses are known to be exclusively localized to or predominantly affecting male genitalia. Awareness of such conditions aids in the efficient management of such patients. This chapter focuses on various dermatoses affecting external male genitals. The diseases affecting the scrotum have been discussed in a separate chapter. This chapter primarily focuses on dermatoses affecting the penis. The clinical approach to penile dermatoses has been summarized in **Table 19.1**.[1–5]

### Vitiligo

- Male genitalia may be affected exclusively or as a part of widespread disease as sharply demarcated patches of milk-white skin that have no evidence of texture change, inflammation, or scales (**Figure 19.1**).

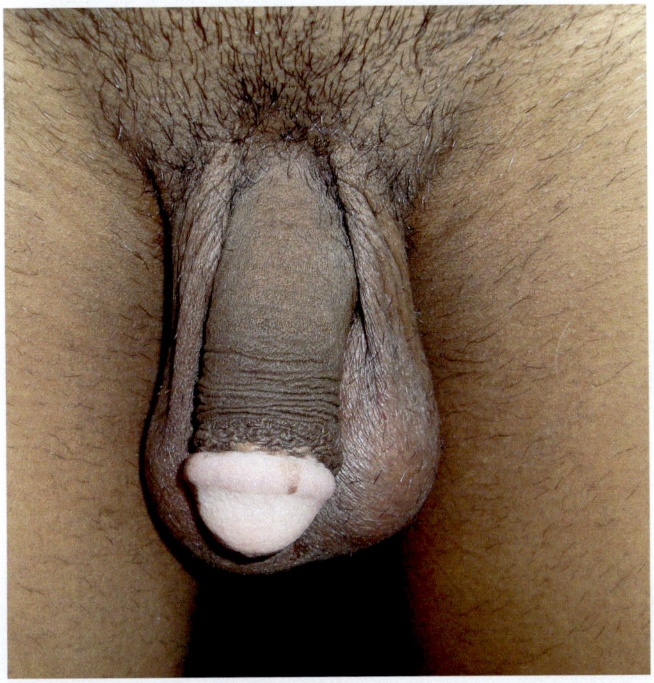

Figure 19.1 Well-demarcated depigmented patch.

- DD: Lichen sclerosus et atrophicus, and post-inflammatory hypopigmentation.

### Melanocytic nevus

- A melanocytic nevus may be congenital or acquired.
- Acquired types have been further classified as junctional, intradermal, or compound.
- Melanocytic nevi of genital region are rare and usually present as an asymptomatic lesion, varying in color from brown to jet black.
- Acquired lesions are typically less than a centimeter in diameter, whereas congenital melanocytic nevi vary in size and can be small (≤1 cm), intermediate (1–3 cm), or large/giant (≥3 cm).
- Junctional melanocytic nevi present as brown to brownish-black macular or thin papular lesions. Compound melanocytic nevi are tan to light-brown papules; and intradermal melanocytic nevi present as papules with no significant pigmentation (**Figure 19.2**).
- One subtype of genital melanocytic nevus, known as atypical genital nevus, is characterized by the presence of atypical melanocytes and may resemble melanoma and dysplastic melanocytic nevus on histopathology but exhibits a benign behavior.
- DD: Dysplastic nevus, and cutaneous melanoma.

### Lentigines

- Lentigines are foci of macular hyperpigmentation in which the number of epidermal melanocytes is increased.
- Benign genital lentiginosis is an uncommon, idiopathic cutaneous abnormality consisting of irregular hyperpigmented macules and patches (**Figure 19.3**).
- This totally flat hyperpigmentation sometimes displays marked irregularity of browns, tans, and black that mimic melanoma.
- DD: Post-inflammatory hyperpigmentation, and malignant melanoma.

DOI: 10.1201/9781351054225-49

Table 19.1 Clinical approach to dermatoses of male genitalia

| Morphology | Feature | Diseases |
|---|---|---|
| Macule/ Patch | Depigmented/ hypopigmented | Vitiligo |
| | Hyperpigmented | Melanocytic nevus<br>Lentigines<br>Dyspigmentation of median raphe |
| | Erythematous | Balanoposthitis<br>Plasma cell balanitis<br>Fixed drug eruption<br>Circinate balanitis<br>Seborrheic dermatitis<br>Irritant contact dermatitis<br>Diaper dermatitis |
| Papule | White | Molluscum contagiosum<br>Lichen nitidus |
| | Hyperpigmented | Melanocytic nevus<br>Lichen planus<br>Bowenoid papulosis |
| | Red | Scabies<br>Dermatophytosis<br>Allergic contact dermatitis<br>Hemangioma<br>Angiokeratoma |
| | Yellowish | Sebaceous hyperplasia |
| | Flesh-colored | Pearly penile papule<br>Skin tag<br>Syringoma<br>Granuloma annulare |
| Plaque | Red | Hemangioma<br>Psoriasis<br>Erythroplasia of Queyrat<br>Extramammary Paget's disease<br>Genitourinary tuberculosis<br>Leprosy<br>Lymphoma |
| | Flesh-colored | Condyloma lata |
| | Depigmented | Lichen sclerosus |
| | Hyperkeratotic/ verrucous | Porokeratosis<br>Pseudoepitheliomatous, keratotic, and micaceous balanitis<br>Buschke-Lowenstein tumor<br>Verrucous carcinoma<br>Verruciform xanthoma |
| | Pigmented | Acanthosis nigricans<br>Bowen's disease<br>Melanoma<br>Basal cell carcinoma |
| Nodule | | Squamous cell carcinoma<br>Lymphoma<br>Epidermoid cyst<br>Steatocystoma multiplex<br>Scrotal calcinosis<br>Penile thrombophlebitis<br>Peyronie's disease<br>Mucoid penile cyst |
| Vesicle | Long standing/ persistent | Lymphangioma<br>Median raphe cyst* |
| | Recurrent/ short duration | Erythema multiforme<br>Genital herpes<br>Irritant contact dermatitis |
| Pustule | | Candidiasis<br>Dermatophytosis |
| Erosion | | Pemphigus vulgaris<br>Bullous pemphigoid<br>Cicatricial pemphigoid<br>Stevens-Johnson syndrome and toxic epidermal necrolysis<br>Acrodermatitis enteropathica |
| Ulcer | Painless | Chancre<br>Squamous cell carcinoma<br>Melanoma<br>Basal cell carcinoma |
| | Painful | Genital herpes<br>Aphthous ulcer<br>Chancroid<br>Donovanosis<br>Dermatitis artefacta<br>Vasculitis<br>Crohn's disease<br>Pyoderma gangrenosum<br>Calciphylaxis<br>Malakoplakia |
| Cyst* | | Median raphe cyst |
| Sinus | | Actinomycosis<br>Scrofuloderma<br>Hidradenitis suppurative |
| Edema | | Lymphedema<br>Paraphimosis<br>Priapism<br>Penile fracture |
| No skin lesion | | Phimosis<br>Hypospadias<br>Gonorrhea |

*Clinically, it looks like a clear fluid containing vesicle.*

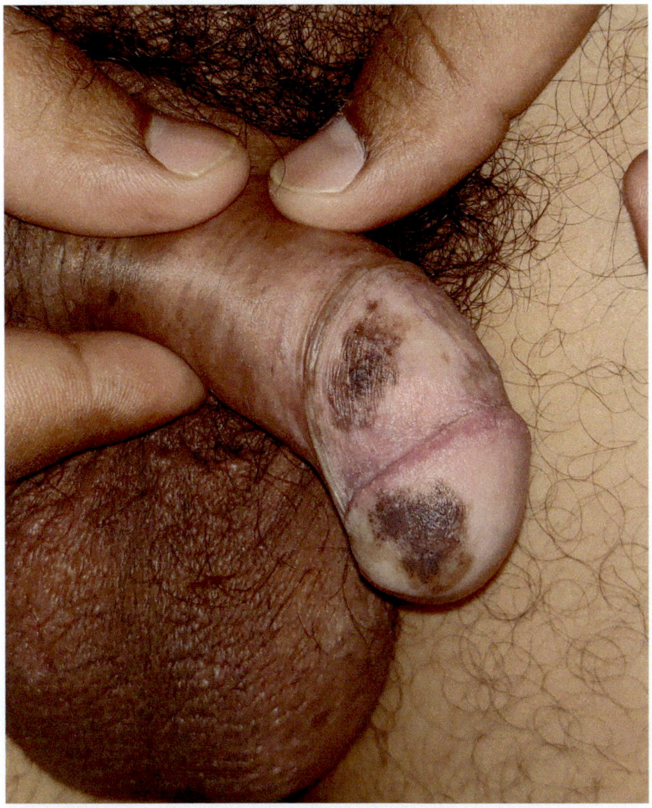

Figure 19.2 "Kissing" melanocytic nevus on the penis. (Courtesy: Dr. Santoshdev P Rathod, Ahmedabad, India.)

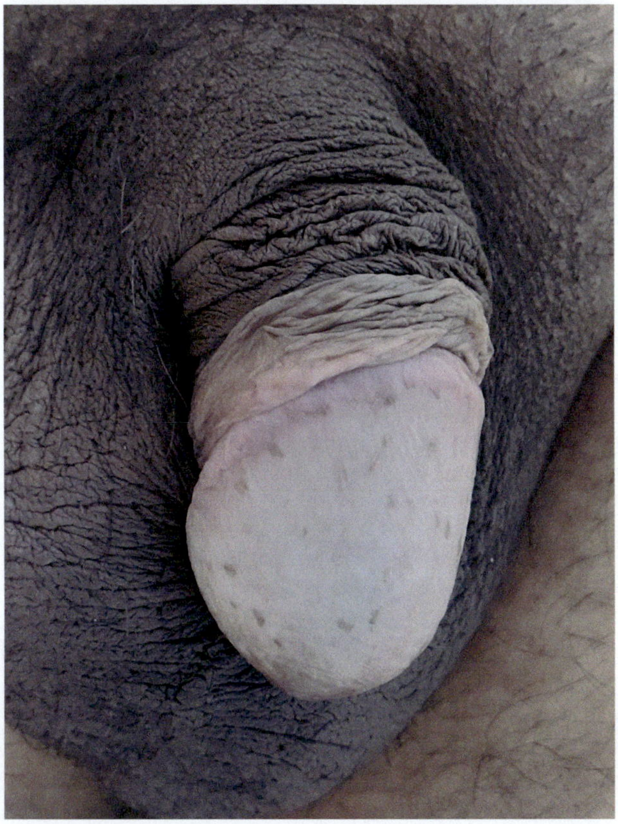

Figure 19.3 Multiple hyperpigmented macules of lentigines. (Courtesy: Dr. Santoshdev P Rathod, Ahmedabad, India.)

## Dyspigmentation of median raphe

- Dyspigmentation of median raphe is a normal variant of median raphe of the penis and usually presents as a pigmentary problem.
- The median raphe may be hyperpigmented or hypopigmented.
- It is one of the most common physiological variations.
- **DD:** Post-inflammatory hyperpigmentation.

## Balanoposthitis

- Balanoposthitis is defined as inflammation of the glans penis (balanitis) and prepuce (posthitis) in uncircumcised males and presents as moist macular erythema.
- Infections (such as *Candida* species), mechanical factors, trauma, contact dermatitis, and dermatoses (such as genital herpes, Zoon's balanitis, fixed drug eruption, lichen sclerosus et atrophicus, and Erythroplasia of Queyrat) are frequently responsible for its appearance.
- Candidal balanoposthitis is characterized by pustules and tiny erosions, white scrapable sloughs, and fissures. Sometimes, prepuce is edematous and transiently adhered to glans (**Figure 19.4a**).
- Genital herpes presents with painful, tiny vesicles and erosions (**Figure 19.4b**).
- Zoon's balanitis is characterized by a well-circumscribed, bright-red patch with a characteristic

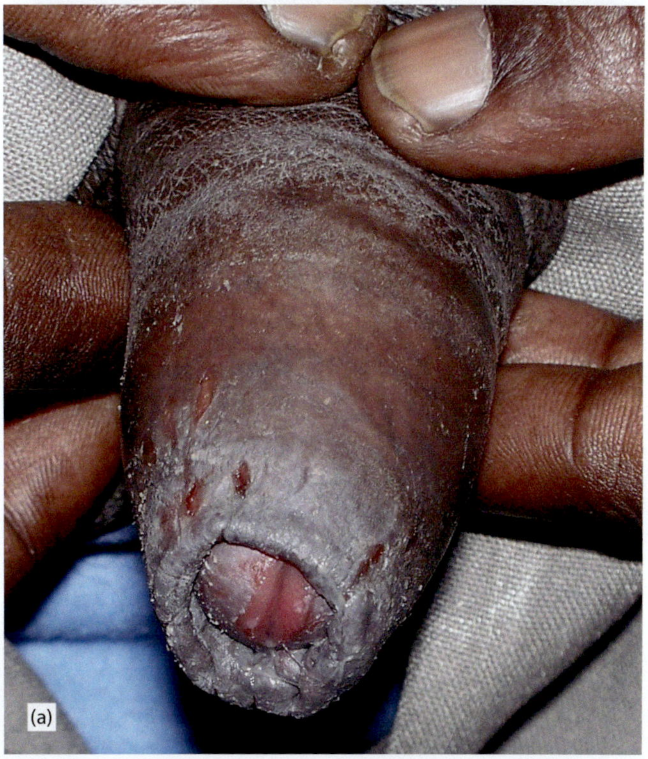


Figure 19.4 **(a)** Glans penis in candidiasis appears erythematous and eroded. Prepuce cannot be retracted and shows fissures and whitish slough. (*Continued*)

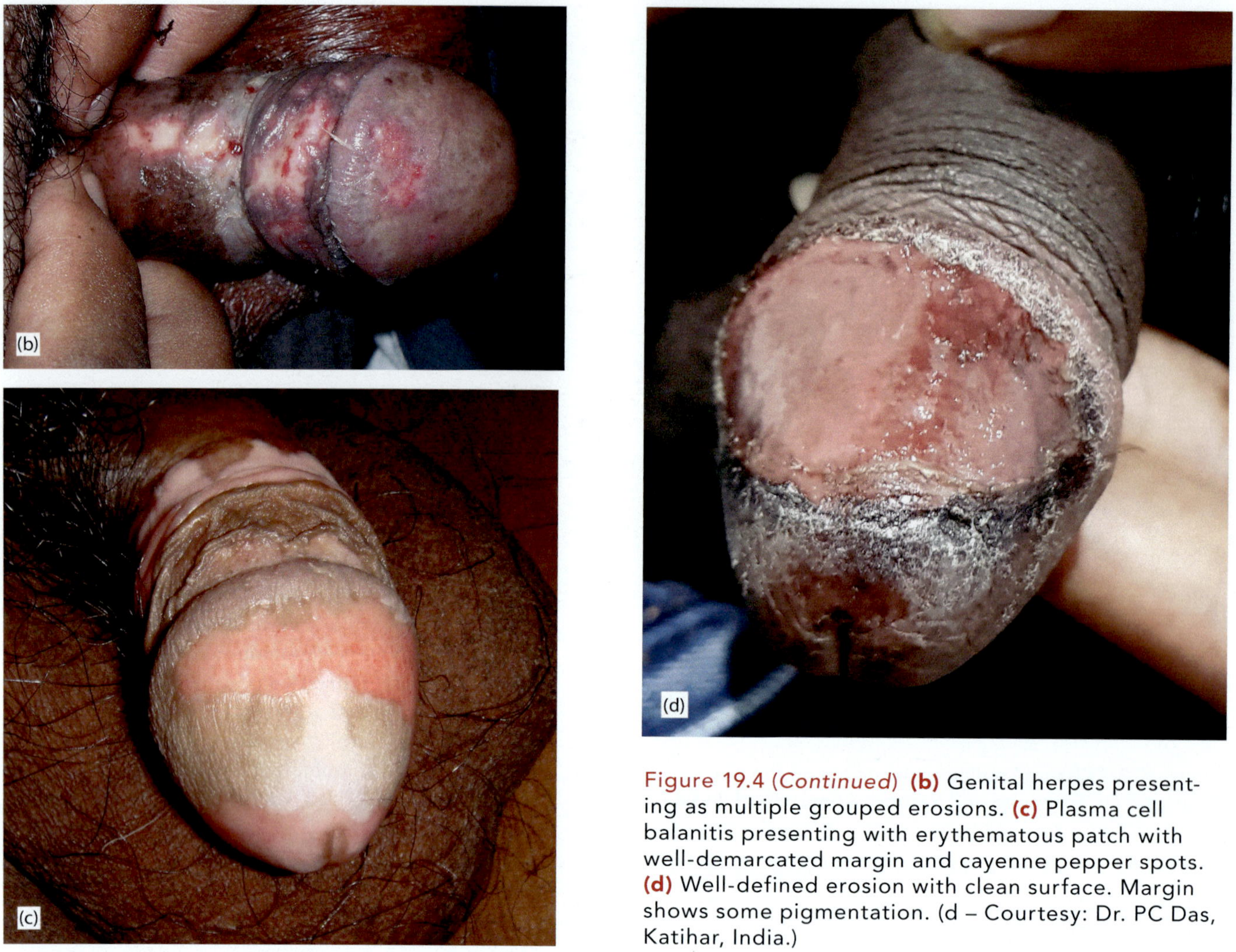

Figure 19.4 (*Continued*) **(b)** Genital herpes presenting as multiple grouped erosions. **(c)** Plasma cell balanitis presenting with erythematous patch with well-demarcated margin and cayenne pepper spots. **(d)** Well-defined erosion with clean surface. Margin shows some pigmentation. (d – Courtesy: Dr. PC Das, Katihar, India.)

glazed appearance and multiple pinpoint redder spots – "cayenne pepper spots" (**Figure 19.4c**).

- Fixed drug eruption presents as well-demarcated erythematous areas that may ulcerate and follows intake of certain specific drugs (**Figure 19.4d**).
- Lichen sclerosus et atrophicus presents as white indurated plaques on the glans and may involve the prepuce, which becomes thickened, fissured, and non-retractile.
- Erythroplasia of Queyrat is a premalignant lesion and presents as red, velvety appearance with sharp margins, and a granular surface.
- DD: Bowen's disease, psoriasis, and intertrigo.

## Plasma cell balanitis (Zoon's balanitis)

- Plasma cell balanitis is an inflammatory disease affecting the glans and prepuce, with chronic-relapsing course and benign behavior.
- It is found at all postpubertal ages, and there seems to be no racial predilection.
- It is clinically characterized by a solitary, asymptomatic erythematous, or erythematous-brownish, sharply marginated patch on the glans and/or the inner foreskin, 1.5 cm or more in diameter, with a bright, smooth, and sometimes erosive surface.
- When occurring on the glans, it is seen only in uncircumcised men (**Figure 19.5a,b**).
- DD: Lichen planus, psoriasis, candidiasis, and squamous cell carcinoma in situ.

## Fixed drug eruption

- Fixed drug eruption is a peculiar cutaneous eruption that characteristically recurs at the same site following the administration of the offending drug or occasionally a member of the same group of drug.
- Genital lesions are commonly caused by tetracyclines.
- The lesions may be single or multiple, round or oval, well-marginated, erythematous, edematous patches that resolve with a violaceous or hyperpigmented patches (**Figure 19.6a**). Bullous lesions may develop occasionally (**Figure 19.6b**).

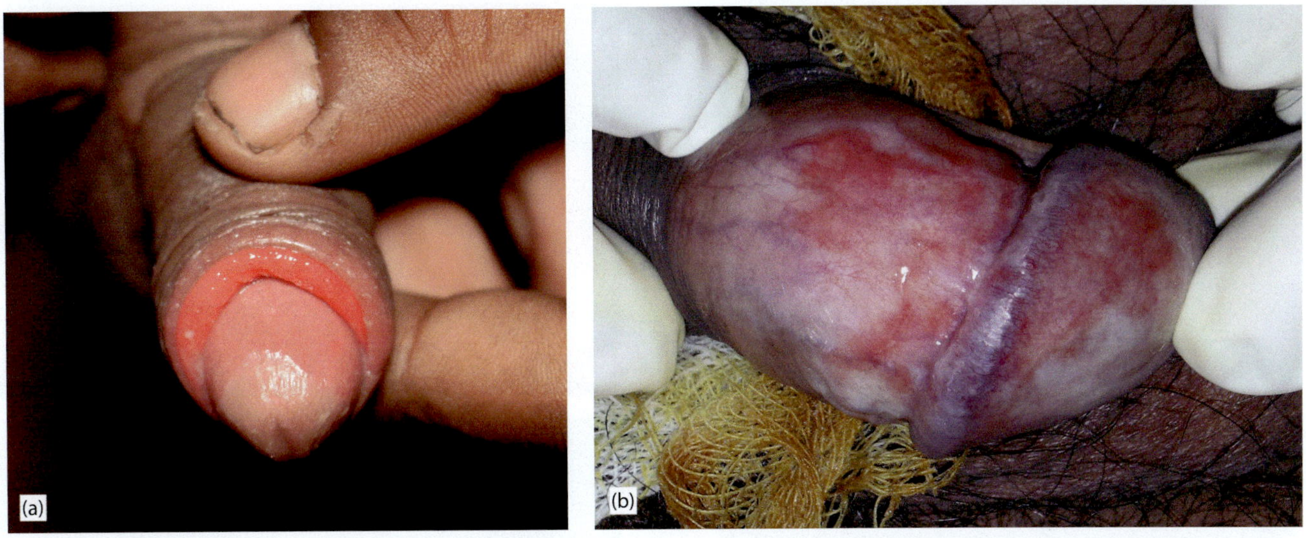

Figure 19.5 **(a)** Plasma cell balanitis presenting as well-demarcated, moist erythema over glans and inner prepuce. **(b)** Another case of plasma cell balanitis.

- They may be asymptomatic or accompanied by localized burning, stinging, or intense pruritus.
- DD: Erythema multiforme, genital herpes.

## Circinate balanitis

- Circinate balanitis is one of the most common and diagnostically significant mucocutaneous findings in reactive arthritis (Reiter's disease).
- Circinate balanitis is usually seen in association with other findings of reactive arthritis (urethritis, conjunctivitis, and arthritis). Rarely, it can present as an isolated finding.
- It starts as small vesicles or pustules in uncircumcised males that rupture, leaving painless superficial erosions that can coalesce to form a

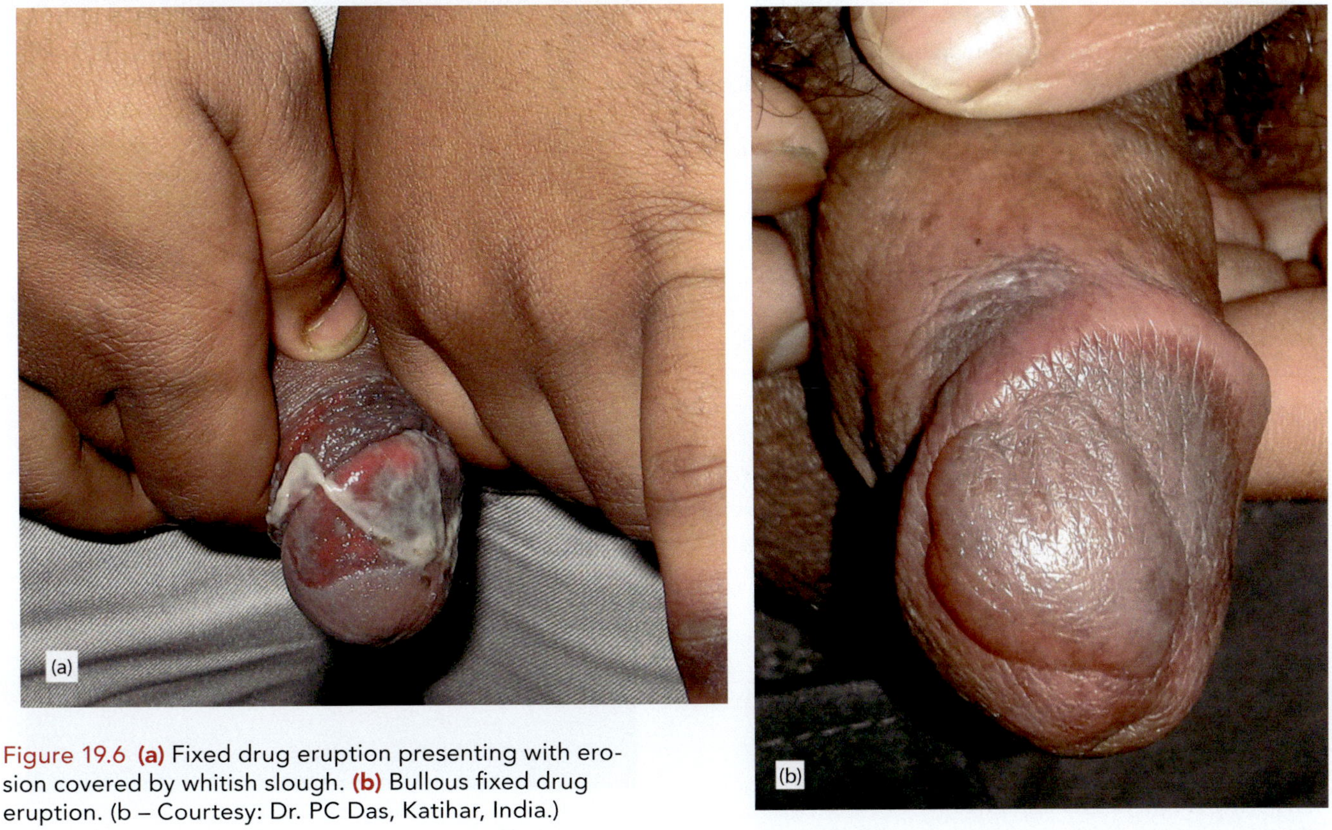

Figure 19.6 **(a)** Fixed drug eruption presenting with erosion covered by whitish slough. **(b)** Bullous fixed drug eruption. (b – Courtesy: Dr. PC Das, Katihar, India.)

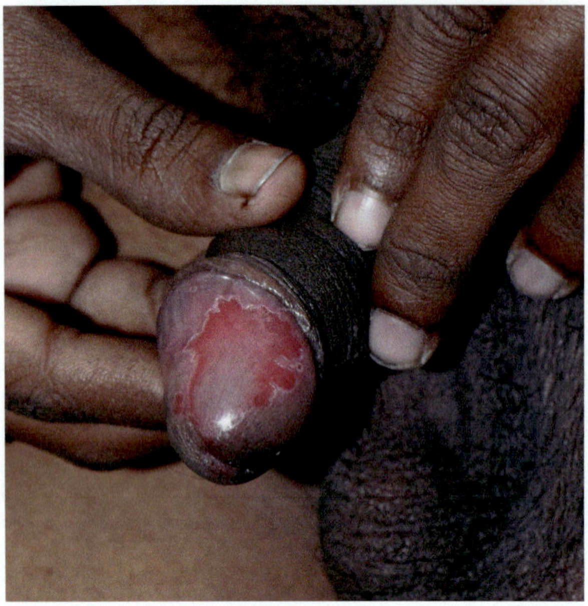

Figure 19.7 Circinate balanitis presenting with erosion with serpiginous margin.

sharply demarcated, characteristic serpiginous lesion (**Figures 19.7** and **19.8a,b**).

- In circumcised males, hyperkeratotic papules and plaques are noted.
- DD: Candidiasis, balanoposthitis, and pustular psoriasis.

## Seborrheic dermatitis

- Occasionally, its severe forms can involve the genital skin. Spread of the eruption to the genitalia is much more common in infants than in adults.
- In addition, this condition is most severe in those who cannot shampoo regularly, such as the homeless and those with neurologic disease or other infirmities that interfere with activities of daily living.
- In the genital area, it is accentuated within the skin folds. A classic but not unique characteristic of genital seborrheic dermatitis is a glazed, shiny texture in the affected skin.
- DD: Atopic dermatitis, allergic contact dermatitis, irritant contact dermatitis, fungal infection, psoriasis, and cutaneous candidiasis.

## Irritant contact dermatitis

- Irritant contact dermatitis (ICD) is an eczematous reaction that develops in response to an exogenous substance that can cause an inflammatory reaction whenever applied to the skin of any individual.
- Mild (and chronic) ICD is usually manifested by irritation, pain, soreness, rawness, and poorly demarcated, slightly scaly erythematous patches or plaques with little or no edema. Often there is a dry, glazed, fissured, chapped appearance.
- Severe (and acute) ICD is manifested by a rapid appearance of erythema, edema, and sometimes, blistering (**Figures 19.9** and **19.10**).
- Poorly keratinized skin, such as the modified mucous membranes of the glans penis and the inner aspect of

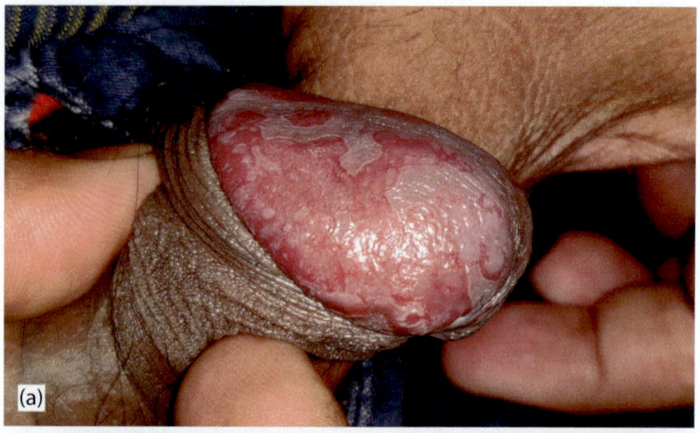

(a)

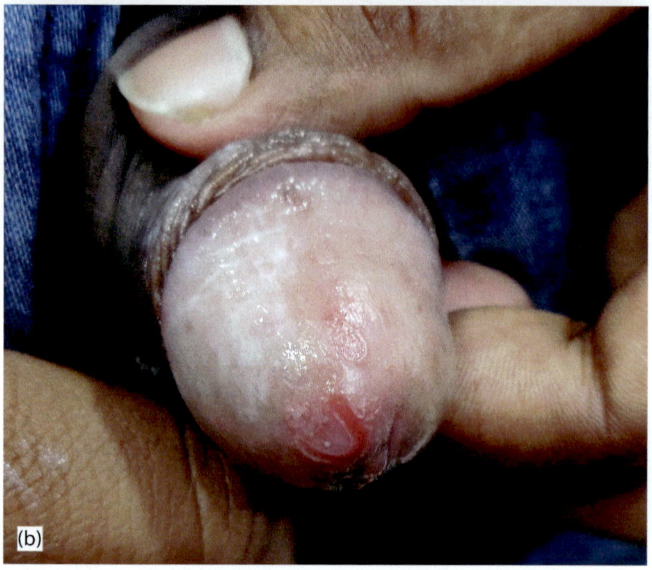

(b)

Figure 19.8 **(a)** Circinate balanitis presenting with erosion with serpiginous margin. **(b)** Circinate balanitis presenting with annular erosion in HLA B27 positive male. (a,b – Courtesy: Soumyajit Roychoudhury, Consultant Dermatologist, Berhampore, India.)

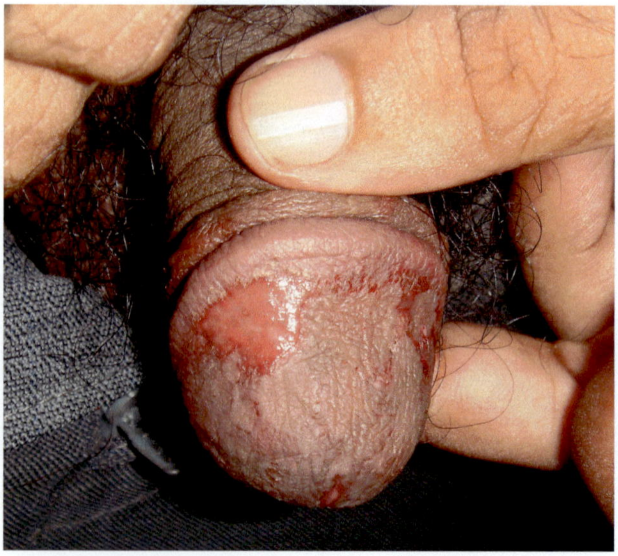

Figure 19.9 Mild irritant contact dermatitis presenting as erythema and erosions on the glans penis.

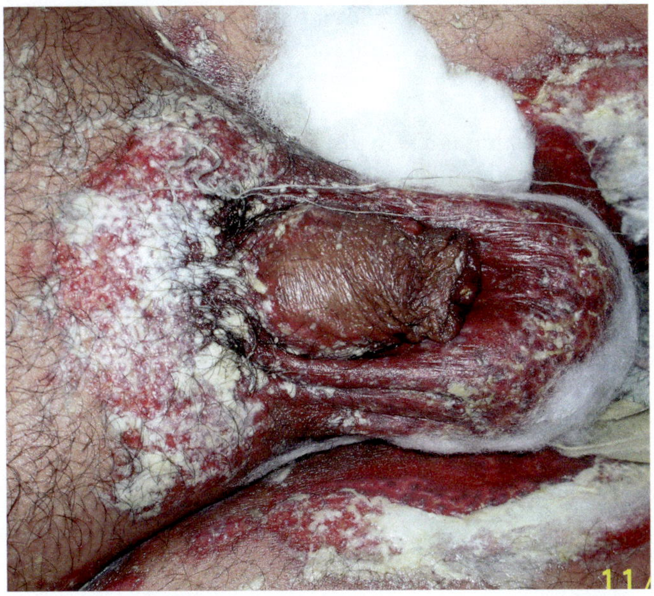

Figure 19.10 Severe irritant contact dermatitis with widespread erosion of penile, scrotal, and surrounding skin.

the prepuce, become very fragile, and blister roofs are shed quickly, forming erosions or even ulcers.

- On the more resilient keratinized skin of shaft of the penis, blisters may remain visible for a day or two before they become unroofed, leaving erosions or ulcers.
- DD: Allergic contact dermatitis, fixed drug eruption.

## Diaper dermatitis

- Diaper dermatitis affects warm, moist areas of groin, including genitalia and gluteals. The **sk**in changes are similar to those of ICD.
- A severe form of irritant dermatitis is termed diaper dermatitis of Jacquet, granuloma gluteale infantum, or pseudo wart, characterized by sharply marginated red

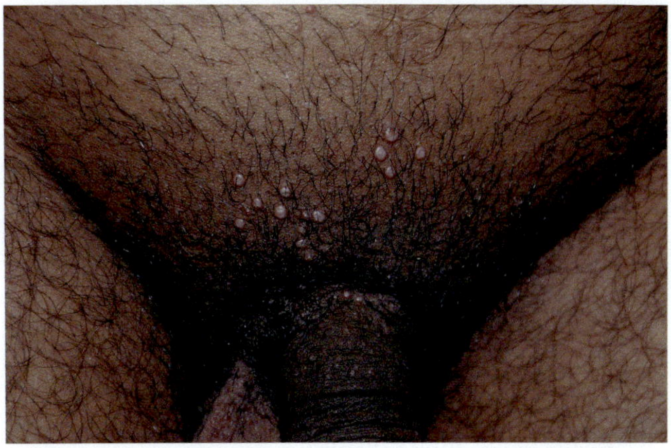

Figure 19.11 Umbilicated white papules of molluscum contagiosum at the root of the penis.

nodules, often with overlying erosion that confers an umbilicated appearance.

- DD: Candidal intertrigo, psoriasis, seborrhea, atopic dermatitis, allergic contact dermatitis, acrodermatitis enteropathica, Langerhans cell histiocytosis, and granuloma gluteale infantum.

## Molluscum contagiosum

- Molluscum contagiosum can be sexually transmitted or may be acquired non-sexually and affects the genitals of children and adults frequently.
- The lesions are characteristic, and patients present with smooth-surfaced, firm, dome-shaped papules with central umbilication.
- Their color can vary from pearly white or pink to yellow. Lesions are usually small, 2–5 mm in diameter, though occasionally much larger (giant mollusca more than 1.5 cm) lesions may be noted, especially in immunocompromised persons (**Figures 19.11** and **19.12a,b**).

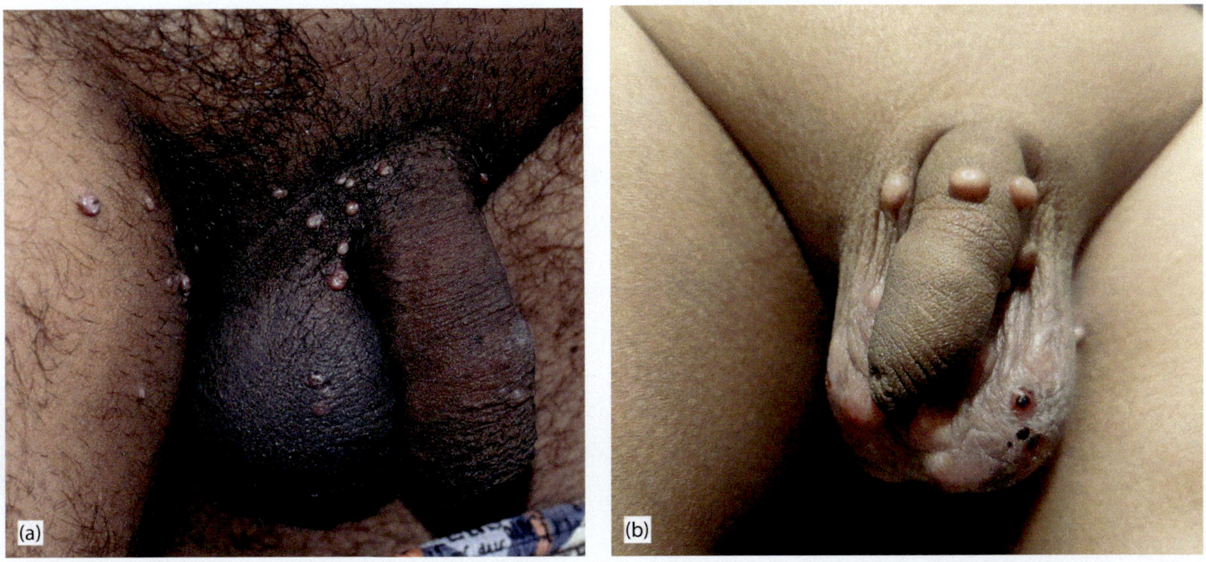


Figure 19.12 **(a)** Molluscum contagiosum on the penis and the scrotum. **(b)** Umbilicated papules of molluscum contagiosum on the penis and scrotum in a child. (b – Courtesy: Dr. Dependra Kumar Timshina, Remedy Clinics, Siliguri, India.)

- The lesions occur in clusters and may be noted in linear arrangement (pseudo koebnerization).
- DD: Lichen nitidus, cutaneous cryptococcosis, and verruca vulgaris.

## Lichen nitidus

- Lichen nitidus may involve genitalia, and the shaft of the penis is characteristically involved.
- The primary lesions consist of multiple 1- to 3-mm, sharply demarcated, round or polygonal, flat-topped, skin-colored shiny papules that often appear in groups (**Figure 19.13a,b**).
- They are most often asymptomatic, though some patients report mild pruritus.
- The condition remits spontaneously after several years.
- DD: Lichen planus, lichen striatus, lichen spinulosus, bowenoid papulosis, and warts.

## Lichen planus

- Lichen planus is a skin disease that exhibits variable morphologies on genital skin.
- Erosive lichen planus is a common non-infectious erosive condition occurring on the penis and almost non-existent in circumcised men.
- Itchy red papules are more common than erosions in men, and moist skin often exhibits white skin lesions (**Figure 19.14a–c**).
- Penile lichen planus are less often eroded, but when erosions occur, they are very painful.
- Men with erosive penile lichen planus experience scarring, with phimosis if uncircumcised, or obliteration of the sharp distinction of the glans from the shaft in the circumcised penis.

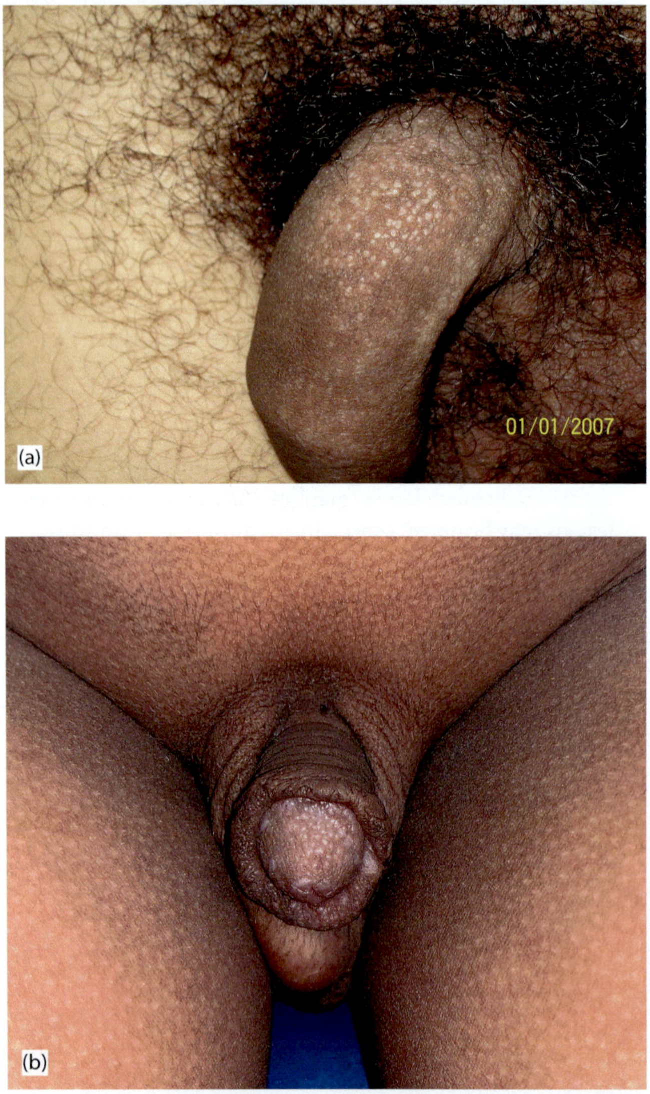


Figure 19.13 **(a)** Shiny papules of lichen nitidus on the shaft of the penis. **(b)** Lichen nitidus on the glans penis of a young boy. (a – Courtesy: Dr. Santoshdev P Rathod, Ahmedabad, India.)

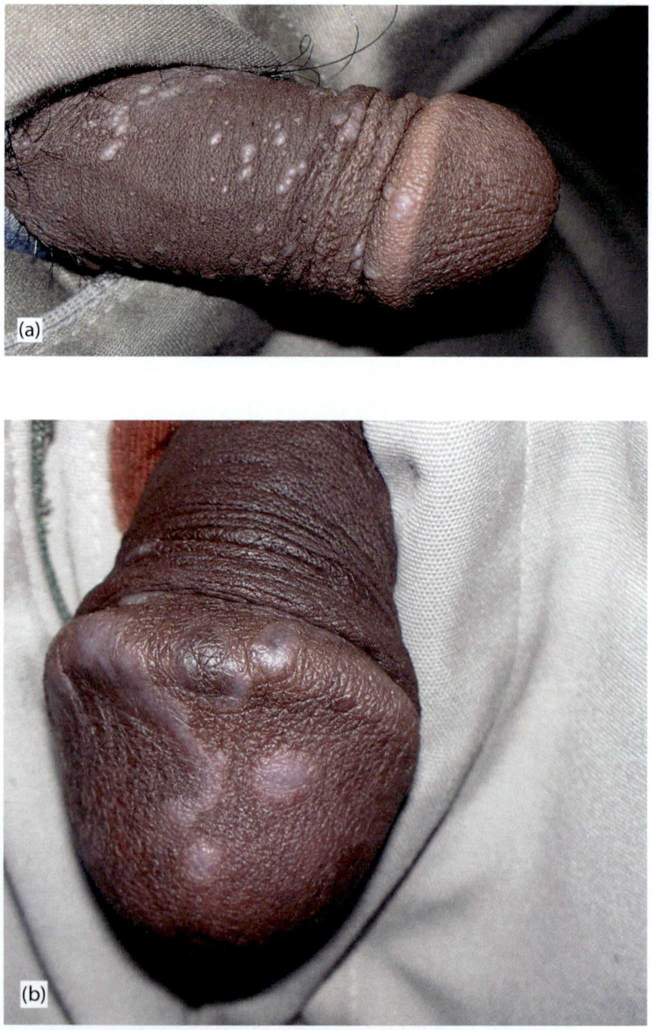


Figure 19.14 **(a)** Violaceous papules of lichen planus. **(b)** Violaceous papules and plaque of lichen planus. *(Continued)*

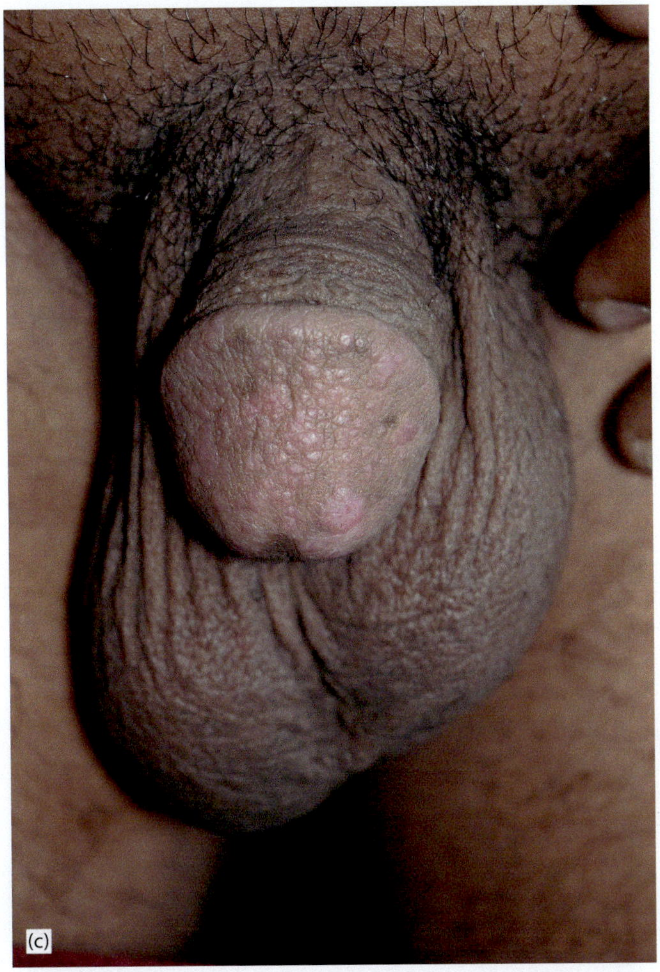

Figure 19.14 (*Continued*) **(c)** Violaceous papules and plaque of lichen planus affecting the glans penis.

- DD: Pemphigus vulgaris, cicatricial pemphigoid, toxic epidermal necrolysis, severe erosive candidiasis, psoriasis, and irritant contact dermatitis.

## Bowenoid papulosis

- Bowenoid papulosis represents an intraepithelial neoplasia located on the shaft of penis, occurring mostly in sexually active males aged 20 to 40 years. Human papillomavirus (HPV) types 16, 18, 31, and 39 play an etiologic role.
- The papules may occasionally become pruritic or inflamed, with pain and tenderness.
- It presents with multiple, small, asymptomatic, well-demarcated red, pink, or skin-colored papillomatous papules and plaques on shaft of penis (**Figure 19.15a,b**).
- DD: Condyloma acuminata, seborrheic keratosis, lichen planus, and Bowen's disease.

## Scabies

- Scabies is a parasitic infestation causing intense pruritus that is worse at night.

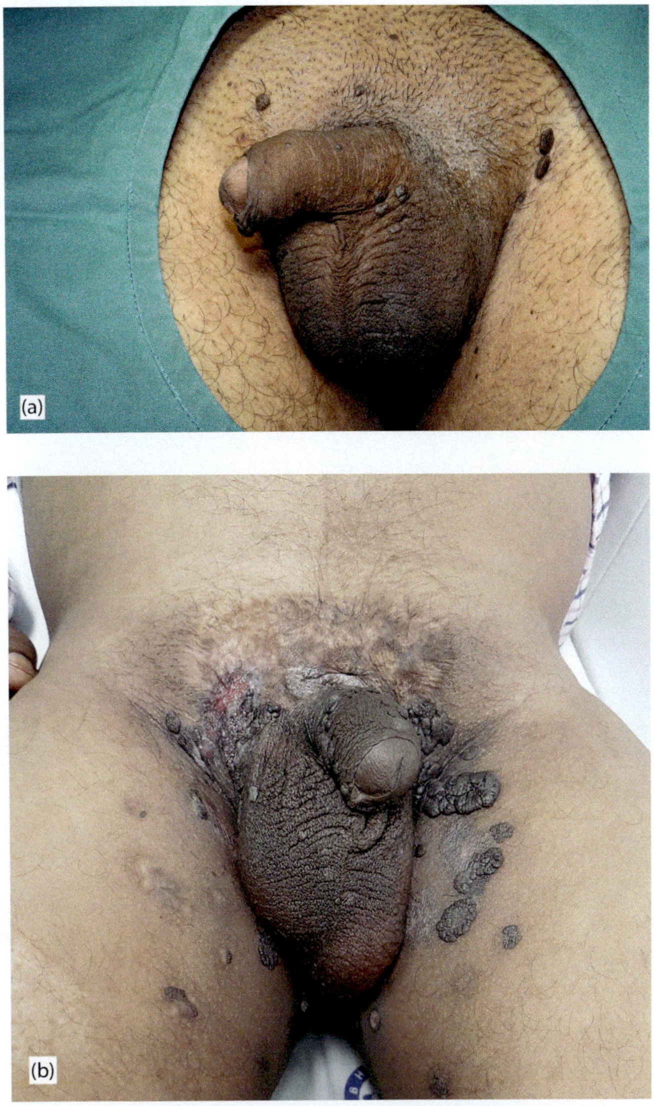

Figure 19.15 **(a)** Smooth-surfaced pigmented papules of the bowenoid papulosis. **(b)** Bowenoid papulosis with papules and plaques over penis, scrotum, and groin. (a – Courtesy: Dr. Sushil S Savant, Mumbai, India; b – Courtesy: Dr. Santoshdev P Rathod, Ahmedabad, India.)

- Classical scabies presents with small, erythematous papulovesicular eruptions and excoriated papules on the penis and scrotum. The lesions may get secondarily infected (**Figure 19.16a–c**). The pathognomonic lesions "burrows" may be found on the penis.
- Nodular scabies is sequelae of hypersensitivity reaction to a mite and its products and presents as extremely pruritic reddish brown nodules (**Figure 19.16d**).
- DD: Impetigo, insect bite, papular urticaria, and lymphomatoid papulosis.

## Dermatophytosis

- External genital involvement is being seen with increasing frequency in dermatophyte infections.

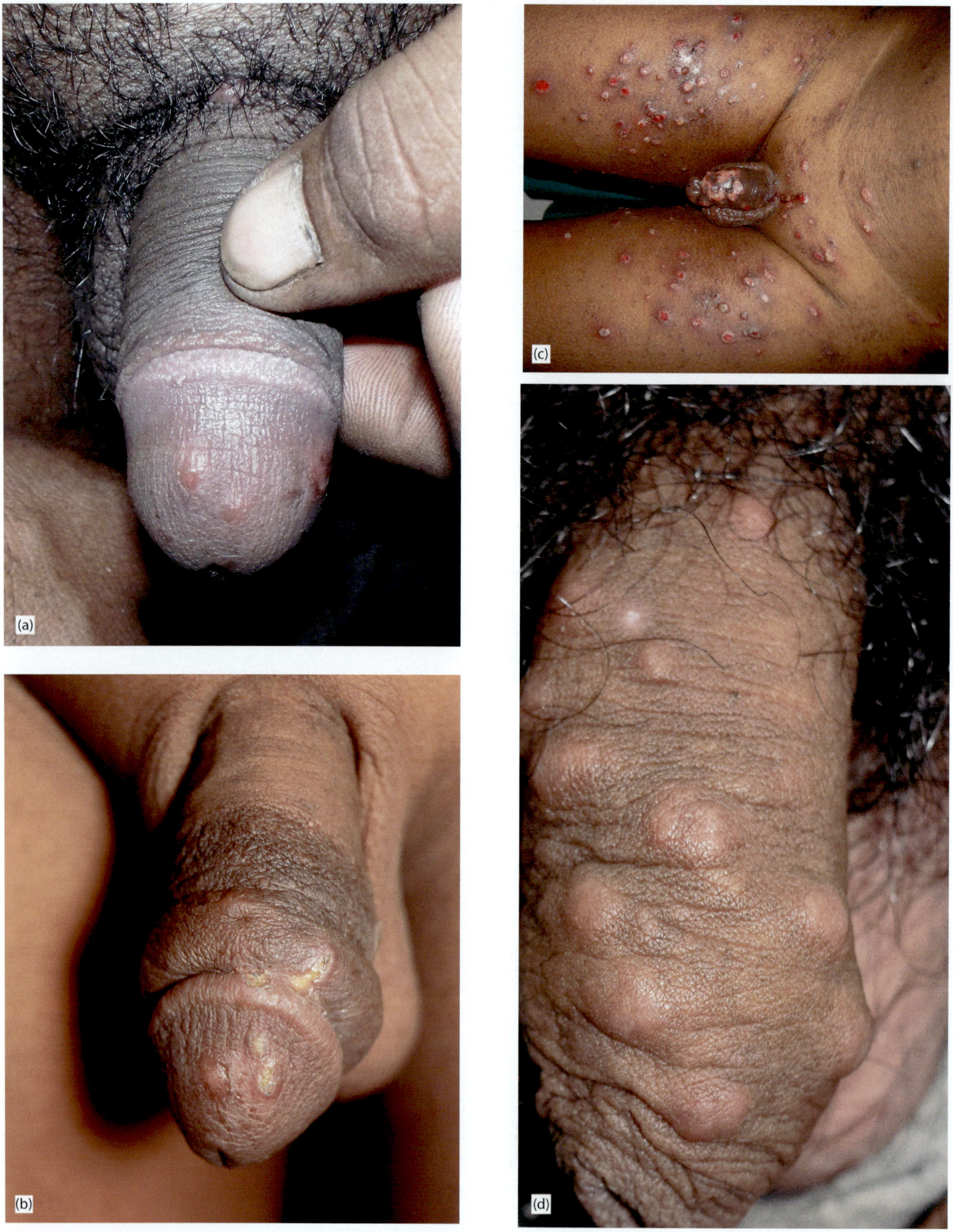


Figure 19.16 **(a)** Excoriated papules of scabies on the glans penis. **(b)** Excoriations with secondary infection in scabies. **(c)** Widespread erosions in a child with scabies. **(d)** Erythematous nodular lesions of nodular scabies.

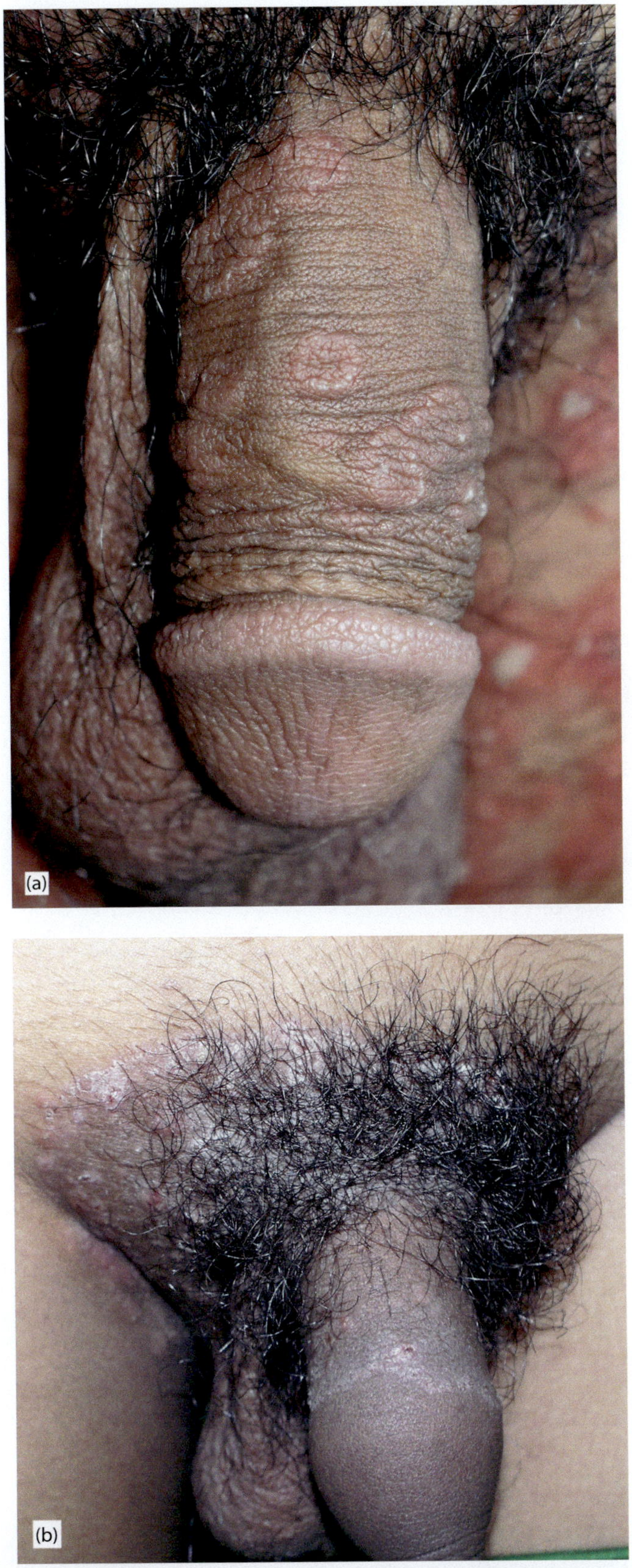


Figure 19.17 **(a)** Multiple annular lesions of dermatophyte infection on the shaft of penis. Tiny pustules at the margin may be identified. Note presence of tinea cruris. **(b)** Annular lesion with papules and scales at the margin.

- Its classical presentation is polycyclic annular lesions, with papules, pustules, and scales at the margin, and central clearing (**Figure 19.17a,b**).
- Atypical manifestations include no central clearing, presenting with only fine powdery scales, and tinea pseudoimbricata (concentric rings) and is commonly seen in people who have applied topical corticosteroids for a while.
- DD: Nummular dermatitis, annular psoriasis, impetigo, pityriasis rosea and allergic contact dermatitis.

## Allergic contact dermatitis

- Allergic contact dermatitis is a delayed type IV sensitivity to specific sensitizing agents or allergens. Only certain individuals exposed to a potential allergen develop allergic contact dermatitis at the time of their next contact with the allergen.
- It is characterized by the presence of pruritic, poorly marginated, bright-red, edematous patches and papules (**Figure 19.18**). Sometimes minute vesicles stud the surface of the erythematous patch. Oozing and scaling are other variable findings.
- Pruritus might result in the development of the itch–scratch cycle and the clinical signs of lichen simplex chronicus, especially seen on the scrotum.
- Both the penis and the scrotum may be affected.
- DD: Candidiasis, and dermatophytosis.

## Hemangioma

- Hemangioma is a true neoplasm of endothelial cells that line the blood vessels and is the most common benign soft-tissue tumor of infancy and childhood, occurring in greater frequency in whites, premature infants, twins, and children born to mothers of high maternal age.
- Hemangiomas involving genitalia comprise a rare clinical entity and have been mostly reported in the pediatric age group and much more rarely reported in adults.
- On genitals, these tumors can involve glans, penile shaft, or scrotum. It usually manifests as an

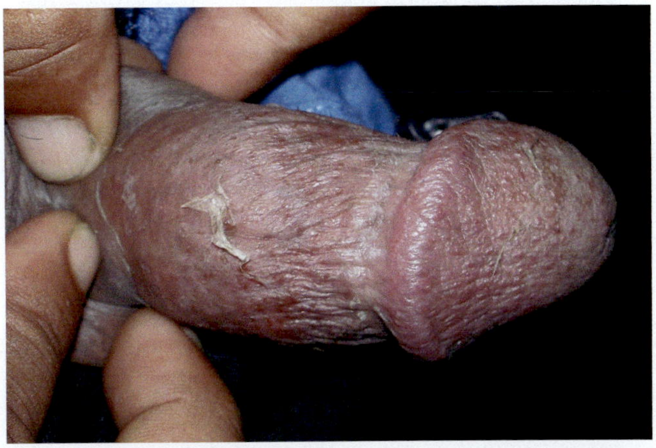

Figure 19.18 Allergic contact dermatitis presenting with multiple erythematous papules and scaling involving the glans and shaft of the penis.

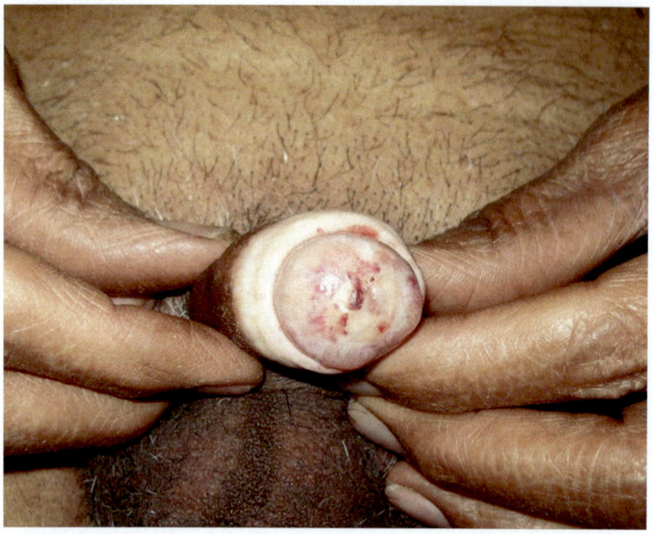

Figure 19.19 Hemangioma affecting the glans penis. (Courtesy: Dr. Santoshdev P Rathod, Ahmedabad, India.)

asymptomatic pale patch, then grows rapidly and finally appears as a port-wine-stain–like lesion.

- They are well-known for rapid growth during the first weeks to months of a child's life followed by a spontaneous but slow involution. As the lesion regresses, the color of the lesion fades from a bright red to a dull red and then a grey-white hue develops at the center of the lesion and spreads to the periphery (**Figure 19.19**). At this stage, the tumor becomes soft in texture followed by a reduction in the volume.
- Lesions may be single or multiple and are usually painless but can be associated with pain, ulceration and bleeding.
- DD: Angiokeratoma, verruca.

## Angiokeratoma

- Angiokeratomas are benign proliferations of dilated thin-walled blood vessels in the upper dermis with overlying epidermal hyperkeratosis.
- The clinical variants of angiokeratoma can be divided into a widespread form that includes angiokeratoma corporis diffusum (Fabry disease), associated with deficiency of Galactosidase A, and localized forms that include solitary angiokeratoma, angiokeratoma circumscriptum neviforme, angiokeratoma of Mibelli, and angiokeratoma of Fordyce.
- The individual lesion presents as an asymptomatic, 2- to 5-mm, blue-to-red papule or plaque with scaly surface. Early lesions are soft, red, and easy compressible (**Figure 19.20**); later, they become blue, keratotic, and non-compressible.
- They may bleed spontaneously, after scratching, on trauma, and following sexual intercourse.
- Angiokeratoma of Fordyce is the most common type of angiokeratoma, seen over the scrotum.
- Malignant transformation has not been seen.
- DD: Condylomata acuminata, cherry hemangioma, granuloma pyogenicum, and verrucous hemangioma.

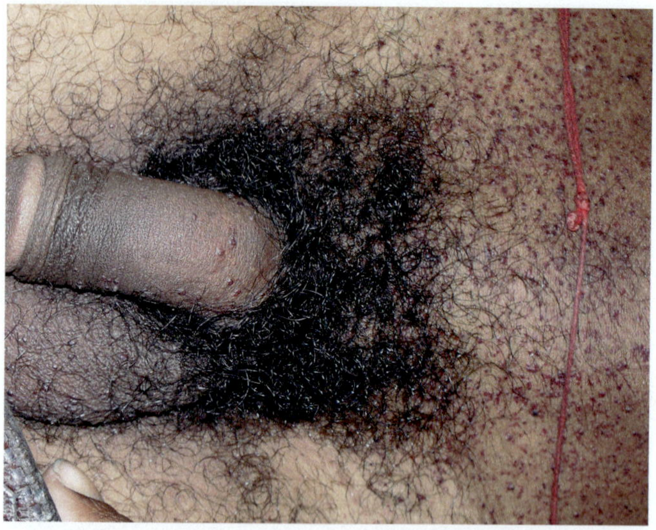

Figure 19.20 Erythematous papular lesions of angiokeratoma in a case with angiokeratoma corporis diffusum.

## Sebaceous hyperplasia

- Sebaceous hyperplasia is a benign hamartomatous condition of epidermal appendage tumors with sebaceous differentiation affecting mainly the adults of middle age or older.
- Occasionally it occurs on scrotum, foreskin, or the shaft of penis.
- It consists of single or multiple, asymptomatic, small, yellow papules, sometimes with a central depression (**Figure 19.21**).

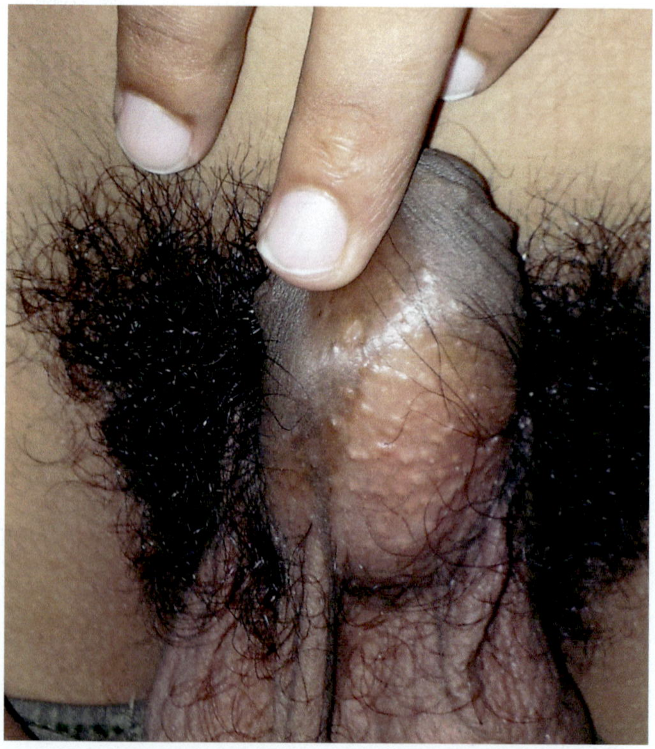

Figure 19.21 Multiple yellowish papules of sebaceous hyperplasia.

- DD: Condyloma acuminate, furuncle, millium, lichen nitidus, and pearly penile papules.

### Pearly penile papule

- Pearly penile papules are small, benign lesions that appear typically in parallel rows on the corona of the glans penis in late adolescence or early adulthood.
- Older males and circumcised males have lower prevalence.
- The lesions are asymptomatic, but patients seek consultation because of concerns of sexually transmitted diseases and of interference with sexual activity.
- The lesions present as pink or white, smooth, dome-shaped or filiform papules, orienting around the corona of the glans penis usually in one or more rows.
- They are most prominent along the dorsal surface of the corona and may encircle the glans entirely. Rarely, lesions may be found on the shaft of penis (**Figure 19.22a–c**).
- DD: Warts (**Figure 19.22d**), condyloma acuminata, Tyson's glands, and molluscum contagiosum.

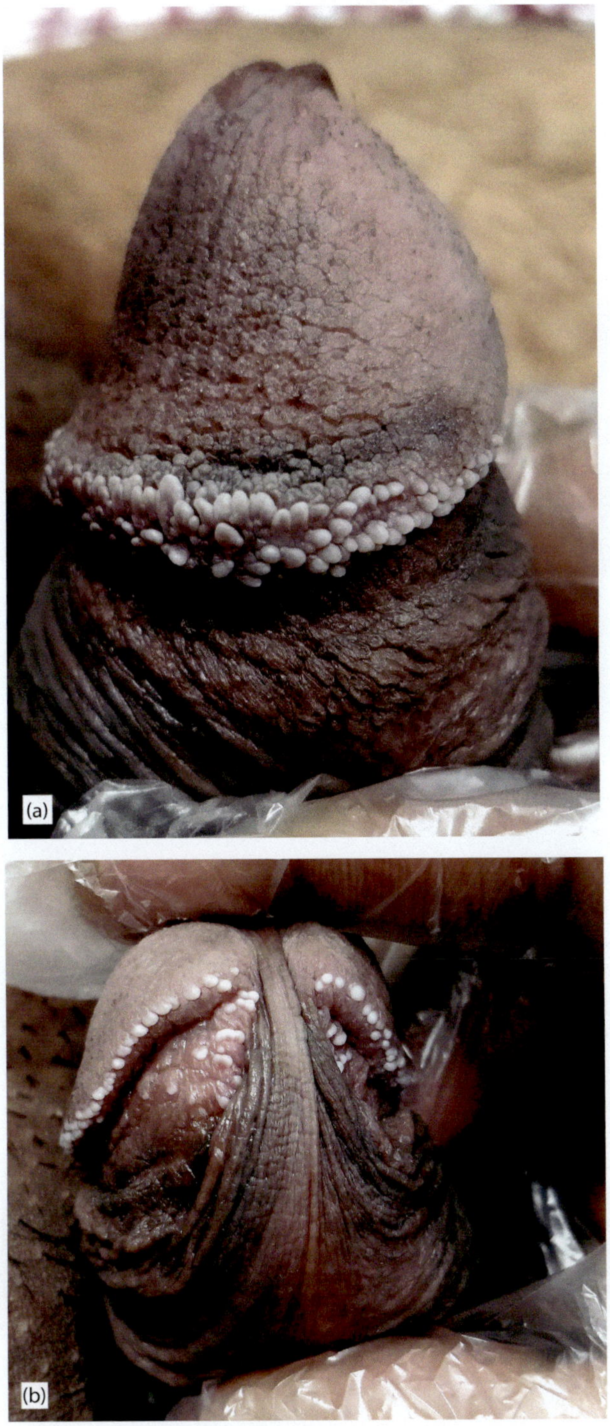


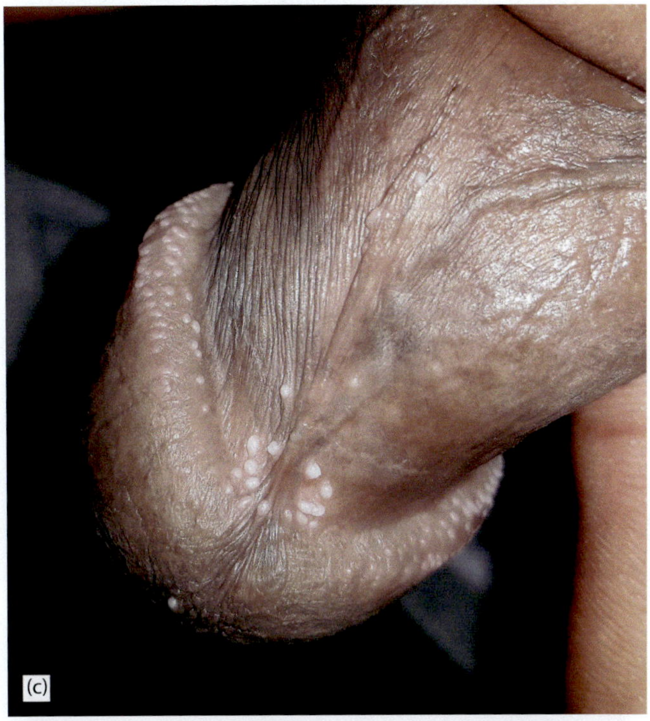


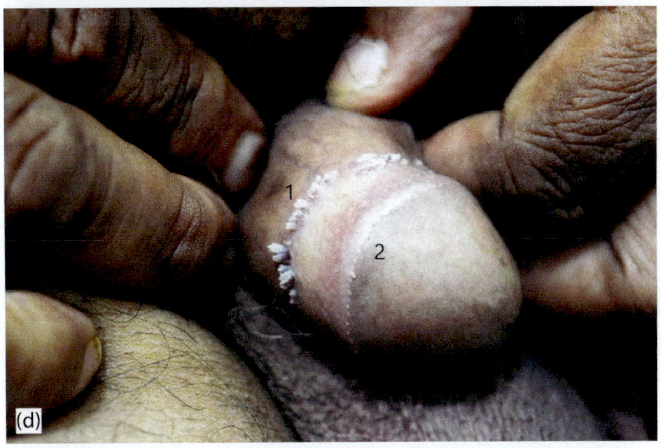


Figure 19.22 **(a)** Flesh-colored papules arranged in parallel rows on the corona of the glans penis (close-up image). **(b)** Pearly penile papules on the ventral aspect (close-up image). **(c)** Pearly penile papules on the ventral aspect of the penis. **(d)** Warts arranged circumferentially around the shaft of the penis **(1)** and pearly penile papules **(2)** in a young male. (a,b – Courtesy: Dr. Deverashetti Srinivas, Nizamabad, India; c – Courtesy: Dr. PC Das, Katihar, India.)

## Skin tag

- Genital skin tags are sessile or pedunculated fleshy growths may have several different shapes and colors, including wrinkled or smooth textures, and dark or light hues.
- Lesions in men are typically around the scrotum, penile shaft, or penis head.
- Tags are benign and hidden away most of the time.
- DD: Anogenital wart.

## Psoriasis

- The genital skin is involved in up to 40% of psoriasis patients.
- In many cases, genital psoriasis is part of more generalized plaque psoriasis or occurs in the setting of inverse psoriasis.
- Lesions on the genital area are brightly erythematous, often less well-demarcated and devoid of the typical psoriatic scales, due to maceration.
- While in uncircumcised males, the non-scaly plaques are most common under the prepuce and on the proximal glans, in circumcised ones, they are usually present on the glans and corona and may be more scaly than those usually seen in genital skin (**Figure 19.23a–d**).
- Fissures, pruritus, and/or burning in the affected area, ranging from minimal to marked, may be observed.
- DD: Balanitis, lichen planus, candidiasis, and extramammary Paget's disease (**Figure 19.23e**).

## Erythroplasia of Queyrat

- Erythroplasia of Queyrat is a premalignant condition of the visible mucous membranes of penis and is usually seen in middle-aged and older uncircumcised men. Etiology is not well known, but chronic irritative triggers are believed to play an important role.

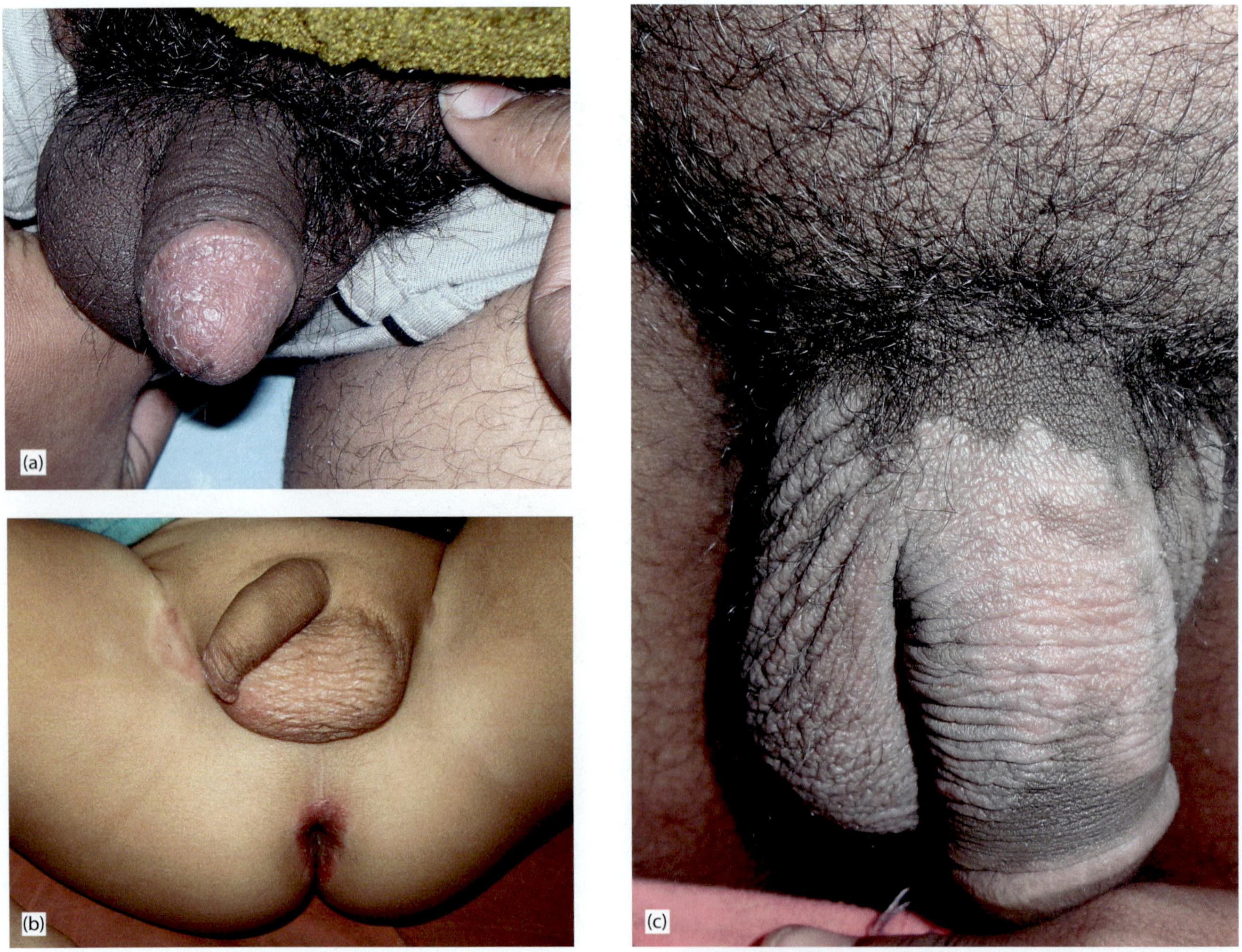


Figure 19.23 **(a)** Erythematous, scaly plaque of psoriasis on the glans penis. **(b)** Flexural psoriasis in a child. **(c)** Dry, scaly erythematous patch of psoriasis. (*Continued*)

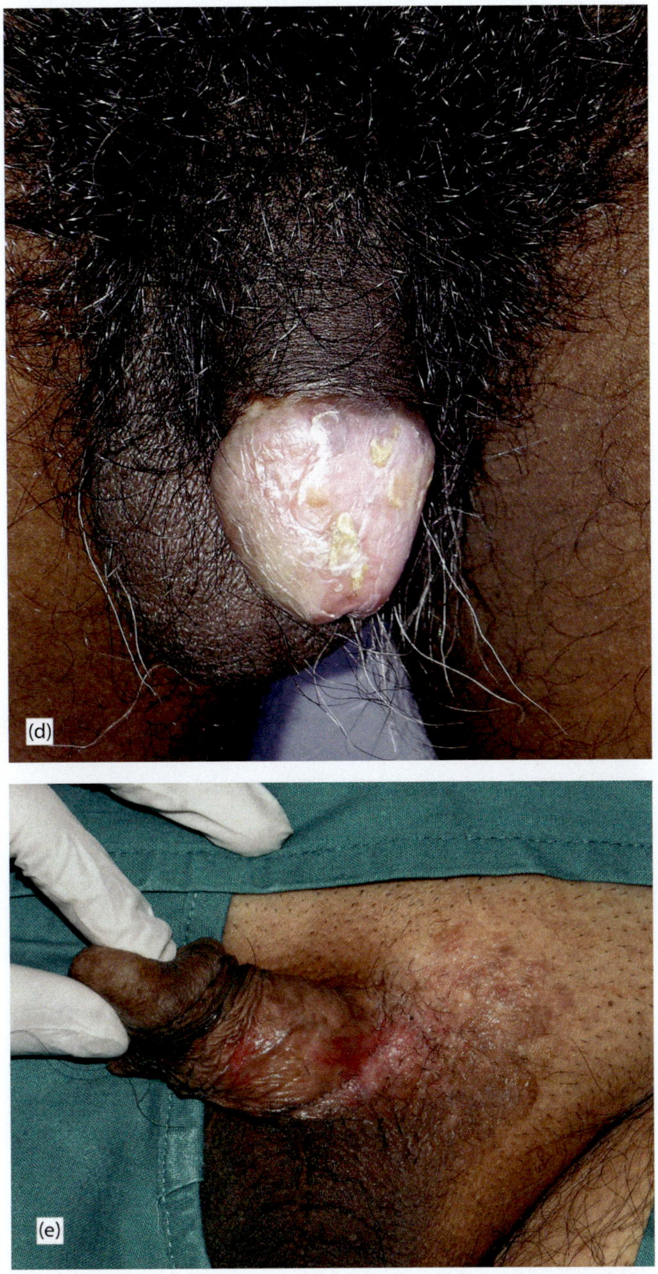


Figure 19.23 (*Continued*) **(d)** Psoriasis of the glans penis. **(e)** Extramammary Paget's disease presenting as erythematous atrophic patch in the genitocrural region. (b – Courtesy: Dr. Santoshdev P Rathod, Ahmedabad, India; e – Courtesy: Dr. Sushil S Savant, Mumbai, India.)

- It presents as asymptomatic, single erythematous patch, with a clear-cut border and lucent surface on glans penis or inner foreskin, which shows slow growth (**Figure 19.24a,b**).
- DD: Allergic/irritant contact dermatitis, balanitis xerotica obliterans, balanoposthitis, basal cell carcinoma, cicatricial pemphigoid, drug-induced bullous disorder, lichen planus, mucosal candidiasis, and plaque psoriasis.

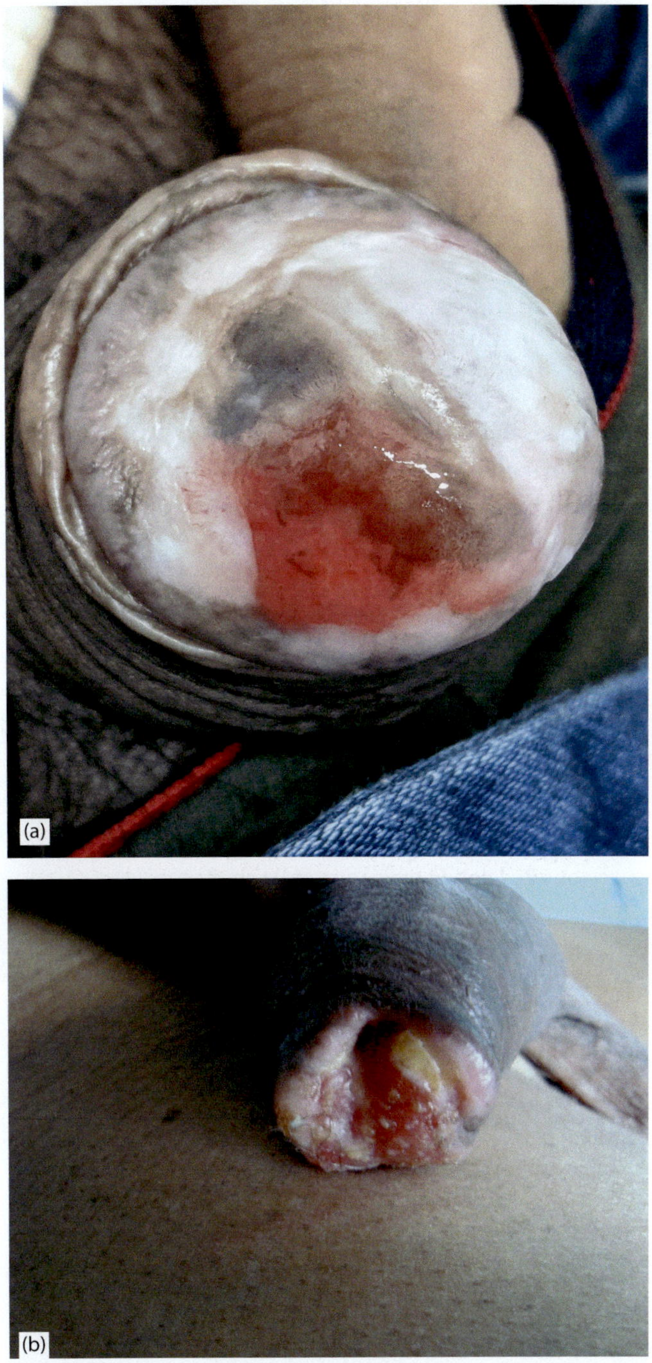


Figure 19.24 **(a)** Erythroplasia of Queyrat presenting as well-defined erythema. **(b)** Erythroplasia of Queyrat progressing to ulcer. (a – Courtesy: Dr. Deverashetti Srinivas, Nizamabad, India; b –Courtesy: Dr. Santoshdev P Rathod, Ahmedabad, India.)

## Genitourinary tuberculosis

- Genitourinary tuberculosis is the second most common extra-pulmonary tuberculosis. An isolated involvement of genital organs has been documented in up to 30% of the cases.
- Penile tuberculosis is usually primary and may be acquired sexually from infected partner.

- Involvement of the testis results from direct extension from the epididymis. Testicular tuberculosis may present with painless or painful scrotal mass, abscess, fistula, and multiple pus-discharging sinuses on the posterior surface of the scrotum.
- Penile tuberculosis usually presents with single or multiple superficial ulcers with or without inguinal lymphadenopathy. Nodules or fungating mass are rarer presentations.
- Papulonecrotic tuberculid is another form of penile affection, which presents as asymptomatic, symmetric, dusky-red papules and pustules over the glans penis. The lesions occur in crops and heal with atrophic scarring (**Figures 19.25** and **19.26**).
- DD: Syphilitic ulcer, carcinoma, granuloma inguinale, and human immunodeficiency virus (HIV) infection.

### Leprosy (Hansen's disease)

- Leprosy may be missed in external genitals unless specifically looked for.
- Genital lesions are mostly observed in multibacillary cases having extra-genital lesions too. Isolated genital involvement is very rare in literature.
- Clinically, patches, plaques, and/or nodules may be observed, depending on the spectrum of leprosy (**Figure 19.27**).
- There are few cases of histoid leprosy in which nodular lesions developed over the penile shaft.

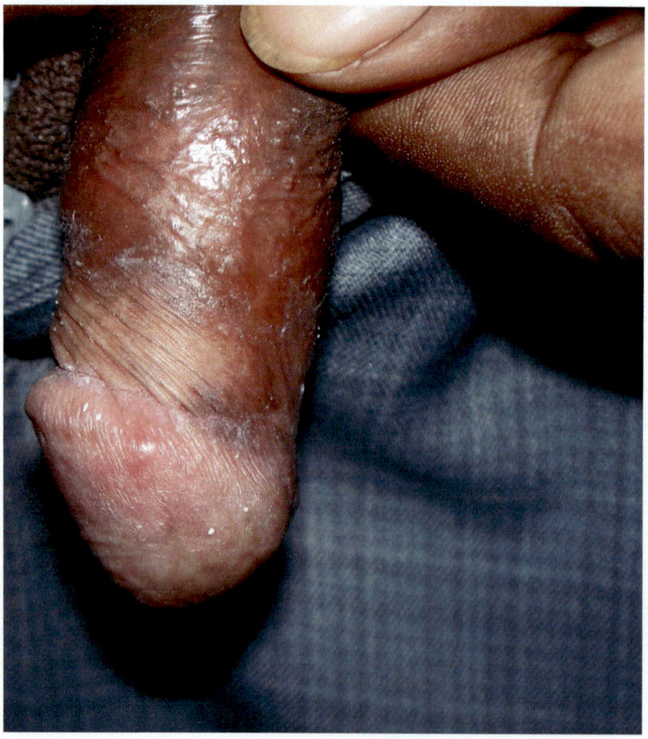

Figure 19.25 Erythematous papule of papulonecrotic tuberculid.

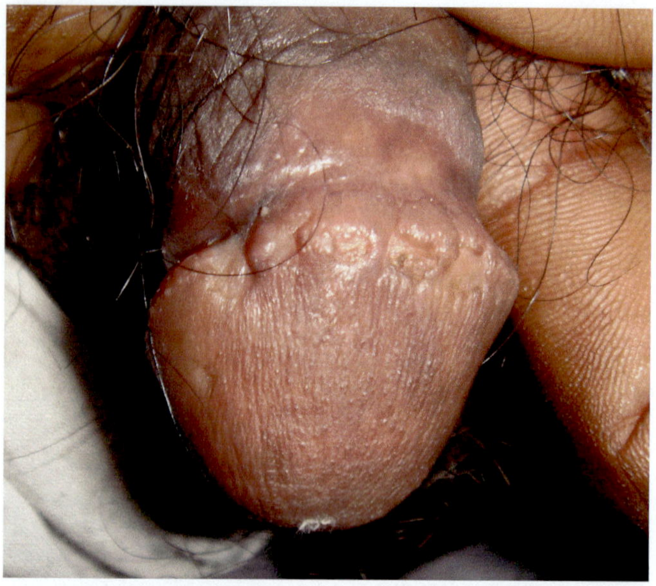

Figure 19.26 Papulonecrotic tuberculid lesions healing with atrophic scars.

- Lesions of erythema nodosum leprosum have been reported in genital region too.
- DD: Psoriasis, sarcoidosis, and syphilis.

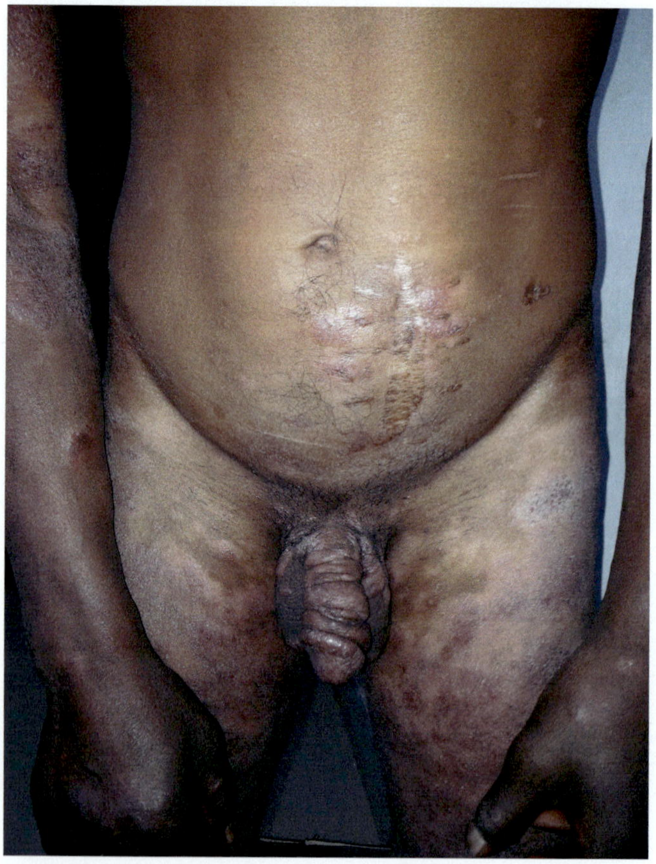

Figure 19.27 Erythematous nodules and plaques on the penis in a case of lepromatous leprosy.

## Lymphoma

- B-cell non-Hodgkin lymphoma affects middle-aged and older individuals and is the most common subtype of lymphoma of the genitalia.
- Other lymphoma types that may involve the genitalia include extranodal marginal-zone lymphoma, follicular lymphoma, and anaplastic large cell lymphoma.
- The lymphoma can result in the formation of a nodular mass and presents with an itching sensation.
- In some cases, pelvic pain and other general signs and symptoms, such as anemia, fatigue, and appetite loss, are noted.
- Patients also present with non-healing ulcers, and male patients, rarely, present priapism.
- DD: Squamous cell carcinoma.

## Lichen sclerosus et atrophicus (hypoplastic dystrophy)

- Lichen sclerosus et atrophicus occurs at all ages.
- Major symptoms are pruritus and eventual pain with more advanced disease. Glans involvement may result in narrower urine stream during micturition (**Figure 19.28a**).
- It is most often characterized by well-demarcated, hypopigmented plaques of fragile skin.
- Usually, at least some areas of the skin show fine crinkling, and fragility is often manifested by purpura or erosions (**Figure 19.28b**).
- Uncircumcised males generally experience phimosis as a presenting abnormality (**Figure 19.28c**).
- DD: Vitiligo, eczema, mucous membrane pemphigoid, and erosive lichen planus.

## Porokeratosis

- Porokeratosis is clinically characterized by annular plaques having central atrophy and raised keratotic border with groove.
- It usually presents as asymptomatic or, rarely, pruritic, solitary or multiple annular skin lesions of a few millimeters to centimeters in size.

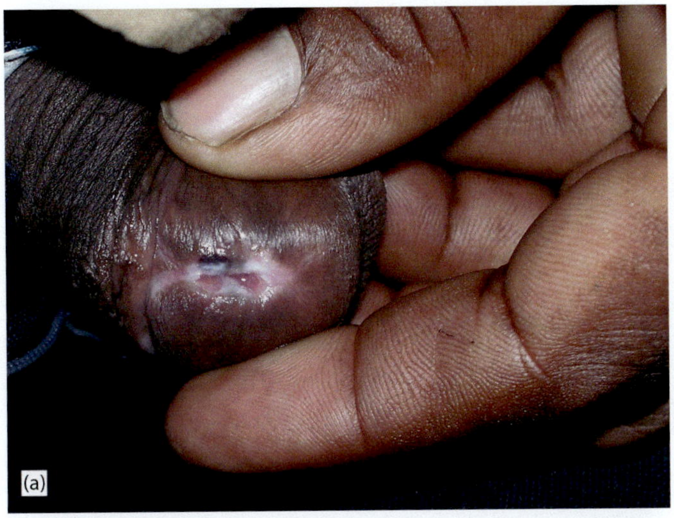


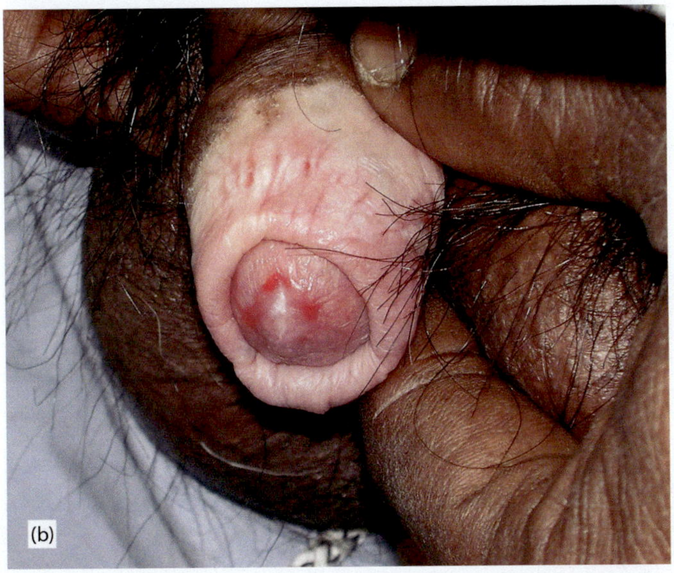


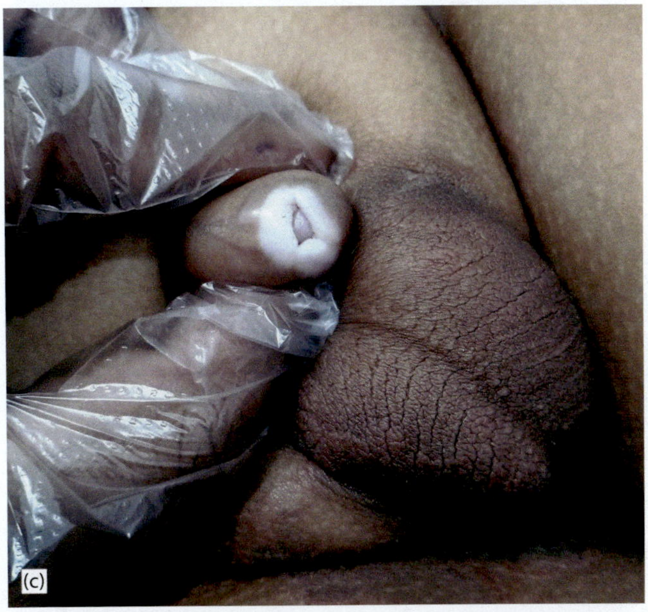


Figure 19.28 **(a)** Lichen sclerosus affecting the skin surrounding urinary meatus. **(b)** Lichen sclerosus causing induration of the prepuce resulting in inability to retract phimosis, fissures, and erosions. **(c)** Lichen sclerosus causing phimosis in a child. (c – Courtesy: Dr. Deverashetti Srinivas, Nizamabad, India.)

- Most commonly, it affects the scrotum and penis (**Figure 19.29a,b**).
- Porokeratosis ptychotropica is a rare clinical variant commonly seen in the genitogluteal region and on the buttocks. Clinically, it presents as itchy, solitary or multiple, coalescing verrucous or scaly plaques with satellite lesions.
- DD: Annular lichen planus.

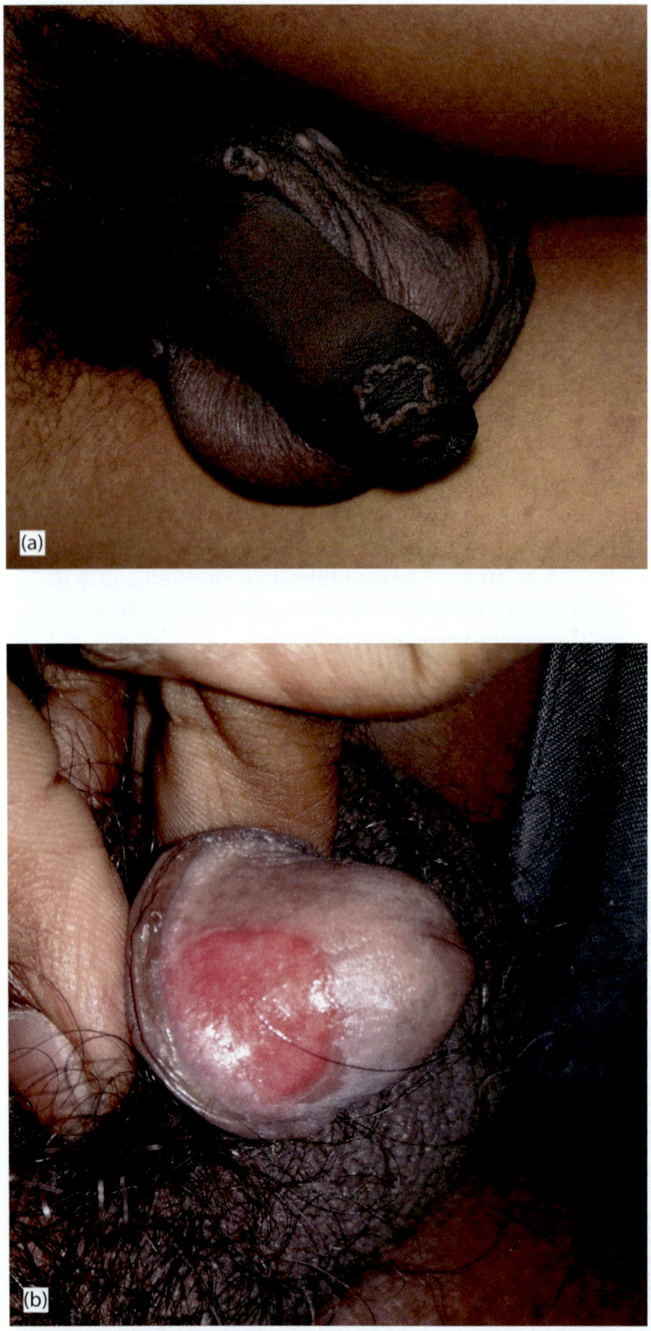

Figure 19.29 **(a)** Porokeratosis (Mibelli type) presenting with annular plaque with keratotic margin. **(b)** Porokeratosis (Mibelli type) presenting as dry erythematous plaque on the glans penis. (b – Courtesy: Dr. Santoshdev P Rathod, Ahmedabad, India.)

## Pseudoepitheliomatous, keratotic, and micaceous balanitis

- Pseudoepitheliomatous, keratotic, and micaceous balanitis is a rare condition affecting the glans penis and is usually seen in older, uncircumcised men.
- It presents as solitary, well-demarcated, hyperkeratotic plaque over the glans penis, with an overlying thick adherent micaceous scale.
- The condition is generally asymptomatic but fissuring, maceration, irritation, and interference with sexual activity may be associated (**Figure 19.30a,b**).
- It needs close monitoring as progression to verrucous carcinoma and squamous cell carcinoma is known.
- DD: Penile horn, penile psoriasis, giant condyloma, verrucous carcinoma, squamous cell carcinoma, and keratoacanthoma.

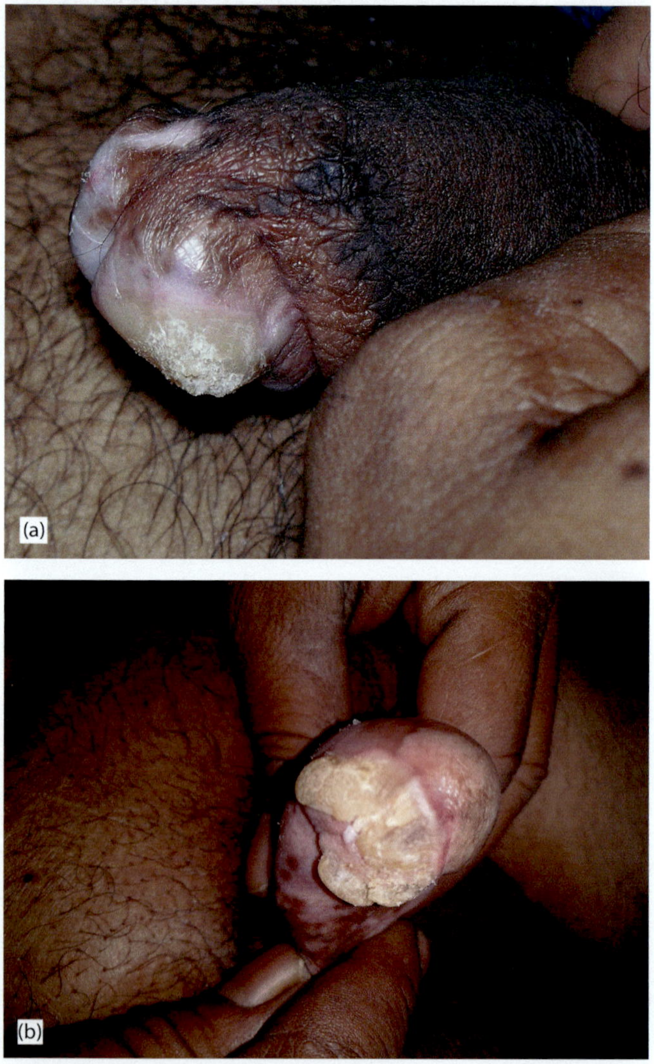

Figure 19.30 **(a)** Well-demarcated, hyperkeratotic plaque of pseudoepitheliomatous, keratotic, and micaceous balanitis. **(b)** Pseudoepitheliomatous, keratotic, and micaceous balanitis with thick keratinous overgrowth on the glans penis. (b – Courtesy: Dr. Santoshdev P Rathod, Ahmedabad, India.)

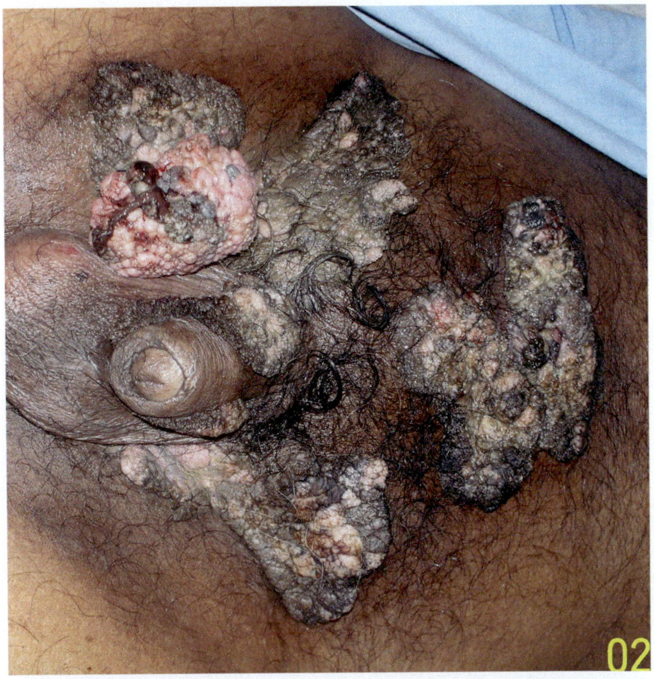


Figure 19.31 Giant cauliflower-like plaques and nodules with verrucous surface in Buschke-Lowenstein tumor.

## Buschke-Lowenstein tumor

- Buschke-Lowenstein tumor is a localized variant of verrucous carcinoma typically associated with HPV types 6 and 11. The tumor is slow-growing and highly destructive to contiguous tissues but seldom metastasizes.
- It presents as an asymptomatic polypoid or cauliflower-like growth on the genitals and surrounding areas that grows to a large size (**Figure 19.31**). Maceration and secondary infections are common.
- DD: Squamous cell carcinoma, genital warts, and primary rectal adenocarcinoma.

## Verrucous carcinoma

- Verrucous carcinoma is a relatively uncommon locally aggressive, low grade, slow-growing well-differentiated squamous cell carcinoma with minimal metastatic potential.
- It presents with a polypoid or exophytic nodule with a verrucous surface. Long-standing cases may progress to an ulcer.
- It may progress locally to cause perianal infection, fistula formation, and local lymphadenopathy.
- Symptoms include pruritus, bleeding, pain, tenesmus, fecal incontinence, discharge, change in bowel habits, etc. (**Figure 19.32**).
- DD: Genital warts.

## Squamous cell carcinoma

- Squamous cell carcinoma (SCC) is the commonest neoplasm of the genital tract and penis and may be invasive cancer and noninvasive or preinvasive lesions.

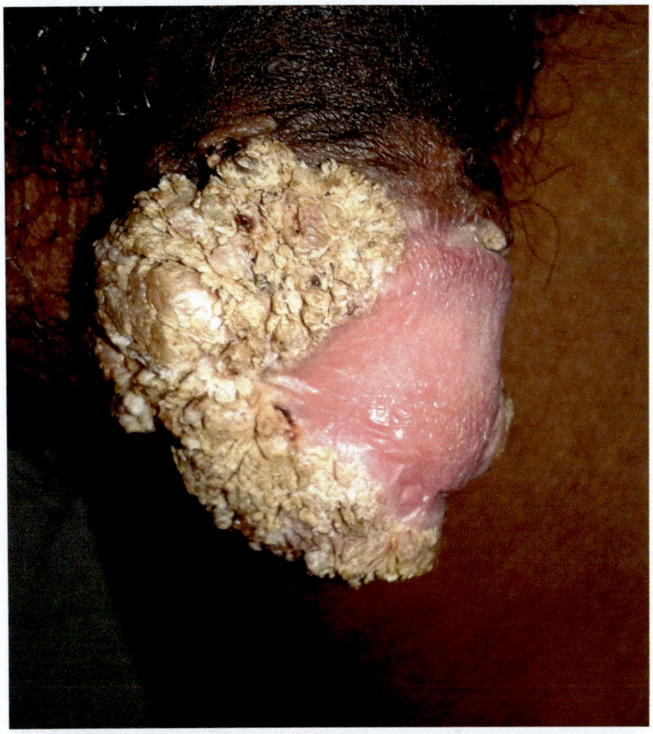

Figure 19.32 Verrucous carcinoma on the glans penis. (Courtesy: Dr. PC Das, Katihar, India.)

The term "invasive" refers to tumors in which the malignant cells have penetrated the underlying basement membrane and have infiltrated into the stroma.
- The risk factors include phimosis, chronic balanoposthitis, chronic irritation, lichen sclerosus et atrophicus, and lichen planus.
- It usually presents as an asymptomatic or itchy, painful, indurated papule or nodule that may ulcerate (**Figure 19.33a,b**).
- Metastasis to regional lymph nodes has been reported in 60% cases of penile SCC.
- DD: Basal cell carcinoma, Kaposi sarcoma, donovanosis, and pyoderma gangrenosum.

## Epidermoid cyst

- Penile epidermoid cysts are uncommon.
- They appear as solitary or, uncommonly, multiple, round, usually small, mobile bumps. They occur in various sizes.
- They are usually white or yellow, though people with darker skin may have pigmented cysts.
- Lesions may be asymptomatic, but rupture may result in significant discomfort.
- DD: Cutaneous lipoma, steatocystoma multiplex.

## Steatocystoma multiplex

- Steatocystoma multiplex is an uncommon but distinct clinical condition characterized by the formation of numerous cutaneous sebum-containing cysts called steatomas, steatocystomas, or sebocysts.

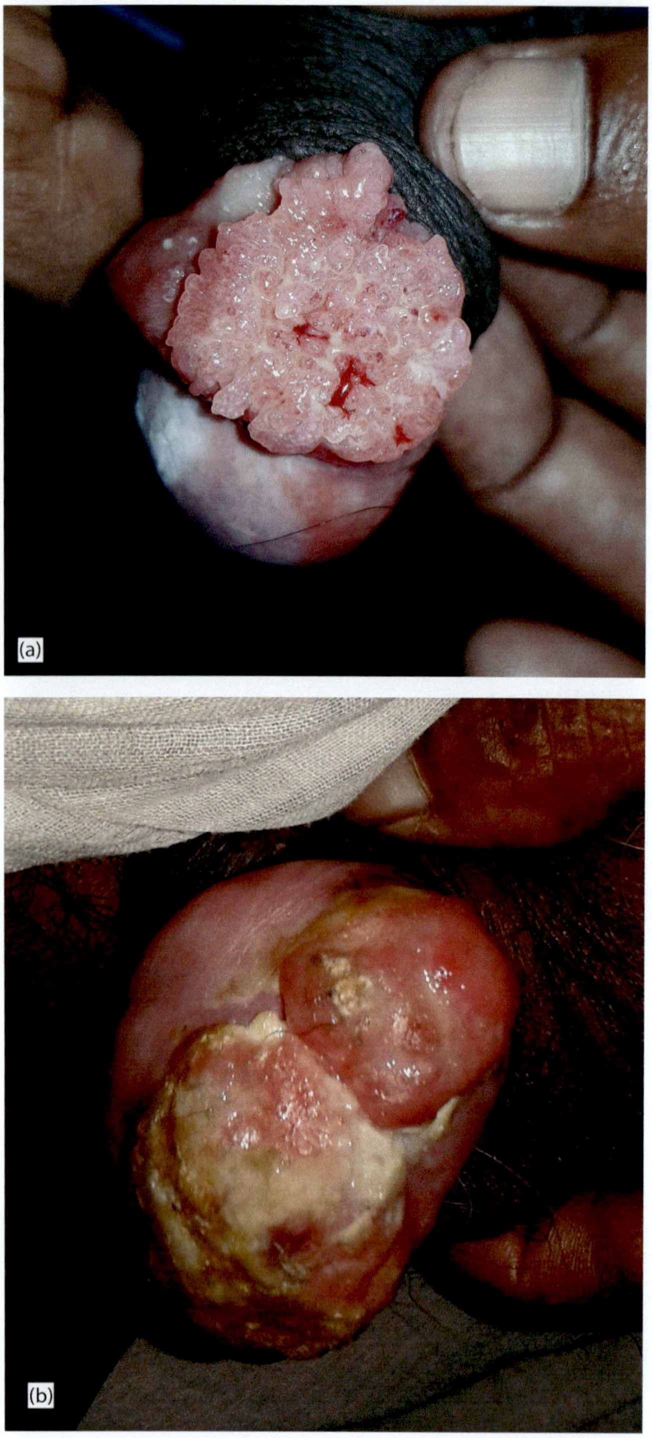

Figure 19.33 **(a)** Squamous cell carcinoma presenting with exophytic nodule on the glans penis. **(b)** Squamous cell carcinoma presenting as noduloulcerative lesions on the glans penis. (a – Courtesy: Dr. PC Das, Katihar, India.)

- In familial cases, it is an autosomal dominant genodermatosis usually appearing at birth or early in life.
- The cysts may be seen on the penis and scrotum. The cysts are always multiple and vary from 1 to 20 mm in diameter.

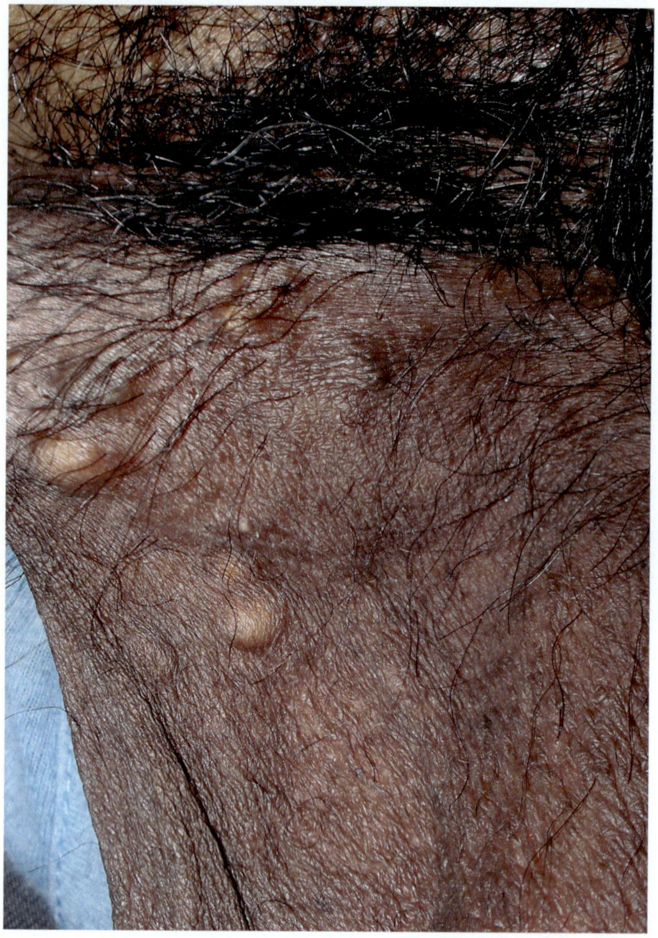

Figure 19.34 Multiple tense cystic lesions on the scrotum.

- The lesions are usually asymptomatic, but occasionally they can become infected and painful (**Figure 19.34**).
- DD: Epidermoid cyst, lipoma, calcinosis cutis.

## Scrotal calcinosis

- Idiopathic scrotal calcinosis is a benign condition, mainly seen in men aged 20 to 40 years.
- The pathogenesis of SC is controversial as to whether the disease is idiopathic or the result of dystrophic calcification of existing structures, including epidermal cyst, eccrine epithelial cyst, and degenerated dartos muscle.
- Clinically, it consists of hard, yellowish nodules within the dermis of scrotal skin.
- Nodules vary in size (from 1 mm to several centimeters) and number (solitary or multiple).
- The nodules are usually asymptomatic, and patients seek medical advice mainly for cosmetic reasons.
- A few cases may have itching or discharge from the calcified masses (**Figure 19.35**).
- DD: Scrotal cyst.

## Penile thrombophlebitis

- Superficial thrombophlebitis of the dorsal vein of the penis (penile Mondor's disease) is a rare disease

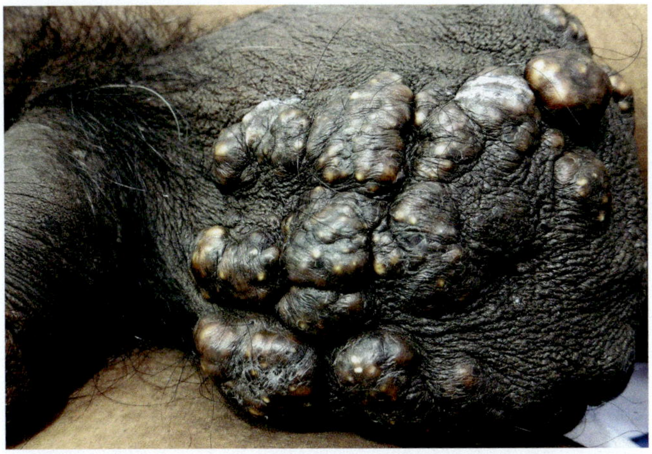

Figure 19.35 Firm nodules of scrotal calcinosis. (Courtesy: Dr. Deverashetti Srinivas, Nizamabad, India.)

presenting with pain and induration of the dorsal part of the penis.

- The possible causes comprise trauma, neoplasms, excessive sexual activity, or abstinence. This disease almost always limits itself.
- The patient consistently presents with a rope-like cord on the dorsum of the penis. The cord is a thrombosed dorsal vein that has become thickened and adherent to the overlying skin.
- The patients have a significant amount of pain, which can be either episodic or constant.
- Some patients may develop irritative voiding symptoms.
- DD: Peyronie's disease, sclerosing lymphangitis.

## Peyronie's disease

- Peyronie's disease is a superficial penile fibromatosis resulting from the growth of fibrous plaques in the penile soft tissues. Specifically, scar tissue forms in the tunica albuginea surrounding the corpora cavernosa.
- It is characterized by palpable nodules in the region of the tunica albuginea enclosing the corpora cavernosa and the penile septum, which may be associated with pain and deformity on erection and a variable degree of erectile dysfunction and decreased girth. DD: Congenital penile curvature, penile dorsal vein thrombosis, thrombophlebitis, systemic sclerosis, bubonulus, penile fracture.

## Mucoid penile cyst

- Mucoid penile cysts are uncommon benign lesions affecting mainly young men and manifesting on the ventral surface of glans penis. They most likely arise from ectopic urethral mucosa sequestrated in the penile skin during embryologic development.
- Most of them are present at birth, but usually they are detectable only in adolescence.
- The cyst commonly presents as a small, soft, and freely movable mass around the glans, mainly on the penile ventral surface.
- Mostly they are asymptomatic but can be complicated by infection or trauma or can make coitus difficult.
- DD: Epidermal cyst, median raphe cyst, lipomas, steatocystoma, dermoid cyst, pilonidal cyst, Tyson's glands cyst.

## Lymphangioma circumscriptum

- Lymphangioma circumscriptum is a benign proliferation of lymphatics and is broadly classified into two major groups based on the depth of involvement and size of the abnormal lymph vessels.
- It can become evident at any age, but the greatest incidence occurs at birth or early in life.
- Genitals, including scrotum and penis, may be affected. Clinically, it presents as multiple discrete or grouped vesicles that may be either translucent or red to blue (or black). A verrucous surface may be seen.
- Usually the condition is asymptomatic, but sometimes it is associated with oozing of the lymphatic fluid from the vesicle and with pain and pruritus.
- Complications include hemorrhage, ulceration, secondary infection, and, rarely, malignant transformation such as lymphangiosarcoma and squamous cell carcinoma.
- DD: Angiokeratoma, condylomataaccuminata, molluscum contagiosum, bacillary angiomatosis and nevi.

## Median raphe cyst

- Median raphe cysts are considered to be a developmental anomaly resulting from abnormal or incomplete development of paired genital folds and can present along the midline of the ventral side of the male genital area, anywhere from tip of penis to anal orifice. Rarely, they may present as cordlike or canaliform induration on the median raphe (**Figure 19.36a,b**).
- They may present at birth or may remain asymptomatic and unrecognized till early adulthood.
- The cyst grows in size with advancing age and may become symptomatic owing to infection and trauma.
- DD: Dermoid cyst, pilonidal cyst, epidermal inclusion cyst, urethral diverticulum, steatocystoma.

## Erythema multiforme

- Erythema multiforme is an acute, immune-mediated, mucocutaneous condition commonly caused by herpes simplex virus infection and certain medications, characterized by classical iris or target lesions.
- Earliest lesions are usually bilaterally symmetrical, round, erythematous, edematous papules surrounded by areas of blanching that may resemble insect bite or papular urticaria.
- These papules may enlarge and develop concentric alteration in morphologic features and color, resulting in target lesions.
- Typical target lesions have a central dusky erythema, purpura, or blister; a middle ring of pale edema; and

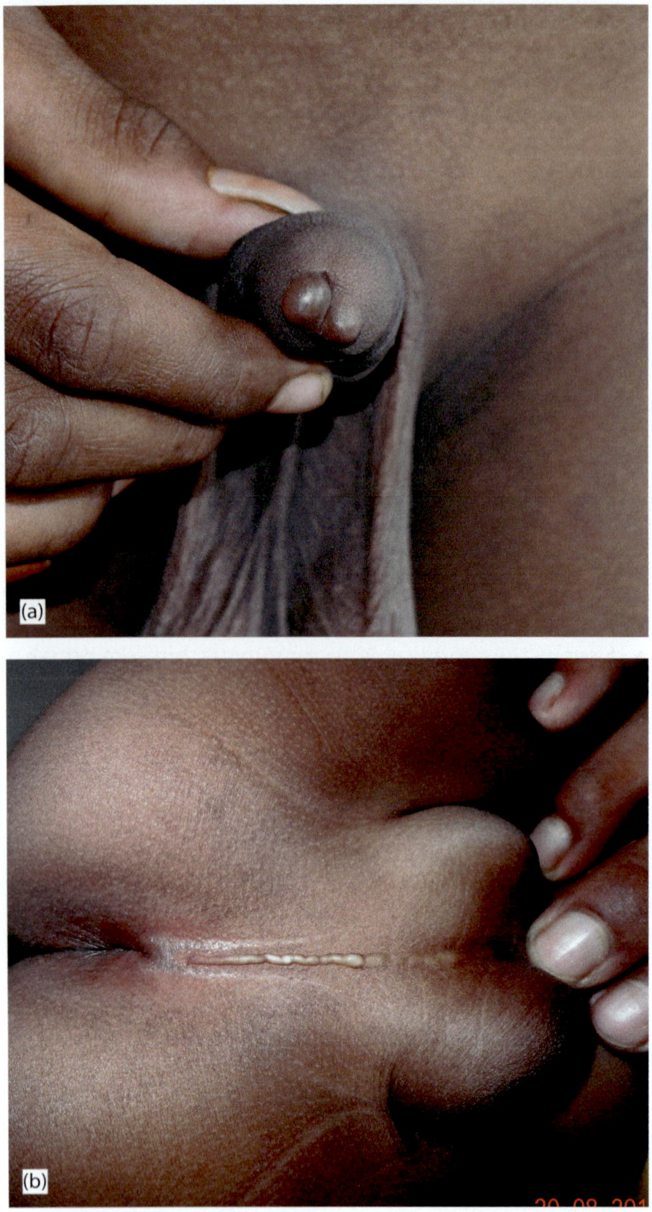


Figure 19.36 **(a)** Median raphe cysts presenting as tense cystic swellings on the glans penis. **(b)** Median raphe cysts presenting as midline cord like swelling in the groin.

an outer well-defined ring of erythematous halo. In atypical lesions, these areas manifest as round, palpable, edematous lesions with only two zones or a poorly defined border or both.

- DD: Pemphigus vulgaris, bullous pemphigoid, and paraneoplastic pemphigus.

## Herpes genitalis

- Genital herpes is a viral infection caused by a DNA virus, *Herpes simplex* virus (HSV) type 2. Incubation period is 5 to 14 days.
- In primary infection, symptoms typically occur within 3 to 7 days after exposure but with a longer duration of 10 to 14 days. Before the onset of lesions, systemic symptoms (fever, malaise) and local symptoms (pain, tenderness, burning and tingling) may precede the development of genital lesions. Genital lesions typically occur on the glans or shaft of penis and start with painful, grouped vesicles appearing on an erythematous base, which progress to pustules, erosions, and/or ulcerations. Inguinal lymphadenopathy may be associated. Crusting of lesions followed by resolution of lesions occurs over the next couple of days (**Figure 19.37a,b**).

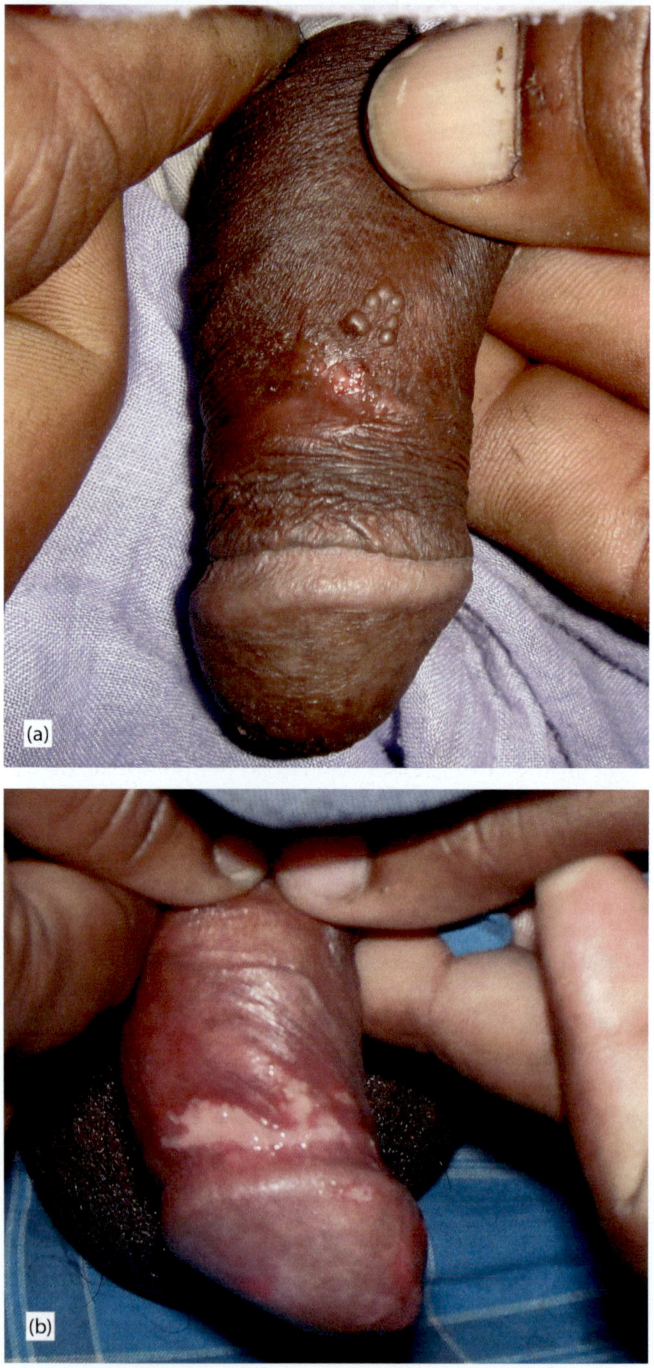


Figure 19.37 **(a)** Genital herpes presenting as grouped vesicles and erosions. **(b)** Grouped erosions in genital herpes.

- Genital herpes usually recurs. During reactivation, a similar prodrome of fever and flu-like symptoms with localized burning, itching, and tingling may occur, but these are often seen with decreased severity. The genital lesions are usually fewer, and duration of disease is less compared to those of primary infection.
- DD: Trauma, syphilitic chancre (non-purulent, usually single, indurated, painless ulcers lymphadenopathy), chancroid ulcers (purulent, often multiple painful ulcers with soft, undermined edges), lymphogranuloma venereum (transient papular, herpetiform vesicle, erosion, or ulcer).

## Candidiasis

- *Candida* species are normal flora and may cause symptomatic infection. Risk factors of candidiasis include older age, diabetes, prolonged antibiotic therapy, and immunosuppression.
- Patients present with mild glazed erythema, satellite pustules and erosions, and moist curd-like accumulations, and sometimes ulceration of the glans penis and fissured prepuce are seen. Peripheral pustular and papular lesions may be noted. Mild burning pain and pruritus are often associated (**Figure 19.38a–e**).
- DD: Pustular psoriasis, impetigo, dermatophytosis.

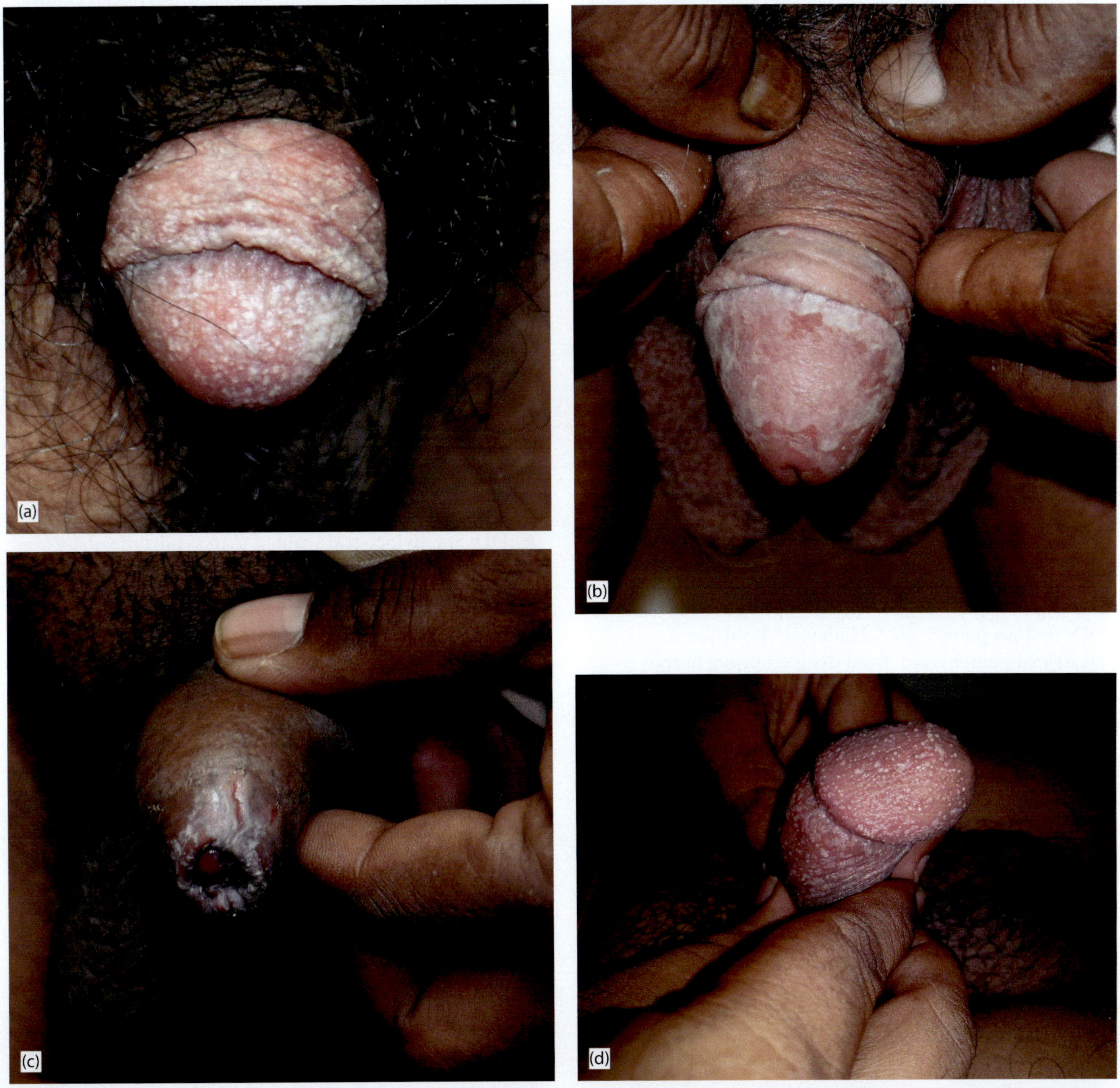


Figure 19.38 **(a)** Candidiasis presenting as whitish slough present on the glans and inner prepuce. **(b)** Candidiasis presenting as erosions and whitish membrane like structure. **(c)** Candidiasis presenting with phimosis, fissures, and accumulation of whitish slough. **(d)** Numerous superficial pustules in candidiasis. (*Continued*)

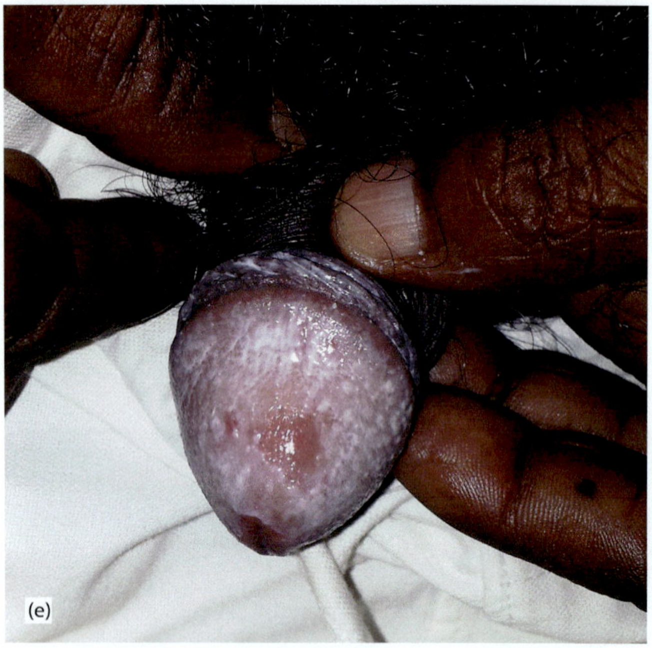


Figure 19.38 (*Continued*) **(e)** Whitish, easily scrapable slough on the glans penis in candidiasis. (d – Courtesy: Dr. Santoshdev P Rathod, Ahmedabad, India.)

## Pemphigus vulgaris and vegetans

- Penile involvement is usually seen along with mucocutaneous disease, but it may occur as early manifestation of the disease too, followed by development of cutaneous lesions in due course.
- Pemphigus vegetans is uncommonly seen and presents as warty lesions in intertriginous areas, including genital region. It has two clinical subtypes: the Neumann type, with poor prognosis, usually begins with bullae; the Hallopeau type, with excellent prognosis and longer remission, usually begins with grouped pustules.
- DD: Bullous pemphigoid, Hailey-Hailey disease, cicatricial pemphigoid, fixed drug eruption, herpes genitalis, genital aphthosis, and Behçet's disease for pemphigus vulgaris, (genital wart, herpes genitalis, and condylomata lata for pemphigus vegetans).

## Bullous pemphigoid

- Localized variants with involvement limited to genital region, including localized penile and scrotal bullous pemphigoid, have been reported.
- DD: Pemphigus vulgaris, erythema multiforme, mucous membrane pemphigoid.

## Cicatricial pemphigoid (mucous membrane pemphigoid)

- Genital regions are involved in 50% of patients.
- In the genital region, it may present as non-specific erosions, skin fragility, and sometimes intact blisters over clinically hair-bearing skin. Scarring may result in phimosis.
- DD: Erosive lichen planus, bullous pemphigoid, lichen sclerosus et atrophicus.

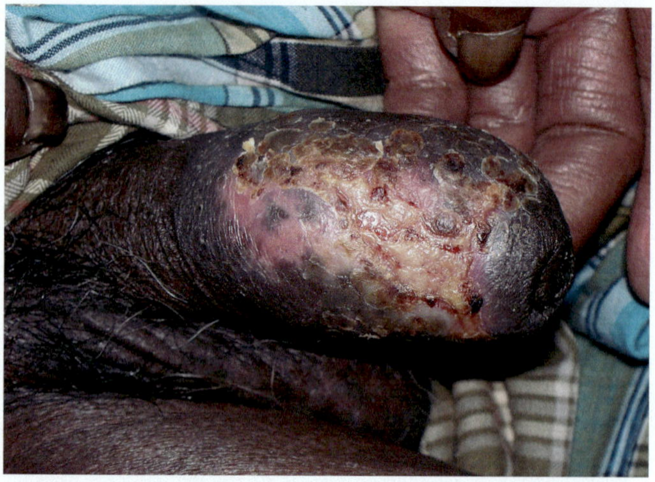

Figure 19.39 Erosions on the penis in a case of Stevens-Johnson syndrome.

## Stevens-Johnson syndrome and toxic epidermal necrolysis

- Stevens-Johnson syndrome (SJS) and toxic epidermal necrolysis (TEN) are severe life-threatening conditions after exposure to drugs (95% of cases) or infections.
- The most common drugs implicated are sulfonamides, penicillin, quinolones, cephalosporin, acetaminophen, carbamazepine, phenobarbital, phenytoin, valproic acid, oxicam group of non-steroidal anti-inflammatory drugs, antitubercular, allopurinol, and antiretrovirals.
- SJS and TEN manifest as erythematous or violaceous patches, atypical targetoid lesions, bullae, erosions, and ulcers involving the skin and mucosa, including genitalia (**Figure 19.39**).
- DD: Staphylococcal scalded skin syndrome, drug-induced pemphigoid and pemphigus, acute graft versus host disease, and paraneoplastic pemphigus.

## Acrodermatitis enteropathica

- Acrodermatitis enteropathica is caused by zinc deficiency and may occur as a rare autosomal recessive disease, in nutritional deficiency states or, less commonly, iatrogenically post-parenteral nutrition.
- The classic presentation is a triad of periorificial and acral dermatitis, diarrhea, and alopecia. The dermatitis consists of erythematous, well-demarcated, and scaling plaques or, sometimes, vesicopustular plaques and crusting, which is most pronounced around the mouth, eyes, and genital area (**Figure 19.40**).
- Secondary infections with staphylococcus and candida are common.
- DD: Diaper dermatitis, flexural psoriasis, other nutritional deficiency dermatosis.

## Chancre

- Chancre seen in primary syphilis is a sexually transmitted infection caused by a spirochaete bacterium, *Treponema pallidum*, subspecies *pallidum*. Incubation period is 9 to 90 days; the average is three weeks.

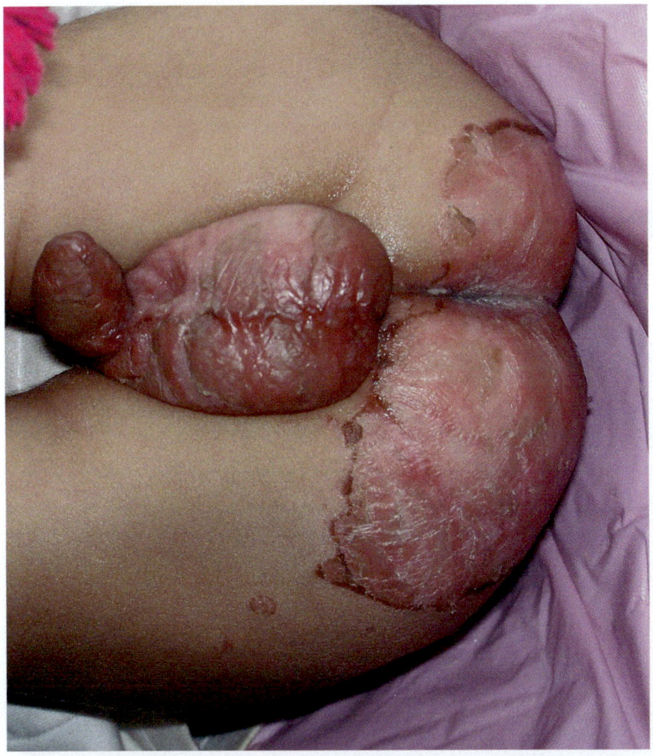

Figure 19.40 Acrodermatitis enteropathica with perianal, scrotal, and ventral penile involvement.

- The primary syphilis presents as a single, indolent, round or oval, indurated painless ulcer or chancre with regional lymph nodes enlargement.
- The lesion starts as a small red papule or crusted superficial erosion that becomes a round or oval, indurated, typically well-circumscribed ulceration and which is firm on palpation (**Figure 19.41a–c**).
- A hard chancre present on the inner surface of the prepuce may snap back on a retracted prepuce (Dory flop sign).
- Common sites are the glans penis, coronal sulcus, prepuce, frenulum, and shaft of penis.
- DD: Herpes genitalis (recurrent painful vesicles, erosions or ulcers), Fixed drug eruption, Behçet's disease.

## Aphthous ulcer (aphtha, aphthous stomatitis, or canker sore)

- Aphthous ulcer is encountered infrequently on the genitalia.
- Genital lesions that are seen in men are secondary and usually occur in the setting of Behçet's disease. Most, but not all patients, with genital aphthous ulcers also have a history of oral aphthae.
- Aphthous ulcers of the genitalia tend to be larger and deeper than those occurring in the mouth.
- The base of the ulcers can be bright red or may be covered with either gray, necrotic material or heme-colored eschar (**Figure 19.41d**).

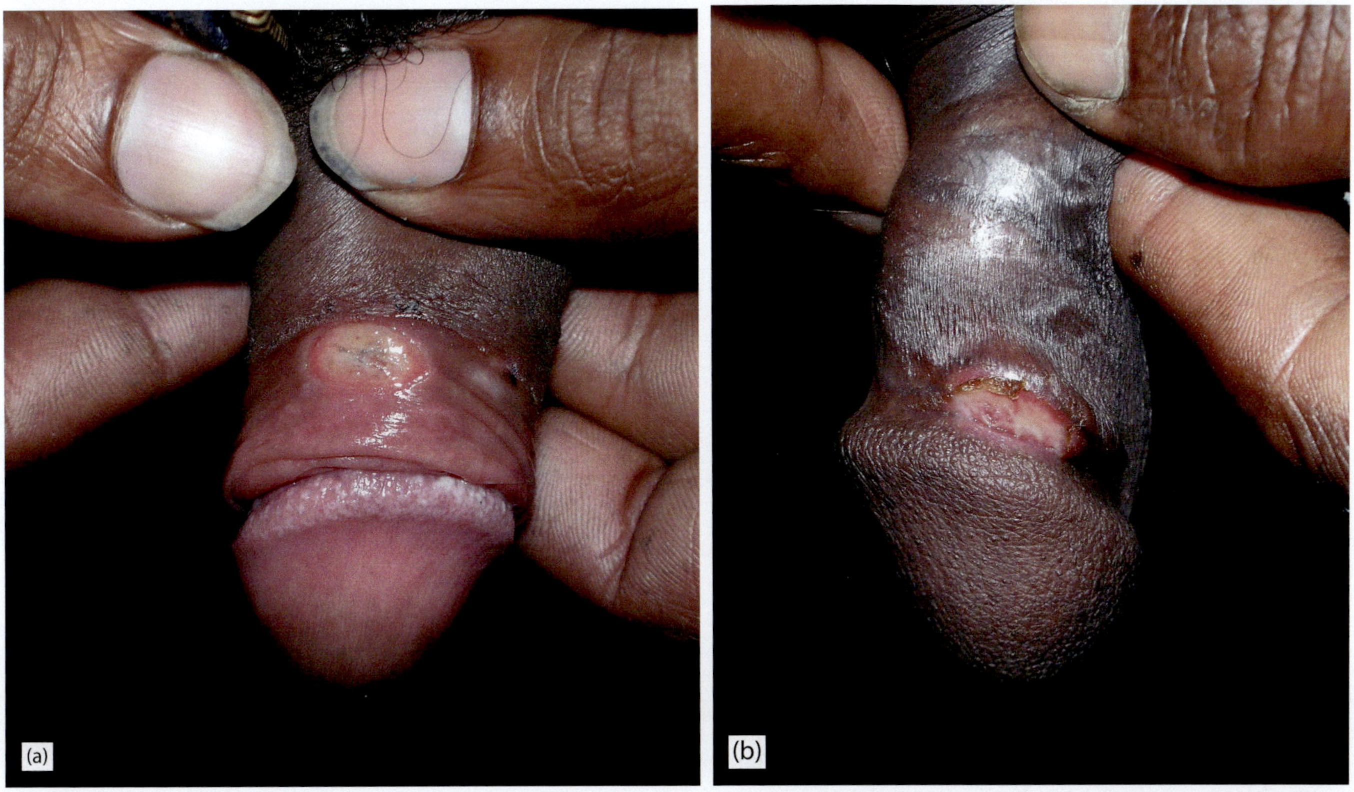


Figure 19.41 **(a)** Chancre on inner prepuce presenting as solitary well-demarcated, ulcer with clean floor and indurated base. **(b)** Chancre on the inner prepuce. (*Continued*)

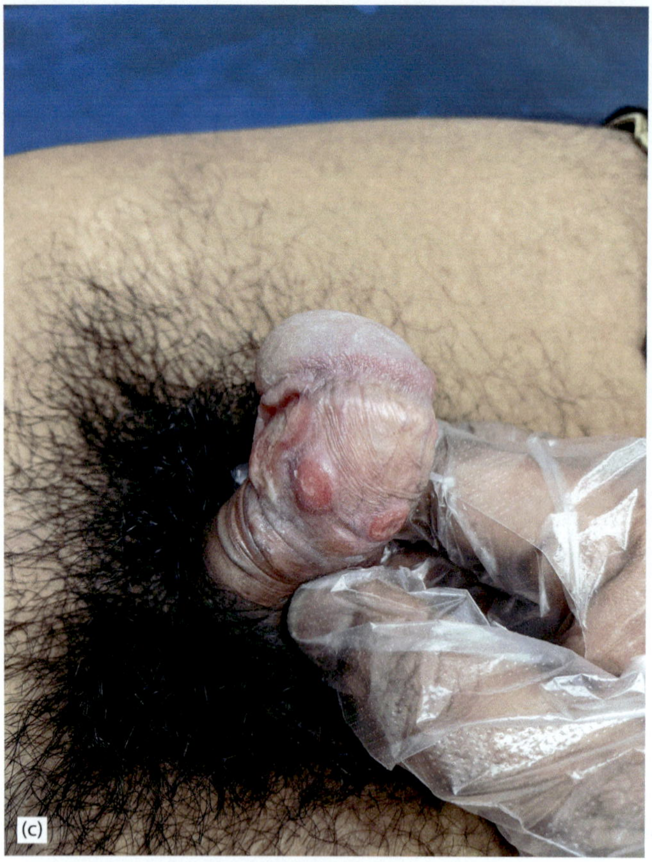


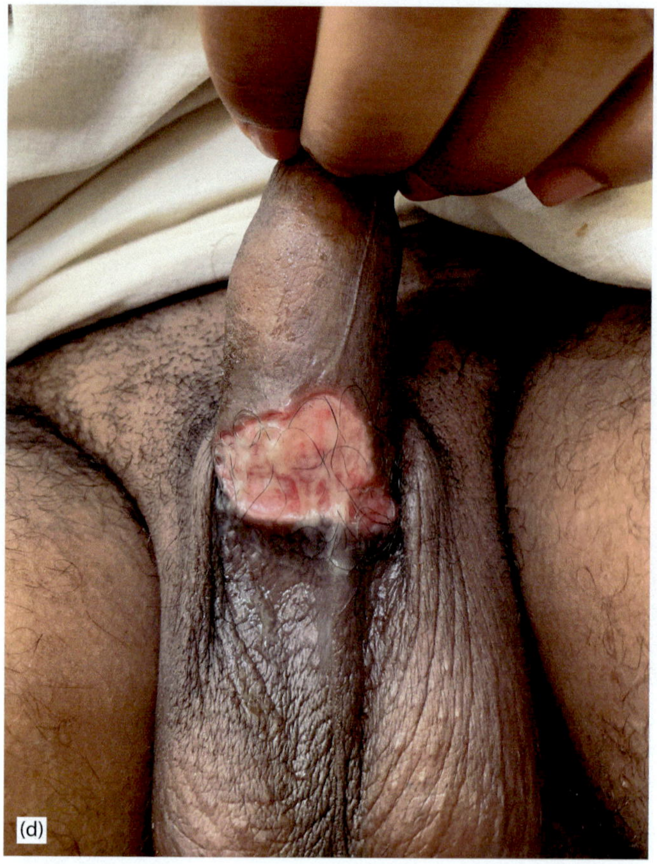


Figure 19.41 (*Continued*) **(c)** Multiple chancres. **(d)** Large painful aphthous ulcer in a patient with Behcet's disease. (c – Courtesy: Dr. Deverashetti Srinivas, Nizamabad, India; d – Courtesy: Dr Rajeev Ranjan, Ara, India.)

- Genital ulcers are extremely painful, and their appearance is sometimes preceded by, or accompanied by, low-grade fever, malaise, gastrointestinal, and/or respiratory symptoms.
- Larger genital lesions may heal with scarring.
- It tends to occur more often on the scrotum than on the penis.
- DD: Behçet's disease, primary syphilis, chancroid.

## Chancroid (soft chancre, ulcus molle)

- It is a sexually acquired infection caused by a gram-negative bacillus, *Haemophilus ducreyi*. Incubation period is three to ten days (average seven days).
- Chancroid presents as multiple painful ulcers on genitalia.
- A lesion starts with a small inflammatory papule surrounded by erythema, rapidly progresses to a pustule, and finally develops into a foul-smelling painful ulcer.
- Ulcers are sharply circumscribed, with a purulent base, soft, undermined edges, and purulent exudates present on the floor of the ulcer; removal of the exudate may bleed on scrapping or gentle manipulation (**Figure 19.42a,b**).
- The base of the ulcer is non-indurated.
- Common sites involved are external or internal surface of prepuce, the frenulum, the coronal sulcus, and occasionally the shaft of penis and external urinary meatus.

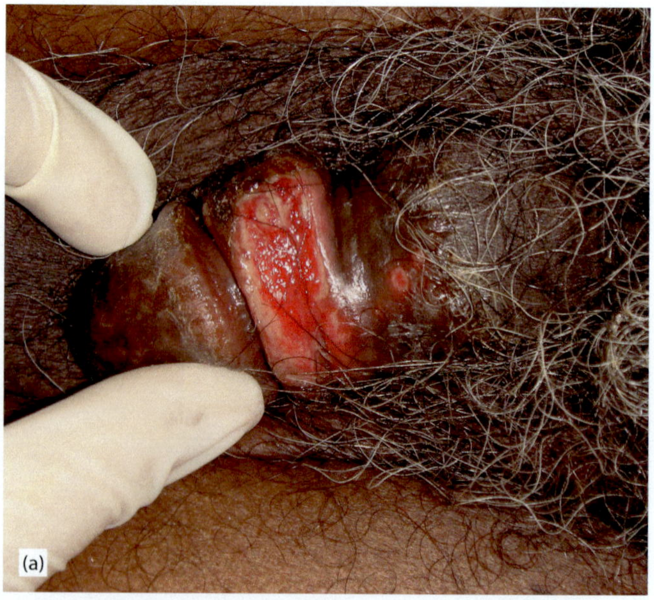


Figure 19.42 **(a)** Chancroid – solitary large ulcer with hemorrhagic floor. Smaller shallow ulcer is present in the vicinity. (*Continued*)

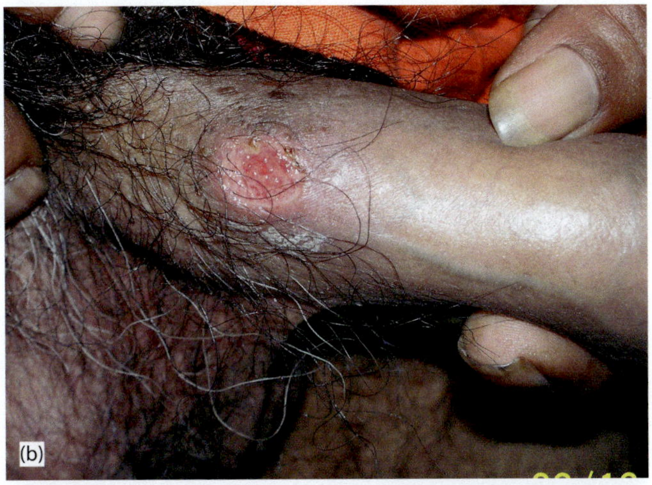

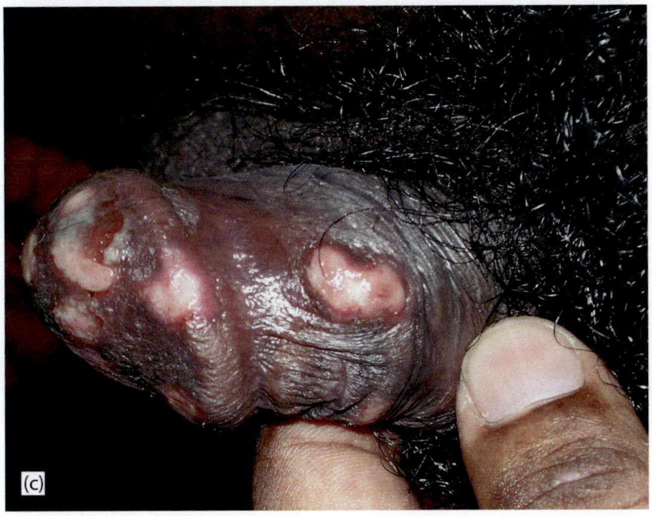

Figure 19.42 (*Continued*) **(b)** Solitary ulcer of chancroid on the shaft of the penis. **(c)** Multiple dwarf type of chancroid ulcers.

- If untreated, inguinal buboes may rupture to form inguinal ulcers.
- Usually, unilateral painful inguinal lymphadenitis may develop along with the genital ulcer.
- Clinical variants include giant, large serpiginous ulcer, phagedenic, transient, follicular, papular, dwarf (**Figure 19.42c**), pseudo granuloma inguinale.
- Complications include phimosis, paraphimosis, urethral fistula, and phagedenic ulcerations.
- DD: Genital herpes (recurrent painful vesicles, erosions, or ulcers), primary chancre (non-purulent, usually single, indurated, painless ulcers), chancroid (purulent, often multiple painful ulcers, soft, undermined edges).

## Donovanosis

- Donovanosis is a rare chronic, progressive ulcerative bacterial infection caused by a gram-negative bacilli, *Klebsiella granulomatis*. The incubation period is one day to one year (average 17 days).
- The disease begins as single or multiple firm papule or nodule that ulcerate eventually.
- The ulcer is usually painless or mildly painful and slowly progresses over weeks to months; it is beefy-red in color and bleeds easily on touch. Foul-smelling exudate due to extensive tissue damage is present.
- The most common sites include the glans penis, prepuce, frenulum, and coronal sulcus.
- Complications are phimosis or lymphoedema of distal tissue in active phase of the disease.
- Recurrence in healed areas is common.
- Morphological variants are classical granulomatous, hypertrophic, sclerotic or cicatricial, destructive necrotic (phagedenic).
- DD: Syphilis (non-purulent, usually single, indurated, painless ulcer, lymphadenopathy), chancroid (purulent, often multiple painful ulcers, soft, undermined edges, painful suppurative lymphadenopathy), herpes genitalis (recurrent painful vesicles, erosions or ulcers).

## Crohn's disease

- Crohn's disease is an inflammatory granulomatous disease that can affect sites distant from the gastrointestinal tract (non-contiguous form or metastatic Crohn's disease) genitalia.
- Genital involvement can present in several different forms. Interestingly, the severity of the cutaneous findings may not correlate with the severity of the bowel symptoms.
- It can occur as a result of direct extension from areas near the bowel, such as the anus or a colostomy site, or it can appear on the genitalia as a solitary lesion.
- Genital lesions usually appear as non-healing ulcers, but they can present as a papule, plaque, or swelling.
- Penile and scrotal edema may occur.
- Linear fissures can develop within intertriginous folds. This sign, termed "knife cut," is a very distinctive finding.
- DD: Hidradenitis suppurativa, Langerhans cell histiocytosis, herpes genitalis in an immunosuppressed patient, syphilis, granuloma inguinale, chancroid, traumatic ulceration.

## Pyoderma gangrenosum

- It usually starts with one or more inflammatory pustules, papules, or nodules that break down to form an ulcer. Most cases of genital localized pyoderma gangrenosum are not complicated with associated systemic diseases in both male and female cases. But, genital cases with extragenital skin lesions tend to have associated systemic diseases (**Figure 19.43a,b**).
- Most commonly associated diseases are inflammatory bowel disease (especially Crohn's disease), rheumatoid arthritis, lupus erythematosus, hematopoietic malignancy, and various gammopathies.

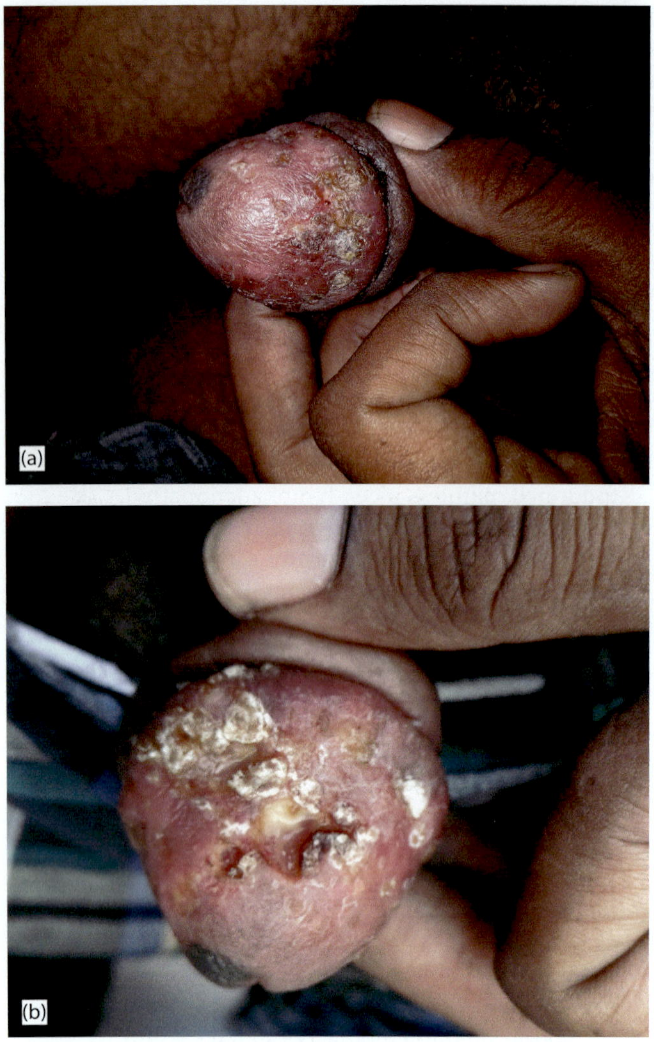

Figure 19.43 **(a)** Pyoderma gangrenosum of the penis presenting as crusted ulcers. **(b)** Rapid progression in the size of ulcers in one month. (a,b – Courtesy: Dr. Santoshdev P Rathod, Ahmedabad, India.)

- DD: Syphilis, herpes simplex, mycobacterial infection, amebiasis, squamous cell carcinoma, cutaneous Crohn's disease, ulcerating sarcoidosis, aphthous ulceration, Behçet's disease, Fournier gangrene.

## Dermatitis artefacta

- Dermatitis artefacta is a factitious disorder in which the patient creates skin lesions in order to satisfy an internal psychological need.
- It has been associated with obsessive-compulsive spectrum disorder, depression, psychosis, and severe personality disorders.
- Its clinical expression is variable in morphology as well as distribution.
- Inconclusive, bizarre, irregular rectilinear outlines and geographical patterning are cardinal (**Figure 19.44**).
- Simultaneous occurrence of artefactual genital ulcers in a couple, "folie à deux," has been described.
- DD: Neurotic excoriations, traumatic ulcer.

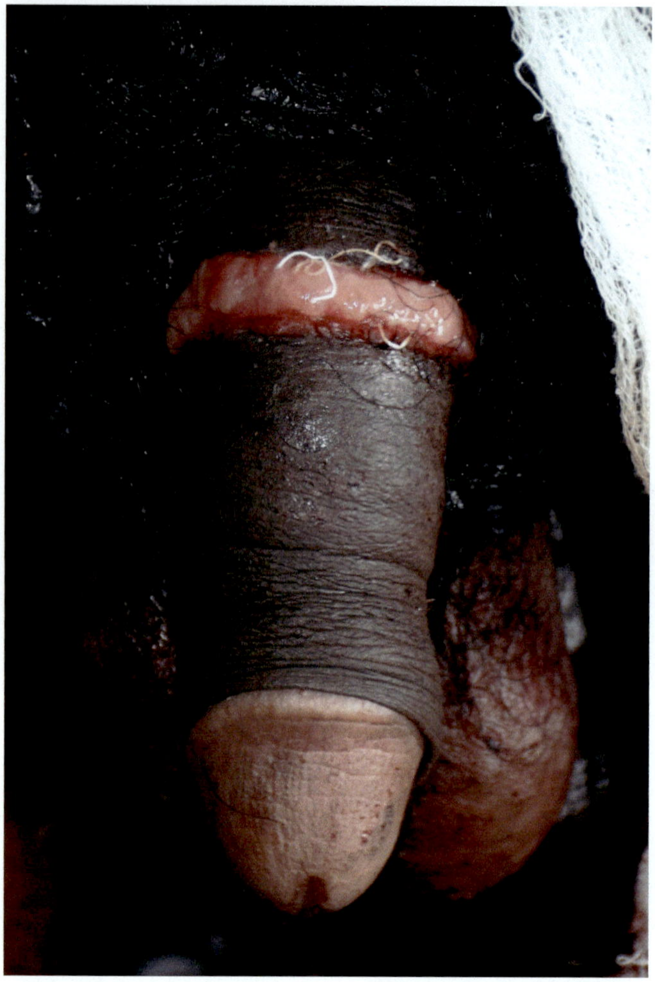

Figure 19.44 Ulceration with granulation tissue affecting the shaft of the penis in circumferential manner in dermatitis artefacta.

## Malakoplakia

- Malakoplakia is an acquired granulomatous disorder, which mainly occurs in the genitourinary tract, accounting for 60% to 70% of the cases.
- Its appearance is associated with organ transplantation, connective-tissue disorders, neoplasm, diabetes mellitus, and chronic debilitating/immunodeficiency disorders such as HIV infection, hepatitis C, sarcoidosis, and chronic immunodeficiency.
- The lesions may present as ulcerations, abscesses, erythematous papules, subcutaneous nodules, or masses and are associated with non-healing surgical wounds and draining fistulas.
- The lesions may present over the perianal area and scrotum.
- DD: Tuberculosis, Whipple disease, lepromatous leprosy, fungal infection (cryptococcus), parasite infection (leishmaniasis), Langerhans cell histiocytosis, fibrous histiocytoma, lymphoma, granular cell tumor, xanthoma, foreign body granuloma, hemophagocytic syndromes, sarcoidosis.

## Actinomycosis

- Primary genital involvement is rare and follows trauma or human bite.
- The condition is characterized by the clinical triad of painless subcutaneous nodules, sinuses, and discharge.
- Penile lesions are mostly situated in the region around the corona and are commonly associated with pilonidal sinus.
- DD: Crohn's disease, abscess, and tuberculosis.

## Lymphedema

- Genital lymphedema is an edematous disease of the genitalia due to abnormal lymph circulation.
- Congenital forms are associated with Turner, Noonan, Klinefelter, yellow nail, and intestinal lymphangiectasia syndromes.
- Swelling due to lymphedema in the early phases is painless.
- The tissue is soft and may pit when depressed.
- As the condition becomes chronic, the skin and subcutaneous tissue may have a woody, indurated texture as the tissue becomes fibrotic. The penis may assume a distorted shape. (**Figure 19.45a,b**).
- Patients experience a sensation of heaviness and/or tension, swelling, urinary troubles, and/or lymphorrhea of the lesion.
- The skin may exhibit warty excrescences or blisters, and it may weep lymphatic fluid (**Figure 19.45c**).
- If the cause is infection, subcutaneous abscesses and sinus formation may be apparent.
- DD: Venous thrombosis or insufficiency, Fournier gangrene, lymphangioma circumscriptum, angioedema.

## Priapism

- Priapism is a persistent and often painful erection that lasts for several hours, even in the absence of stimulation or after stimulation has ended.

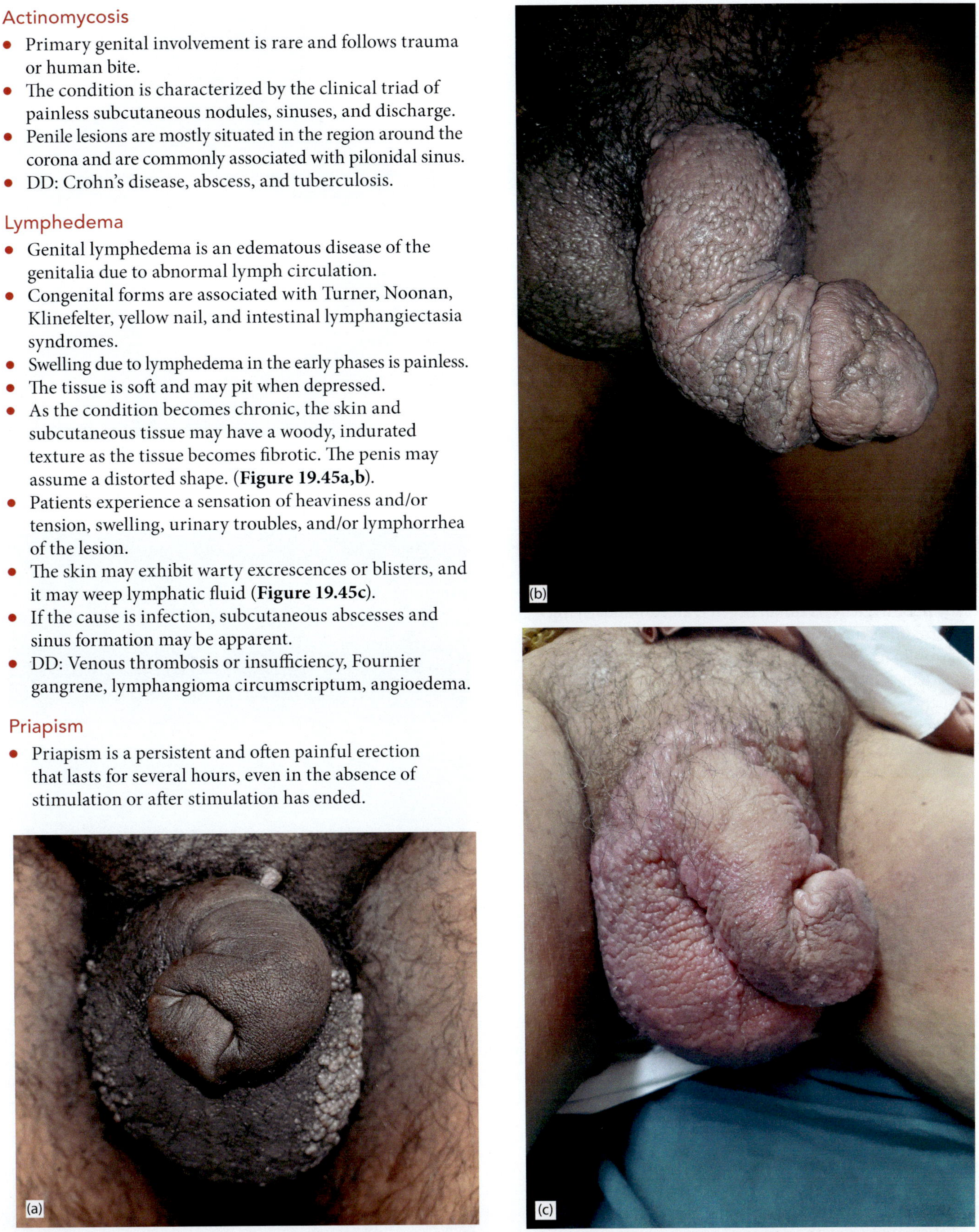


Figure 19.45 **(a)** Penile swelling (and deformity) and scrotal lymphangiectasia in filariasis. **(b)** Saxophone penis in lymphatic filariasis. Note surface changes due to chronic lymphedema. **(c)** Lymphatic cysts in a case of acquired lymphedema due to surgery for inguinal hernia. (b – Courtesy: Dr. PC Das, Katihar, India; c – Courtesy: Dr Hiral Shah, Baroda Medical College, Vadodara, India.)

- During priapism, the shaft of the penis is rigid and inflexible, but the glans of the penis is usually soft.
- DD: Peyronie's disease, penile implant.

## Penile fracture

- Penile fracture is a tear in the tunica albuginea of the penis.
- Its most common etiology is a direct blow to the erect penis during intercourse or masturbation. Erection thins out the tunica and makes it more susceptible to injury.
- Patients complain of a cracking or popping sound, immediate pain, rapid detumescence, penile swelling, and penile deviation away from the injury.
- Urethral injury may occur in 15–22% of fractures.
- Location of the fracture can often be identified by physical examination in which focal tenderness and overlying hematoma with contralateral penile deflection may be present.
- DD: Congenital penile curvature, penile dorsal vein thrombosis, thrombophlebitis, Peyronie's disease.

## Phimosis

- Phimosis is the inability of the prepuce to be retracted behind the glans penis in uncircumcised males.
- It is normally seen in younger male children and resolves in most cases by three years of age.
- Adult phimosis is usually pathological and is caused by poor hygiene, trauma, neglect, and an underlying dermatosis including candidiasis, lichen sclerosus et atrophicus, non-specific balanoposthitis in diabetic patient, penile lymphedema, and malignant conditions such as erythroplasia of Queyrat and squamous cell carcinoma.
- Congenital or physiological phimosis is clinically asymptomatic and is often associated with ballooning of the foreskin during voiding.
- Pathological phimosis is symptomatic, and skin irritation, dysuria, bleeding, and occasionally urinary retention are noted.
- Prepucial skin appears inflamed and edematous and sometimes shows white circumferential scarring and fissures, and patients complain of pain during sexual activity (**Figure 19.46**).
- DD: Paraphimosis, squamous cell carcinoma.

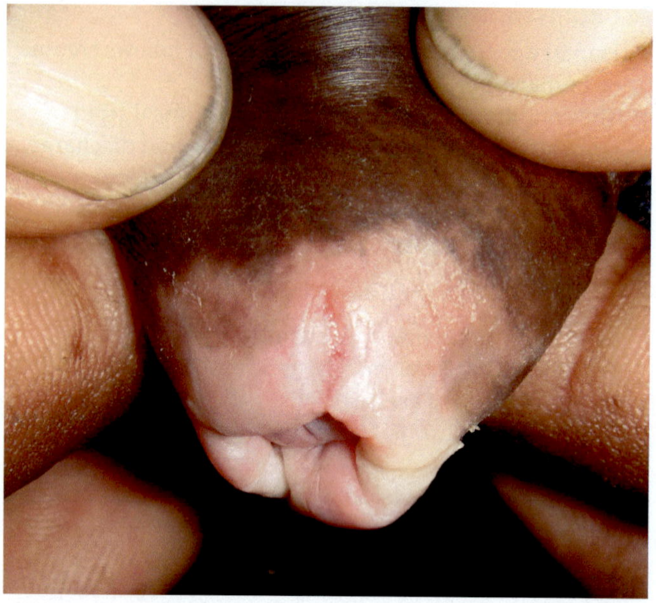

Figure 19.46 Phimosis in lichen sclerosus.

## Paraphimosis

- Paraphimosis is an emergency condition in which the retracted prepuce cannot be returned to its normal anatomic position. It is important to recognize this condition promptly, as delay in management can result in gangrene and amputation of the glans penis.
- It develops when the retracted prepuce is left retracted for several hours. The common causes include trauma, infections, and sexual activity.
- Patients present with acute onset of painful swelling of the glans penis and prepuce. A constricting band of edematous prepuce is noted directly behind the swollen glans penis. The rest of the penile shaft appears normal (**Figure 19.47a,b**).

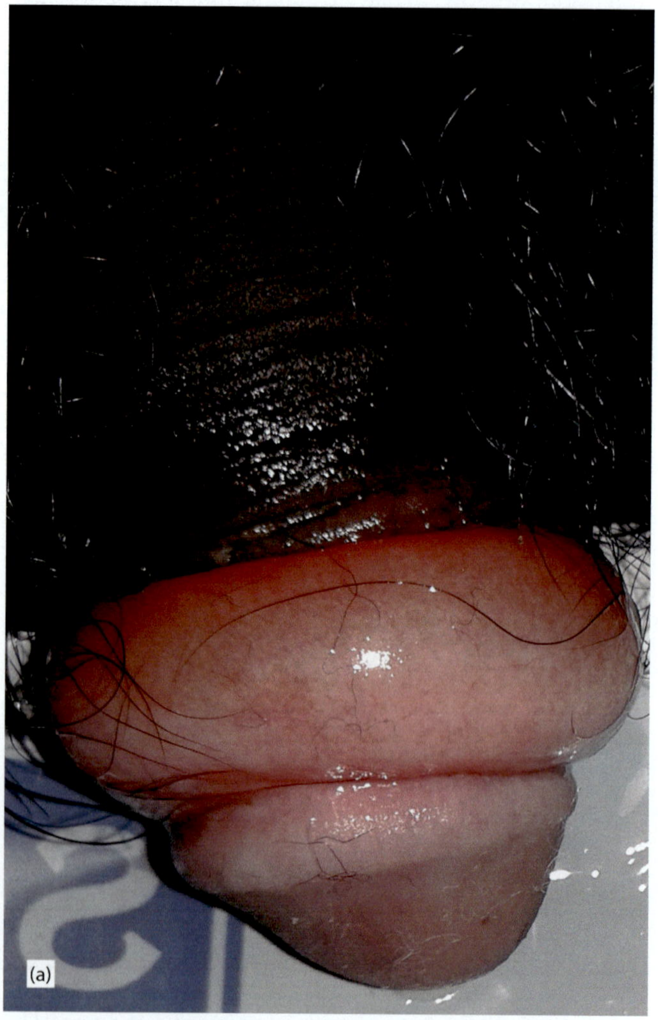

Figure 19.47 **(a)** Paraphimosis in a young male after sexual activity. *(Continued)*

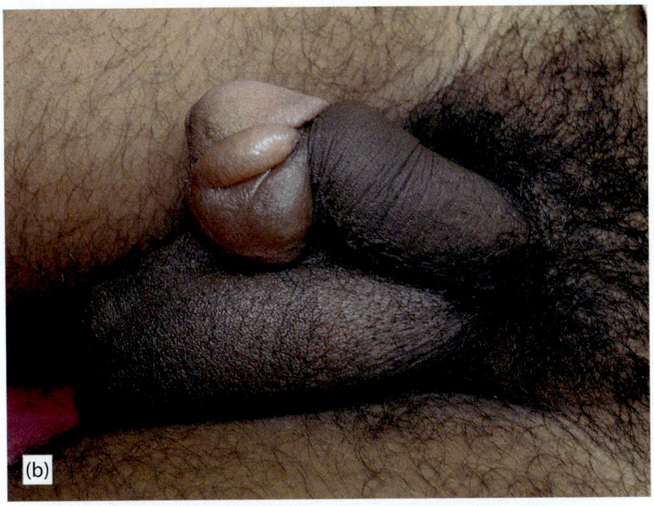

Figure 19.47 (*Continued*) **(b)** Edematous swelling in paraphimosis.

- If left untreated, necrosis and subsequent auto-amputation of the distal penis may occur.
- DD: Phimosis.

## Hypospadias

- Hypospadias is an abnormality of the anterior urethral and penile development in which an abnormal urethral opening is ectopically located on the ventral penis.
- The urethral opening may be located as far down as the scrotum or perineum, extending up to the navicular fossa.
- It is often associated with a ventral curvature of the penis (chordee) and/or a defective ventral foreskin.
- It is characterized by abnormal urethral opening on the ventral penis and is usually asymptomatic.
- Distal hypospadias without curvature does not cause any functional limitations.
- Proximally, one can impair control of the urine stream.
- An accompanying curvature can hinder sexual intercourse.
- DD: Trauma, ambiguous genitalia.

## Gonorrhoea

- Gonorrhea is a sexually acquired infection caused by *Neisseriagonorrhoeae*. The incubation period is two to five days.
- The most common clinical manifestation is acute anterior urethritis with dysuria and profuse purulent urethral discharge (**Figure 19.48a,b**).
- It starts with scanty, mucopurulent or mucoid discharge. As it progresses, the discharge becomes thick, purulent, and profuse, with intense burning and pain during micturition as well as increased frequency and urgency.
- Occasionally it can present as a disseminated form in immunocompromised patients with fever, acral cutaneous pustules, arthritis, and tenosynovitis.
- Complications include posterior urethritis, inflammation of Cowper's and Tyson's glands, gonococcal pyoderma, epididymitis, acute or chronic prostatitis, vesiculitis, and periurethral abscess.
- DD: Urinary tract infection.

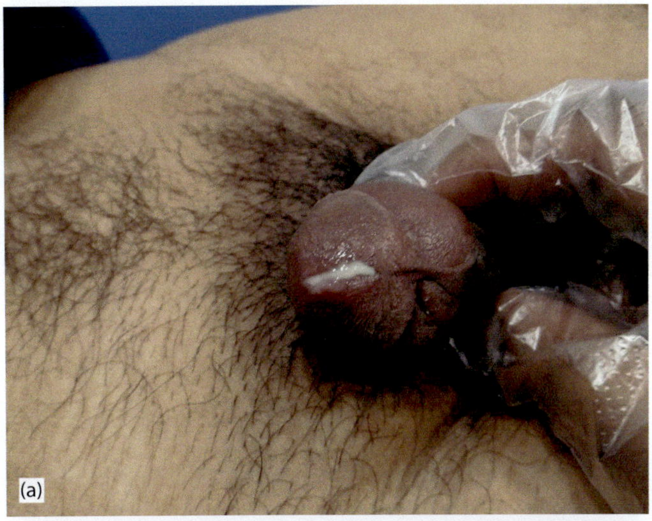

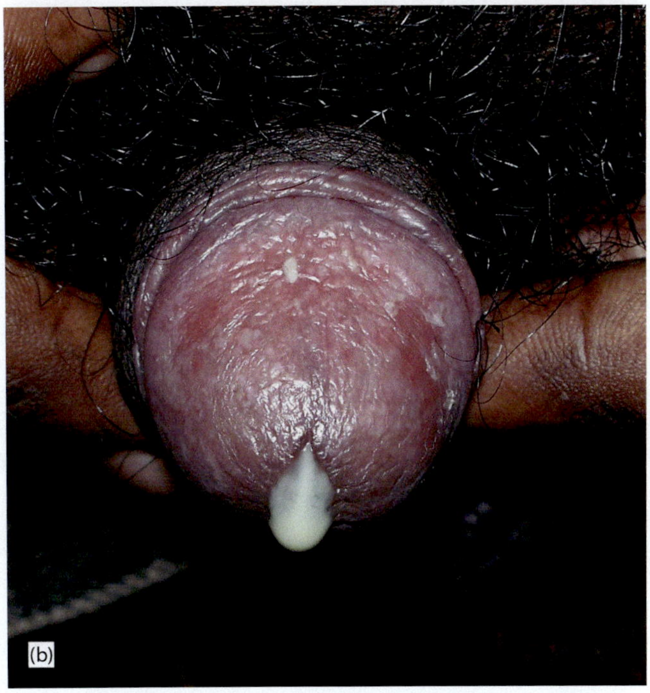

Figure 19.48 **(a)** Gonorrhea presenting with purulent discharge. **(b)** Gonorrhea with copious purulent discharge. (a – Courtesy: Dr. Deverashetti Srinivas, Nizamabad, India.)

## Genital foreign body (corpus alienum)

- Foreign body or corpus alienum is the presence within the body of an object that originates outside the organism.
- Male genital foreign bodies include injections of paraffin, mineral oil, and silicone in the subcutaneous tissue of the penis in order to increase the penile girth.

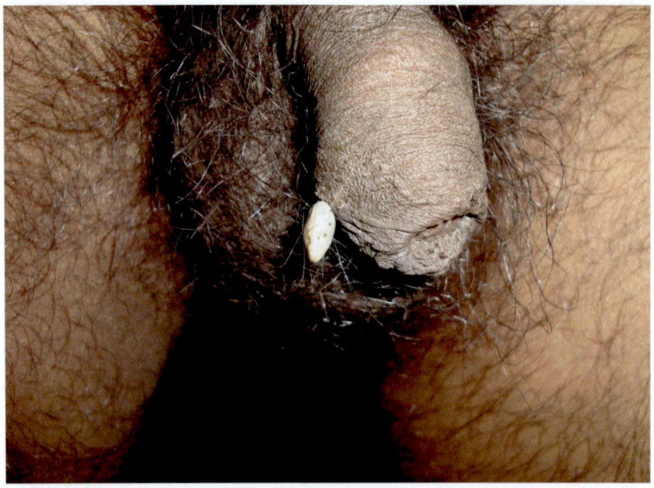

Figure 19.49 Penile foreign body. (Courtesy: Dr. Santoshdev P Rathod, Ahmedabd, India.)

- It presents as irregular, indurated nodules with varying degrees of sclerosis (**Figure 19.49**).
- The prepuce, penile shaft, scrotum, and pubis are the sites most commonly involved; however, oily substances can migrate to subcutaneous tissues, muscles, and lymph nodes.
- Its complications include penile necrosis, infection, phimosis, erectile dysfunction, penile deformity, fistulization, and acute urinary retention.

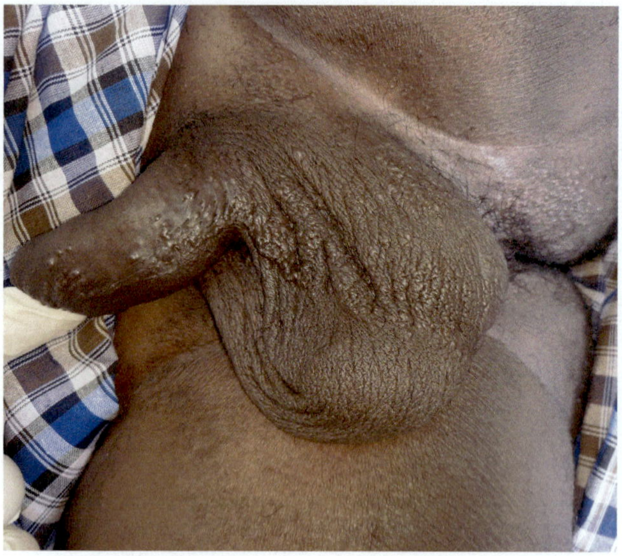

Figure 19.51 Herpes zoster affecting the penis, scrotum, and perineum. (Courtesy: Dr. Santoshdev P Rathod, Ahmedabd, India.)

- DD: Other causes of subcutaneous nodules of the male genitalia, scleroderma, infiltrative lesions in storage disease, malignancies such as squamous cell carcinoma, and infectious disease.

## Additional images – Figures 19.50a,b, 19.51, 19.52, 19.53, and 19.54

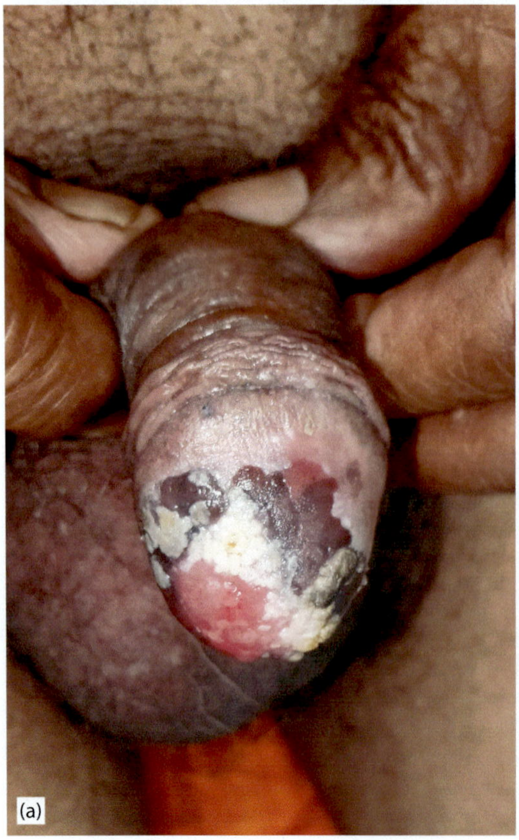

(a)

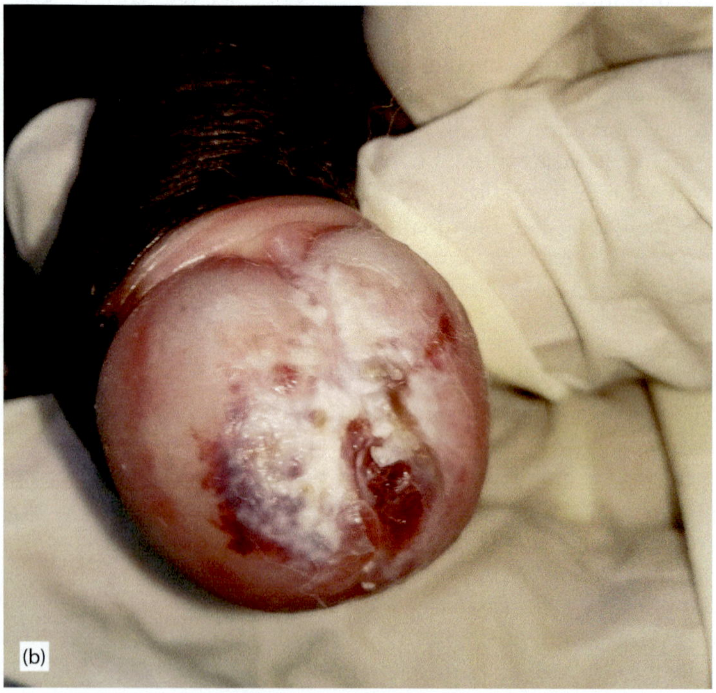

(b)

Figure 19.50 **(a)** Bowen's disease of the glans penis. **(b)** Bowen's disease of the glans penis. (a – Courtesy: Dr. Swetalina Pradhan, AIIMS Patna, India; b – Courtesy: Dr. Santoshdev P Rathod, Ahmedabd, India.)

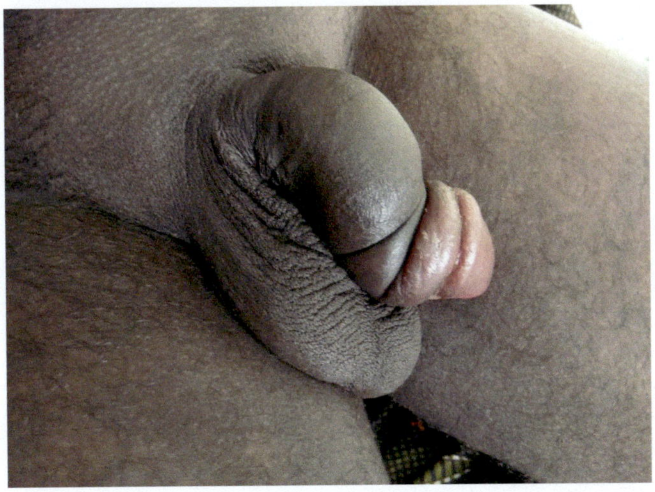

Figure 19.52 Edematous, distorted penis in lymphogranuloma venereum. (Courtesy: Dr. Santoshdev P Rathod, Ahmedabd, India.)

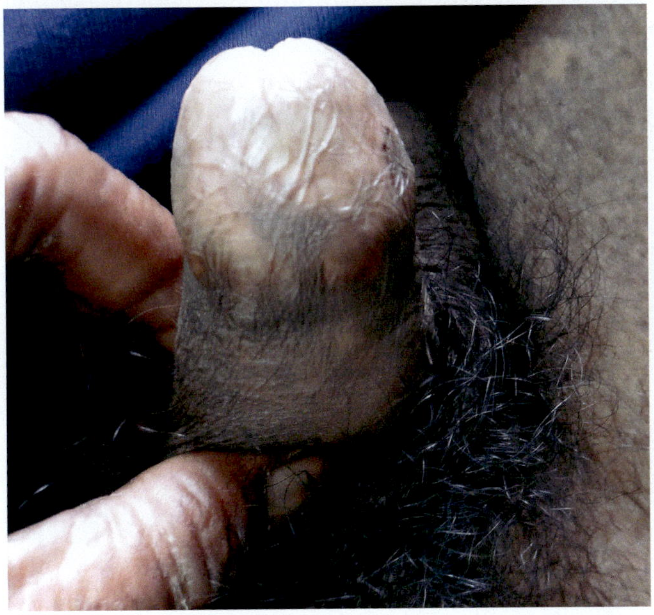

Figure 19.53 Atrophy of the skin of glans penis due to topical corticosteroid abuse. (Courtesy: Dr. Santoshdev P Rathod, Ahmedabd, India.)

## REFERENCES


1. Kumar P, Khare S, Rathod SP, Nimisha E, Khoja M, Kulkarni S, Tiwary AK, Madke B. The Genital, Perianal, and Umbilical Regions. In: Smoller BR, Bagherani N, editors. Atlas of Dermatology, Dermatopathology and Venereology. 1st edition. Switzerland: Springer Nature; 2020. P. 1–80.


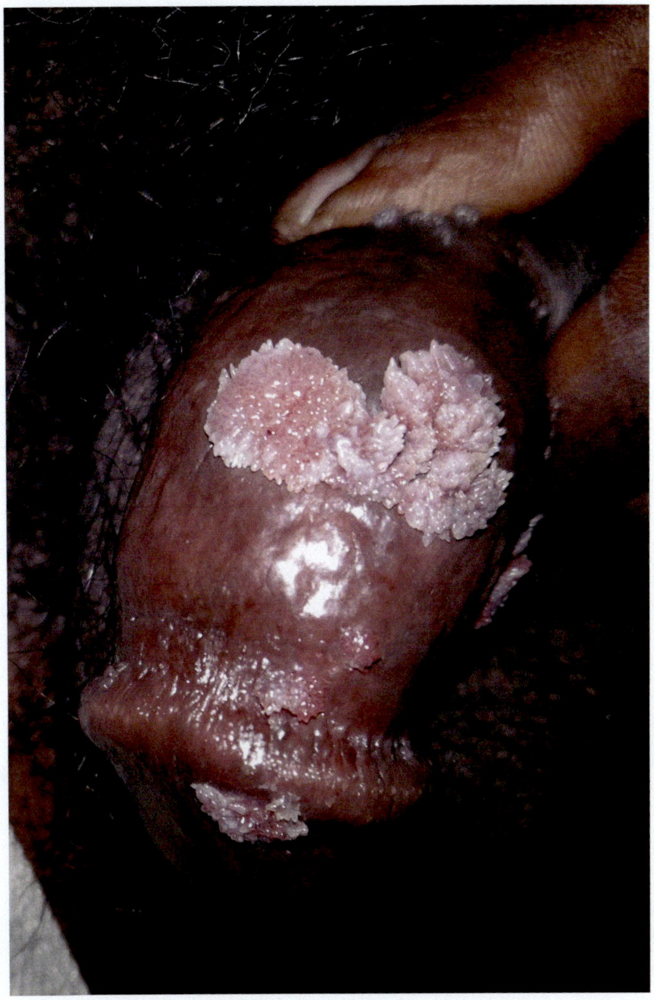

Figure 19.54 Penile warts.


2. Shim TN, Ali I, Muneer A, Bunker CB. Benign male genital dermatoses. BMJ 2016;354:i4337.
3. Yura E, Flury S. Cutaneous lesions of the external genitalia. Med Clin North Am 2018;102(2):279–300.
4. Bunker CB, Porter WM. Dermatoses of the Male Genitalia. In: Griffiths CEM, Barker J, Bleiker T, Chalmers R, Creamer D, editors. Rook,s Textbook of Dermatology. 9th edition. West Sussex: John Wiley & Sons; 2016. P 111.1–111.41.
5. Bunker CB. Diseases and Disorders of the Male Genitalia. In: Goldsmith LA, Katz SI, Gilchrest BA, Paller AS, Leffell DJ, Wolff K, editors. Fitzpatrick's Dermatology in General Medicine. 8th edition. McGraw Hill; 2012; 852–877.

# E28

# Female genitalia

MADHULIKA MHATRE, ASEEM SHARMA

## ABSTRACT

By convention, female genital dermatoses have been classified as venereal and non-venereal. This approach clubs entities with totally different morphological presentations together (e.g., genital herpes, and genital warts) which does not help much in making a clinical diagnosis. This chapter has classified female genital dermatoses based on morphology, according to the theme of the atlas.

The text of this chapter is available online at https://routledgetextbooks.com/textbooks/9781032399669/



DOI: 10.1201/9781351054225-50

# E29

# Nipple areola complex

AMARKANT JHA AMAR, SHIVANI SHARMA

## ABSTRACT

The nipple-areolar complex is best considered a separate anatomical region of the breast and may be affected by many developmental physiological variations and pathological conditions (including various benign or malignant lesions). Many clinical conditions are unique to this anatomical region, and awareness of such conditions helps clinicians in making a diagnosis.

The text of this chapter is available online at https://routledgetextbooks.com/textbooks/9781032399669/

DOI: 10.1201/9781351054225-51

# E30

# Scrotum

DILIP KUMAR SA

## ABSTRACT

This is an overview of various dermatoses that are predominantly seen on the scrotum. Clinical classification has been done according to the types of skin lesions. The salient features of both common and rare conditions of scrotum have been described.

The text of this chapter is available online at https://routledgetextbooks.com/textbooks/9781032399669/



DOI: 10.1201/9781351054225-52

# E31

# Seborrheic area

POOJA NUPUR

## ABSTRACT

Seborrheic areas include the scalp, eyebrows, nasal alae, chin and beard area, center of the chest, axilla, back, and groins. These areas contain numerous sebaceous glands, which secrete sebum and contribute to the skin surface lipids. Any perturbation of the sebaceous lipid barrier makes these areas susceptible to various infections (e.g., pityriasis versicolor) and inflammatory conditions (e.g., seborrheic dermatitis). Some other conditions too show a predilection for seborrheic area. This chapter discusses dermatoses showing predilection for seborrheic areas.

The text of this chapter is available online at https://routledgetextbooks.com/textbooks/9781032399669/

DOI: 10.1201/9781351054225-53

E32

# Intertriginous areas

POOJA NUPUR, SHAHID HASSAN

## ABSTRACT

Intertriginous areas are some of the most commonly affected sites for dermatologic disorders of the face for which the majority of patients consult a physician. A variety of skin diseases may involve these areas as a part of primary cutaneous diseases or secondary to the underlying systemic diseases. At first glance, many of the intertriginous dermatoses may appear similar. However, a thorough history and physical examination may further narrow the differential diagnosis considerably or help us reach a specific diagnosis.

The text of this chapter is available online at https://routledgetextbooks.com/textbooks/9781032399669/



DOI: 10.1201/9781351054225-54

20

# Nails

PIYUSH KUMAR

## INTRODUCTION

The nail unit is a specialized structure situated on the dorsal aspect of the distal-most part of each finger and toe. The nail unit consists of a nail plate, four modified epithelial tissues (proximal nail fold, nail matrix, nail bed, and hyponychium), lateral nail folds, and dermal tissue under the nail bed (**Box 20.1** and **Figures 20.1** and **20.2**). The nail is firmly anchored to the underlying bone of the digit with the help of the nail folds, dermal tissue of the nail bed, and fibrous tissues merging with the periosteum and tendons. The detailed discussion on the anatomy is beyond the scope of this chapter.

Nail involvement in various diseases results in recognizable abnormalities of one or more components of the nail unit in varying combinations. The diagnosis of nail diseases rests on identification of these abnormalities. Nail unit abnormalities (nail unit signs) have been discussed as abnormalities of nail plate (size, thickness, curvature,

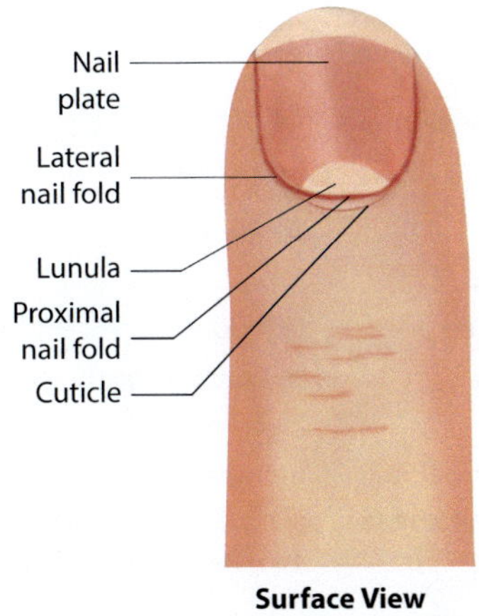


Figure 20.1 Surface view of the nail unit. (Courtesy: Dr. Sunil Kothiwala; Reprinted by permission from Taylor and Francis Group LLC Books Nail Disorders: A Comprehensive Approach by Archana Singal, Shekhar Neema, Piyush Kumar [COPYRIGHT] 2019.)

**BOX 20.1: The nail apparatus**

- **Nail plate** – It is a horny rectangular translucent plate made up of hard keratin plate which appears pink due to vascular structures underneath. The proximal semilunar whitish area is termed as **lunula**. The surface of nail plate is generally convex in both longitudinal and horizontal directions. Histologically, nail plate has three horizontal layers – thin dorsal lamina, thick intermediate layer and thin ventral lamina.
- **Nail folds** – The nail folds (proximal and paired lateral nail folds) are soft tissues that partially cover the nail plate. The proximal nail fold keratinizes to produce cuticle.
- **Cuticle** – It is a thin, translucent fold of skin extending onto proximal nail plate.
- **Hyponychium** – It is an epithelial tissue underlying the free edge of the nail plate and is distally continuous with the volar skin of the digit.
- **Matrix** – It is the germinal part of the nail unit and is mostly covered by the proximal nail fold (except for lunula). It keratinizes to produce the major bulk of the nail plate – the proximal part of the nail matrix gives rise to the ventral nail plate, and the distal nail matrix contributes to the intermediate nail plate (**Figure 20.3**). Understanding this fact is crucial in determining the exact site of nail matrix pathology and nail matrix biopsy.
- **Nail bed** – The nail bed consists of specialized epithelium, two to three cells thick, with underlying connective tissue in close proximity to the periosteum. The connective tissue is devoid of subcutaneous fat but is rich in nerves, blood vessels, and glomus bodies.

DOI: 10.1201/9781351054225-55

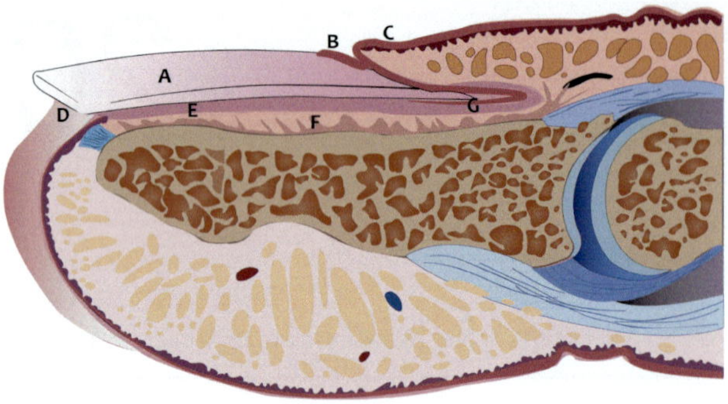


Figure 20.2 The longitudinal section of the nail unit: **(a)** Nail plate, **(b)** Cuticle, **(c)** Proximal nail fold, **(d)** Hyponychium, **(e)** Nail bed, **(f)** Terminal phalanx bone, **(g)** Nail matrix. (Courtesy: Dr. Sunil Kothiwala.)

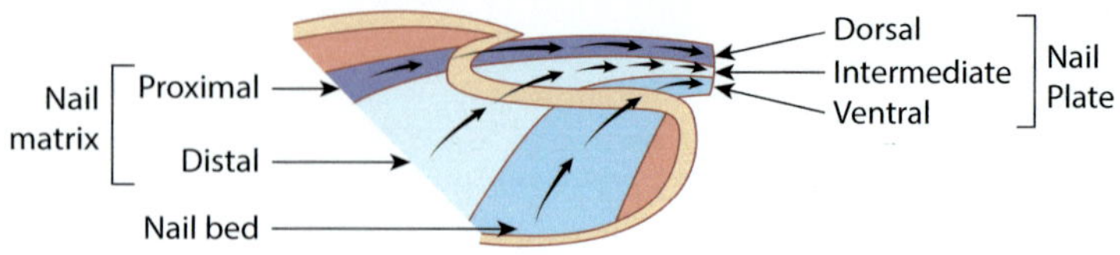


Figure 20.3 Formation of nail plate by nail matrix and nail bed.

surface changes, adhesion, and color), and surrounding soft tissues **Table 20.1**.[1–6]

## Abnormalities of nail plate size

### Anonychia/Micronychia

- Anonychia is complete absence of nails in single or multiple digits (**Figure 20.4**).

Table 20.1 Various nail signs

| Affected part of the nail unit | Features | Nail sign |
|---|---|---|
| Nail plate | Absent | Anonychia |
| Abnormalities of nail-plate size | Small | Micronychia, onychoatrophy |
| | Large | Macronychia |
| | Width > length | Brachyonychia (racquet nail) |
| | Deformed | Onychodystrophy |
| Abnormalities of nail-plate thickness | Increased | • Complete nail involvement – pachyonychia, onychochauxis, onychogryphosis<br>• Partial nail involvement – onychomatricoma (usually single nail) |
| | Decreased | • Complete nail affected – nail-plate thinning, haplalonychia<br>• Partial nail involvement – traumatized nails, worn-down nails |
| Abnormalities of nail-plate curvature | Flat (loss of normal curvature) | Platonychia |
| | Concave/spoon-shaped (reversal of normal curvature) | Koilonychia |
| | Increased transverse and longitudinal curvatures | Clubbing |
| | Increased transverse curvature | Pincer nails, Tile-shaped nails, plicated nails |
| | Increased longitudinal curvature | Parrot beak nails |
| Abnormalities of nail-plate surface | Longitudinal indentation | • Single/few – Longitudinal groove, median canaliform dystrophy of Heller<br>• Numerous (affecting entire nail plate) – onychorhhexis |
| | Longitudinal elevation | • Single/few – Longitudinal ridge (complete length of nail plate affected) and beads (partial nail plate affection)<br>• Numerous – trachyonychia |
| | Transverse indentation | • Single or few – Beau's line<br>• Numerous – habit tic deformity |
| | Focal defect/indentation | Pits |
| Nail plate fragility | Increased | Brittle nails |
| Abnormalities of nail-plate adhesions | Distal separation of different layers of nail plate | Onychoschizia |
| | Distal separation of nail plate from nail bed | Onycholysis |
| | Proximal separation of nail plate from nail bed | Onychomadesis |
| | Abnormal adhesions | Dorsal and ventral pterygium |

*(Continued)*

Table 20.1 Various nail signs (*Continued*)

| Affected part of the nail unit | Features | Nail sign |
|---|---|---|
| Abnormalities of nail-plate color | Nail plate loses translucency and appears colored | Chromonychia |
| | White | Leukonychia (true, apparent, and pseudo) |
| | Red | Erythronychia |
| | Brown-black | Melanonychia |
| | Others | Yellow nails, green nails |
| Alterations in lunula | | • Red lunula<br>• Macro Lunula<br>• Triangular lunula |
| Nail folds changes | Inflamed | Paronychia, onychocryptosis |
| | Pigmentation | • Hutchinson's sign<br>• Pseudo-Hutchinson's sign |
| Subungual changes | Collection of keratin material | Subungual hyperkeratosis |
| | Collection of blood | • Large – subungual hematoma<br>• Tiny, linear – splinter hemorrhage |

- It could be congenital or acquired; congenital forms may be a syndromic (e.g., ectodermal dysplasia) or isolated disorder.
- Acquired forms may be permanent or transient. Transient anonychia can occur in various inflammatory processes.
- Micronychia (**Figure 20.5**) is too-small nail plates.
- Some important acquired causes of anonychia/micronychia include burn, trauma/surgery, lichen planus, Stevens-Johnson syndrome, and epidermolysis bullosa (junctional and dystrophic types).

## Onychoatrophy

- Onychoatrophy is faulty underdevelopment of the nail in which there is reduction in size and thickness of the nail unit (**Figure 20.6**).

## Macronychia

- The nail plate is too large (**Figure 20.7**).
- Macronychia occurs from an underlying bone abnormality.

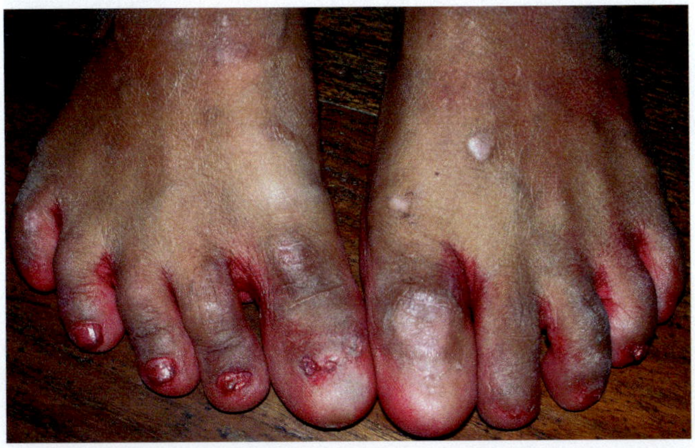

Figure 20.4 Anonychia of great toenails in epidermolysis bullosa.

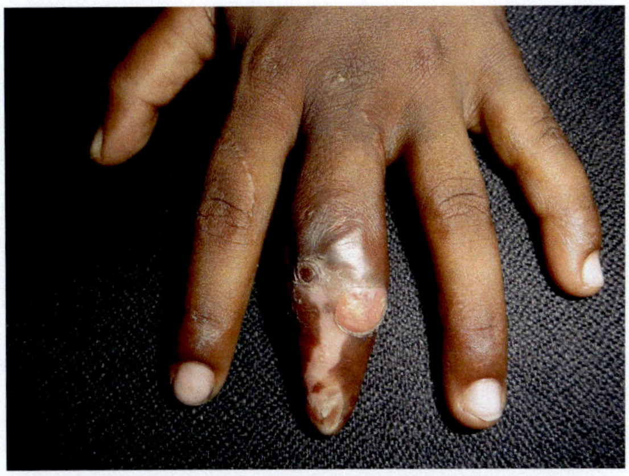

Figure 20.5 Micronychia of middle finger in leprosy.

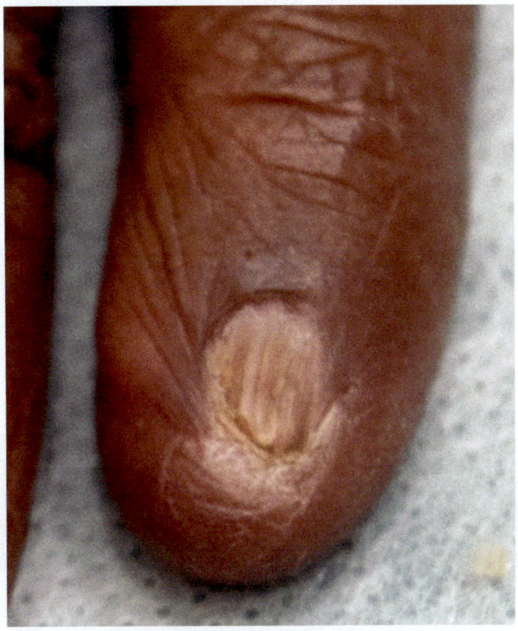

Figure 20.6 Onychoatrophy in a case of lichen planus.

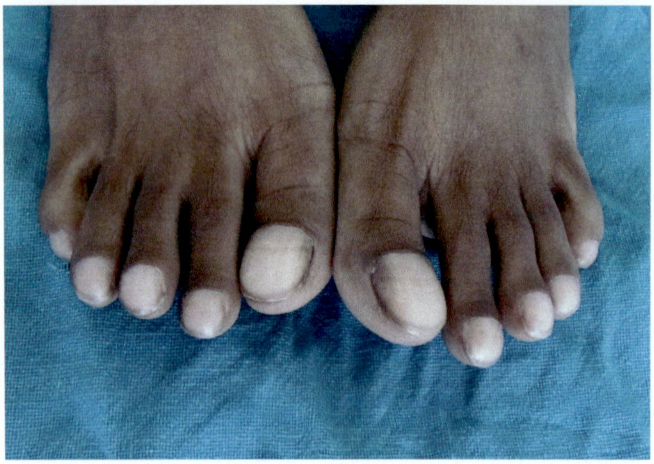

Figure 20.7 Macronychia.

### Brachyonychia/racquet nail

- Racquet nails refers to short nails in which the width of the nail plate and nail bed is greater than the length. It occurs due to shortening of the bone of the terminal phalanx.
- Usually thumbs are affected (**Figure 20.8**).

### Onychodystrophy/dystrophic nail

- Onychodystrophy refers to nails that become misshapen or thickened or that exhibit a partially destroyed nail plate (**Figure 20.9a,b**).

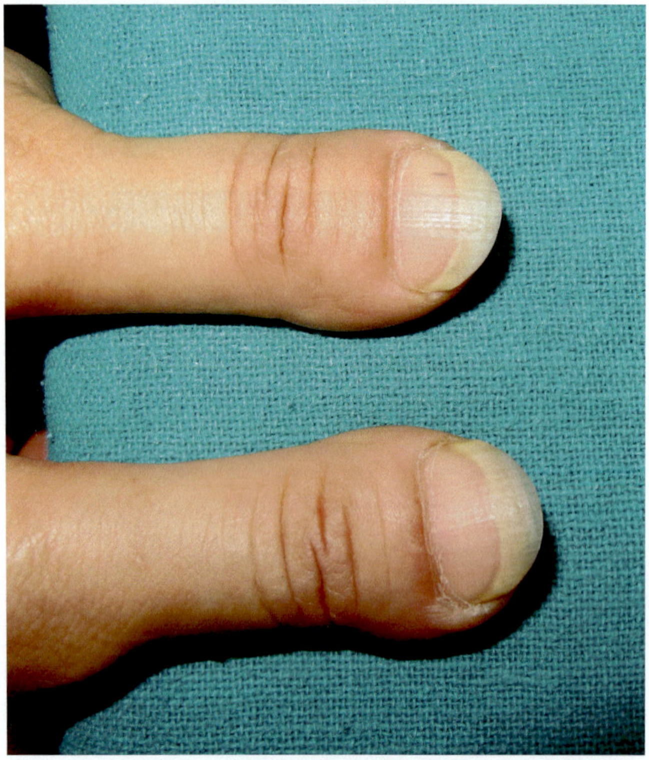

Figure 20.8 Racquet nail – short nail plate with length less than the width.

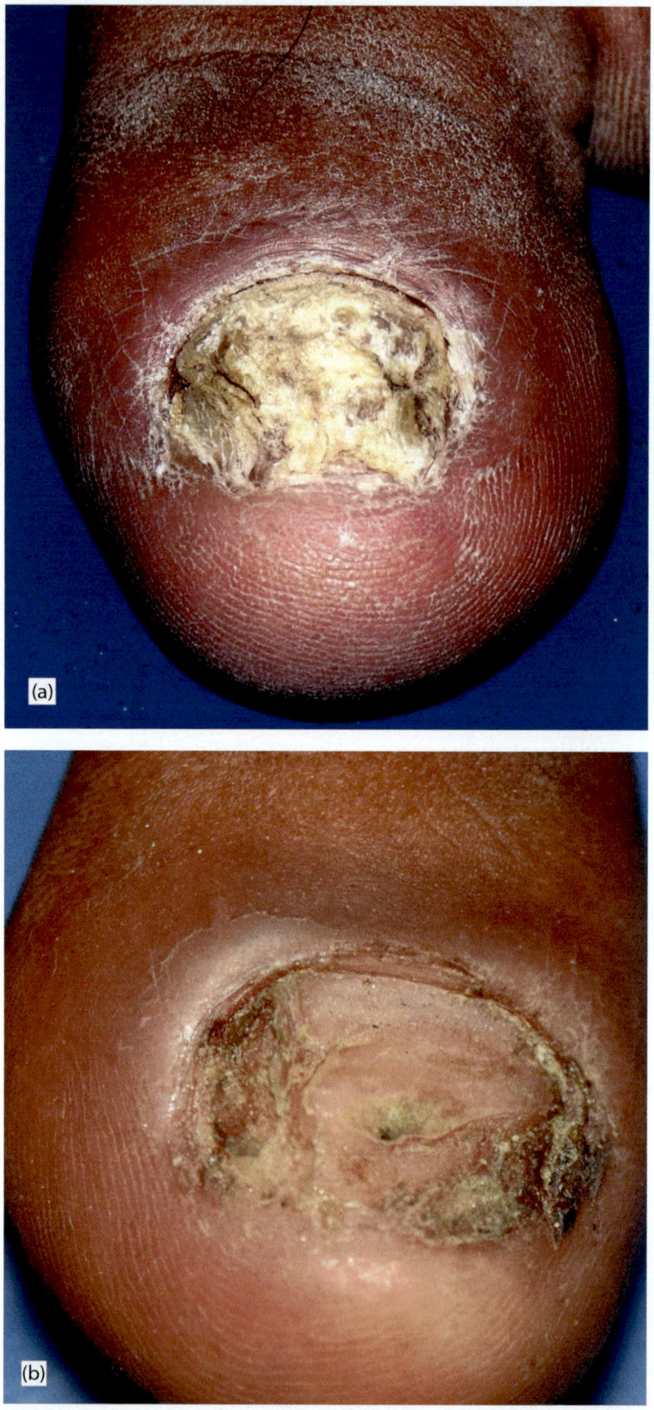

Figure 20.9 **(a,b)** Onychodystrophy of toenail.

## Abnormalities of nail plate thickness

### Nail-plate thickening

- Normal nail plate gains thickness as it grows distally. The vascular supply, subungual hyperkeratosis, and drugs may influence nail thickening.
- Nail-plate thickening may be congenital or acquired. Acquired thickening may occur as a result of reduced nail growth or inflammatory disorders of the nail

bed. Subungual hyperkeratosis due to onychomycosis, pachyonychia congenita, pityriasis rubra pilaris, or psoriasis also results in nail-plate thickening.

- Nail thickening is also commonly seen in elderly and in patients with foot deformities due to chronic trauma and friction.
- Thickened nail plates may assume different morphologies.
    - Pachyonychia – It refers to a thickened nail with an increased transverse curvature (**Figure 20.10a**).
    - Onychochauxis – It is characterized by a thickened nail with yellowish discoloration without any change in the curvature of the nail plate (**Figure 20.10b**).
    - Onychogryphosis – It is characterized by nail-plate thickening with gross hyperkeratosis and increased curvature of the nail plate (**Figure 20.10c,d**). It most commonly affects the great toes of elderly patients with poor foot care and podiatric abnormalities.

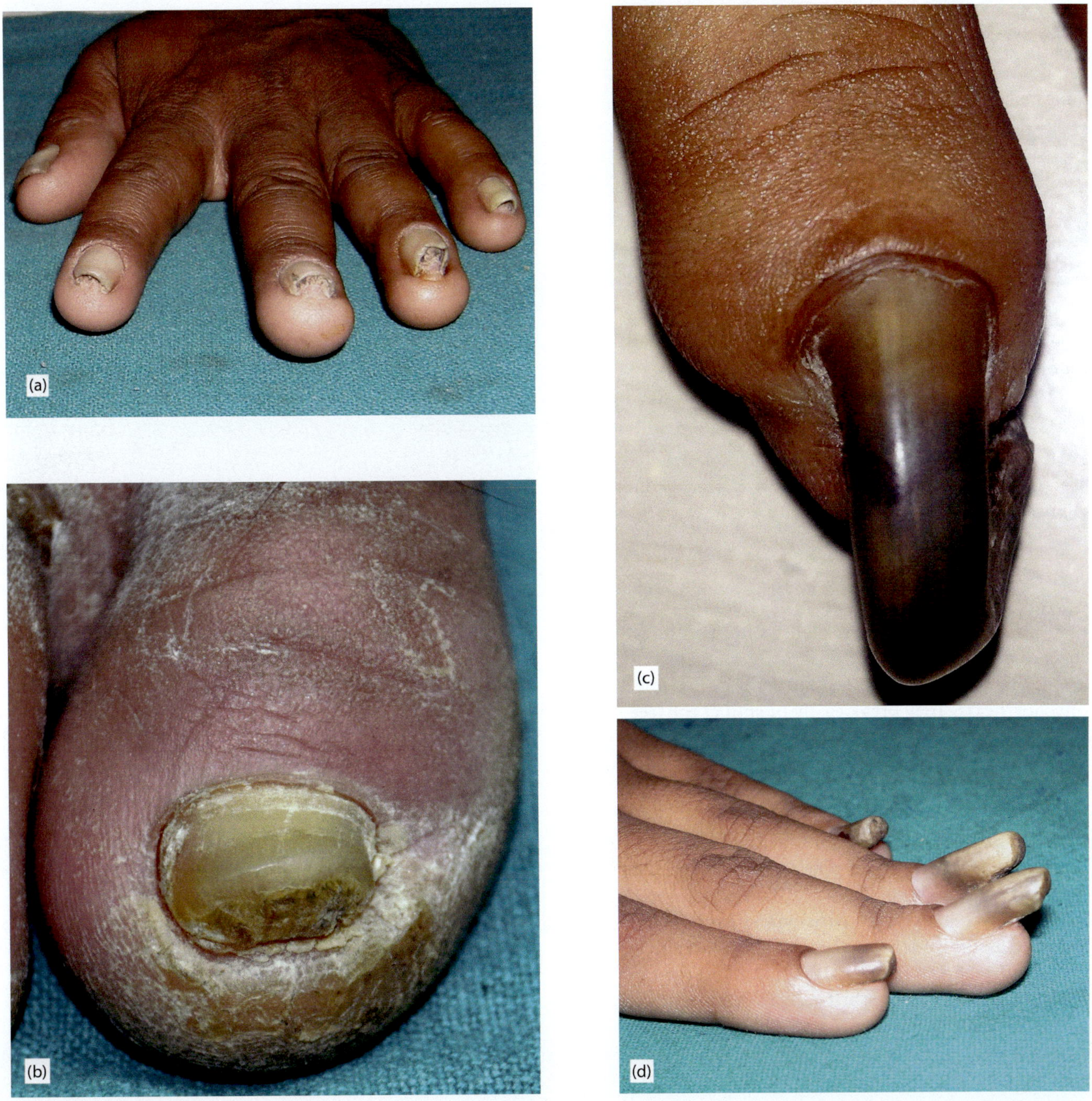


Figure 20.10 **(a)** Pachyonychia. **(b)** Onychochauxis. **(c)** Oyster-like onychogryphosis. **(d)** Ram's horn dystrophy (onychogryphosis). (*Continued*)

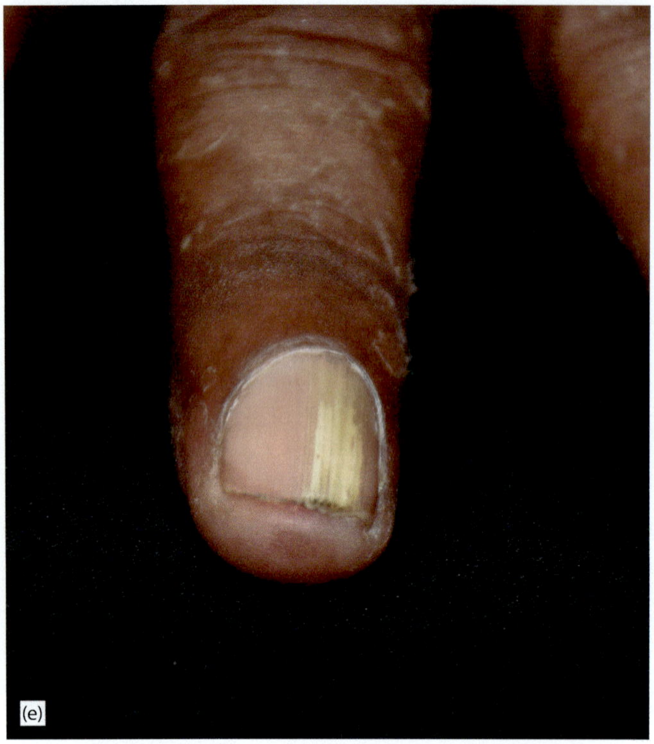

Figure 20.10 (*Continued*) **(e)** Longitudinal yellow discoloration and thickening of the nail plate in onychomatricoma.

- Partial nail-plate thickening of a single digit may be seen in nail matrix tumors such as onychomatricoma (**Figure 20.10e**).

## Nail-plate thinning

- Nail-plate thinning is defined as thickness of the nail plate less than 0.5 mm. Nail-plate thinning results from diseases affecting the proximal nail matrix and is often associated with fissuring, ridging, and onychorrhexis. They break easily or split at the free edge of the nail plate.
- They are seen in amyloidosis, hemiplegia, occupational contact with chemicals, trachyonychia, and lichen planus (**Figure 20.11a**).
- In lichen planus, uniform thinning is due to atrophy of proximal nail matrix and is referred to as "angel wing" deformity.
- In hapalonychia (egg shell nails), nail plates become thin and assume a semitransparent, bluish-white hue (**Figure 20.11b**). Such nails may be observed in malnutrition, chronic arthritis, leprosy, myxoedema, acroasphyxia, peripheral neuritis, hemiplegia, and cachexia etc.
- Focal nail plate thinning may be seen in traumatized nails, onychoschizia, and worn-down nails (**Figure 20.11c**).

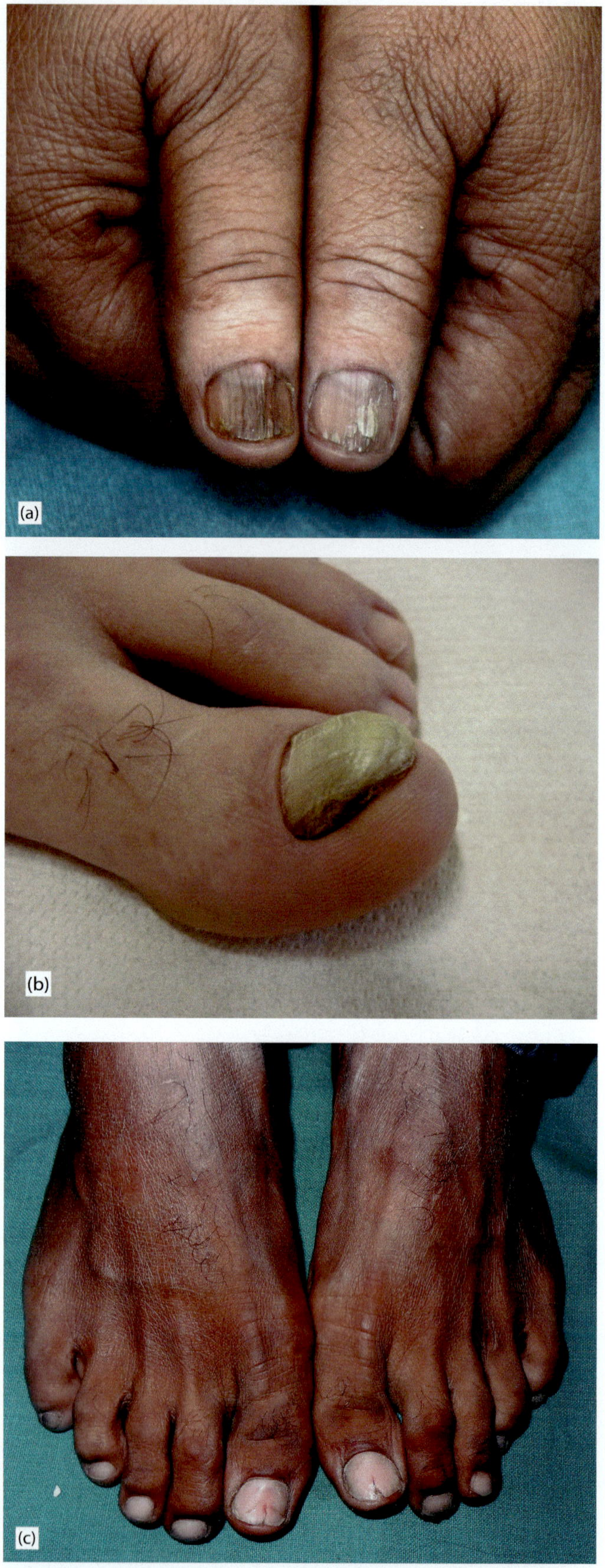

Figure 20.11 **(a)** Nail plate thinning in lichen planus. **(b)** Egg shell nail. **(c)** Distal triangular thinning in worn-down nails.

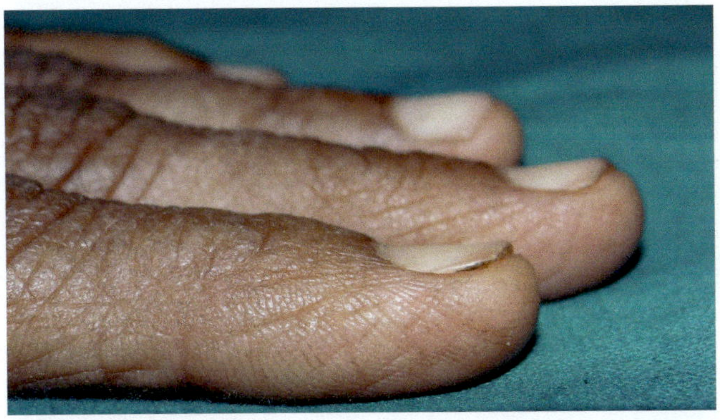

Figure 20.12 Flat nail plates.

## Abnormalities of nail plate curvature

### Platonychia

- The transverse curvature of the nail plate is lost, resulting in an abnormally flat nail (**Figure 20.12**). It may be an early feature of koilonychia.

### Koilonychia (spoon nails) (derived from Greek word *koilos* meaning hollow)

- It is a common nail dystrophy in which the dorsal surface of nail plate becomes flat or truly concave. It is believed that anoxia and atrophy of the distal matrix are responsible for development of koilonychias.
- Koilonychia is the converse of clubbing. It is more visible when viewed from the side. When a drop of water is put on the surface, it will not roll off. It should be noted that nails in koilonychia are brittle. It is commonly seen in fingernails rather than toenails.
- Physiological koilonychias is seen in healthy infants and children who have thin and soft nails and improves spontaneously in due course.
- Two types of koilonychia are described – familial form and acquired form.
- Iron deficiency is the most common cause of acquired koilonychias. It may develop before clinical or laboratory signs of anemia manifest (**Figure 20.13**).

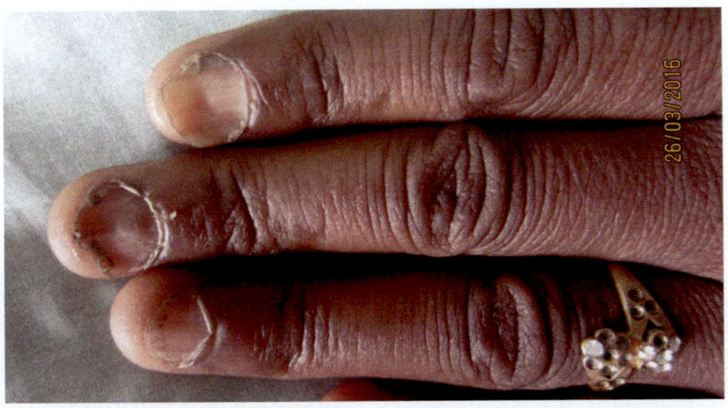


Figure 20.13 Koilonychia in iron deficiency anemia.

Table 20.2 Koilonychia

| Koilonychia | Causes |
|---|---|
| Physiological | • Healthy infants<br>• Old age |
| Familial | • Syndromic – LEOPARD syndrome, nail–patella syndrome<br>• Isolated |
| Acquired koilonychias | • Dermatological diseases – lichen planus, psoriasis, lichen striatus, keratoderma, Darier disease, Raynaud's disease<br>• Systemic diseases – iron deficiency anemia, hemochromatosis, polycythemia vera, malnutrition, systemic lupus erythematosus, pellagra, thyroid diseases |
| Occupational koilonychias | • Toenails – rickshaw pullers, farmers<br>• Fingernails – dentists, construction workers, butchers, and automotive workers |
| Others | • Trauma |

- Various causes of koilonychias have been summarized in **Table 20.2**.

### Clubbing (Hippocrates fingers, acropachy)

- Clubbing refers to increased transverse and longitudinal curvatures of the nail plate along with hypertrophy of the soft tissue of nail pulp (**Figure 20.14a**).
- It can be hereditary (autosomal dominant with variable penetrance) or acquired and may be unilateral or bilateral (**Figure 20.14b**, **Table 20.3**).
- Clinical changes are present in nails and fingertips. Nails bulge along both the longitudinal as well as transverse axes. Changes are prominent in the three radial digits. Tissues around the terminal phalanx become hypertrophied and appear as "drum sticks" (**Figure 20.14c**). It is insidious in onset. Sometimes abrupt clubbing can be seen in lung carcinoma.
- Three geometric assessments exist, namely Lovibond's angle, Curth's angle, and Schamroth's window (**Figure 20.14d**).
    - Lovibond's angle is found at the junction between the nail plate and proximal nail fold. Normally it is less than 160°. It is altered to more than 180° in clubbing.
    - The angle at the distal interphalangeal joint is called Curth's angle and is normally 180°. It is reduced to 160° in clubbing.
    - Schamroth's window is formed when the dorsal aspects of fingers on opposite hands are apposed. In clubbing, this window is closed (**Figure 20.14e**).

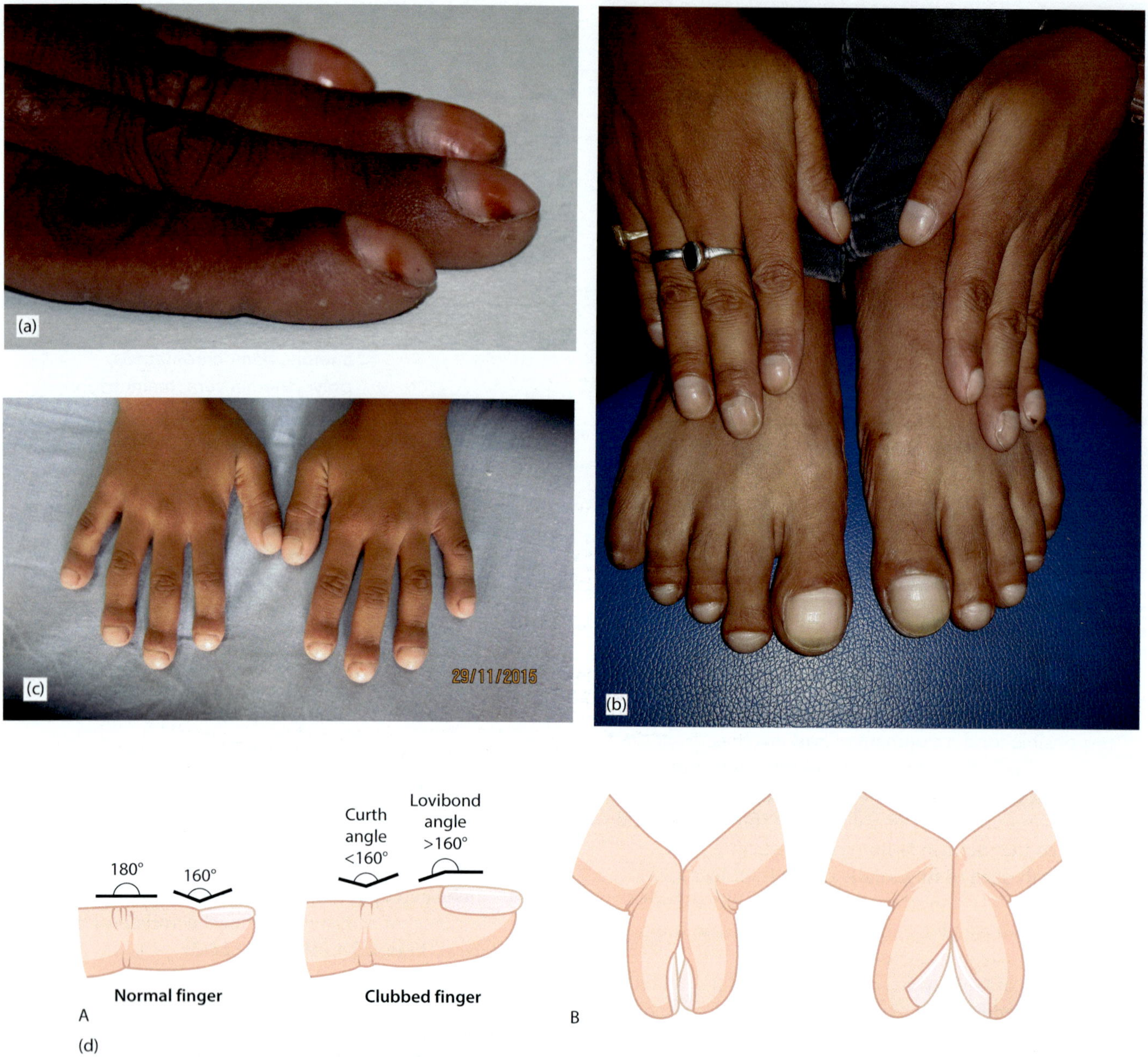


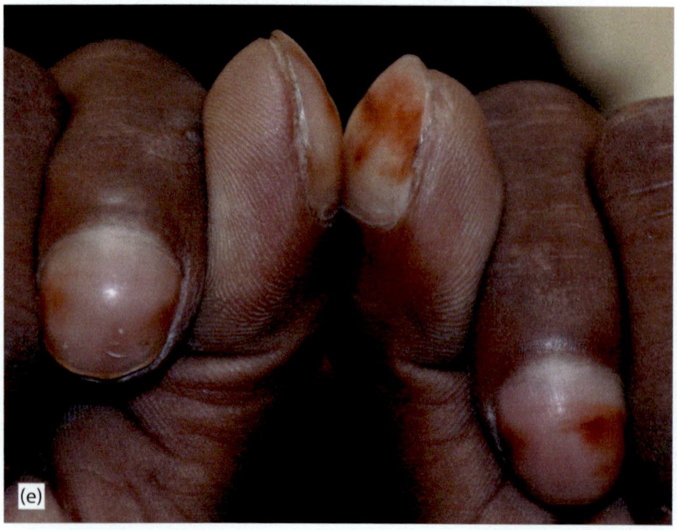


- Clubbing should be differentiated from pseudoclubbing, in which Lovibond's angle is preserved. Pseudoclubbing may be seen in nail bed tumors or in diseases of distal phalangeal bone.

## Transverse overcurvature of the nail

- Nail curvature may exceed the normal limits, resulting in nail-plate abnormalities. These deformities may be associated with ingrowing nails, but inflammatory edema is absent. Three types have been recognized.

Figure 20.14 **(a)** Clubbing of finger nails. **(b)** Familial clubbing. **(c)** "Drum sticks" appearance in clubbing. **(d)** Geometric assessments for clubbing. **(e)** Closed Schamroth's window in clubbing. (b – Courtesy: Dr. PC Das, Katihar, India.)

Table 20.3 Clubbing

| Unilateral clubbing | Bilateral clubbing |
|---|---|
| • Idiopathic<br>• Arterial aneurysms and fistula<br>• Hemiplegia<br>• Pancoast tumor<br>• Local injury | • Pulmonary disease – lung cancer, cystic fibrosis, empyema, pleural mesothelioma, lung hydatid cysts, pulmonary metastases<br>• Cardiac disease – Cyanotic congenital heart disease, other causes of right-to-left shunting, and bacterial endocarditis<br>• Gastrointestinal disease – ulcerative colitis, Crohn's disease, primary biliary cirrhosis, cirrhosis of the liver, hepatopulmonary syndrome<br>• Dermatological disease – pachydermoperiostosis<br>• Malignancies – thyroid cancer; Hodgkin disease; chronic myeloid leukemia; polyneuropathy, organomegaly, endocrinopathy, monoclonal gammopathy, and skin changes (POEMS) syndrome<br>• Endocrinological diseases – acromegaly, thyroid acropachy, secondary hyperparathyroidism<br>• Other conditions – pregnancy, sickle cell disease, alcoholism, HIV infection<br>• Drugs – hypervitaminosis A, heroin abuse, laxative abuse, heavy metal poisoning, angiotensin II receptor blocker |

- Pincer nail (trumpet, arched, or omega nail): This is characterized by transverse overcurvature, the degree of which increases distally (**Figure 20.15a,b**), resulting in pinching of the underlying nail bed and pain, even at rest. This condition may be inherited or acquired after prolonged use of ill-fitting shoes or high-heeled shoes. Acquired pincer nails usually affect great toes. However, if fingernails are affected, inflammatory osteoarthritis or subungual exostosis should be looked for.
- Tile-shaped nail: There is an increase in the transverse curvature, but, unlike with pincer nails, lateral margins remain parallel (**Figure 20.15c**). This is an acquired form and associated with degenerative osteoarthritis affecting nails of fingers and toes.
- Plicated nail: The surface is flat, but the lateral margins are sharply angled, forming vertical sides that are parallel (**Figure 20.15d**). This is due to injury to the distal phalanx and nail unit by psoriasis and total destructive onychomycosis.

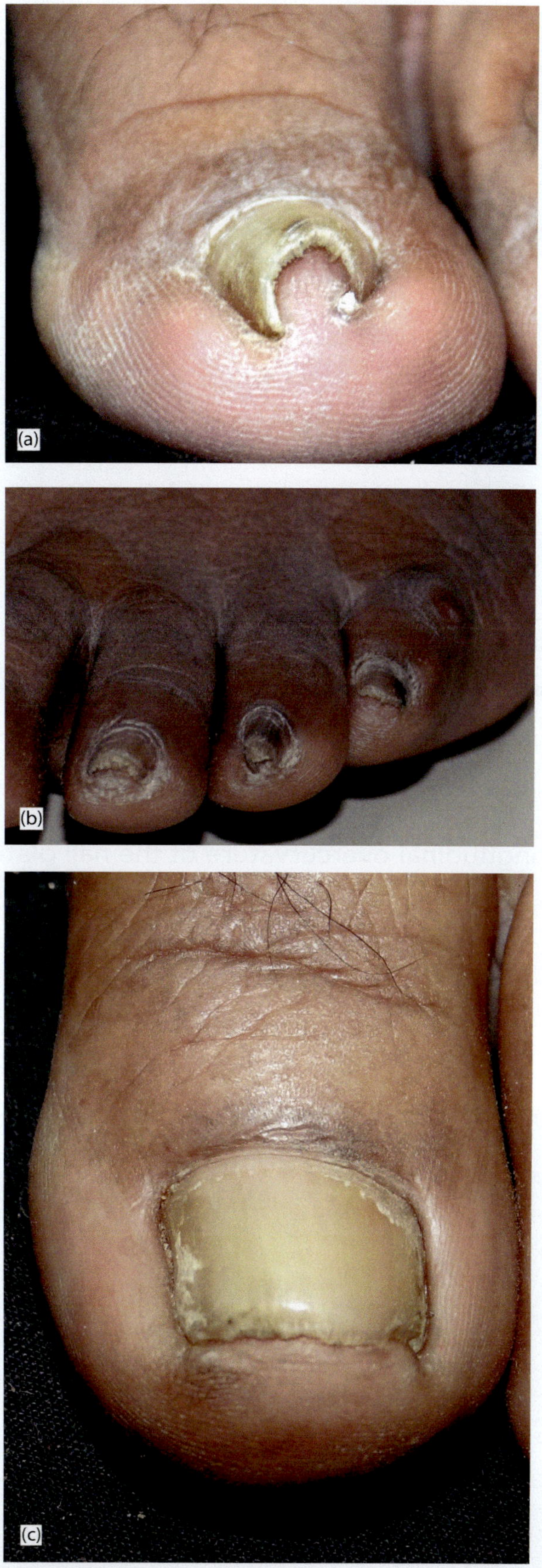


Figure 20.15 **(a,b)** Pincer nail. **(c)** Tile-shaped nails showing increased transverse curvature. Note the parallel lateral margins. (*Continued*)

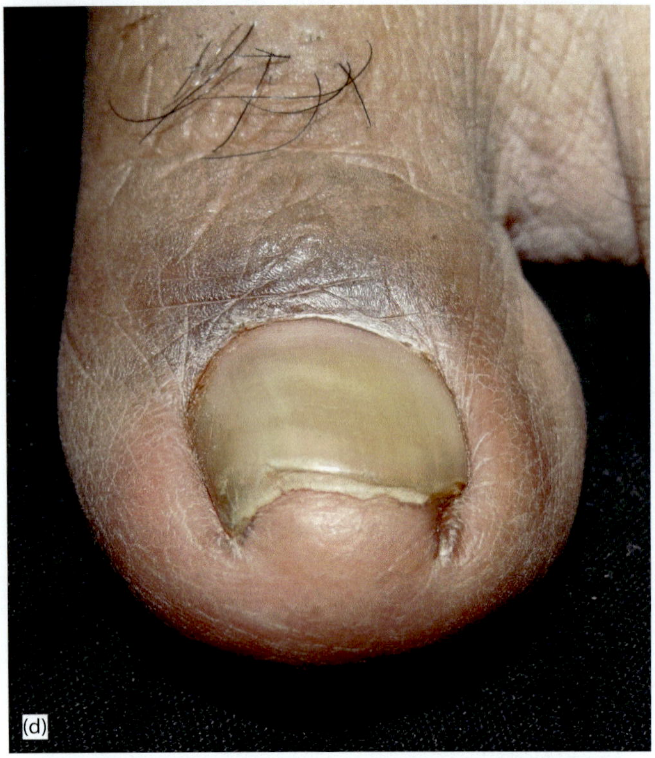

Figure 20.15 (*Continued*) **(d)** Plicated nail surface due to over curvature of nail plate. Vertical growth of lateral margins is evident. (c,d – Courtesy: Dr. Balachandra S. Ankad.)

## Longitudinal overcurvature of the nail plate

### Nail beaking (Parrot beak nails)

- It is a condition where the distal nail plate bends around the tip of the digit; it is usually seen in fingernails (**Figure 20.16**).
- It is usually seen in systemic sclerosis and leprosy, where there is shortening of the terminal phalanges.

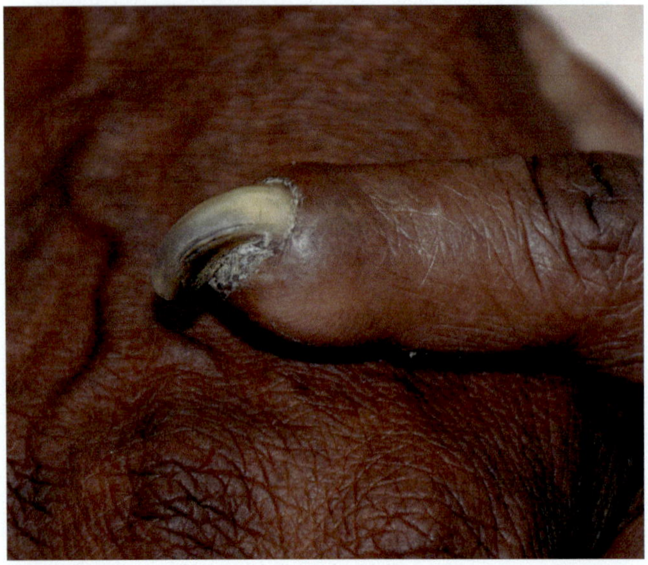

Figure 20.16 Nail beaking in a case of leprosy, with shortening of the digit.

## Abnormalities of nail-plate surface

### Longitudinal grooves

- Longitudinal grooves (LG) are canal-like longitudinal defects on the nail surface (**Figure 20.17a**). The depth of the groove may be complete or partial. It should be differentiated from ridges, which are linear elevations on the surface.
- Longitudinal grooves occur due to long-standing nail abnormalities, causing defects in the nail matrix growth. LG can be solitary or multiple, with different clinical implications.
    - Single (or a few) longitudinal groove affecting one or multiple nails – This occurs due to the pressure effect of space occupying lesions (SOL) like wart, myxoid cyst, or periungual fibromas (Koenen tumor) on the nail matrix. The groove is deep and wide. SOL can be visualized at the proximal portion of longitudinal

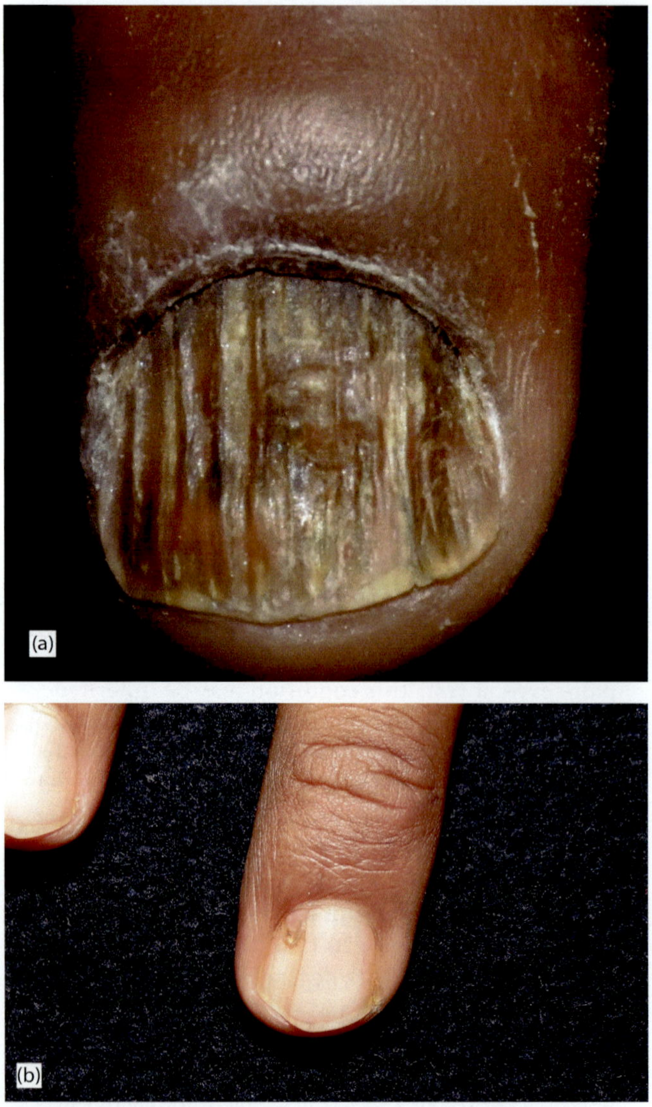

Figure 20.17 **(a)** Longitudinal grooves on the nail plate. **(b)** Solitary longitudinal groove with an angiofibroma visible at its proximal end. (*Continued*)

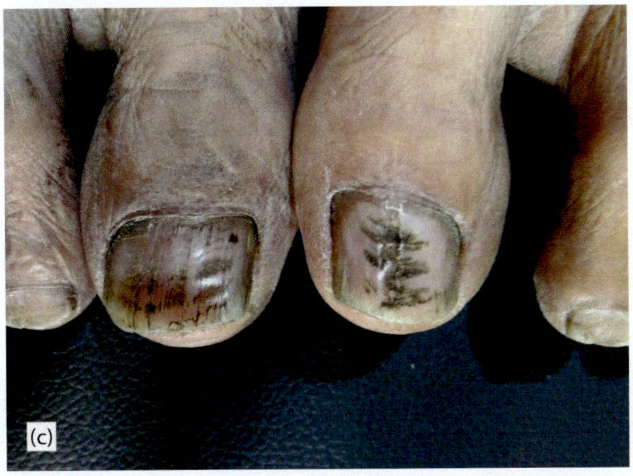

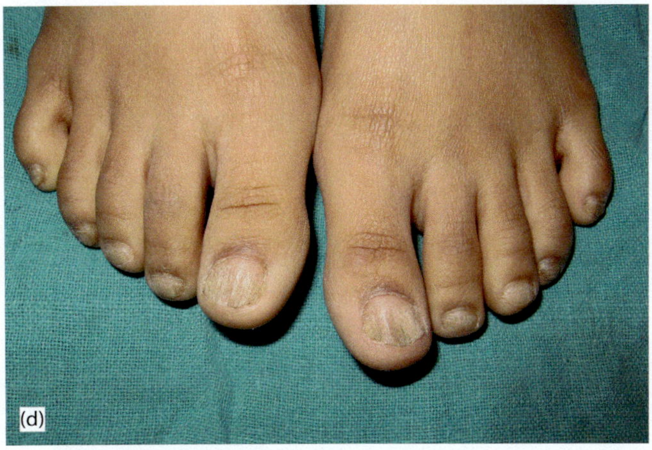

Figure 20.17 (*Continued*) **(c)** Median canaliform deformity of Heller. **(d)** Onychorrhexis.

canal (**Figure 20.17b**). It may also result from repeated cuticle manipulation as in habit tic deformity.
  - Multiple longitudinal grooves – Multiple LG may be observed in various physiological (young children, old age) and pathological conditions (lichen planus, Darier disease, rheumatoid arthritis).
- Some specific examples of longitudinal grooves include the following:
  - Median canaliform dystrophy of Heller (MCDH) is most distinctive form of LG. This uncommon condition consists of central or paracentral, longitudinal groove or split that starts at the cuticle or mid-way along nail plate and extends up to free edge of nail plate (**Figure 20.17c**). This longitudinal groove is associated with multiple small transverse fissures or grooves extending from the groove towards the periphery (but do reaching the edge of nail plate) – a "fir-tree" appearance. Usually thumbs and toes are affected symmetrically, but other digits too may be affected. The exact etiology of this condition is not known; it may be idiopathic or may develop after repeated self-inflicted trauma (impulse control disorder).
  - Onychorrhexis is another LG in which a series of shallow and narrow furrows are present, running parallel to each other and involving the entire surface of the nail (**Figure 20.17d**). The common conditions causing onychorrhexis are included in **Table 20.4**.

Table 20.4 Onychorrhexis

| Etiology | Diseases |
|---|---|
| Medical causes | Hypothyroidism, bulimia, anemia, anorexia nervosa |
| Dermatological | Psoriasis |
| Trauma | Repeated injuries like keyboard players |
| Chemical trauma | Excessive exposure to soaps and detergents, Nail polish removers |
| Miscellaneous | Exposure to cold, genetic, old age |

## Longitudinal ridges and beads

- Longitudinal ridges (continuous elevations running from the cuticle to the free edge of nail plates) and beads (elevations running for a short distance on the nail plate surface) are minor changes and may not indicate any disease (**Figure 20.18a,b**). However, they may become prominent with age. Some known associations include leprosy and other neuropathies, rheumatoid arthritis,

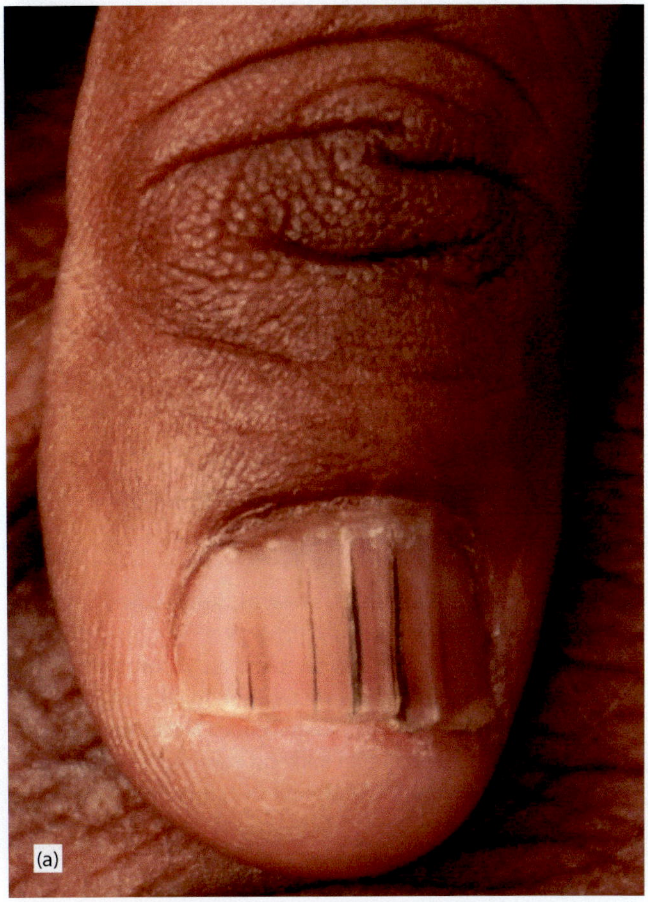

Figure 20.18 **(a)** Longitudinal ridges. (*Continued*)

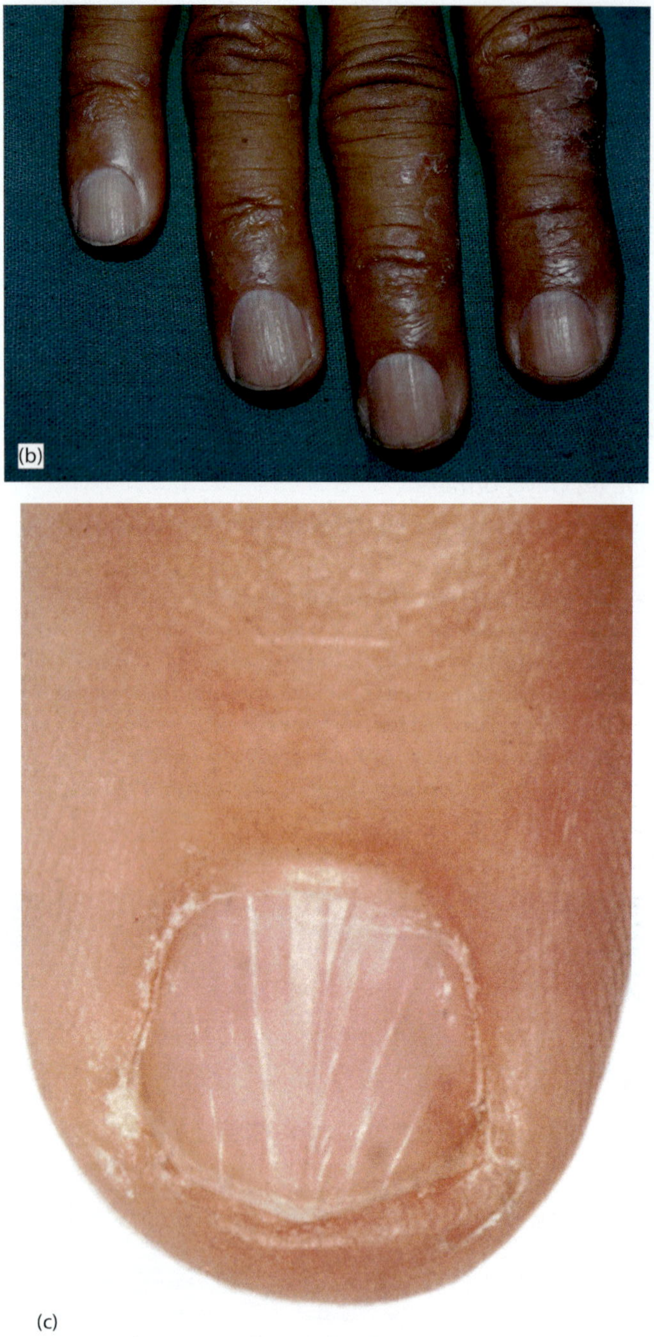


Figure 20.18 (*Continued*) **(b)** Longitudinal beads. **(c)** Chevron nail.

collagen vascular diseases, systemic amyloidosis, and nutritional deficiency.

- Chevron nail/herringbone nail is an uncommon example of patterned longitudinal ridges seen in children; they resolve in adulthood. The ridges arise from the proximal nail fold and converge in a V-shaped pattern towards the midpoint distally (**Figure 20.18c**).

## Trachyonychia (rough nails, twenty-nail dystrophy, from the Greek word *trakos* for rough)[7]

- Trachyonychia refers to gray, rough nail plates that lose luster and appear as "sandpapered nails" or "sand-blasted nails." The term "twenty-nail dystrophy" is misleading, as any number of nails may be affected and hence, trachyonychia is the preferred term (**Figure 20.19a**).
- Two clinical types are recognized. Both types may have associated koilonychia, onychoschizia, and hyperkeratosis of the cuticles.
  - Opaque trachyonychia – It is a severe type and is characterized by rough, thin, brittle nails with excessive longitudinal ridging (**Figure 20.19b**).

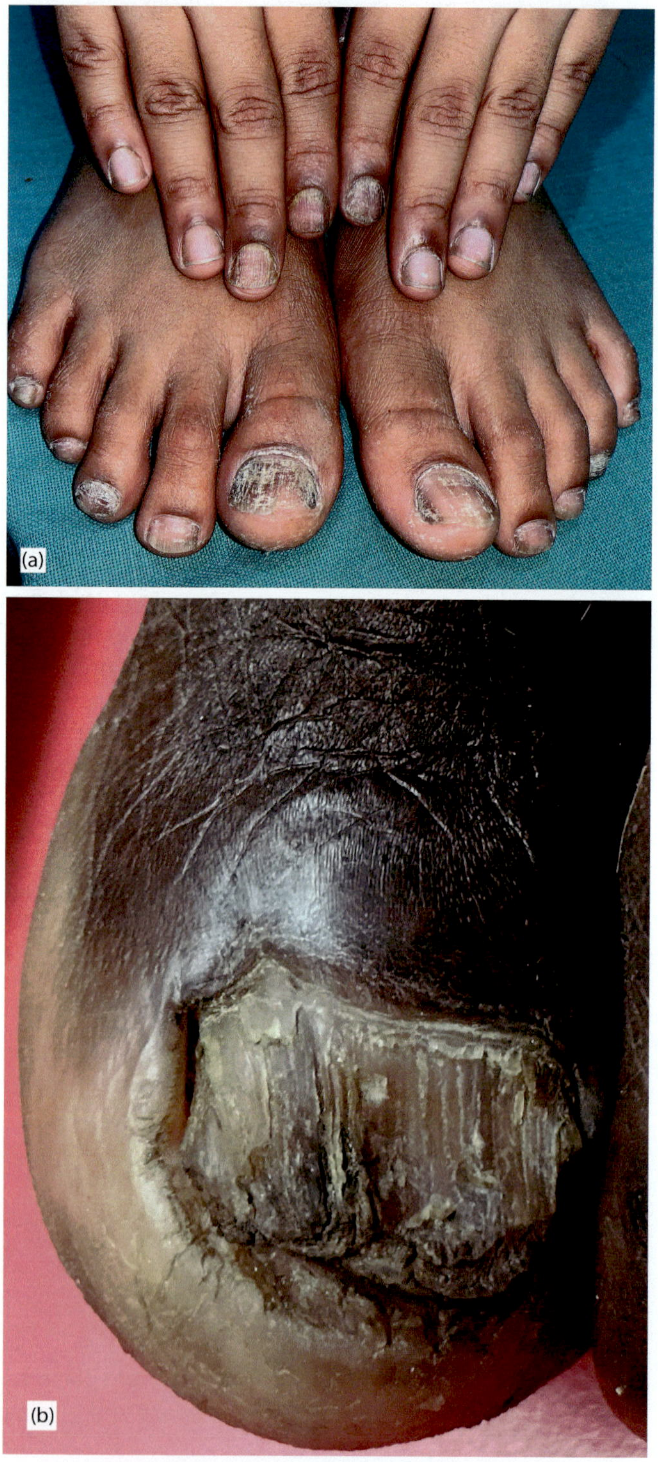


Figure 20.19 **(a)** Multiple, but not all, digits affection in trachyonychia. **(b)** Opaque trachyonychia. (*Continued*)

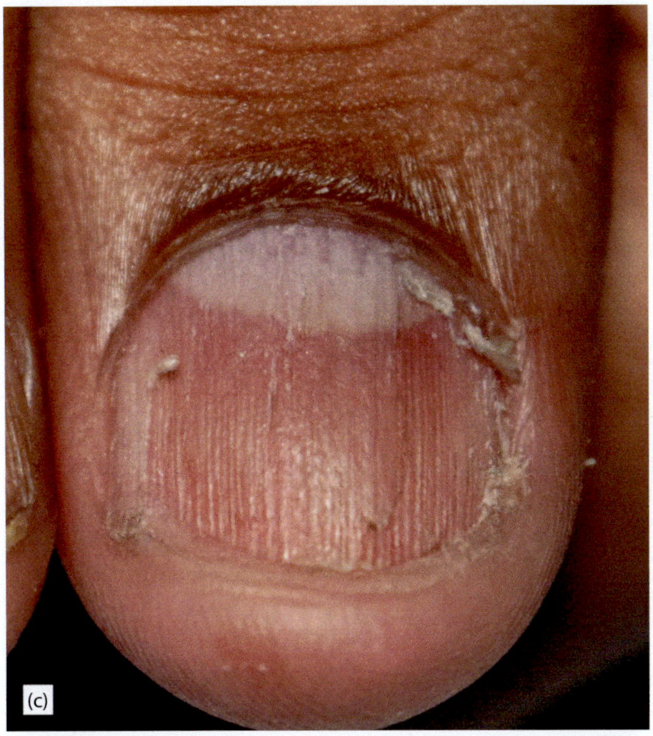

Figure 20.19 (*Continued*) **(c)** Shiny trachyonychia.

- Shiny trachyonychia – It is a less severe type and presents as shiny nails with superficial ridging and numerous pits. The nail is less thin and fragile compared to opaque trachyonychia (**Figure 20.19c**).
- The common causes of trachyonychia include alopecia areata, lichen planus, and psoriasis.
- It is more common in children, where it may show spontaneous resolution over years, and is mostly idiopathic. In adults, the disease runs a longer course. However, it does not cause permanent nail changes or scarring even when it is associated with lichen planus.

## Transverse grooving (TG)

- Transverse grooves are horizontal indentations on the nail surface, caused by injury to the nail matrix, resulting in transient cessation of nail growth. TG moves distally when the nail matrix resumes its function, and it ultimately disappears.
- **Beau's lines** are transverse grooves that may affect a few, multiple, or all digits (**Figure 20.20a,b** and **Table 20.5**). The depth and width of the groove give clues to the severity and duration of illness respectively. The distance of the groove from the proximal nail fold gives an estimate of the timing of injury in the past. Multiple Beau's lines indicate a repetitive injury to the nail matrix, as in chemotherapy. These lines are non-specific but serve as "retrospective indicators" of many pathological states. The thumb nail supplies information for the previous five to six months, whereas the great toe may give evidence of past disease for up to two years.

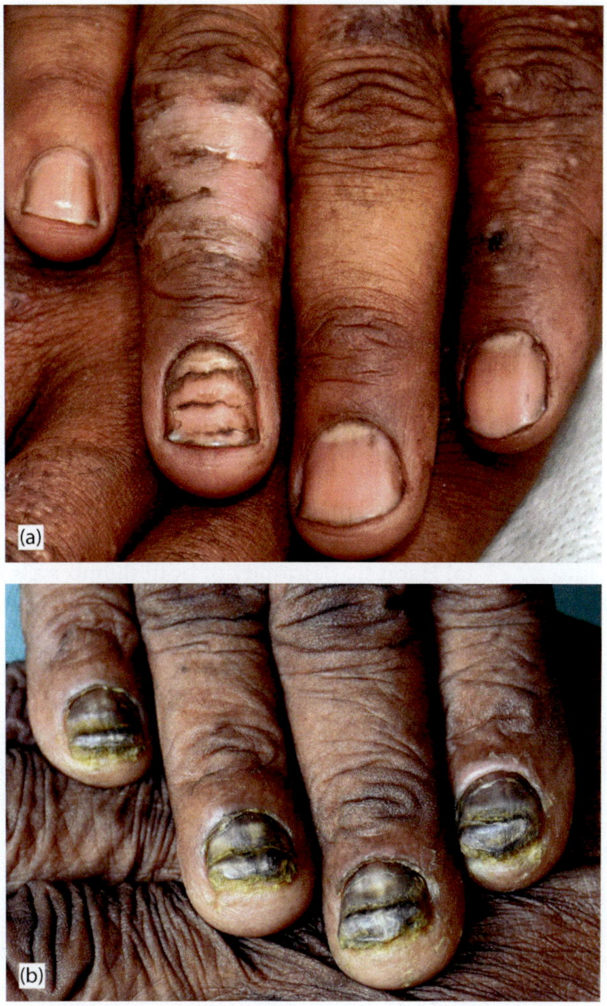

Figure 20.20 **(a,b)** Multiple Beau's lines.

Table 20.5 Beau's lines

| Single or a few digits | Multiple digits affected |
|---|---|
| • Trauma<br>• Paronychia<br>• Psoriasis<br>• Eczema | • Physiological – infants, cyclically with menstruation<br>• Systemic diseases – coronary thrombosis, pulmonary embolism, renal failure, Kawasaki disease, zinc deficiency, malnutrition<br>• Dermatological diseases – autoimmune vesicobullous diseases (pemphigus vulgaris, epidermolysis bullosa acquisita, pemphigoid gestationis, linear IgA disease, etc.), pustular psoriasis, Stevens-Johnson syndrome<br>• Infections – measles; mumps; pneumonia; hand, foot, and mouth disease<br>• Drugs – retinoids, metoprolol, anti-mitotic agents, dapsone hypersensitivity syndrome<br>• Others – severe exposure to cold |

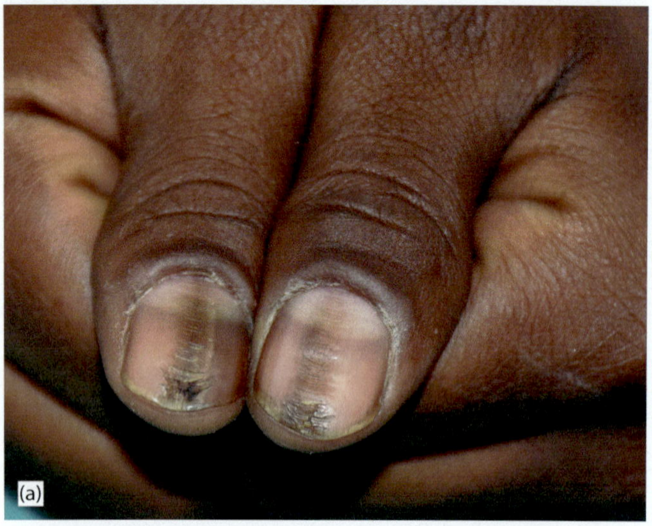


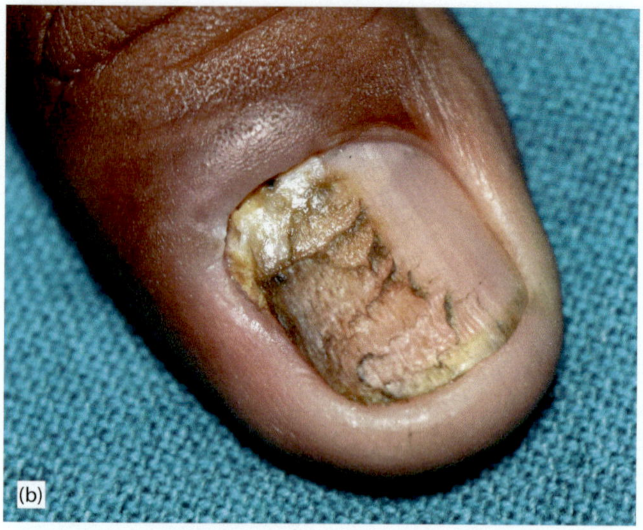


Figure 20.21 **(a)** Habit tic deformity of both thumb nails caused by proximal nail fold pushed back repeatedly. **(b)** Thumb nail showing severe changes of habit tic deformity.

- Sometimes a very deep Beau's line may develop as a result of complete cessation of nail matrix activity (for more than two weeks duration) and cause total division of the nail plate, resulting in latent onychomadesis.

## Habit tic deformity

- Habit tic deformity (washboard nails) is caused by repetitive external trauma to the nail matrix and is clinically characterized by transverse grooves and parallel ridging, both running from the nail fold to the distal edge of the nail; the surface changes resemble a washboard (**Figure 20.21a,b**).
- Thumbs are most commonly affected.

## Pitting (pits, erosions, onychia punctata)

- Pits are appreciable as punctate indentations on the nail plate and occur due to defective keratinization of the proximal matrix, with persistence of foci of parakeratotic cells in the nail plate (**Figure 20.22a**). As the nail plate grows beyond the proximal nail fold, abnormal parakeratotic keratinocytes are lost, leaving behind tiny depressions or pits on the surface. Pits commonly affect fingernails more than toenails.
- Pits are seen in various inflammatory conditions (**Table 20.6**). Trauma is the most common cause of pits affecting a single digit.

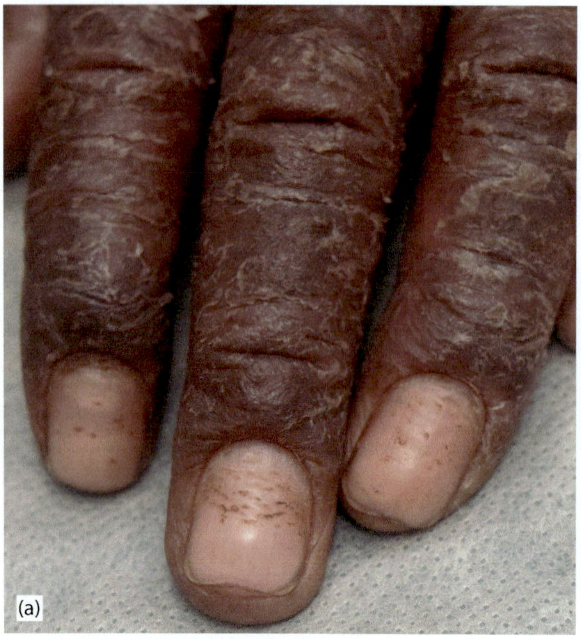


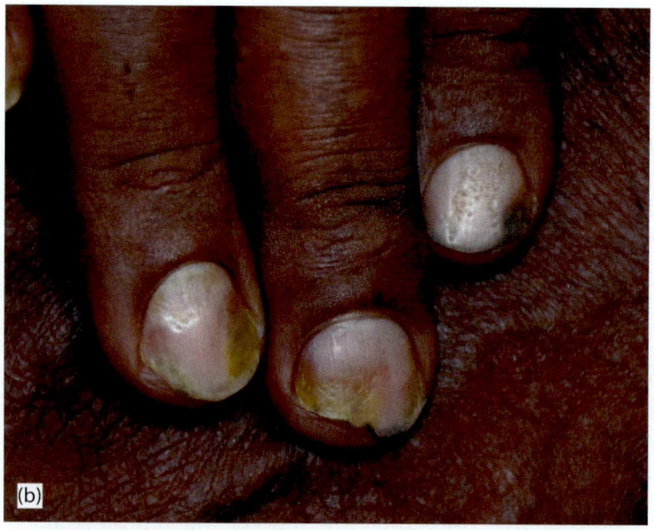


Figure 20.22 **(a)** Nail pitting in a case of erythroderma. **(b)** Coarse, irregularly arranged nail pits in psoriasis. *(Continued)*

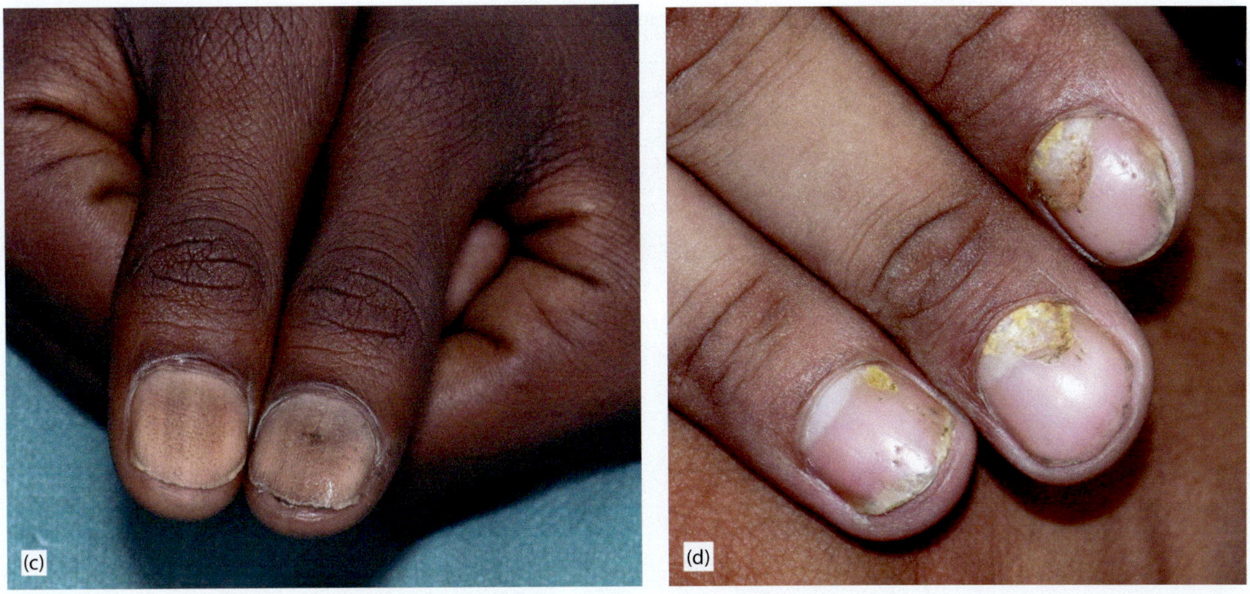

Figure 20.22 (*Continued*) **(c)** Shallow, regularly arranged nail pits. **(d)** Elkonyx in psoriasis.

- Pits vary in depth, size, shape, and number, depending on the etiology.
  - In psoriasis, they are irregular, coarse, and randomly placed on the surface. The presence of more than 20 pits is suggestive of psoriasis (**Figure 20.22b**).
  - In alopecia areata, pits are small and shallow, arranged in a regular and uniform pattern or in a grid-like pattern (Glen-plaid or Scotch-plaid pattern) (**Figure 20.22c**).
  - Sometimes a single, larger and deeper pit is noted in psoriasis and is called an elkonyxis (**Figure 20.22d**). Occasionally, it is also seen in secondary syphilis, Reiter's syndrome, after etretinate, and in isotretinoin therapy.
  - In eczema, coarse and irregular pits are seen in affected fingernails.
  - In Reiter's syndrome and secondary syphilis, pits are seen in lunula, giving a mottled appearance to the lunula.
  - In diabetes mellitus, pits are seen as small craters on the middle and ring fingers and are referred to as Rosenau's depressions.
- Occasional pits may appear in normal individuals.

Table 20.6 Nail pitting

| Etiology | Diseases |
|---|---|
| Dermatological diseases | • Single (/few) digit – chronic paronychia, lichen nitidus, lichen striatus, parakeratosis pustulosa<br>• Multiple digits – psoriasis, alopecia areata, eczema, lichen planus, Reiter's disease, pityriasis rosea, pityriasis rubra pilaris, pemphigus vulgaris, chemical dermatitis, dermatomyositis |
| Systemic diseases | Diabetes mellitus, systemic lupus erythematosus, sarcoidosis, rheumatoid arthritis |
| Others | Drug induced erythroderma, trauma |

## Increased nail plate fragility

### Brittle nails

- Brittle nails are clinically characterized by onychoschizia and onychorrhexis (**Figure 20.23**).

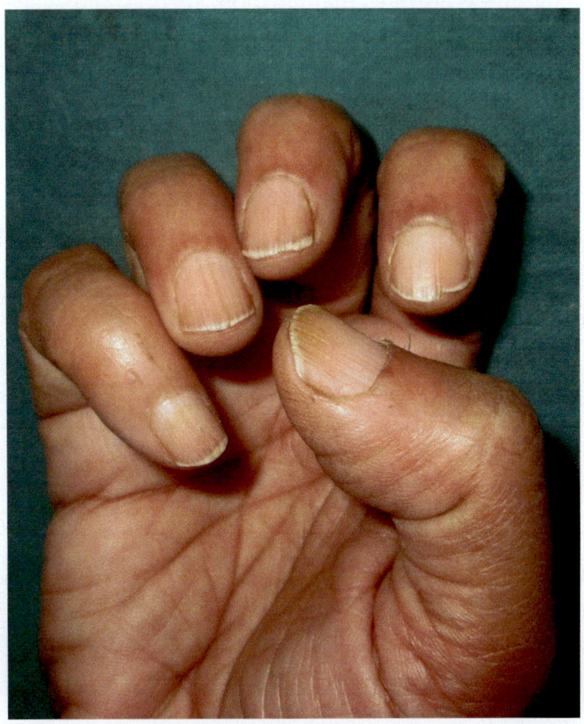

Figure 20.23 Brittle nails in a homemaker.

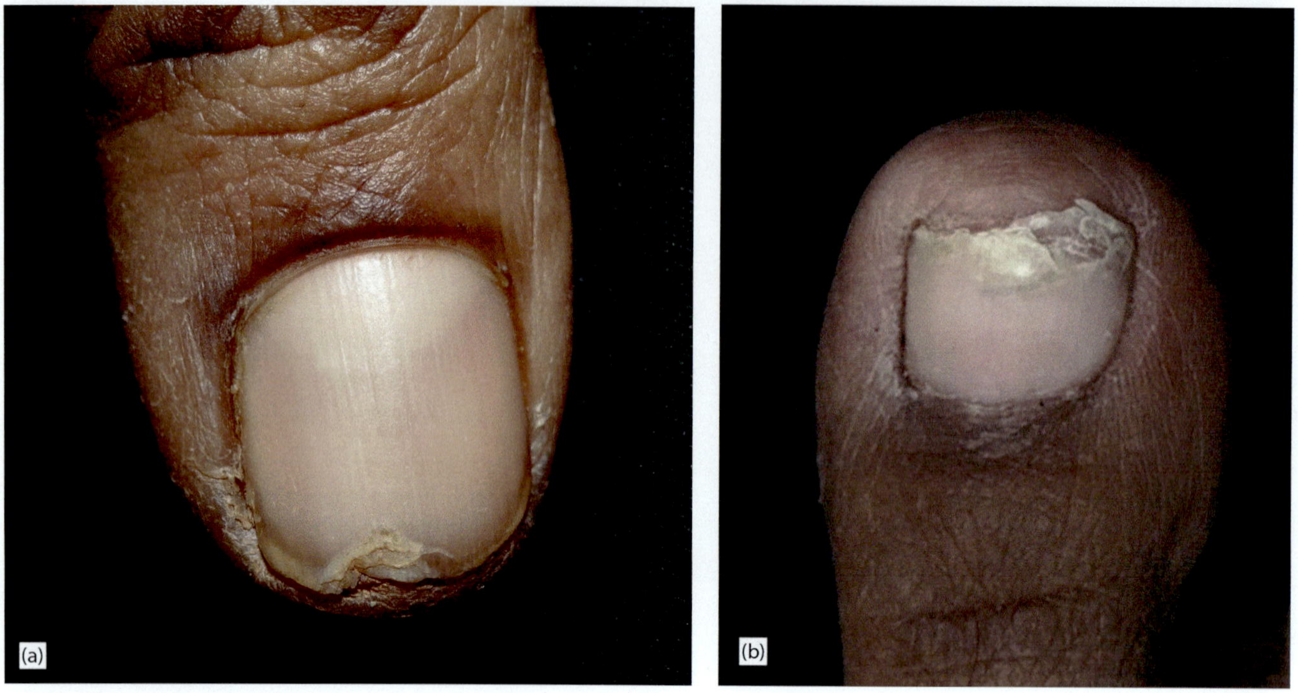


Figure 20.24 **(a)** Onychoschizia of finger nail. **(b)** Onychoschizia of toe nail.

- It may be idiopathic and is common in women. Local causes including damage by alkalis, solvents, sugar solutions, and hot water may be contributory.
- Dermatological diseases like eczema, lichen planus, and onychomycosis may present with brittle nails.
- Systemic causes include endocrinopathies, tuberculosis, Sjögren's syndrome, malnutrition, anemia, and peripheral neuropathy.

## Abnormalities of nail plate adhesions

### Onychoschizia (Lamellar nail dystrophy, peeling of nails)

- It is splitting of nail plate at the free edge in fingers and toes. The nail is formed in layers analogous to skin layers, and in this condition it is split horizontally into layers (**Figure 20.24a,b**).
- Repeated soaking of nails in water followed by drying is considered crucial in development of onychoschizia. Hence, it is commonly seen in those who are involved in such activities – house cleaners, nurses, hairdressers, etc. Nail cosmetics and exposure to chemicals (solvents, thioglycolates) also predispose a person to development of onychoschizia.

### Onycholysis

- Onycholysis is the separation of the nail plate from the underlying nail bed and/or lateral nail folds, starting at the distal end and progressing proximally (**Figure 20.25a**). The detached part of

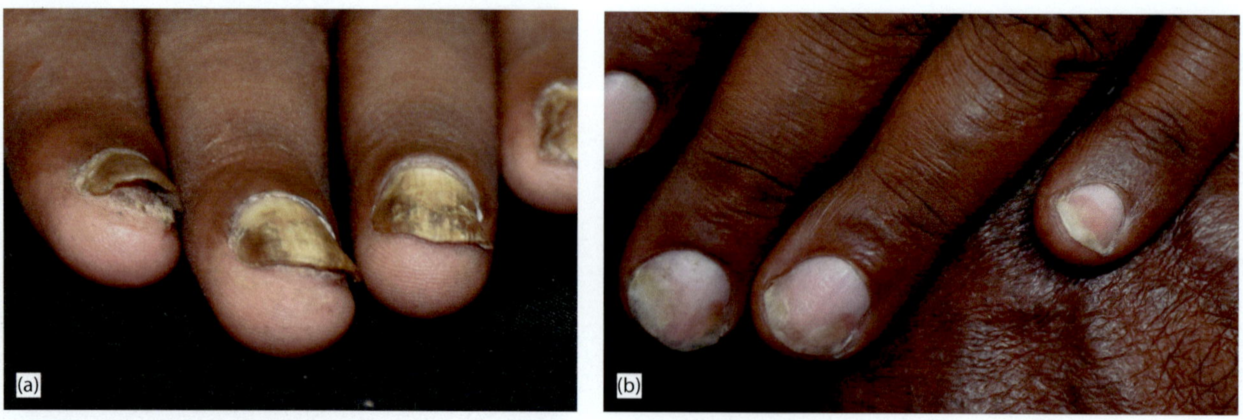


Figure 20.25 **(a)** Onycholysis. **(b)** Onycholysis in nail psoriasis. Note distal nail plate appearing white (area of onycholysis) and erythema proximal to it.

the nail plate loses translucency and appears white (or yellowish) (**Figure 20.25b**). Sometimes, the area may be colonized by *Pseudomonas* spp, producing a greenish hue.
- Additional findings provide important diagnostic clues and include proximal erythematous border (psoriasis vide **Figure 20.25b**), yellowish discoloration (onychomycosis vide **Figure 20.25a**), green discoloration (*Pseudomonas* spp. colonization) and red discoloration (photo-onycholysis).
- The causes of onycholysis are summarized in **Table 20.7**.

## Onychomadesis

- It is spontaneous separation of nail plate from the nail bed, starting from its proximal portion. It

Table 20.7 Onycholysis

| Single nail affection | Few nails/Multiple digits affected |
|---|---|
| • Trauma<br>• Foreign body implantation<br>• Nail bed tumors – both benign and malignant | • Dermatological causes – psoriasis, onychomycosis, eczema, pachyonychia congenita, lichen planus, pemphigus vulgaris and vegetans, reactive arthritis, lichen striatus, contact dermatitis from various nail cosmetics<br>• Systemic causes – anemia (iron deficiency), diabetes mellitus, hyperthyroidism and hypothyroidism, peripheral arterial diseases, pellagra, erythropoietic porphyria, porphyria cutanea tarda, histiocytosis X, sarcoidosis, scleroderma, amyloid and multiple myeloma<br>• Trauma – pedicure/manicure, mechanical trauma<br>• Chemical exposure – paint removers, dicyandiamide, thioglycolate, solvents, color developers<br>• Photo-onycholysis – tetracyclines, psoralens, fluoroquinolones, oral contraceptives, griseofulvin<br>• Drugs (not through photo-onycholysis) – chemotherapy, retinoids, hydroxylamine<br>• Others – pregnancy, prolonged maceration<br>• Idiopathic and familial forms |

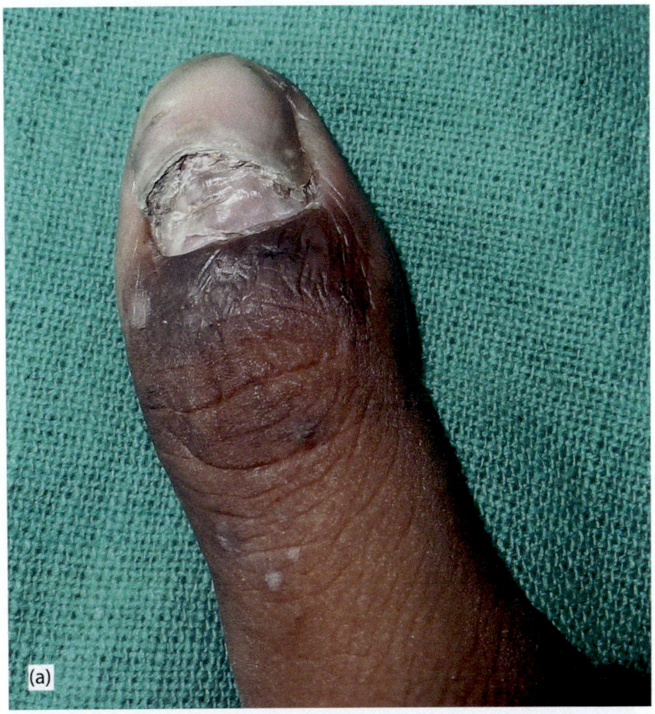


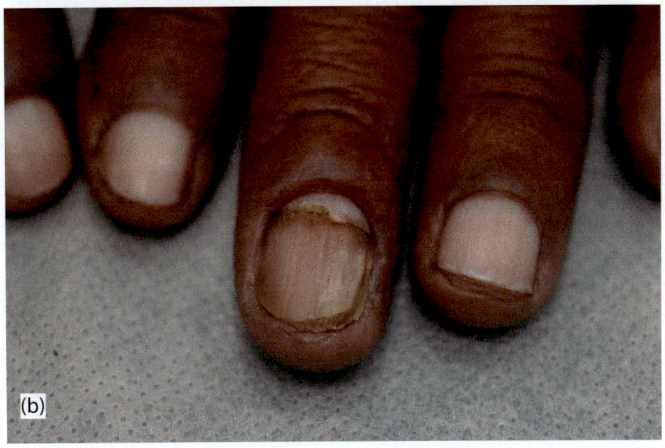


Figure 20.26 **(a,b)** Onychomadesis.

results from complete cessation of growth of the proximal nail matrix lasting for more than two weeks (**Figure 20.26a,b**).
- Onychomadesis and Beau's lines are caused by the same set of conditions; the difference lies in severity and duration of the insult.
- Sometimes total loss of nail is observed due to destruction of the matrix following trauma and lichen planus.

## Pterygium (from the Greek word *pterygion* meaning wing)

- Pterygium refers to a nail abnormality caused by abnormal adhesions between two components of the nail units. Two types are recognized – dorsal

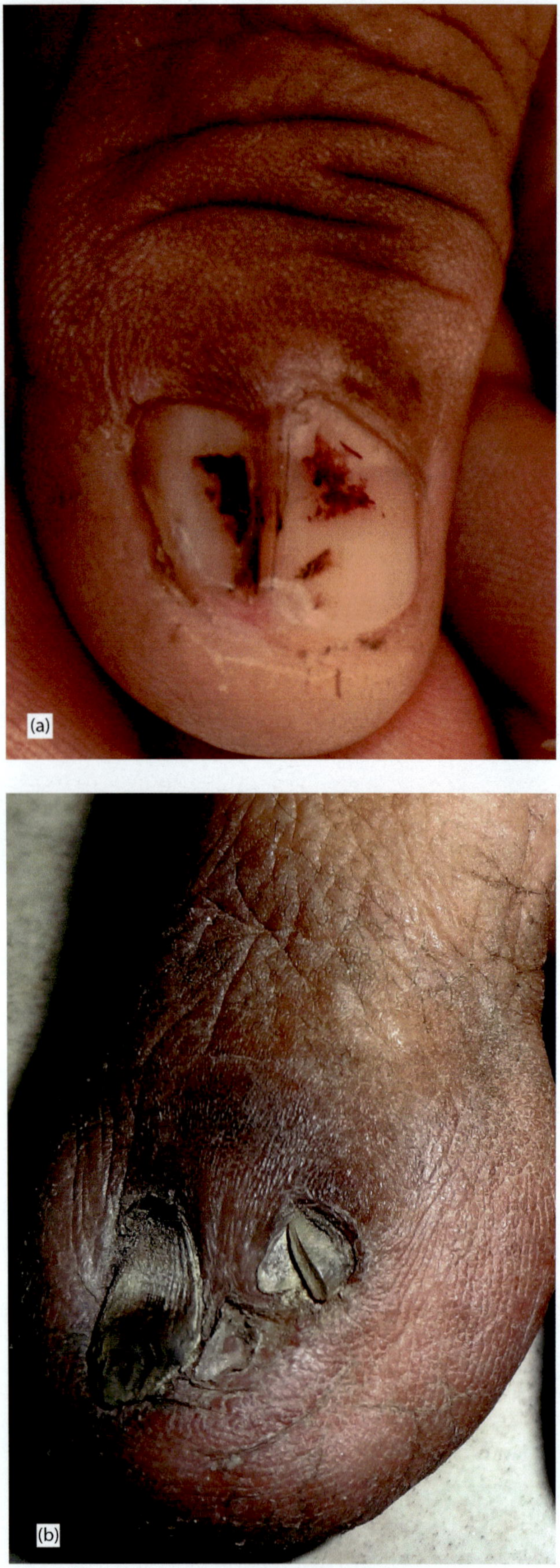

(pterygium unguis) and ventral (pterygium inversus unguis).

- Dorsal pterygium: It is characterized by linear or "wing-like" fibrotic tissue that causes the proximal nail matrix to adhere to the nail matrix and nail bed. Usually the nail plate gets divided into two halves, and sometimes, in severe cases, the whole nail plate is lost (**Figure 20.27a,b**). It indicates severe nail disease and is due to destruction of nail matrix. It is a specific, end-stage finding in lichen planus and a hallmark of severe disease. However, it is also observed in other conditions, such as burns, trauma, radiation dermatitis, cicatricial pemphigoid, graft-versus-host disease, and toxic epidermal necrolysis.
- Ventral pterygium: In this condition, hyponychium gets attached to the undersurface of the nail plate, causing obliteration of distal nail groove (**Figure 20.27c**). It is usually asymptomatic but may cause pain during trimming of the affected nails. The common causes include trauma, systemic sclerosis, lupus erythematosus, and leprosy. Rarely, the condition may be idiopathic or familial.

## Abnormalities of nail plate color

### Chromonychia

- The nail plate normally appears as a "pink translucent" structure, and any deviation from the normal appearance is termed chromonychia. The complete nail plate or its part may be affected.
- Chromonychia can be exogenous or endogenous. Exogenous chromonychia (**Figure 20.28a**) occurs after exposure to dyes (e.g., silver nitrate, potassium permanganate) and decorative use of henna, and the

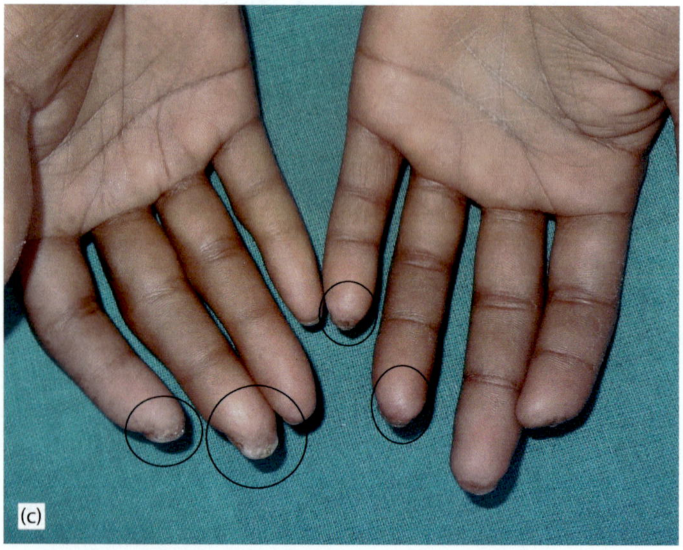

Figure 20.27 **(a)** Dorsal pterygium due to trauma. **(b)** Dorsal pterygium in nail lichen planus. **(c)** Ventral pterygium in multiple digits (circled) in a case of systemic sclerosis.

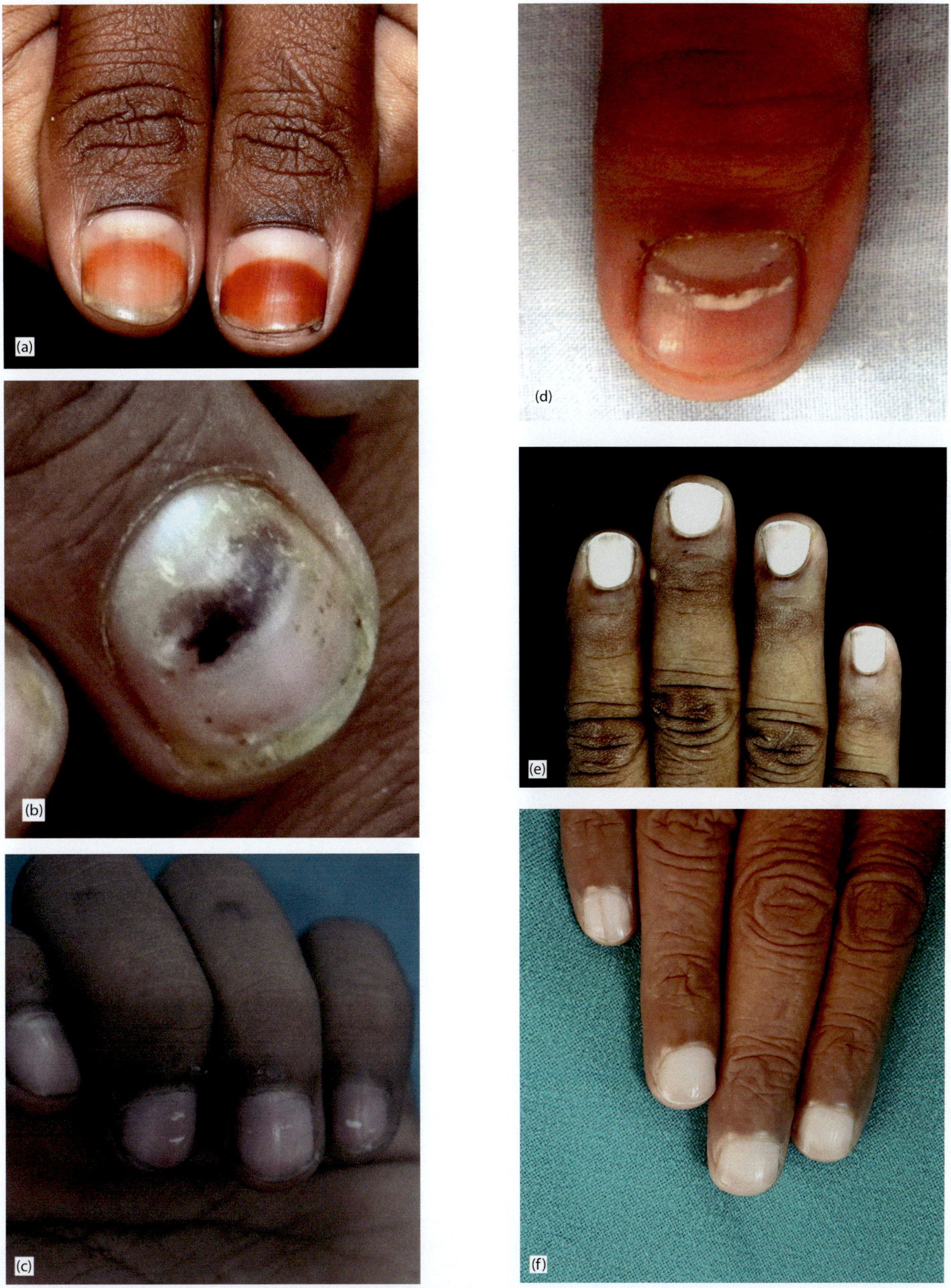


Figure 20.28 **(a)** Exogenous chromonychia after henna application. Note that proximal margin of chromonychia follows the shape of proximal nail fold. **(b)** Endogenous chromonychia due to subungual hematoma. Note that proximal margin of chromonychia follows the lunula. **(c)** Punctate leukonychia in a child. **(d)** Mees' lines. **(e)** Total leukonychia. **(f)** Terry's nails. (*Continued*)

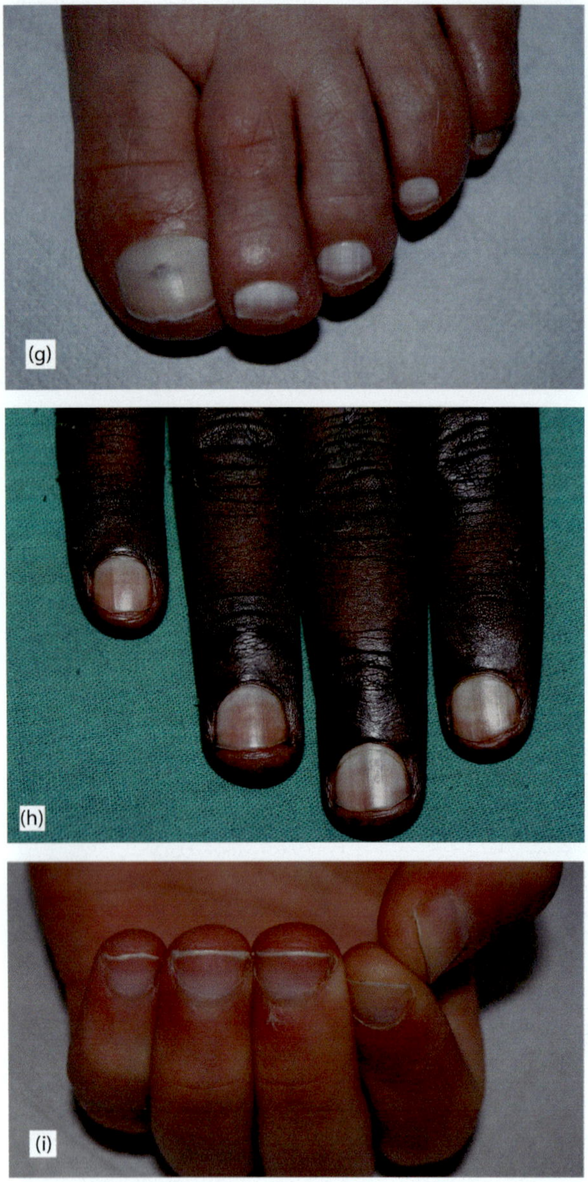


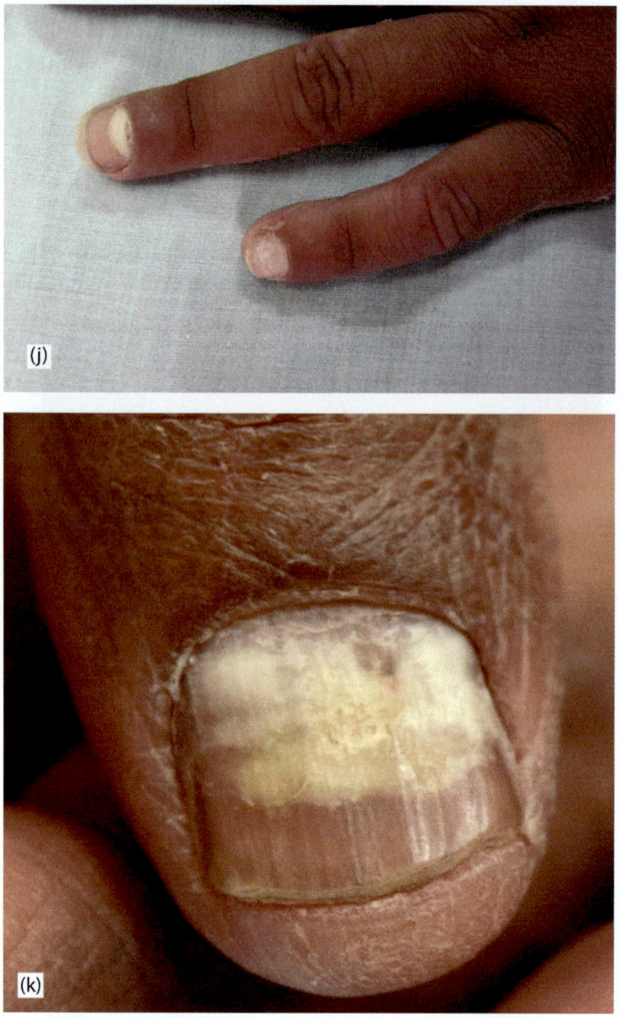


Figure 20.28 (*Continued*) **(g)** Terry's nails. **(h)** Half and half nails. **(i)** Half and half nails. **(j)** Muehrck's nails. **(k)** Apparent leukonychia in onychomycosis. (g,i – Courtesy: Michela Starace, Aurora Alessandrini, and Bianca Maria Piraccini.)

proximal margin of chromonychia follows proximal the nail fold. In contrast, the proximal margin of endogenous chromonychia (**Figure 20.28b**) parallels the lunula.

- Various clinical forms of chromonychia have been established – white nails (leukonychia), yellow nails, green nails, red nails (erythronychia), and brown-black nails (melanonychia) (**Tables 20.8** and **20.9**).

Table 20.8 Leukonychia

| Types | Features | Examples |
|---|---|---|
| **True leukonychia** | Nail matrix diseases result in parakeratotic nuclei retained within the nail matrix.<br>True leukonychia (partial) moves distally as the nail grows.<br>It does not fade on pressure. | Four types are known<br>• Punctate – idiopathic, trauma, psoriasis) (**Figure 20.28c**)<br>• Transverse – trauma, heavy metal poisoning (e.g., Mees' lines – single or multiple, transverse, narrow whitish line running along the width of the nail and parallel to lunula, **Figure 20.28d**), chemotherapy<br>• Longitudinal – Darier disease, Hailey-Hailey disease<br>• Total – congenital (**Figure 20.28e**) |

(*Continued*)

Table 20.8 Leukonychia (*Continued*)

| Types | Features | Examples |
|---|---|---|
| **Apparent leukonychia** | Whitening of nail plate is because of abnormal subungual tissues. Apparent leukonychia develops because of pallor of nail bed due to anemia and vascular impairment. It disappears or fades on pressure. | • Terry's nails describes a nail with a proximal white and distal normal-appearing (or brown) nail plate. It is seen in liver cirrhosis and congestive heart failure (**Figure 20.28f,g**). • Half and half nails (Lindsay's nails) are seen in uremic patients in whom proximal white and distal brownish discoloration is noted (**Figure 20.28h,i**). • Muehrcke's nails are seen in hypoalbuminemia (< 2gm/dl) and in patients receiving chemotherapy as paired (or multiple) bands of white lines. A pink line lies between the white lines (**Figure 20.28j**). Usually, the second, third, and fourth fingernails are affected, and thumbs are spared. Correction of the hypoalbuminemia reverses the sign. |
| **Pseudo leukonychia** | Pseudo leukonychia is whitening of nail plate and nail bed due to the external origin. | • Onychomycosis (**Figure 20.28k**), keratin granules. |

Table 20.9 Chromonychias

| Chromonychia | Features | Diseases |
|---|---|---|
| Erythronychia | Focal | Glomus tumor (**Figure 20.29a**) |
| | Longitudinal band | Onychopapilloma (single nail), Darier disease (alternate longitudinal leukonychia and erythronychia (**Figure 20.29b**), Hailey-Hailey disease |
| Yellow nails | Distal, focal, varying shades | Onychomycosis (**Figure 20.29c**) |
| | Complete | Yellow nail syndrome (**Figure 20.29d,e**) |
| Green nails | Associated onycholysis | *Pseudomonas* colonization (**Figure 20.29f**) |
| Brown-black color | Longitudinal 1- to 3-mm lines | Splinter hemorrhage (**Figure 20.29g**) |
| | Focal or complete | Subungual hematoma (**Figure 20.29h**), Fungal melanonychia |
| | Band-like pigmentation | Melanonychia (**Figure 20.29i**) |

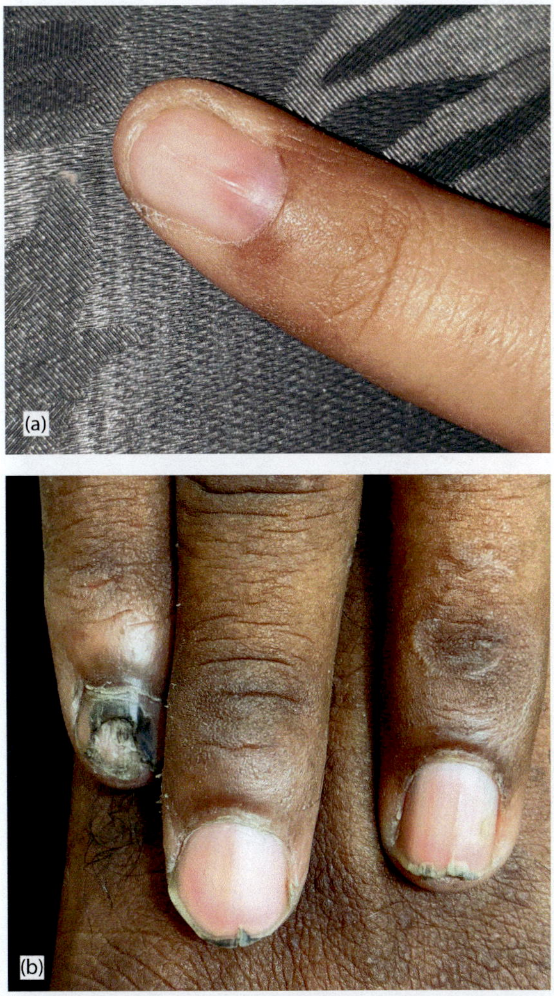

Figure 20.29 **(a)** Focal erythronychia and swelling in glomus tumor of nail bed. **(b)** Longitudinal erythronychia in Darier disease. (*Continued*)

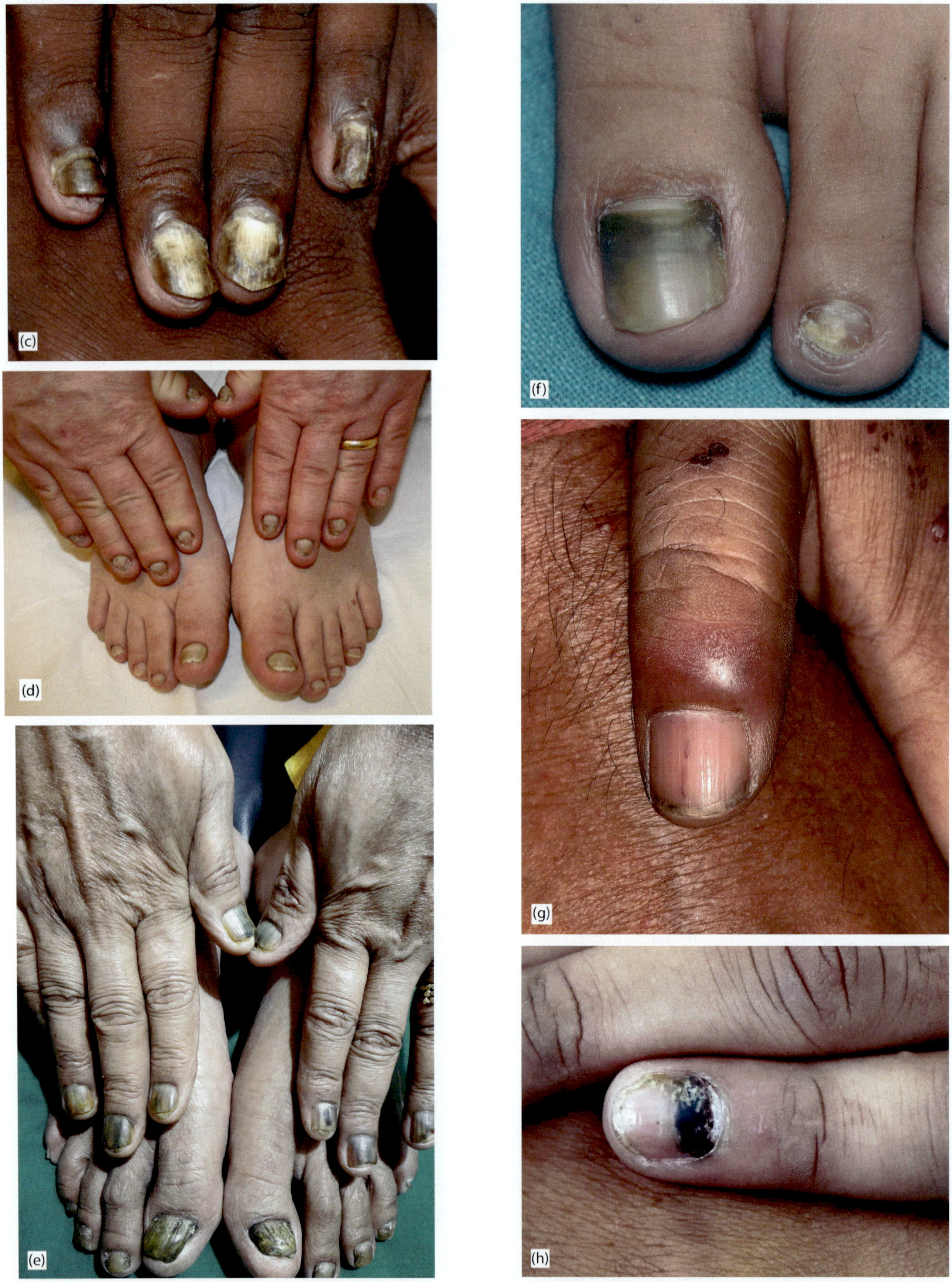


Figure 20.29 (*Continued*) **(c)** Onychomycosis with yellow and other discolorations. **(d)** Yellow nail syndrome. **(e)** Yellow nail syndrome. **(f)** *Pseudomonas* spp colonization causing green nails. **(g)** Splinter hemorrhage in a case of herpes zoster. **(h)** Subungual hematoma following intramatricial injection. (*Continued*)

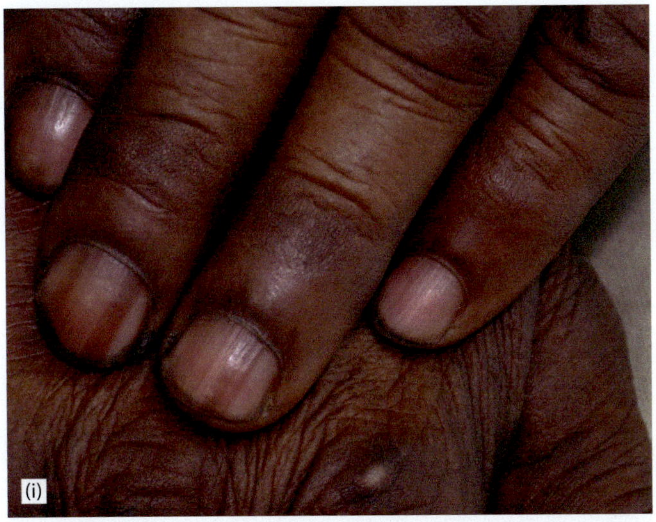


Figure 20.29 (*Continued*) **(i)** Multiple bands of longitudinal melanonychia. (a – Courtesy: Dr. Rajesh Kumar Mandal, North Bengal Medical College and Hospital, Darjeeling, India; d – Courtesy: Michela Starace, Aurora Alessandrini, and Bianca Maria Piraccini; e – Courtesy: Dr. Anil Patki, Pune, India.)

### Longitudinal melanonychia

- Longitudinal melanonychia appears as linear streaks or bands of brown-black pigmentation (**Figure 20.30**).
- Nail melanocytes are quiescent and generally do not produce melanin. Nail pigmentation may occur as a result of activation of melanocytes (trauma- or drug-induced), nevus (benign proliferation of melanocytes), or melanoma. Hence, pigmentation of the nail is a warning and should be critically evaluated.
- Clinical suspicion of nail unit melanoma (NUM) is raised by ABCDEF rule (**Table 20.10**).

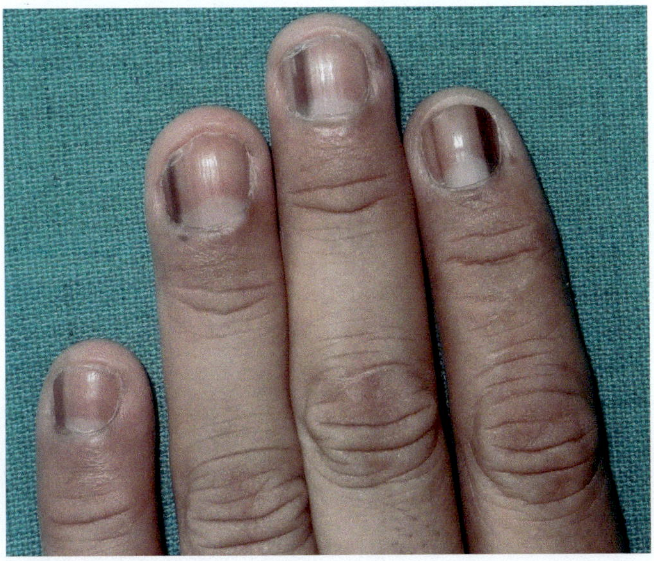

Figure 20.30 Longitudinal melanonychia affecting multiple nails in a young lady.

Table 20.10 ABCDEF rule

| ABCDEF mnemonic | Features |
|---|---|
| A | • Age peak – elderly population (40–70 years of age)<br>• Predisposed race – **A**sians, **A**fricans, **A**frican-**A**mericans, and Native **A**mericans |
| B | • Brown-black pigment<br>• Breadth (width) – > 3–5 mm<br>• Border – irregular |
| C | • Change – rapid increase in width and growth rate of nail band; nail dystrophy does not improve with "adequate treatment" |
| D | • Digit involved – single more often than multiple, dominant hand, thumb more often than big toe, which is more often than index finger |
| E | • Extension – pigmentation of proximal and/or lateral nail folds (Hutchinson's sign) |
| F | • Family history – previous melanoma or dysplastic nevus syndrome |

- Hutchinson's sign should be differentiated from pseudo-Hutchinson's sign, in which pigmentation of periungual tissue occurs due to conditions other than melanoma.
- Dermoscopy picks up early pigmentation of the proximal nail fold and is referred to as "micro-Hutchinson's sign."

## Alterations in lunula (Table 20.11)

Table 20.11 Lunula – change in color and shape

| Changes in lunula | Diseases |
|---|---|
| Red lunula (**Figure 20.31a**) | Alopecia<br>Lichen planus |
| Blue lunula (**Figure 20.31b**) | Raynaud's disease |
| Macro Lunula | Habit tic deformity |
| Triangular lunula (**Figure 20.31c**) | Nail patella syndrome |

## Nail folds changes

### Paronychia

- Paronychia is inflammation of the nail folds, with erythema, swelling, and pain. Two types are recognized
    - Acute paronychia is usually infective in nature and is most commonly caused by *Staphylococcus aureus*, followed by streptococci and pseudomonas organisms. Other responsible agents include gram-negative organisms, herpes simplex virus, and yeasts. Acute paronychia develops following trauma/injury to the nail folds and presents as

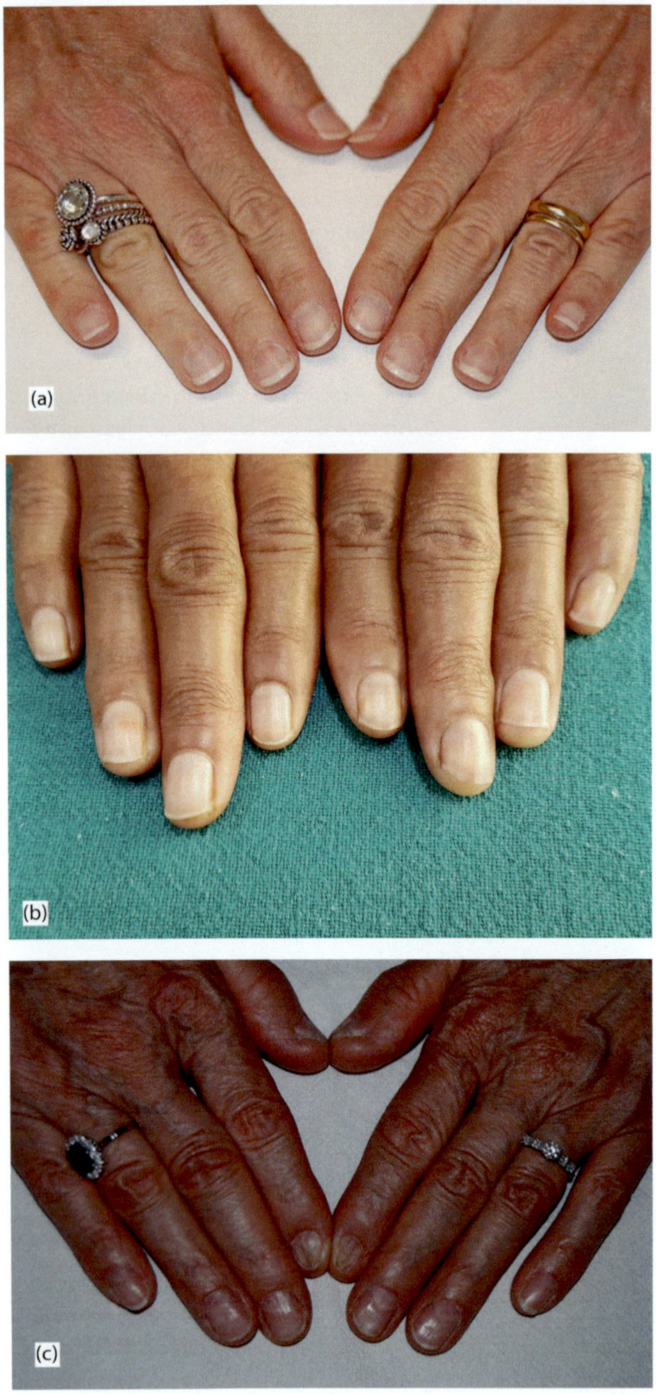

Figure 20.31 **(a)** Red lunula. **(b)** Blue lunula. **(c)** Triangular lunula.

a painful, erythematous swollen nail fold with collection of pus (**Figure 20.32a**).

- Chronic paronychia (persisting more than six weeks) is usually multi-factorial in origin and presents as periodically inflamed and painful nail folds. The cuticle is usually lost, and in long-standing cases, the nail plate becomes dystrophic, with pronounced transverse ridges (**Figure 20.32b,c**).

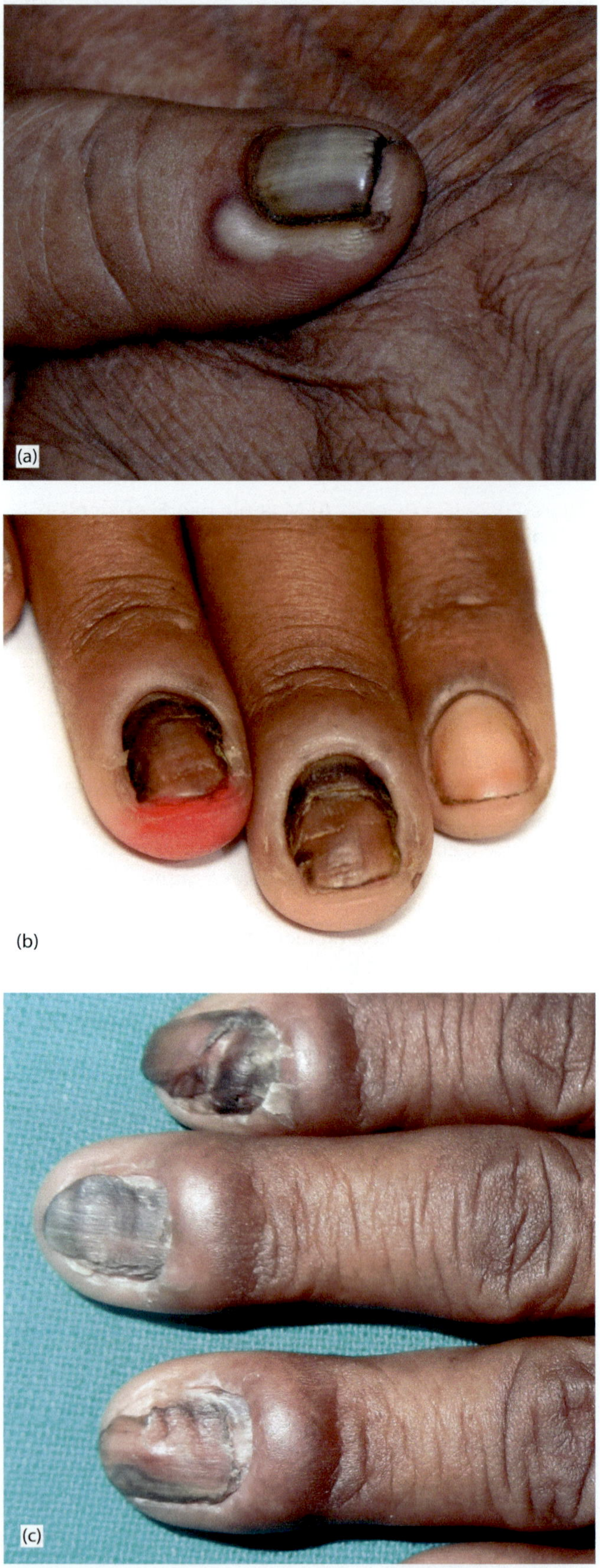

Figure 20.32 **(a)** Acute paronychia with pus formation. **(b)** Chronic paronychia. Note loss of cuticle. **(c)** Long standing chronic paronychia with dystrophic nails.

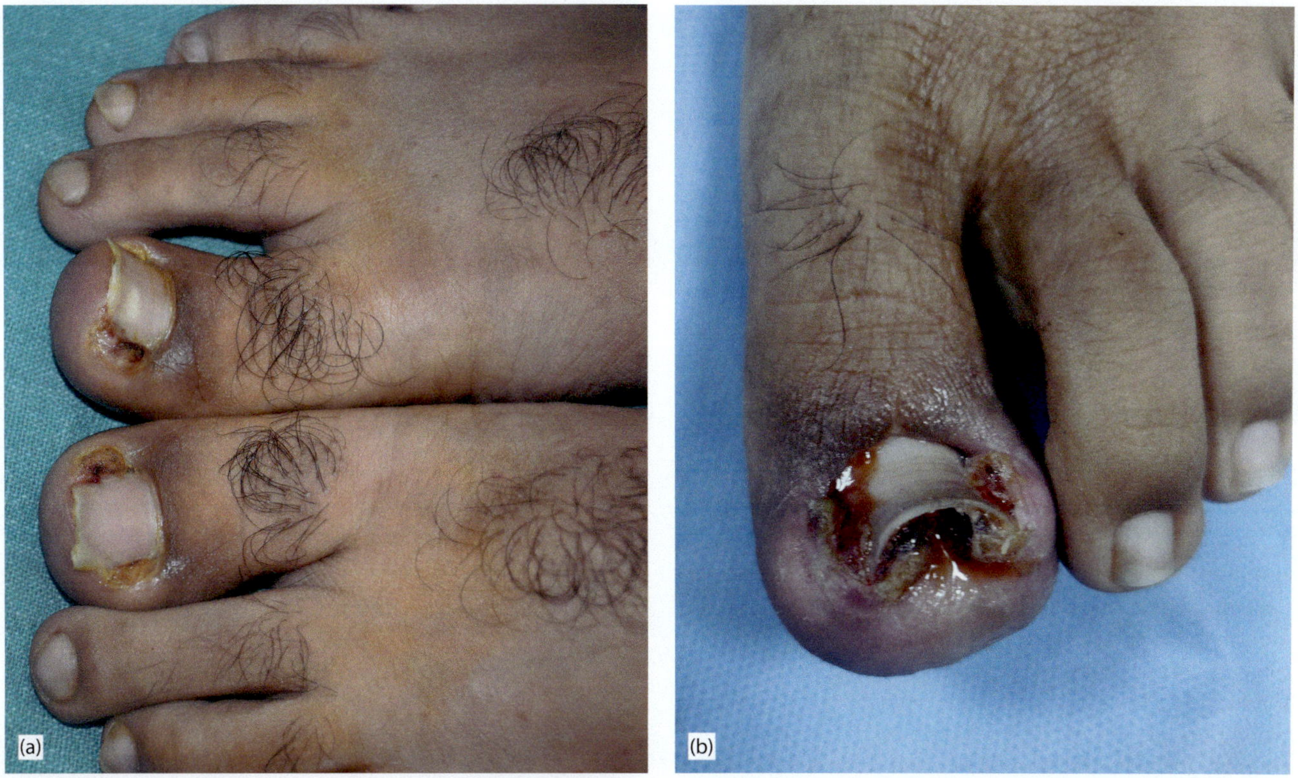


Figure 20.33 **(a)** Ingrown nails affecting both great toes. Note overgrowth of lateral nail folds. **(b)** Ingrown nail with serosanguinous discharge and swelling of lateral nail folds. (b – Courtesy: Dr. Dependra Kumar Timshina, Remedy Clinic, Siliguri, India.)

## Ingrown nails/onychocryptosis

- In onychocryptosis, the lateral edges of nail plate penetrate into the soft tissue of the lateral nail folds, causing periungual inflammation and pain (**Figure 20.33a,b**).

## Hutchinson's sign

- Hutchinson's sign refers to the periungual extension of brown-black pigmentation from longitudinal melanonychia onto the proximal and lateral nail folds (**Figure 20.34**). It is an important indicator of subungual melanoma.

## Pseudo-Hutchinson's sign

- It refers to the pigmentation of nail folds (along with nail-plate pigmentation) in non-melanoma conditions (e.g., ethnic pigmentation, Laugier-Hunziker-Baran syndrome, Bowen's disease, minocycline-induced pigmentation, etc.) (**Figure 20.35**). In pseudo-Hutchinson's sign, the cuticle remains translucent.

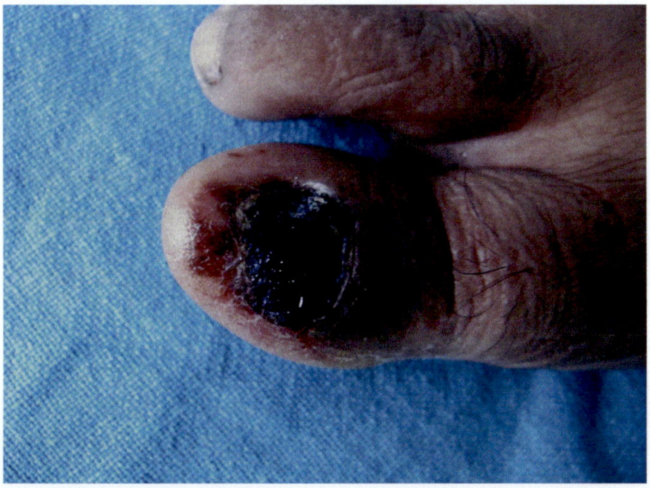

Figure 20.34 Subungual melanoma with pigment spreading to surrounding tissue.

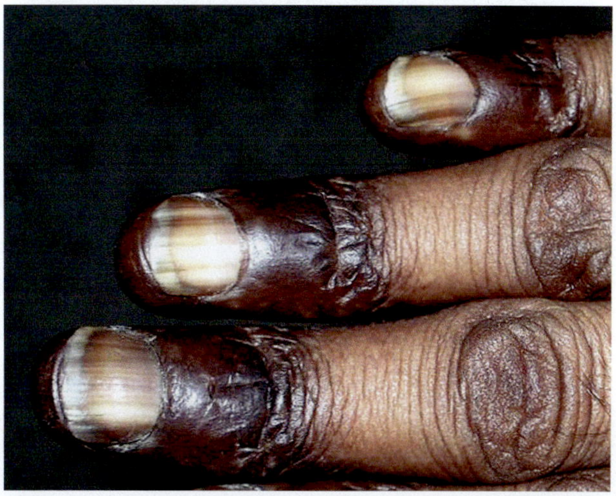

Figure 20.35 Pseudo-Hutchinson's sign in Laugier-Hunziker-Baran syndrome.

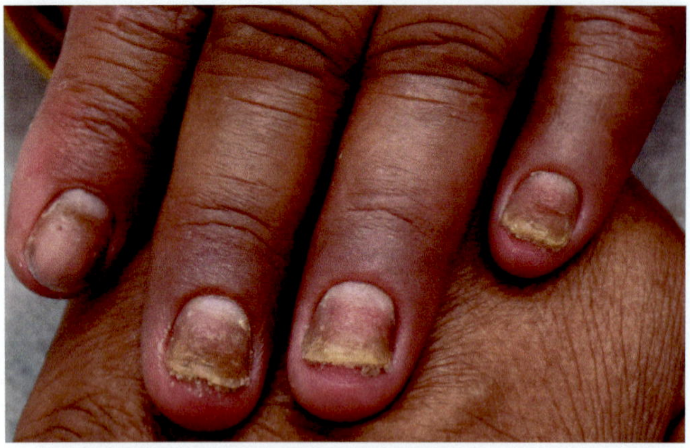

Figure 20.36 Subungual hyperkeratosis.

## Subungal changes

- Subungal hyperkeratosis results from accumulation of keratin material under the nail plate as a result of nail bed hyperkeratosis. As a result of subungual hyperkeratosis, the nail plate loses its translucency and appears yellowish-white in color (**Figure 20.36**). Common causes include psoriasis, dermatophyte infection, and eczema.
- Subungual hematoma is a transient condition characterized by a painful collection of blood under the nail plate and occurs as a result of traumatic injury to the digit. The nail plate loses its translucency, and the color changes over time from the initial red-purple to dark brown and black as the blood clots (**Figure 20.37**).

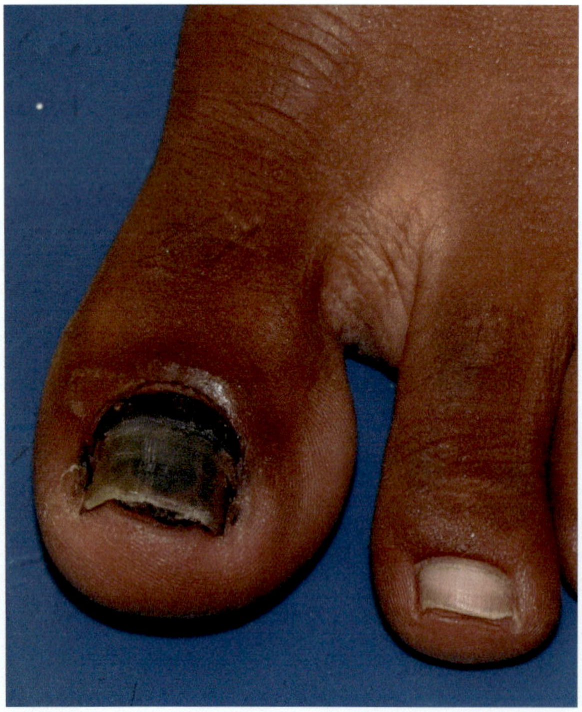

Figure 20.37 Traumatic subungual hematoma of great toe.

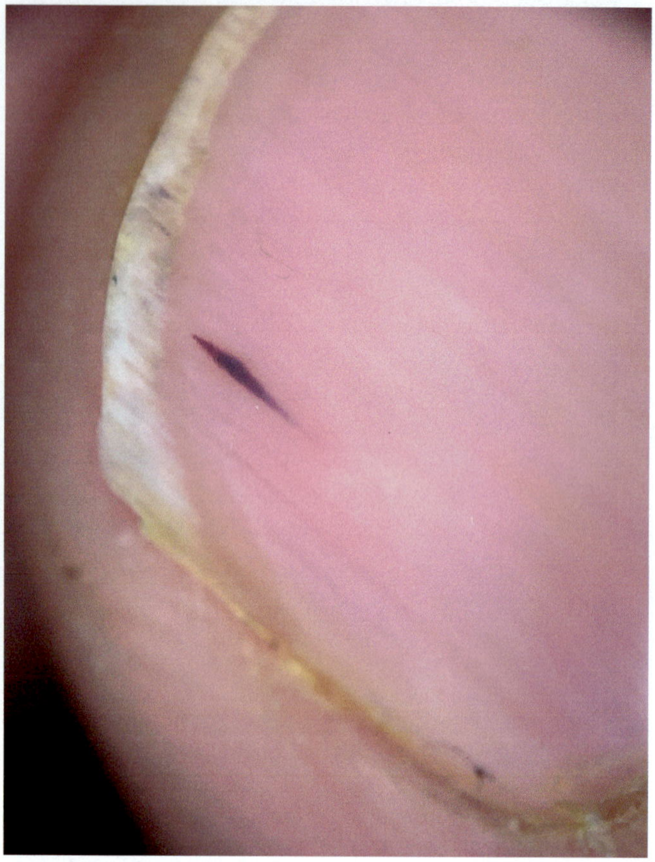

Figure 20.38 Onychoscopic view of distal splinter hemorrhage.

Gradually, the color fades and the nail plate assumes its normal appearance.
- Splinter hemorrhage refers to a micro-hemorrhage from nail bed capillaries due to local trauma or microemboli. It presents as longitudinal 1- to 3-mm red, brown, or black lines under the nail plate (**Figure 20.38**). It may be solitary or multiple, and asymptomatic or tender. Splinter hemorrhage may be caused by trauma (usually distal in location) or may be seen in various dermatological (psoriasis) and systemic (proximal in location, infective endocarditis, meningococcal disease, antiphospholipid syndrome, systemic lupus erythematosus, Raynaud's disease, and cutaneous vasculitis) conditions.
- Glomus tumor is a painful tumor of the nail unit that usually affects the first and second finger nails. The pain is disproportionate to the clinical signs and is typically paroxysmal in nature, with associated cold sensitivity. There is often a pinpoint tenderness. Glomus tumor may be visible as a red-purple subungual mass, while bigger masses may be associated with onycholysis, nail plate thinning, and fissuring (**Figure 20.39**).

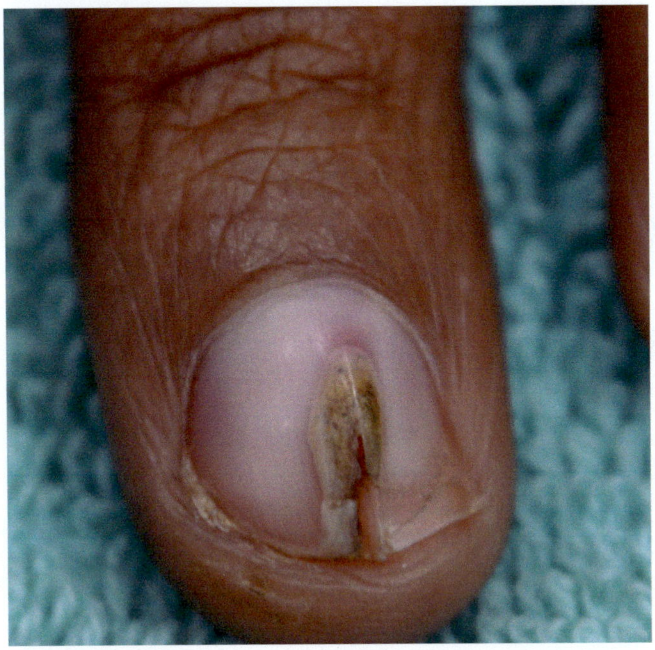

Figure 20.39 Large nail bed glomus tumor with nail plate splitting. (Courtesy: Soumyajit Roychoudhury, Behrampore, India.)


## ACKNOWLEDGMENT

The author would like to thank the editors and publisher (CRC Press) of the book Nail Disorders: A Comprehensive Approach for allowing the use of images and content from the book. The author would like to thank Prof. Archana Singal (Figures 20.10a, 20.10c, 20.10d, 20.11b, 20.13, 20.17d, 20.19c, 20.23, 20.28c, 20.28d, 20.28f, 20.28h, 20.28j, 20.31b, 20.34); Dr. Michela Starace (Figures 20.7, 20.18c, 20.29d, 20.31a, 20.31c); Prof. Balachandar Ankad (Figures 20.12, 20.18b, 20.24a, 20.28e), Prof. Bela J Shah (figure 20.14c); and Prof. Eckart Haneke (Figure 20.29f) for their invaluable contributions.


## REFERENCES


1. de Berker D. Nail anatomy. Clin Dermatol 2013;31:509–515.
2. Lal NR, Kumar P, Barkat R. Nail Unit Signs. In: Singal A, Neema S, Kumar P, editors. Nail Disorders: A Comprehensive Approach. 1st edition. New York: CRC Press/Taylor & Francis Group; 2019. P. 21–48.
3. Ankad BS, Beergouder SA. Nail Plate Abnormalities. In: Singal A, Neema S, Kumar P, editors. Nail Disorders: A Comprehensive Approach. 1st edition. New York: CRC Press/Taylor & Francis Group; 2019. P. 147–164.
4. Starace M, Alessandrini A, Piraccini BM. Chromonychia. In: Singal A, Neema S, Kumar P, editors. Nail Disorders: A Comprehensive Approach. 1st edition. New York: CRC Press/Taylor & Francis Group; 2019. P. 165–175.
5. Rich P. Overview of Nail Disorders. In: Stratman E, Corona R, editors. UpToDate [Internet]. Waltham (MA): UpToDate Inc; 2019 [cited 2019 Dec 10]. Available from: https://www.uptodate.com/contents/overview-of-nail-disorders
6. Singal A, Arora R. Nail as a window of systemic diseases. Indian Dermatol Online J 2015;6:67–74.
7. Haber JS, Chairatchaneeboon M, Rubin AI. Trachyonychia: Review and Update on Clinical aspects, histology, and therapy. Skin Appendage Disord 2017;2(3–4):109–115.

# SECTION 4

# Skin in systemic diseases

PC DAS, PIYUSH KUMAR

Skin is the interface between the internal milieu of the body and the environment. The health of an individual can be easily judged by their skin, and it is rightly said to be the mirror of the human body. Hence, careful dermatological examination can provide important clues to various systemic diseases. Dermatologists need to develop a keen eye to look for and identify these clues. There are numerous dermatological signs that are harbingers, or telltale signs, of various systemic diseases. Some of these dermatological signs, such as pallor, jaundice, cyanosis and clubbing, are non-specific, but they are still useful as they always trigger a search for systemic illness. Some other cutaneous signs are specific enough to allow a clinical diagnosis. Some notable examples include pretibial myxoedema in Graves' disease, Gottron papules in dermatomyositis, hypertrichosis lanuginosa acquisita, and erythema gyratum repens in internal malignancy, etc.

Most of the systemic diseases, be they infectious, metabolic, genetic, neoplastic, autoimmune, or environmental, have some form of skin involvement at some stage of the disease process. Many of the systemic diseases – involving systems ranging from the central nervous system to kidneys and internal malignancies – have dermatological manifestations that not only help in diagnosis of internal diseases but also cause suffering to patients and require treatment in their own right. The treatment of systemic diseases also results in dermatologic toxicity, which requires expert management by dermatologists.

Dermatologists should be aware of dermatologic manifestation of internal disease, dermatological manifestation of internal malignancy, and cutaneous toxicity of various drugs. In-depth knowledge of cutaneous manifestations and a high index of suspicion can place dermatologists in a unique position where they can diagnose systemic diseases early and prevent needless suffering. The ensuing few chapters emphasize the dermatological presentations of systemic diseases.

DOI: 10.1201/9781351054225-56

# 21

# Nutritional deficiency disorders

CHIRAG DESAI, PIYUSH KUMAR

## INTRODUCTION

The human body requires many nutrients (**Table 21.1**) on a regular basis for a variety of biological functions. Though many or all organ systems are affected when one or more nutrients are deficient, the skin (and its appendages) and mucosa are affected early in most cases. These skin and mucosal changes are "tell-tale" signs of nutritional deficiency, and some of them are specific enough to allow a clinical diagnosis of deficiency of a particular nutrient. Thus, recognition of mucocutaneous, hair, and nail changes can be an important tool for diagnosing various nutritional deficiencies. This chapter discusses clinical diagnosis of various nutritional deficiencies based on presentation (**Table 21.2**) and other clues (**Table 21.3**). As the causative factors responsible for various nutrient deficiencies are common (**Box 21.1**), multiple nutritional deficiencies tend to co-exist. This should be kept in mind while dealing with a patient with suspected nutritional deficiency. Also, these dermatoses mimic many common dermatoses and should be considered as clinical differentials, especially in people who are at risk of developing nutritional deficiencies (vide **Box 21.1**) and who develop mucocutaneous lesions consistent with nutritional disorders (vide **Table 21.2**).[1–4] Some of the nutrient deficiency states do not have a prominent cutaneous involvement (e.g., thiamine deficiency causing beri beri) and will not be discussed here.

### Atrophic glossitis

- Atrophic glossitis (AG) refers to the absence of filiform or fungiform papillae on the dorsal surface of the tongue, causing a soft and smooth appearance (**Figure 21.1a**).
- This change is non-specific and may be seen in the deficiency of various nutrients, usually several of them rather than one at a time. Deficiency of riboflavin (vitamin $B_2$), niacin (vitamin $B_3$), pyridoxine (vitamin $B_6$), folate, cobalamin (vitamin $B_{12}$), iron, and zinc may cause atrophic glossitis.
- Affected patients complain of pain and a burning sensation.
- Clinically, the tongue appears beefy red with a smooth, glossy surface. Angular cheilitis is frequently associated.
- DD: Candidiasis, lichen planus, median rhomboid glossitis, migratory glossitis.

Table 21.1 Different nutrients required for humans

| | | |
|---|---|---|
| Macronutrients | Energy-yielding | • Carbohydrates<br>• Proteins<br>• Fats (saturated fats, monounsaturated fats, polyunsaturated fats, essential fatty acids) |
| | Non-energy–yielding | • Water<br>• Fiber |
| Micronutrients (all are non-energy–yielding) | Vitamins | • Water soluble – vitamins B complex and vitamin C<br>• Fat soluble – vitamins A, D, E and K |
| | Minerals | Sodium, potassium, calcium, magnesium, chloride and phosphorus |
| | Trace elements | Zinc, selenium, molybdenum, chromium, copper, iodine, iron, manganese and fluorine |

DOI: 10.1201/9781351054225-57

Table 21.2 Clinical approach to dermatoses seen in various nutritional disorders

| Presenting feature | Deficient nutrient/condition | Nutrient excess (toxicity)/ condition |
| --- | --- | --- |
| Glossitis (red) | Niacin, pyridoxine, riboflavin, vitamin $B_{12}$, folate, vitamin $B_1$, biotin, iron | |
| Angular stomatitis | Riboflavin, niacin, pyridoxine, folate, vitamin $B_{12}$, Iron, zinc, marasmus | Vitamin A |
| Xerosis | Vitamin A, essential fatty acids, | Hematochromatosis, selenium |
| Scaling/exfoliation | • Generalized – PEM, vitamin A<br>• Acral – niacin<br>• Scalp – biotin (early),<br>• Periorificial – biotin (early) | Vitamin A |
| Follicular papules | Vitamin A, vitamin C, EFA, copper | Vitamin A |
| Skin and mucosa; hyperpigmentation | Vitamin $B_{12}$ (Addisonian pattern), folate, vitamin A (face and neck), kwashiorkor (extremities) | Hemochromatosis, vitamin A |
| Hypopigmentation of skin | Copper, selenium | |
| Eczematous changes | • Acral areas – zinc, biotin<br>• Seborrheic areas – niacin, riboflavin, pyridoxine<br>• Periorificial areas – zinc, biotin<br>• Intertriginous areas – biotin<br>• Sun exposed areas – niacin | • Scalp – selenium toxicity<br>• Genitals – selenium toxicity |
| Purpuric lesions | Vitamin C (perifollicular petechiae), vitamin K, Essential fatty acids (traumatic) | Vitamin E |
| Edema | Protein (generalized), thiamine (pedal edema), vitamin C ("woody edema" of lower legs), niacin (sunburn like), iron | |
| Photosensitivity | Niacin | Pyridoxine (acral blistering) |
| Yellowish discoloration | | β-carotene |

Table 21.3 Clues for the diagnosis of nutritional disorders.

| Signs | Deficient nutrient |
| --- | --- |
| Pallor | Iron, folate, vitamin $B_{12}$, copper |
| Atrophic lingual papillae | Niacin, iron, riboflavin, folate, vitamin $B_{12}$, pyridoxine |
| Transversely depigmented hairs | PEM (flag sign), copper, EFA |
| Easily pluckable hairs | PEM |
| Sparse, thin hairs | PEM, zinc, biotin, vitamin A |
| Corkscrew hairs (flattened and curled) | Vitamin C |
| Koilonychia | Iron |
| Beau's lines | PEM |
| Brittle nails | EFA, Iron, (selenium excess) |
| Bleeding gums | Vitamin C, riboflavin, Vitamin K |
| Reduced taste sensation | Vitamin A, zinc |
| Muscle pain | Vitamin C, thiamine, selenium |
| Muscle wasting | PEM |
| Bone tenderness | Vitamin C, vitamin D, calcium, phosphorus |
| Delayed wound healing | Zinc, PEM, vitamin C |
| Genital lesions | Zinc, riboflavin, vitamin $B_3$, folate |
| Night blindness | Vitamin A |
| Conjunctival erythema and Corneal vascularization | Riboflavin |
| Conjunctival xerosis | Vitamin A |
| Hemorrhagic disease of the newborn (HDN) | Vitamin K |
| Peripheral neuropathy | Vitamin $B_1$, pyridoxine (both excess and deficiency), Vitamin $B_{12}$, Zinc |

*Abbreviations:* EFA, essential fatty acids; PEM, protein energy malnutrition.

## BOX 21.1: Factors responsible for deficiency of nutrients

- **Inadequate intake** (poverty, old age, alcoholics, anorexics, people with psychiatric morbidities, etc.)
- **Impaired absorption** (inflammatory bowel disease, celiac disease and tropical sprue, short bowel syndrome, etc.)
- **Impaired metabolism**
- **Increased requirement** (infancy and adolescence, pregnancy, lactation, concurrent infection, malignancy)
- **Increased excretion**
- **Increased destruction**

### Angular cheilitis (AC) (Angular stomatitis, perlèche/perlèche)

- Angular cheilitis is an inflammatory condition that affects either or both angles of the mouth.
- AC may develop due to inadequate dentures, loss of vertical dimension of the mouth in older people, contact allergy, nutritional deficiencies, hypersalivation, marionette lines, and atopic or seborrheic dermatitis. *Candida albicans*, *Staphylococcus aureus*, and β-hemolytic streptococci infection too may cause AC.
- Patients may complain of discomfort, pain while opening the mouth, and a burning sensation.
- AC typically presents with erythema, painful cracking, scaling, bleeding, and ulceration at the corners of the mouth (**Figure 21.1b**). AC due to nutrient deficiency is associated with atrophic glossitis.

### Riboflavin (vitamin $B_2$) deficiency (oral-ocular-genital syndrome)

- Risk factors – pregnancy, lactation, phototherapy for hyperbilirubinemia (in premature infants), advanced age, low income, depression, alcoholics, hypothyroidism, and phenytoin therapy.
- The clinical findings include the following:
  - Oral – tongue (atrophic and magenta in color) and lips (chapping and fissuring of the lips, angular cheilitis) involvement.
  - Ocular – photophobia and blepharitis angularis; cataracts may develop.

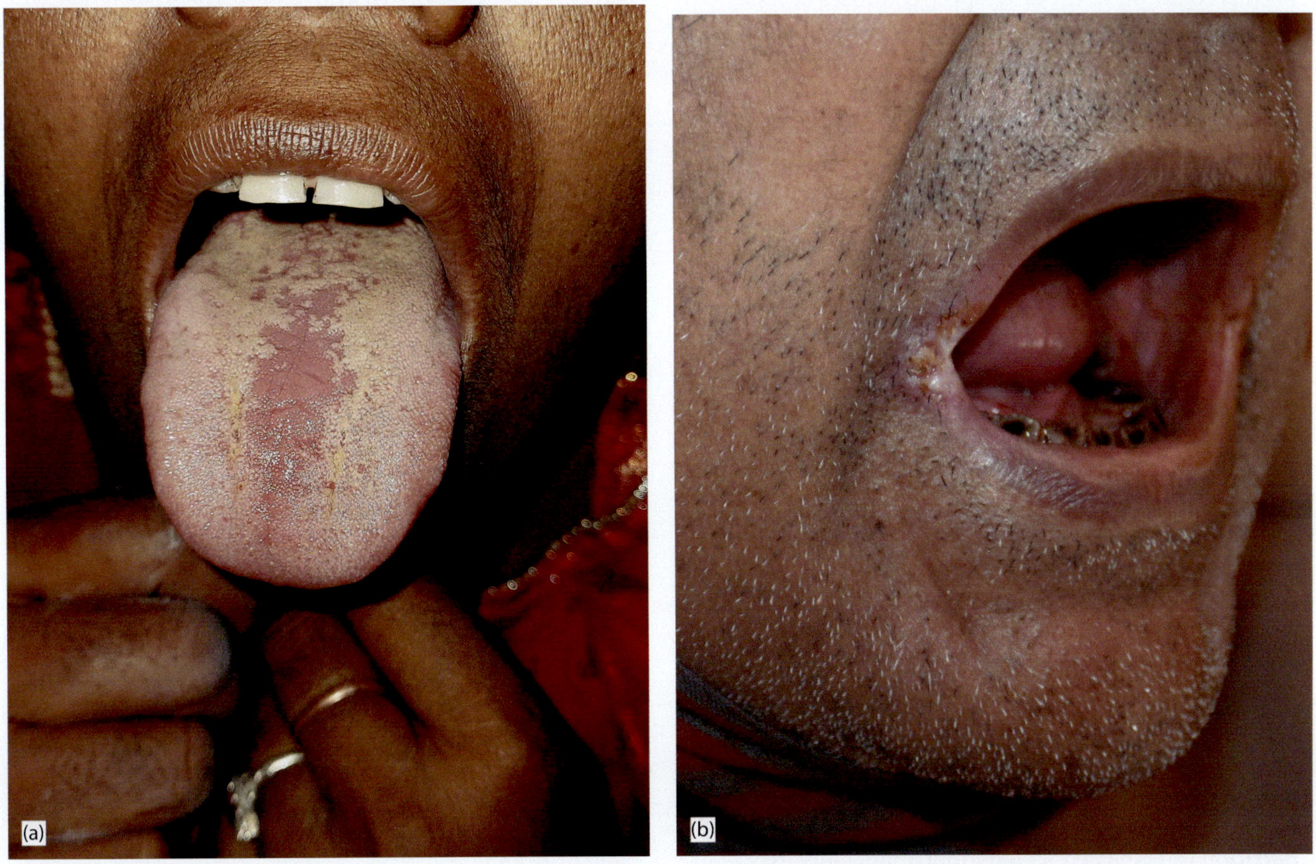

Figure 21.1 **(a)** Loss of papilla in the central part of the tongue. **(b)** Erosion and crusting at the angle of mouth in angular cheilitis.

**BOX 21.2: Genital involvement in riboflavin deficiency**

- Mild: Pruritic dermatitis on sweating
- Moderate: Acute dry phase with erythema, confluent red papule that spreads to involve the perianal area and inner thighs
- Severe: Balanitis and phimosis

  - Genital – males affected more than females; clinical findings vary according to the severity of the condition (**Box 21.2**).
- Cutaneous features include seborrheic dermatitis-like changes and dyssebacia.
- Extracutaneous findings include anemia, peripheral neuropathy, depression.
- DD: Erythema multiforme, fixed drug eruption, zinc deficiency.

## Protein energy malnutrition (PEM)

- PEM is a group of malnutrition disorders that include marasmus, kwashiorkor, and marasmic kwashiorkor (having features of both).
- Marasmus is primarily caused by a deficiency in calories and energy, whereas kwashiorkor is thought to result from protein deficiency. Protein deficiency results in characteristic edematous appearance of kwashiorkor and is absent in marasmus.
- PEM is common in the developing countries of Asia and Africa, and is mostly seen in children and older population.
- Predisposed groups include children from low socioeconomic status, adults with HIV, alcohol and substance abuse, history of gastric bypass surgery, and anorexia nervosa.
- In marasmus, the child appears lethargic and cachetic, with marked loss of subcutaneous fat and muscle wasting. Patients have dry, wrinkled, loose skin and have a "Monkey facies" due to loss of buccal fat. Adults with marasmus may develop additional follicular hyperkeratosis and folliculitis.
- In kwashiorkor, the child appears edematous, with a moon facies and a swollen abdomen. The typical skin change is termed "crazy pavement dermatosis, or mosaic skin" – the skin becomes pigmented and dry, and develops irregular fissures revealing pale areas. The fragile skin peels away in large sheets in an irregular pattern (flaking paint appearance). These changes are characteristically noted over friction- and trauma-prone areas. Other cutaneous findings include erythema, thinning, petechiae, ecchymoses, and purpura. The child is often irritable (**Table 21.4**, **Figure 21.2a–d**).
- In PEM, hairs lose pigmentation and become dry, lusterless, sparse, and brittle. Also, they can be pulled out easily. In patients who have periods of adequate nutrition interspersed with malnutrition, hairs may show alternating dark and pale areas (flag sign). Nail plates become thin and soft and may show Beau's lines. AG, AC, and dry, chapped lips are commonly associated findings. Eyes may show xerophthalmia.

## Vitamin A deficiency

- Risk factors include persons with fat malabsorption, cystic fibrosis, pancreatic insufficiency, cholestasis, people with small-bowel bypass surgery, vegans, refugees, recent immigrants, persons with alcoholism, preschool children with low socioeconomic status.
- The clinical findings include diffuse dryness of skin with pruritus and fine scaling, phrynoderma, dry hair with hyperpigmentation of the hair cast, increased nail fragility, and keratinization of the mucosa.
- Phrynoderma presents as asymptomatic or mildly pruritic, discrete but grouped follicular papules of various sizes with central keratotic plugs that block the follicle openings. The lesions usually appear first on the

Table 21.4 Protein energy malnutrition: kwashiorkor and marasmus

| Features | Kwashiorkor | Marasmus |
|---|---|---|
| Age group | 6 months–5 years | Less than 1 year |
| Predominant etiology | Protein deficiency > Energy deficiency | Energy deficiency |
| Dermatosis, flaky-paint | Flaky-paint dermatosis, crazy pavement dermatitis | Wrinkled, dry skin |
| Hair changes | Common, "Flag sign" and "salt and pepper" appearances | Less common |
| Subcutaneous fat | Reduced | Extreme loss |
| Pitting edema | Present on extremities and face | Absent |
| Face | May be edematous, moon face | Drawn in, monkey-like |
| Growth retardation | Present (–2 SD) | Present (–3 SD) |
| Wasting | Present but not severe | Severe |
| Appetite | Poor | Usually good |
| Mental changes | Very common (irritability, apathy) | Uncommon |
| Anemia | Severe (sometimes) | Present, less severe |
| Response to treatment | Relatively faster | Slower |

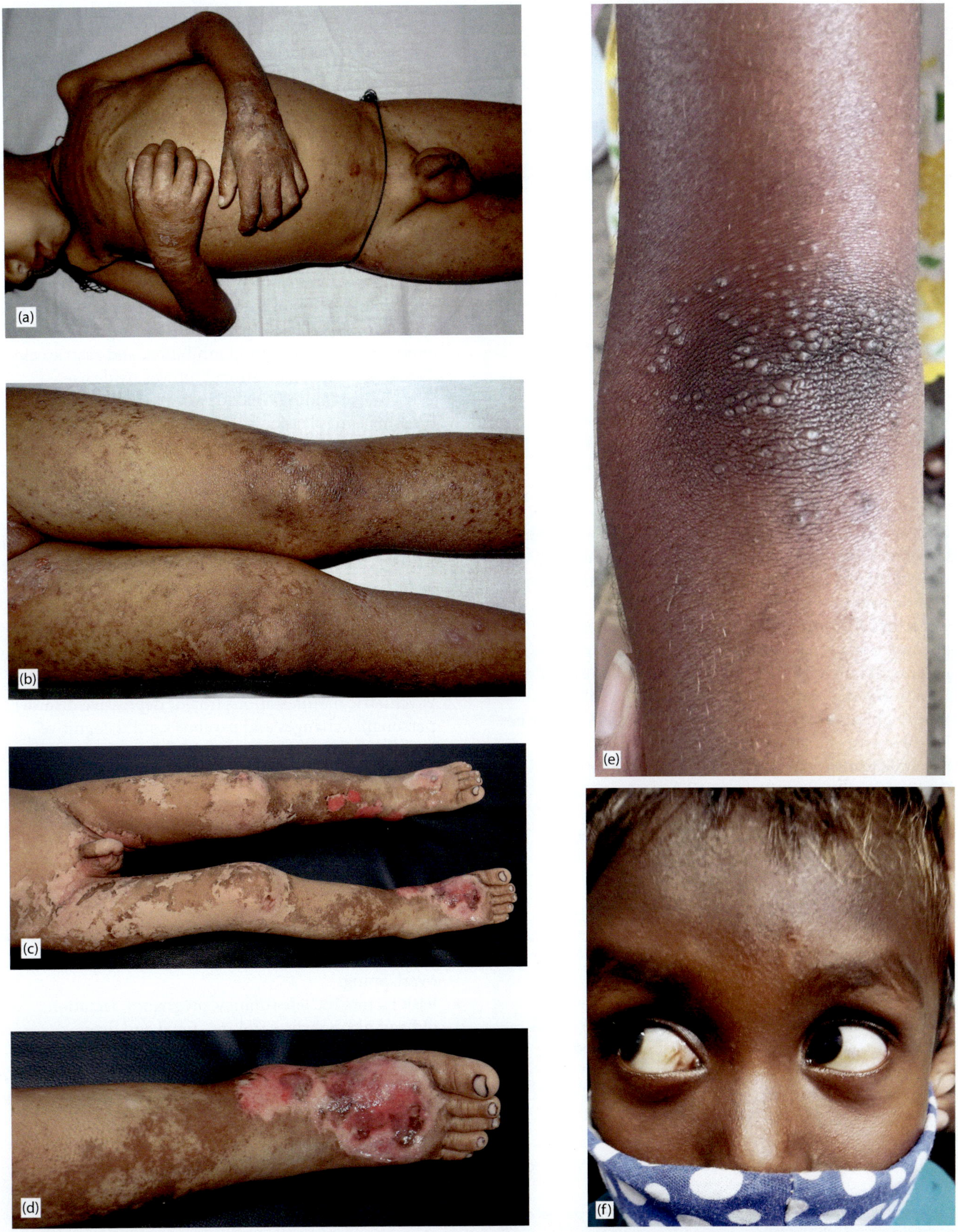


Figure 21.2 **(a)** Generalized exfoliation in a boy with bulging belly, and edema of hands. **(b)** Red-brown areas of epidermal damage and exfoliation in the same patient (Figure 21.2a). **(c)** Skin exfoliation as flaky paint dermatosis and erosions on the legs. **(d)** Close-up of the lesions. **(e)** Follicular papules of phrynoderma on the elbow. **(f)** Bitot's spots. (e – Courtesy: Dr. Anup Kumar Tiwary, Consultant Dermatologist, Yashoda Hospital and Research Center, Ghaziabad, India; f – Courtesy: Dr. Pradeep Kumar Jha, Consultant Ophthalmologist, Darbhanga, India.)

**BOX 21.3: Bitot's spots**

- Bitot's spots are slightly elevated, white lesions seen on the bulbar conjunctiva near the limbus, at the three o'clock or nine o'clock positions. Bitot's spots are more common on the temporal side (**Figure 21.2f**).
- It does not disappear completely, even after the treatment of vitamin A deficiency. Hence, it is not a sign of active VAD.

back of the elbows (**Figure 21.2e**) and the front of the knees, and can spread to involve the extremities, upper forearms, and thighs. Occasionally the abdomen, back, and buttocks may be affected. The face is rarely affected, and hands and feet are spared.
  - It may be seen in the deficiency of vitamin A (commonly), vitamin E and essential fatty acids.
  - DD: Keratosis pilaris, lichen spinulosus.
- Ocular findings include poor adaptation to darkness (nyctalopia), xerophthalmia, Bitot's spots (**Box 21.3**), keratomalacia, corneal perforation, and blindness.

### Essential fatty acids deficiency

- Essential fatty acids (EFA), linoleic acid (LA) and alpha-linolenic acid (ALA), deficiency is rare and is usually seen in infants and children with low EFA in their diet. EFA deficiency is frequently seen with PEM.
- Other risk factors include malabsorption states, pancreatic insufficiency, bariatric surgery, long-term parenteral nutrition, and extreme dietary fat restriction.
- Skin is dry and scaly with some degree of erythema. Intertriginous areas may develop erosions. Hairs may be less pigmented or alopecia may develop.
- Systemic features include growth failure, poor wound healing, increased capillary fragility, and increased susceptibility to infections.
- DD: PEM, vitamin A deficiency, atopic dermatitis.

### Hypervitaminosis A

- Risk factors inclute hepatic and renal compromise, excessive intake of preformed vitamin A.
- Patients complain of joint and bone pain and headache.
- Patients develop loss of hair and coarseness of remaining hair, loss of eyebrows, exfoliative cheilitis, fissuring of corner of mouth and nostrils, generalized exfoliation, pigmentation of face (and neck), and follicular keratotic papules.
- Chronic cases may develop clubbing.

### Vitamin $B_{12}$ deficiency

- Risk factors include strict vegetarianism and veganism, pernicious anemia, malabsorption, atrophic gastritis, surgical resection of the terminal ileum, celiac disease, bariatric surgeries, long-term use of drugs such as metformin, proton-pump inhibitors, and gastric acid-blocking agents, recreational nitrous oxide use.
- The clinical findings include atrophic glossitis (Hunter's glossitis), angular cheilitis, lemon-yellow waxy pallor, hyperpigmentation especially in dark-skinned patients, and brittle hair with premature whitening (**Figure 21.3a,b**).
- Hyperpigmentation is usually generalized with accentuation in flexural areas, palms, and soles, and in areas of pressure, such as the terminal phalanges, knees, and elbows. Mucosal and nail pigmentation too may be observed (**Figure 21.3c,d**).
- Extracutaneous findings include anemia (macrocytic type), neurological findings (**Box 21.4**) (peripheral nervous system and spinal cord involvement), psychiatric manifestations (major depressive disorder, personality changes and psychosis, mild cognitive impairment or dementia), optic nerve atrophy.
- Subacute combined degeneration of the spinal cord (Lichtheim's disease) characterized by patchy losses of myelin in the dorsal and lateral columns may develop in untreated cases.

### Folate deficiency

- Folate and vitamin $B_{12}$ play their roles in a common biochemical pathway, homocysteine remethylation, and hence the clinical picture of their deficiency states is overlapping.
- Risk factors include infancy, pregnancy, lactation, old age, alcoholism, smoking, renal and liver disease, malabsorption states, folate antimetabolites (methotrexate and trimethoprim), malignancy, vitamin $B_{12}$ deficiency (increased urinary loss of folate).

**BOX 21.4: Neurological manifestations in vitamin $B_{12}$ deficiency**

1. Sensory impairment in gloves-and-stocking pattern
2. Diminished vibration sense and proprioception in the legs, varying degrees of ataxia, positive Romberg sign
3. Deep tendon reflexes (DTRs) that may be exaggerated, diminished, or absent
4. Motor involvement and spastic paraparesis autonomic bladder, bowel, or sexual symptoms
5. Positive Babinski sign

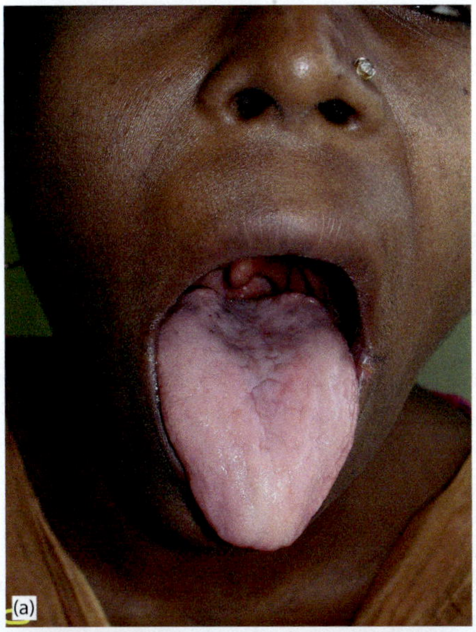

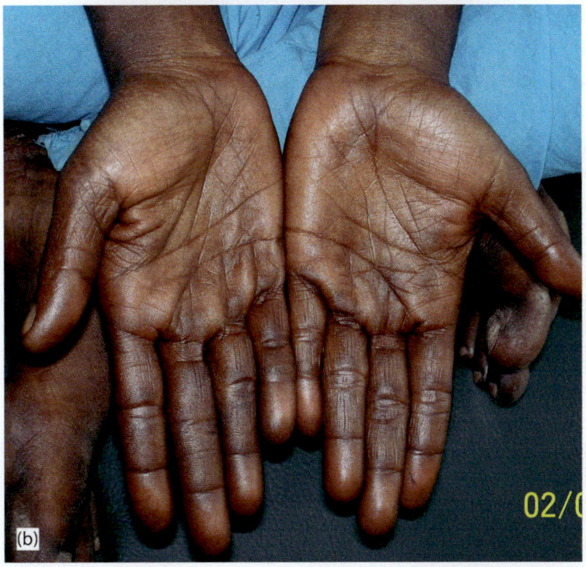

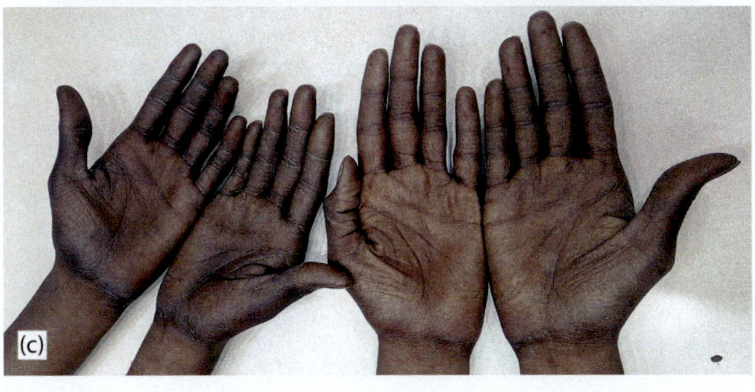

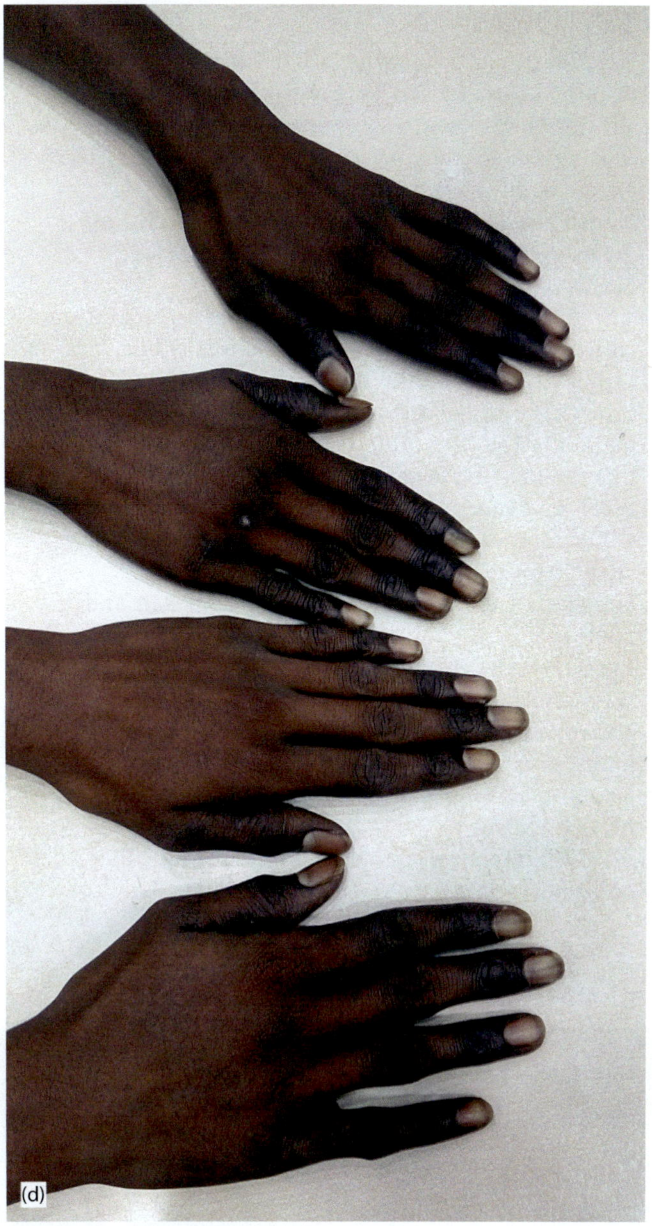

Figure 21.3 **(a)** Atrophic glossitis and angular cheilitis in vitamin $B_{12}$ deficiency. **(b)** Diffuse pigmentation of both palms in vitamin $B_{12}$ deficiency. **(c)** Vitamin $B_{12}$ deficiency in two sisters with diffuse pigmentation of palms. **(d)** Same patients (Figure 21.3c) with increased pigmentation over the knuckles. (c – Courtesy: Dr. Deverashetti Srinivas, Nizamabad, India; d – Courtesy: Dr. Deverashetti Srinivas, Nizamabad, India.)

- Patchy hyperpigmentation of the skin and mucous membranes is present, particularly at the dorsal surfaces of the fingers, toes, and creases of palms and soles.
- Patients may complain of unexplained temperature elevation (< 102°F) and significant weight loss.
- The tongue is swollen and sore and appears beefy-red or shiny, usually around the edges and tips initially. Angular stomatitis is often co-existing. Perineal eczematous lesions and ulcerations may develop.
- Systemic features include gastrointestinal (anorexia, nausea, vomiting, abdominal pain, and diarrhea after meals) and neuropsychiatric (cognitive impairment, dementia, and depression) manifestations.
- DD: Vitamin $B_{12}$ deficiency, Addison's disease.

## Hemochromatosis

- Hereditary hemochromatosis (HH) is an adult-onset disorder characterized by inappropriately high iron absorption resulting in progressive iron overload, causing dysfunction of certain organs – the liver, heart, pancreas, pituitary, joints, and skin.
- HH shows a clear male predilection. In addition, males present earlier and develop more severe disease.
- The cutaneous hallmark is skin hyperpigmentation, which starts early in the disease and may be a presenting feature. Patients develop a diffuse brownish-bronze or, at times, slate-gray pigmentation pronounced over sun-exposed areas like the face. Hyperpigmentation may affect mucosa, teeth, and scars too.
- Other cutaneous findings include ichthyosiform changes (over sun-exposed areas), skin atrophy, koilonychia, and hair loss (including body hair and pubic hair).
- Extracutaneous findings include liver disease (hepatomegaly, and cirrhosis), diabetes mellitus, arthropathy (most commonly affected joints are MCP joints, proximal interphalangeal joints, knees, and wrists), cardiomyopathy, amenorrhea, impotence, hypogonadism.
- DD: Drug-induced pigmentation, actinic reticuloid, beta thalassemia.

## Hypozincemia (Zinc deficiency)[5]

- Acquired form is mostly seen where there are predisposing factors such as pregnancy, lactation, extensive cutaneous burns, generalized exfoliative dermatoses, food faddism, parenteral nutrition, anorexia nervosa, intestinal malabsorption syndromes (inflammatory bowel disease), cystic fibrosis, alcoholism, HIV infection, malignancy, uremia, and chronic renal disease.
- The inherited form (acrodermatitis enteropathica, AE) is mostly seen in children.
- AE typically presents at weaning, with a clinical triad of dermatitis, diarrhea, and alopecia. Initially, the patients develop erythematous, dry, and scaly patches (scald-like appearance) around orifices (perioral and perianal area) and over trauma-prone sites (hands and feet). If left untreated, lesions progress to vesiculobullous, erosive, and crusted lesions. Mucosal findings include angular cheilitis, and glossitis. Patients may develop paronychia and nail dystrophy, and loss of scalp hair, eyebrows, and eyelashes in severe cases. Children are usually irritable and inconsolable (**Figure 21.4a–c**).
    - Ocular involvement is common and manifests as conjunctivitis, blepharitis, punctate keratopathy, and photophobia.

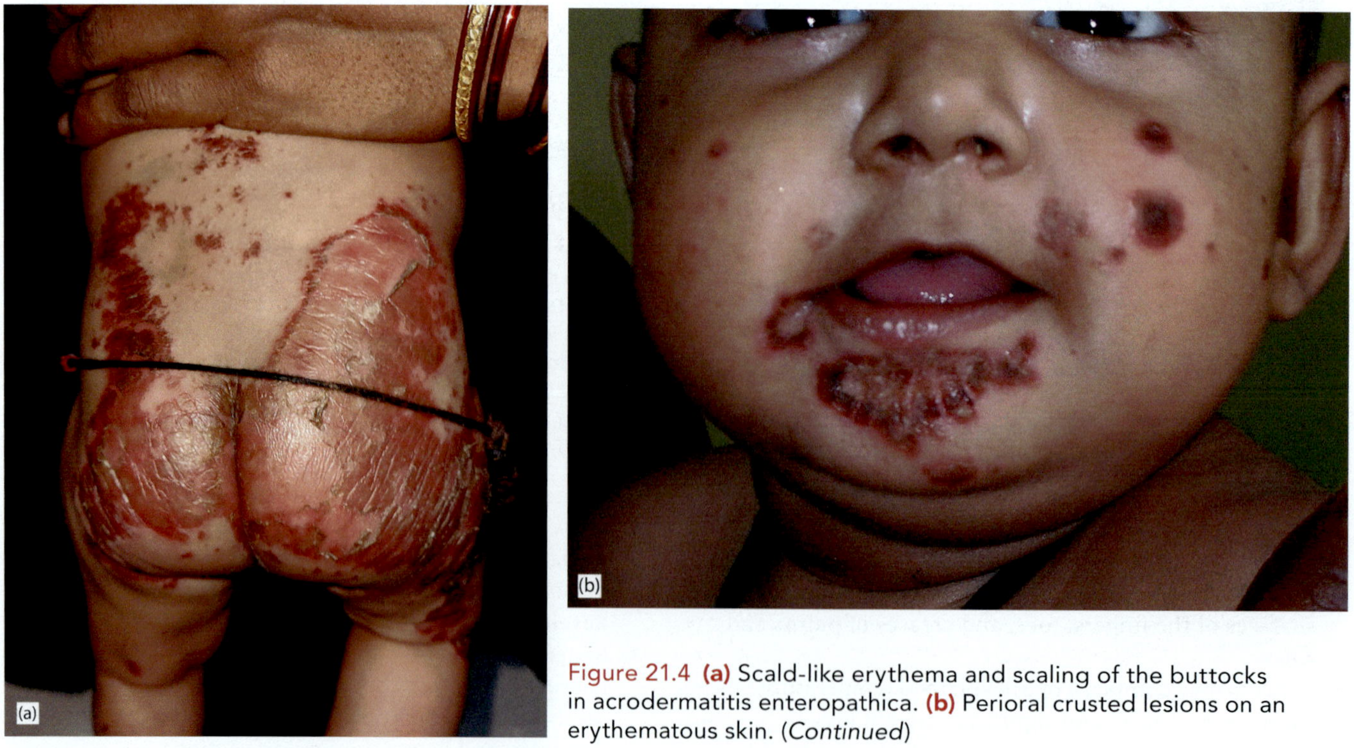


Figure 21.4 **(a)** Scald-like erythema and scaling of the buttocks in acrodermatitis enteropathica. **(b)** Perioral crusted lesions on an erythematous skin. (*Continued*)

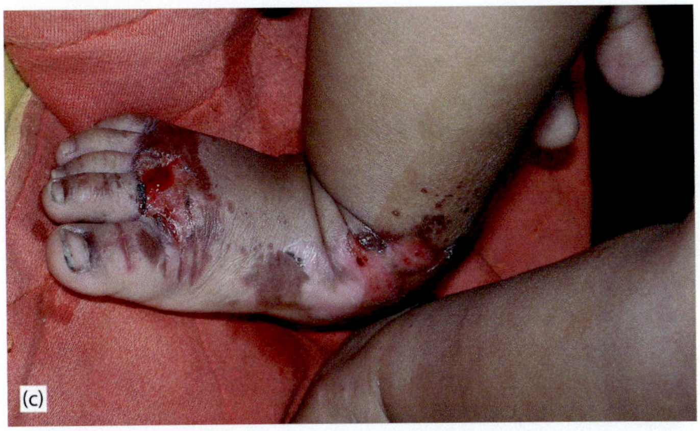


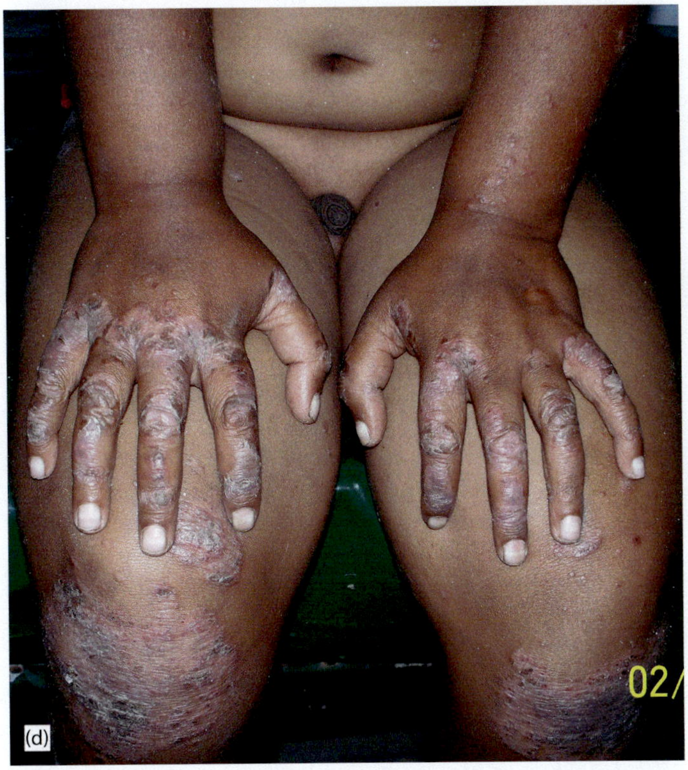


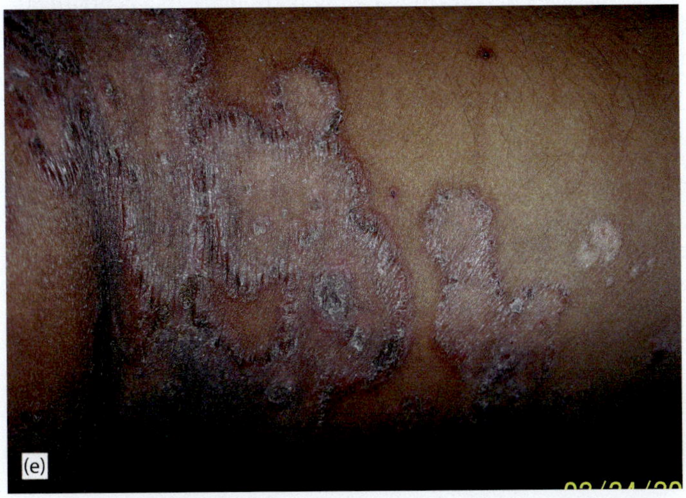


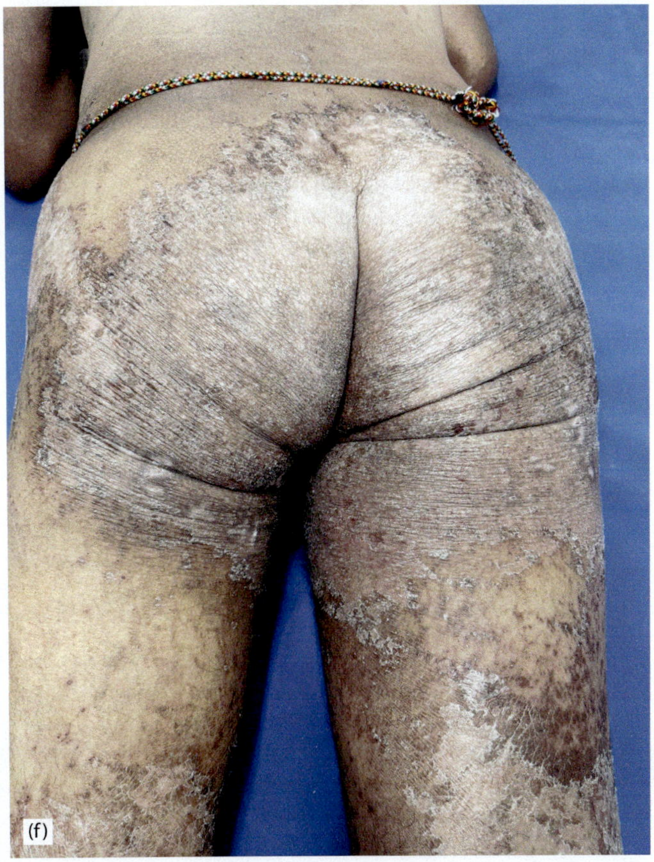


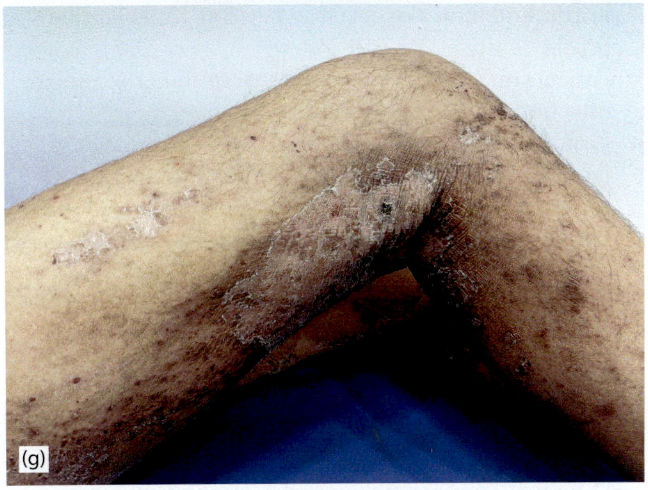


Figure 21.4 (*Continued*) **(c)** Dusky erythematous patches with central erosions on the foot. **(d)** Erythematous, scaly and crusted plaques over trauma prone areas in a case of hypozincemia due to Nephrotic syndrome. **(e)** Close up of lesions over upper thigh- central area heal while the peripheral area shows erythema, scaling and crusting. Without treatment central area, once healed, develops erythematous crusted lesions again. **(f)** Scaly crusted lesions on the buttock and lower extremities in a chronic alcoholic patient. In alcoholic patients, multiple nutritional deficiencies often co-exist and hence, dermatoses cannot be attributed to the deficiency of any one nutrient. **(g)** close up of lesions. (f,g – Courtesy: Dr. Deverashetti Srinivas, Nizamabad, India.)

- The skin changes in acquired form are usually similar but milder and of slower onset. The patients develop eczematous scaly plaques that can develop into vesicles, bullae, or pustules. Periorificial and acral trauma-prone areas are typically affected (**Figure 21.4d–g**).[6]
- Long-standing cases may show frequent infections, delayed wound healing, growth retardation, anorexia, anemia, photophobia, hypogonadism, delayed puberty, and altered mental status.
- DD: Biotin deficiency, essential fatty acid (EFA) deficiency, vitamin $B_2$ (riboflavin) deficiency, necrolytic migratory erythema (NME), pseudo glucagonoma syndrome.

## Biotin deficiency

- Nutritional deficiency of biotin is uncommon. The clinical manifestations of biotin deficiency result more commonly from the deficiencies of enzymes involved in biotin homeostasis (e.g., biotinidase deficiency).
- Risk factors include chronic alcoholism, smoking, inflammatory bowel disease, long-term anticonvulsants therapy, and consumption of excessive amounts of raw eggs.
- Cutaneous findings include dry skin, seborrheic dermatitis-like eruptions and erythematous eczematous rash in periorofacial locations. Hairs become fine and brittle, and total alopecia may develop. Nails may be brittle.
- Patients may exhibit increased susceptibility of fungal infections, especially candidiasis.
- Prominent systemic symptoms include neurological findings (developmental delay, hypotonia, seizures, progressive spastic paresis, myelopathy, encephalopathy, ataxia, etc.), gastrointestinal features (nausea, anorexia), and sensorineural hearing loss.
- DD: Zinc deficiency.

## Pyridoxine (vitamin $B_6$) deficiency

- Risk factors include old age, cirrhosis, chronic renal failure, hemodialysis, peritoneal dialysis, phototherapy for hyperbilirubinemia, drugs (hydralazine, isoniazid, D-penicillamine, pyrazinamide), alcoholism, tobacco smoking, and pregnancy.
- The clinical findings include stomatitis, atrophic glossitis, angular cheilitis, and seborrheic dermatitis-like eruption.
- Extracutaneous findings include neurological findings (distal-limb numbness and weakness, impaired vibration and proprioception, preserved pain and temperature, sensory ataxia, generalized seizures), anemia, cardiovascular (atherosclerosis, early myocardial infarction, recurrent venous thromboembolism), psychiatric (depression).
- Secondary niacin deficiency can result from a deficiency of pyridoxine, which is essential for metabolism of tryptophan and niacin. Hence, patients with prolonged pyridoxine deficiency invariably develop features of pellagra.
- DD: Pellagra, folate deficiency, isoniazid toxicity.

## Pellagra (Vitamin $B_3$ or Niacin deficiency)

- Risk factors include alcohol abuse; diet composed mainly of corn, millet, or sorghum; carcinoid tumors; Hartnup disease; Crohn's disease; anorexia nervosa, restricted diet in atopic dermatitis for food allergy; drugs (isoniazid, 5-fluorouracil).
- The clinical presentation encompasses four Ds: diarrhea, photosensitive dermatitis, and dementia. Death (a fourth D) occurs in untreated cases.
- Cutaneous lesions are typically present on photo-exposed areas. The dorsum of the hands with lesions extending over forearms (glove or gauntlet pattern), feet (usually not extending proximal to malleoli-boot pattern), neck (casal necklace – broad collar-like lesions in cervical dermatomes with C3 and C4 innervation, sometimes with a cravat-like extension anteriorly over the sternum to the level of the nipples), and face (in distribution of the trigeminal nerve) are most commonly affected. Pressure-prone areas like shoulders, elbows, forearms, and knees may be involved in some cases. The symmetry and the line of demarcation from unaffected skin are particularly striking.
- The early skin lesions mimic sunburn. The lesions appear as bilaterally symmetrical erythematous, edematous lesions on photo-exposed areas. Severe cases may develop blisters that may rupture, leaving large denuded areas. The lesions eventually heal with a dusky, brown-red pigmentation. Additionally, patients may develop erythematous, scaly lesions on trauma- and friction-prone areas (**Figure 21.5a–d**).
- The late lesions are characterized by thickened, pigmented skin with a dry, scaly, and fissured surface (parchment-like appearance). Blisters and other acute changes may recur. Healing takes place in a centrifugal manner.
- The tongue may show changes, such as pseudomembranous furs, erosions, and ulcers, but later becomes atrophic. Other findings include angular stomatitis and bleeding from the gingiva. The lips may be inflamed, chapped, or fissured. Genitalia may show erosions and ulcerations.
- Gastrointestinal involvement results in diarrhea, loss of appetite, nausea, vomiting, epigastric discomfort, abdominal pain, and increased salivation.
- Neuropsychiatric manifestations include headache, irritability or apathy, anxiety, delusions, hallucinations, stupor, photophobia, tremor, ataxia, spastic paresis, fatigue, depression and dementia.
- DD: Phototoxic reaction, zinc deficiency, Hartnup syndrome, porphyria cutanea tarda.

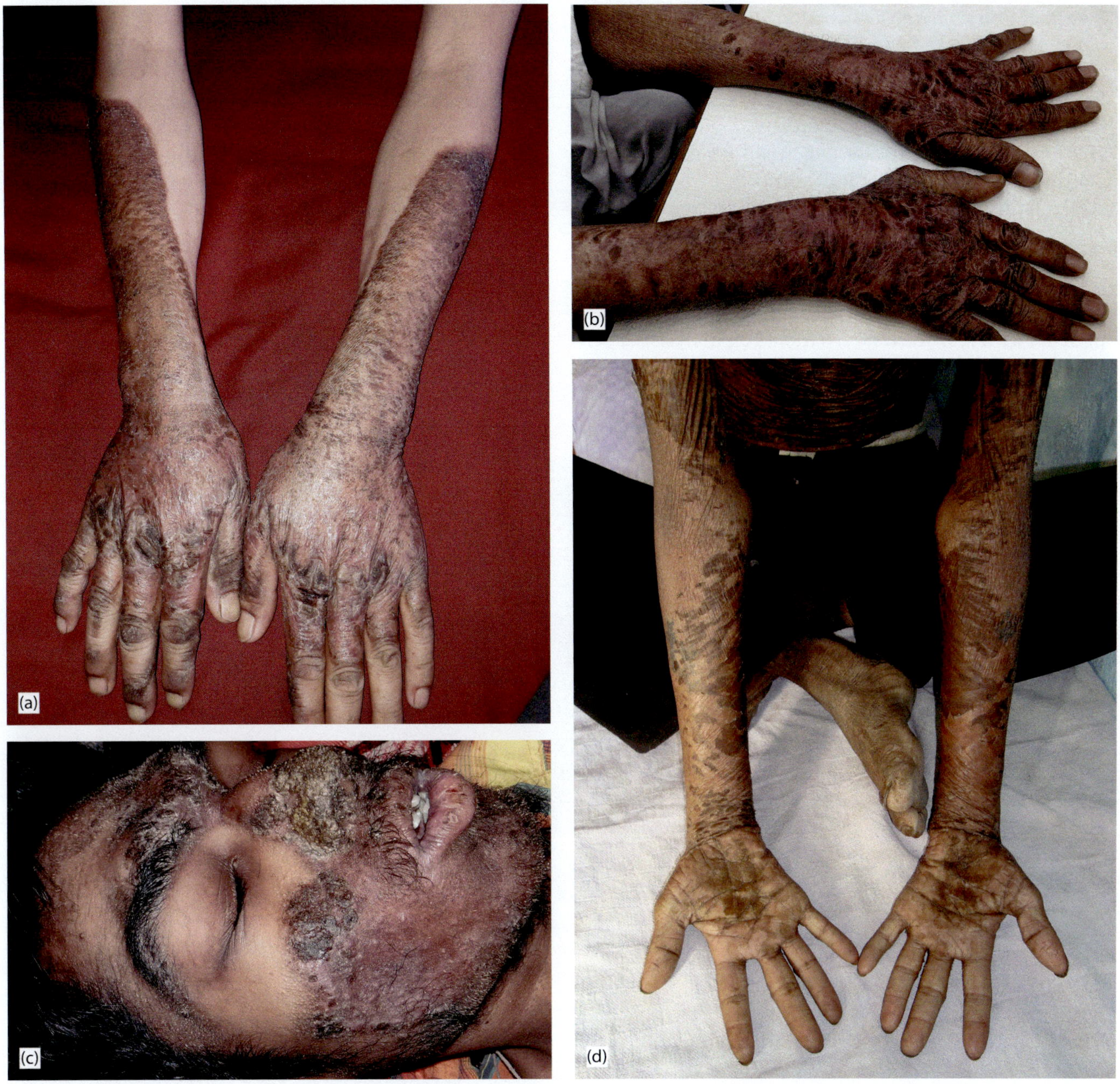


Figure 21.5 **(a)** Bilateral, symmetrical involvement of extensor forearms and dorsum of hands in pellagra. **(b)** Bilaterally symmetrical erythematous, scaly patch in pellagra palms. **(c)** Erythematous patch with crusting at places. **(d)** A severe case of pellagra with extensive involvement of trunk and upper extremities. (a – Courtesy: Dr. Dependra Kumar Timshina, Remedy Skin Clinic, Siliguri, India; b – Courtesy: Dr. Deverashetti Srinivas, Nizamabad, India; c – Courtesy: Dr. Hiral Shah, Baroda Medical College, Vadodara, India; d – Courtesy: Dr. Santoshdev Rathod, SVPIMSR Smt. NHL Municipal Medical College, V.S. Hospital, Ahmedabad, India.)

## Vitamin K deficiency

- Risk factors include neonates, malabsorption (biliary cirrhosis, cystic fibrosis, malabsorption syndromes), anorexia nervosa, drugs (coumarins, salicylates, cephalosporin, cholestyramine, warfarin, salicylates, anticonvulsants), chronic illness, malnutrition, alcoholism, parenchymal liver disease, massive transfusion, chronic kidney disease, and hemodialysis.
- Vitamin K has its major roles in coagulation, bone development, and cardiovascular health.
- There is often a history of profuse bleeding on trivial trauma, epistaxis, hematoma, gastrointestinal bleeding, menorrhagia, hematuria, and gum bleeding.

- Petechiae and ecchymosis, hematomas, and/or oozing of blood at surgical and puncture sites may be evident on clinical examination.
- Infants may develop intracranial bleeding signs – vomiting, poor intake, and seizures.
- DD: von Willebrand disease, deficiency of various clotting factors, scurvy, immune thrombocytopenia (ITP) and thrombotic thrombocytopenic purpura (TTP).

## Scurvy

- Predisposed groups include alcoholics, psychiatric patients with restricted diet, patients on dialysis, people who eat primarily at fast food restaurants, cigarette smokers, refugees and people of low socioeconomic status, pregnant and lactating women, people with type 1 diabetes or with disease of the small intestine.
- The cardinal clinical features consist of four Hs – hemorrhage, hyperkeratosis, hypochondriasis, and hematologic abnormalities.[7,8]
  - Hemorrhages: The bleeding may be superficial (typically perifollicular in location and affects the legs and buttocks where hydrostatic pressure is the greatest) or deep (subcutaneous bleeds presenting as nodules). Spontaneous bleeding may occur from the gums or may be subconjunctival, intra-articular, subungual, and intramuscular hemorrhages. Periosteal hemorrhages in long bones are very painful and cause pseudoparalysis. Affected babies present in a typical immobilized posture with semiflexion of the hips and the knees ("pithed frog").
  - Hyperkeratotic papules: Perifollicular keratotic follicular papules and curling of central hairs (corkscrew like hair) are other characteristic cutaneous findings (**Figure 21.6a,b**).
  - Hypochondriasis.
  - Haematological abnormalities: anemia.
- Other important cutaneous findings include alopecia, increased capillary fragility, poor wound healing, and breakdown of old scars.
- Extracutaneous findings include hypotension, hemopericardium (may cause sudden death), intraocular and retrobulbar bleeding, spongy friable gum with bluish-purple hue, and loose teeth. Scorbutic rosary (beading at the costochondral junctions) and sternum depression are other characteristic bony features.

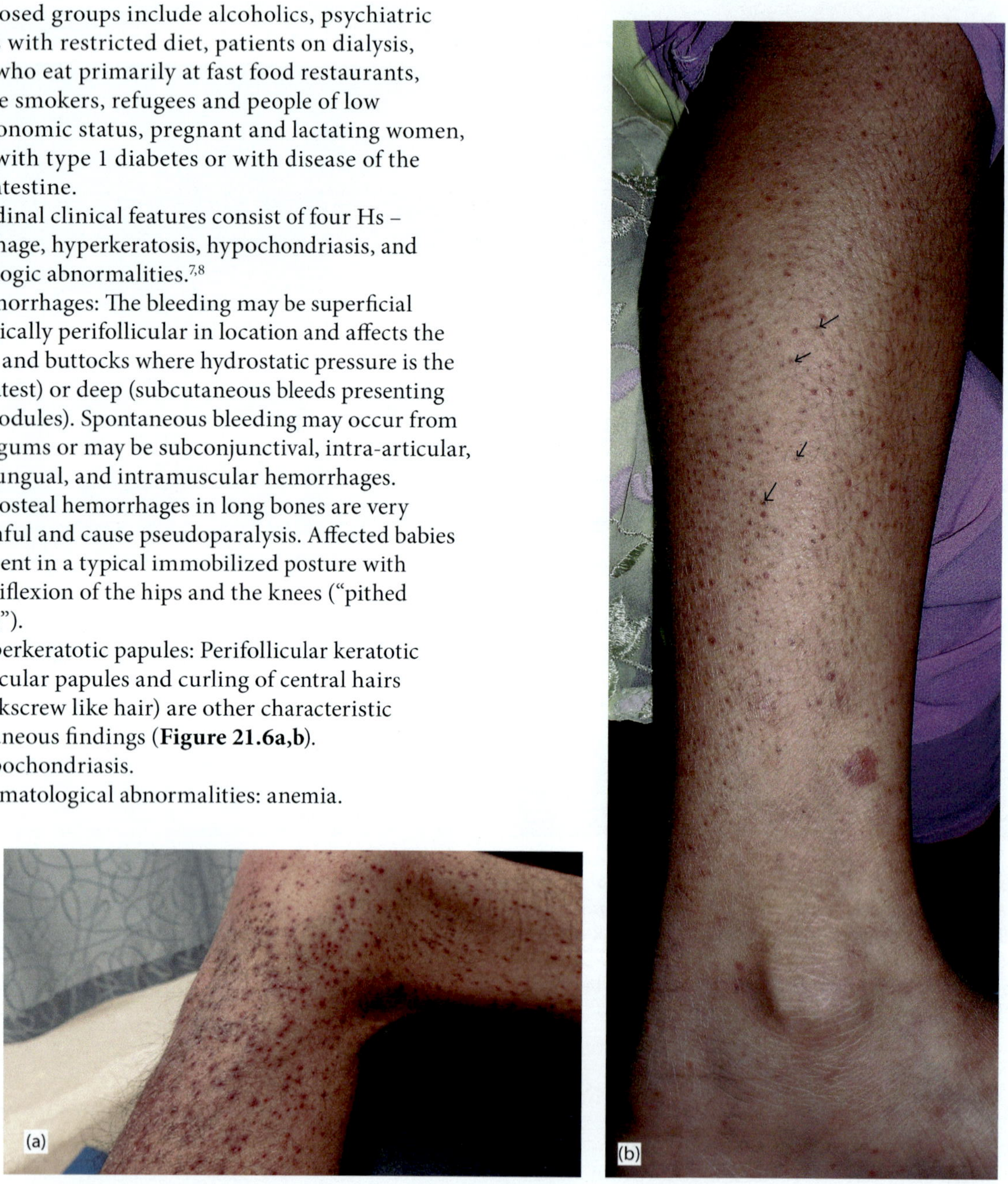


Figure 21.6 **(a)** Perifollicular petechiae in scurvy. **(b)** Perifollicular hemorrhagic lesions on leg of 17-year-old girl. Note twisted broken "corkscrew hairs" (arrow). (a – Courtesy: Dr. Carolina Rincon-Cordoba and Prof Pablo Fernandez-Penas, Westmead Hospital, Sydney; b – With permission from Journal of Pakistan Association of Dermatologists 2011; 21 (3): 202–206.)

- DD: Child abuse. bleeding disorders, hematologic malignancies.

## Carotenemia and Carotenoderma

- Risk factors include excessive ingestion (mango, orange, papaya, carrots, green beans, asparagus, broccoli, cucumber, butter, eggs, milk, etc.), hypothyroidism, diabetes mellitus, pancreatic insufficiency, hepatic disorders, anorexia nervosa, and renal diseases (nephrotic syndrome).
- Patients develop yellow-orange coloration of the skin (carotenoderma), particularly noticeable in palms, soles, forehead, the tip of the nose, and nasolabial folds. Mucosa and sclera are typically spared (**Figure 21.7**).
- Female patients may develop amenorrhea.
- DD: Jaundice (sclera is involved).

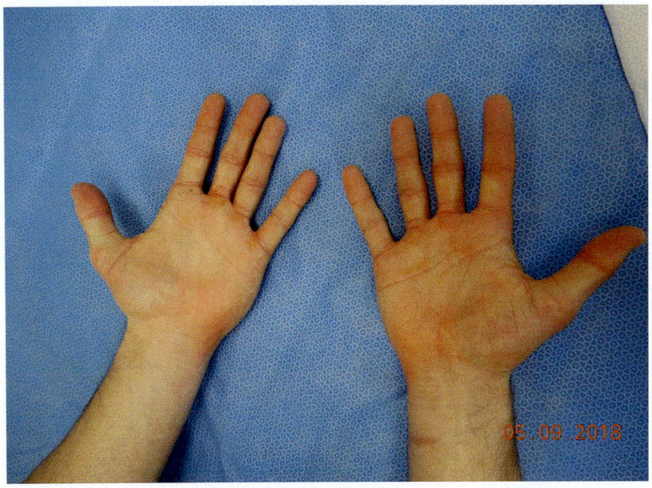

Figure 21.7 Orange palm in carotenemia. (Courtesy: Dr. Carolina Rincon-Cordoba and Prof Pablo Fernandez-Penas, Westmead Hospital, Sydney.)

## Minerals

Minerals of dermatological significance have been summarized in **Table 21.5**.

Table 21.5 Minerals of dermatological importance

| Mineral | Risk groups | Mucocutaneous features | Hair and nail finding | Systemic findings |
|---|---|---|---|---|
| Zinc | Risk group – Premature infants<br>• Inherited (Onset – days to weeks after birth if bottle-fed, or after weaning if breastfed)<br>• Acquired – Low zinc level in mothers milk, alcohol, malabsorption, inflammatory bowel disease, HIV infection, anorexia nervosa, medications like penicillamine, diuretics, valproate | • Mucosa – angular cheilitis, stomatitis<br>• Cutaneous – impaired wound healing, secondary infection (*Candida albicans*, *Staphylococcus aureus*), periorificial and acral dermatitis, psoriasiform dermatitis on extremities | • Hair – alopecia,<br>• Nails – nail dystrophy, paronychia | • Gastrointestinal – diarrhea, dysgeusia<br>• Neuropsychiatric – irritability, emotional, apathetic, listless<br>• Ocular – photophobia, blepharitis, conjunctivitis, abnormal dark adaptation<br>• Others – growth retardation, hypogonadism in males, fatal if untreated |
| Selenium | Patients receiving total parenteral nutrition, low soil content, low-birth-weight infants | Keshan disease (selenium deficiency)<br>• Cutaneous – hypopigmentation of skin | Keshan disease<br>• Hair – hypopigmentation of the hair<br>Thinning and curling (pseudo-albinism)<br>Nails – white nail beds, terry-like nails, Leukonychia | Keshan disease<br>• Cardiovascular system – myocarditis, cardiomyopathy, cardiomegaly, chronic congestive heart failure<br>• Musculoskeletal – muscular pain and weakness<br>• Gastrointestinal tract – hepatic congestion, liver necrosis mesenteric lymphadenosis<br>• Hematology – erythrocyte macrocytosis |

*(Continued)*

Table 21.5 Minerals of dermatological importance (*Continued*)

| Mineral | Risk groups | Mucocutaneous features | Hair and nail finding | Systemic findings |
|---|---|---|---|---|
| | | Selenium toxicity<br>• Cutaneous – reddish hue, swelling, blisters, occasionally ulcer which heal slowly | Selenium toxicity<br>• Hair – dry, brittle rapid loss of hair<br>• Nails – brittle with white horizontal streaking on the surface, nail loss | Selenium toxicity:<br>• Neuropsychiatric – depression dizziness, peripheral anesthesia hyperreflexia, seizures<br>• Gastrointestinal tract – nausea, vomiting, diarrhea hypersalivation, garlic breath odor, hemorrhagic gastritis<br>• Kidney – acute tubular necrosis |
| Copper | Risk group – infants<br>• Causes – low copper level in milk/diet, protein energy malnutrition (PEM) and excessive zinc intake | • Cutaneous – hypopigmentation of skin | • Hair – hypopigmentation of hair | • Musculoskeletal – osteoporosis, fracture, periosteal reaction,<br>• Myeloneuropathy<br>• Ocular – permanent vision loss |
| | Menkes disease (kinky-hair disease) – infants after 2–3 months | Menkes disease<br>• Cutaneous – follicular hyperkeratosis, soft inelastic depigmented skin at the nape of neck, pudgy cheeks, a Cupid's bow of the upper lip | Menkes disease<br>• Hair – alopecia with hair-shaft abnormalities including pili torti, monilethrix, and trichorrhexis<br>• Horizontal eyebrows | Menkes disease<br>• Musculoskeletal – depressed nasal bridge, bony abnormalities like osteoporosis, diaphyseal periosteal reaction, subperiosteal new bone formation, increased risk of fracture<br>• Ocular – ptosis<br>• Central nervous system – growth retardation, lethargy, hypothermia, seizures, developmental delay, failure to thrive<br>• Hematology – anemia,<br>• Renal – hydronephrosis,<br>• Others – high-arched palate, delayed tooth eruption, reduced facial movements |
| Iron | Active menstruating women, vegetarians | • Mucosa – glossitis, angular cheilitis, aphthous ulcer<br>• Cutaneous – pruritis | • Hair – telogen effluvium, lusterless dry focally narrow and split hair shaft<br>• Nails – koilonychia, fragile longitudinal ridging, brittle nails | • Ocular – blue sclerae |

(*Continued*)

Table 21.5 Minerals of dermatological importance (*Continued*)

| Mineral | Risk groups | Mucocutaneous features | Hair and nail finding | Systemic findings |
|---|---|---|---|---|
| | | Plummer-Vinson syndrome<br>• Mucosa – glossitis, smooth atrophy of tongue, thin lip, reduced mouth opening<br>• Cutaneous – dry and wrinkled skin | Plummer-Vinson syndrome<br>• Nails – koilonychia | Plummer-Vinson syndrome<br>• Hematology – microcytic anemia<br>• Orogastric – dysphasia |
| | | Iron overload-<br>• Cutaneous – bronze pigmentation of the skin, ichthyosis | | Iron overload<br>• Cardiovascular system-Cardiomyopathy<br>• Liver – cirrhosis<br>• Endocrinology – diabetes mellitus |

## REFERENCES


1. Galimberti F, Mesinkovska NA. Skin findings associated with nutritional deficiencies. Cleve Clin J Med 2016;83(10):731–739.
2. Heath ML, Sidbury R. Cutaneous manifestations of nutritional deficiency. Curr Opin Pediatr 2006 Aug;18(4):417–422.
3. Lekwuttikarn R, Teng JMC. Cutaneous manifestations of nutritional deficiency. Curr Opin Pediatr 2018 Aug;30(4):505–513.
4. Jen M, Yan AC. Syndromes associated with nutritional deficiency and excess. Clin Dermatol. 2010 Nov-Dec;28(6):669–685.
5. Kumar P, Lal NR, Mondal AK, Mondal A, Gharami RC, Maiti A. Zinc and skin: A brief summary. Dermatol Online J 2012 Mar 15;18(3):1.
6. Kumar P, Anand V, Mallik SK. Hyperkeratotic scaly lesions. Indian Pediatr 2012;49: 935.
7. Kumar P, Debbarman P, Mondal AK, Lal NR, Mondal A, Gharami RC, Maiti A. Perifollicular hemorrhagic lesions and broken twisted hairs on legs. J Pak Assoc Dermatol 2011;21(3):202–206.
8. Tiwary AK, Kumar P. Nutritional Disorders of Skin. In: Lahiri K, De A, editors. Postgraduate Dermatology. New Delhi: Jaypee Brothers;2021. pp. 571–86.

# E33

# Endocrine disorders

VIKAS PATHANIA, SUNMEET SANDHU

## ABSTRACT

Endocrine diseases cause alterations in cutaneous biology because of deficiency or excess of a particular hormone. The mucocutaneous changes may be specific to a particular endocrine disease or may be non-specific, but the constellation of cutaneous and systemic manifestations guide the physicians to the diagnosis.

The text of this chapter is available online at https://routledgetextbooks.com/textbooks/9781032399669/


DOI: 10.1201/9781351054225-58

# E34

# Renal disorders

DEPENDRA KUMAR TIMSHINA, VISHAL GOLAY

## ABSTRACT

Cutaneous manifestations are not uncommon in renal dysfunction, ranging from non-specific hyperpigmentation or pruritus to specific skin or nail changes. Chronic kidney diseases are very common in the population. Careful examination of the skin and nails of kidney patients can provide timely clinical clues about underlying kidney diseases. In this chapter, we discuss the clinical features and differential diagnosis of common cutaneous conditions seen in patients of various renal disorders.

The text of this chapter is available online at https://routledgetextbooks.com/textbooks/9781032399669/

DOI: 10.1201/9781351054225-59

E35

# Autoimmune rheumatic diseases

ANUP KUMAR TIWARY

## ABSTRACT

Autoimmune rheumatic disorders are a vast group of chronic inflammatory conditions that characteristically and invariably involve joints, ligaments, tendons, muscles, blood vessels, subcutaneous tissue, and skin to a variable extent. Though autoimmune rheumatic diseases can present with a diverse range of cutaneous and systemic manifestations, skin manifestations can guide treating physicians in making a clinical diagnosis. This chapter aims at discussing cutaneous signs that can be useful in making clinical diagnosis of various autoimmune rheumatic diseases.

The text of this chapter is available online at https://routledgetextbooks.com/textbooks/9781032399669/


DOI: 10.1201/9781351054225-60

# E36

# Hereditary disorders of connective tissue

RAVI HIREMAGALORE, PIYUSH KUMAR

## ABSTRACT

Inherited-connective tissue disorders arise from mutations in genes coding for molecules such as collagen, elastin, fibrillin, etc., which form the bulk of connective tissues of various organs such as skin, bones, joints, heart, blood vessels, etc. Thus, such disorders can present with a myriad of clinical features, depending on the major organs involved. This chapter discusses the clinical approach to the diagnosis of various hereditary disorders of connective tissues.

The text of this chapter is available online at https://routledgetextbooks.com/textbooks/9781032399669/

DOI: 10.1201/9781351054225-61

E37

# Hepatic diseases

GAUTAM KUMAR SINGH

## ABSTRACT

Mucocutaneous changes are quite common in patients with liver diseases. Many of these changes, though common, are non-specific; not only can they be seen in patients without liver diseases, but also they generally do not point to a specific underlying liver disease. However, they can be telltale signs of underlying liver disease, and they contribute to morbidity, requiring a physician's attention. This chapter discusses various dermatoses associated with underlying liver diseases.

The text of this chapter is available online at https://routledgetextbooks.com/textbooks/9781032399669/

 DOI: 10.1201/9781351054225-62

# E38

# Cardiovascular diseases

PREEMA SINHA, ANWITA SINHA

## ABSTRACT

Many cardiovascular diseases are associated with both non-specific and specific cutaneous findings and signs. For example, pedal edema is a non-specific sign, raising the possibility of underlying cardiovascular disease. On the other hand, Osler nodes and erythema marginatum are characteristic of infective endocarditis and acute rheumatic fever respectively. Awareness and identification of dermatoses associated with cardiovascular diseases are useful for both dermatologists and internists.

The text of this chapter is available online at https://routledgetextbooks.com/textbooks/9781032399669/

DOI: 10.1201/9781351054225-63

# E39

# Neurocutaneous conditions

SATYAKI GANGULY

## ABSTRACT

Both the central nervous system and skin are derived from embryonic ectoderm. Mutations affecting the formation, migration, and differentiation of these cells give rise to a group of diseases, collectively called neurocutaneous syndrome. Mucocutaneous manifestations are telltale signs and provide crucial clinical clues to the diagnosis of these conditions. This chapter discusses the clinical approach to the diagnosis of various neurocutaneous syndromes based on predominant cutaneous findings.

The text of this chapter is available online at https://routledgetextbooks.com/textbooks/9781032399669/



DOI: 10.1201/9781351054225-64

# 22

# Psychocutaneous disorders

SWETALINA PRADHAN, GAURAV DASH

## INTRODUCTION

Psychocutaneous disorders are commonly encountered in dermatology. Patients usually have a primary psychiatric disease with cutaneous manifestations. Most patients are apprehensive about visiting a psychiatrist, but they do visit a dermatologist for treatment of their skin problems. Therefore, dermatologists can play a key role in the management of these disorders. Most of the time clinical diagnosis is challenging, as these disorders mimic a variety of dermatological conditions. In this chapter we discuss clinical clues to diagnose such conditions and how to clinically differentiate them from other disease entities.

### When to suspect psychocutaneous disorders? [1,2]

- Psychocutaneous disorders may be suspected when the history of the patient does not match the lesions.
- They are mostly seen in emotionally unstable patients, more commonly in adolescent or middle-aged females.
- They are commonly seen in patients with other psychiatric illnesses or with a history of emotional or physical abuse.
- They are clinically suspected when there are bizarre lesions at various stages of healing over approachable areas without proper history.

The clinical approach to various psychocutaneous disorders is summarized in **Figure 22.1**, and some of these conditions are discussed here.[1–4]

### Prurigo simplex (chronic prurigo of adults, prurigo mitis, subacute prurigo, and Hebra prurigo)

- Prurigo simplex is characterized by intense itching that is relieved only when the patient scratches the lesion until it bleeds.
- The condition is mostly seen in middle-aged and elderly persons of both genders. Most patients have neurotic behavior patterns and overreact to the pruritus.
- The trunk and extensor aspects of the extremities are common sites. Other areas include the face, neck, and buttocks (**Figure 22.2a,b**).
- The primary lesion is an erythematous papule with a tiny vesicle in the center. The lesions appear in crops and tend to be symmetrically distributed. The lesions are so pruritic that they are immediately attacked and are rarely observed by physician.
- Secondary lesions are what one usually observes, which include excoriations and crusts. Lesions heal with

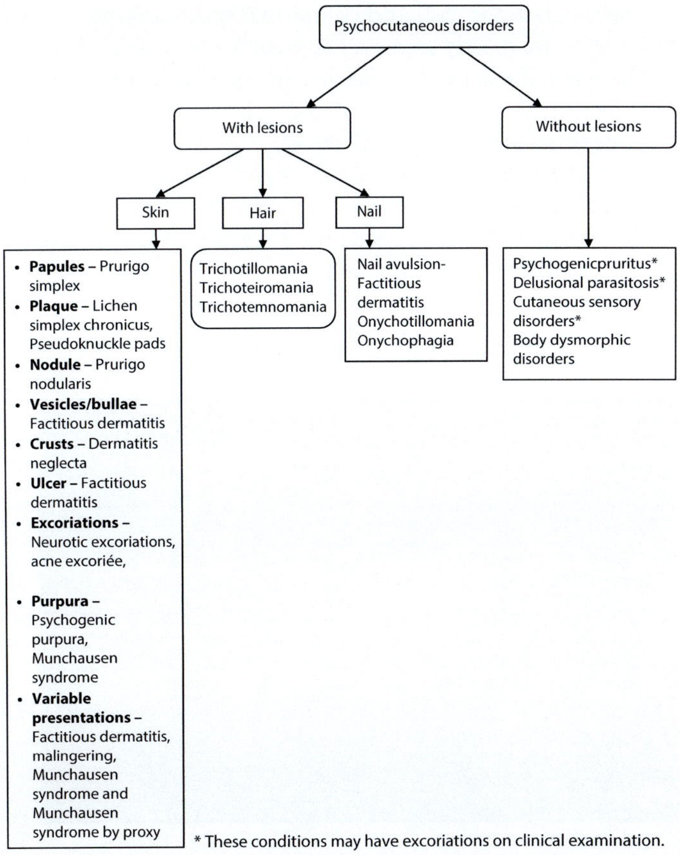


Figure 22.1 Clinical approach to psychocutaneous disorders.

DOI: 10.1201/9781351054225-65

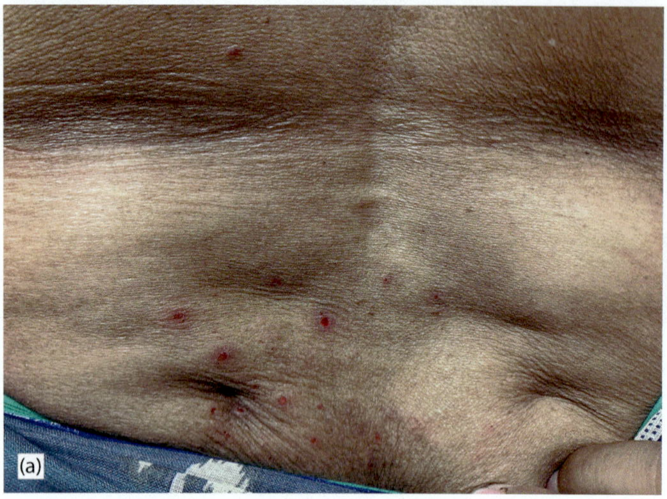


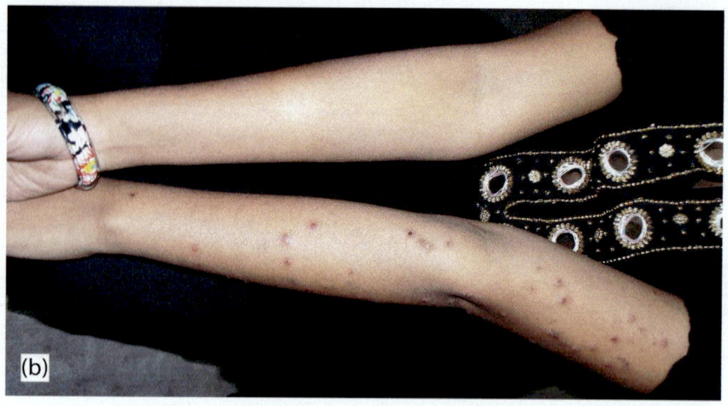


Figure 22.2 **(a)** Excoriated papules of prurigo simplex in a middle aged lady. **(b)** Prurigo simplex affecting extensor aspect of upper extremity. (a,b – Courtesy: Dr. Piyush Kumar, Katihar, India.)

hypopigmented, atrophic scars with hyperpigmented margins.
- DD: Scabies, atopic dermatitis, insect-bite reactions, papular urticaria, dermatitis herpetiformis, contact dermatitis, pityriasis lichenoides et varioliformis acuta (PLEVA).

## Lichen simplex chronicus

- Well-developed lesions present as circumscribed lichenified plaques (pigmented, thickened, and slightly scaly) with excoriations on the surface with characteristic accentuation of normal skin marking.
- Lesions are mostly seen over approachable areas such as the scalp, the nape of the neck, legs, extensor aspects of the arms, scrotum (in males) and vulva (in females), and anogenital areas (**Figure 22.3a–c**).
- These lesions are characterized by paroxysmal itching and scratching.
- DD: Psoriasis (well-defined raised erythematous plaques with loose whitish scales on the surface), hypertrophic lichen planus (well-defined lichenified plaque with central depigmentation and atrophy).

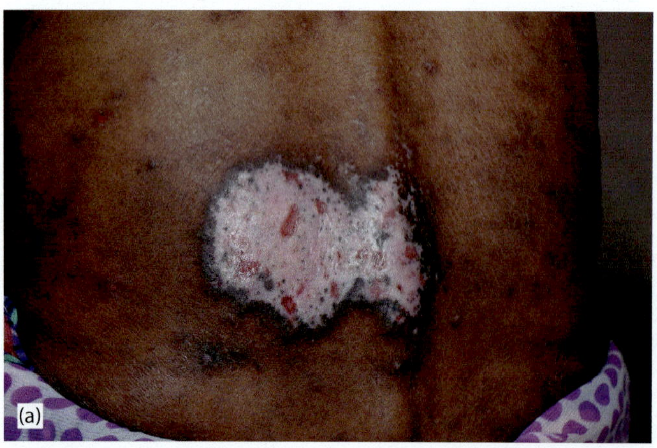


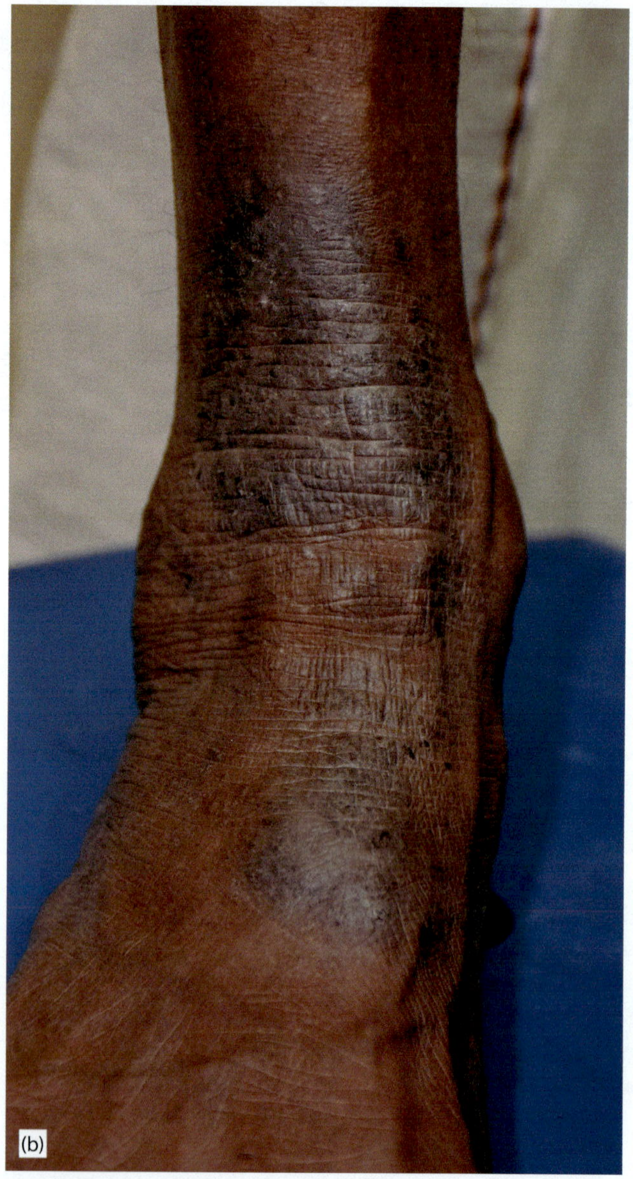


Figure 22.3 **(a)** Lichenified plaque on the back. The margin is well defined and hyperpigmented, and the surface is remarkable for erosions. **(b)** Lichen simplex chronicus over extensor aspect of ankle and dorsum of foot. (*Continued*)

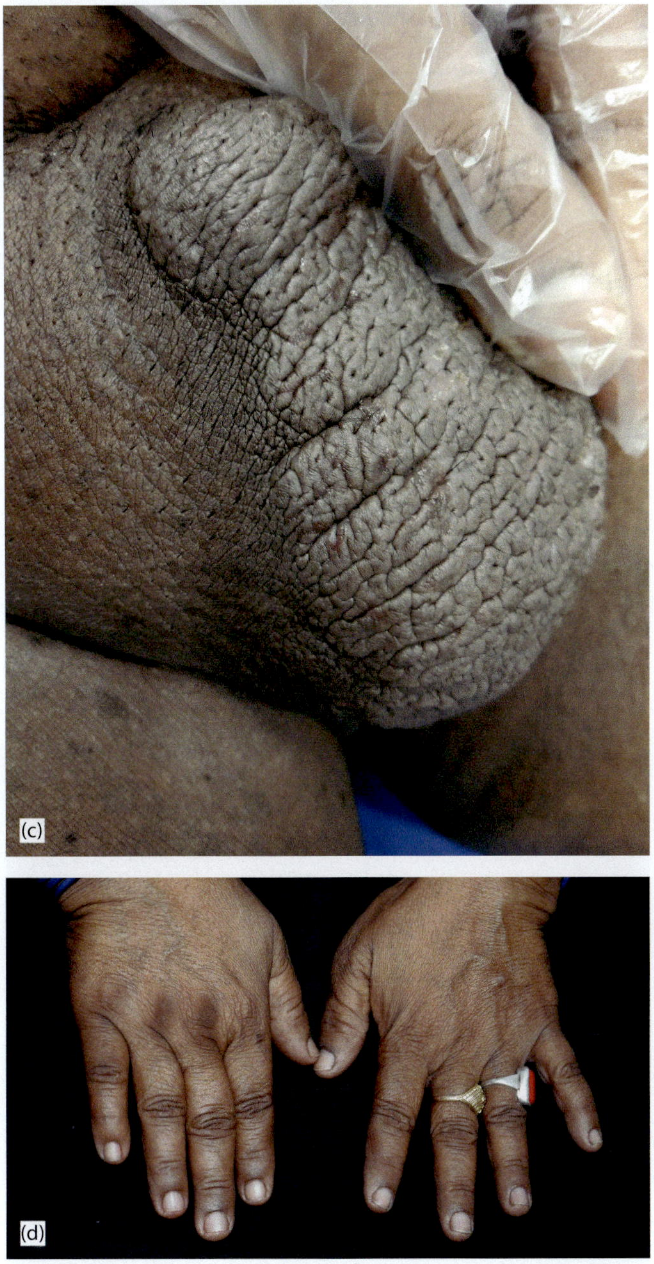


Figure 22.3 (*Continued*) **(c)** Lichen simplex chronicus affecting the scrotum. Note the well-defined margin of the lesion. **(d)** Unilateral lichenified plaques of pseudo knuckle pads. (a,b,d – Courtesy: Dr. Piyush Kumar, Katihar, India; c – Courtesy: Dr. Deverashetti Srinivas, Nizamabad, India.)

## Pseudo-knuckle pads

- Pseudo-knuckle pads occur after repeated trauma or friction.
- Commonly seen in children with obsessive behavior as "chewing pads" and in adults as an occupational disorder.
- Common sites are the dorsal surface of the fingers (knuckles) and hand joints.
- It presents as a hypertrophic lesion on the joints, usually unilaterally (**Figure 22.3d**).

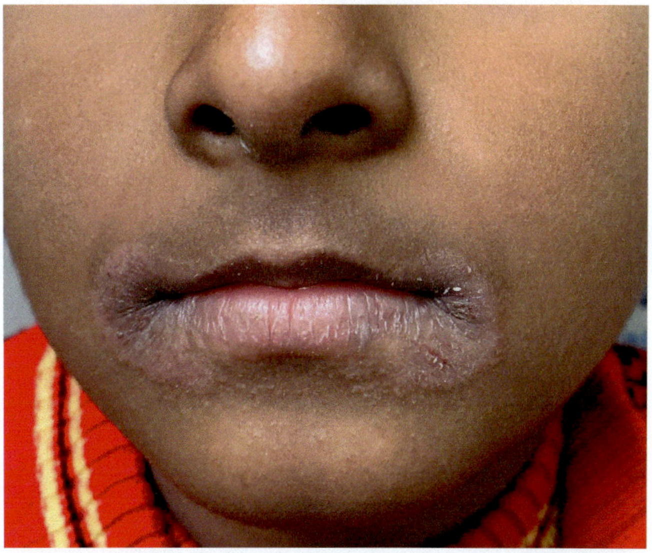

Figure 22.4 A young girl with factitious cheilitis presenting with erythema and scaling of the lips and surrounding area. (Courtesy: Dr. Piyush Kumar, Katihar, India.)

- In purging types of anorexia and bulimia nervosa, callosities develop over the knuckles of the dominant hand due to constant friction with the incisors during induced vomiting. This is known as Russell's sign.
- DD: True knuckle pads (unrelated to trauma).

## Factitious cheilitis

- Factitious cheilitis is commonly seen in children with compulsive disorders.
- The main mechanism is repeated licking of lips, with or without biting.
- Patient presents with irritant contact dermatitis, crusting, and ulceration of lips (**Figure 22.4**).
- DD: Actinic cheilitis.

## Prurigo nodularis

- Nodules are distributed chiefly on extremities, especially on the anterior aspect of the thighs and legs.
- Hyperpigmented, hyperkeratotic nodules and/or plaques with injury or excoriation occur on the surface. The margins of individual lesions are often pigmented (**Figure 22.5a,b**).
- Lesions heal with scarring, and new lesions keep appearing insidiously.
- There is paroxysmal itching severe enough to be relieved only by scratching to the point of damage.
- Background skin has excoriation and lichenified changes.
- DD: Lichen planus hypertrophicus (**Table 22.1**).

## Obsessive-compulsive disorder (OCD)

- It is a common anxiety disorder in which patients have repeated and unwanted thoughts or ideas that compel them to act upon to provide a sense of temporary relief.

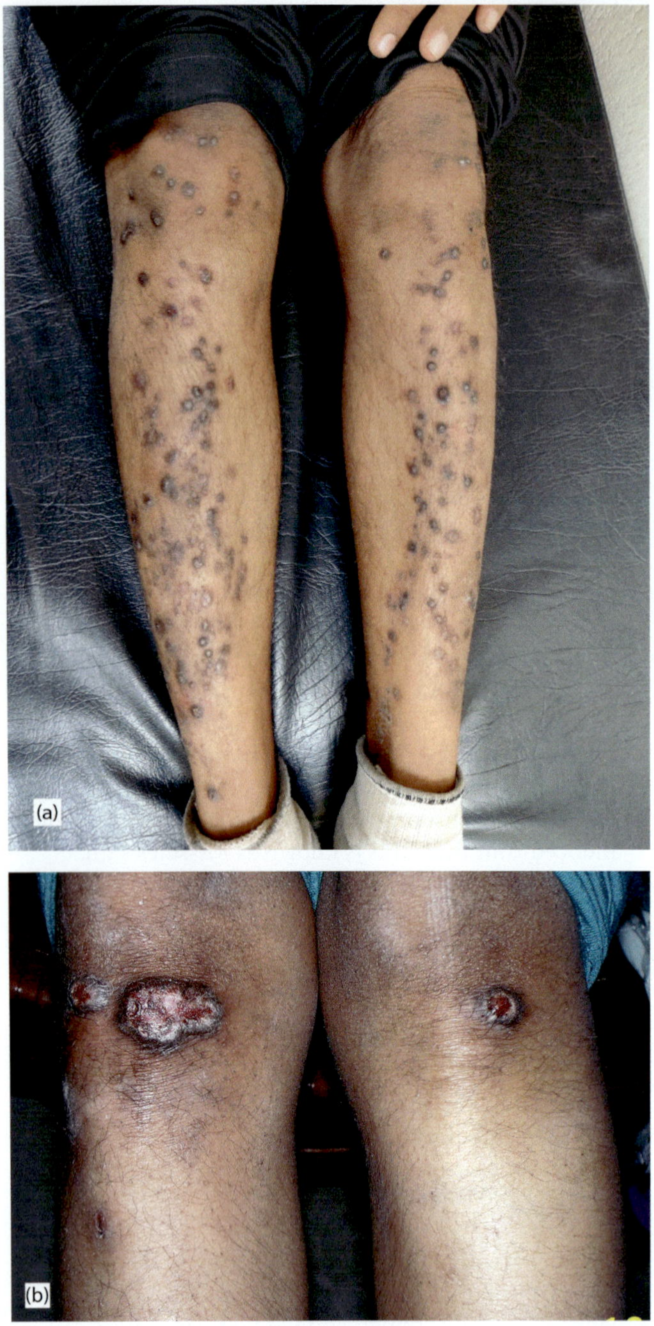

Figure 22.5 **(a)** Multiple nodules of prurigo nodularis on extensor aspect of both shins. **(b)** Prurigo nodularis presenting as well-defined plaques with eroded top and pigmented margin. (b – Courtesy: Dr. Piyush Kumar, Katihar, India.)

- Obsession of cleanliness leads to repeated hand washing, using detergents and other chemicals to clean the house, repeated bathing, excess use of soap and shampoo.
- Commonly seen in young and middle-aged women.
- Excess hand washing and use of water often leads to candidiasis or irritant contact dermatitis due to overuse of soaps and detergents (**Figure 22.6a,b**).
- Irritant contact dermatitis due to OCD of cleanliness is also known as "washing eczema."

Table 22.1 Lichen planus hypertrophicus and prurigo nodularis

| Features | Lichen planus hypertrophicus | Prurigo nodularis |
|---|---|---|
| Excoriations | Not seen | Present |
| Itching | Patients usually rub the lesions | Very severe itching, may lead to injury marks on the surface |
| Perilesional lesions | Perilesional papules of lichen planus may be seen | No such lesions seen |
| Background skin | Appears normal | Has excoriations and lichenified changes |

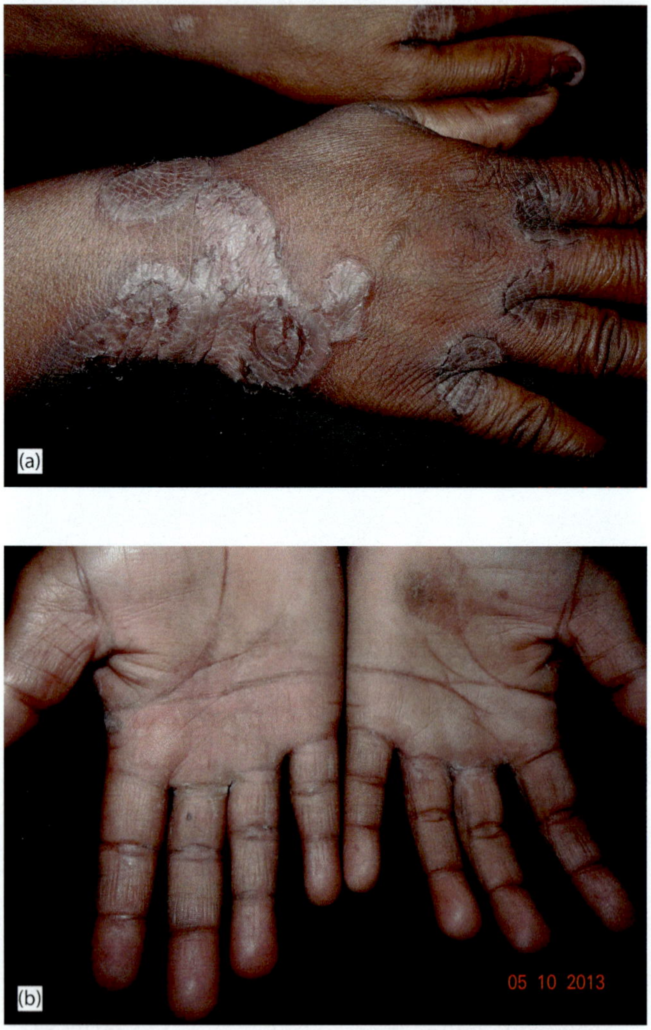


Figure 22.6 **(a)** A middle-aged lady with compulsive hand washing presenting as candidiasis- dorsal aspect. **(b)** Candidiasis of the palmar aspect. Note preferential involvement of creases. (a,b – Courtesy: Dr. Piyush Kumar, Katihar, India.)

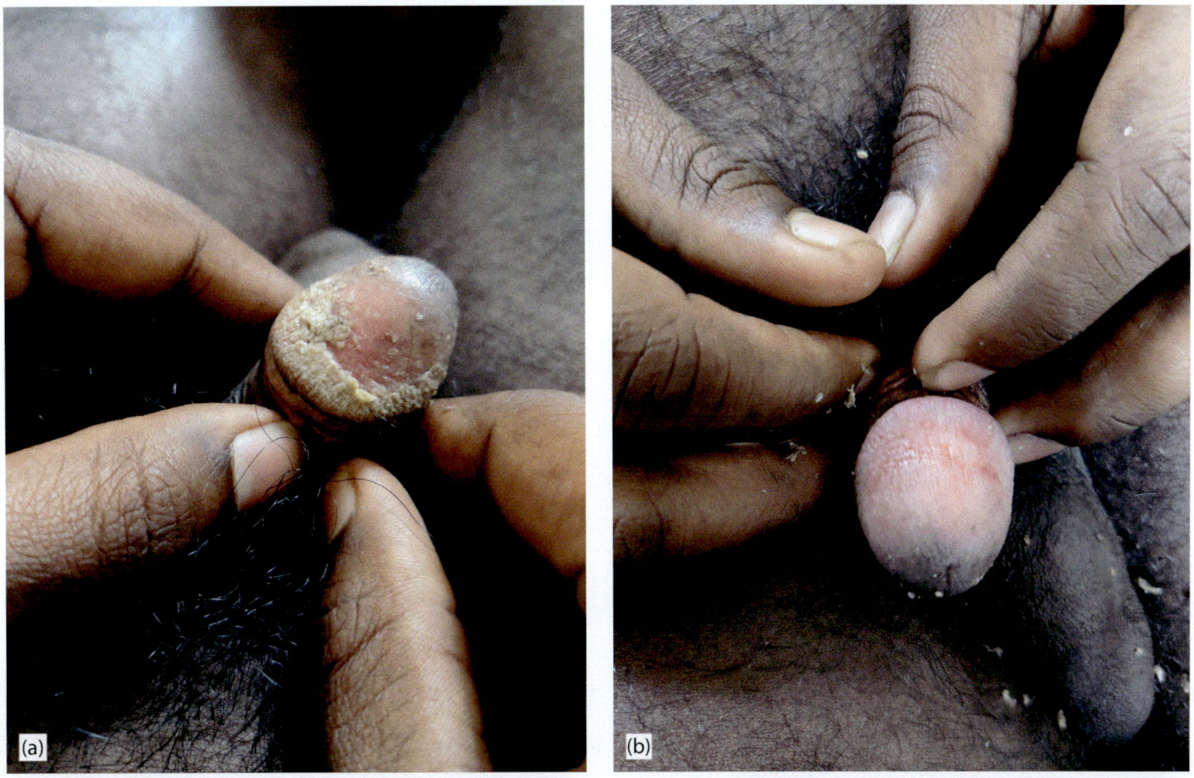


Figure 22.7 **(a)** Keratinous debris on the glans penis and inner prepuce in a case of dermatitis neglecta. **(b)** Clearance of keratinous material after cleaning with ethyl alcohol swab.

## Dermatitis passivata (dermatitis neglecta)

- It is commonly seen in geriatric or demented patients who suffer from self-neglect.
- Lesions are usually found on the upper central chest, over the back.
- The cessation of normal skin cleansing will produce an accumulation of keratin and dirty debris that forms a thick carapace with time (**Figure 22.7a,b**).
- It's extreme form has been called the Diogenes syndrome.

## Dermatitis artefacta

- It is a factitious disorder in which patients inflict cutaneous lesions upon themselves to satisfy a psychological need of which they are usually not consciously aware.
- Usually seen in adolescent women.
- Patients present with various kinds of lesions, such as purpura, blisters, ulcers, and erythema only over approachable sites. These lesions are polymorphic and bizarre in shape with geometric borders and angulated edges surrounded by normal skin, or they assume patterns that do not conform to any recognized skin disease morphology (**Figure 22.8a–c**).
- The patient usually gives a hollow history with unclear initiation or evolution of lesions.

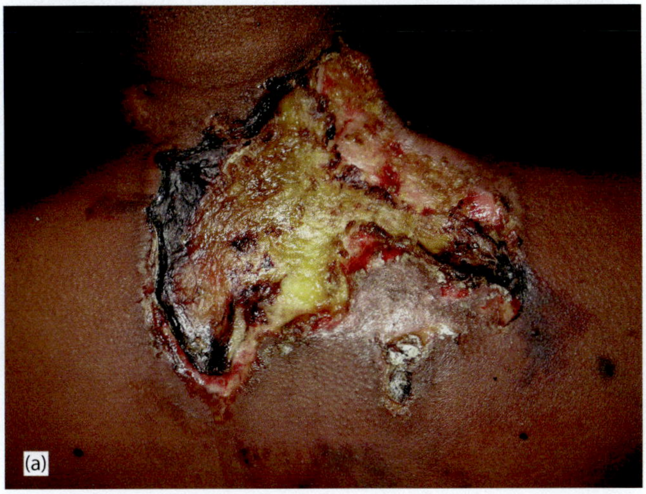


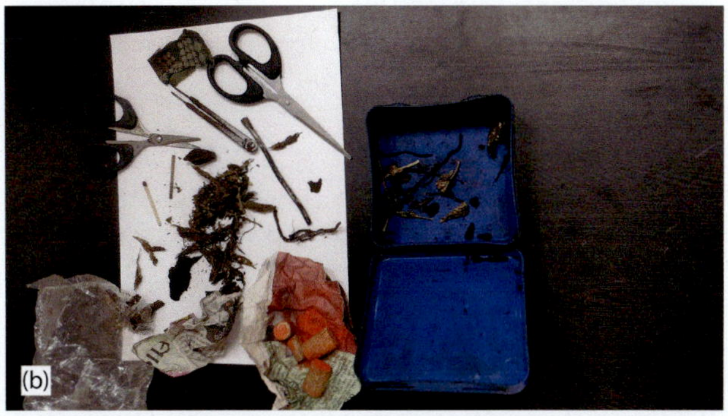


Figure 22.8 **(a)** Geographic-shaped ulcer on the upper back. The patient injured himself with scissors and other sharp objects. **(b)** Sharp objects and medicinal herbs found in possession of the patient. *(Continued)*

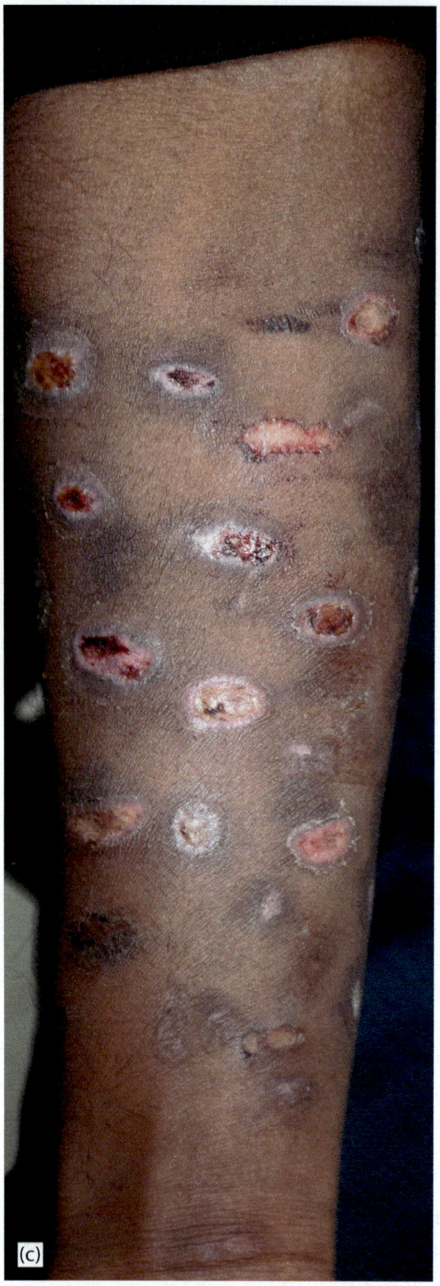

Figure 22.8 (*Continued*) **(c)** Ulcers of different depths in dermatitis artefacta. The guy developed these lesions after getting separated from his girlfriend. (c – Courtesy: Dr. Piyush Kumar, Katihar, India.)

## Neurotic Excoriations

- It is an obsessive-compulsive disorder characterized by a repetitive and compulsive desire to pick, scratch, or rub the skin.
- It is most commonly seen in middle-aged women.
- It is associated with depression.
- The face is the most commonly affected site. Other sites include accessible areas like the extensor aspects of the forearms, arms, legs, thighs, face, and upper trunk. Unreachable areas such as the central mid-upper back are spared.
- Multiple lesions are seen in various stages of evolution. There may be small superficial erosions to deep ulcerations with linear/angular or circular/oval shapes varying from 2 mm to several cm caused by repeated picking or scratching.
- The lesions heal with post-inflammatory hyperpigmentation and leave behind hypo- or hyperpigmented scars.
- DD: Prurigo simplex, atopic dermatitis.

## Acne excoriée

- Patients usually have mild acne, but they pick and squeeze the lesions, leading to scarring.
- It presents as excoriations on a background of acne lesions (**Figure 22.9a,b**).
- Most frequently seen in young women.
- DD: Facial picking disorder (where there are no acneiform lesions originating the picking habit), trigeminal trophic syndrome, dermatitis artefacta.

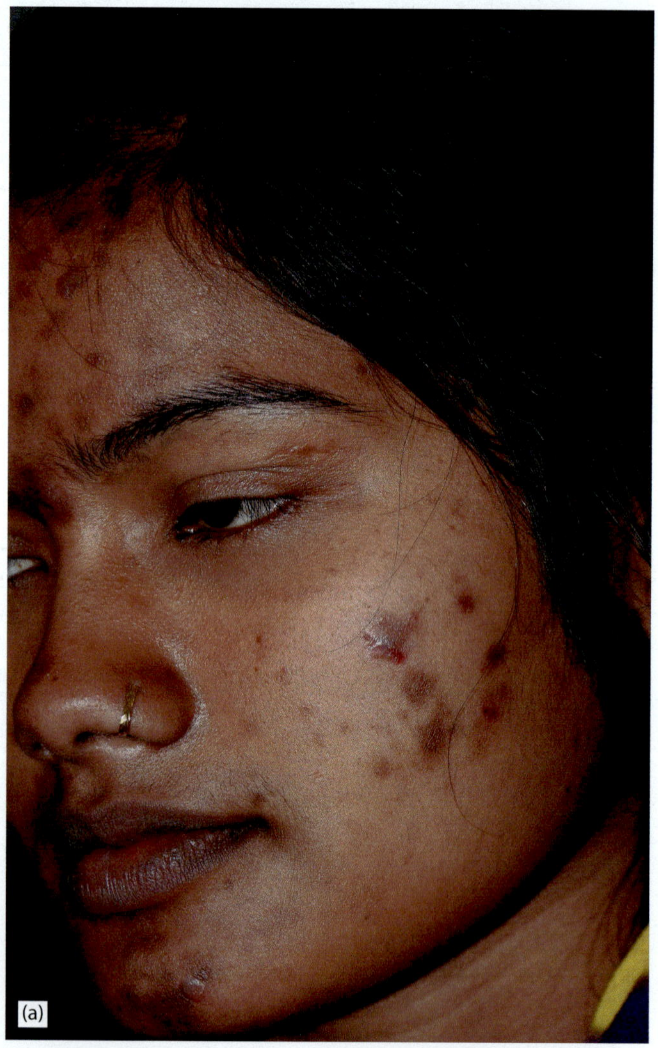

Figure 22.9 **(a)** Punctate excoriations on the face in a young female with acne vulgaris. Older lesions have healed with post-inflammatory hyperpigmentation. (*Continued*)

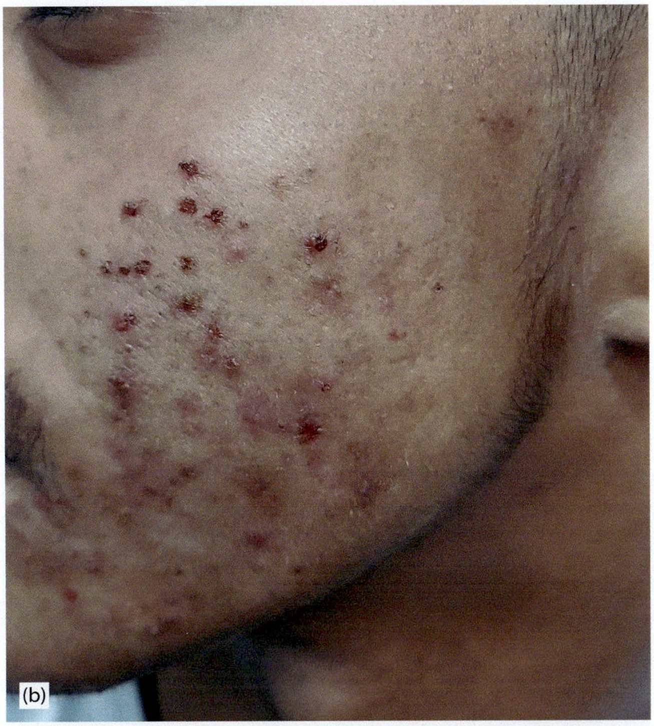


Figure 22.9 (*Continued*) **(b)** Acne excoriae presenting as erosions and crusting. (a,b – Courtesy: Dr. Piyush Kumar, Katihar, India.)

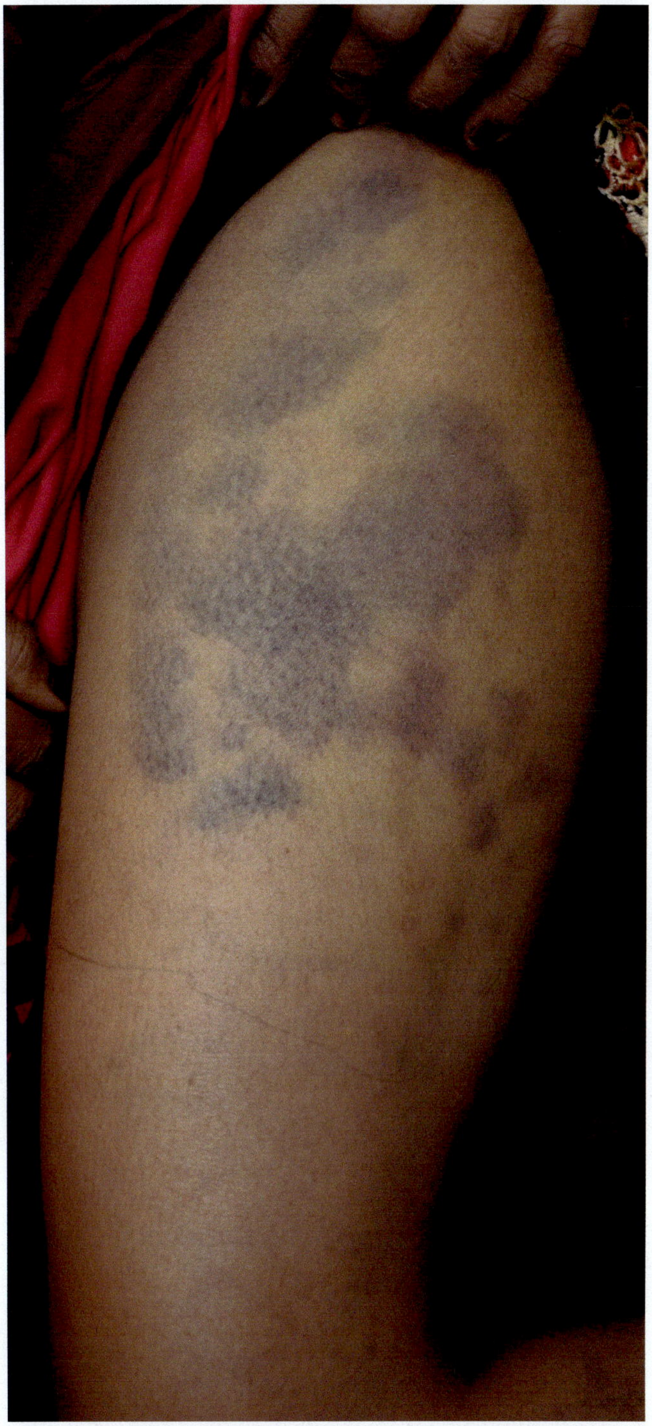

Figure 22.10 Painful purpuric lesions on the thigh of a lady. (Courtesy: Dr. Piyush Kumar, Katihar, India.)

## Psychogenic purpura syndrome

- Also known as Gardner-Diamond syndrome, autoerythrocyte sensitization, or painful bruising syndrome.
- It occurs more common in emotionally unstable middle-aged females.
- Patients present with bizarre, recurrent, tender purpuric or ecchymotic lesions spontaneously or after mental or physical stress (**Figure 22.10**).
- Extremities are a common site.
- Lesions are often preceded by a tingling or burning sensation.

## Munchausen syndrome

- It is a factitious disorder.
- Munchausen syndrome has also been called "hospital addiction," "polysurgical addiction," and "professional patient syndrome."
- It is seen mostly among medical students and health care professionals.
- Essential features are recurrent nature of illness, similarity in pattern of presentation, visiting different hospitals with the same complaint, dropping off treatment once deception is discovered.
- Patients mostly present with abdominal or neurological complaints. Dermatological complaints are rare.
- Symptoms or behaviors are present only when the patient is aware of being observed. There may be controlling, hostile, angry, disruptive, or attention-seeking behavior during hospitalization.
- Patients are pathological liars and have pseudologia fantastica (uncontrollable lying characterized by the fantastic description of false events).
- On the skin, patients present with bizarre lesions on accessible areas, usually self-inflicted by sharp objects or chemicals. Lesions may be ulcerative, erythematous, or

gangrenous; there may be subcutaneous emphysema or lymphedema.
- Other symptoms may be unexplained bleeding, repetitive urinary tract infection, non-healing wounds, repeated infections at different sites, and skin and genital injuries.
- Multiple hospitalizations often lead to iatrogenic general medical conditions (e.g., multiple scars because of unnecessary surgeries or adverse drug reactions). Individuals with the chronic form of this disorder can have a "gridiron abdomen" caused by multiple surgical scars.

## Munchausen by proxy

- The victims are usually infants or toddlers.
- Usually the mother or caregiver inflicts lesions on another person in order to satisfy a subconscious psychological need.
- Risk factors include single parent, previous abuse, disturbed family, frequent visits to the doctors, frequent accidents, poverty, overcrowding, and young parents.
- Skin lesions in form of non-healing wounds, hemorrhages, blisters, bruising, and excoriations may be seen.
- Associated systemic features, such as fever, abdominal pain, diarrhea, vomiting, and septicemia from infection of induced cutaneous ulcerations, may be seen.
- Bruises at "punishment" sites such as the face, ears, and head of a child less than one year old, black eyes, and bruising on the buttocks/lower back and outer thighs should raise suspicion.
- The pattern of bruising in form of fingertip marks, striate finger stripe effects from slapping, or pinch marks as opposing crescent-shaped lesions can give a clue to diagnosis.
- Kicks to the lower body show as irregular, large, deep bruises. Belt and strap damage appears on the trunk as parallel curved marks.
- The people administering the harm refuse treatments and hospital admission and may become hostile and abusive.

## Trichotillomania, trichotemnomania, trichoteiromania

- Trichotillomania is a body-focused repetitive behavior disorder, better termed trichotillosis.
- Two peaks of preponderance are seen: one in childhood, mainly between the ages of 5 and 12 years, and other as chronic cases who present as adults but who started hair-pulling activities in adolescence or early adult life.
- There is equal sex predilection in children; in adolescents and adults, female predominance is seen.
- There is an irresistible compulsion of hair pulling, resulting in a short-lived sense of relief and gratification when hair has been pulled out.
- The hair is twisted or plucked out in patches, mainly in areas accessible to the dominant hand. It leads to a kind of traumatic alopecia, with the patch containing hair of uneven length described as "irregularly irregular" in a wave-like or centrifugal pattern (**Figure 22.11a**).
- In extreme cases only hair on the occiput is seen, which is known as a Friar Tuck or tonsure pattern (**Figure 22.11b**).
- Clinically, three zones are seen on scalp:
  Zone 1 – uninvolved hair
  Zone 2 – missing hair due to recent pulling
  Zone 3 – regrowing short hair of various lengths
- The eyelashes, eyebrows, and facial and pubic hair may also be primarily affected.
- Trichotemnomania is another psychocutaneous disorder that involves intentional cutting of hair.

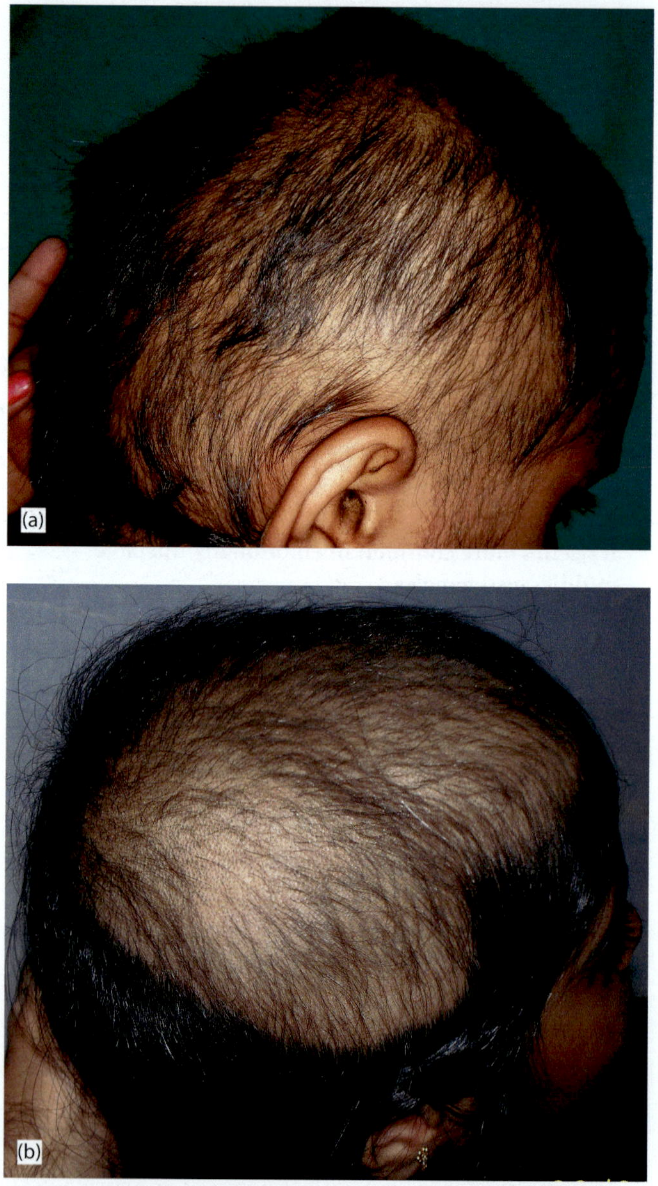


Figure 22.11 **(a)** Trichotillomania in a young girl. Note varying length of the hairs. **(b)** Trichotillomania – Friar Tuck sign. *(Continued)*

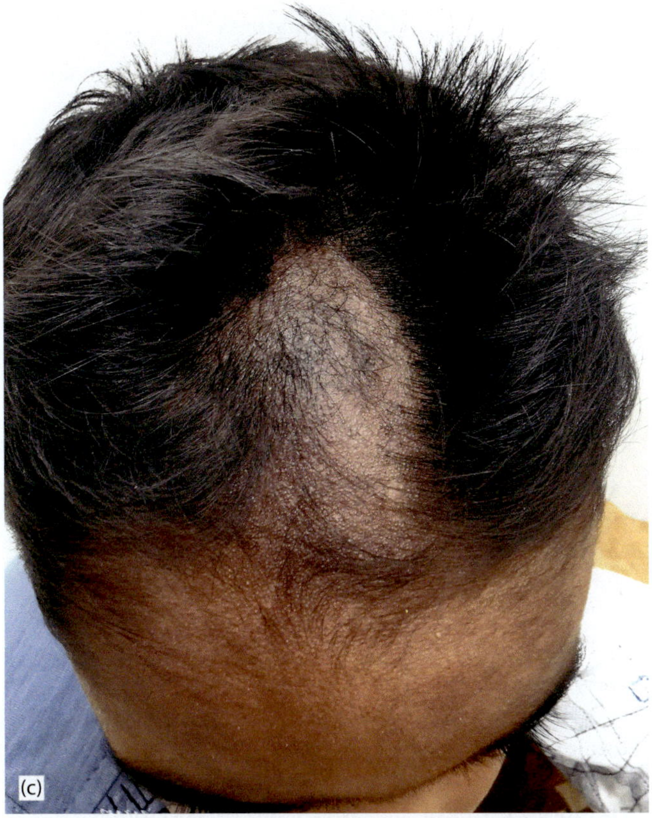

Figure 22.11 *(Continued)* **(c)** Trichoteiromania presenting as localized alopecia. Note lichenified scalp in the affected area. (b – Courtesy: Dr. Piyush Kumar, Katihar, India; c – Courtesy: Dr. Deverashetti Srinivas, Nizamabad, India.)

- In trichoteiromania the patient manipulates the hair by rubbing or scratching, leading to frictional damage, split ends, and traumatic alopecia (**Figure 22.11c**).
- DD: Alopecia areata (localized area of hair loss without any textural change; new hairs are fine and exclamation mark hairs present), tinea capitis (localized loss of hair with surface change in the form of scaling and dermatitis).

## Onychophagia, onychotillomania, onychotemnomania

- Onychophagia is a body-focused repetitive behavior disorder that involves chronic, seemingly uncontrollable nail biting and chewing.
- It usually begins in childhood and is most commonly seen during adolescence.
- Onychophagia may be associated with thumb-sucking or secondary irritant dermatitis, infection, inflammation, or malformation of digits (**Figure 22.12a,b**).
- Onychotillomania involves nail pulling, which may be so severe as to lead to complications like paronychia, trauma of cuticles.

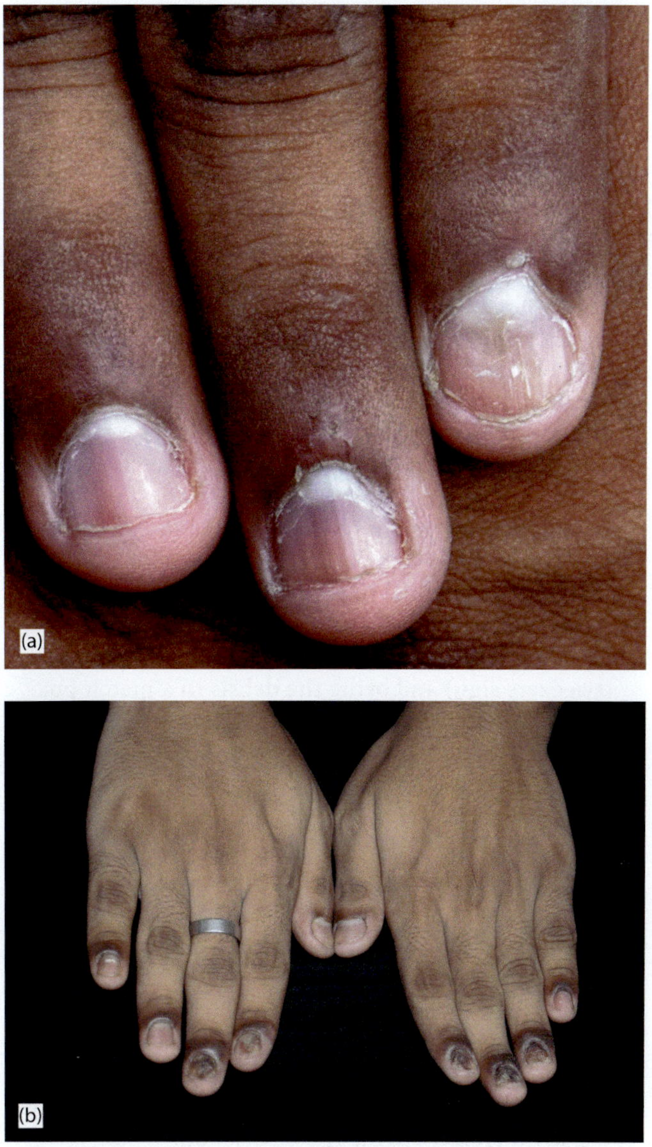

Figure 22.12 **(a)** Onychophagia in a young male. Note damage to proximal nail fold and hang nails. **(b)** Loss of cuticle, proximal nail fold pigmentation and onychophagia. (a,b – Courtesy: Dr. Piyush Kumar, Katihar, India.)

- Onychotemnomania involves nail cutting to the point of pain or injury to the surrounding area.

## Delusional parasitosis

- It is also known as Ekbom syndrome or pseudoparasitica dysaesthesia.
- It is a primary psychiatric condition in which the patient believes they are infested with mites, parasites, bacteria, worms, insects, or animate material even though no infesting organism or material can be found by the clinician. This may disable the patient to such an extent that they often find themselves unemployed, end up in debt (in an attempt to rid their home of the infesting organisms), repeatedly buy new furniture and

carpets, and repeatedly wash or clean their bodies to get rid of infections.

- Most of the patients are more than 50 years old, with a female preponderance.
- Patients complain of localized or generalized itching, burning, or crawling felt on the skin, most often persistent in nature and disabling.
- Skin manifestations are variable, ranging from none to excoriation, lichenification, prurigo nodularis, erosions, and sometimes ulcerations.
- Patients often bring evidence of the parasitic infection in the form of clothing, lint, skin crusts, or other debris, which is delusionally misinterpreted as entire organisms, body parts, larvae, or ova. This is often collected in a matchbox. This is called "matchbox sign" or specimen sign.
- A variant of delusional parasitosis is Morgellons disease, in which the patient has a fixed belief that fibers are embedded in their body. It presents as an itching, pricking, or biting sensation. The patients dig and pick their skin with nails and tweezers (tweezers sign) and bring the debris in a match box (matchbox sign).
- DD: A genuine infestation, generalized pruritus, dermatitis herpetiformis.

## Psychogenic pruritus

- This is also known as somatoform pruritus or functional itch disorder.
- Patient presents with intense chronic (more than six weeks) pruritus not associated with any known cause.
- There are no primary lesions. Secondary lesions such as excoriations, scars, pigmentation, and lichenification may be present.
- The intensity of pruritus may vary with stress and usually increases during rest or inaction.

## Psychogenic dysesthesia

- This is also known as persistent somatoform pain disorder of regional cutaneous/mucosal dysesthesia.
- There is burning, stinging, or itching in skin and mucous membrane without any visible lesions or systemic abnormalities (**Table 22.2**).
- Associated psychiatric disturbances like depression or anxiety may be seen.

Table 22.2 Psychogenic dysesthesias

| Dysethesias | Clinical features |
|---|---|
| **Vulvodynia** | • Patients complain of pain and burning in the vulva in the absence of organic causes.<br>• Patient may even abstain from sexual relations. |
| **Glossodynia** | • Burning sensation in the mouth without organic causes, such as diabetes mellitus, iron deficiency, deficiency of vitamins B2, B6, and B12, folic acid, or allergy to dental material.<br>• The symptoms are aggravated by foods and liquid and during the end of the day. |
| **Trichodynia** | • Unexplained pain of hair is almost always associated with sleep dysesthesia.<br>• It is commonly seen in people who complain of hair loss. |
| **Coccydynia** | • Chronic and disabling pain occurs in or around the coccyx. |
| **Notalgia paresthetica (Figure 22.13a,b)** | • There is itching and paresthesia in the interscapular region, which may extend to the shoulders, chest, and back. |

## Body dysmorphic disorder

- It is also called dermatologic hypochondriasis, beauty hypochondriasis, or dysmorphophobia.
- It is usually seen in adolescent women.
- It is described as "rich in symptoms but poor in signs."
- There is preoccupation with a real or an imagined defect in physical appearance; or if there is a slight physical anomaly, concern is out of proportion to the anomaly.
- Females are often more obsessed with facial defects and weight issues, whereas males are more concerned with genitalia and muscle mass.
- There is an imagined defect in appearance in the face (excessive facial hair, presumed scarring, wrinkling, excessive facial redness associated with burning sensation, large nose, wrinkles) or scalp (excessive hair loss, thinning hair), shrinking of genitals, or discomfort in the genital areas, extending to the thigh.

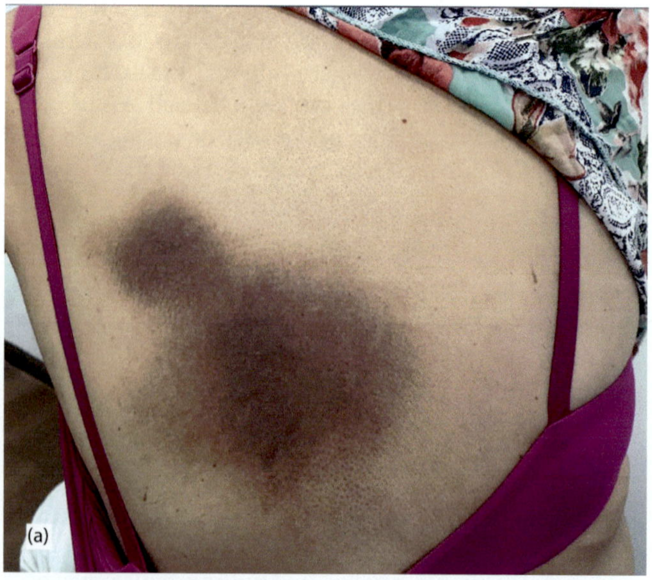


Figure 22.13 **(a)** Unilateral, pigmented patch in the scapular region in notalgia paresthetica. (*Continued*)

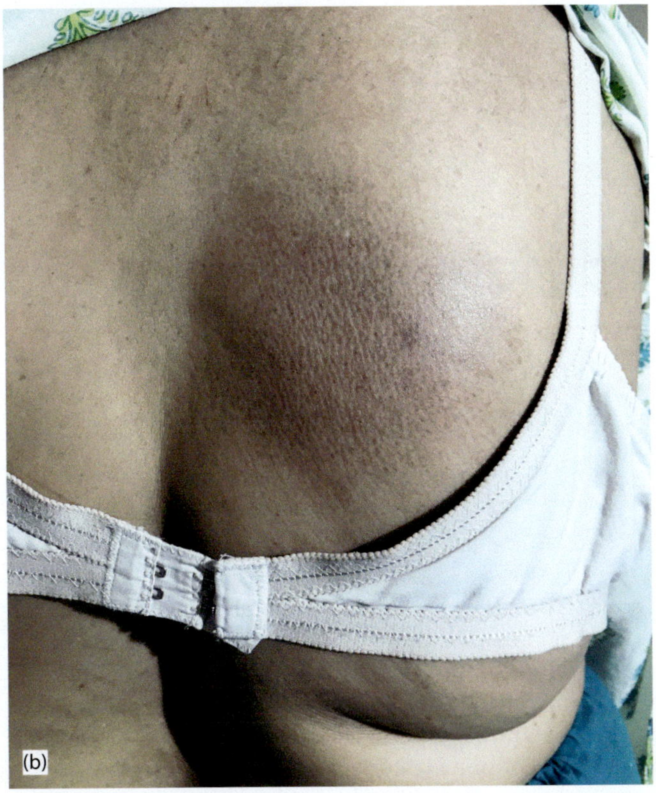


Figure 22.13 (*Continued*) **(b)** Unilateral erythematous and pigmented patch on the back in notalgia paresthetica. (a,b – Courtesy: Dr. Chirag Desai, Mumbai, India.)

- The affected individuals often spend an excessive amount of time in front of a mirror or repeatedly checking for perceived imperfections.
- This causes significant distress, frequently leading to social isolation or functional impairment.

## REFERENCES


1. Kuhn H, Mennella C, Magid M, Stamu-O'Brien C, Kroumpouzos G. Psychocutaneous disease. J Am Acad Dermatol 2017;76(5):779–791.
2. Yadav S, Narang T, Kumaran MS. Psychodermatology: A comprehensive review. Indian J Dermatol Venereol Leprol 2013;79:176–192.
3. Al Hawsawi K, Pope E. Pediatric psychocutaneous disorders: A review of primary psychiatric disorders with dermatologic manifestations. Am J Clin Dermatol 2011;12(4):247–257.
4. Vhiriac A, Brzezinski P, Pinteala T, Chiriac AE, Foia L. Common psychocutaneous disorders in children. Neuropsychiatr Dis Treat 2015;11:333–337.

E40

# Dermatoses in HIV-infected persons

SANTOSHDEV P RATHOD

## ABSTRACT

Human immunodeficiency virus/acquired immunodeficiency syndrome (HIV/AIDS) has a great potential to affect skin, mostly due to immunosuppression and antiretroviral therapy. It may range from non-specific pruritus to extensive/disseminated skin infections threatening life. Immunosuppression can alter the typical morphologies of various infectious skin lesions such as molluscum contagiosum, warts, deep mycosis, tuberculosis, syphilis, chancroidal genital ulcers, and herpes. Non-infectious dermatoses, such as psoriasis, seborrheic dermatitis, granuloma annulare and skin malignancies, may have a more rapid course, generalized distribution, and resistance to treatment. Occasionally, immune restoration after starting antiretroviral drugs may reactivate varicella zoster virus and exaggerate the inflammation in various other dermatoses. Thus, it is imperative to know the common dermatoses and their altered clinical course observed in AIDS patients. Knowing the expected cutaneous side effects of antiretroviral drugs is another prerequisite to allow the replacement of one drug with another without compromising the efficacy.

The text of this chapter is available online at https://routledgetextbooks.com/textbooks/9781032399669/



DOI: 10.1201/9781351054225-66

# E41

# Internal malignancy

SHEKHAR NEEMA, DIPALI RATHOD

## ABSTRACT

Underlying systemic changes may be often signaled by a skin manifestation. Any symptomatic and non-metastatic condition associated with a neoplasm constitutes a paraneoplastic syndrome. Also, some neoplastic diseases affecting the internal organs may further trigger several cutaneous manifestations. However, recognition of some typical paraneoplastic dermatoses may lead to the early diagnosis of a neoplasm and in future may determine a better prognosis. According to the various clinical presentations, age, and gender of patients, the underlying neoplasms may be different. This places great responsibility on the dermatologists in diagnosing malignancies depending upon the presenting cutaneous signs and symptoms and referring the affected patient to the concerned specialty for appropriate management. Although these dermatoses are relatively unusual, in this chapter we discuss the various paraneoplastic cutaneous manifestations. We aim to highlight the clinical manifestations of these dermatoses to provide assistance in the early diagnosis and management of these rare, but life-threatening conditions. Careful evaluation of the clinical features and performing the necessary investigations related to respective neoplasms is of utmost importance for the diagnosis of the paraneoplastic conditions.

The text of this chapter is available online at https://routledgetextbooks.com/textbooks/9781032399669/

DOI: 10.1201/9781351054225-67

E42

# Nails in systemic disease

BALACHANDAR S ANKAD, BALAKRISHNA NIKAM

## ABSTRACT

Different parts of the nail unit exhibit specific changes in many internal diseases, and hence, certain nail changes may serve as indicators of systemic diseases. Thus, knowledge of nail changes can equip dermatologists to suspect and diagnose unapparent systemic disorders.

The text of this chapter is available online at https://routledgetextbooks.com/textbooks/9781032399669/



DOI: 10.1201/9781351054225-68

# SECTION 5

# Miscellaneous

DOI: 10.1201/9781351054225-69

# E43

# Head and neck mass

SASI KIRAN ATTILI

## ABSTRACT

The head and neck form a distinct area of body incorporating numerous important anatomic structures. Space-occupying lesions arising out of these structures are considered under the topic "head and neck mass." *Space-occupying lesion* means any nodule, tumor, plaque, or cyst of significant dimension causing disfigurement. Obviously, such masses may have their origin not only in the skin but rather more frequently in the subcutaneous structures and eye, nose, oral cavity, etc. The former group of cutaneous conditions is considered in this chapter.

The text of this chapter is available online at https://routledgetextbooks.com/textbooks/9781032399669/



DOI: 10.1201/9781351054225-70

# E44

# Red face

ABHISHEK JHA, SHIVANI SHARMA

## ABSTRACT

Dermatoses of the face presenting with prominent erythema are called "red face." Apart from redness, other morphologies of skin lesions are usually evident. Analysis of these skin lesions in the background of facial erythema helps to reach differentials.

The text of this chapter is available online at https://routledgetextbooks.com/textbooks/9781032399669/

DOI: 10.1201/9781351054225-71

# E45

# Leonine facies

SOURABH JAIN

## ABSTRACT

Leonine facies can be seen in a wide range of benign and malignant conditions, associated with chronic disease course and/or bad prognosis. Rarely, leonine facies can be a presenting feature of previously undiagnosed critical conditions such as Sézary syndrome or leukemia cutis. Thus, recognizing leonine facies can be an important, easily appreciable clinical clue to the diagnosis of various conditions needing immediate medical attention. This chapter discusses the clinical approach to the diagnosis of various conditions commonly associated with leonine facies.

The text of this chapter is available online at https://routledgetextbooks.com/textbooks/9781032399669/


DOI: 10.1201/9781351054225-72

# E46

# Linear lesions

ANUPAM DAS, PREETI SHARMA

## ABSTRACT

Linear lesions are frequently encountered in the day-to-day practice of dermatology. These lesions may follow the lines of Blaschko, lymphatics, blood vessels, or dermatomes. They may vary in morphology from a papule to vesicle to plaque, etc. Many common dermatoses such as lichen planus, psoriasis, etc. may sometimes present in a linear distribution. Knowledge about common linear lesions as well as atypical presentation of common dermatoses may help in making a faster and more accurate diagnosis. In this chapter we have tried to classify linear lesions on the basis of the morphology, and the common ones have been discussed in detail.

The text of this chapter is available online at https://routledgetextbooks.com/textbooks/9781032399669/

DOI: 10.1201/9781351054225-73

# 23

# Annular lesions

PIYUSH KUMAR, RASHMI ROY

## INTRODUCTION

Clinical diagnosis is an art of identifying, compiling, and analyzing clues present in history and clinical examination findings. Recognition of additional clues such as annular configuration may help a physician in arriving at a clinical diagnosis or bring a physician closer to the diagnosis.

> "The next time you see a circle in the sky, in a drawing, or on the skin, pause and consider its significance."
>
> —*Robert Jackson*[1]

The list of dermatoses assuming an annular configuration is exhaustive. A detailed discussion on the pathomechanisms behind the formation of annular configuration is beyond the scope of this chapter, and readers are requested to go through the excellent texts by R Jackson and Sharma et al.[1,2] Certain dermatoses appear annular because of different stages of the disease process at different sites of a particular lesion. For example, healing lesions of discoid lupus erythematosus may have an atrophic center while the margin is still active and erythematous (or sometimes, pigmented). Similarly, the center of bullous impetigo may heal with epithelization while the margin is still active as erosion or pustule. The discussion on dermatoses that appear annular during the evolution of lesions or that assume an annular morphology only occasionally has not been attempted. The chapter aims to focus on entities commonly presenting with annular lesions.

The clinical diagnosis of annular lesions rests on a particular shape (**Box 23.1**) and clinical characteristics of the border (**Table 23.1**).[2–5] Certain additional clues have been included in **Table 23.2**. Various dermatoses that commonly present with annular lesions are discussed below.[2–5]

### Actinic lichen planus (lichen planus actinicus, lichen planus subtropicus, lichen planus tropicus, summertime actinic lichenoid eruption)

- This is Common in Africa, the Middle East, and the Indian subcontinent.
- There is no gender predilection, and it affects adults as well as children.
- The disease is exacerbated in spring and summer.
- The lesions present in four morphologic patterns: annular, dyschromic, classic plaque-like, and pigmented.
- It presents as hyperpigmented plaques surrounded by hypopigmented border over sun-exposed sites such as the face, V area of the chest, neck, back of the hand, lower extensor forearms (**Figure 23.1a,b**).
- Pruritus is mild or absent.
- The disease may be seen with lichen planus pigmentosus, which does not involve sun-exposed areas. Mucous membrane involvement is much less. The Koebner phenomenon is not seen.

**BOX 23.1: Annular and related morphology**

**Annular**: Ring-shaped lesion. Usually, plaques present with annular configuration, but other lesions, such as macular, papules, nodular, vesicles, or pustules, may present in annular configuration.
**Arcuate**: Incomplete annular lesion, arc-shaped lesion.
**Polycyclic**: Polycyclic lesions are formed by coalescing of the adjacent annular or arcuate lesions.
**Target/Iris lesions**: The lesion has three zones – a central dusky-red macule (or vesicle) surrounded by pallor, which in turn is surrounded by erythema. Typically seen in erythema multiforme.


DOI: 10.1201/9781351054225-74

Table 23.1 Clinical diagnosis of annular lesion

| Border | Features | Dermatoses |
|---|---|---|
| Patch | Hypopigmented | Actinic lichen planus (perilesional halo with pigmented center), halo nevus, Wornoff ring, steroid-induced perilesional hypopigmentation |
| | Hyperpigmented | Discoid lupus erythematosus (during healing) |
| | Erythematous | Dermatophyte infection (steroid-modified), figurate erythemas, fixed drug eruption, bullous impetigo (healing phase), necrolytic migratory erythema, livedo reticularis, circinate balanitis (vulvitis), annular lichenoid dermatitis of youth |
| Papule | Scaly | Dermatophyte infection |
| | Non-scaly | Granuloma annulare |
| | Keratotic | Elastosis perforans serpiginosa |
| Plaque | Erythematous | • Scales present – annular psoriasis, pityriasis rosea, subacute cutaneous lupus erythematosus, neonatal lupus erythematosus, secondary syphilis<br>• Scales absent – urticaria and urticaria multiforme, granuloma annulare, annular giant cell elastolytic granuloma, necrobiosis lipoidica, annular tufted angioma<br>• Variable scaling – Hansen's disease, Jessner's lymphocytic infiltration, annular sarcoidosis<br>• Crust/hyperkeratotic areas – lupus vulgaris |
| | Pigmented | Lichen planus, basal cell carcinoma |
| | Keratotic | • With a groove/canal – porokeratosis<br>• without a groove – annular lupus vulgaris, annular tuberculosis verrucosa cutis |
| | Targetoid appearance | • Acute hemorrhagic edema of infancy |
| Nodules | | Keratoacanthoma centrifugum marginatum |
| Vesicles & Bullae | | Linear IgA dermatosis/chronic bullous disease of childhood, cutaneous larva migrans, neutrophilic figurate erythema, necrolytic migratory erythema |
| Pustules | | Dermatophyte infection, bullous impetigo, subcorneal pustular dermatosis, pustular psoriasis, circinate balanitis, pseudo-circinate balanitis |
| Scales | | • Leading scale – dermatophyte infection<br>• Trailing scale – pityriasis rosea, erythema annulare centrifugum (figurate erythema)<br>• Double edged scales – ichthyosis linearis circumflexa<br>• Transient lesions – erythrokeratodermia variabilis |
| Purpura | | Purpura annularis telangiectodes of Majocchi, acute hemorrhagic edema of infancy, Henoch-Schönlein purpura, suction (traumatic) purpura, neutrophilic figurate erythema |

Table 23.2 Clinical clues for the diagnosis of annular lesions

| Clue | Dermatoses |
|---|---|
| **Arcuate lesions** | Elastosis perforans serpiginosa, lupus vulgaris, Jessner's lymphocytic infiltration, keratoacanthoma centrifugum marginatum, circinate balanitis, ichthyosis linearis circumflexa |
| **Serpiginous lesions** | Cutaneous larva migrans |
| **Polycyclic lesions** | Dermatophyte infection |
| **Predominantly affected sites** | • Photoexposed area – actinic lichen planus, subacute cutaneous lupus erythematosus, neonatal lupus erythematosus, basal cell carcinoma<br>• Flexures – subcorneal pustular dermatosis, necrolytic migratory erythema, annular lichenoid dermatitis of youth<br>• Genitalia – erythema multiforme, circinate balanitis<br>• Acral areas – necrolytic migratory erythema, granuloma annulare (dorsal surface), secondary syphilis (palmar/plantar surface)<br>• Lower legs – necrobiosis lipoidica, purpura annularis telangiectodes of Majocchi, Henoch-Schönlein purpura<br>• Trauma prone areas – lupus vulgaris and tuberculosis verrucosa cutis, necrolytic migratory erythema, cutaneous larva migrans |
| **Rapidly spreading lesions** | Dermatophyte infection, granuloma annulare, figurate erythema, necrolytic migratory erythema |
| **Transient/Migratory lesions** | Urticaria, cutaneous larva migrans, circinate balanitis, ichthyosis linearis circumflexa, erythrokeratodermia variabilis |
| **Reverse Koebnerization** | Granuloma annulare |

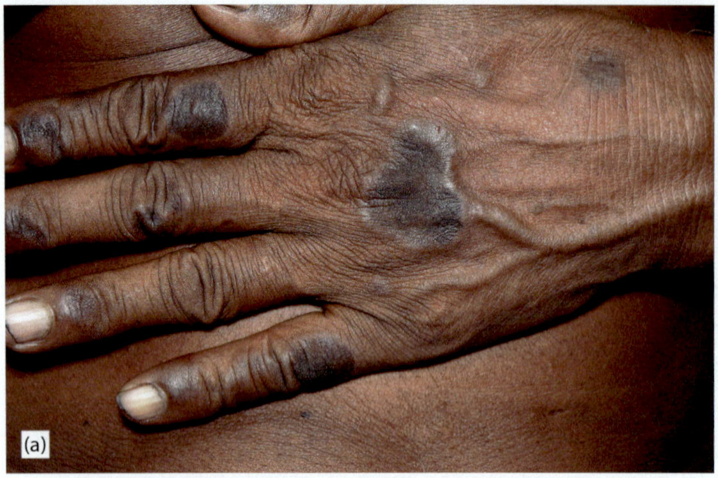


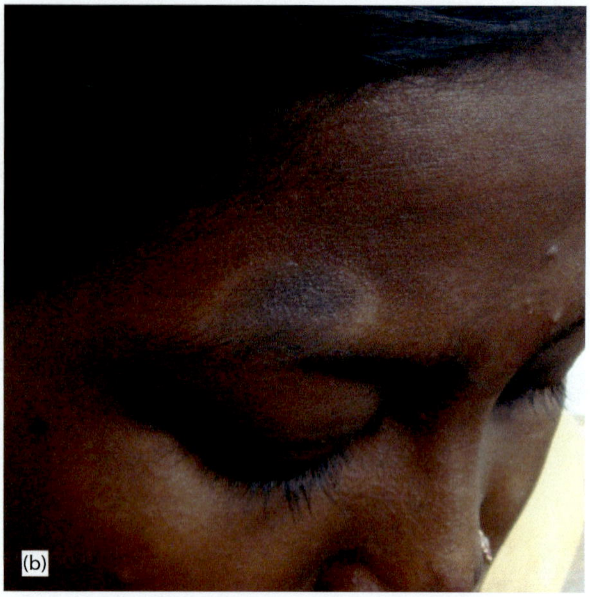


Figure 23.1 **(a)** Actinic lichen planus seen as pigmented patch and plaque with palo halo. **(b)** Actinic lichen planus on the forehead.

- DD: Discoid lupus erythematosus (active lesion – erythematous plaque with adherent scales; healing lesion – depigmented atrophic center with pigmented margin), sarcoidosis, halo nevus, steroid-induced perilesional hypopigmentation.

## Figurate erythema (gyrate erythema)

- These are a group of reactive conditions seen in a variety of benign or malignant conditions and are clinically characterized by annular erythema with trailing scales.
- Classically, this group includes erythema annulare centrifugum, erythema marginatum, erythema migrans and erythema gyratum repens (**Table 23.3**).
- DD: Tinea corporis (itchy, polycyclic lesions with papules, pustules, and scales at the margin), annular psoriasis, annular urticaria (transient lesions without any scales), granuloma annulare, Hansen's disease (annular lesions of borderline tuberculoid and mid-borderline), erythrokeratodermia variabilis (transient gyrate or circinate erythematous patches which fade or migrate within few hours, additional fixed erythematous hyperkeratotic plaques), purpuric annular dermatoses (**Table 23.4**).

## Erythema annulare centrifugum (EAC)

- It is the most common type of figurate erythema and may affect any age group, with a peak incidence in the fifth decade of life.
- It has been reported in many infectious entities such as dermatophytes, candida, Epstein-Barr virus, pox virus, HIV, varicella, parasites and bacteria. Certain drugs (cimetidine, NSAIDS, antimalarials), Crohn's disease, hypereosinophilic syndrome and pregnancy also act as causative factors.

Table 23.3 Figurate erythemas

| Diseases | Age of presentation | Common sites | Progression of lesion (rate) | Course of disease | Associated diseases (selected) |
|---|---|---|---|---|---|
| **Erythema annulare centrifugum** | Affect any age group<br>Peak at fifth decade of life | Favors thighs, hips, and trunk | Up to 6 cm in diameter or more in 1–2 weeks | Lesion persists for weeks to months<br>Total duration ranges from days to decades | Crohn's disease, autoimmune endocrinopathies, hypereosinophilic syndrome, neoplasm |
| **Erythema migrans** | Bimodal age of onset<br>One peak at 5–19 years and second at 55–70 years | Lower extremities, axillae, groin, and popliteal fossa in adults and trunk in children | Lesion begins after tick bite and can progress up to 15 cm | Lesion lasts for 4–6 weeks | *Borrelia burgdorferi* infection |
| **Erythema marginatum** | Children 5–15 years<br>Can also affect the adult population | Trunk, axillae, and proximal extremities | 2–12 mm over 12 hours | Lesion lasts from hours to a few days | Rheumatic fever |
| **Erythema gyratum repens** | Commonly affects adults | Trunk and other large body surface areas | 1 cm per day | Lesion resolves after treatment of the underlying malignancy | Lung, breast, and esophagus cancer pulmonary tuberculosis |

Table 23.4 Purpuric annular lesions

| Annular purpuric conditions | Commonly affected age group and site | Clinical features |
|---|---|---|
| Purpura annularis telangiectodes of Majocchi | • Mostly in young adults<br>• Common in females<br>• Bilateral lower legs affection is common<br>• Arms and trunk may be involved | • Annular lesions with pinpoint petechiae at the margin. The center may show atrophy and telangiectasia.<br>• The lesion may persist for years. |
| Acute hemorrhagic edema of infancy | • Typically affects children between 4 and 24 months of age | • Triad of fever, large purpuric plaques, and acral edema.<br>• Bilaterally symmetrical purpuric plaques on the extremities and face, with relative sparing of trunk.<br>• Purpuric plaques have targetoid appearance.<br>• Systemic features are minimal.<br>• The disease runs an acute self-limiting course. |
| Henoch-Schönlein purpura | • Commonly affects children between 3 and 6 years of age | • Papular, purpuric, and urticarial lesions on lower legs. The lesions appear in crops.<br>• Visceral involvement manifests as abdominal pain, vomiting, diarrhea, intussusceptions, bloody stools, joint pain (knees and ankles) and nephritis.<br>• The disease runs an acute self-limiting course, but recurrence may occur. |
| Suction (traumatic) purpura | • May affect any age group<br>• Any site affected<br>• History of suction toys, vacuum cleaners, gas masks, therapeutic cups, and sucking while kissing | • Localized suction to the skin usually produces purpura or sometimes, blisters.<br>• Acute self-limiting condition. |
| Neutrophilic figurate erythema | • Any age group affected<br>• Face, trunk, or extremities affected | • Annular lesions with erythema, vesicles, or purpura at the margin.<br>• The disease runs a self-limiting course with relapse in summers. |

- A rare autosomal dominant form of EAC has been described, which is referred to as "familial annular erythema."
- The initial lesions present as firm pink papules that expand centrifugally, with central clearing in an annular pattern but polycyclic. An incomplete arc pattern is also seen when the expansion is not uniform (**Figure 23.2**).

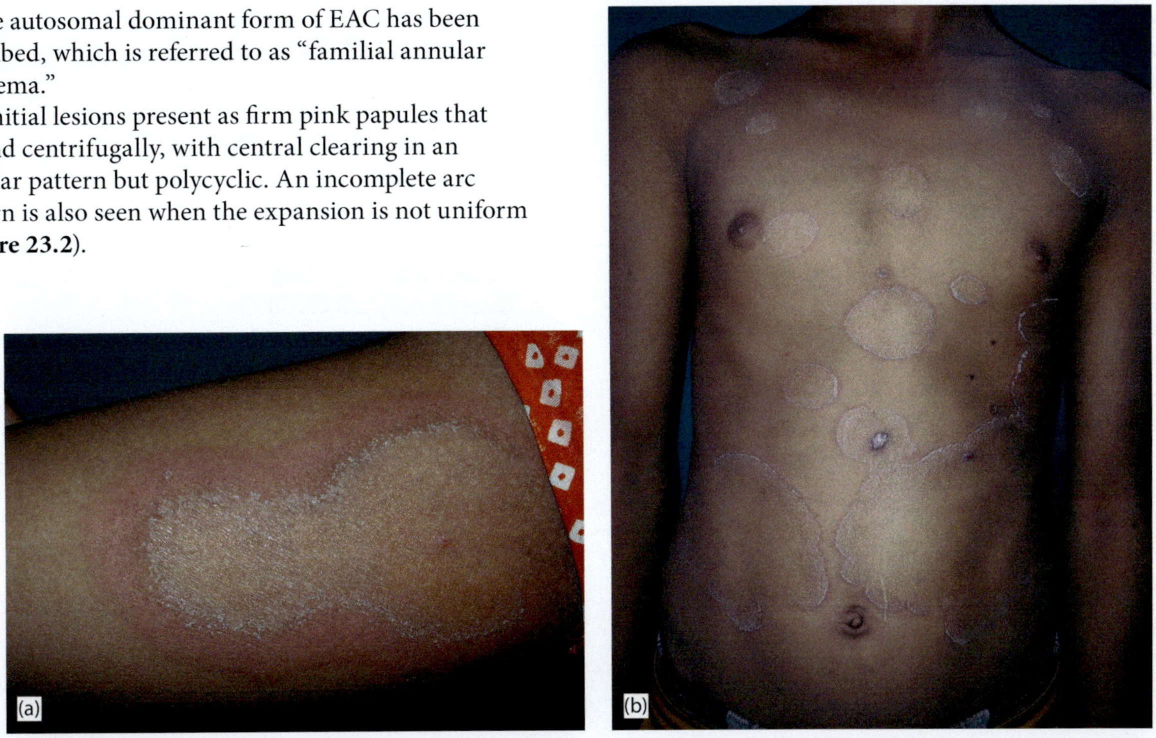


Figure 23.2 **(a)** Erythema annulare centrifugum with annular erythema and trailing scale. **(b)** Multiple lesions of erythema annulare centrifugum on the trunk.

**BOX 23.2: Clinical forms of Erythema annulare centrifugum**

**Superficial form** – It shows minimally elevated lesions with trailing scales at the inner border of the annular erythema due to desquamation. Scaling may not be seen in all of the lesions. Pruritus may be associated. Vesicles may develop occasionally at the margin.
**Deep form** – It shows lesions with elevated edges without scales. Pruritus is absent.

- An individual lesion can expand up to 6 cm or more in diameter in a period of one to two weeks. It can persist for weeks to months without any associated systemic manifestations.
- The lesion can be localized or generalized, rarely involving the palm, sole, mucous membrane, and scalp.
- Two forms of EAC are known (**Box 23.2**).
- The lesions resolve with post-inflammatory hyperpigmentation without any scarring. But recurrences are known. The total duration of disorder ranges from days to decades.

### Erythema marginatum (erythema marginatum rheumaticum or erythema annulare rheumaticum)

- This disorder is a cutaneous manifestation of rheumatic fever. Not all patients with rheumatic fever develop erythema marginatum.
- Mostly children between 5 to 15 years are affected, but adults can also develop the disease.
- The lesion begins as erythematous macules that spreads peripherally and forms annular or polycyclic patches or plaques without scaling. The lesions are asymptomatic and can migrate from 2–12 mm over a period of 12 hours. The skin appears pale or lightly pigmented in areas of previous involvement. The lesions are more prominent in afternoon.
- It commonly involves trunk, axillae, and proximal extremities.
- The lesions last from hours to a few days. Recurrent crops can occur over a number of weeks.
- Carditis, migratory polyarthritis, subcutaneous nodules, and sydenham chorea are the associated findings.

### Erythema migrans (Erythema chronicum migrans)

- It is seen in Lyme disease, an infectious disease following the bite of infected tick. The disease is caused by *Borrelia burgdorferi* spirochetes, which are transmitted by bites from several species of *Ixodes* tick.
- This disorder is seen commonly in the northeast, mid-Atlantic Great Lake regions, and Northern and Eastern Europe.
- The peak incidence is seen in spring and the summer.
- Males and females are equally affected, and there is a bimodal age of onset with one peak at 5 to 19 years and second at 55 to 70 years.
- The lesion starts after the tick bite as a small, red macule or papule at the site. After 7 to 15 days it expands, with annular erythematous plaque around the papule, a raised advancing border without scales, and a central light-colored area resembling a bull's-eye. The lesion is warm to the touch. The color may vary from red to bluish-red. The lesion can become indurated or develop vesicles and may undergo necrosis.
- It commonly affects the lower extremities, axilla and groin, and popliteal fossa in adults and affects the trunk in children.
- The annular erythema can develop up to a diameter of 15 cm.
- The lesion is associated with burning in some cases.
- Pruritus and pain are absent. Localized alopecia may develop at the site of the lesion.
- The lesions last four to six weeks when left untreated.
- Multiple lesions can occur in the same patient due to multiple tick bites.
- Disseminated lesions can appear days to weeks after the appearance of the primary lesion and are smaller in size and with a less indurated center.
- Other features of Lyme disease, such as fever, arthralgia, malaise, fatigue, headache, neck stiffness, myalgia, and lymphadenopathy, are also present.
- DD: Southern tick-associated rash illness. Presents with similar lesions but have negative serology for Lyme disease.

### Erythema gyratum repens

- It is a rare and often paraneoplastic eruption associated with lung, breast, esophagus, and stomach cancer. The cutaneous lesion can develop prior to or after the diagnosis of neoplasm.
- It commonly affects adults.
- The patient presents with pruritic, multiple, concentric polycyclic, annular or circinate erythematous plaques with scales at the advancing age. The lesion assumes a characteristic "wood grain" appearance (or zebra-like pattern). The lesion spreads peripherally with a rate of 1 cm/day.
- DD: Resolving pityriasis rubra pilaris. History of initial classic lesion is present, which resolves and resembles erythema gyratum repens. Can be differentiated histologically.

### Fixed drug eruption (FDE)

- FDE usually presents with a discoid erythematous patch that resolves with post-inflammatory hyperpigmentation. Sometimes, during recurrence,

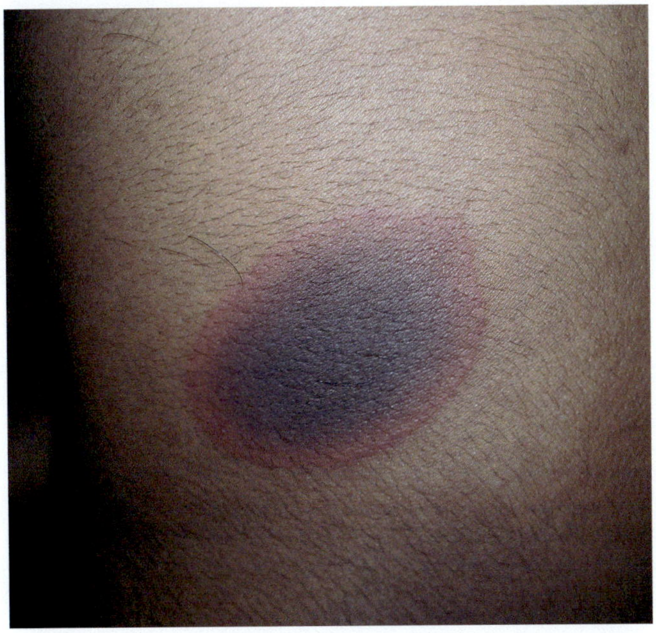

Figure 23.3 Recurrent lesion of fixed drug eruption may appear annular with central pigmentation (from prior episode) and peripheral erythema.

only the margin becomes active and erythematous with a pigmented center, assuming an annular appearance (**Figure 23.3**).

## Bullous impetigo

- Lesions of bullous impetigo start healing from the center with epithelization, and lesions assume an annular configuration for a brief period of time. The still-active margin is clinically characterized by erosion or pustules (**Figure 23.4a,b**).

## Livedo reticularis

- It is a benign condition that occurs after a physiologic vasospastic response to cold exposure or may occur due to various pathological causes (**Box 23.3**).
- The disease commonly affects young children and middle-aged women.
- Lesions present as a transient or persistent blotchy, reddish-blue to purple, net-like reticulated cyanotic

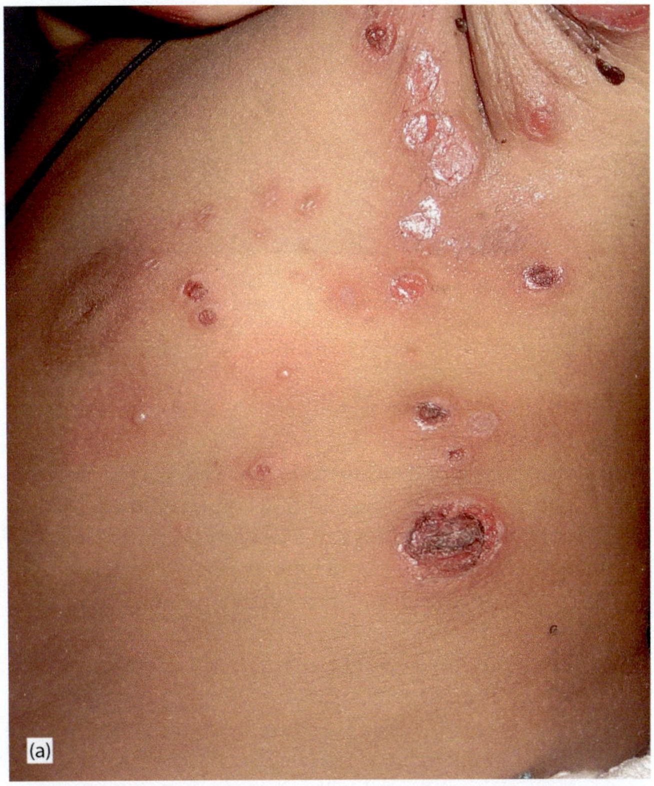

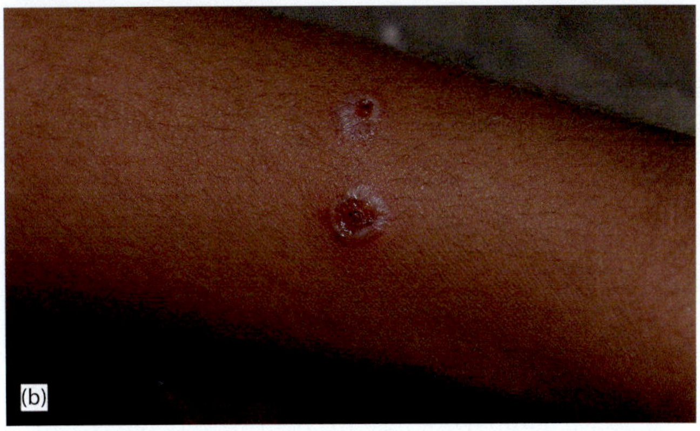

Figure 23.4 During the course of disease, bullous impetigo may appear annular with central erosion or crust and peripheral rim of pus. In late stages, central epithelization and peripheral erosion may be observed.

### BOX 23.3: Causes of livedo reticularis

- Hypercoagulable states like antiphospholipid syndrome, DIC, protein C and S deficiency, Homocystinuria.
- Vasculitis like – cutaneous polyarteritis nodosa, cryoglobulinemic vasculitis, autoimmune CTD vasculitis like- SLE, rheumatoid arthritis, Sjögren's syndrome.
- Calciphylaxis
- Sneddon syndrome
- Embolic states
- Medications, such as amantadine, interferons, heparins.
- Neoplasms
- Neurological disorders, such as complex regional pain syndrome, multiple sclerosis, diabetes mellitus.

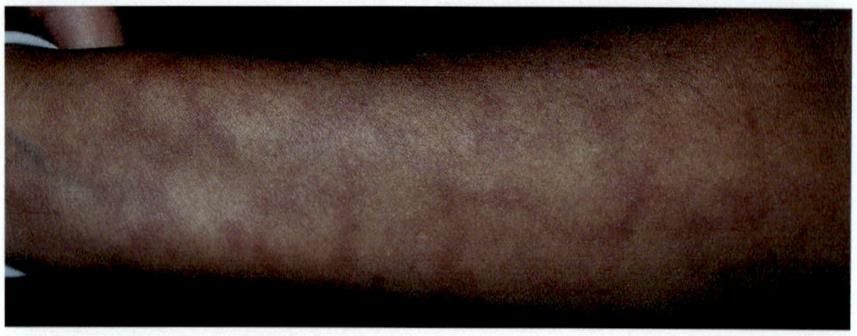

Figure 23.5 Livedo reticularis as fixed erythema in a net-like pattern.

pattern that is symmetric, reversible, and uniform and affects the extremities (**Figure 23.5**).

- Different types of livedo reticularis are recognized:
    - Congenital (cutis marmorata telangiectatica congenital) presents as a persistent reticular vascular pattern limited mostly to one extremity. The lesion is present since birth and complete resolution is seen in few years in some patients.
    - Physiological livedo reticularis (cutis marmorata) is seen in neonates, infants, and young women commonly. It occurs in response to cold exposure. Resolution of the lesion is noted on rewarming.
    - Primary or idiopathic livedo reticularis presents with a widespread fine network affecting the lower extremities. The lesion persists on warming.
    - Livedo reticularis with systemic diseases (**Box 23.3**) is due to vasospasm, autoimmune connective tissue, vessel-wall pathology, or intraluminal pathology.
- DD: Livedo racemosa (symmetric, irreversible and broken pattern), erythema ab igne (develops in response to heat and evolves into a fixed reticulated hyperpigmentation localized to the rea exposed to heat), reticulated erythematous mucinosis, poikiloderma.

## Circinate balanitis

- Circinate balanitis (or circinate vulvitis in females) is a mucosal hallmark of reactive arthritis and, rarely, can be a presenting feature.
- Affected patients develop moist erythema and/or pustules in a serpiginous, arcuate, or annular configuration (**Figure 23.6**).
- Similar lesions have been noted in pustular psoriasis too.
- When patients with secondary syphilis develop similar lesions, the condition is called pseudo circinate balanitis.[6]

## Annular lichenoid dermatitis of youth (ALDY)

- The condition is mostly reported in young males and shows a predilection for the axilla, groin, and flanks.
- ALDY presents as solitary or multiple sharply demarcated annular or arcuate erythematous patches or plaques with central hypopigmentation.
- The lesions heal with post-inflammatory hyperpigmentation.

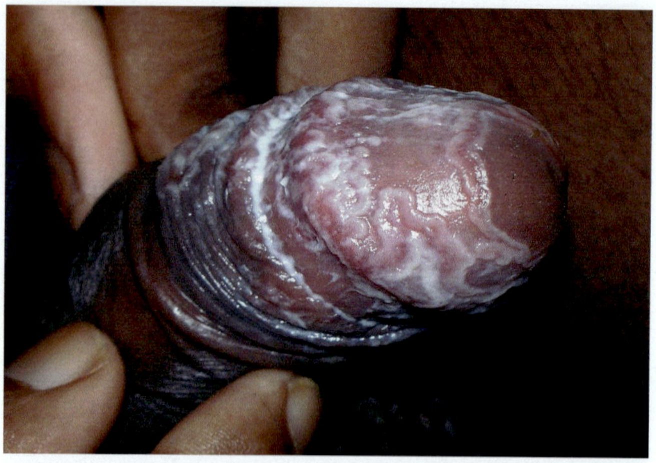

Figure 23.6 Circinate balanitis seen as whitish slough and erythema in a serpiginous pattern.

## Dermatophyte infection

- The clinical presentation of dermatophyte infection is highly variable and depends on a lot of factors. The patients usually present with single or multiple circular, annular, circinate, arcuate, concentric, or oval patches or plaques. Central clearing of the lesions with sharply defined, raised erythematous scaly borders gives them an annular appearance. The lesion spreads in centrifugal fashion from the core, with central clearing and mild scaling, giving them a ring shape, hence the term ringworm.
- It may be localized or generalized and unilateral or bilateral. It is usually asymmetrical when it has bilateral involvement.
- Non-inflammatory types present with itchy, annular, or polycyclic lesions with scales and papules at the margin (**Figure 23.7a,b**).
- Inflammatory types are characterized by itchy polycyclic or annular lesions with erythematous papules, pustules, erosions, crusts, and scales at the margin (**Figure 23.7c,d**).
- Tinea imbricata (tokelau) – It is commonly seen in Southeast Asia, the South Pacific, Central America, and South America and is caused by *Trichophyton concentricum*. It clinically presents as concentric, annular scales, with variable erythema.
- Steroid-modified tinea/tinea incognito – The characteristic clinical features are lost, and hence, diagnosis requires a high index of suspicion. Common clinical features are as follows:
    - The border becomes less prominent or barely appreciable.
    - The lesions become less scaly and more erythematous.
    - The central clearing is less appreciable, with eczematous changes in the central part (**Figure 23.7e**).

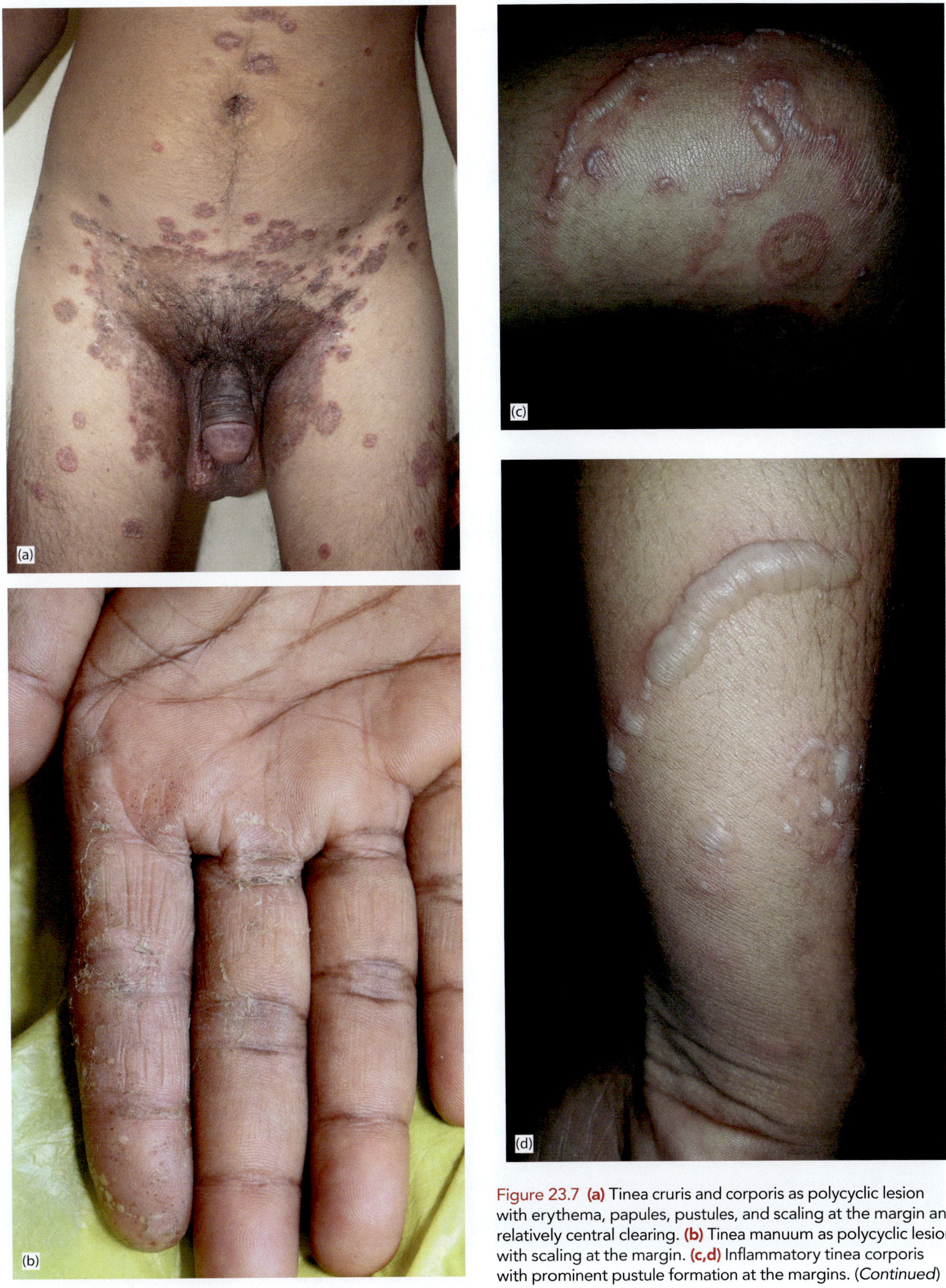


Figure 23.7 **(a)** Tinea cruris and corporis as polycyclic lesion with erythema, papules, pustules, and scaling at the margin and relatively central clearing. **(b)** Tinea manuum as polycyclic lesion with scaling at the margin. **(c,d)** Inflammatory tinea corporis with prominent pustule formation at the margins. (*Continued*)

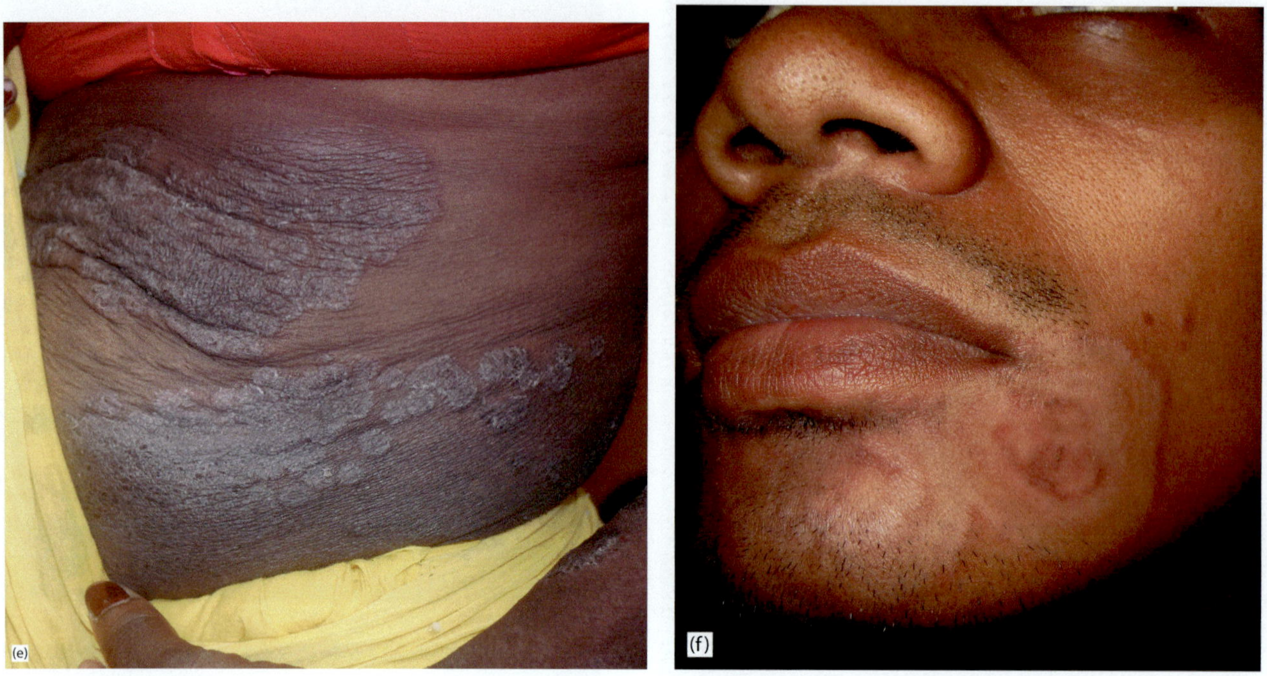


Figure 23.7 (*Continued*) **(e)** Steroid-modified tinea with central eczematous changes. **(f)** Steroid-modified tinea presenting as concentric rings of erythema (tinea pseudoimbricata). (c,d,f – Courtesy: Dr. PC Das, Katihar, India.)

- The lesions may have more inflammatory papules and pustules without much central clearing.
- The lesions may show concentric rings of tinea lesions (Tinea pseudoimbricata) (**Figure 23.7f**).[7]
- The lesions become more widespread.
- DD: Classical tinea lesions (Figurate erythema, pityriasis rosea, secondary syphilis), steroid-modified tinea (nummular eczema, contact dermatitis).

## Granuloma annulare

- The lesion presents as solitary or multiple, skin-colored or erythematous, small grouped papules. The lesions spread with central clearing, forming annular lesions. Papules at the periphery give the lesions their characteristic "beaded" appearance. The lesions are typically non-scaly, and this finding is of diagnostic value (**Figure 23.8a–d**).

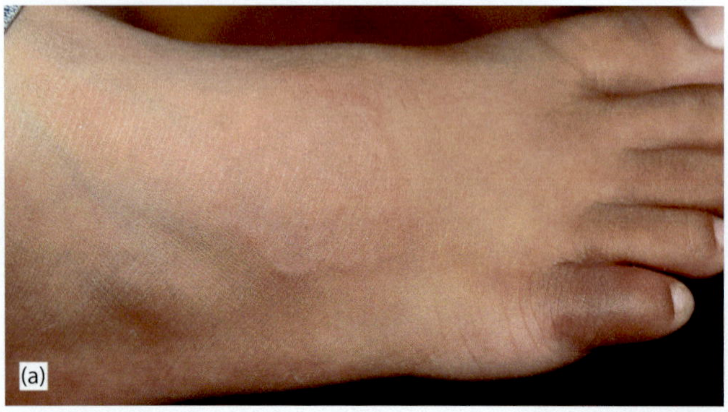


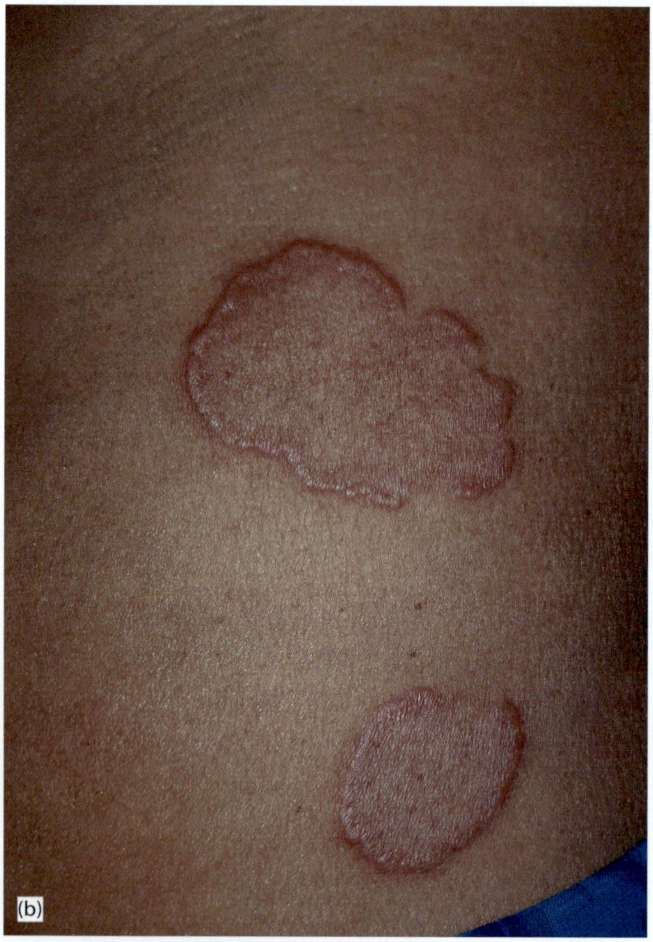


Figure 23.8 **(a)** Granuloma annulare with indurated margin. **(b)** Granuloma annulare with prominent indurated margin. Note beaded appearance of the margin and absence of surface changes. (*Continued*)

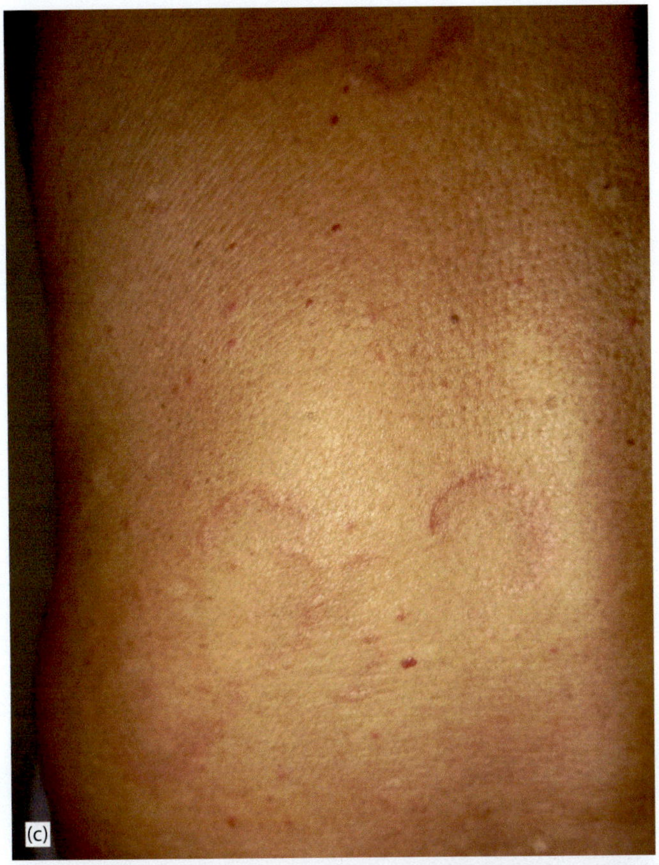

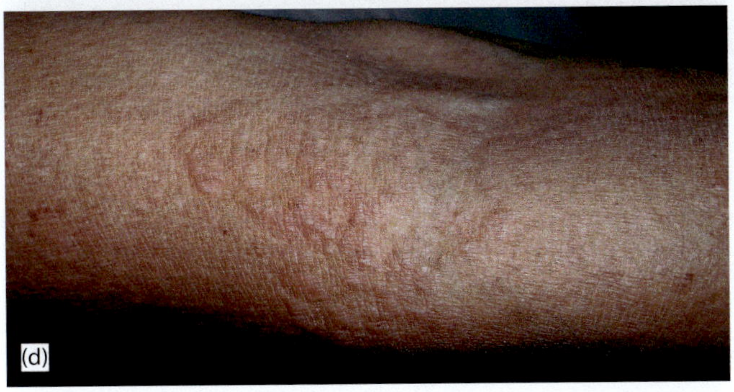

Figure 23.8 (*Continued*) **(c)** Multiple lesions of granuloma annulare on the trunk. **(d)** Multiple papules of granuloma annulare. Lesions have started to assume annular configuration. (b – Courtesy: Dr. PC Das, Katihar, India.)

- Lesions are often in a symmetrical distribution and affect the distal upper extremities, but legs, feet, trunk are also involved. Facial involvement is rare.
- Spontaneous resolution of the lesions is seen.
- Many forms of granuloma annulare are present, and the patient shows only one type during its course of illness except in the subcutaneous form.
- The variants of granuloma annulare are localized granuloma annulare, generalized granuloma annulare, patch-type or macular granuloma annulare, subcutaneous granuloma annulare, perforating granuloma annulare, palmar granuloma annulare, granuloma annulare in HIV patients, granuloma annulare with malignant disease.
- DD: Annular sarcoidosis, Tinea corporis, leprosy, eruptive xanthoma.

## Elastosis perforans serpiginosa (EPS)

- It is a rare skin condition caused by transepidermal elimination of abnormal elastic fibers and focal dermal elastosis. The disease can be inherited or acquired.
- It commonly affects children or young adults.
- It can be seen in association with Down syndrome, Ehlers-Danlos syndrome, osteogenesis imperfecta, Marfan syndrome, pseudo xanthoma elasticum, Rothmund-Thomson syndrome, aerogeria, long-term use of penicillin, chronic renal failure, cutis laxa, diabetes mellitus, Wilson's disease, cystinuria, and scleroderma.
- The lesion of EPS starts as 2- to 5-mm keratotic papules that are arranged in serpiginous or annular patterns. Lesions may enlarge to several centimeters.
- They involve the face, neck, arms, and flexures.
- Spontaneous resolution of the lesion is often observed, or the lesion may persist for many years.
- DD: Tinea corporis, granuloma annulare, annular sarcoidosis, porokeratosis of Mibelli (annular or serpiginous plaque with thready keratotic border with central groove. Center may show hyperpigmentation, atrophy, or hypertrophy).

## Pityriasis rosea

- It is a self-limited inflammatory papulosquamous eruption usually affecting adolescents and young adults between 10 and 35 years.
- The disease is most prevalent in spring and autumn.
- At first a solitary lesion (herald patch or mother patch) appears, mostly over the trunk and enlarges to 2–4 cm over several days. This lesion is salmon-pink or brown, oval patches or plaques with advancing raised margins. The center of the lesion shows small fine scales, and the margin has a large trailing collarette of scales with free edges pointing inward. The scales tend to fold across the line of stretch – "hanging curtain" sign (**Figure 23.9**).
- After some days, similar but smaller lesions (daughter lesions) appear, involving the trunk, neck, and proximal extremities. Rarely eyelids, palms, soles, scalp, or penis may be involved. The lesions appear with their long axis following lines of cleavage on the trunk, arranged in a "fir tree" or "Christmas tree" pattern (**Figure 23.10**). Pruritus is mild to severe.
- The eruption persists for six to eight weeks followed by spontaneous resolution. Occasionally lesions may persist longer. Relapse and recurrences are infrequent.
- Some of the atypical variants are as follows:
    - Inverse pityriasis rosea involves the axilla and inguinal area.

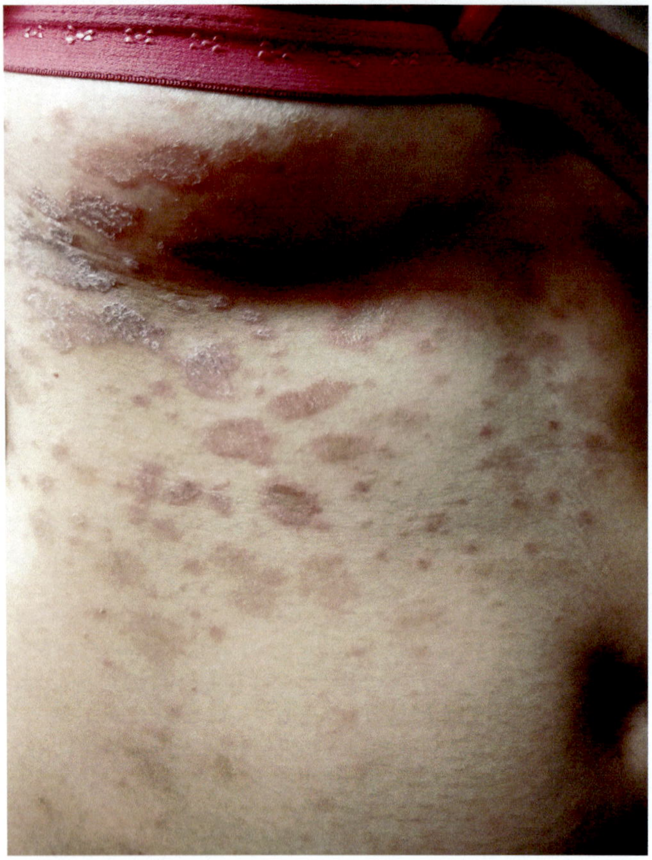

Figure 23.9 Multiple annular lesions of pityriasis rosea on the trunk. (Courtesy: Dr. Niharika Ranjan Lal, ESIPGIMSR, Kolkata, India.)

- Oral variants are asymptomatic, erythematous macules with raised borders and clearing centers. Sometimes aphthous ulcer-like lesions are present.
    - Papular variant has a predilection for the face and scalp and is seen commonly in black children.
    - Purpuric variant has petechiae and ecchymosis along Langer lines of the neck, trunk, and proximal extremities and can be a sign of acute myeloid leukemia.
    - Urticarial, pustular, vesicular, and erythema multiforme-like variants are also present.
    - Herald patches may be absent or multiple.
- DD: Seborrheic dermatitis (yellow greasy scales are present over the lesions), secondary syphilis (split papules and condyloma lata, a history of chancre), tinea corporis, tinea versicolor (perifollicular hypopigmented lesions), guttate psoriasis (raindrop like scaly papules, Koebnerization).

## Subacute cutaneous lupus erythematosus (SCLE)

- It is a subtype of cutaneous lupus erythematosus and commonly affects young to middle-aged women.
- SCLE may present without any systemic involvement.

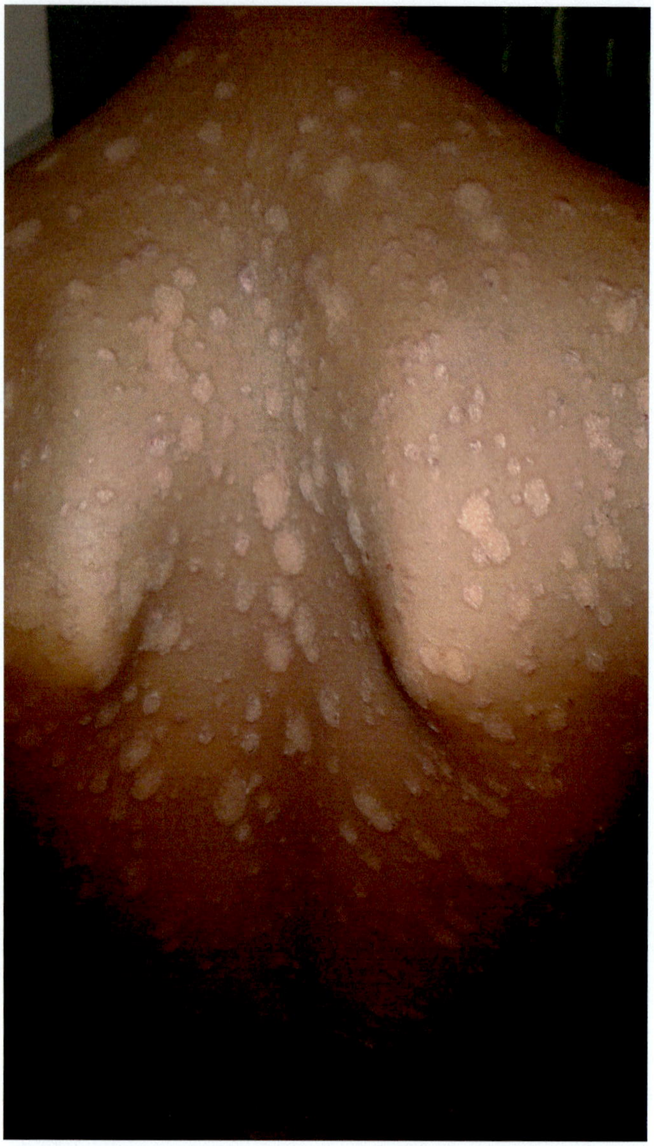

Figure 23.10 Annular lesions of Pityriasis rosea on the back.

- Lesions of SCLE occur on sun-exposed areas and may present in two forms (**Figure 23.11**).
    1. The annular form presents with erythematous, annular scaly plaques with central clearing. They tend to coalesce and form a polycyclic array.
    2. The papulosquamous form presents as eczematous or psoriasiform lesions.
- Induration is minimal, and the lesion heals without scarring. Dyspigmentation or hypopigmentation can develop.
- Patients may have associated arthralgia or arthritis and leukopenia.
- Fifty percent of patients meet the ARA criteria for SLE.
- DD: Pityriasis rosea, secondary syphilis, tinea corporis, erythema annulare centrifugum, classic granuloma annulare.

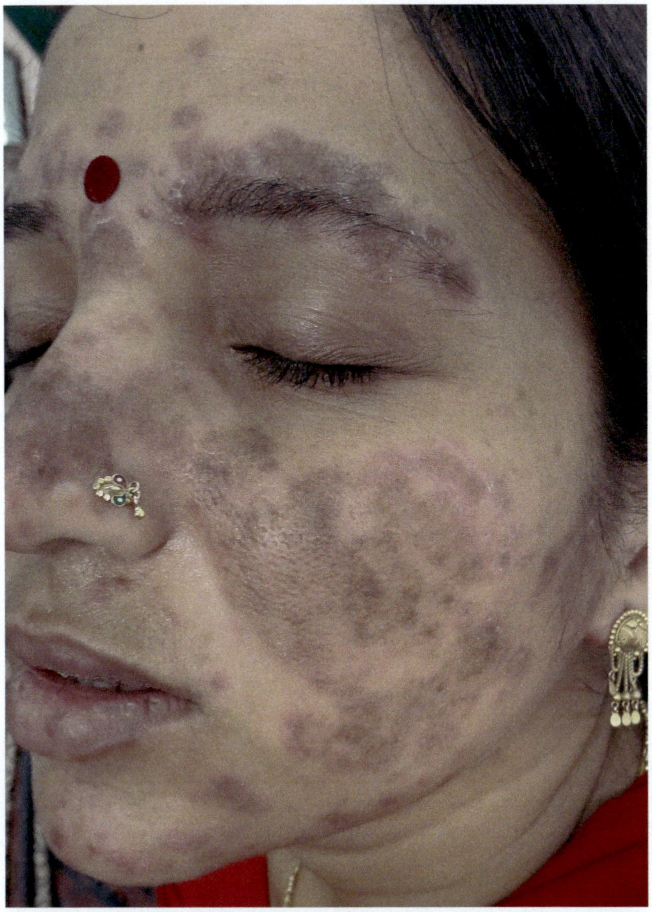

Figure 23.11 Annular scaly plaque of subacute cutaneous lupus erythematosus.

## Neonatal lupus erythematosus

- Neonatal lupus erythematosus is an infantile form of SCLE caused by transplacentally acquired Ro/SSA antibodies.
- It appears to be more common in blacks, Latinos, and Asians.
- The lesion presents as an annular, round or elliptical erythematous macule and scaly plaques, commonly involving the face over the periorbital region and scalp. The extremities can also get involved. It is present since birth or develops within the first few weeks. The mucosa is spared.
- These lesions resolve in six to eight months without scarring, but some cases show dyspigmentation and residual telangiectasia.
- The major associated systemic finding is congenital heart block, with or without cardiomyopathy. The heart block is usually present from birth (or may appear later) and is permanent. Other systemic concerns are thrombocytopenia and hepatobiliary disease, which may present as liver failure during gestation or hyperbilirubinemia in neonates.
- DD: Tinea faciei, seborrheic dermatitis, pityriasis versicolor.

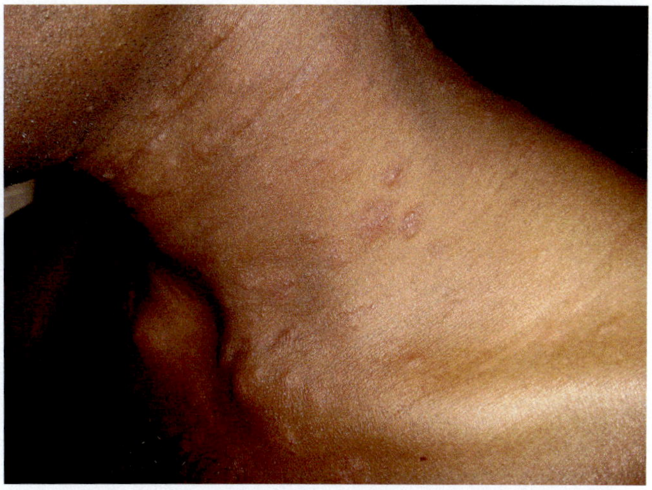

Figure 23.12 Annular and plaque type papulosquamous lesions in secondary syphilis.

## Secondary syphilis

- Secondary syphilis presents typically as generalized, macular, papular or papulosquamous eruptions that are copper-colored, non-pruritic, discrete, and distributed over the flanks, shoulders, extremities and trunk, including palms and soles.
- Atypical lesions, such as annular plaques, pustular, nodular, ulcerative, corymbiform, and SLE-like lesions, can also appear.
- Annular lesions with central hyperpigmentation commonly affect children and dark-skinned people and are observed on the cheeks or around the angle of the mouth. They can also be seen over the penis, feet, and legs. Lesions can range from 1–2 mm to 15 –20 mm (**Figure 23.12**).
- Condyloma lata, syphilitic sore throat, moth-eaten alopecia, painless aphthae, necklace of Venus (diffuse hyperpigmentation of neck with superimposed hypopigmented macules), corona veneris (papular syphilitic lesions along the anterior margin of the scalp or on the back of the neck), and split papules around oral commissures are other presenting features.
- DD: Pityriasis rosea, guttate psoriasis.

## Urticaria

- Urticaria is characterized by wheals and angioedema. Wheals during the course of disease may resolve centrally while peripheral activity is maintained, resulting in annular appearance (**Figure 23.13a**).
- Urticaria multiforme (acute annular urticaria) is considered a morphological variant of acute urticaria and is a benign, self-limited disease.
  - It commonly affects pediatric age groups from infants to children.
  - Viral infections, antibiotics, and immunization are known triggering factors.

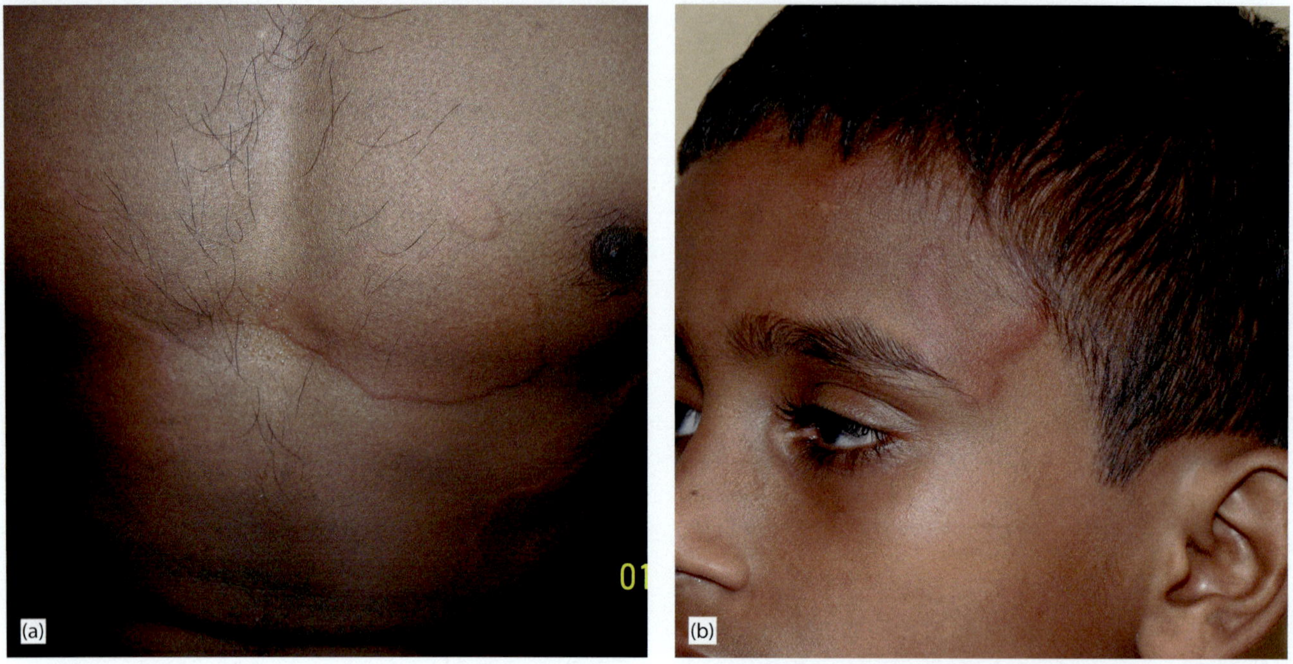

Figure 23.13 **(a)** Annular lesion of urticaria with central blanching. **(b)** Urticaria multiforme with dusky center.

- The lesion presents as itchy, blanchable annular or polycyclic erythematous plaques with an ecchymotic dusky center, followed by central clearing. It commonly affects the face, trunk, and extremities. The individual lesion does not last for more than 24 hours (**Figure 23.13b**).
- Acral edema, dermatographism, and mild fever are seen.
- The disease lasts 2 to 12 days.
- DD: Erythema multiforme (typical target lesions, persists for more than 24 hours, mucous membrane affected), urticarial vasculitis (commonly affects adults, lesions persist for more than 24 hours, burning sensation).

## Annular elastolytic giant cell granuloma (AEGCG) (actinic granuloma, elastolytic giant cell granuloma)

- AEGCG is a rare dermatosis possibly related to ultraviolet rays and infrared radiation exposure.
- The disease commonly affects middle-aged females.
- Initial lesions are single or grouped skin-colored to pink papules that coalesce to form annular plaques. Well-developed lesions present as annular plaques 1–10 cm in diameter with a raised erythematous border and slightly atrophic, hypopigmented center. Surface changes including scales are usually absent. The lesions are present over sun-exposed areas (**Figure 23.14a**).
- Lesions are usually asymptomatic, but pruritus has been seen in many cases.
- Spontaneous remission of the plaques occurs within months to years, and then mottled dyspigmentation or normal appearing skin is left behind.

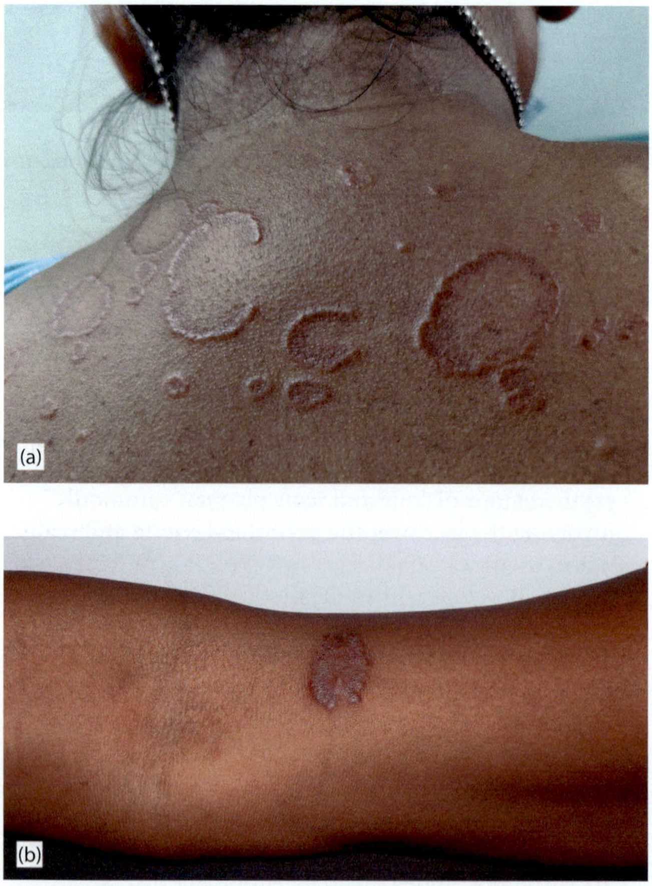

Figure 23.14 **(a)** Annular and arcuate lesions of annular elastolytic giant cell granuloma on the upper back. **(b)** Brown colored annular plaque with central atrophy in necrobiosis lipoidica. (*Continued*)

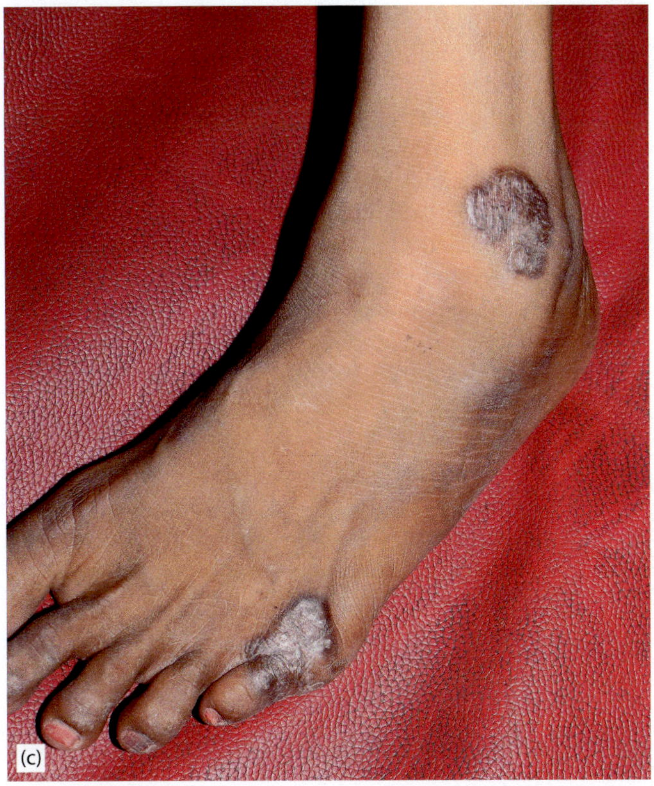


Figure 23.14 (*Continued*) **(c)** Necrobiosis lipoidica presenting with brownish annular plaques. (Courtesy: Dr. Dependra Kumar Timshina, Remedy Clinic, Siliguri, India.)

- DD: Tinea corporis, granuloma annulare, necrobiosis lipoidica (yellowish plaques with telangiectatic center, ulceration), erythema annulare centrifugum (annular erythematous plaque with trailing scales).

## Necrobiosis lipoidica

- The lesion usually starts as small, firm red-brown papules with slight scales that enlarge gradually to form an annular lesion.
- A well-developed lesion is clinically characterized by yellow-brown glistening or telangiectatic plaque with central atrophy and an elevated violaceous well-defined rim (**Figure 23.14b,c**).
- The lesion commonly occurs on shins, but the upper extremities, trunk, face, scalp, palms, and soles can also get affected.
- Decreased sensation to pin prick, fine touch, hypohidrosis, and partial alopecia can be seen in some cases.
- Ulceration and Koebnerization are common.
- Development of squamous cell carcinoma is a late complication.
- DD: Granuloma annulare, lipodermatosclerosis (presents as hardening of the skin on lower limb), necrobiotic xanthogranuloma (yellowish plaques and nodules mostly around periorbital area).

## Annular tufted angioma

- It is a rare form of benign vascular neoplasm and commonly affects children and young adults without any gender preference.
- The disease presentation can be congenital or acquired.
- The lesion presents as mottled red to pink asymptomatic patches or plaques with superimposed angiomatous papules. The lesion grows slowly by lateral expansion, acquiring annular and arciform shapes over a period of months to years (**Figure 23.15**).
- Lesions commonly affect the upper trunk, neck, and proximal part of the extremities.
- Over years lesions stabilize, shrink, or heal, leaving a fibrotic scar. Complete spontaneous regression may be observed in some cases.
- Congenital disease may develop the Kasabach-Merritt phenomenon.
- DD: Infantile hemangioma (grows rapidly during first year of life followed by spontaneous slow involution), Kaposiform hemangioendothelioma (lesion presents with deeper involvement of tissues as bulky deep seated lesion infiltrating multiple tissue planes), Kaposi sarcoma (lesions lack tufting and are multicentric; they are pink to violaceous in appearance).

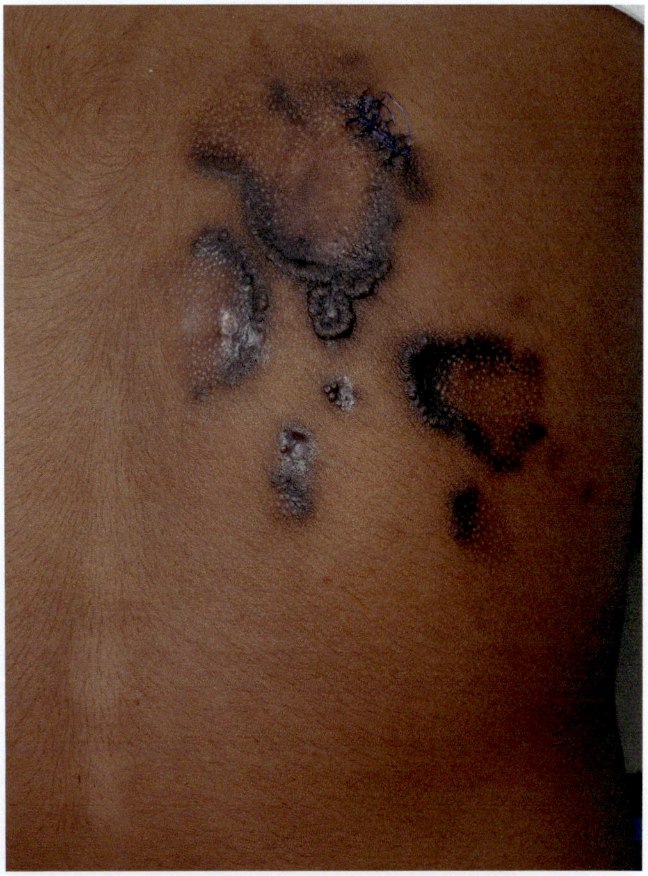

Figure 23.15 Annular tufted angioma presenting as pigmented, indurated plaques in arciform and annular pattern.

## Hansen's disease[8]

- Two forms of leprosy are present, depending upon the degree of immunity – tuberculoid type and lepromatous type. Ridley and Jopling have classified leprosy on the basis of clinical, bacteriological, immunological and histopathological features into five types – tuberculoid (TT), borderline tuberculoid (BT), mid-borderline (BB), borderline lepromatous (BL), and lepromatous leprosy (LL).
- Annular lesions are typically seen in borderline leprosy (BT, BB, BL) and careful analysis of annular morphology serves as an important clinical clue (**Figure 23.16a,b**). Sometimes, TT leprosy may assume annular configuration during the course of the disease.
- Tuberculoid type (TT) – Sometimes, the plaque may heal from the center, resulting in an atrophic center with a sharply defined and elevated border, giving an annular appearance (saucer right way up appearance).
- Borderline tuberculoid (BT) – Annular lesion of BT leprosy is characterized by a raised and well-defined margin raised in one part but with an ill-defined margin merging gradually with normal skin in another part. Satellite lesions can also be seen. The center is dyshidrotic (**Figure 23.16c,d**).

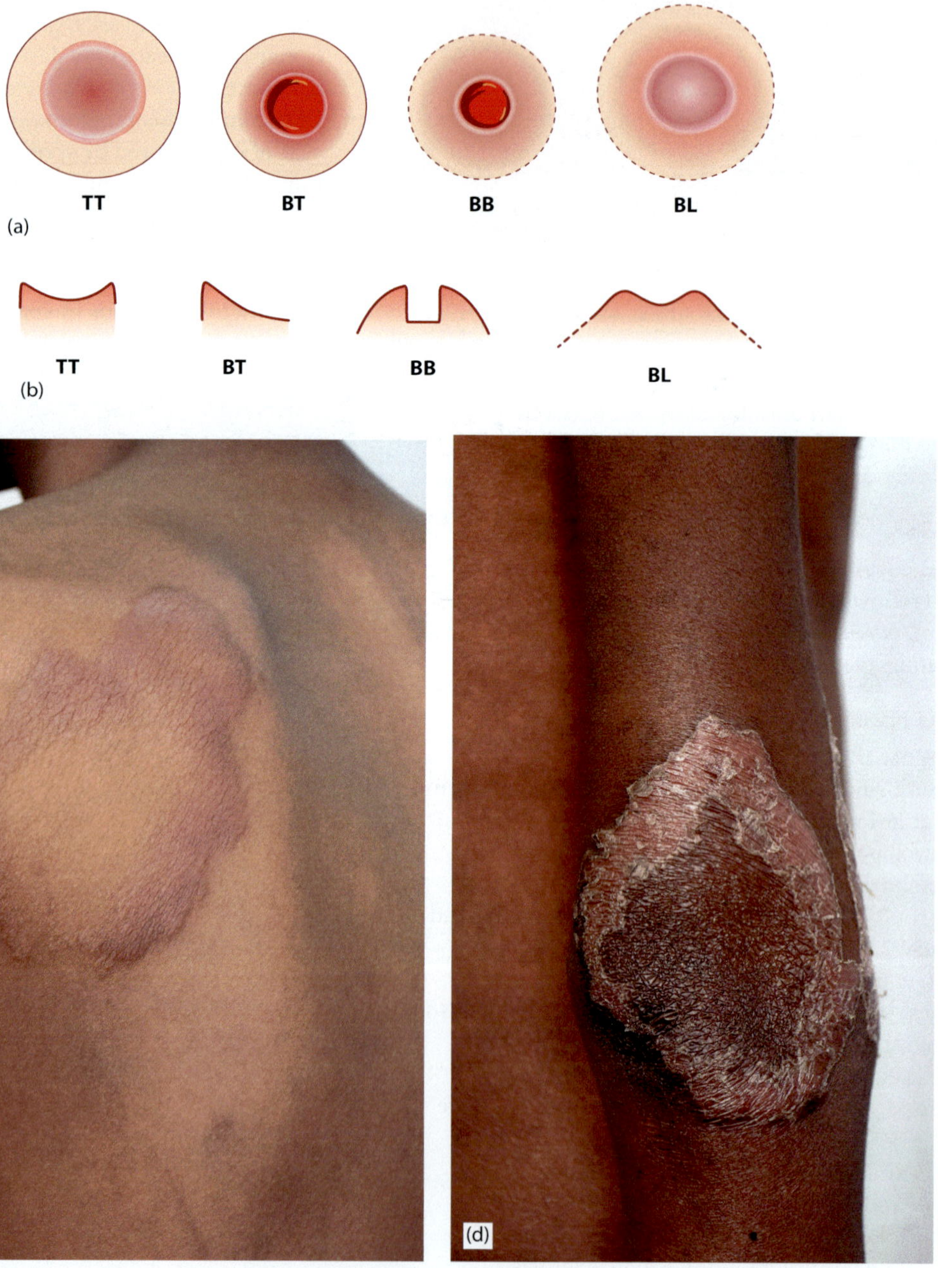


Figure 23.16 **(a)** Schematic diagram: Surface view of annular lesions in leprosy. **(b)** Schematic diagram: Cross-section view of annular lesions in leprosy. **(c)** Annular plaque of BT leprosy with ill-defined borders at the lower pole. **(d)** BT leprosy with type 1 lepra reaction presenting as annular scaly plaque with ill-defined borders at places. (*Continued*)

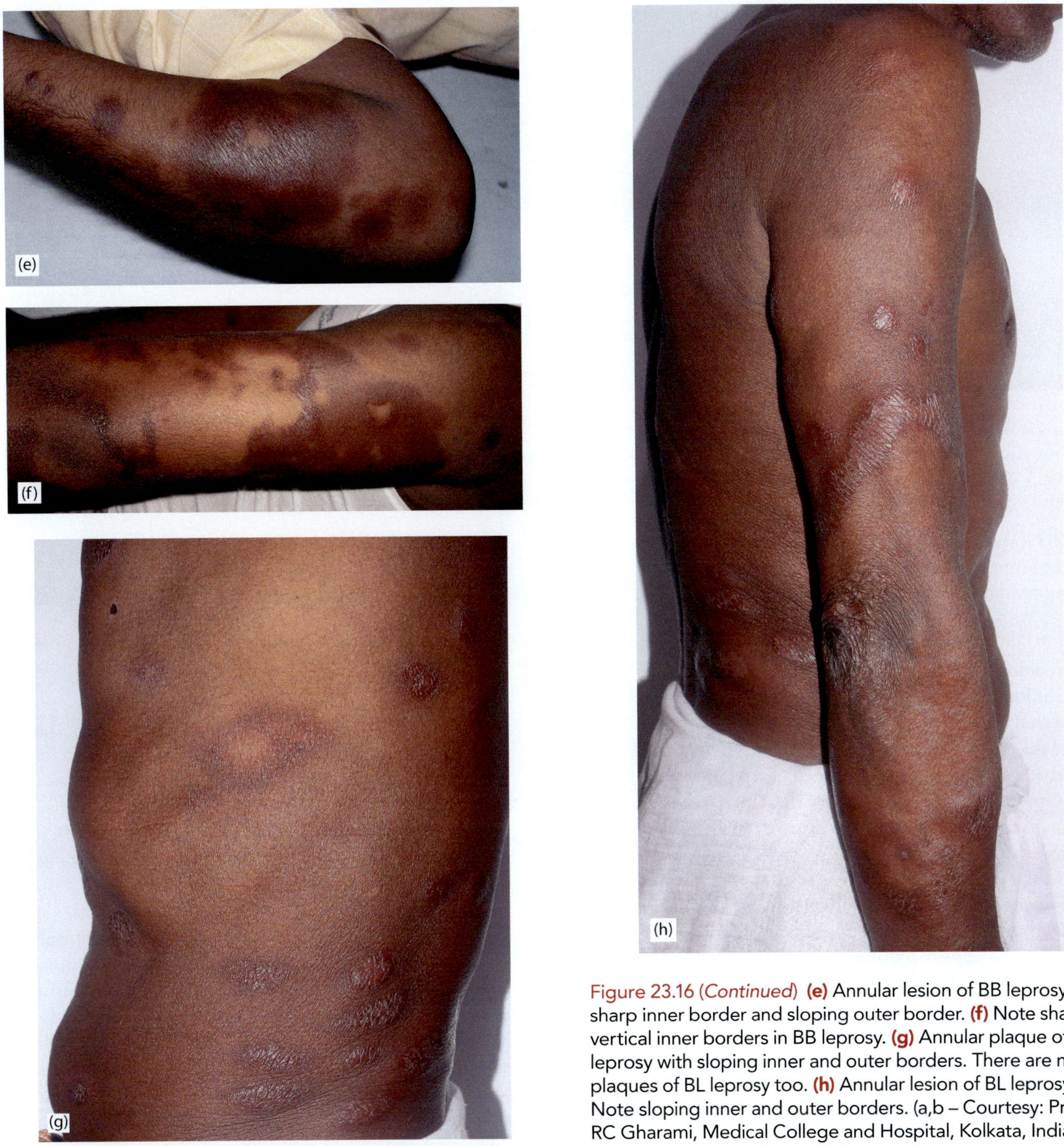

Figure 23.16 (*Continued*) **(e)** Annular lesion of BB leprosy with sharp inner border and sloping outer border. **(f)** Note sharp vertical inner borders in BB leprosy. **(g)** Annular plaque of BL leprosy with sloping inner and outer borders. There are many plaques of BL leprosy too. **(h)** Annular lesion of BL leprosy. Note sloping inner and outer borders. (a,b – Courtesy: Prof RC Gharami, Medical College and Hospital, Kolkata, India.)

- Mid-borderline leprosy (BB) – Annular lesions of the BB leprosy characteristically assume a punched-out (Swiss-cheese) appearance: a sharp clear-cut inner margin with sloping outer edges (**Figure 23.16e,f**).
- Borderline lepromatous (BL) – Annular lesions of BL leprosy are characterized by sloping outer as well as inner margins. However, the center of the lesion is more infiltrated (and elevated) than the periphery, giving an inverted saucer appearance (**Figure 23.16g,h**).
- DD: annular plaques of leprosy (granuloma annulare, annular sarcoidosis, necrobiotic xanthogranuloma, psoriasis).

## Jessner lymphocytic infiltration of the skin

- It is a benign T-cell infiltrative disease that presents as asymptomatic, recurrent arciform or annular plaques over the face.
- The lesion presents as solitary or multiple, asymptomatic, erythematous papules and annular plaques or nodules over the head, neck, and upper back (**Figure 23.17**).
- Individual lesions may disappear in several weeks to months, with complete resolution and no sequelae. Recurrence is common.

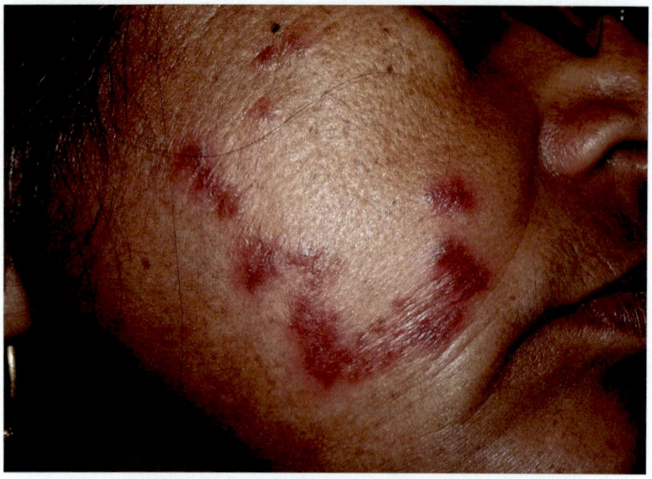

Figure 23.17 Annular erythematous plaque of Jessner's lymphocytic infiltration. (Courtesy: Dr. Hiral Shah, Baroda Medical College and Hospital, Vadodara, India.)

- DD: Granuloma annulare, plaque-type polymorphous light eruption, lupus erythematosus tumidus, cutaneous lymphoid hyperplasia.

## Annular sarcoidosis

- Sarcoidosis is a chronic multisystem inflammatory granulomatous disease that affects both skin as well as internal organs.
- The disease has two peaks of onset, first between 25 and 35 years and second between 45 and 65 years. It commonly affects women more than men.
- The disease is more prevalent in African-Americans than whites.
- Annular lesions in sarcoidosis are uncommon.
- The lesion starts as papules, which may coalesce to form red-brown annular or serpiginous plaques with patchy scales.
- The lesions appear indurated, with central clearing, and they heal with hypopigmentation, atrophy, or scarring (**Figure 23.18**).
- It commonly affects head and neck and is associated with chronic sarcoidosis. Sun-exposed areas are the favored sites.
- Alopecia can result in the center of the lesion.
- DD: Secondary syphilis, discoid lupus erythematosus, annular lichen planus, Hansen's disease.

## Lupus vulgaris (LV)

- LV is a chronic, progressive, common form of cutaneous tuberculosis in adults.
- It commonly affects people with poor socioeconomic status and those with moderate to high immunity.
- The disease affects all age groups and has female preference compared to male in the ratio of 2–3:1.
- It is acquired through hematogenous or lymphatic spread or may develop after direct contiguous spread from other primary sites of infection, usually from bone, joint, and lymph-node infection. The lesion commonly affects the face, neck, and extremities. The nose, earlobes, and cheeks are common sites.

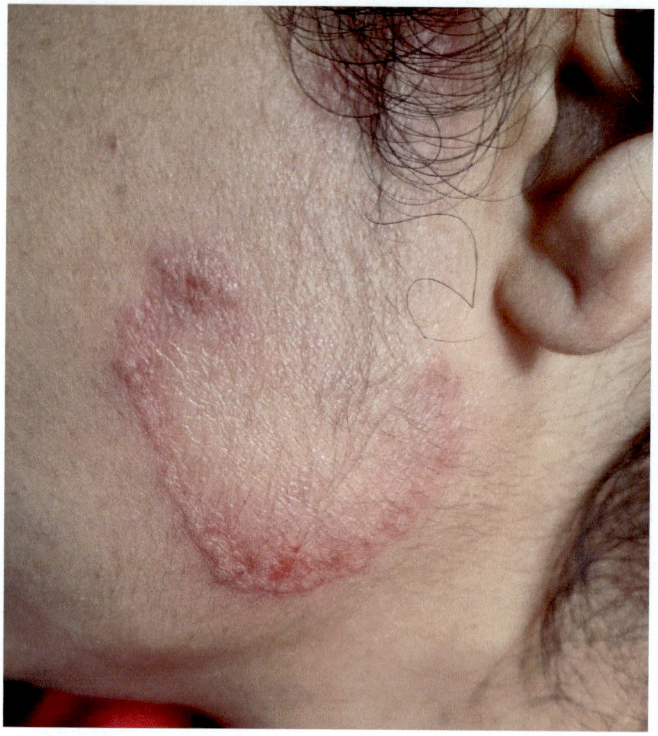

Figure 23.18 Arcuate erythematous plaque of sarcoidosis on the face. (Courtesy: Dr. Rajib Gogoi, Guwahati, India.)

- In developing countries like India, lupus vulgaris is commonly acquired after trauma, and hence trauma-prone areas are frequently affected.
- One of the most characteristic features of LV is peripheral expansion with central healing (with scarring). Because of this feature, LV frequently presents with annular (when spread is uniform in all directions) and serpiginous or arciform (when expansion is not uniform) lesions. LV lesions developing into annular or arciform lesions is a valuable diagnostic clue (**Figure 23.19a–c**).
- LV commonly presents as single annular plaque with a raised hyperkeratotic border with central scarring. The lesion starts as red-brown grouped papule and nodule that shows blanching on diascopy with apple jelly color. The lesion expands by development of new papules at the periphery, which coalesce with the main plaque. As the lesion progresses in one direction, previously involved parts tend to heal with scarring (**Figure 23.19d,e**).
- The disease has a slow rate of progression. The lesion remains limited to a particular area for several years.
- Other clinical variants of LV are ulcerative type, vegetative type, papulonodular type, etc.
- DD: Leprosy, sarcoidosis, discoid lupus erythematosus.

## Annular lichen planus

- It is an uncommon variant of lichen planus.
- These lesions start as purple to polygonal papules that spread peripherally with central clearing. The

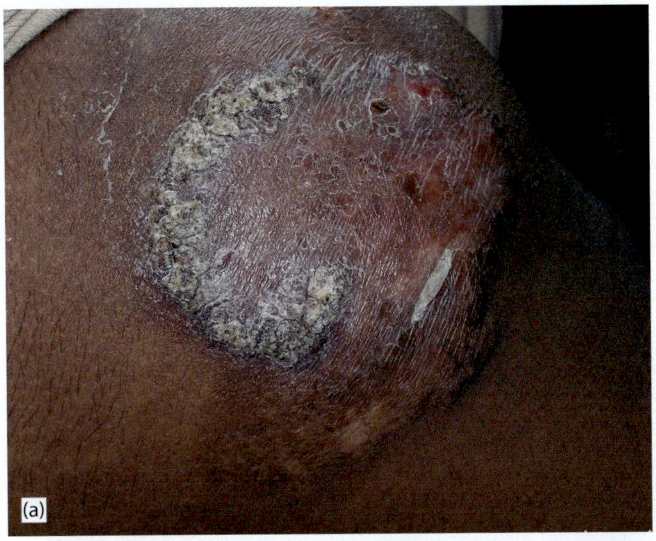

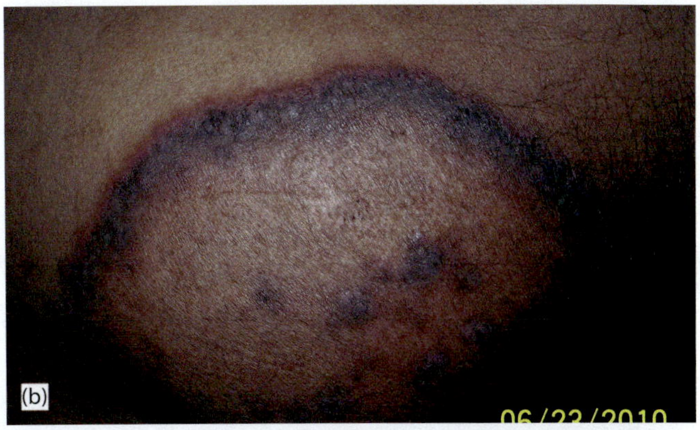

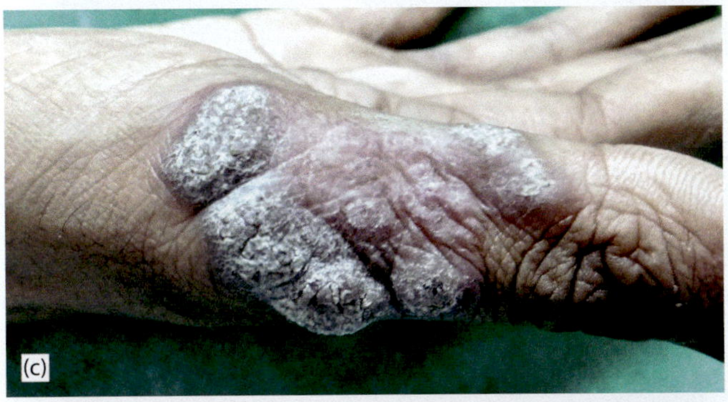

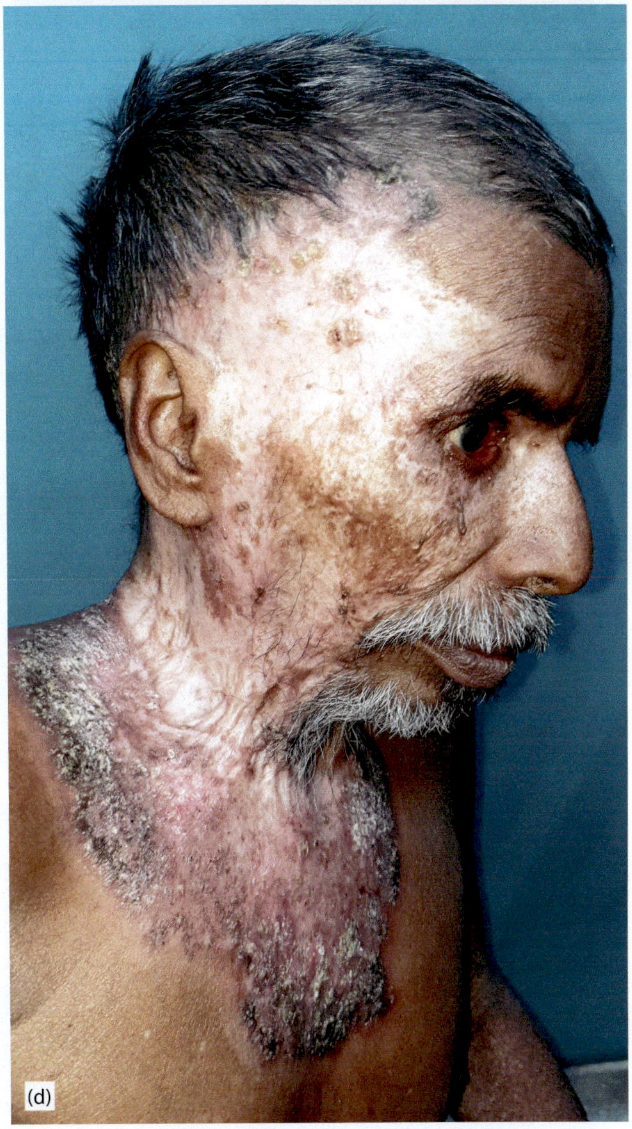

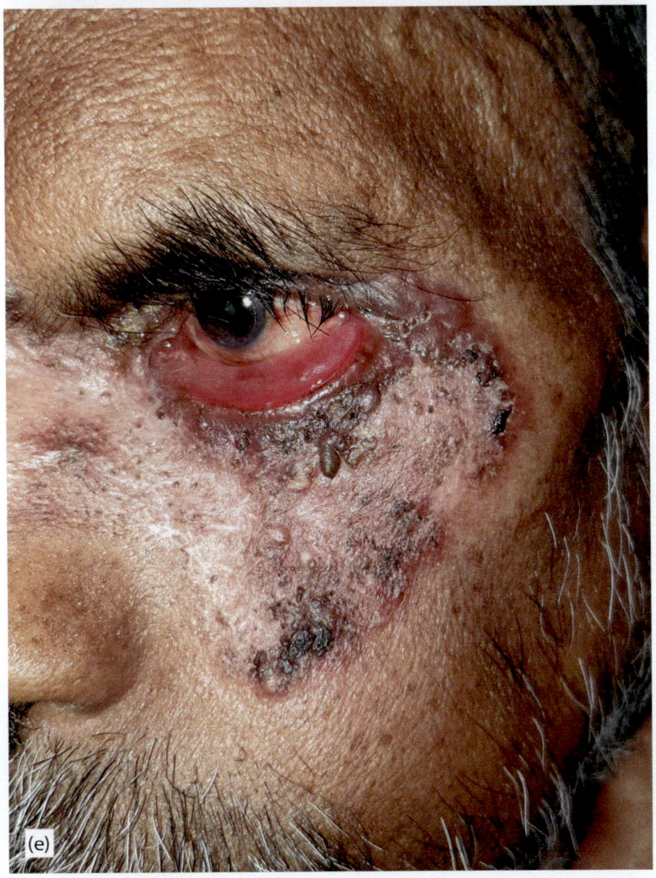

Figure 23.19 **(a)** Arciform crusted plaque in lupus vulgaris. Note atrophic scarring. **(b)** Lupus vulgaris with erythematous indurated border. **(c)** Lupus vulgaris on the hand with hyperkeratotic arciform plaque. **(d)** Giant lesion of lupus vulgaris affecting the contiguous areas of the face, neck, and upper trunk. **(e)** Same patient with lupus vulgaris on face. Note ectropion due to scarring. (c – Courtesy: Dr. Shreya Singh, India; d,e – Courtesy: Dr. Rajesh Kumar Mandal, North Bengal Medical College and Hospital, India.)

raised border is violaceous in color, and the center is hyperpigmented.

- The most commonly affected sites are axilla, penis, extremities, groin, back, buttocks, flanks, neck, and eyelids (**Figure 23.20a–d**).
- DD: Tinea corporis, porokeratosis (elevated thread border with central groove).

## Basal cell carcinoma (BCC)

- Basal cell carcinoma is the most common benign non-melanocytic skin cancer, presenting mostly on sun-exposed areas.
- The incidence of BCC is higher in white populations, but it can affect all races. Fitzpatrick skin types 1 and type 2 are the ones with greater incidence.

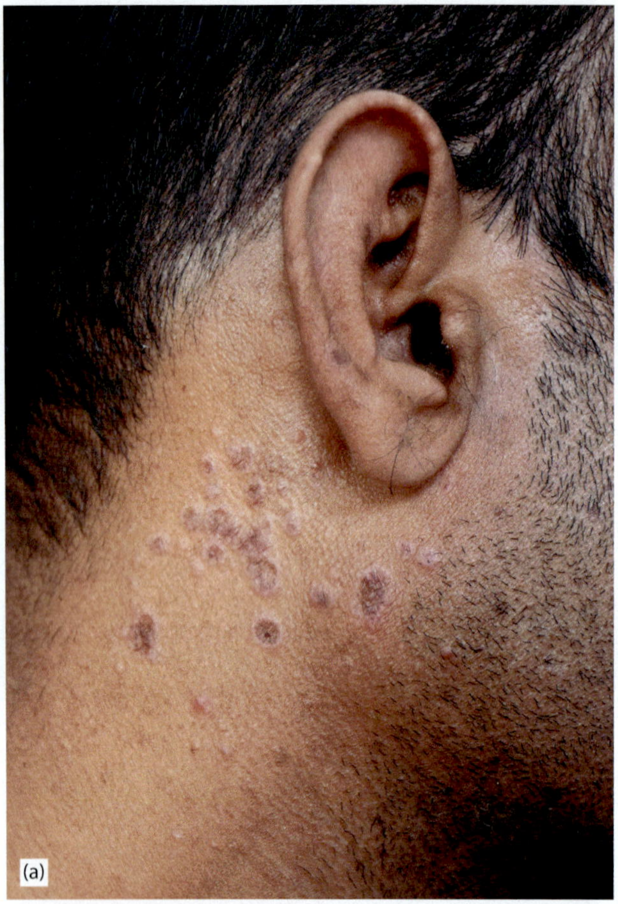

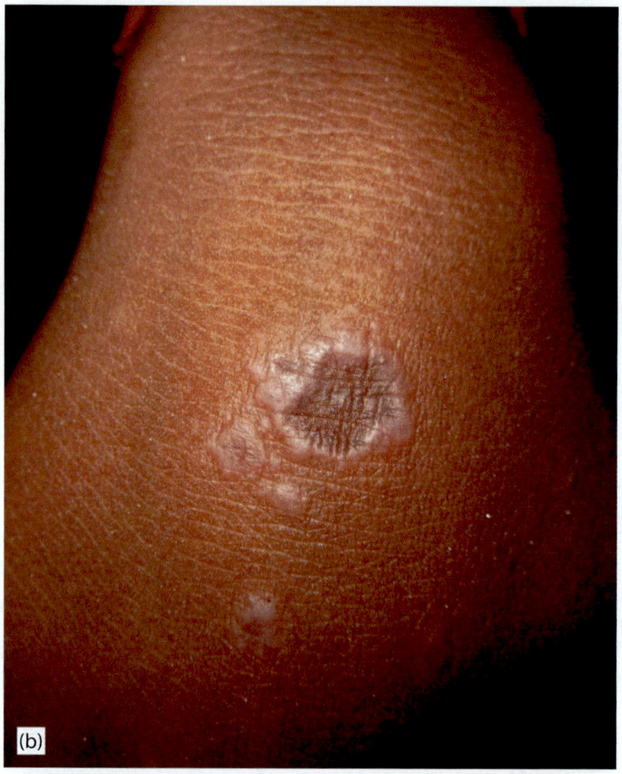

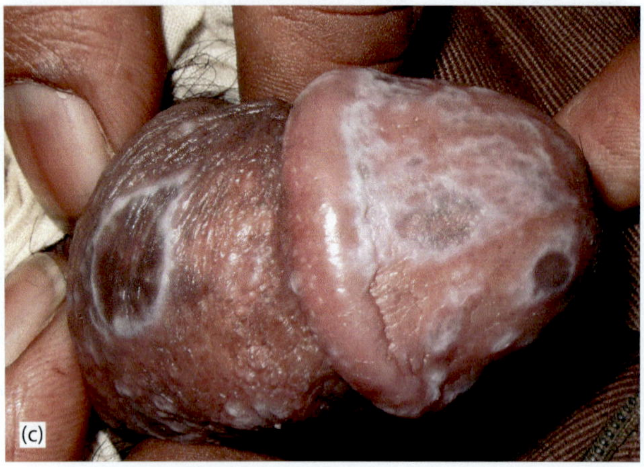

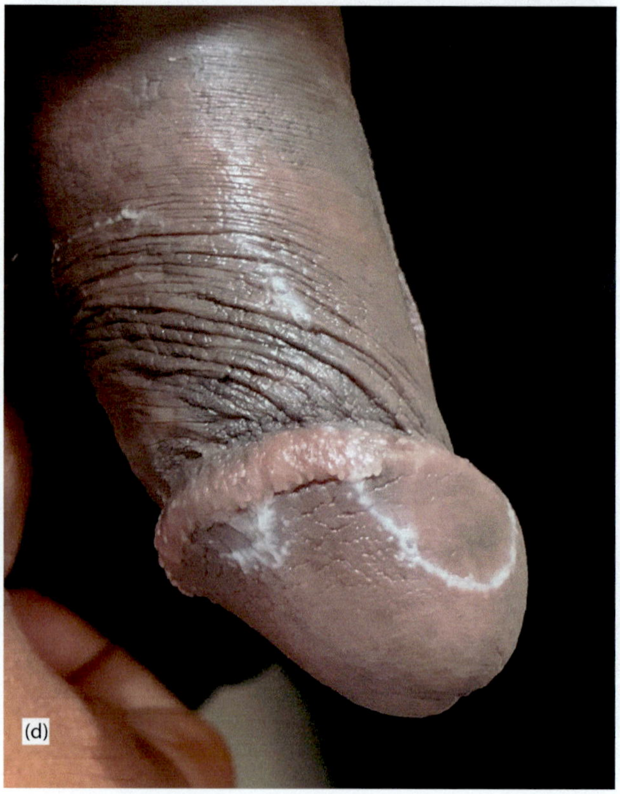

Figure 23.20 **(a)** Lichen planus with annular violaceous plaques with pigmented atrophic center. **(b)** Annular lichen planus on the dorsum of the hand. **(c)** Annular lichen planus on the penis. Note reticulate whitish areas surrounding the lesion. **(d)** Annular lesions of lichen planus are common on mucosa. (d – Courtesy: Dr. Rajeev Ranjan, Ara, India.)

- Men have a higher tendency to develop the disease than women.
- Incidence is higher in older individuals aged 55 to 70 years.
- Annular lesions are appreciable in nodular, superficial spreading and morpheaform types of BCC.
  - Nodular type – It is the most common subtype and starts as a shiny, pearly papule or nodule with a smooth surface with telangiectasia. Over time, the lesion enlarges to form an elevated rolled, waxy border. In colored skin, the border is commonly pigmented. The center may get ulcerated and crusted. The lesion favor the face, especially the cheeks, nasolabial folds, forehead, eyelids, and nose **(Figure 23.21a–c).**
  - Superficial type – The lesion presents as well-circumscribed annular plaque with scales and pigmented, waxy papules on the border. The lesion typically shows some areas of spontaneous regression with atrophy and hypopigmentation. The tumor mostly grows horizontally but may infiltrate deep with induration, infiltration, and ulceration (**Figure 23.21d,e**).
  - Morpheaform type – The lesion presents as a pink to white or yellow waxy, sclerotic plaque that rarely ulcerates. The lesion can be slightly elevated or depressed, fibrotic or firm with ill-defined borders. The typical pearly border is absent for the most parts of the lesion. The lesion is more aggressive, with extensive local destruction.
- DD: Bowen's disease (well-defined erythematous, slightly scaly and crusted, non-infiltrated patch), annular lichen planus, seborrheic keratosis (tan to light-brown to black, sharply demarcated papule or plaque, "stuck on" appearance).

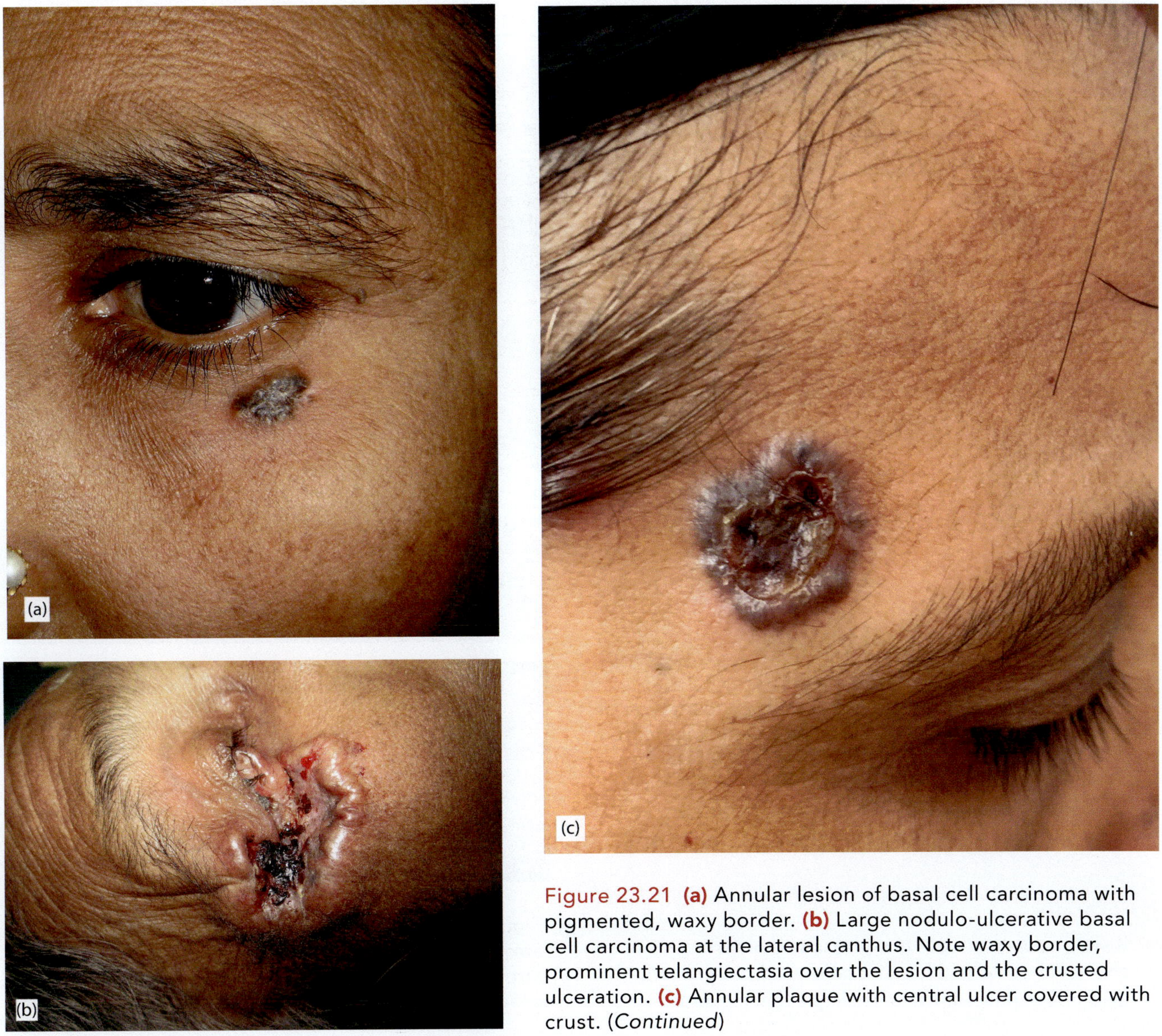

Figure 23.21 **(a)** Annular lesion of basal cell carcinoma with pigmented, waxy border. **(b)** Large nodulo-ulcerative basal cell carcinoma at the lateral canthus. Note waxy border, prominent telangiectasia over the lesion and the crusted ulceration. **(c)** Annular plaque with central ulcer covered with crust. (*Continued*)

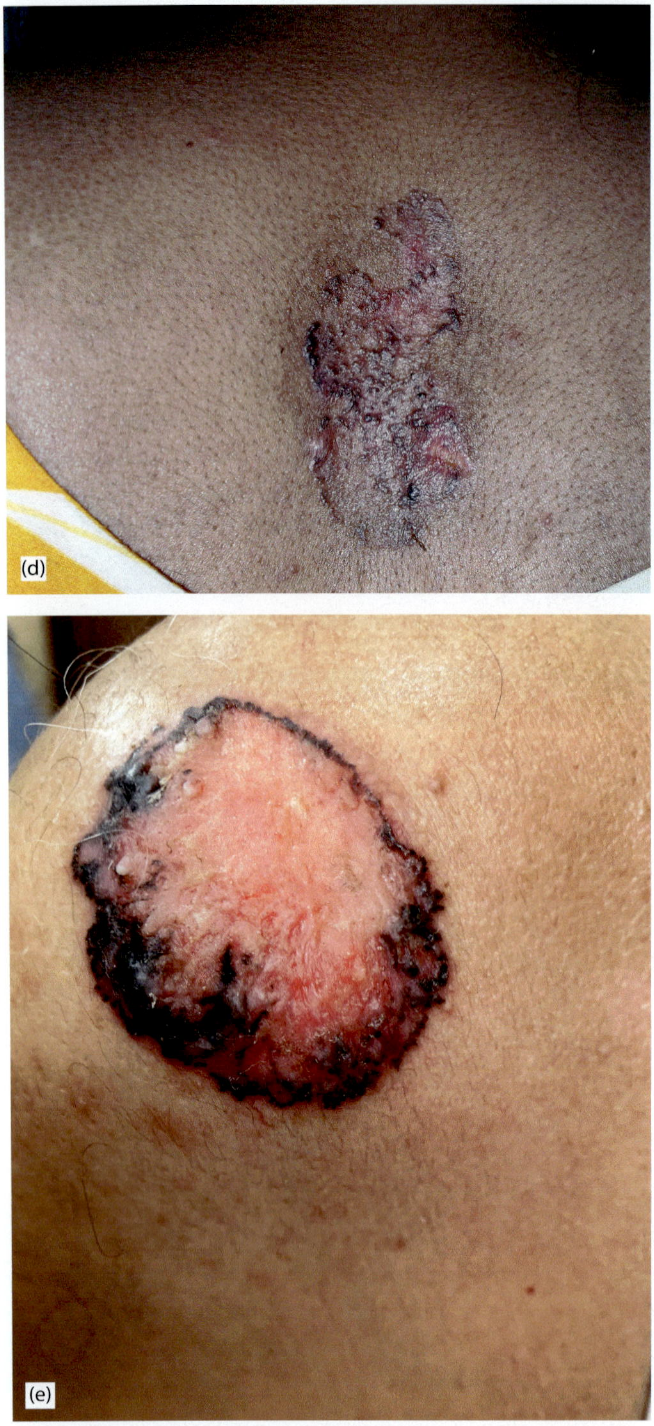


Figure 23.21 (*Continued*) **(d)** Superficial spreading type of basal cell carcinoma. Note central scarring and pigmented papules at the margin. **(e)** Large lesion of Superficial spreading type of basal cell carcinoma. Part of the lesions have evolved into nodular basal cell carcinoma. (c,e – Courtesy: Dr Rajeev Ranjan, Ara, India.)

## Porokeratosis

- It comprises a rare group of diseases that show abnormal epidermal keratinization and present as keratotic papules or annular plaque that expands centrifugally with an elevated border that corresponds to cornoid lamella on histology.
- The disease may be inherited in autosomal dominant patterns except the punctate type.
- Sun exposure, immunosuppression, and radiation therapy act as aggravating factors.
- The lesion starts as an asymptomatic keratotic papule that expands over weeks or months to form an annular plaque with keratotic border. The border has a central groove (resembling the Great wall of China), a diagnostic feature of porokeratosis.
- Commonly known clinical types include (**Figure 23.22a**) the following:
    - Porokeratosis of Mibelli – It appears during infancy or childhood and affects boys more than girls. It commonly affects the distal extremities but may be localized or may be widespread. The lesions may be solitary or multiple, giant (as large as 20 cm) or itchy (especially flexural lesions). Clinically, the Mibelli type shows typical lesions of porokeratosis (described earlier) with the center of lesion showing hyperpigmentation, hypopigmentation, atrophy, or anhidrosis (**Figure 23.22b,c**).

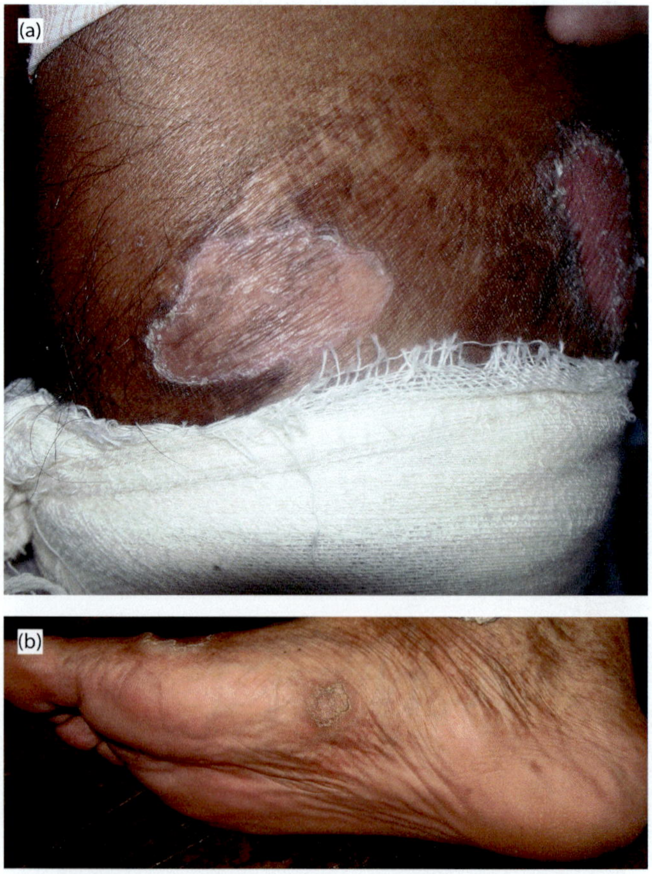


Figure 23.22 **(a)** Porokeratosis: annular lesion with atrophic center and keratotic margin with groove (black arrow). **(b)** Porokeratosis on the sole showing prominent groove. (*Continued*)

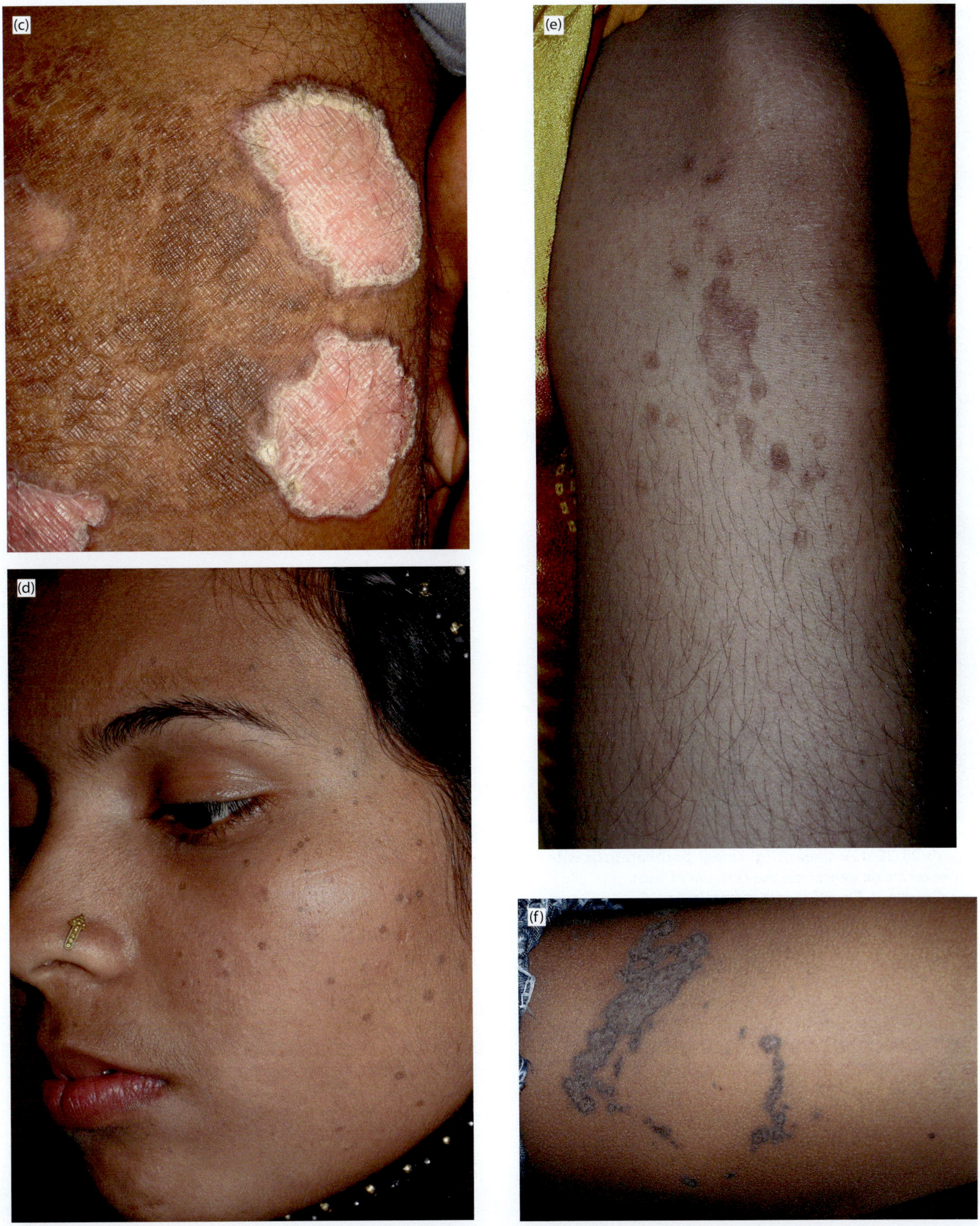


Figure 23.22 (*Continued*) **(c)** Porokeratosis with annular erythematous, scaly plaques. **(d)** Lesions in disseminated superficial actinic porokeratosis are smaller and keratotic ridge is less prominent. **(e)** Disseminated superficial porokeratosis. Like DSAP, the keratotic ridge is usually subtle. **(f)** Linear porokeratosis following Blaschko's lines on the trunk. (*Continued*)

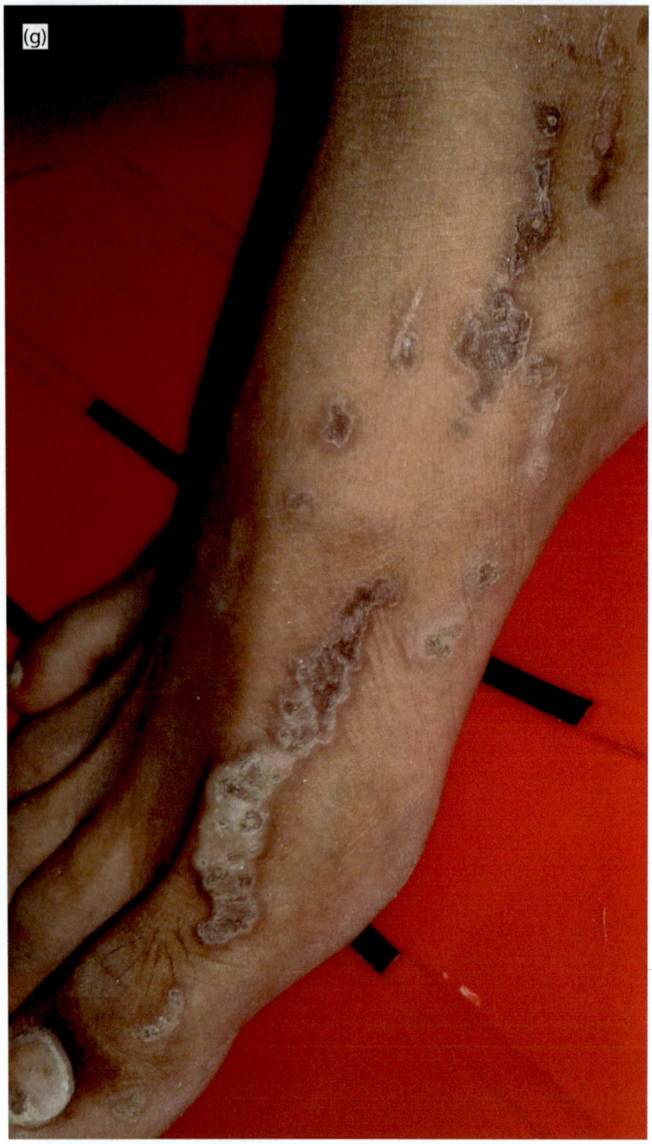


Figure 23.22 (*Continued*) **(g)** Linear porokeratosis with hyperkeratotic center on the dorsum of foot. (g – Courtesy: Dr. PC Das, Katihar, India.)

- Disseminated superficial actinic porokeratosis (DSAP) – It is common in countries with high sun exposure and is usually present in the third to fourth decade of life. Patients develop several small (about 1 cm) annular lesions distributed in a bilaterally symmetric manner on sun exposed sites. The border is not as prominent as that of the Mibelli type, and the central part of the lesion is usually pigmented (**Figure 23.22d**).
- Disseminated Superficial PK (DSP) – The lesions are similar to DSAP, but the lesions appear on sun-covered parts too and the condition has an early onset (**Figure 23.22e**).
- Linear porokeratosis – It arises during infancy or childhood as keratotic papules and erythematous patches and plaques along the lines of Blaschko and has the highest tendency of malignant transformation. In colored skin, lesions often appear pigmented (**Figure 23.22f,g**).
- Punctate porokeratosis – It appears during adolescence and childhood as small, keratotic, sometimes tender papules of 1–2 mm diameter with raised peripheral rims over the palm and soles. Clinically it resembles punctate keratoderma, Darier disease, Cowden syndrome and arsenical keratosis.
- Porokeratosis palmaris et plantaris disseminata – The lesions are similar to punctate porokeratosis, but they affect the trunk, extremities, and mucous membranes in addition to palms and soles. The condition shows male preponderance and usually arises during adolescence and childhood.
- Porokeratosis ptychotropica – It presents as red to brown pruritic papules and plaques involving the intergluteal clefts and buttocks. Central coalescence of lesions with peripherally scattered papules is also seen.

- DD:
    - Porokeratosis of Mibelli – annular lichen planus, granuloma annulare
    - Linear porokeratosis – linear lichen planus, linear epidermal nevus and incontinentia pigmenti.

## Tuberculosis verrucosa cutis

- It is a common form of cutaneous tuberculosis caused by accidental inoculation of *Mycobacterium tuberculosis* in previously sensitized or infected persons with moderate to high cell-mediated immunity. Trauma prone sites are commonly affected.
- The lesion starts as asymptomatic small indurated wart-like papules having an inflammatory rim that slowly progresses in firm reddish-brown verrucous or hyperkeratotic plaques over months to years. Superficial scaling and fissuring with intermittent purulent discharge is seen.
- Sometimes, the lesion may undergo central clearing with scarring and atrophy, giving an annular configuration.
- DD: Majocchi granuloma, lichen simplex chronicus (well-circumscribed plaque resulting from repeated rubbing or scratching), warts, psoriasis, hypertrophic lichen planus.

## Keratoacanthoma centrifugum marginatum

- It is a rare variant of keratoacanthoma.
- The disease commonly affects white adults in their fifth decade of life.
- It starts as solitary or multiple lesions that expand by peripheral extension reaching up to 5–20 cm, with raised, rolled borders and central healing (with atrophic scarring). The margin may show erythematous papulonodular lesions with keratotic plugs; the

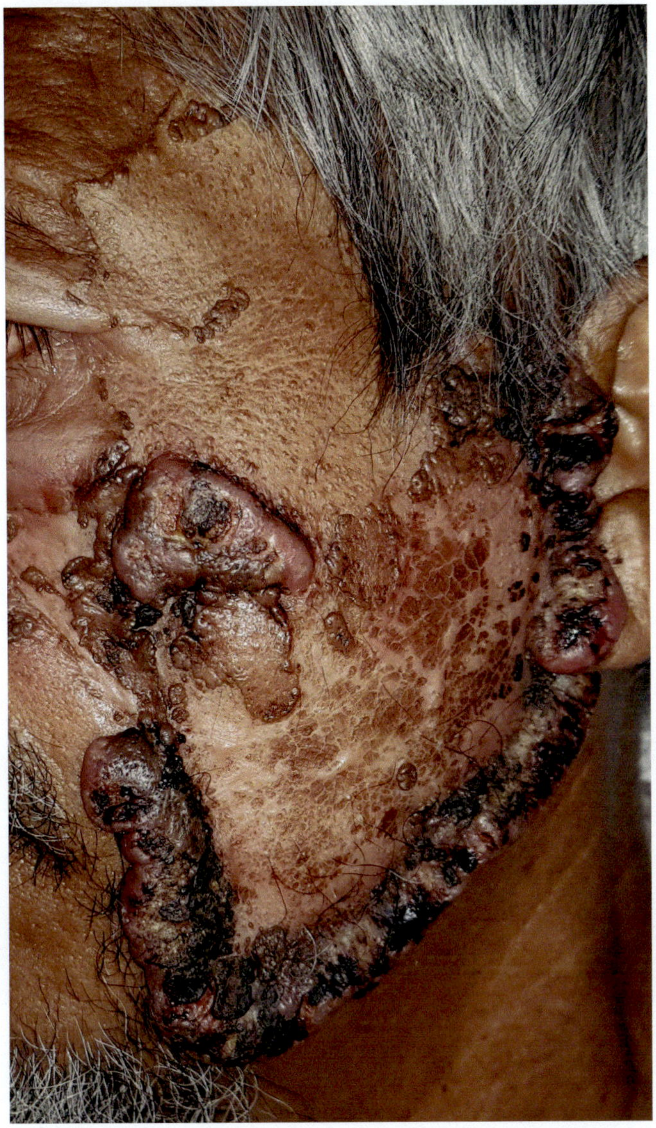

Figure 23.23 Keratoacanthoma centrifugum marginatum with central atrophic scarring and erythematous nodules on the margin. The surface of the nodules are crusted and hyperkeratotic. (Courtesy: Dr. Shahid Hassan, Purnea, India.)

latter mimic lesions of nodular keratoacanthoma (**Figure 23.23**).

- Lesions usually appear on sun-exposed areas.
- The tumor is benign and locally destructive. The lesion does not show a tendency of spontaneous resolution and may progress to huge dimensions.
- DD: Lupus vulgaris, squamous cell carcinoma, botryomycosis.

## Linear IgA bullous dermatosis (LABD)

- LABD (and its childhood counterpart, chronic bullous disease of childhood, [CBDC]) is an immune-mediated, subepidermal, vesiculobullous disease.
- It affects children two to three years of age, the average being four and a half years, and adults above 60 years of age, with slight female preponderance.

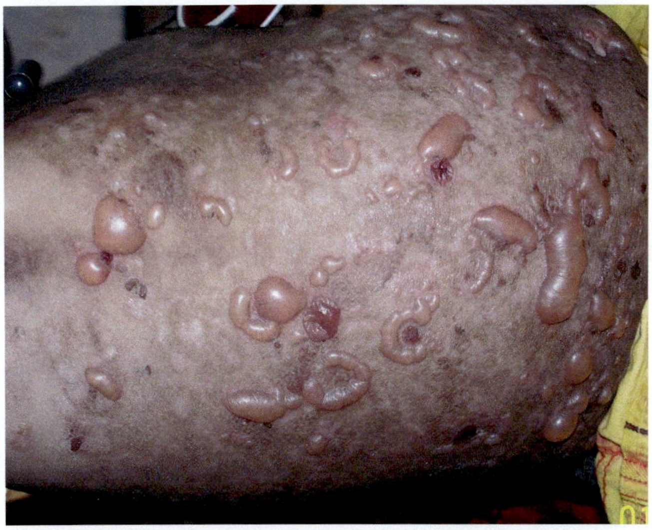

Figure 23.24 Chronic bullous disease of childhood with tense blisters arranged in an annular configuration.

- Patients present with bullae on the erythematous base or on normal-looking skin, commonly over the lower trunk, thighs, buttocks, groin, perioral, and scalp region. New blisters appear at the periphery of crusted old bullae and thus, the bullae appear arranged in annular or rosette pattern ("string of pearls" or "cluster of jewels'). Oral mucosa involvement is seen (**Figure 23.24**).
- The classical clinical appearance (bullae in annular pattern) may be less distinctive in the adult form. LABD usually mimics dermatitis herpetiformis or bullous pemphigoid.
- DD: Dermatitis herpetiformis (itchy, grouped papulovesicles and excoriations over extensors, scalp and trunk), bullous pemphigoid, bullous impetigo, Stevens-Johnson syndrome.

## Cutaneous larva migrans (creeping eruption)

- It is a serpiginous or curvilinear eruption caused by the accidental penetration and migration of animal hookworms (mostly by *Ancylostoma braziliense* or *Ancylostoma caninum*) larvae through the epidermis.
- The disease is endemic the Caribbean, Central America, South America, Southeast Asia, and Africa.
- It occurs commonly in warmer climates, in the people who walk barefoot over contaminated ground, and in manual workers, carpenters, plumbers, etc.
- The disease onset is characterized by slight local itching and small vesicles, followed by formation of serpiginous tracks. Intermittent stinging pain is present.
- Each larva forms a separate tract and migrates at the rate of 1–2 cm/day. The linear lesions are interrupted by papules formed from resting larvae. As the eruption advances, the earlier involved parts begin to fade. If left untreated the larva dies in two to four weeks, leading to spontaneous resolution (**Figure 23.25a**).
- Larvae may remain quiescent for several days or months before they start migrating.

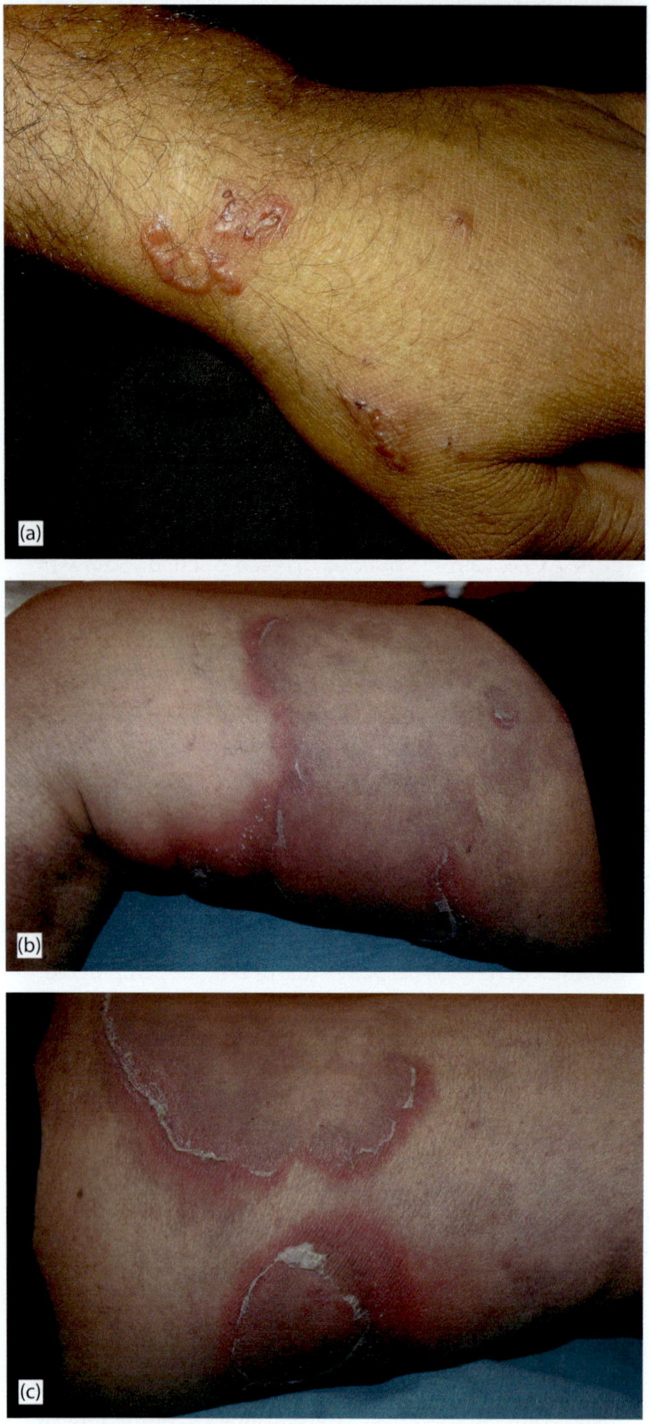


Figure 23.25 **(a)** Linear and serpiginous vesicles in cutaneous larva migrans. **(b,c)** Annular erythematous scaly patches in neutrophilic figurate erythema in an elderly male.

- It commonly affects lower extremities, but buttocks, hands, thighs, and perianal areas can also get involved.
- Purulent manifestations can occur due to secondary infections; erosions and excoriations are seen frequently.
- Migratory pulmonary infiltrates and Löffler syndrome are rarely seen.
- DD: Inflammatory tinea corporis, larva currens ("running" larva) (serpiginous erythematous papules coalescing into urticarial linear plaques caused by *Strongyloides stercoralis*).

## Neutrophilic figurate erythema (NFE)[9]

- NFE presents as an arcuate or annular lesion on face, trunk, or extremities, without any predilection. The lesion spreads centrifugally, and the active margin is clinically characterized by erythema, edema, vesicles and bullae, and purpura with some scaling (**Figure 23.25b,c**). The condition may heal spontaneously but may recur in summers.

## Necrolytic migratory erythema (NME)

- NME is a cutaneous hallmark of glucagonoma, characterized by a triad of weight loss, diabetes mellitus, and NME. Pseudoglucagonoma syndrome has been reported in liver diseases and intestinal malabsorption.
- The cutaneous lesions start as intensely pruritic or painful erythematous scaly patches with centrifugal growth. The lesions are predominantly seen in the periorificial area and in areas with increased pressure or friction (intertriginous areas, buttocks, lower abdomen, and distal extremities). The central part of the lesion develops into flaccid blisters, and the latter get ulcerated and crusted and eventually heal with hyperpigmentation. As the central part of the lesions heal, erythema spreads centrifugally and fresh blisters at the advancing margins. These new blisters too heal in a similar manner.
- The disease runs a chronic relapsing course.
- Associated mucosal changes include angular cheilitis, glossitis, and stomatitis. Nails may show onychoschizia.
- Systemic features found in NME are diarrhea, neuropsychiatric changes, anemia, and hypercoagulability.

## Sneddon-Wilkinson disease (subcorneal pustular dermatosis)

- It is an autoimmune neutrophilic dermatosis with a chronic relapsing course commonly affecting women over 40 years of age. Children and adolescents are also affected.
- It presents as annular or polycyclic lesions commonly involving flexures of the extremities, intertriginous areas, and trunk.
- The initial lesion presents as superficial sterile pustules that progress to flaccid blisters with clear fluid in the upper part and pus in the lower part. These pustules coalesce and form annular lesions. The blisters rupture with superficial scaling, crusting, and secondary hyperpigmentation. New lesions keep coming, and the disease runs a chronic relapsing course.
- DD: IgA pemphigus, pustular psoriasis, bullous impetigo.

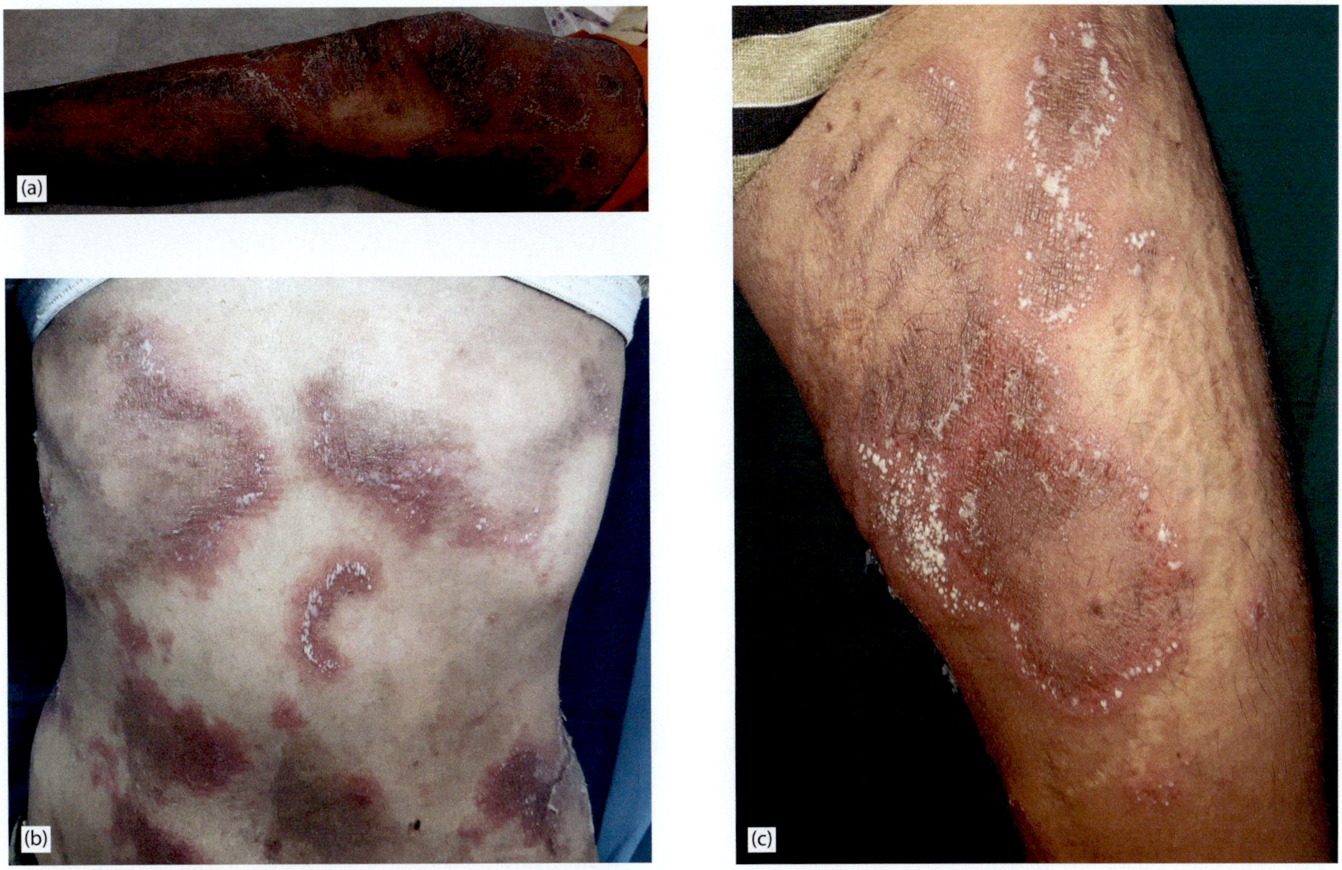

Figure 23.26 **(a)** Annular pustular psoriasis with pustules surrounding central erythematous scaly area. **(b)** Arcuate lesions of pustular psoriasis. **(c)** Annular pustular psoriasis. Note superficial nature of pustules. (b,c – Courtesy: Dr Hiral Shah, Baroda Medical College, Vadodara, India.)

## Annular pustular psoriasis

- It is a rare variant of pustular psoriasis that has a chronic relapsing course with a good prognosis.
- It affects mostly children, but adults are also affected.
- The patient presents with well-circumscribed, annular lesions consisting of erythema, scaling, and pustules at the periphery. The lesions enlarge in centrifugal fashion, with central healing within several days. Lesions heal within days but have a relapsing course (**Figure 23.26a–c**).
- DD: Tinea corporis.

## Ichthyosis linearis circumflexa (ILC)

- It is an inherited autosomal recessive disorder in which migratory annular or polycyclic patches occur.
- The lesion appears in infancy or early childhood.
- The lesion appears as severe generalized exfoliative erythroderma at birth or shortly after. Later the lesion becomes annular, polycyclic, or serpiginous with a double-edged scaly border over the trunk and proximal extremities. Lesions attain their maximum diameter in one week and resolve without atrophy, scarring, or pigmentation (**Figure 23.27**).
- Lesions may clear almost completely in summer.
- Lichenification of the popliteal and cubital fossa with red, scaly face and eyelids are also seen due to coexistence of atopic dermatitis.

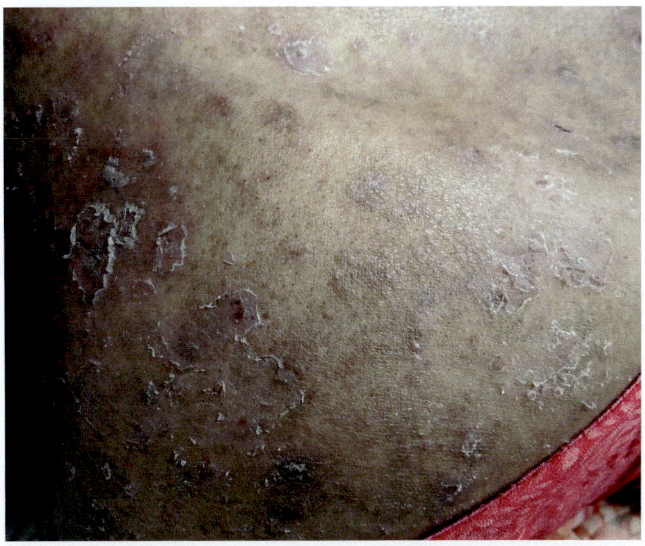

Figure 23.27 Annular and serpiginous double-edged scales in ichthyosis linearis circumflexa. (Courtesy: Dr. Anil Patki, Pune, India.)

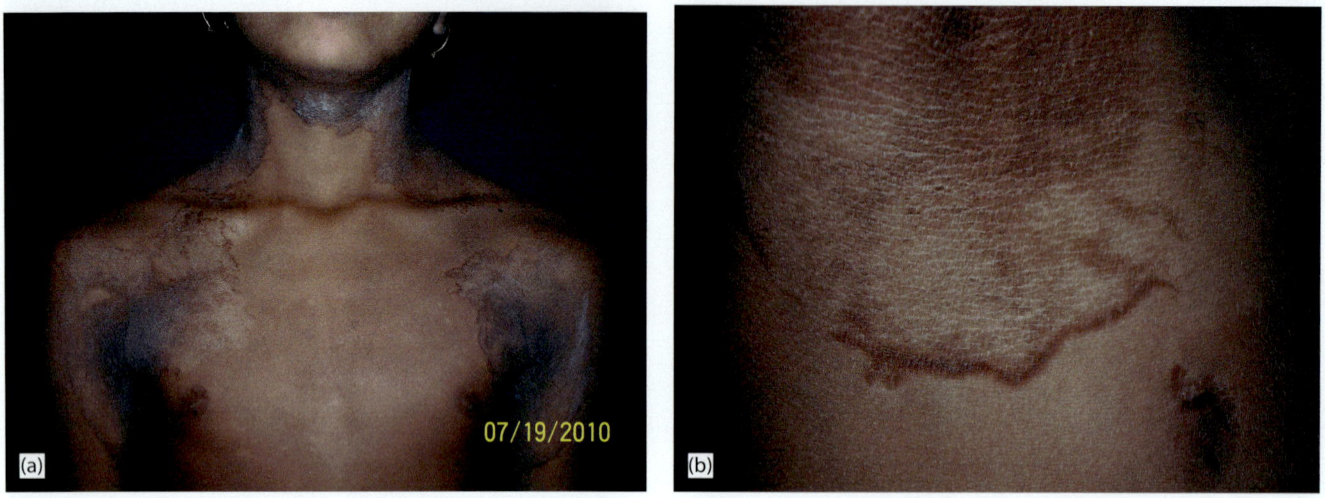


Figure 23.28 **(a)** Bilaterally symmetrical annular scaly plaque with well-defined margins in erythrokeratodermia variabilis. **(b)** Axillary lesion in erythrokeratodermia variabilis.

- The patient also presents with bamboo hairs called trichorrhexis invaginata. Hair may fracture below the surface of the scalp and the patient may appear bald.
- Ichthyosiform dermatitis, hair abnormality, and atopic diathesis together are called Netherton syndrome.
- DD: Erythrodermic atopic dermatitis, Tinea corporis, familial peeling skin syndrome.

### Erythrokeratodermia variabilis

- It is an inherited autosomal dominant disorder that presents as transient erythematous patches and hyperkeratotic plaque.
- Patients usually present at birth or within the first year of life.
- Lesions present as well-defined round to oval, geographic, circinate, annular, or target-like lesions that may coalesce into figurate patches that vary in size, number, and position. Erythema is associated with a burning sensation. Individual lesions persist for only minutes to hours or may sometimes last for days.
- Erythema is sometimes surrounded by a blanched halo.
- Lesions are aggravated by emotional stress, environmental heat or cold, mechanical friction, and sun exposure.
- Well-demarcated, hyperkeratotic or scaly, erythematous plaque evolves simultaneously with or following the development of migratory red scaly patches. The lesion commonly affects the extensors of limbs, buttocks, and trunk in a symmetrical pattern, similar to progressive symmetric erythrokeratoderma (**Figure 23.28a,b**).
- Thickening of palms and soles, with sparing of face, scalp, and flexures, is present.
- The surface of the lesion can be verrucous, velvety, and ridged. It may have collarette-like peeling or psoriasiform scales. Hypertrichosis may be seen.
- Hyperkeratosis with a spiny, hystrix-like appearance is present mostly on lower limbs.
- The lesion shows improvement over time, and the condition stabilizes after puberty, following gradual progression throughout infancy and childhood.
- DD: Progressive symmetric erythrokeratoderma, ichthyosis linearis circumflexa in Netherton syndrome, psoriasis, epidermolytic ichthyosis, Greither syndrome, MEDNIK syndrome.

## REFERENCES


1. Jackson R. Circles: Concerning circles in nature, circles produced by man, and circles in dermatology. Int J Dermatol 1994;33(11):818–825.
2. Sharma A, Lambert PJ, Maghari A, Lambert WC. Arcuate, annular, and polycyclic inflammatory and infectious lesions. Clin Dermatol 2011;29(2):140–150.
3. Narayanasetty NK, Pai VV, Athanikar SB. Annular lesions in dermatology. Indian J Dermatol 2013;58:157.
4. Trayes KP, Savage K, Studdiford JS. Annular lesions: Diagnosis and treatment. Am Fam Physician 2018;98(5):283–291.
5. Unwala R. Approach to the patient with annular skin lesions. In: Stratman E, Ofori AO, editors. UpToDate. Waltham, Massachusetts: UpToDate, 2018. Available from https://www.uptodate.com/contents/approach-to-the-patient-with-annular-skin-lesions. Accessed on November 1, 2019.
6. Daroach M, Vinay K, Kumaran MS. Pseudo circinate balanitis: Great masquerader lives. Postgrad Med J 2019;95(1123):283.
7. Singal A, Jakhar D, Kaur I, Pandhi D, Das S. *Tinea pseudoimbricata* as a unique manifestation of steroid abuse: A clinico-mycological and dermoscopic study from a tertiary care hospital. Indian Dermatol Online J 2019;10:422–425.
8. Bhushan P, Thatte SS. Saucer lesions in leprosy: Anatomy of the controversy. Indian J Dermatol 2016;61:100–102.
9. Wu YH, Hsiao PF. Neutrophilic figurate erythema. Am J Dermatopathol 2017;39(5):344–350.

# 24

# Alopecia

PIYUSH KUMAR, PRIYA RAJBANSH

## INTRODUCTION

Hair, just like nails, is an ectodermal structure and is a visible component of one's self-image and personality. Since ages past hair has been linked to masculinity and femininity, sexuality, and attractiveness. No wonder alopecia impairs psychological well-being and social functioning, and becomes an issue of serious concern, despite causing no serious morbidity in most cases. Hair may be lost in various genodermatoses and acquired dermatoses, systemic illness, traumatic events and as a primary disease of hairs. Some of these processes can result in scarring and irreversible alopecia. Timely diagnosis and efficient treatment can prevent scarring alopecia in most cases. Though there are various tools for diagnosis, many conditions can be diagnosed clinically with reasonable certainty. The clinical diagnosis rests on determination of non-scarring and scarring nature of alopecia, age of onset, pattern and extent of involvement, hair care and grooming practices, presence of various dermatoses and telltale signs (skin lesions), and knowledge of systemic illness, if any (**Table 24.1**). Additional clinical clues include easy pluckability of hairs or presence of fragile, brittle hairs, scalp skin changes, etc. Some of the common and rare conditions causing alopecia are discussed in this chapter.[1–8]

### Alopecia areata

- Alopecia areata (AA) is a non-scarring, polygenic, and autoimmune disorder that is characterized by its relapsing and remitting course. The antibodies in AA are heterogenous and target multiple structures of anagen hairs. It can affect all hair-bearing areas but most commonly affects scalp hairs.
- AA does not show any racial variation and can occur at any age and in either sex, but mostly it is reported to develop before the age of 40. Early onset AA is considered when the mean age of presentation is between 5 and 10 years and is associated with poor prognosis.
- Patients may complain of pruritus or a burning sensation. Patients present with single or multiple, round or oval, spontaneously appearing, alopecic patches. No changes in scalp skin are noted. Active disease is characterized by a positive hair pull test from the margin and the presence of exclamation hairs (hairs tapered near the proximal end). Non-pigmented hairs are spared, and their presence in alopecic patches is an important clinical clue (**Figure 24.1a,b**). Spontaneous regrowth of hairs in the affected area is common and is seen over a period of a few months (**Figure 24.1c**).
- Various clinical patterns of AA are recognized:
  - Patchy/localized AA – Solitary or multiple patches of AA are noted. Sometimes, multiple patches may coalesce to form a reticular pattern (**Figure 24.1d,e**).
  - Alopecia totalis – There is total or near total loss of scalp hairs (**Figure 24.1f**).
  - Alopecia universalis – There is total or near total loss of hair on all hair-bearing sites of the body (**Figure 24.1g**).
  - Ophiasis type – This type is characterized by band-like loss of hair along the temporal and lower occipital areas (**Figure 24.1h**).
  - Sisaipho (ophiasis spelt backwards) type – In this variant, there is extensive loss of hair that spares the sides and the back of the head.
  - Diffuse AA – There is loss of hair from all over the scalp in equal density without any patches (**Figure 24.1i**).
- Nail involvement is seen in severe cases of AA and is associated with poor prognosis. Nail findings include nail pitting, trachonychia, brittle nail, onycholysis, koilonychias, and, rarely, onychomadesis (**Figure 24.1j**).
- AA is found to have association with other autoimmune conditions such as vitiligo, diabetes mellitus, autoimmune thyroid disease, and atopy (atopic dermatitis, allergic rhinitis, asthma) (**Figure 24.1k**).
- DD: Depends on clinical pattern of AA. DD of localized AA includes tinea capitis (h/o infection, lesion on scalp), and trichotillomenia. Diffuse AA mimics telogen effluvium.

DOI: 10.1201/9781351054225-75

Table 24.1 Clinical approach to alopecia

| Nature of alopecia | Features | Diseases |
|---|---|---|
| **Patterned** | **Patchy/ moth-eaten** | • **Non-scarring** – alopecia areata (reticulate type), Tinea capitis, syphilitic alopecia<br>• **Scarring** – Pseudopelade of Brocq |
| | **Frontotemporal** | • **Non-scarring** – androgenetic alopecia (male), tractional alopecia, lupus hair<br>• **Scarring** – frontal fibrosing alopecia, morphea |
| | **Temporal** | • **Non-scarring** – temporal triangular alopecia<br>• **Scarring** – morphea |
| | **Vertex** | • **Non-scarring** – female androgenetic alopecia, lipedematous alopecia<br>• **Scarring** – central centrifugal cicatricial alopecia |
| | **Occipital** | • **Non-scarring** – transient neonatal alopecia, pressure alopecia<br>• **Scarring** – acne keloidalis |
| | **Temporal-occipital region** | • **Non-scarring** – alopecia areata (ophiasis pattern), tractional alopecia, hair shaft disorders with increased hair fragility |
| **Localized** | **Non-scarring** | • **With surface changes** – Tinea capitis, nevus sebaceous<br>• **Without surface changes** – alopecia areata, trichotillomania (excoriations may be seen), tumor alopecia, bubble hairs |
| | **Scarring** | Usually secondary cicatricial alopecia – burn, trauma, folliculitis, morphea, aplasia cutis, etc. |
| **Diffuse/ generalized** | **Non-scarring** | • **Hypotrichosis without brittle hairs** – telogen effluvium, anagen effluvium, loose anagen syndrome, short anagen syndrome<br>• **Hypotrichosis with brittle hairs** – hair shaft disorders<br>• **Complete alopecia** – diffuse alopecia areata, congenital universal atrichia, atrichia with papular lesions, hereditary vitamin D-resistant rickets with alopecia |
| | **Scarring** | • **With papules** – lichen planopilaris, keratosis follicularis spinulosa decalvans, acne keloidalis, alopecia mucinosa<br>• **With plaque** – discoid lupus erythematosus, lichen planus, alopecia mucinosa<br>• **With nodules** – Dissecting cellulitis, furunculosis<br>• **With pustules** – folliculitis decalvans, erosive pustular dermatosis of scalp, furunculosis<br>• **Without any skin lesion** – central centrifugal cicatricial alopecia, pseudopelade of Brocq, end stage of lichen planopilaris and tufted folliculitis |

## Tinea capitis

- Tinea capitis is a common dermatophytic infection of scalp hair follicles and surrounding skin that mainly occurs due to *Trichophyton* and *Microsporum* genera.
- Tinea capitis results from invasion of hair structure by fungus; three modes of invasion are known – endothrix (arthroconidia seen within the hair shaft and cuticle is intact), ectothrix (arthroconidia are seen outside the hair

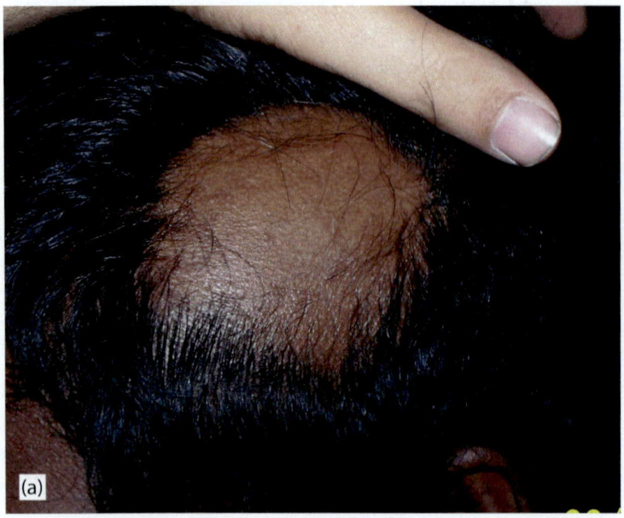

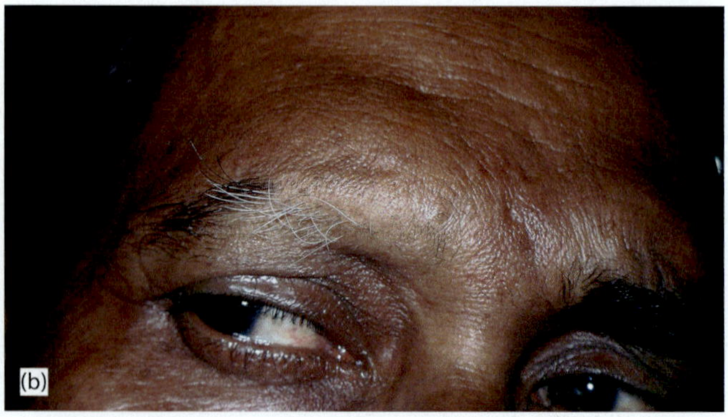

Figure 24.1 **(a)** Single lesion of alopecia areata. Note unremarkable scalp epidermis. **(b)** Alopecia areata affecting medial part of eyebrow. Note gray hairs within alopecic patch. *(Continued)*

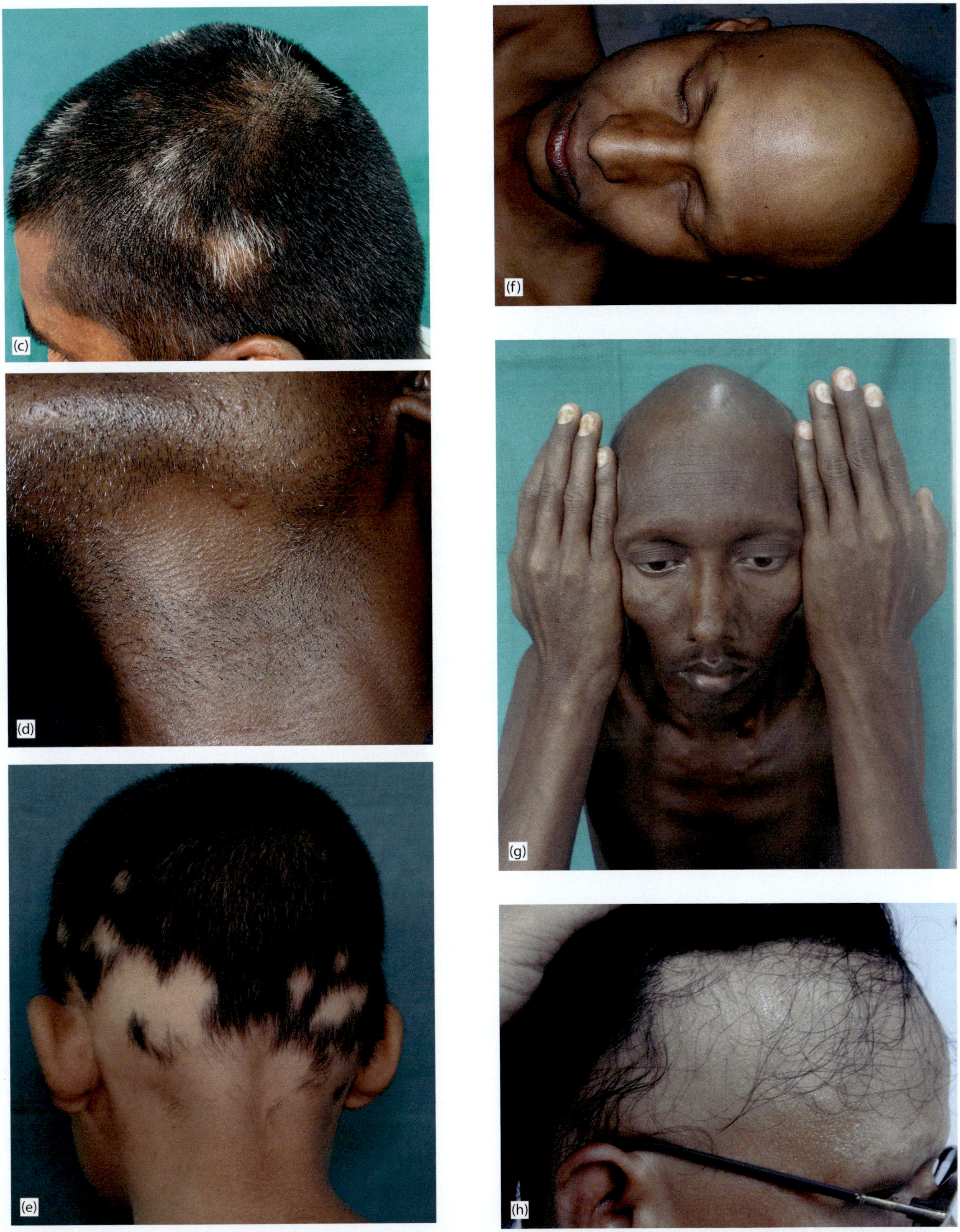


Figure 24.1 (*Continued*) **(c)** Regrowing hairs within the lesions of alopecia areata may be gray. **(d)** Alopecia areata in the beard area. **(e)** Reticular alopecia areata. **(f)** Alopecia totalis progressing to alopecia universalis. Note that right eyebrow is still appreciable. **(g)** Alopecia universalis with nail changes. **(h)** Ophiatic alopecia areata. (*Continued*)

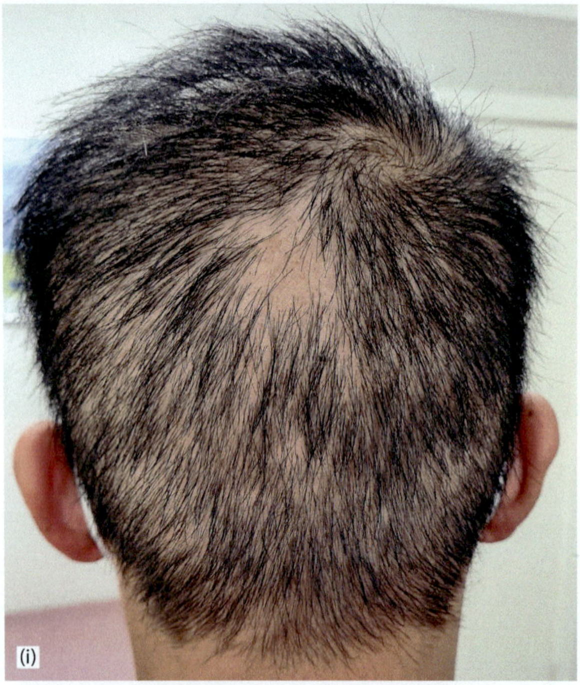


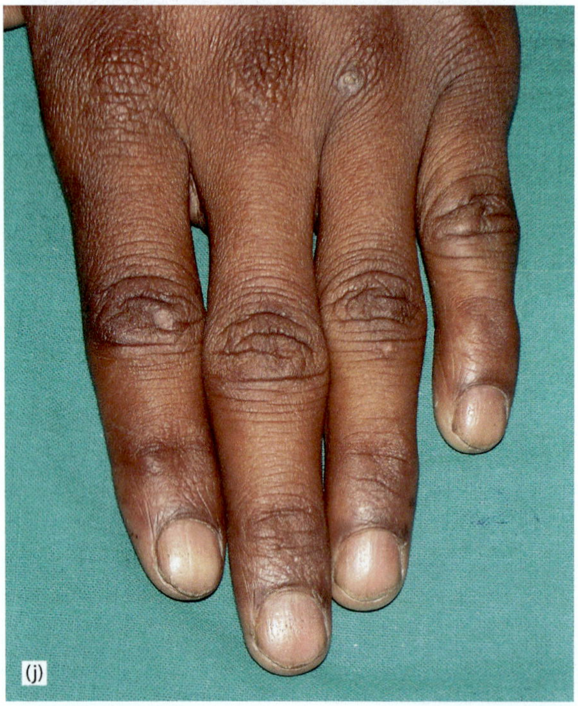


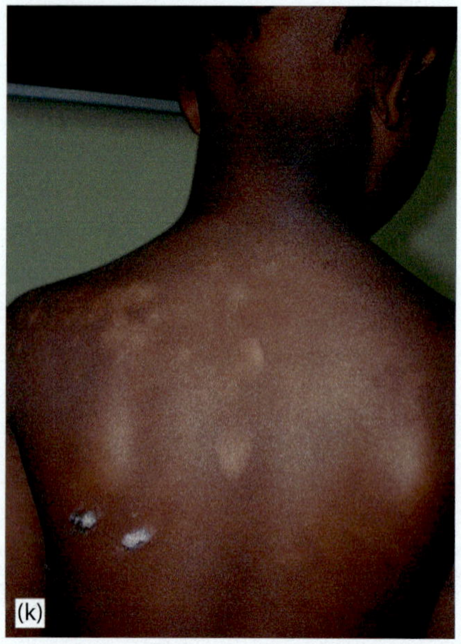


Figure 24.1 (*Continued*) **(i)** Diffuse alopecia areata. **(j)** Regular, shallow nail pitting in a case of alopecia totalis. **(k)** A child with alopecia areata of the occipital region with segmental vitiligo and lichen planus. (i – Courtesy: Dr. Tanumay Raychaudhury, Skin and Cancer Foundation, The University of Sydney, Australia.)

shaft and cuticle is lost), and favus (hyphae and air bubbles are observed within the hair shaft). As a result of fungal invasion, the hair shaft becomes brittle and may break near the scalp ("black dot"). Also, affected hairs may become dystrophic and distorted (comma or corkscrew hairs).

- The condition is particularly prevalent in the tropics, in children of African descent, and in children aged 3 to 14 years, without any sex predilection. Rarely, adults too may be affected, and in adults, female preponderance is noted.
- There may be a history of dermatophytic infection in family members.
- The clinical picture consists of varying degrees of scaling, hair loss, and inflammation and can be broadly divided into two groups – non-inflammatory and inflammatory types.
- Non-inflammatory types (seborrheic form) – This type of infection is usually caused by anthropophilic organisms such as *Microsporum audouinii* or *M. ferrugineum*. It clinically presents with single or multiple, well-circumscribed or diffuse patches of scaling and hair loss.
    - Gray patch – The characteristic presentation is patchy, well-circumscribed, circular hair loss with fine scaling. The hairs in affected areas appear dull gray due to arthrospores coating the hairs (**Figure 24.2a,b**).
    - Diffuse scale type – It presents with diffuse, seborrheic dermatitis like scaling with decreased hair density (**Figure 24.2c**).
    - Black dot type – It is an endothrix infection, caused by various species of *Trichophyton* (*T. tonsurans*, *T.violaceum*). The characteristic finding is multiple patchy hair loss with fine scaling and grouped black dots (**Figure 24.2d,e**). The black dots appear due to breakage of hairs near the scalp. Black dot type is most non-inflammatory in nature, but some patients may develop follicular pustules and nodules.
- Inflammatory type – Such infections are usually caused by zoophilic or geophilic pathogens, such as *M. canis*, *M. gypseum*, and *T. verrucosum*. Patients

may complain of itching, pain, and tenderness. The severity of infection varies from follicular pustules to kerion. Patients often have associated posterior cervical lymphadenopathy.

- Pustular form – It is a milder infection and presents with patchy alopecia and scattered follicular papules and pustules (**Figure 24.2f**).
- Kerion – It is a severe clinical presentation of inflammatory variant and occurs mainly due to *T. verrucosum* or *T. mentagrophytes*. Well-developed kerion presents as single or multiple, painful, crusted, boggy, matted tender plaque or mass along with purulent discharge. Hairs are matted in this region and easily pluckable.

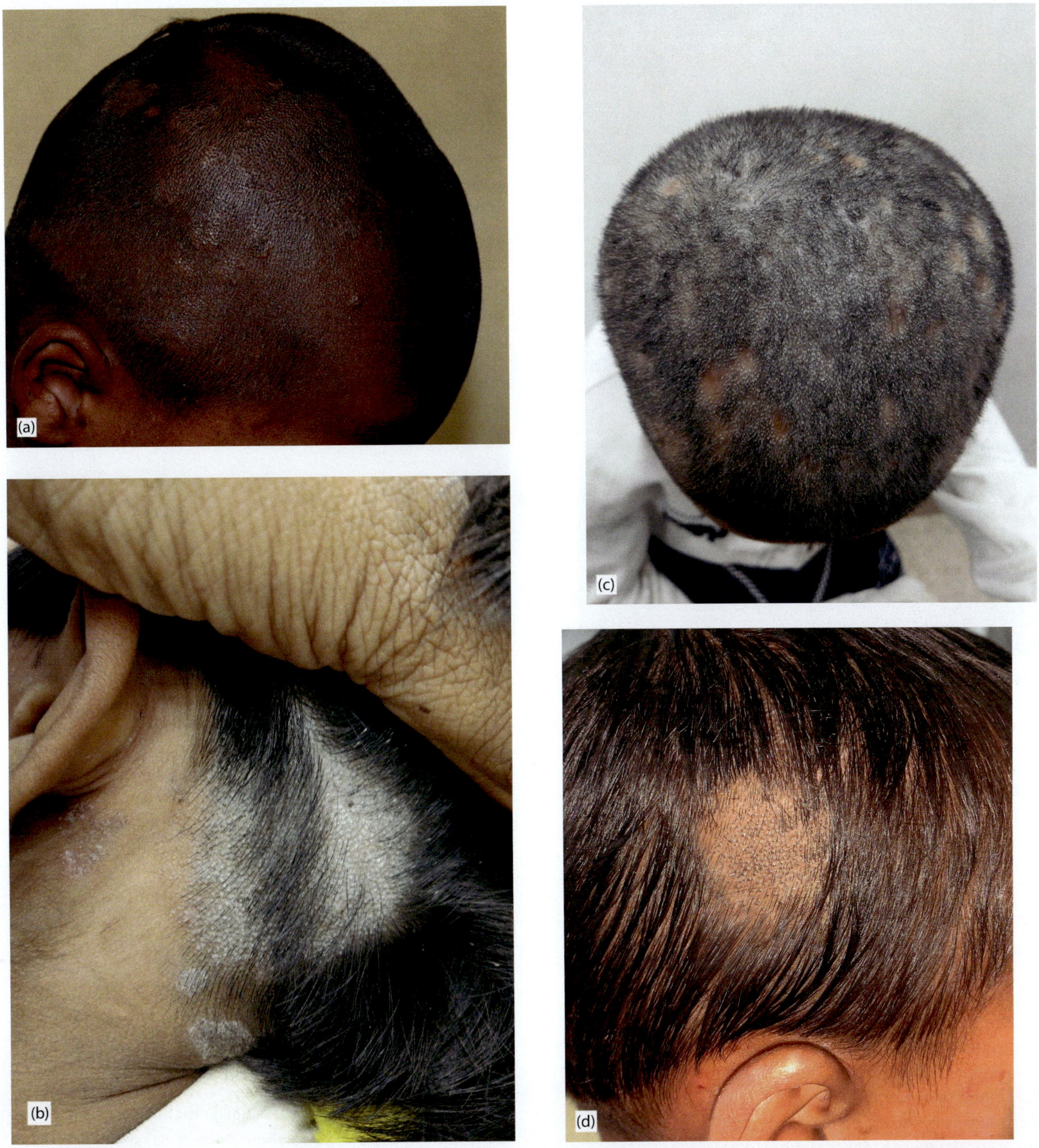


Figure 24.2 **(a)** Gray patches of tinea capitis. **(b)** Gray patch of tinea capitis. **(c)** Diffuse scaling in tinea capitis **(d)** Black dot type of tinea capitis. (*Continued*)

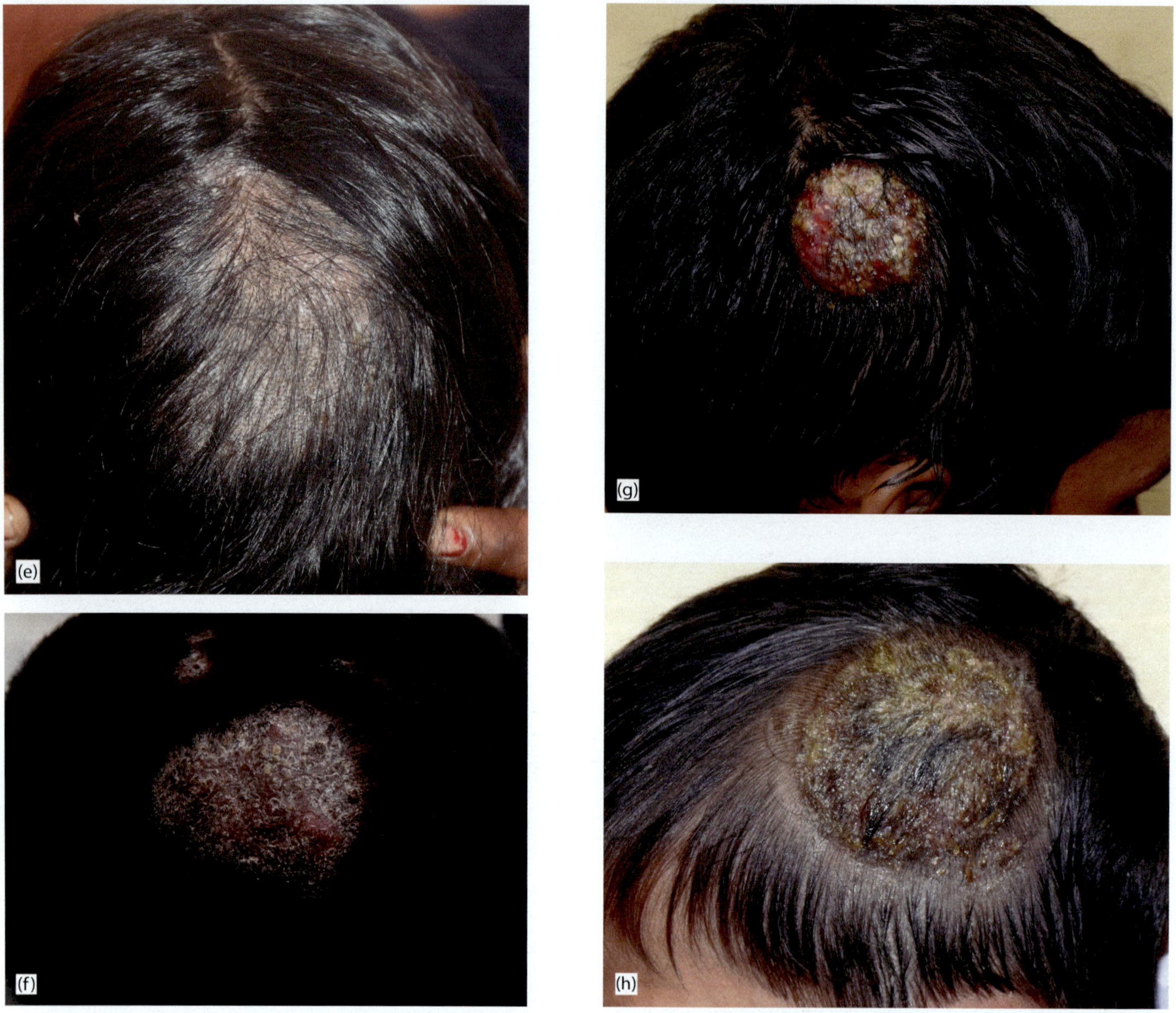


Figure 24.2 (*Continued*) **(e)** Black dot tinea capitis with alopecia. **(f)** Inflammatory tinea capitis seen as alopecic patch with erythematous papules, pustules and a few nodules over an erythematous skin. **(g)** Kerion as erythematous, boggy plaque with alopecia. Surface is remarkable for pustules and crusts. **(h)** Kerion in a young boy. (a,b – Courtesy: Deverashetti Srinivas, Nizamabad, India.)

  The condition is potentially scarring, and if not treated in time, it may heal with scarring alopecia (**Figure 24.2g,h**).
  - Favus – It is also the inflammatory variant of tinea capitis, which is caused by *T. schoenleinii* infection. The classical presentation is a thick, yellow, cup-shaped crust (called scutula), composed of hyphae and skin debris. Adjacent scutula may coalesce to form a large mass of pale powdery crusts. Untreated cases lead to cicatricial alopecia.
- Inflammatory tinea capitis, especially kerion, may be associated with dermatophytid reactions – eczematous lesions consisting of papules, vesicles, and pustules and scaling. The dermatophytid reaction may be localized or generalized, and when localized, helix, antihelix, and retroauricular regions are frequently affected (ear sign).
- DD: depends on the clinical presentation of tinea capitis **(Table 24.2).**

Table 24.2 Differential diagnosis of tinea capitis

| Type of tinea capitis | Clinical differential diagnosis |
|---|---|
| Gray patch | Scalp psoriasis, trichotillomania, |
| Diffuse scaly type | Seborrheic dermatitis, scalp psoriasis |
| Mild inflammatory type | Bacterial folliculitis, pustular psoriasis |
| Kerion | Folliculitis decalvans, bacterial abscess |

## Syphilitic alopecia[9]

- Syphilitic alopecia (SA) is non-scarring, inflammatory alopecia caused by immune response against *Treponema pallidum* that have invaded the hair bulge epithelium and peribulbar capillaries. It may be seen with mucocutaneous lesions of secondary syphilis (symptomatic) or, rarely, without any mucocutaneous features of secondary syphilis (essential SA).
- It can occur in any age group but is most frequently found in sexually active people.
- There may be a history of unprotected sex with multiple partners, and painless genital ulcer.
- Clinically, four morphological types are recognized:
  - Moth-eaten or patchy – This is the most common variant of SA and typically presents with patchy loss of hair of irregular shape and size over the parieto-occipital region. These patches are not completely devoid of hairs, and margins of lesions are not well defined. The scalp skin does not show any sign of inflammation. This variety of SA can also occur on other hair-bearing areas of body such as the beard, axilla, pubis, legs, and trunk (**Figure 24.3a,b**).
  - Diffuse SA – It is characterized by diffuse loss of hair without any obvious patches and mimics telogen effluvium (**Figure 24.3c**).

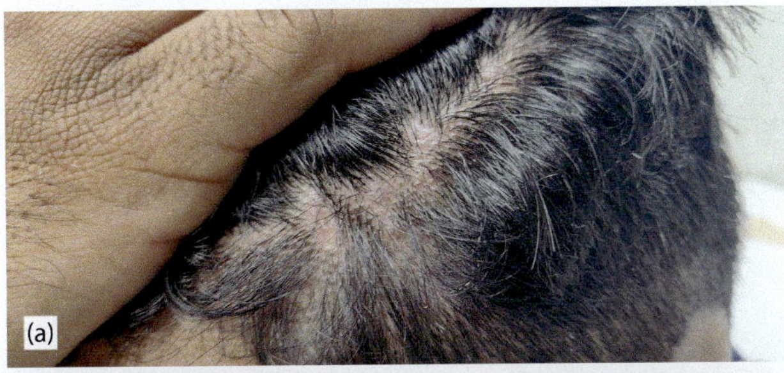
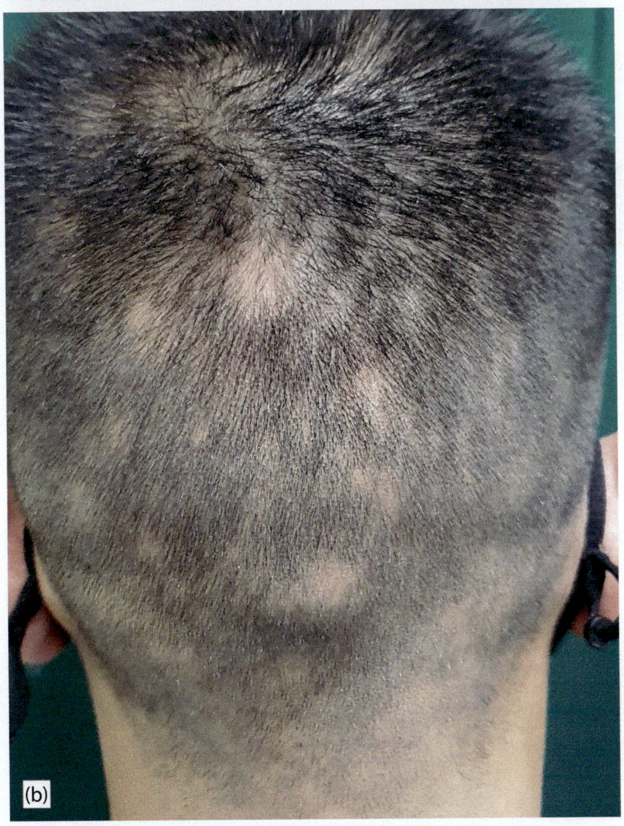
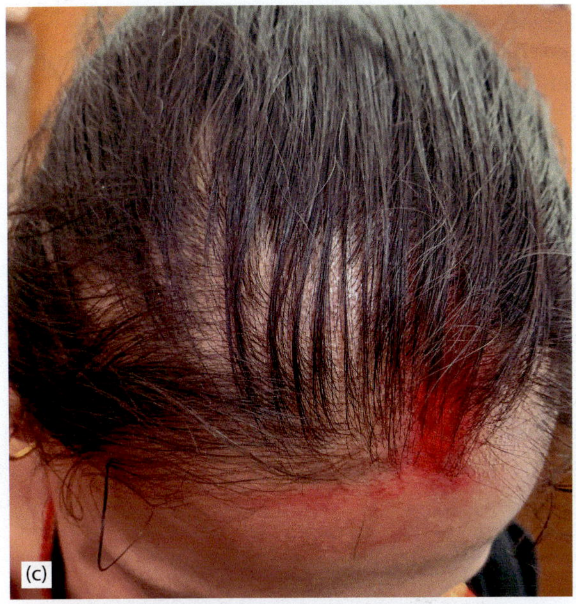
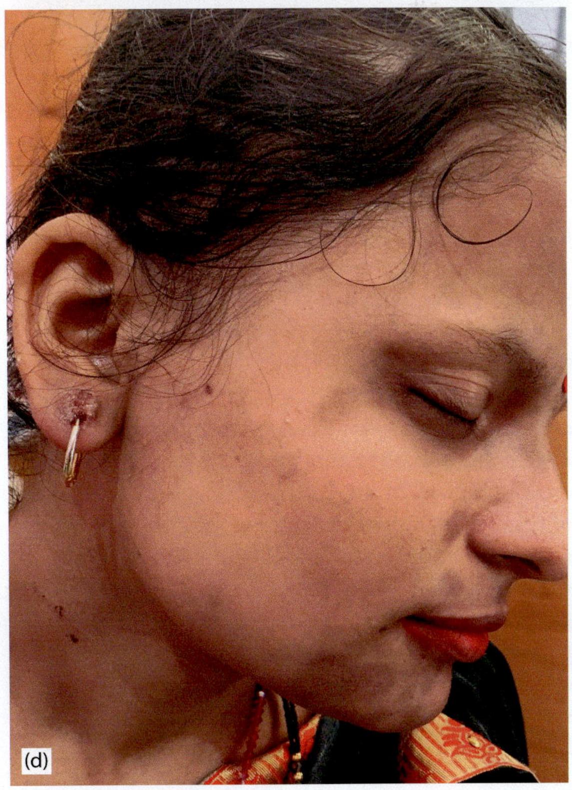

Figure 24.3 **(a)** "Moth-eaten" alopecia in secondary syphilis. **(b)** Moth-eaten alopecia in secondary syphilis. **(c)** Diffuse hair loss in a female with secondary syphilis. **(d)** Loss of lateral eyebrows in secondary syphilis. Note eroded papule on the ear and hyperpigmented patches on the face. (a – Courtesy: Prof. Santoshdev P Rathod, Smt. NHL Municipal Medical College, SCL General Hospital, Ahmedabad, India; b – Courtesy: Dr. Shekhar Neema, Armed Forces Medical College, Pune, India.)

    - Mixed type – Here the features of both patchy and diffuse alopecia are found.
    - Alopecia of the eyebrows ("omnibus sign") – This involves loss of the lateral third of eyebrows (**Figure 24.3d**).
- In primary syphilis, alopecia is extremely rare and is found in only cases having primary chancre over the scalp.
- Non-scarring alopecia is seen in secondary syphilis, whereas scarring alopecia is a feature of tertiary syphilis.
- The different clinical variants of SA are associated with various cutaneous and systemic findings, such as malaise, low-grade fever, lymphadenopathies, and anorexia, and cutaneous findings such as generalized non-pruritic papulo-squamous rashes predominantly over trunk. Other finding includes palmoplantar pigmented lesion, mucosal ulceration, and condyloma lata.
- DD: Tinea capitis (history of scalp infection), telogen effluvium, trichotillomenia (hair texture changed, fractured hairs), alopecia areata.

## Androgenetic alopecia (male pattern baldness) and female androgenetic alopecia/female pattern hair loss (FAGA/FPHL)

- Androgenetic alopecia (AGA) occurs due to genetically determined sensitivity of hair follicles of scalp to the androgen dihydrotestosterone (DHT). Under the influence of DHT, there is progressive thinning of hairs, characteristically over the frontal and vertex region.
- In AGA, the anagen phase of hairs is shortened and there is gradual, progressive conversion of terminal hairs (large, thick, pigmented) into vellus hairs (short, fine, non-pigmented) in the characteristic pattern (involvement of vertex and frontal region with sparing of occipital and parietal regions, called Hippocratic wreath).
- AGA is most common in Caucasian people, followed by Asians. It normally affects middle-aged and elderly people but can occur any time after puberty and, rarely, in prepubertal children (six to ten years of age). Its incidence increases with increasing age. Men outnumber women.
- There is gradual bitemporal recession of anterior hairline (professor's angle), with loss of hairs on vertex in affected men. Positive family history is present (**Figure 24.4a–c**).
- The Hamilton-Norwood classification is used to evaluate the severity of male pattern hair loss.
- In females, FAGA results in diffuse hair loss over the crown (**Figure 24.4d–h**). There is a gradual thinning of the central hair with widening of the part width, rather than an area of marked baldness. The part width is markedly increased in the frontal region, with progressive decline in width posteriorly (Christmas tree pattern). The frontal hairline is often preserved. The clinical diagnosis of FAGA, especially in early cases, may be difficult, and trichoscopy is a very valuable tool for making a diagnosis.

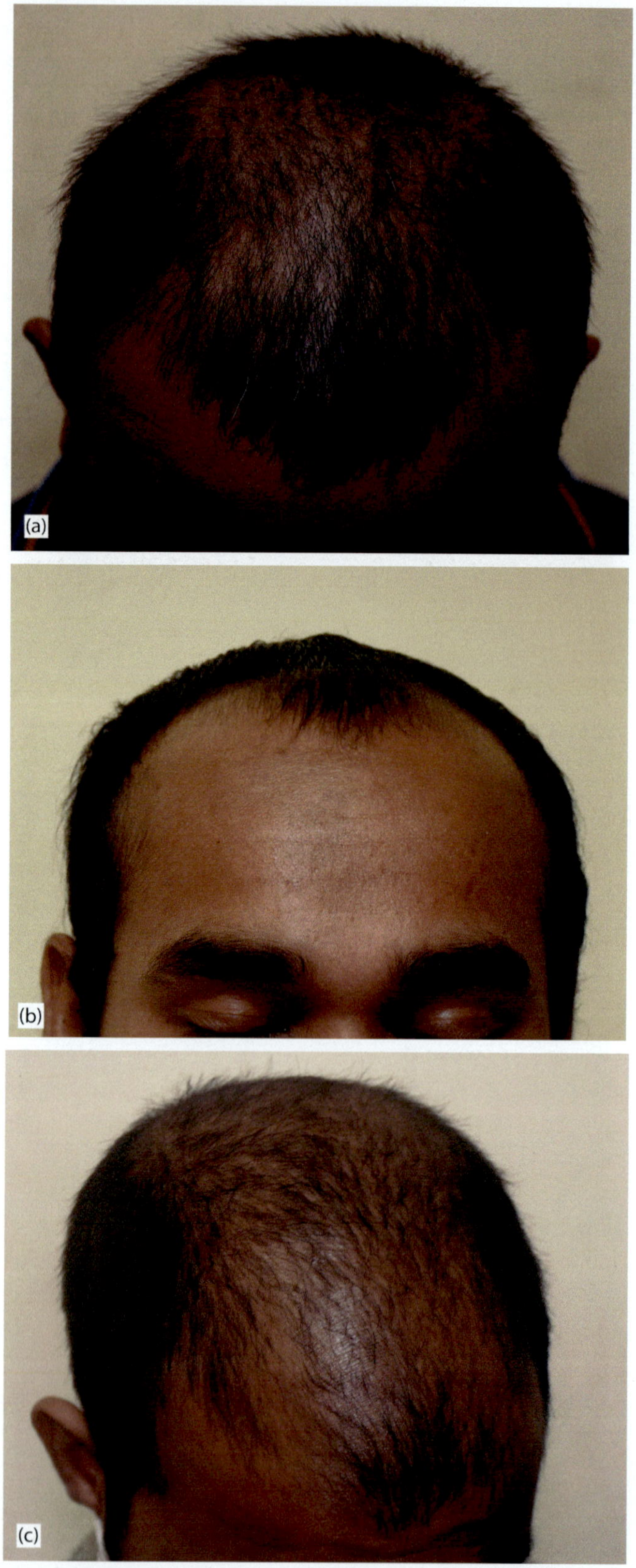


Figure 24.4 **(a)** Bilateral temporal recession of anterior hairline and reduced density of hairs on the vertex in androgenetic alopecia. **(b)** Advanced androgenetic alopecia in a young male. **(c)** Androgenetic alopecia with diffuse hair loss in frontal and vertex region. Hairs from parietal regions are relatively preserved. (*Continued*)

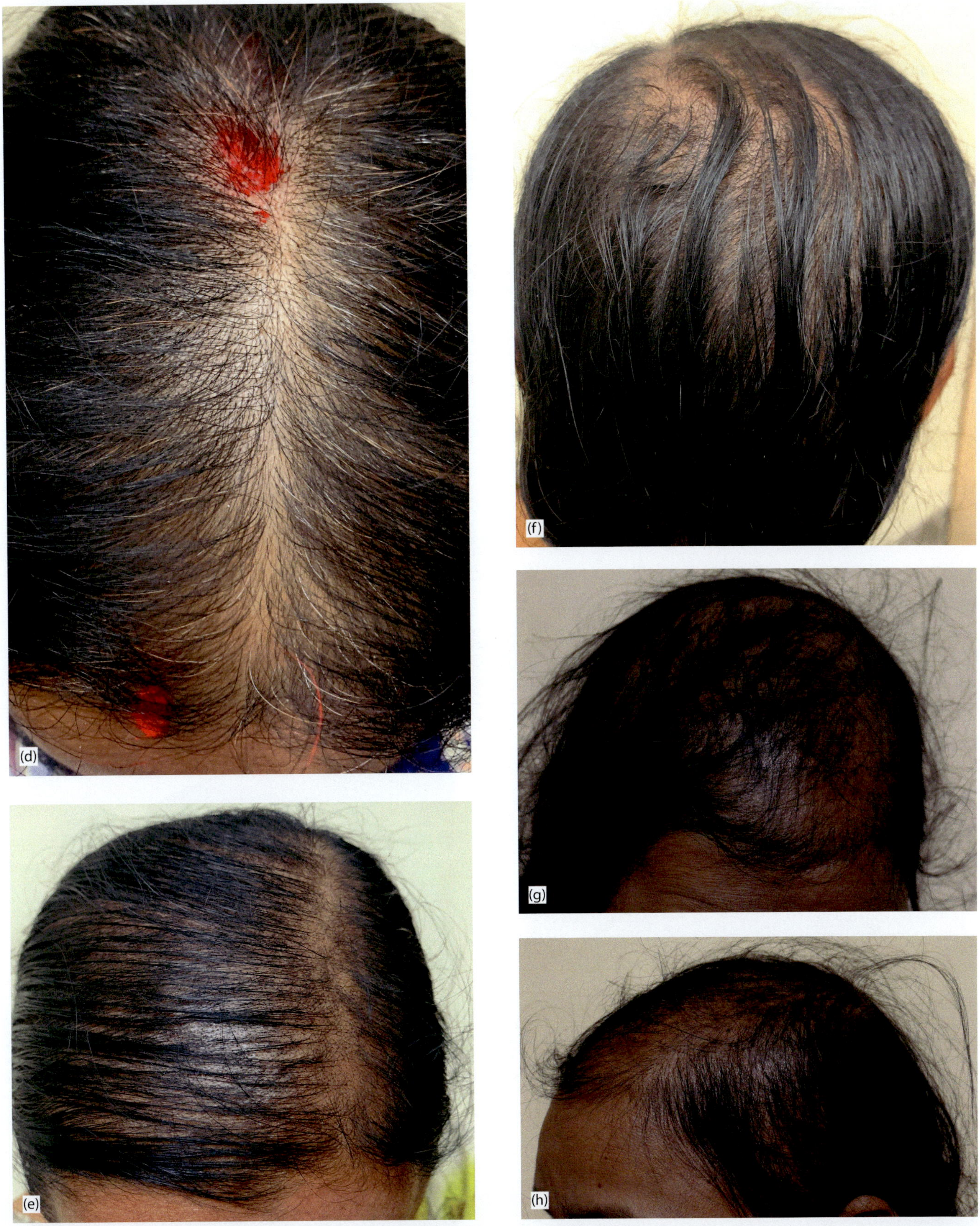


Figure 24.4 (*Continued*) **(d,e)** Female androgenetic alopecia in a middle-aged lady. **(f,g)** A middle-aged lady with advanced female androgenetic alopecia. Top view **(f)** and lateral view **(g)**. **(h)** Advanced female androgenetic alopecia with extensive hair loss.

Table 24.3 Traumatic hair styling by different population

| Traumatic hair styles | Population who commonly practice it |
|---|---|
| Braids, cornrows, hair weave | Afro-Caribbean men, women, and children |
| Dreadlocks | African men and women, Indian sadhus, Western fashion and counterculture |
| Ponytail | Asian and Hispanic women, athlete women |
| Turban | Sikh men |
| Hijab | Muslim women |
| Bun | Indian women, ballerinas |
| Nurse's cap | Nurses in developing and Asian countries |
| Excessive long hairs | Women |

- The severity of FAGA can be assessed by the Ludwig classification and Sinclair scale.
- DD: Telogen effluvium (equal density of hair over all areas of scalp), loose anagen syndrome (specific age group), diffuse alopecia areata (exclamation sign on dermoscopy).

## Traction alopecia[10]

- Traction alopecia (TA) is an acquired disorder of gradual, progressive hair loss resulting from traumatic hair styles (**Table 24.3**) that cause repetitive pressure or tension on the hair roots. It has been observed in many races.
- It can occur in any age group, and the incidence increases with age, but young adult females predominate.
- There may be a history of use of chemical relaxers, extensions, and curlers. Also, affected patients may have a history of chronic use of hair wefts, hair pins, or clips.
- Also, patients may give a history of headache that is relieved when hairs are loosened.
- TA starts with perifollicular erythema, which progresses to follicular papules and pustules formation. Other findings are hair casts, reduction in hair density and replacement with vellus hairs, and the presence of broken hairs in the affected areas. If left untreated, the disease may progress to cause scarring alopecia. TA to start with is non-scarring alopecia and may progress to scarring alopecia if patients do not adopt non-traumatic hair care practices.
- The pattern of hair loss in TA is variable and correlates with distribution of the traction. The following patterns are commonly observed:
    - Marginal TA – The hair density is reduced over the frontotemporo parietal area. A strip of thin hair ("the fringe sign") is retained at the margin of alopecic patch (**Figure 24.5a–e**).

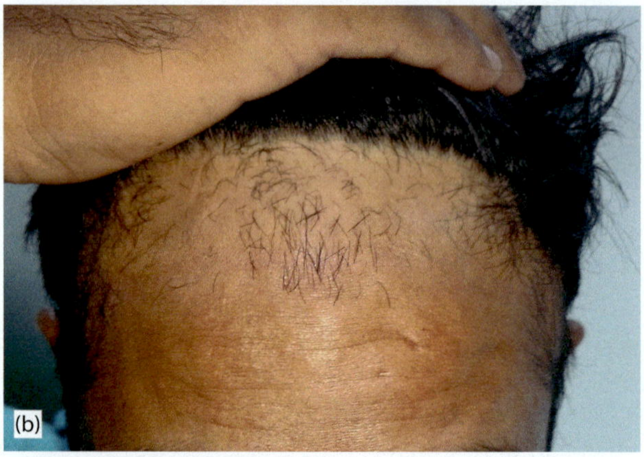
(b)

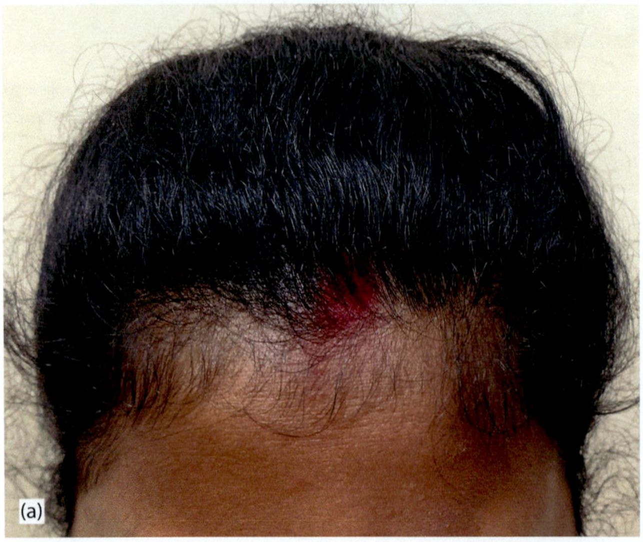
(a)

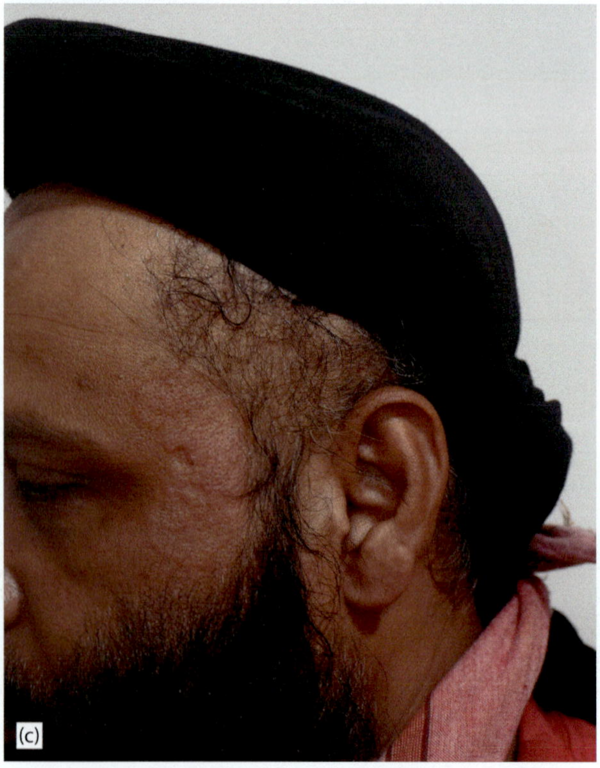
(c)

Figure 24.5 **(a)** Traction alopecia with fringe sign. **(b)** Traction alopecia in a Sikh male. **(c)** A Sikh male wearing turban regularly has developed marginal traction alopecia of parietal region. *(Continued)*

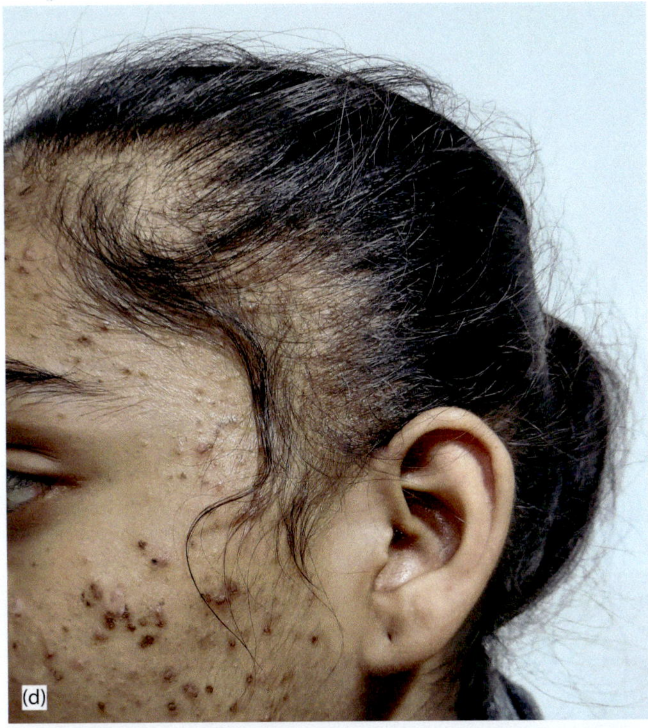

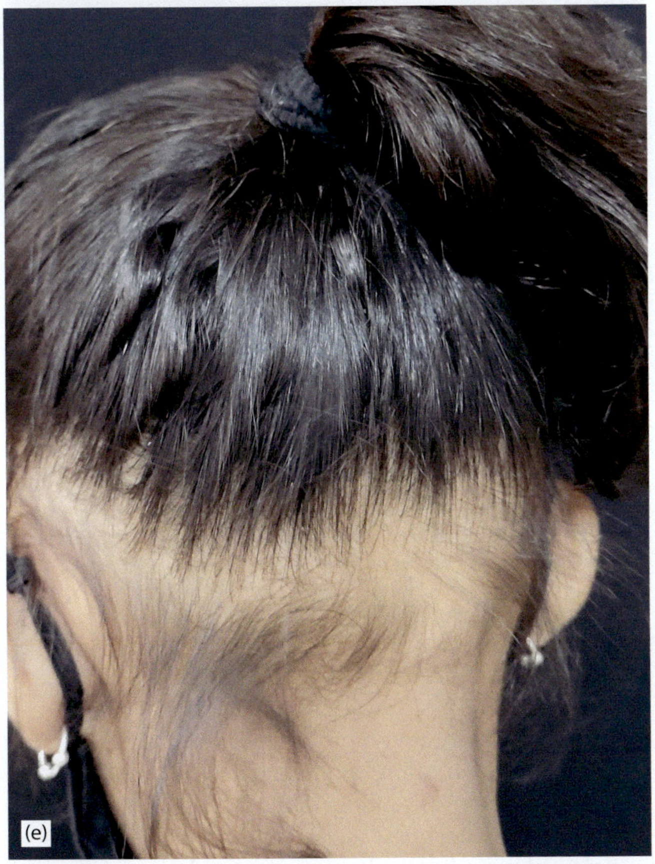

Figure 24.5 (*Continued*) **(d)** Traction alopecia in a young girl who keeps hairs in a tight bun. **(e)** Marginal tractional alopecia is not always restricted to frontotemporal region. (b – Courtesy: Dr. Dhiraj Kumar, Patna, India; e – Courtesy: Dr Shekhar Neema, Armed Forces Medical College, Pune, India.)

- The non-marginal variant of TA has also been reported after hair wefts, hair pins, or clips use. Some notable examples of non-marginal TA include the following:
  a. Horseshoe pattern of T – It is seen in persons using wefted hair extensions.
  b. Chignon alopecia – It occurs in women with long hair making a tight ponytail or tight bun.
  c. Band like alopecia – A band-like hair loss in the frontotemporal line, commonly seen in Sikhs because they tie their hair in a bun over the vertex.
- The presence of swelling and tenderness at the site of tight braiding is an ominous sign and indicates impending scalp necrosis.
- DD: Androgenetic alopecia, telogen effluvium, trichotillomenia.

## Lupus hair

- Lupus hair is a distinct non-scarring alopecia seen in patients with chronically active systemic lupus erythematosus (SLE). Some authors consider it a variant of telogen effluvium, while others believe it a result of retarded hair growth.
- Lupus hair presents as short, fragile, coarse, and dry hairs along the anterior hairline. Sometimes, background erythema may be appreciated. Other peripheral scalp regions too can be affected but are less obvious (**Figure 24.6a–c**).
- The presence of lupus hair in SLE suggests disease activity and exacerbations.

## Frontal fibrosing alopecia[11]

- Frontal fibrosing alopecia (FFA) is a variant of LPP and is clinically characterized by progressive band-like hair loss affecting the frontotemporal zone of scalp.
- The prevalence is not known, but the disease appears to be common among people from Europe, the United

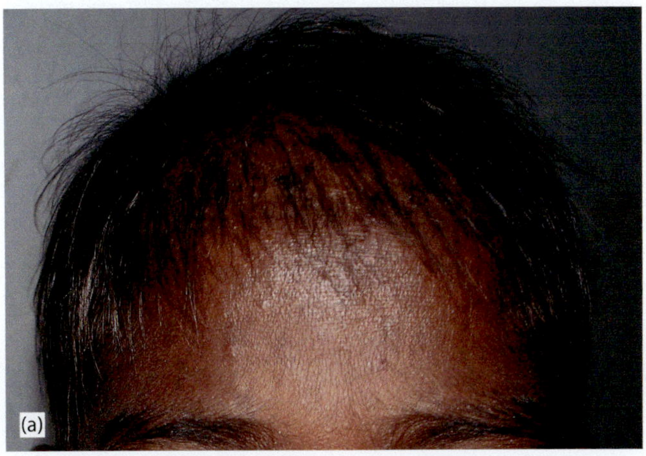

Figure 24.6 **(a)** Hair loss with frontal, short, broken hairs (lupus hairs) in systemic lupus erythematosus. (*Continued*)

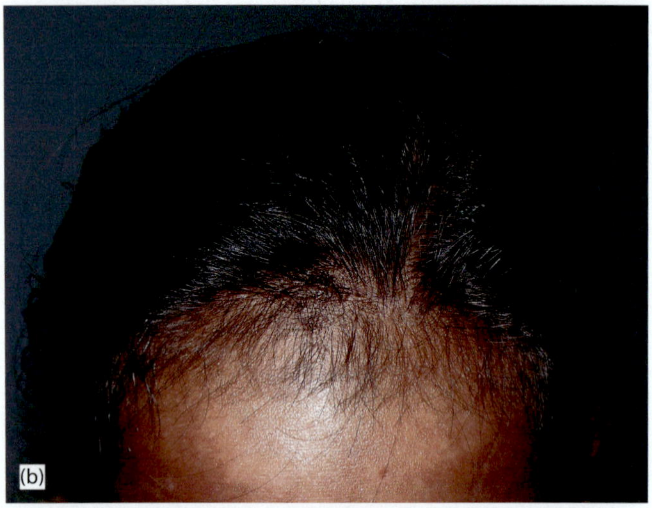

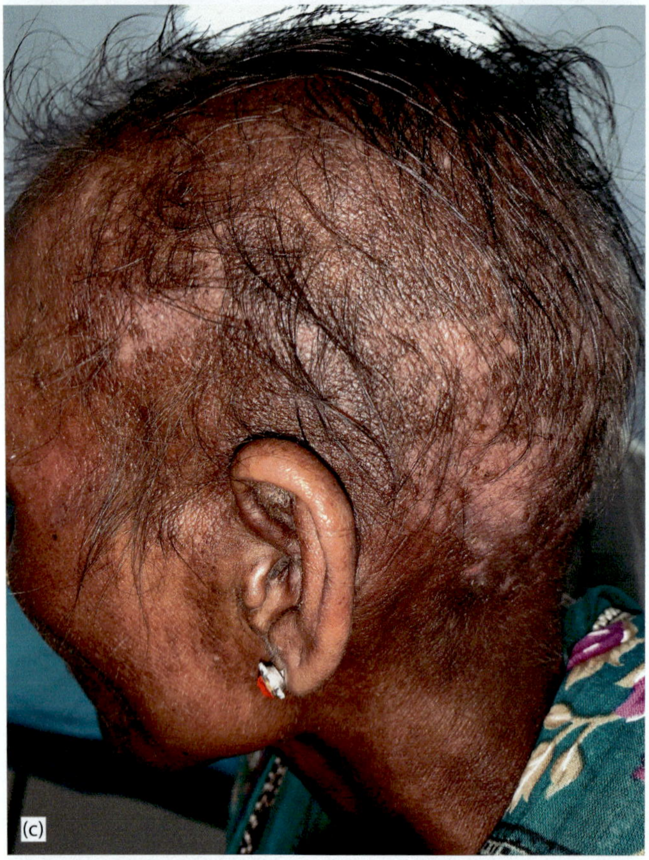

Figure 24.6 (*Continued*) **(b)** Lupus hairs. **(c)** Extensive hair loss during an exacerbation of systemic lupus erythematosus.

States, and Japan. Typically, postmenopausal women are affected. Affection of young female or males is uncommon.

- FFA is characterized by asymptomatic, progressive recession of the frontotemporal (anterior) hairline due to scarring alopecia, along with the loss of eyebrows. This recession of the hairline is typically bilateral and symmetrical (**Figure 24.7a,b**).

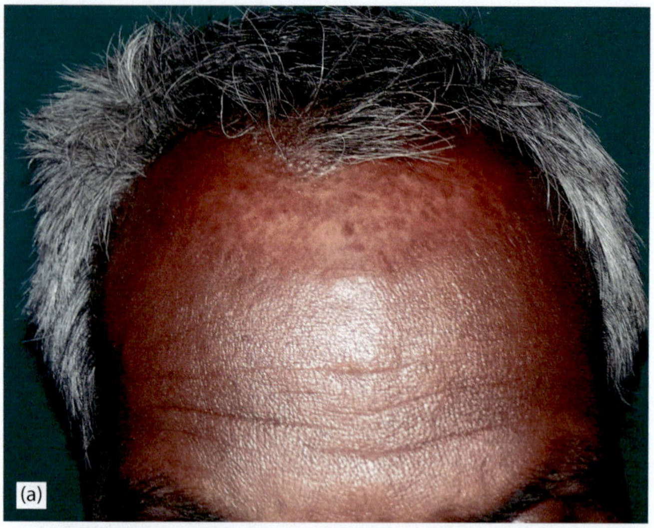

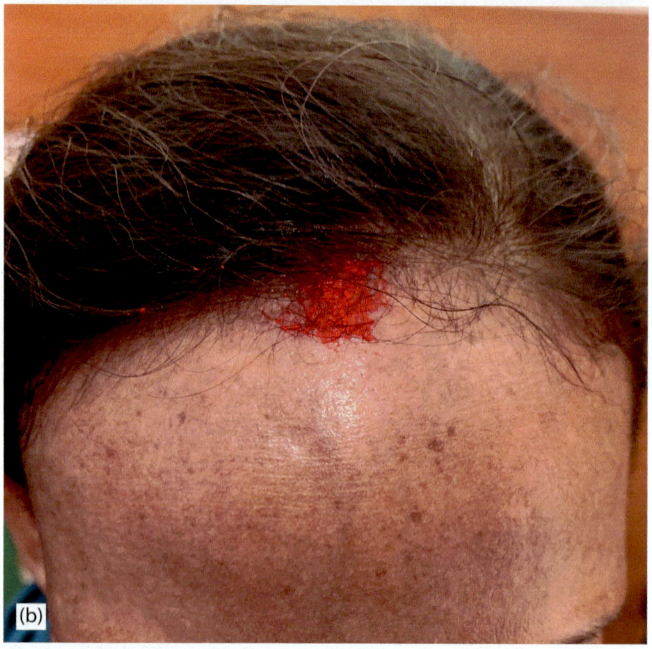

Figure 24.7 **(a)** Frontal fibrosing alopecia in a 56-year-old male. **(b)** Frontal fibrosing alopecia in a female with lichen planus pigmentosus. (a – Courtesy: Dr. Hiral Shah, Baroda Medical College, Vadodara, India.)

- These recessions of hair can extend up to the preauricular and retro-auricular regions of scalp. The frontal recession varies from 1 cm to 6 cm (observing contraction of the frontalis muscle allows differentiation of forehead from scalp and allows quantification of hairline regression) and can extend up to occipital region. The affected skin is pale, shiny and devoid of follicles (including vellus hairs), and hairs at the edge may show erythema and perifollicular papules in active stage of disease. The hair pull test is positive on the affected area during the active stage of disease.

- Presence of "lonely hair" is another important clinical clue. In the alopecic area, isolated terminal hair may persist and may show perifollicular erythema. Sometimes, terminal hairs at the original hairline may be spared (pseudo fringe sign) and are associated with good prognosis.
- Alopecia of eyebrows sometimes precedes the frontal alopecia and typically involves the lateral third of eyebrows.
- Patients may have associated lichen planus pigmentosus.
- DD: Androgenetic alopecia, alopecia areata.

### Temporal triangular alopecia (congenital triangular alopecia, Brauer nevus)

- Triangular temporal alopecia (TTA) is a non-scarring and patterned hair loss characterized by replacement of normal terminal hairs by vellus hairs. The condition is non-progressive and remains unchanged throughout life.
- TTA can be present since birth or be acquired thereafter. The onset is usually in childhood, but, rarely, adults too may present with recent onset of disease.
- As the name suggests, the classical site of affection is the frontotemporal area, but it can occur over temporoparietal or occipital area too.
- Patients present with unilateral or, uncommonly, bilateral, triangular, oval, or lanceolate (with the tip of lancet points superiorly and posteriorly) patches of hair loss, with or without small islands of dark, terminal hairs within the patch. The affected area appears hairless, but fine vellus hairs may be appreciated by the naked eye or on trichoscopy. The underlying skin shows no visible changes (**Figure 24.8a–c**).
- The diagnostic criteria has been proposed by Inui et al. TTA is diagnosed if the following features are present:
  - A triangular or lanceolate alopecic patch located over the frontotemporal region or other regions of the scalp
  - Trichoscopy showing normal hair follicles with vellus type hair

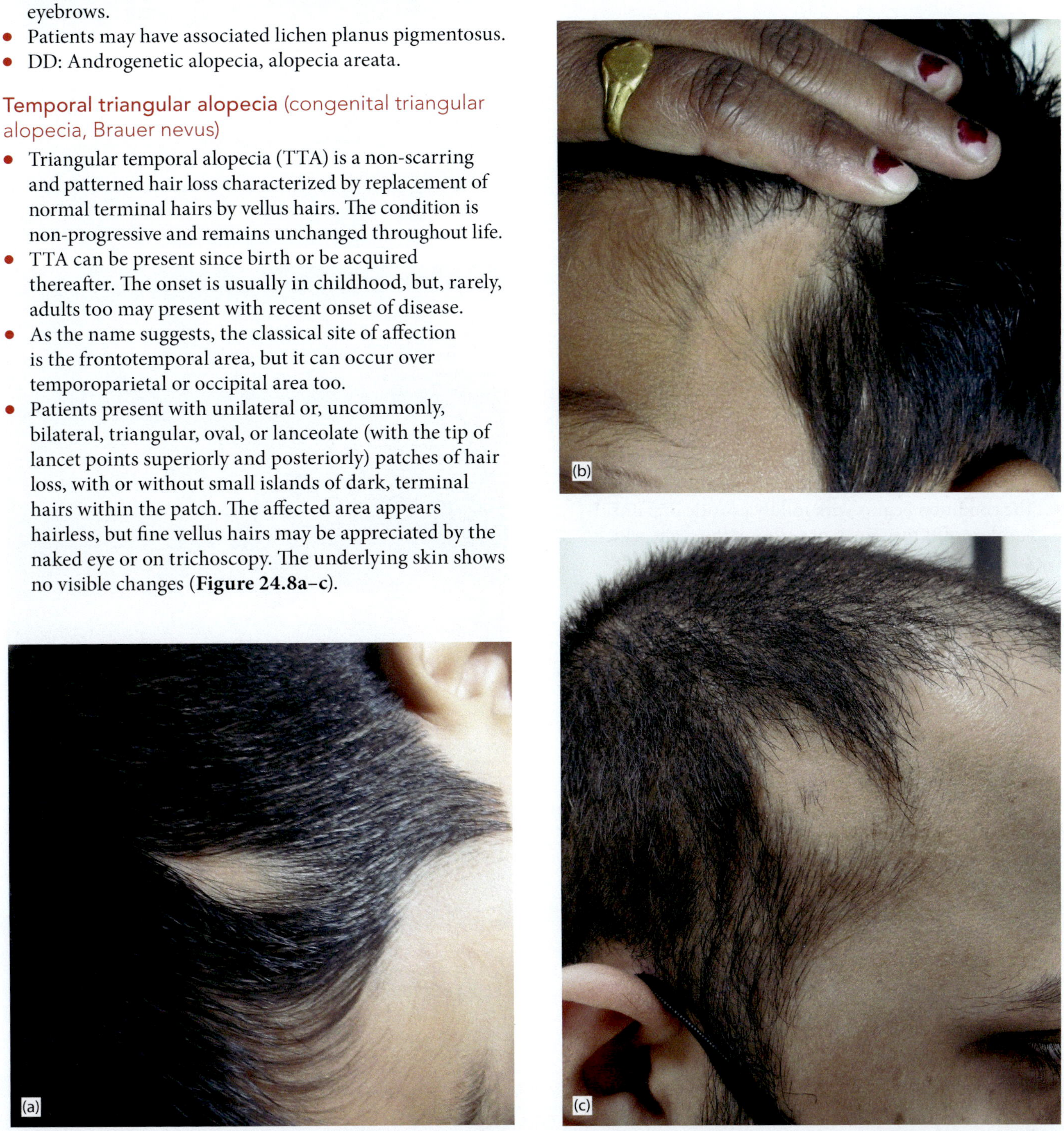


Figure 24.8 **(a)** Lanceolate-shaped alopecic patch in temporal triangular alopecia. **(b)** Temporal triangular alopecia in a child. **(c)** Temporal triangular alopecia. (a,b – Courtesy: Dr. Anil Patki, Pune, India; c – Courtesy: Dr. Ganesh Avhad, Mumbai, India.)

- Absence of fractured hairs, black dots or yellow dots with preserved follicular orifices on trichoscopic examination
- Lack of significant hair growth six months after confirming the presence of vellus hairs

- DD: Alopecia areata (exclamation hair on dermoscopy), pressure alopecia, tinea capitis (history of infection), trichotillomenia (texture of hair changed).

### Lipedematous Alopecia

- This disorder is characterized by a thick, boggy scalp due to expansion of the subcutaneous fat layer. The condition is most commonly seen in women with colored skin, and the vertex is usually affected. The condition may be associated with vertex alopecia.

### Central centrifugal cicatricial alopecia (CCCA) (hot comb alopecia, follicular degeneration syndrome)

- CCCA is an idiopathic, primary, scarring alopecia characterized by progressive loss of hair starting at crown or vertex region and progressing in a centrifugal manner.
- It can affect any population but is predominantly seen in colored skin, with a female preponderance The disease typically starts in the second or third decade of life.
- A history of hair straightening, traumatic hair styles, hair lengthening, etc., may be present.
- The condition begins with mildly pruritic or painful hair loss over the crown or vertex of the scalp, which gradually progresses in a centrifugal manner and extends up to the side of the scalp. However, the severity of the disease remains the maximum at the vertex. The condition is characterized by slowly progressive scarring alopecia, and the symmetrical forward progress of hair loss resembles female pattern hair loss (**Figure 24.9a,b**).
- The scalp skin appears shiny, shows nil/minimal inflammation or scaling, and may show a few short, brittle hairs. Also, as in much of scarring alopecia, polytrichia may be seen (a group of hairs coming out of one follicle).
- A minority of patients suffering from rapidly progressive disease or bacterial super infection can have pustules and crusts.
- DD: Female pattern hair loss, male pattern hair loss, lichen planopilaris, telogen effluvium.

### Neonatal occipital alopecia (NOA) (transient neonatal hair loss)

- It is non-scarring alopecia caused by synchronized physiologic telogen effluvium after a prolonged anagen phase (under the influence of maternal hormones) since the prenatal period. Earlier, the condition was attributed to friction from sleeping in a supine position.
- It can affect any race and typically occurs after two to three months after birth.

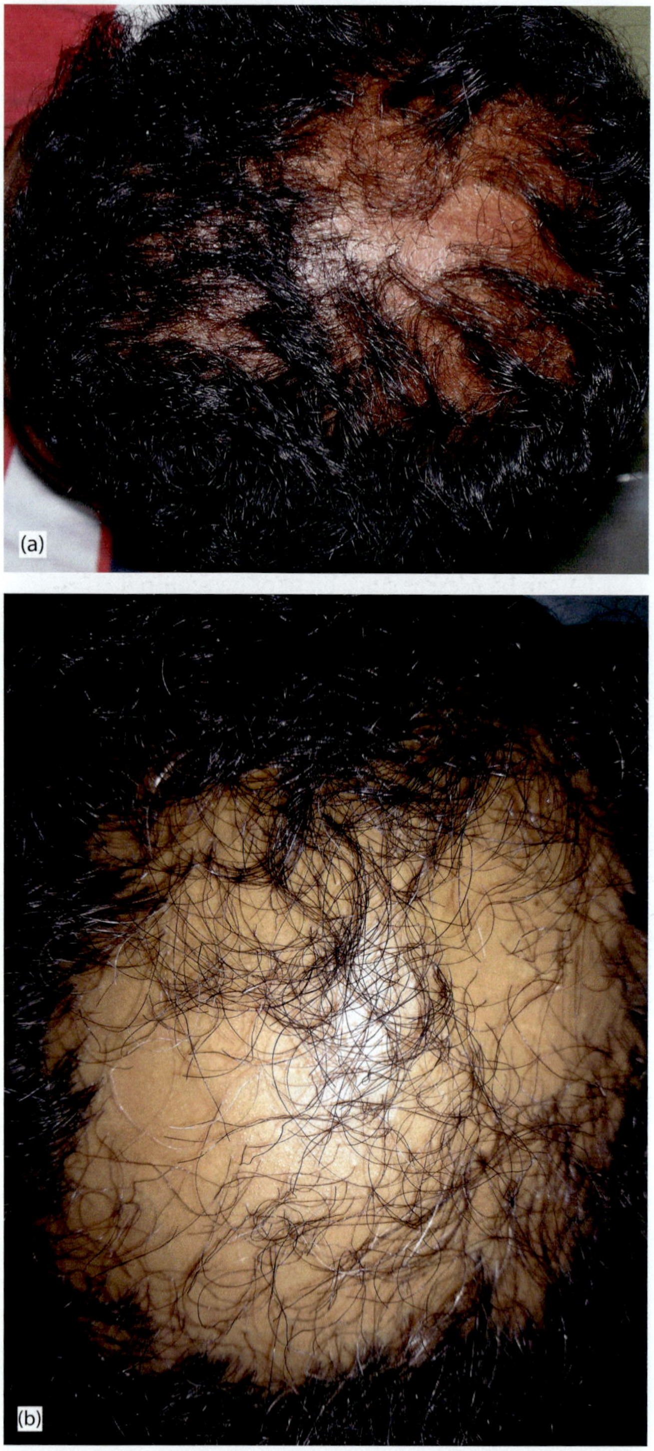

Figure 24.9 **(a)** Central cicatricial scarring alopecia – vertex of scalp is affected and alopecic patch is progressing peripherally. **(b)** Extensive scalp involvement in central cicatricial scarring alopecia. (b – Courtesy: Dr. Shashank Bansod, Nagpur, India.)

- NOA characteristically involves the occipital area. The frontotemporal region is now increasingly recognized to be affected simultaneously or independently (**Figure 24.10a,b**).
- Affected infants present with a linear band or oval area of alopecia over the occipital area. The lower end of this

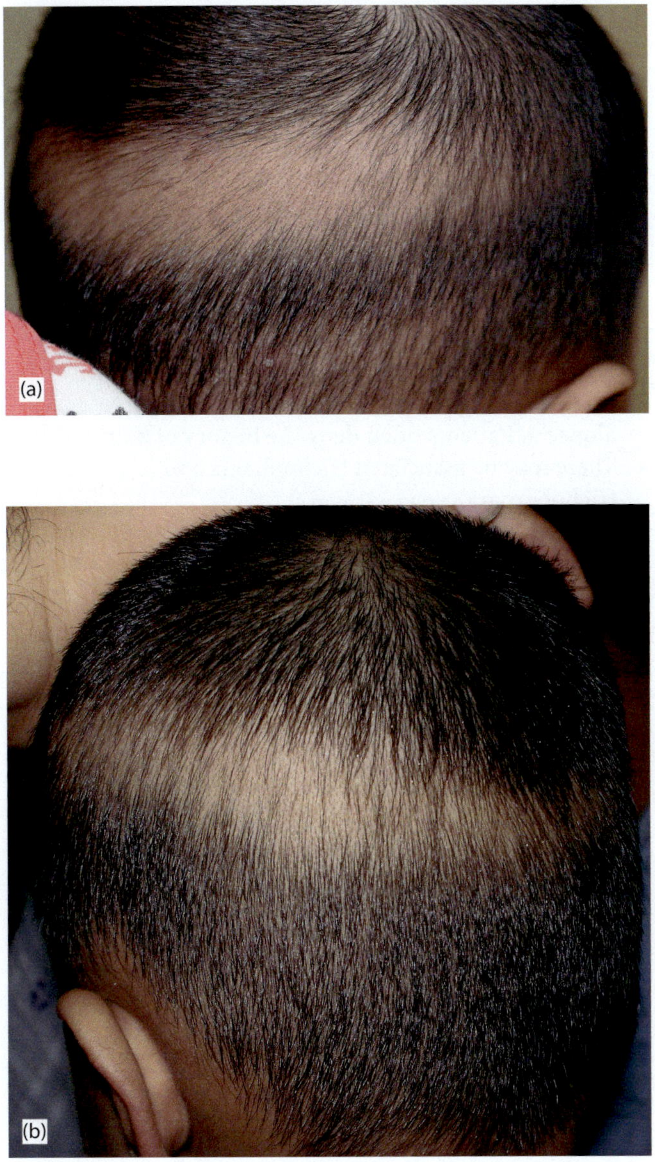
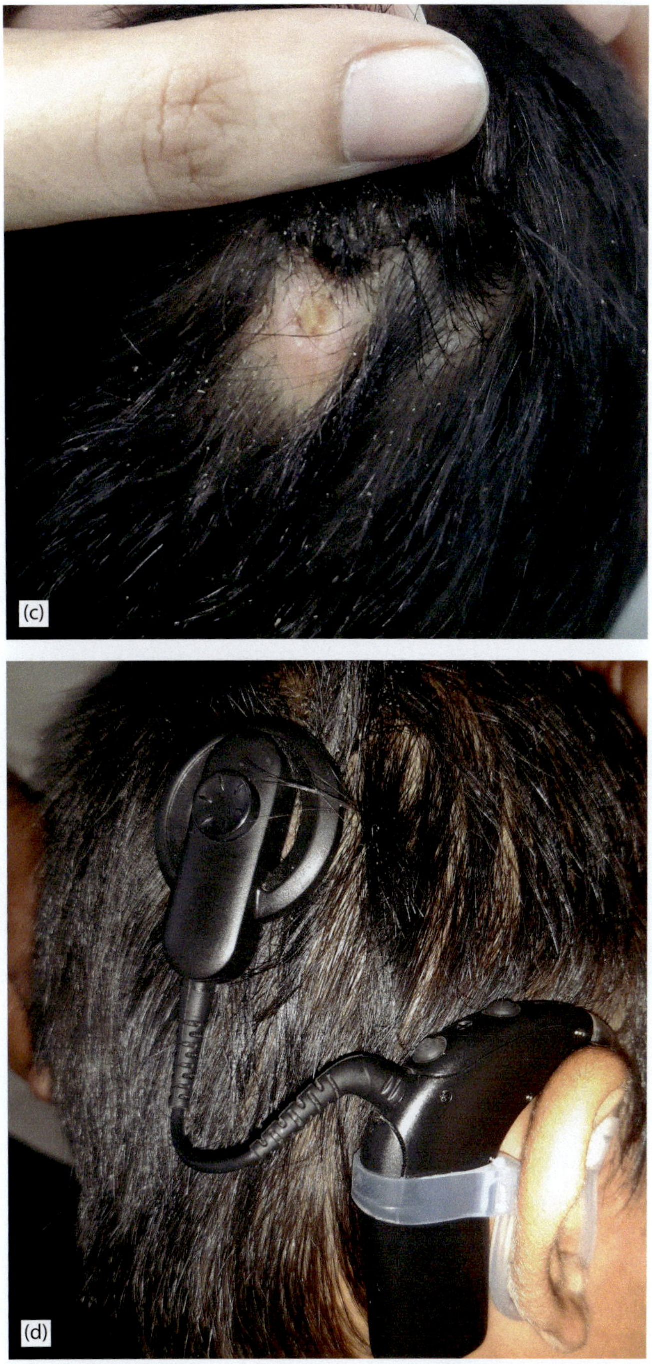

Figure 24.10 **(a)** Band-like neonatal occipital alopecia. **(b)** Neonatal occipital alopecia. **(c)** Focal alopecia and ulcer in a child using cochlear implant. **(d)** External unit of cochlear implant causes continuous pressure. (c,d – Courtesy: Dr. Hiral Shah, Baroda Medical College, Vadodara, India.)

alopecic patch has a sharp margin, but the upper margin merges with the hairs of vertex and is less distinct.
- The condition is self-limiting, and spontaneous resolution is noted.
- DD: Alopecia areata, temporal triangular alopecia, telogen effluvium.

## Pressure alopecia

- Pressure alopecia results from ischemic damage to the scalp in patients undergoing prolonged surgery or in bedridden patients. The alopecia may be non-scarring or scarring, depending on the severity of ischemia.
- It usually presents as a solitary, roughly oval patch at the site of greatest pressure, usually the upper occiput (**Figure 24.10c,d**).
- DD: Alopecia areata, trichotillomania.

## Acne keloidalis

- The condition is mostly seen in males and in people with colored skin.
- It is clinically characterized by follicular pustules and smooth, firm papules on the occipital scalp and posterior neck. With time, lesions heal with scarring alopecia (**Figure 24.11a,b**).

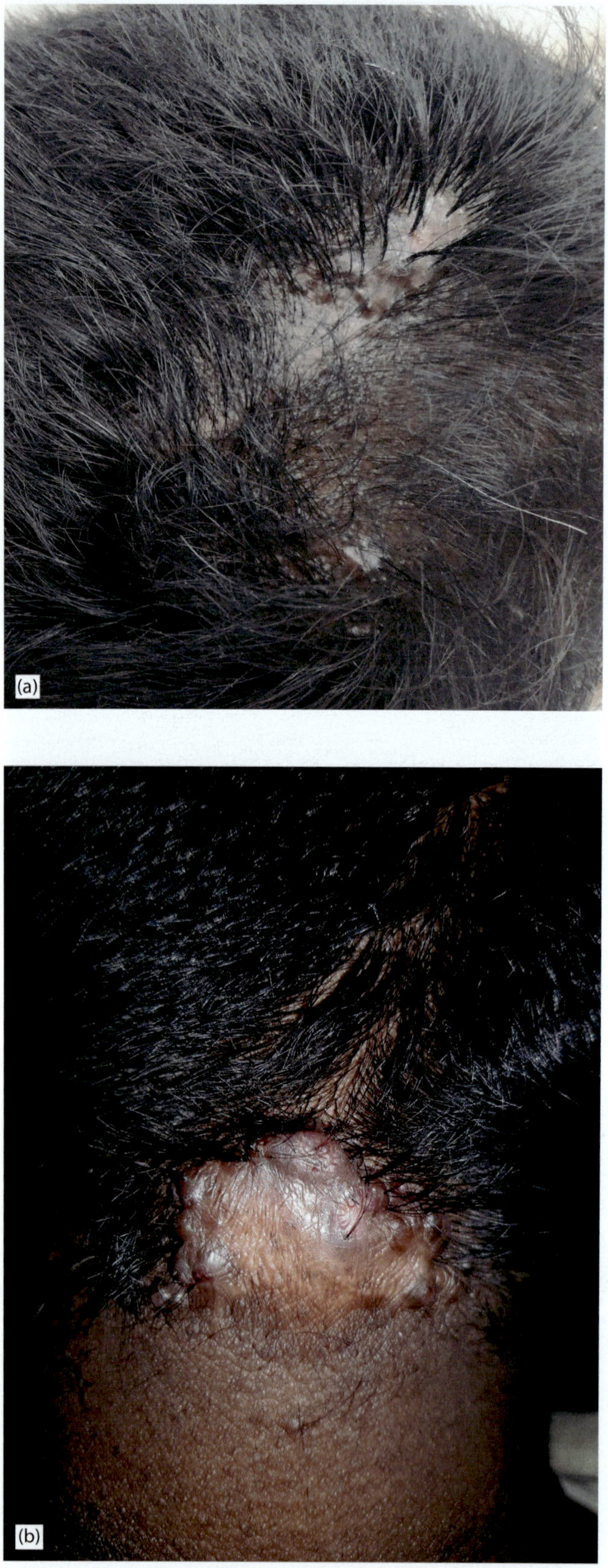


Figure 24.11 **(a)** Keloidal lesions and scarring alopecia in acne keloidalis. **(b)** Acne keloidalis nuchae with scarring alopecia. (a – Courtesy: Deverashetti Srinivas, Nizamabad, India; b – Courtesy: Dr PC Das, Katihar, India.)

- Occasionally, papules may coalesce to form hairless, keloid-like plaques.

## Nevus sebaceous (see Chapter E20: Scalp)

- Nevus sebaceous presents with hairless, yellowish plaque on the scalp in infants or children. Later lesions assume a verrucous appearance and may develop various tumors.

## Trichotillomania

- Trichotillomania is a psychocutaneous disorder (an impulse control disorder) characterized by an irresistible urge to pull out one's hair, leading to alopecia. Patients often deny the history of hair pulling.
- There may be associated trichophagia and trichobezoars.
- Affected patients may have other associated psychiatric disorders such as anxiety disorder, attention-deficit disorder, obsessive-compulsive disorder, mood disorder, tic disorder, and body-focused repetitive behaviors (e.g., skin picking, nail biting).
- It can occur in any age group but is more common among the children. The age of onset usually lies between 5 and 12 years of age, without any gender predilection. However, trichotillomania can also have adult onset, which is more common in females.
- Patients may complain of some kind of discomfort in the affected area, such as itching, pain, etc. There may be a history of disease aggravation during the stressful periods. Also, there may be a history of distress, impairment of social or academic functioning, and impact to family relationships.
- The scalp is the most affected site, but other areas, including eyebrows and eyelashes, can be involved.
- The presentation is variable – it ranges from localized patches to complete scalp involvement, and from decreased density to complete alopecia. Patients commonly present with single or multiple, geometric-shaped patches with incomplete, non-scarring alopecia. The hairs in the affected area are characteristically of different lengths in an irregular pattern. The hairless patch is usually seen over easily accessible sites. In severe cases, complete scalp involvement and even involvement of eyebrows and eyelashes may be noted (**Figure 24.12a–c**).
- Clinically, different zone of hairs can be identified:
    - Long normal texture hair in the periphery of scalp
    - Patchy hair loss with or without spots of bleeding
    - Short, thin, regrowing hairs within the patch
- Sometimes the vertex of the scalp may be involved and marginal hairs are spared; such a presentation is called tonsure trichotillomania or Friar Tuck (a fictional character in legends about Robin Hood) sign (**Figure 24.12d**).
- The hair pull test is negative.
- Clinical diagnosis in suspected cases can be confirmed by creating a "hair growth window" – a small area in the affected area is shaved on a weekly basis to

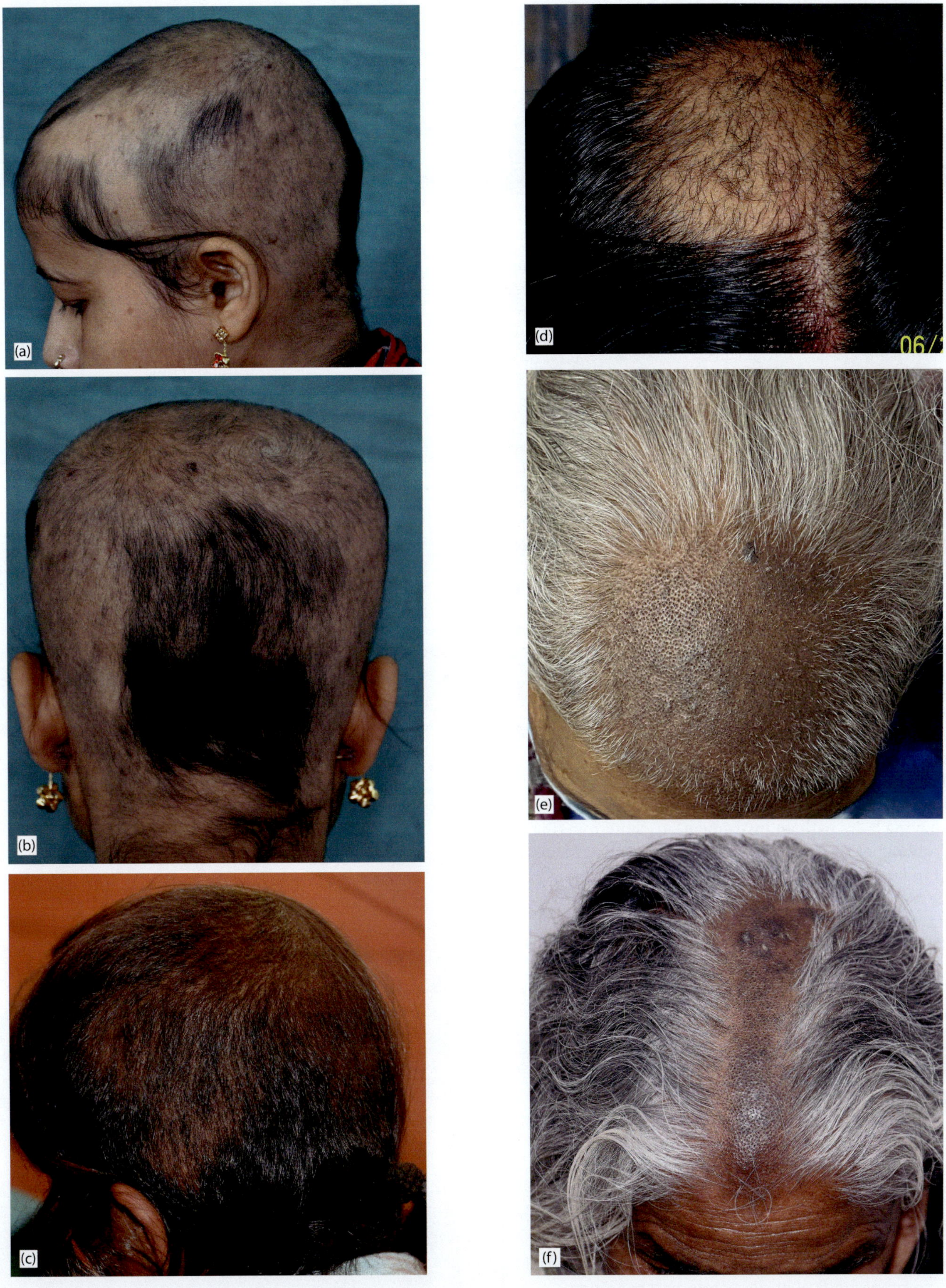


Figure 24.12 **(a)** Extensive hair loss in trichotillomania. **(b)** In same patient, hairs in mid-occipital area are spared. **(c)** Different lengths of hairs in trichotillomania. **(d)** Friar Tuck type of trichotillomania. **(e)** Trichoteiromania causing patchy alopecia in an elderly female. **(f)** Trichoteiromania in an elderly female. Note prurigo nodularis like lesions on the scalp. (*Continued*)

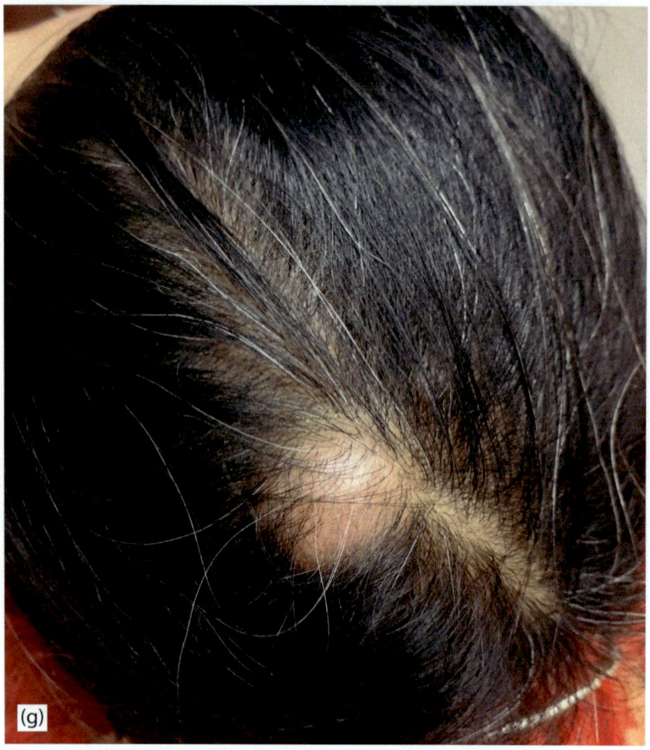


Figure 24.12 (*Continued*) **(g)** Benign cystic lesion causing localized alopecia. (e – Courtesy: Prof. Bhushan Madke, Jawaharlal Nehru Medical College, Datta Meghe Institute of Medical Sciences, India.)

demonstrate the dense regrowth of hair within the affected area. DSM-5 criteria are used to diagnose this condition (**Box 24.1**).

- It needs to be differentiated from other compulsive hair disorders such as trichotemnomania (cutting or shaving hairs with an instrument), trichoteiromania (rubbing of hairs, leading to fracturing of hair shafts) (**Figure 24.12e,f**), trichorrexomania (cutting of hairs by nails), and trichodagnomania (compulsive biting of hairs of accessible areas).
- DD: Tinea capitis, alopecia areata, traction alopecia.

**BOX 24.1: Diagnostic criteria (DSM-5) for trichotillomania**

1. Recurrent habit of pulling one's own hair, eventually leading to alopecia
2. Repeated attempt to reduce or stop the hair pulling behavior
3. The hair pulling behavior leads to clinically significant distress, impairment of social, occupational, or other important area of functioning
4. Repetitive hair pulling or alopecia is not attributed to other medical or dermatological condition
5. Hair pulling cannot be better explained by the symptom of another mental disorder

Table 24.4 Causes of secondary scarring alopecia

| Causes | Example |
|---|---|
| Physical and chemical injury | Burns (**Figure 24.13a,b**), acid or alkali burns, ionizing radiation |
| Infections | Bacterial (**Figure 24.14a**), viral and fungal infections |
| Granulomatous diseases | Sarcoidosis |
| Autoimmune and inflammatory diseases | Vesicobullous disorders, morphea (**Figure 24.14b,c**), systemic sclerosis, graft-versus-host disease, psoriasis, |
| Benign and malignant tumors | Primary tumors, metastases, lymphoproliferative diseases, organoid nevi |
| Genodermatoses | Aplasia cutis congenita, ectodermal dysplasias, epidermolysis bullosa |
| Others | Amyloidosis |

## Tumor alopecia

- Many benign or malignant tumors on the scalp may replace normal appendageal structures during their growth and may cause localized alopecia (**Figure 24.12g**).
- Alopecia neoplastica refers to hair loss seen in metastatic scalp tumors.

## Secondary scarring alopecia

- Secondary scarring alopecia results from non-specific damage to the tissue, including hair follicles. The conditions responsible for secondary scarring alopecia are diverse and are summarized in **Table 24.4**.

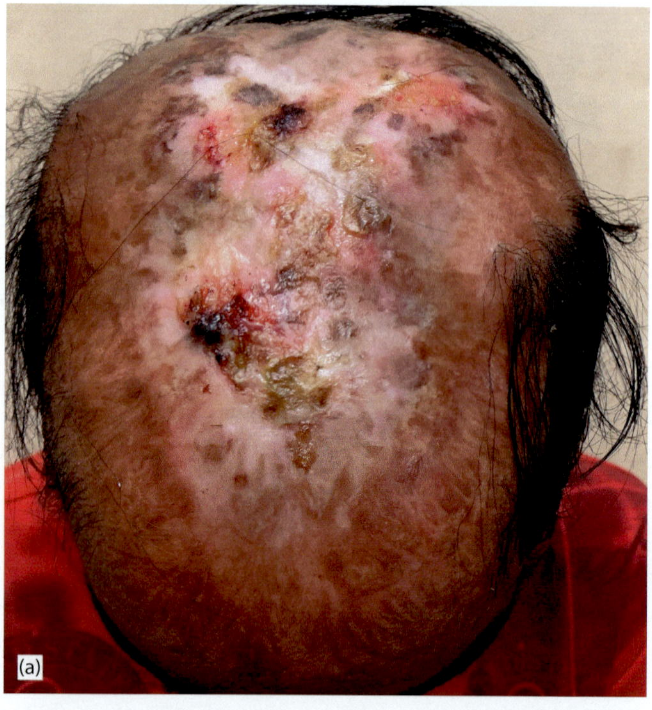


Figure 24.13 **(a)** Scarring alopecia due to burn. There are non-healing ulcers and crusted ulcers on the scalp. (*Continued*)

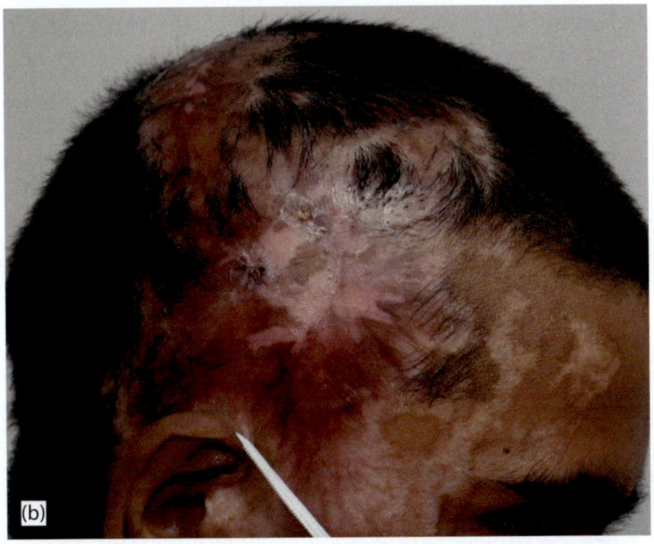

Figure 24.13 (*Continued*) **(b)** Scarring alopecia following burn.

## Aplasia cutis congenita (ACC)

- ACC is a rare cutaneous malformation that is characterized by the congenital absence of skin. The scalp is the most commonly affected site.
- ACC presents as solitary (or rarely, multiple), well-demarcated, circular, linear, oval, or stellate atrophic patches with hair loss on the scalp, usually lateral to midline. The size of the lesion varies from 0.5–10 cm. Often there is distorted hair growth around the scalp lesion (hair collar sign).
- ACC can be membranous or non-membranous, with membranous being the most common type (**Figure 24.15**).
- If the lesion occurs in first week of gestation, the lesion heals completely before birth and presents as atrophic, membranous, and fibrotic patch of alopecia.
- ACC can also present as ulcer of variable depth and heals spontaneously within the first year of life
- DD: Traumatic ulcer.

## Telogen effluvium (TE)

- Telogen effluvium (TE) occurs with excessive shedding of normal telogen hair in response to physiologic and pathologic stress (**Table 24.5**). Drugs such as retinoids, anticoagulants, antithyroid, cimetidine, enalapril and discontinuation of oral contraceptive pills too are associated with TE.
- Chronic telogen effluvium (CTE) is a diffuse hair loss of the scalp that persists for more than six months and

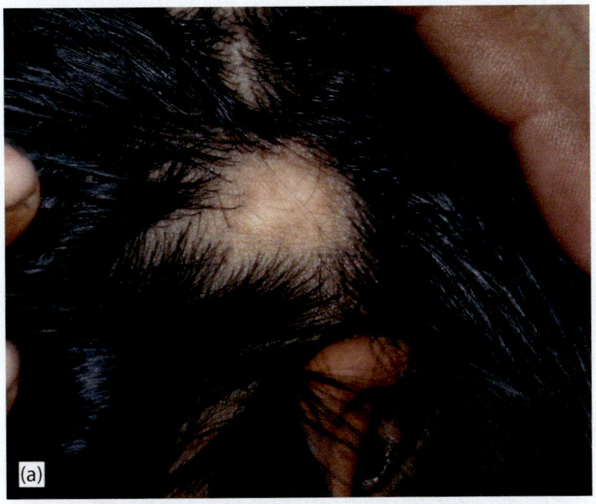

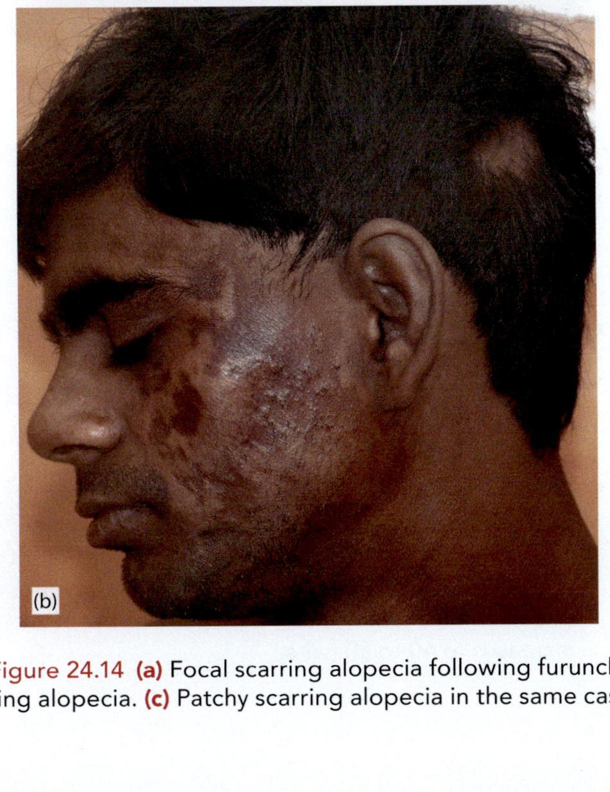

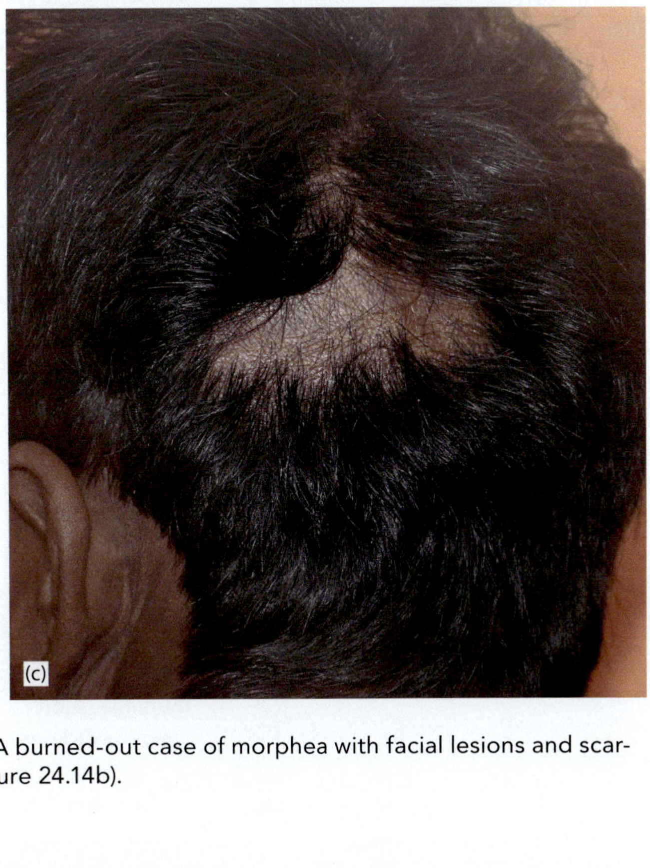

Figure 24.14 **(a)** Focal scarring alopecia following furuncle. **(b)** A burned-out case of morphea with facial lesions and scarring alopecia. **(c)** Patchy scarring alopecia in the same case (Figure 24.14b).

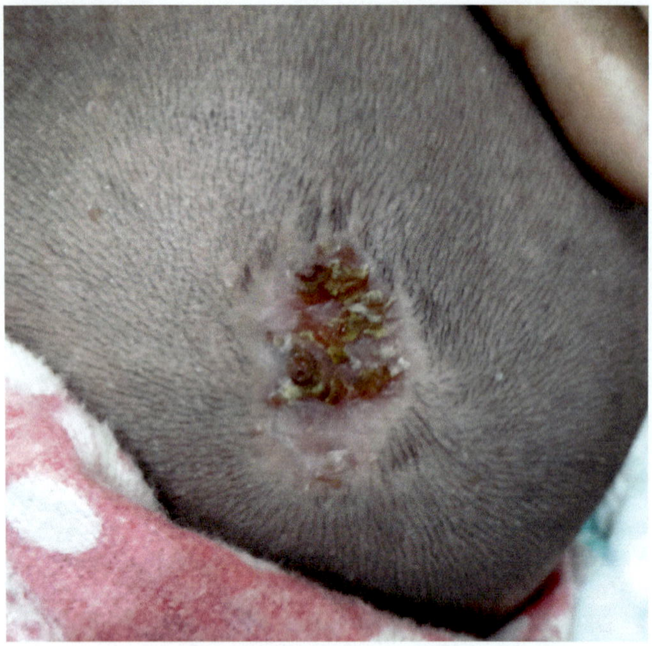

Figure 24.15 Aplasia cutis with focal alopecia, atrophy, and crusted ulcer. (Courtesy: Dr. Hiral Shah, Baroda Medical College, Vadodara, India.)

Table 24.5 Different types of telogen effluvium

| Type of telogen effluvium | Feature | Examples |
|---|---|---|
| Immediate anagen release | Premature apoptosis of hair bulb leads anagen hairs into catagen and telogen phase. | Physiologic or pathologic stress, high fever |
| Delayed anagen release | Hairs are in prolonged anagen phase during gestation and decreased hormones level at delivery cause them to enter catagen and telogen phase. | Postpartum TE (telogen gravidarum) |
| Immediate telogen release | Telogen phase is shortened. | Minoxidil use |
| Delayed telogen release | Hairs remain in prolonged telogen phase and are shed when finally teloptosis (termination of telogen phase with hair shedding) occurs. | Seasonal hair loss, hair loss associated with travel from low-daylight to high-daylight areas |
| Short anagen phase | Anagen phase is shortened. | Hereditary hypotrichosis, ectodermal dysplasia, short anagen syndrome |

is commonly seen in middle-aged females. The disease may run a chronic relapsing and remitting course over several years.

- TE normally affects women between 30 and 60 years of age but can occur in any age and sex.
- TE usually develops approximately two to three months after the triggering event.
- The patient complains of excessive shedding of hairs (**Box 24.2**) while combing or washing. On examination, there is excessive thinning of scalp hairs that involves the whole scalp. Bitemporal recession is seen. Characteristically, any patch or area with complete alopecia is not noted (**Figure 24.16a,b**).
- The shed hairs have a visible depigmented club shaped bulb.
- Spontaneous recovery is common and is seen usually within six months if the precipitating factor has been taken care of. Short regrowing hairs are found on frontal and other areas of scalp in resolving TE.
- Both hypothyroidism and hyperthyroidism can cause TE. Hairs become sparse, dry, and brittle. In hyperthyroidism, hairs become extremely thin and sparse.
- Nutritional deficiency of iron and zinc may be associated with TE; however, studies have shown conflicting results.
- DD: Androgenetic alopecia (hair loss follows a pattern: more thinning over frontal and vertex area), diffuse alopecia areata, anagen effluvium.

**BOX 24.2: Objective assessment of hair loss**

There are certain parameters to evaluate the hair loss in TE:

- Hair pull test – gently grasp about 40 hairs between the thumb and index finger and pull; a count of four to six club hairs is abnormal for unwashed hair whereas two to three hairs is considered abnormal for washed hair.
- Trichogram (forcible hair pluck) – shows the mixture of telogen and anagen hairs, and tells about the anagen to telogen ratio. If the quantity of telogen hairs exceeds 20% of total hair, then it is considered abnormal shedding.
- One-minute combing test – the patient is asked to comb their hair for one minute before washing on three consecutive days, over a cloth or white floor. A count of greater than 10 hairs found on the cloth or floor is abnormal, where as in TE the count increases to 40 to 50 hairs.

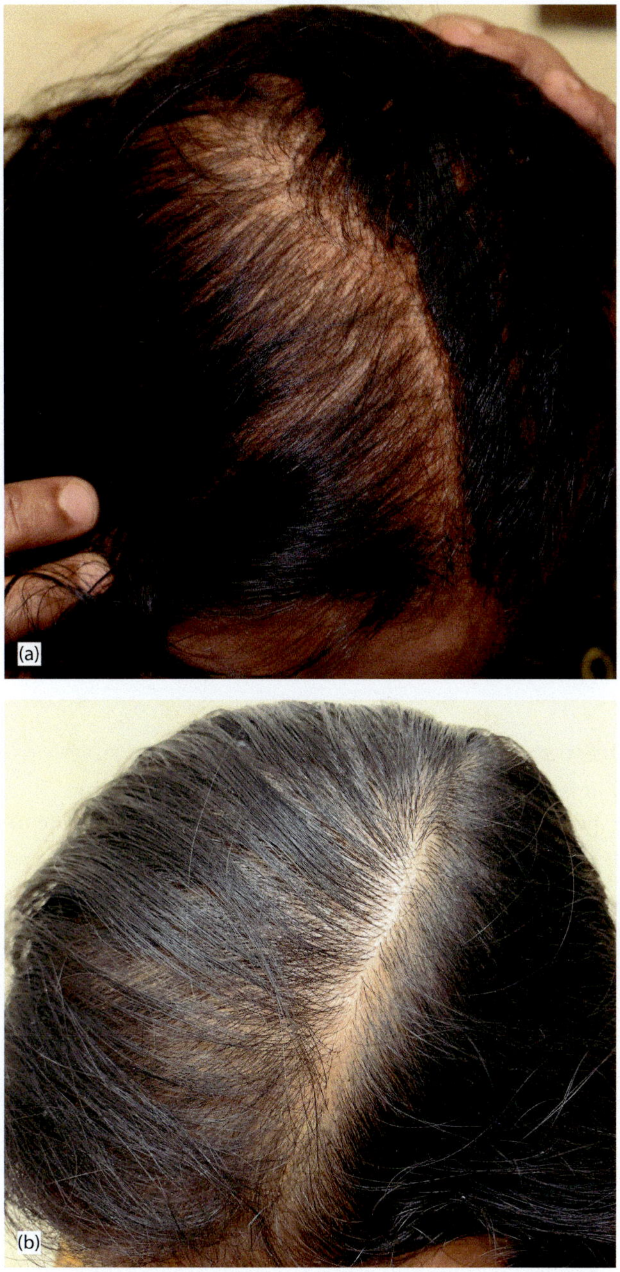

Figure 24.16 **(a)** Telogen effluvium with reduced hair density. **(b)** Chronic telogen effluvium in a middle-aged lady.

## Anagen effluvium (AE) (chemotherapy-induced alopecia)

- It is non-scarring alopecia that commonly occurs after administration of chemotherapeutic drugs. These drugs cause impairment of mitotic or metabolic activity of hair matrix cells, leading to loss of anagen hairs. In addition, there is constriction of hair shafts (Pohl-Pinkus constriction).
- AE can follow administration of chemotherapeutic agents (e.g., doxorubicin, nitrosoureas, cyclophosphamide) and other drugs (isoniazid, levodopa, colchicine, and cyclosporine), or may also occur in conditions like alopecia areata, secondary syphilis, pemphigus vulgaris, radiation, malnutrition due to inflammatory insult to the hair matrix cells.
- The condition does not show any racial or gender predilection.
- The patient presents with shedding of hairs within two week of chemotherapy. The shed hairs are anagen hairs – full pigmented hairs with inner and outer root sheath. Here the hair loss doesn't follow any pattern and involves the whole scalp. Scalp skin examination is characteristically unremarkable. Other sites, such as eyebrows, armpits and the genital area, may be affected (**Figure 24.17a–c**).

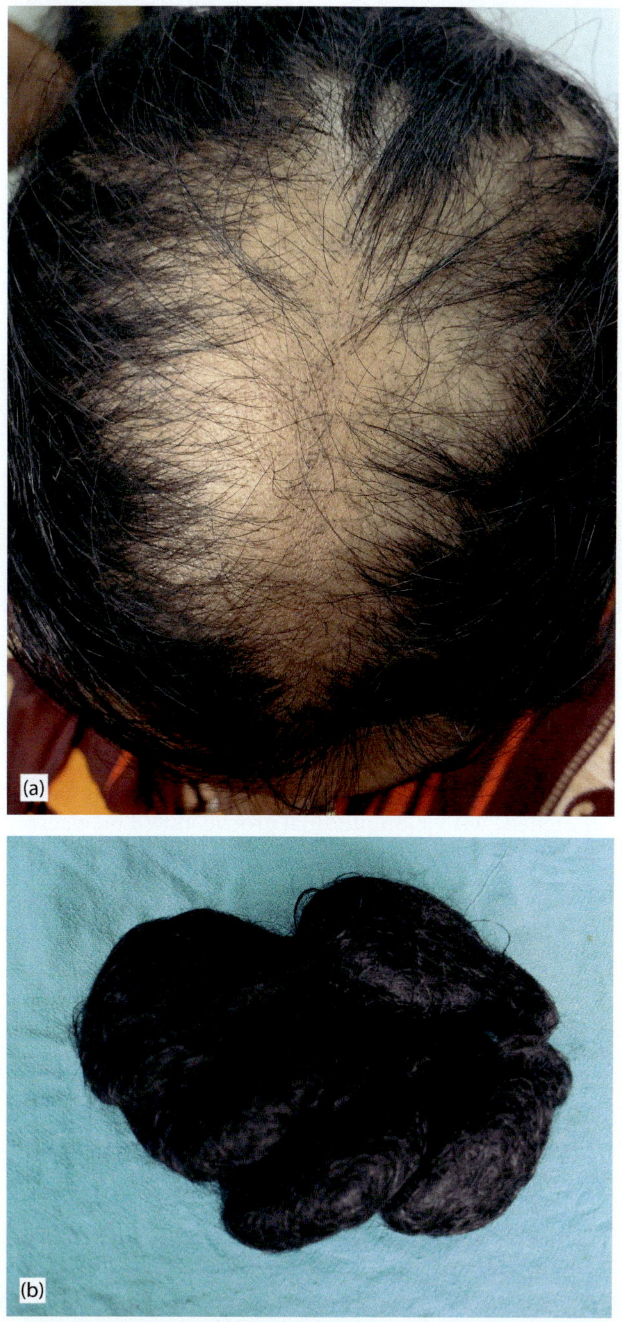

Figure 24.17 **(a)** Anagen effluvium due to azathioprine in a lady with vitiligo vulgaris. **(b)** Clump of shed hairs brought by same patient. (*Continued*)

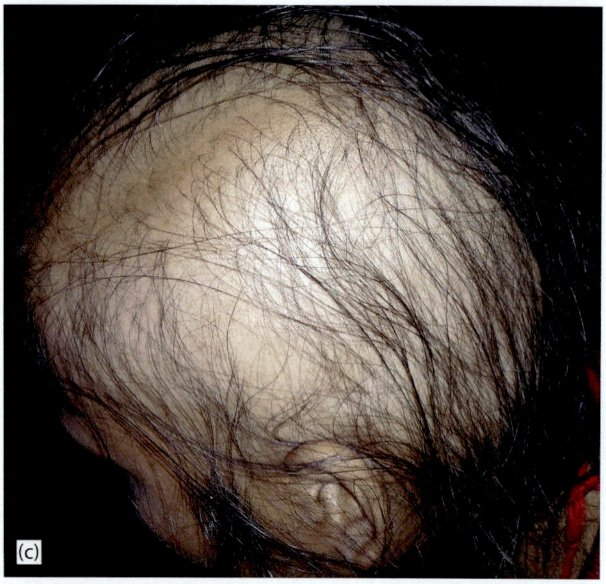


Figure 24.17 *(Continued)* **(c)** Another case of anagen effluvium due to azathioprine.

- The condition is reversible, and hair regrowth is noted upon discontinuation of the offending agent.
- DD: Telogen effluvium (no history of chemotherapy), androgenetic alopecia (follows a characteristic pattern), loose anagen syndrome (particular age group involved), trichotillomenia.

### Loose anagen hair syndrome (LAHS)

- LAHS is a rare, sporadic, or autosomal dominant condition causing premature keratinization of the outer root sheath, inner root sheath, and cuticle of the hair shaft. The end result is a malformed hair that can be extracted painlessly with little effort. The hair assumes a distorted shape (triangular, quadrangular, or flattened) with a longitudinal groove, noted on electron microscopy.
- The condition is common in whites and the most common presenting age group is children, though adults too may present with LAHS. Female preponderance is noted. Parents complain of thin, sparse hair, less growth of hair that requires less frequent haircuts, or dry lusterless unmanageable hairs of the child. There may be a history of easily and painlessly pluckable hairs.
- Clinical examination reveals dry, lusterless, thin hairs and diffuse (or patchy) non-scarring alopecia without any inflammation or scalp skin changes. Gentle traction results in painless extraction of hairs, which, on light microscopy, are shown to be anagen hairs with distorted hair bulbs (bent at an acute angle to hair shaft) and baggy, ruffled cuticle ("rumpled sock" appearance). Hairs may be of varying lengths (**Figure 24.18**).
- DD: Diffuse AA, trichotillomenia, telogen effluvium.

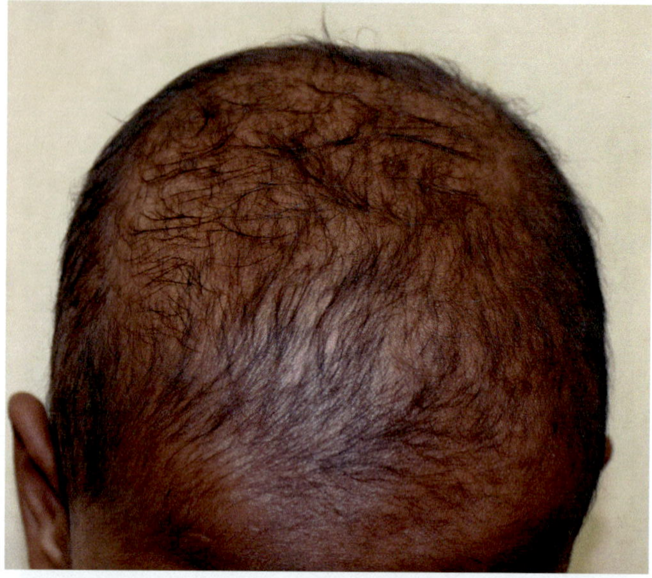

Figure 24.18 Loose anagen hair syndrome with reduced hair density and length.

### Short anagen syndrome (SAS)

- It is a congenital hair condition characterized by persistently short hair since birth, which occurs due to a shortened anagen phase.
- Females are more commonly affected, but it can affect males also.
- Typical presentation is in two- to five-year-old white girls. The condition is apparently rare in Africans and Asians.
- The parents complain that the child has very short hairs that do not grow long even though the hairs have never been cut.
- The hairs in these children are normal in texture and density.
- The hair pull test is negative in SAS, which helps to differentiate it from other hair shedding conditions such as telogen effluvium and loose anagen syndrome, where the hair pull test is positive.
- DD: Telogen effluvium, loose anagen syndrome.

### Hair shaft disorders (Table 24.6)

### Diffuse alopecia areata (alopecia areata incognita)

- Diffuse AA is a rare clinical variant of AA, characterized by abrupt onset of extensive hair loss. The condition is usually seen in young adults and shows a female preponderance. Here, there is generalized loss of hair involving the entire scalp over a period of a few weeks. In this condition the non-pigmented hairs are initially spared, so the patient may complain of rapid graying of hairs. The hair pull test is positive.
- Along with the thinning of scalp hair, nail findings can also be appreciated in this condition. Nail findings include regular nail pitting, brittle nails, trachonychia (sandpaper like roughness), and onycholysis.

Table 24.6 Hair shaft disorders causing alopecia

| Disease | Features | Clinical presentation | Comments |
|---|---|---|---|
| Monilethrix (beaded hairs) (**Figure 24.19a,b**) | • Autosomal dominant condition<br>• Periodic thinning of the hair shaft resulting in beaded appearance of the hair<br>• Presents in infancy | • Scalp involvement may be localized (occiput) or widespread. Occasionally, eyelashes, eyebrows, pubic, axillary, and limb hair may be involved.<br>• Hairs are dry, lusterless, and brittle.<br>• Keratosis pilaris (on scalp, nape of the neck, and extensor surfaces extremities) and koilonychias are often associated. | • Persists lifelong, may regress during puberty.<br>• Beading may not be evident to naked eye and may require dermoscopy or light microscopy for better visualization. |
| Pili torti | • Hair shaft flattened at irregular intervals and twisted 180° along its axis<br>• Onset in second or third year of life<br>• Late onset after puberty is known. | • Sparse and brittle hairs are strikingly sparkling in reflected light.<br>• Occiput and temporal areas are most severely affected. | • Twisting of the hair shaft is best appreciated on light microscopy.<br>• Pili torti may be an isolated condition or a part of different syndromes (Menkes syndrome, Rapp-Hodgkin syndrome, trichothiodystrophy etc.).<br>• Retinoid therapy too can cause acquired pili torti. |
| Trichorrhexis invaginata (Bamboo hairs) | • Occurs due to abnormal keratinisation leading to structurally weak hair shafts at certain points along its length. Harder (normal) adjacent segments of the hair shaft invaginate into structurally weak segments, creating a ball and socket appearance.<br>• Onset after one year | • Hairs are sparse, short, lusterless, and brittle.<br>• Changes are most pronounced on friction-prone areas – occiput and temporal areas. | • Classically seen in Netherton syndrome (ichthyosiform erythroderma, ichthyosis linearis circumflexa, atopic diathesis, and bamboo hairs). |
| Trichorrhexis nodosa (TN) | • May be congenital or acquired after various traumatic hair care practices (hair straightening, overuse of hair dryer, frequent swimming in chlorinated water, excessive traction)<br>• Characterized by small nodes at irregular intervals throughout the length of the hair shaft.<br>• Acquired form common in females and in middle-aged or older persons. | • Hairs are short, lusterless and brittle.<br>• Acquired TN is of three types:<br>  • Proximal – Common in dark-skinned individuals who use chemical hair relaxers.<br>  • Distal – Common in Asians and whites; associated with traumatic hair care practices.<br>  • Localized – seen in pruritic scalp dermatoses. | • Congenital form may be seen in argininosuccinic aciduria, Menkes disease, and trichothiodystrophy.<br>• Acquired TN is reversible after avoidance of hair trauma. |
| Bubble hairs | • Results from thermal damage (from hair dryers, heating tongs or hot curls) to hairs in genetically predisposed persons. | • There is a localized area of sparse, dry and brittle hairs. | |

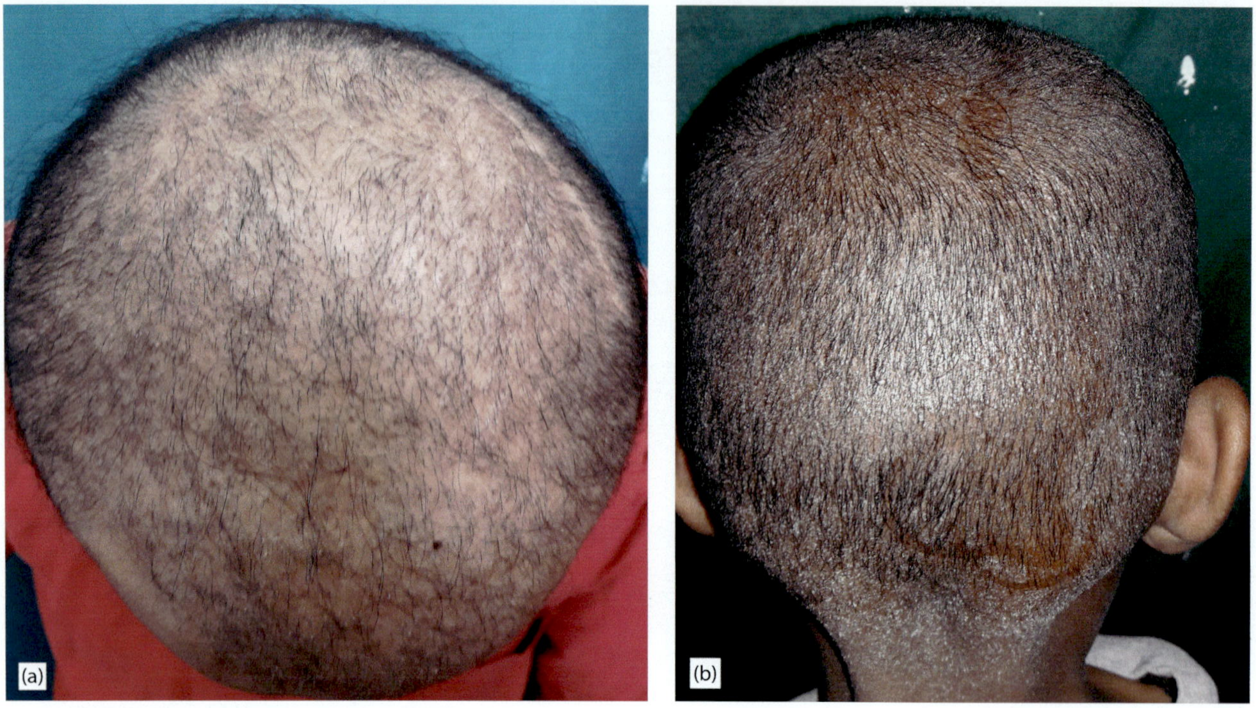


Figure 24.19 **(a)** Short broken hairs, dry lusterless hairs, and reduced hair density in monilethrix. **(b)** Monilethrix in a young girl. Her father too had monilethrix. (a,b – Courtesy: Dr. Hiral Shah, Baroda Medical College, Vadodara, India.)

- DD: Telogen effluvium, anagen effluvium (history of chemotherapy), androgenetic alopecia (follows a typical pattern).

### Atrichia with papular lesions (APL)

- APL is a rare autosomal recessive disorder caused by mutations in the hairless (HR) gene, leading to failure of catagen hairs to re-enter the anagen phase. The condition manifests as irreversible alopecia universalis with papular lesions.
- There may be a history of consanguineous marriage of parents.
- The affected child may have a normal or sometimes, scant hair growth at birth. Hairs are gradually lost by the age of five to six months and are never regained.
- Clinical examination reveals hair loss and multiple skin-colored, keratotic papules (**Box 24.3**). These papules keep increasing in number as the child grows and may involve the entire body (**Figure 24.20a,b**).

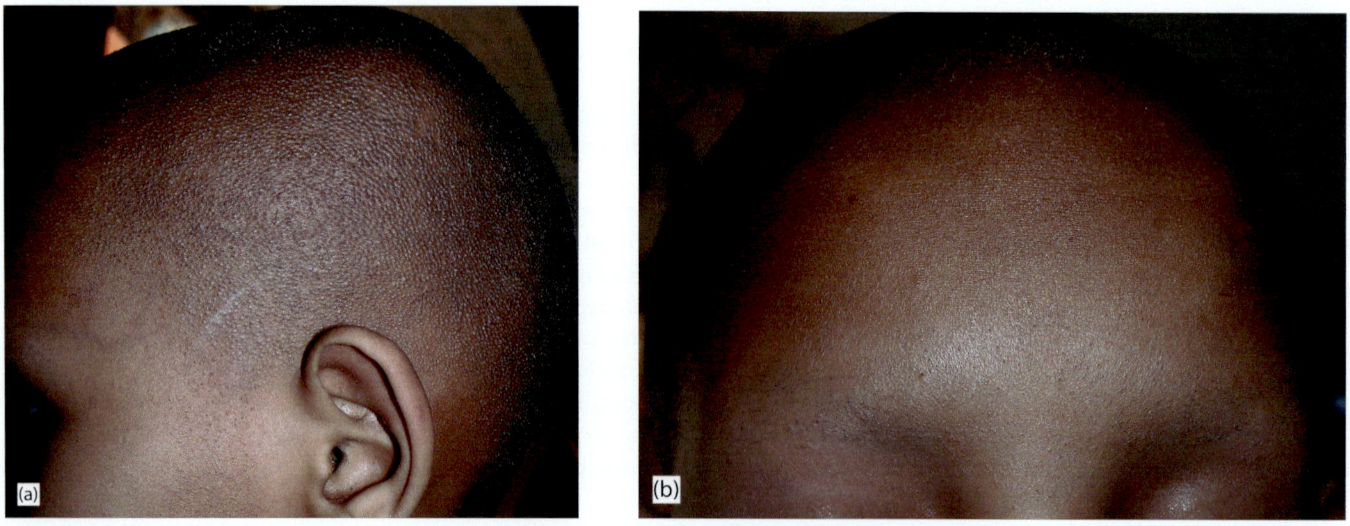


Figure 24.20 **(a)** Atrichia with papules. **(b)** Loss of eyebrows in the same patient.

**BOX 24.3: Diagnosis of atrichia with papular lesions**

MAJOR CRITERIA (four out of five required)

1. Permanent or complete absence of scalp hair by the first few months of life
2. Few to widespread smooth, whitish, or milia-like papules on the face, scalp, arms, elbows, thighs, or knees from infancy or childhood
3. Replacement of mature hair follicle structure by follicular cyst, filled with cornified material in scalp histology
4. Mutation in human hairless gene through genetic testing
5. Clinical or molecular exclusion of vitamin D-dependent rickets

MINOR CRITERIA

1. Family history consanguinity
2. Absence of secondary axillaries, pubic or body hair growth and/or sparse eyebrows and eyelashes
3. Normal growth and development including normal bone, teeth, nail, and sweating
4. Whitish hypopigmented streaks on scalp
5. Lack of response to any treatment modality

- The patients have normal growth and development.
- DD: Alopecia areata (universalis type), KFSD, vitamin D-dependent rickets.

### Hereditary vitamin D-resistant rickets with alopecia

- It is an autosomal recessive condition that occurs due to mutation of the vitamin D receptor (VDR) gene, which leads to unresponsiveness of the mutant receptor to active form of vitamin D3 (1, 25-dihydroxyvitamin D3).
- The condition is characterized by alopecia, hypocalcemia, hypoparathyroidism, increased 1, 25-dihydroxyvitamin D3, and early onset rickets. Alopecia can be present since birth or may develop in later life.
- Alopecia is one of the earliest symptoms and is associated with poorer prognosis. There is complete loss of scalp hair, eyebrows, eyelashes, and other body hairs, and it is resistant to all treatment modalities.
- DD: Alopecia universalis, atrichia with papular lesions.

### Lichen planopilaris

- Lichen planopilaris (LPP) is an inflammatory, primary cicatricial alopecia and is considered a follicular variant of lichen planus. Many patients may show co-existing lichen planus of skin, mucosa, or nails.
- The disease is common in females, and the most commonly presenting age group is 40 to 60 years.
- Patients may complain of itching, burning, pain, and tenderness.
- The alopecic patches may be single or multiple, focal or diffuse, and occur anywhere on the scalp. Smaller areas may coalesce to form larger irregular areas. Hairs at the margin of these lesions show perifollicular erythema and perifollicular scale. The hair pull test may be positive during active disease. The disease may have an insidious or explosive course and results in scarring alopecia (**Figure 24.21a–g**).
- The lesions of cutaneous lichen planus may present before, during, or after the scalp involvement.
- Graham-Little-Piccardi-Lasseur syndrome is considered a variant/sub-type of LPP and is characterized by LPP of scalp, non-cicatricial alopecia of the axillae and the perineum, and follicular hyperkeratosis of the trunk and extremities. The onset of these lesions may occur in any order.
- Frontal fibrosing alopecia is another variant of LPP.
- DD: Discoid lupus erythematosus, Alopecia areata, frontal fibrosing alopecia.

### Keratosis follicular spinulosa decalvans (See Chapter 6: Facial papules)

- KFSD is a rare X-linked follicular syndrome usually presenting in infancy. The disease is clinically characterized by widespread follicular keratotic papules; scarring alopecia of the scalp, eyebrows, and eyelashes; and photophobia.
- DD: Atrichea with papular lesion, lichen planopilaris.

### Discoid lupus erythematosus

- DLE can occur in any age group but is most commonly seen between 20 and 40 years of age. It is two to three times more common in females than males. It affects all races.
- The classical lesion of DLE presents as erythematous to violaceous scaly atrophic plaque with follicular

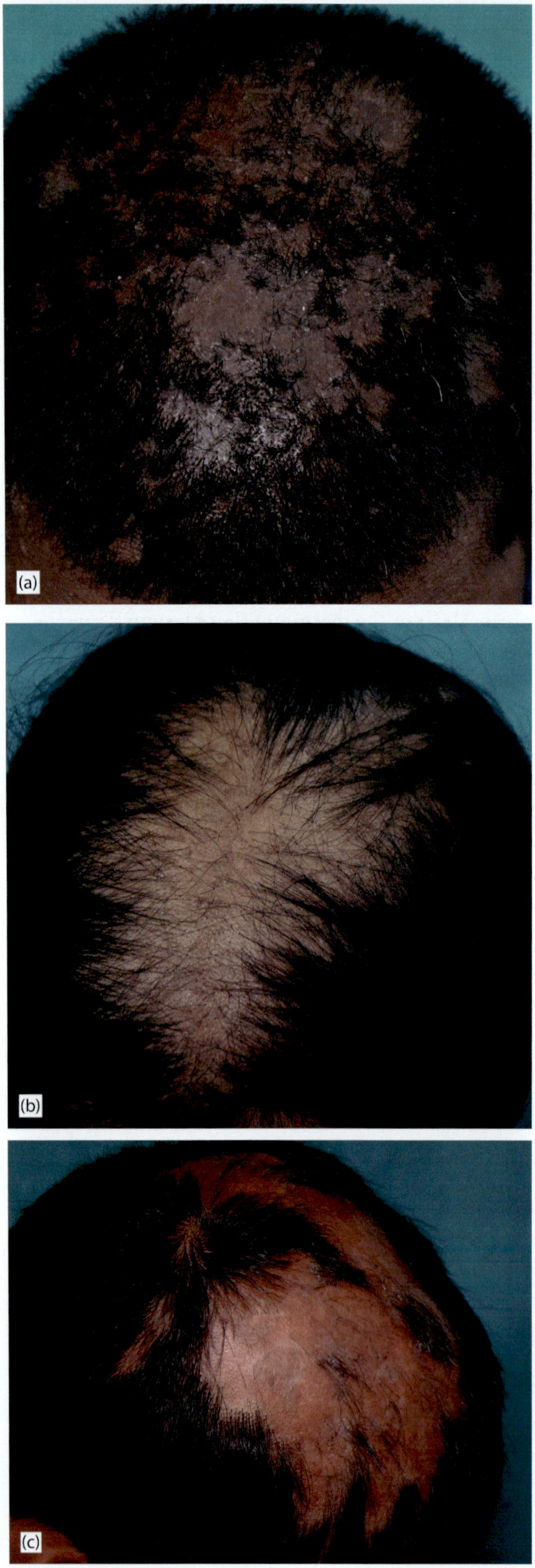


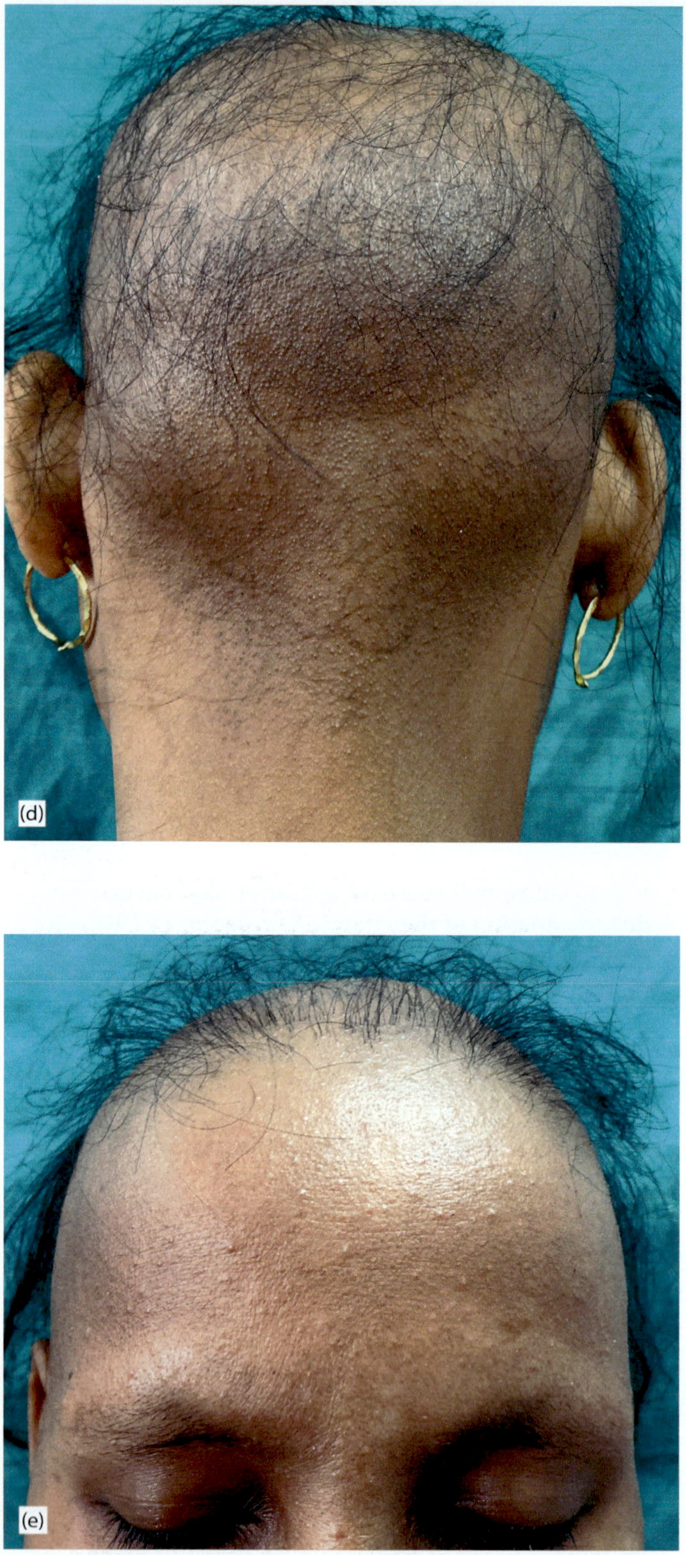


Figure 24.21 **(a)** Lichen planopilaris seen as scarring alopecia and pigmentation of the scalp. **(b)** Lichen planopilaris in a young female. Note perifollicular pigmentation. **(c)** Lichen planopilaris with lesions of annular lichen planus on the scalp. **(d)** A case with extensive scarring alopecia due to lichen planopilaris. Note follicular keratotic papules. **(e)** Same case with frontal hair loss. (*Continued*)

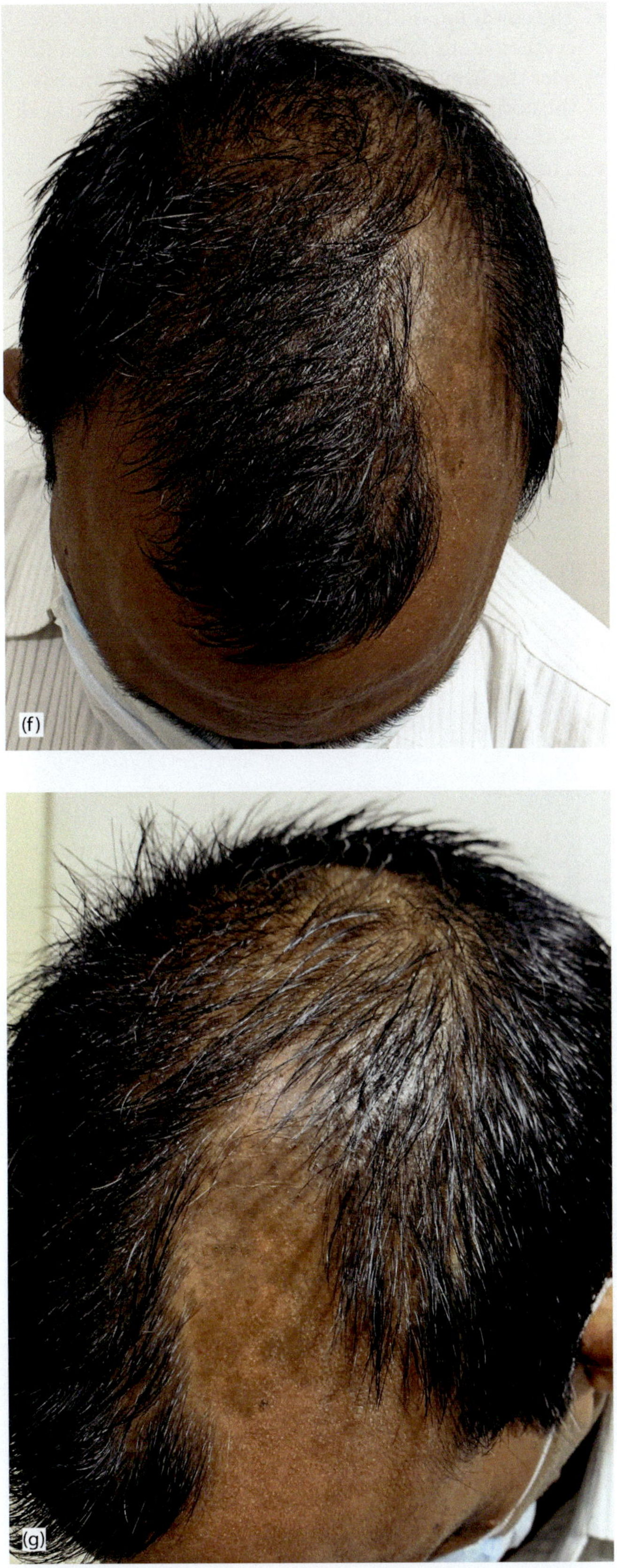


Figure 24.21 (*Continued*) **(f,g)** A male having androgenetic alopecia had a pigmented patch of scarring alopecia due to lichen planopilaris on the left parietal region.

plugging. When DLE lesions are present on the scalp or other hair-bearing areas, scarring alopecia develops within the lesion (**Figure 24.22a,b**).

- DD: Lichen planopilaris, secondary scarring alopecia (due to trauma and burn, etc.).

## Alopecia mucinosa (follicular mucinosis)

- The hallmark of alopecia mucinosa is accumulation of mucin within the hair follicle and sebaceous glands. It can be a primary disease or may occur secondary to both benign (lupus erythematosus, angiolymphoid

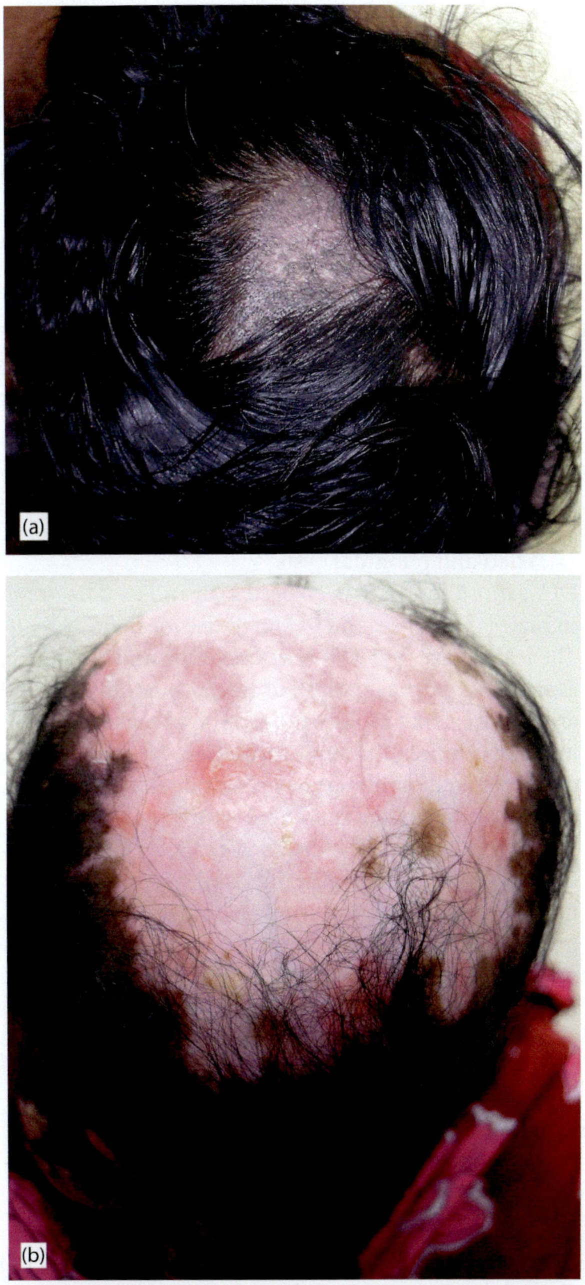


Figure 24.22 **(a)** Plaque of discoid lupus erythematosus with lesional alopecia. **(b)** Extensive scarring alopecia due to discoid lupus erythematosus.

hyperplasia) and malignant (cutaneous T-cell lymphoma, Hodgkin lymphoma, etc.) conditions.
- It is a rare condition with no racial predilection. Both the sexes are affected, with male predominance.
- The primary localized type mainly affects young adults under 40. The primary generalized type predominantly affects people over 40. The secondary alopecia mucinosa, either with benign or malignant association, generally affects people in the fifth to seventh decade of life.
- The patient presents with hair loss in hair-bearing areas. Alopecia in the early part of the disease is reversible and is accompanied by pruritic, erythematous, follicular papules and scaly plaque over scalp. Occasionally mucinous material can be expressed from the active lesion. As the disease progresses, follicular units are destroyed, and dilated follicular orifices with keratin plug can be appreciated.
- The primary AM lesions usually resolve spontaneously within two years with scarring alopecia.
- DD: Tinea capitis, Lichen planopilaris, folliculitis decalvans.

## Dissecting cellulitis (DC) (perifolliculitis capitis abscedens et suffodiens/Hoffman disease)

- It is an uncommon suppurative condition of the scalp resulting from the occlusion of the pilosebaceous unit. It may be a part of follicular occlusion triad or tetrad
  - Follicular occlusion triad – acne conglobata, hidradenitis suppurativa, dissecting cellulitis
  - Follicular occlusion tetrad – follicular occlusion triad and pilonidal cysts
- DC is more common in colored skin and usually presents in males in their second to fourth decade of life.
- The lesions are typically seen on vertex and occiput. The lesions start as painful follicular pustules and nodules that rapidly progress to abscess and intercommunicating sinus formation. Nodules may coalesce to form tubular or linear ridges with loss of hair. Seropurulent discharge with a foul smell is frequently present. The disease runs a chronic, relapsing course and heals with scarring alopecia and keloids.
- One of the prominent features is sinus formation; pressure on one site elicits pus discharge from a distant site on the scalp.
- Sometimes, arthritis, keratitis, and pyoderma gangrenosum are seen in association.
- DD: Kerion, folliculitis decalvans, tufted folliculitis.

## Folliculitis decalvans (FD)

- Folliculitis decalvans is a neutrophilic inflammatory disorder characterized by follicular pustules and nodules that eventually lead to scarring alopecia. *Staphylococcus aureus* has been frequently identified in the lesions, but its role in development of FD is not clear.
- It can occur at any age and in either sex but is most commonly found among young adults and middle-aged people, between 30 and 60 years of age.
- The condition initially presents as painful or pruritic, erythematous follicular papules, pustules, and nodules over the frontal and vertex area and progress towards the occipital area. The pustules come in crops and heal with erythematous scarring with alopecia.
- The lesions usually progress in one direction by peripheral extension. Well-developed lesions are characterized by multiple erythematous papules and pustules over the margin of alopecic patch, with atrophic, shiny scarring at the center (**Figure 24.23a,b**).

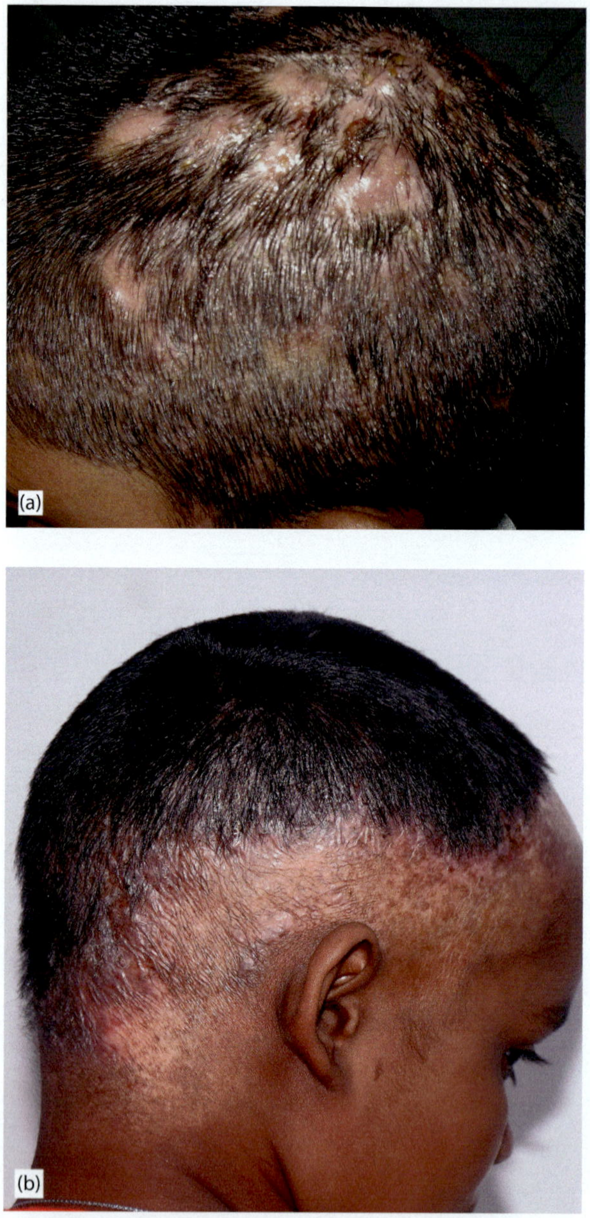


Figure 24.23 **(a)** Erythematous nodules with pustules and lesional alopecia in folliculitis decalvans. **(b)** Lesions in folliculitis decalvans showing progression towards central scalp in this girl. Pustules and nodules appear at active margin, leaving scarring behind.

- The most common site is scalp, but it can involve other hair-bearing sites of body.
- Tufted folliculitis is a variant of folliculitis decalvans in which multiple hairs emerge from a single dilated follicular opening in a "doll's hair" pattern. These tufts of hairs are present within the areas of scarring alopecia with complete loss of hairs. The areas of scarring and tufted folliculitis are usually well circumscribed. Varying degrees of edema, erythema, and tenderness are noted.
- DD: Dissecting cellulitis, bacterial folliculitis.

### Erosive pustular dermatosis of scalp (EPDS) (erosive pustulosis of scalp)[12]

- EPDS is an idiopathic, inflammatory disorder of chronically sun-damaged skin. It may also occur after trauma, surgical procedures, burn injuries, etc.
- The disease appears to be common in light-skinned persons and is mostly seen in elderly people, with a female predilection.
- The classical site of affection is the scalp, especially bald areas, but similar disease has been observed on legs too. Hence, some authors prefer to use "erosive pustular dermatosis."
- The lesions start as itchy or painful, non-follicular pustules that progress to lakes of pus and get covered with yellow-brown crusts. The surrounding skin is atrophic. The disease runs a chronic, relapsing and remitting course and ultimately heals with scarring alopecia.
- The disease may be associated with co-existing actinic keratosis or squamous cell carcinoma and the latter should be specifically sought for.
- DD: Folliculitis decalvans, dissecting cellulitis, localized cicatricial pemphigoid.

### Pseudopelade of Brocq

- It is rare idiopathic, chronic, slowly progressive, non-inflammatory patchy scarring alopecia of scalp that mimics alopecia areata. (The French term for AA is *Pelade*.)
- It appears to be more common in light-skinned populations and in females. The usual age of presentation is between 30 and 50 years.
- Patient presents with randomly distributed, irregularly shaped, smooth-surfaced, atrophic, flesh-colored or white alopecic patches over the vertex and occiput of the scalp. The pattern of involvement is called "footprint in snow." In progressive cases hairs can be plucked from the affected area with a gentle pull (**Figure 24.24**).
- The disease usually progresses insidiously but may burn out spontaneously at any stage.
- DD: CCCA, alopecia areata.

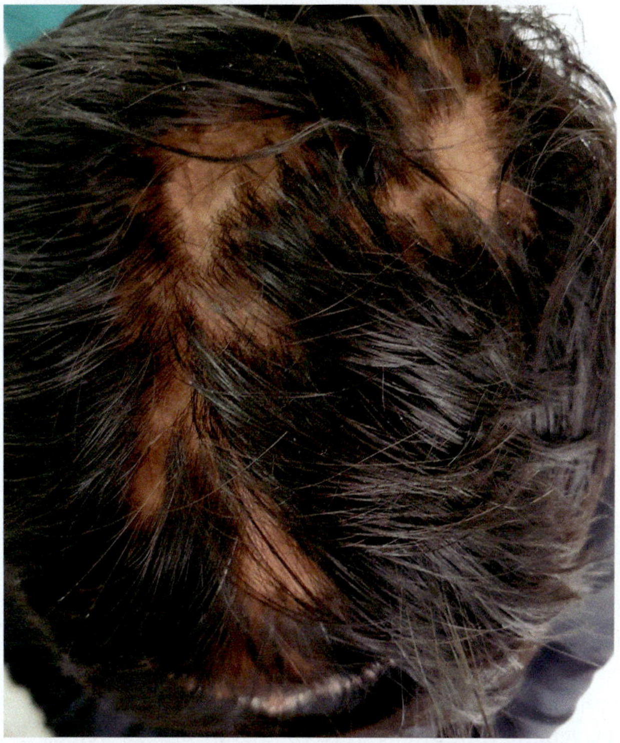

Figure 24.24 Random and irregular patches of scarring alopecia in pseudopelade of Brocq. (Courtesy: Dr. Aman Goyal, Haryana, India.)

## REFERENCES


1. Shapiro J, Hordinsky M. Evaluation and diagnosis of hair loss. In: Callen J, Ofori AO, editors. [UpToDate] 2019. https://www.uptodate.com/contents/evaluation-and-diagnosis-of-hair-loss. Accessed on 25.04.2020.
2. Springer K, Brown M, Stulberg DL. Common hair loss disorders. Am Fam Physician 2003;68(1):93–102.
3. Trüeb RM. Systematic approach to hair loss in women. J Dtsch Dermatol Ges 2010;8(4):284–97.
4. Xu L, Liu KX, Senna MM. A practical approach to the diagnosis and management of hair loss in children and adolescents. Front Med (Lausanne) 2017;4:112.
5. Kanti V, Röwert-Huber J, Vogt A, Blume-Peytavi U. Cicatricial alopecia. J Dtsch Dermatol Ges 2018;16(4):435–461.
6. Bolduc C, Sperling LC, Shapiro J. Primary cicatricial alopecia: Other lymphocytic primary cicatricial alopecias and neutrophilic and mixed primary cicatricial alopecias. J Am Acad Dermatol 2016;75(6):1101–1117.
7. Singh G, Miteva M. Prognosis and management of congenital hair shaft disorders with fragility - Part I. Pediatr Dermatol 2016;33(5):473–480.
8. Singh G, Miteva M. Prognosis and management of congenital hair shaft disorders without fragility - Part II. Pediatr Dermatol 2016;33(5):481–487.
9. Piraccini BM, Broccoli A, Starace M, Gaspari V, D'Antuono A, Dika E, Patrizi A. Hair and scalp manifestations in secondary syphilis: Epidemiology, clinical features and trichoscopy. Dermatology 2015;231(2):171–176.
10. Billero V, Miteva M. Traction alopecia: The root of the problem. Clin Cosmet Investig Dermatol 2018;11:149–159.
11. Melo DF, de Mattos Barreto T, de Souza Albernaz E, Haddad NC, Tortelly VD. Ten clinical clues for the diagnosis of frontal fibrosing alopecia. Indian J Dermatol Venereol Leprol 2019;85:559–564
12. Wilk M, Zelger BG, Hauser U, Höpfl R, Zelger B. Erosive pustular dermatosis of the scalp: Reappraisal of an underrecognized entity. J Dtsch Dermatol Ges 2018;16(1):15–19.

E47

# Hypertrichosis and hirsutism

B SHINY SHULAMITE

## ABSTRACT

Entities presenting with surplus hair over the body may be categorized into hypertrichosis or hirsutism, depending upon distribution characteristics and sex of the affected person. Hypertrichosis may be seen in either sex and in any age group, and the excess hair may be anywhere or everywhere over the body. Hirsutism occurs in females only, and the excess hair is noted typically in androgen-dependent areas. Causes of hypertrichosis encompass physiological causes, endocrine causes, various genetic conditions, different syndromes as well as malignancies. Hirsutism presents usually at puberty and is androgen hormone-influenced, which may be idiopathic or due to benign or malignant ovarian, adrenal, or pituitary causes.

The text of this chapter is available online at https://routledgetextbooks.com/textbooks/9781032399669/



DOI: 10.1201/9781351054225-76

25

# Vascular lesions

SUNIL KUMAR GUPTA

## INTRODUCTION

Cutaneous vascular lesions comprise a wide spectrum of entities, ranging from birthmarks to benign tumors to malignant tumors. They may be localized or generalized, innocuous looking or disfiguring, and may cause significant morbidity and sometimes death. Considering the variations in clinical presentation, it is important for physicians to suspect (**Box 25.1**) and diagnose various cutaneous vascular lesions. The clinical approach to the diagnosis of various vascular lesions is outlined in **Table 25.1** and the salient points are discussed below.[1–9]

### Salmon patch

- It is a capillary malformation (**Table 25.2**) occurring in about 30–40% of newborns.
- Clinically, it presents with irregular bright-red macules/ patches with or without fine telangiectasia. The margin is poorly defined.
- The lesions are often triangular or rhomboid in shape.
- The most common site is the face, particularly the forehead, glabella (angel's kiss), and upper eyelid and the nape of neck ("stork bites") (**Figure 25.1**). Sometimes the sacral area is also involved and is associated with occult spinal dysraphism.
- Facial lesions tend to fade by the end of infancy and are seldom detected after the age of six; however, the neck and body lesions tend to be persistent.

**BOX 25.1: Common clinical presentations of cutaneous vascular lesions**

- Red or blue patch, papule, or plaque
- Lesion bleeds spontaneously or on minor trauma
- Compressible swelling
- Reticulate erythema or blotchy skin color
- Painful red or blue lesions
- Telangiectasia
- Soft tissue overgrowth, hypertrichosis
- Pulsatile lesion, bruit

- DD: Port-wine stain and congenital medial fronto-facial capillary malformation.

### Port-wine stains (PWS)

- This is A capillary malformation that appears at birth and remains unchanged throughout life.
- It is usually unilateral and segmental; it may be localized or extensive, involving the whole limb.
- They are low-flow vascular malformations that may occur on any part of the body but commonly affect the face in the distribution of the trigeminal nerve (V1, V2, V3).
- Lesions are initially pale pink and later turn bluish or violaceous. The margin is well defined (**Figure 25.2a,b**).

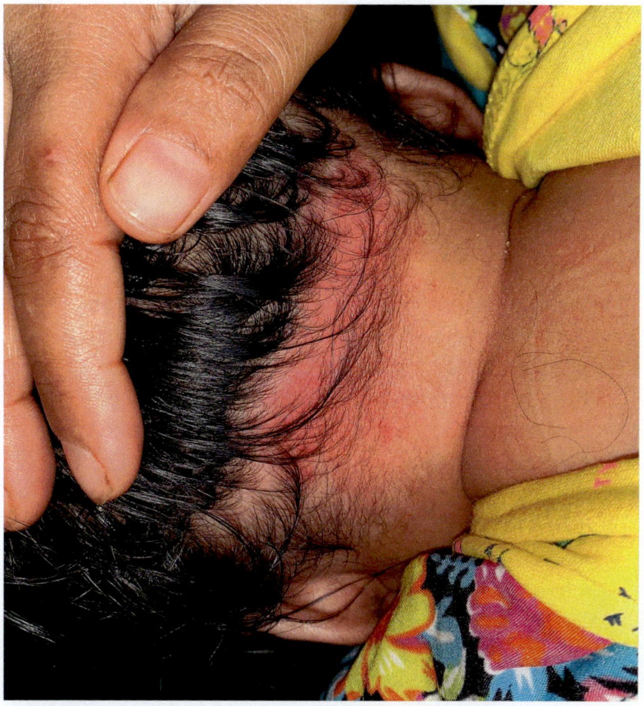

Figure 25.1 Bright red salmon patch in an infant.

DOI: 10.1201/9781351054225-77

Table 25.1 Clinical approach to vascular lesions

| Morphology | Diseases |
|---|---|
| Macules/patches | • Fades – salmon patch<br>• Persists/grows – port-wine stain, infantile hemangioma (early), angioma serpiginosum |
| Papules | • Localized – granuloma pyogenicum (lobular capillary hemangioma)<br>• Linear – angioma serpiginosum<br>• Disseminated<br>  ◦ Older population, asymptomatic person – cherry angioma<br>  ◦ Symptomatic person (fever, lymphadenopathy, etc.) – bacillary angiomatosis, verruga peruana |
| Papules, plaques, or nodules | Infantile hemangioma, congenital hemangioma, tufted angioma, hemangiopericytoma, reactive angioendotheliomatosis<br>• Hyperkeratotic/crusted surface – angiokeratoma, verrucous hemangioma, lymphangioma circumscriptum<br>• Commonly seen in head and neck region – angiolymphoid hyperplasia with eosinophilia, Kimura disease<br>• History/features of chronic venous insufficiency or arteriovenous shunt – acroangiodermatitis<br>• Immunosuppressed patients – Kaposi sarcoma<br>• Targetoid appearance – targetoid hemosiderotic hemangioma (hobnail hemangioma)<br>• Ulcerated plaque – ulcerated infantile hemangioma, angiosarcoma, Dabska tumor |
| Red or blue nodules | • Usually solitary, painful – glomus tumor<br>• Usually multiple, asymptomatic – glomangioma |
| Fluid-filled lesions | • Solitary – venous lake<br>• Clear fluid – lymphangioma circumscriptum<br>• Blood – angiokeratoma, verrucous hemangioma |
| Compressible swelling | Venous lake, venous malformation, arteriovenous malformation |
| Reticulate erythema/ blotchy skin | • Transient, improve on warming – cutis marmorata, livedo reticularis<br>• Persistent – cutis marmorata telangiectatica congenita<br>• Localized – nevus anemicus |
| Telangiectasia | See Chapter E18 |
| Purpura | See Chapter 14 |

Table 25.2 Vascular malformations

| Simple | Combined |
|---|---|
| • Capillary malformations port-wine stain, telangiectasia<br>• Venous malformations<br>• Glomuvenous malformations<br>• Lymphatic malformations – macrocystic, microcystic | • Capillary lymphatic malformations (CLM) – angiokeratomas<br>• Capillary venous malformations (CVM) – cutis marmorata telangiectatica congenital<br>• Arteriovenous malformation (AVM)<br>• Capillary AVM (CAVM) |

*Note:* Vascular malformations result from an error in vascular development in the embryonic period and have been classified on the basis of the nature of the vessels affected.

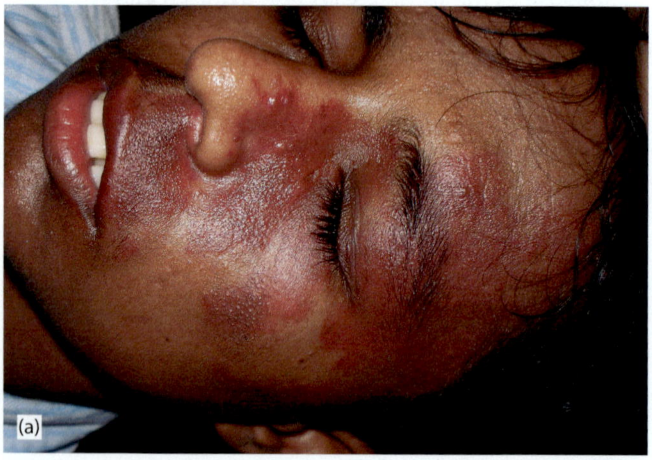


Figure 25.2 **(a)** Bright red patch of port-wine stain. Note well-defined margin of the lesion. (*Continued*)

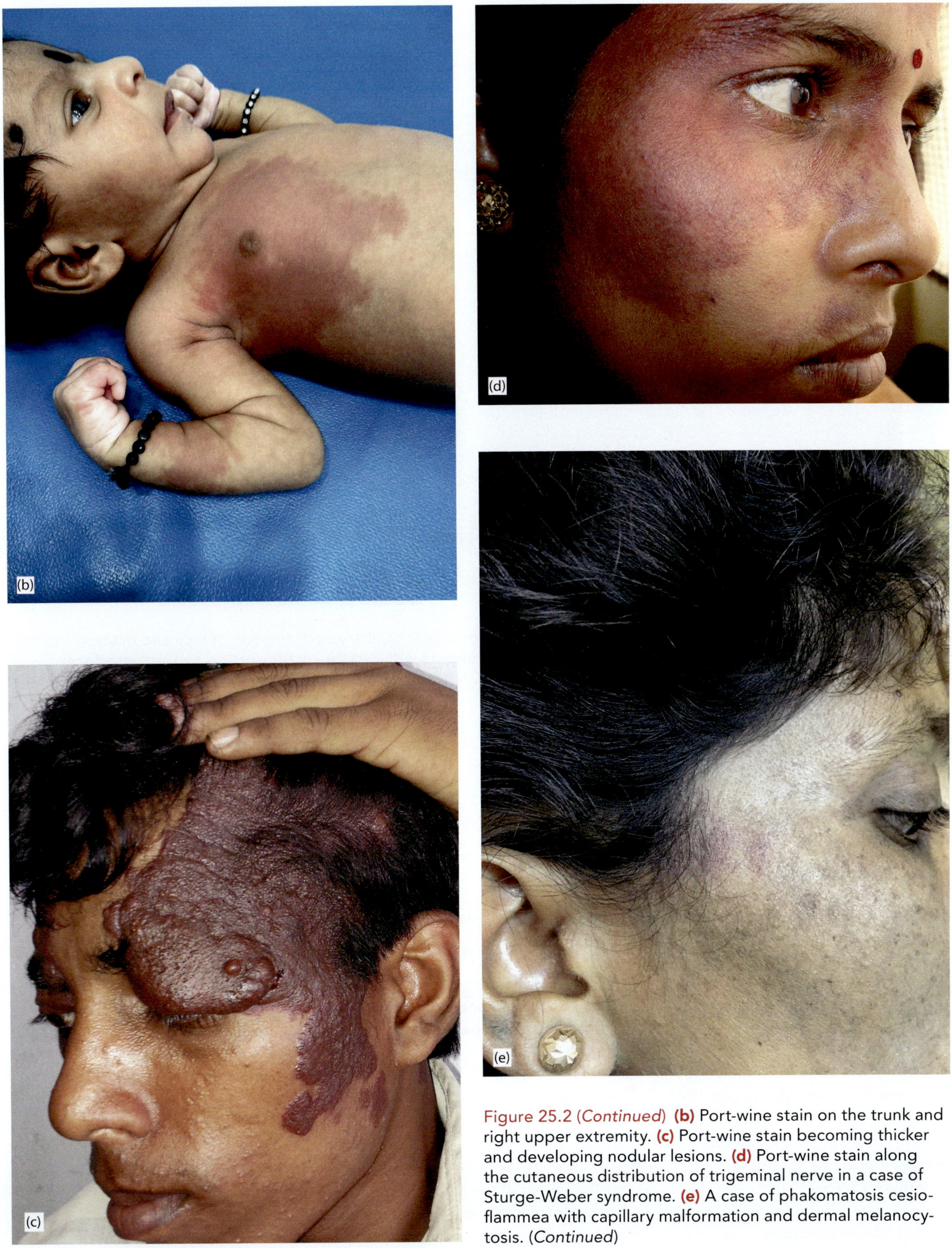


Figure 25.2 (*Continued*) **(b)** Port-wine stain on the trunk and right upper extremity. **(c)** Port-wine stain becoming thicker and developing nodular lesions. **(d)** Port-wine stain along the cutaneous distribution of trigeminal nerve in a case of Sturge-Weber syndrome. **(e)** A case of phakomatosis cesioflammea with capillary malformation and dermal melanocytosis. (*Continued*)

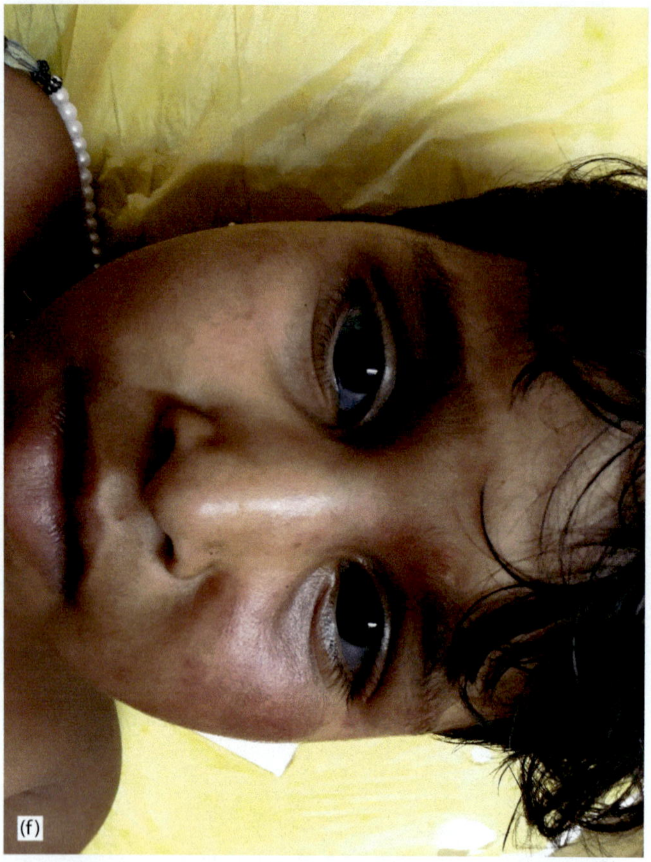


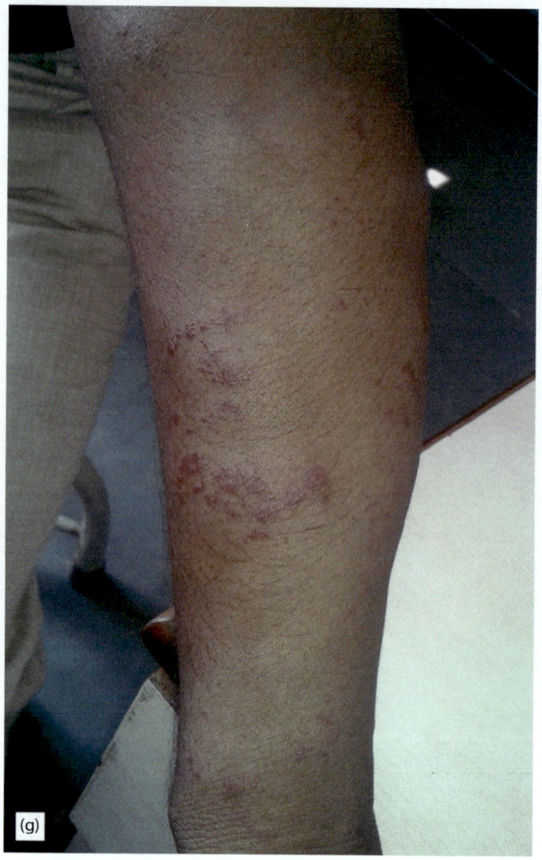


Figure 25.2 (*Continued*) **(f)** A case of phakomatosis cesioflammea with capillary malformation of face and bilateral dermal melanocytosis of bulbar conjunctiva. **(g)** Klippel-Trenaunay syndrome with capillary malformation and increased soft-tissue swelling. (a,c – Courtesy: Dr. Piyush Kumar, Katihar, India; b – Courtesy: Dr. Deverashetti Srinivas, Nizamabad, India; e,f – Courtesy: Dr. Balaganpathy R, Trichy, India.)

- Long-standing lesions sometimes develop vascular blebs or pyogenic granuloma-like lesions. Underlying soft tissues and bones may show hypertrophic changes (**Figure 25.2c**).
- For associated syndromes see **Table 25.3** and **Box 25.2**.
- DD: Infantile hemangioma, tufted angioma, early arteriovenous malformation.

## Granuloma pyogenicum (lobular capillary hemangioma, LCH)

- Granuloma pyogenicum is a misnomer; they are neither infectious nor granulomatous. Lobular capillary hemangioma (LCH) is the preferred diagnostic term.

Table 25.3 Syndromes associated with port-wine stain (capillary malformation)

| Syndrome | Capillary malformation | Other features |
|---|---|---|
| Sturge-Weber syndrome | Capillary malformation affecting the V1 and V2 cutaneous distribution of trigeminal nerve (**Figure 25.2d**) | Intracerebral calcification and early onset seizures, mental retardation, migraine, headache, cognitive impairment, hemiplegia, vision abnormalities and neonatal glaucoma |
| Beckwith-Wiedemann syndrome (BWS) (exomphalos-macroglossia-gigantism syndrome) | Centrofacial capillary malformations | Exomphalos, macroglossia and gigantism, hypoglycemia |
| Phakomatosis pigmentovascularis | Capillary malformation | **Box 25.2** |
| Klippel-Trenaunay syndrome (**Figure 25.2g**) | Mixed capillary venous malformation of the limb with lymphatic malformation | Soft-tissue and bony hypertrophy of the affected limb, and varicose veins |
| Parkes Weber syndrome | Capillary malformation with arteriovenous malformation | Soft-tissue and bony hypertrophy of the affected limb |

**BOX 25.2: Phakomatosis pigmentovascularis**

- The term phakomatosis refers to a developmental malformation simultaneously affecting the eyes, skin, and central nervous system.
- Rare group of disorders characterized by the combination of a capillary malformation with pigmented nevi and are traditionally classified into the following types:
  - Type 1: Port-wine stain/capillary malformation (CM) + Epidermal nevus
  - Type 2: CM + dermal melanocytosis + nevus anemicus
  - Type 3: CM + nevus spilus + nevus anemicus
  - Type 4: CM + Nevus spilus + nevus anemicus + dermal melanocytosis
  - Type 5: Cutis marmorata telangiectatica congenita + dermal melanocytosis
- Each of the above types are further divided into:
  A. Only cutaneous involvement
  B. Presence of extracutaneous involvement
- Recent classification by Happle includes
  - Phakomatosis cesioflammea: CM + dermal melanocytosis (**Figure 25.2e,f**)
  - Phakomatosis spilorosea: CM + nevus spilus
  - Phakomatosis cesiomarmorata: CMTC + dermal melanocytosis
  - Unclassifiable forms of phakomatosis

- It presents as a solitary, glistening, raspberry-like red or blue-black papule or nodule, often at the site of injury (**Figure 25.3a–c**).
- It is prone to bleeding and ulceration after slight manipulation.

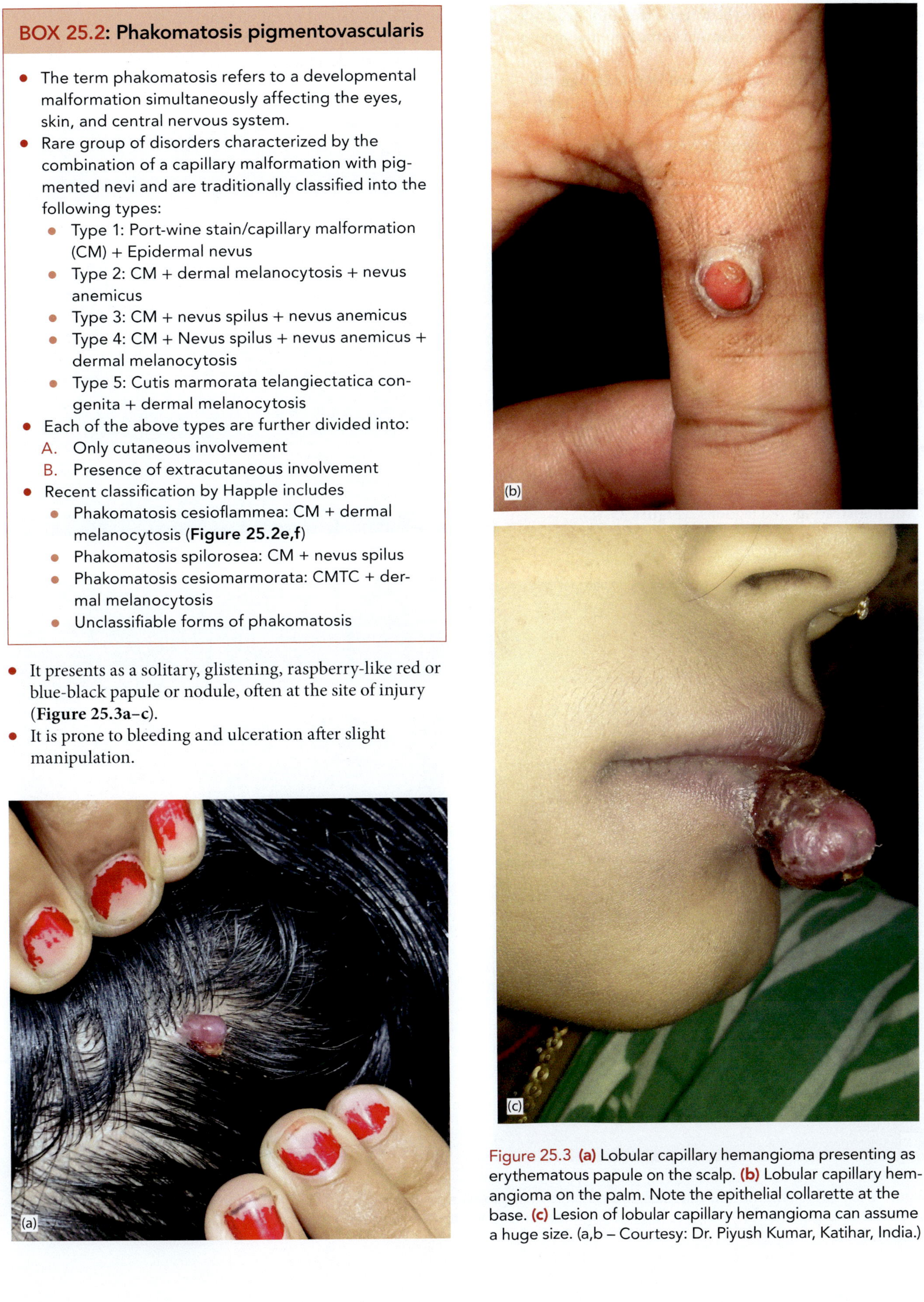


Figure 25.3 **(a)** Lobular capillary hemangioma presenting as erythematous papule on the scalp. **(b)** Lobular capillary hemangioma on the palm. Note the epithelial collarette at the base. **(c)** Lesion of lobular capillary hemangioma can assume a huge size. (a,b – Courtesy: Dr. Piyush Kumar, Katihar, India.)

- The common sites are the fingers, feet, lips, head and upper trunk, and the mucosal surfaces of the mouth and perianal area.
- It is common in both sexes and in middle age, but oral lesions are more common in females during pregnancy.
- DD: Infantile hemangioma, vascular malformation, and Kaposi sarcoma.

## Angioma serpiginosum

- It is a rare cutaneous vascular nevus of superficial capillaries, characterized by minute puncta (ectatic capillaries) in clusters or in a serpiginous pattern.
- Clinically present as minute copper-red to vividly red satellites that spread into circles and gradually coalesce, producing the irregular serpiginous pattern (**Figure 25.4a,b**).
- Common sites are the lower limbs and buttocks; it is initially unilateral, but it can be more widespread.
- The lesions may not blanch completely under pressure.
- Dermoscopy can be helpful in diagnosis by demonstrating "red lagoons" (**Figure 25.4c**).
- DD: Unilateral nevoid telangiectasia, angiokeratoma circumscriptum neviforme, purpuric dermatosis.

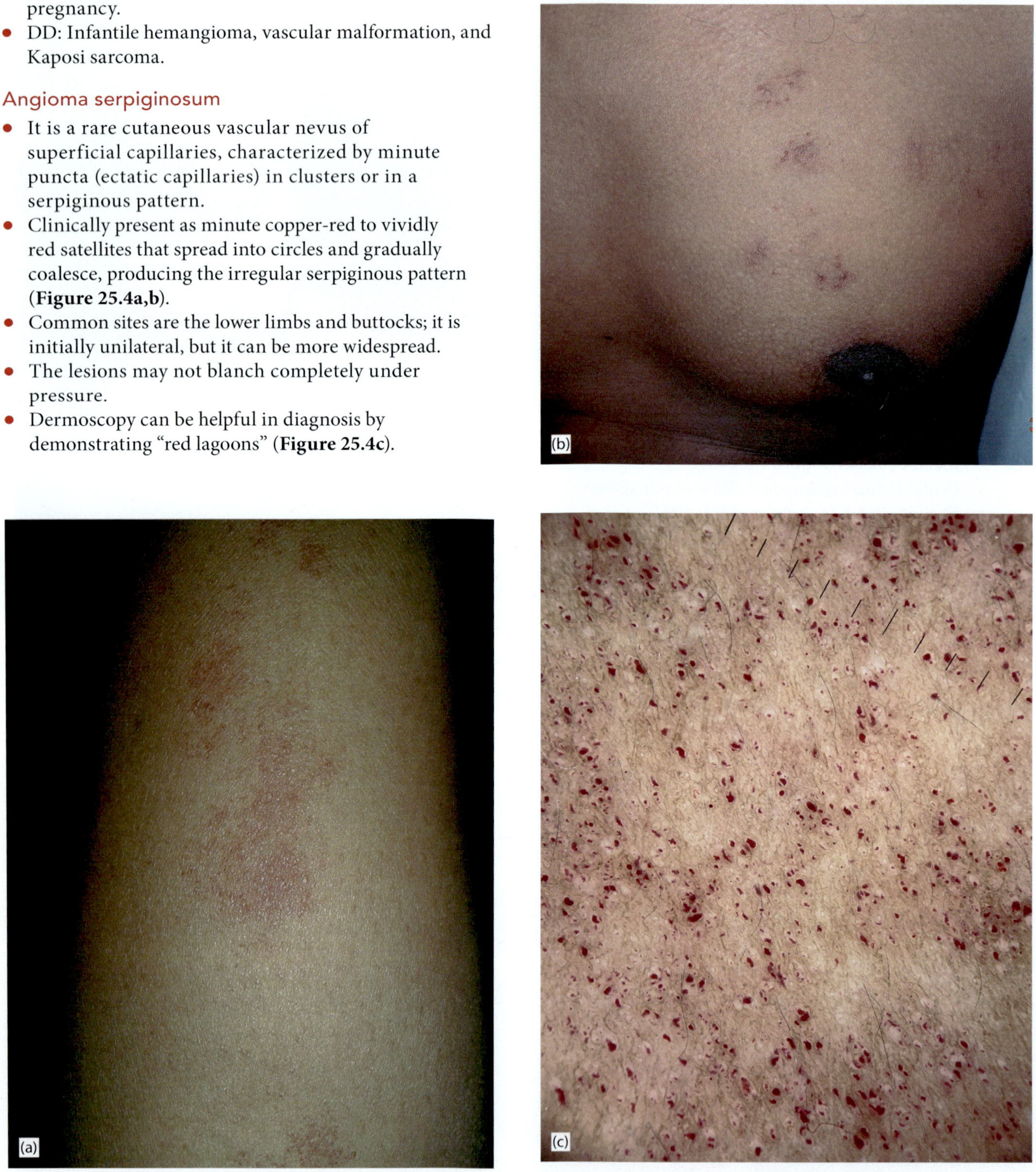


Figure 25.4 **(a)** Erythematous macules and patches in angioma serpiginosum. **(b)** Erythematous macules and papules in angioma serpiginosum. **(c)** Dermoscopy of angioma serpiginosum showing red lagoons. (b,c – Courtesy: Dr. Piyush Kumar, Katihar, India.)

## Cherry angioma (Campbell de Morgan spots)

- These are the most common cutaneous vascular proliferations.
- They present as tiny cherry-red blanchable macules or papules in middle or older age group (**Figure 25.5a**).
- The most common site is the trunk.
- They may be single, discrete or multiple, and widespread.
- They are composed of dilated venules and usually do not undergo spontaneous involution.
- DD: angiokeratoma, spider angioma (**Figure 25.5b**), pyogenic granuloma, amelanotic melanoma.

## Bacillary angiomatosis

- It is a vascular, proliferative form of *Bartonella* infection, caused by *B. henselae* and *B. quintana,* that occurs primarily in AIDS and immunocompromised patients.
- It is characterized by the development of solitary or multiple red, purple, or flesh-colored friable angiomatous papules, nodules or large, pedunculated, polypoid exophytic masses.
- Sometimes constitutional symptoms such as fever, chills, malaise, night sweats, anorexia, and weight loss are also associated with it.
- DD: Pyogenic granulomas, angiokeratoma, molluscum contagiosum, Kaposi sarcoma, deep fungal infections, verruga peruana.
- Oroya fever and verruga peruana represent two stages of infection with *Bartonella bacilliformis* and are endemic in Peru.
    - First stage (Oroya fever) – Characterized by sudden onset of pyrexia, accompanied by a rapidly progressive, hemolytic anemia, hepatosplenomegaly, and generalized lymphadenopathy, and a petechial or ecchymotic rash may develop.
    - Second stage (verruga peruana) – It may develop without previous Oroya fever or may follow it by weeks or months. The eruption is composed of erythematous papules, which appear in crops and often become nodular or pedunculated. They are most numerous on the face, neck, and limbs but may also involve mucous membranes. Characteristically they may be present in different stages of evolution in the same patient.

## Infantile hemangioma (IH)

- This is the most common benign vascular neoplasm of infancy, occurring in 1–3% of newborns. It usually appears during the first month of life and is characterized by rapid proliferation followed by slow involution.

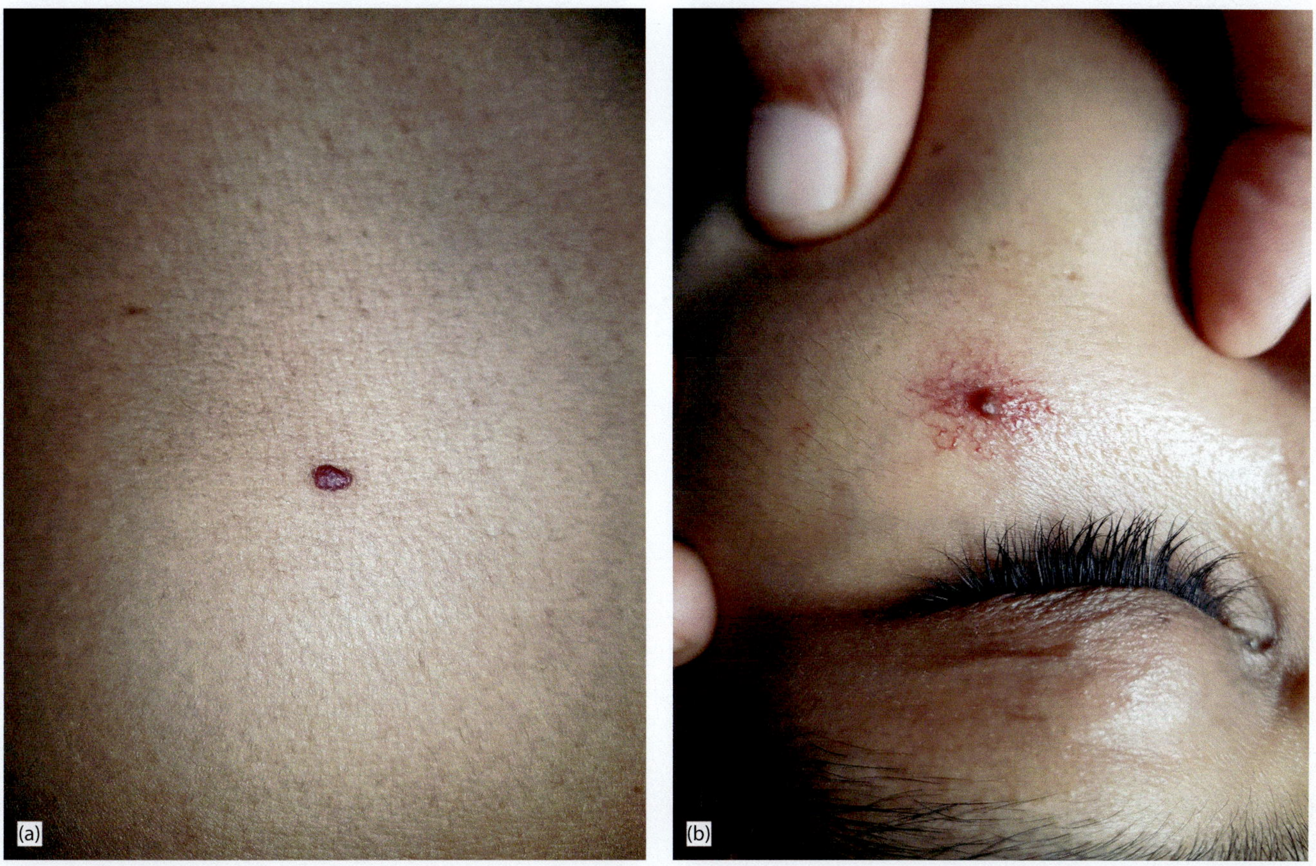


Figure 25.5 **(a)** Bright-red papule of cherry angioma on the chest. **(b)** Spider angioma with a central red papule with radiating vessels. (a,b – Courtesy: Dr. PC Das, Katihar, India.)

- The origin is from invading angioblasts differentiating towards placental phenotype or from embolized placental cells.
- Caused by unknown somatic mutation leading to increased endothelial expression of angiogenic growth factors such as VEGF, IGF, and bFGF.
- More than 50% of hemangiomas correspond to sites of embryological fusion lines and facial developmental metameres.
- Hemangiomas may appear as telangiectatic macules or blanched spots that may not be recognized at birth. Nodules develop by two to four weeks of age, marking the 6- to 12-month proliferative phase characteristic of hemangiomas (**Figure 25.6a,b**). A stationary phase predominates until 15 months of age. The involuting phase then begins, with the development of pale gray regions within the nodules and diminished firmness.
- Full regression occurs in 50% of patients by age five, in 70% by age seven and in 90% by age nine. Deep

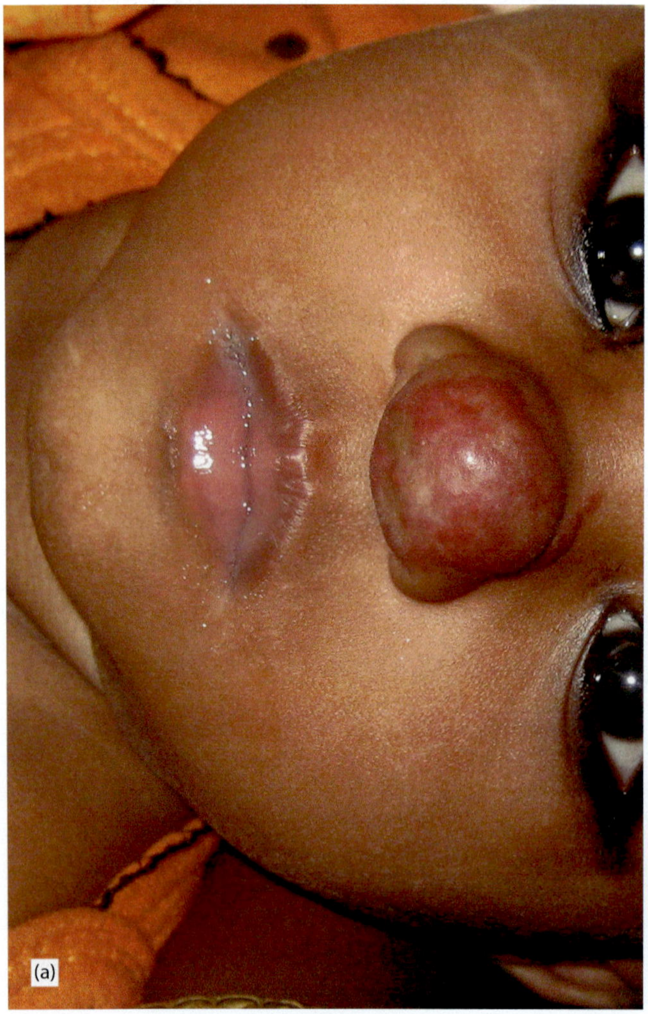

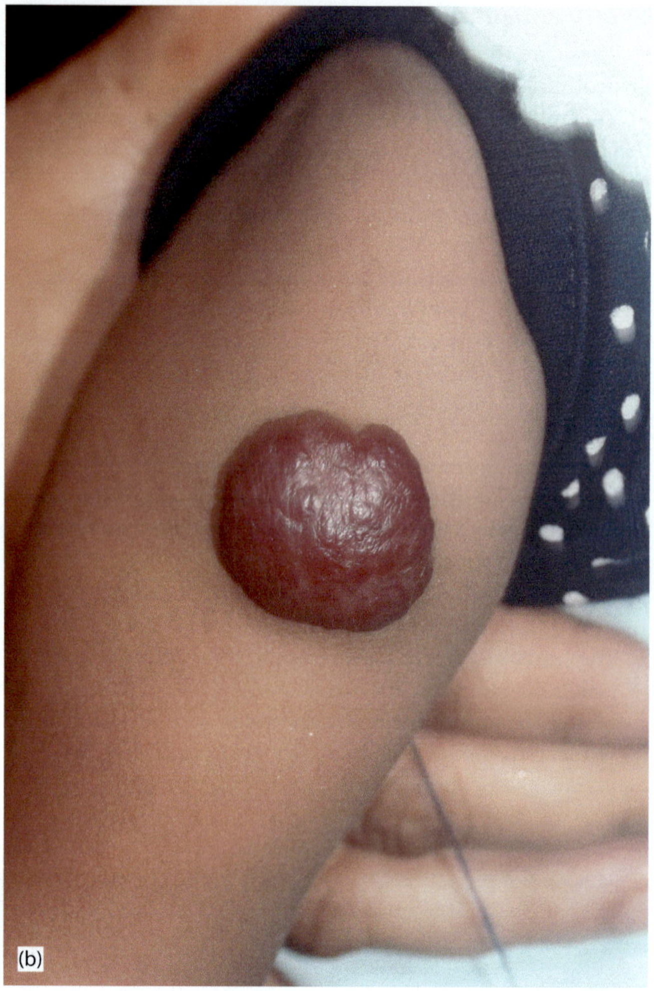

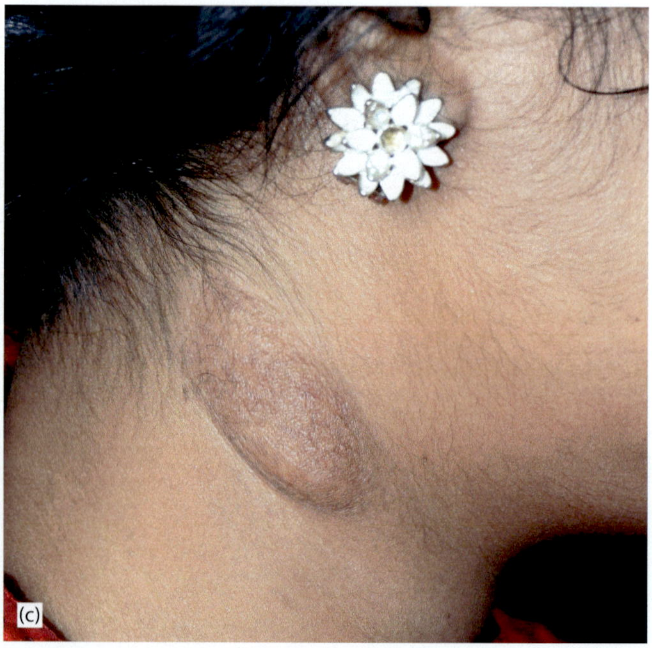

Figure 25.6 **(a)** Infantile hemangioma on the tip of nose. **(b)** A well-developed lesion of infantile hemangioma on the arm. **(c)** Healing of infantile hemangioma results in localized atrophy with wrinkled skin surface. (*Continued*)

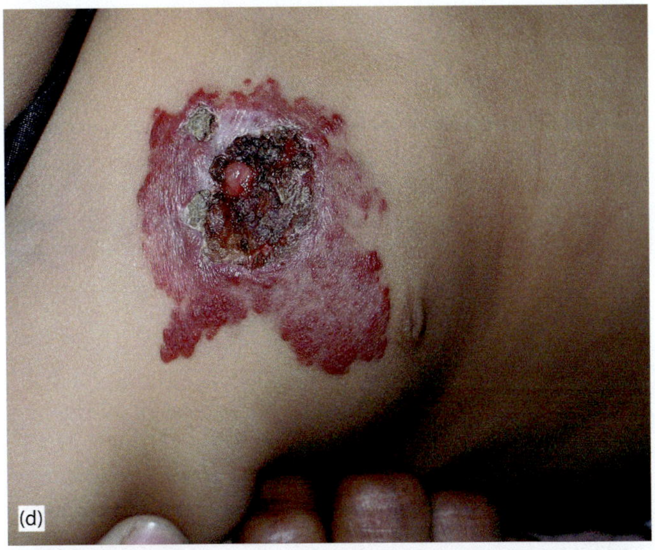


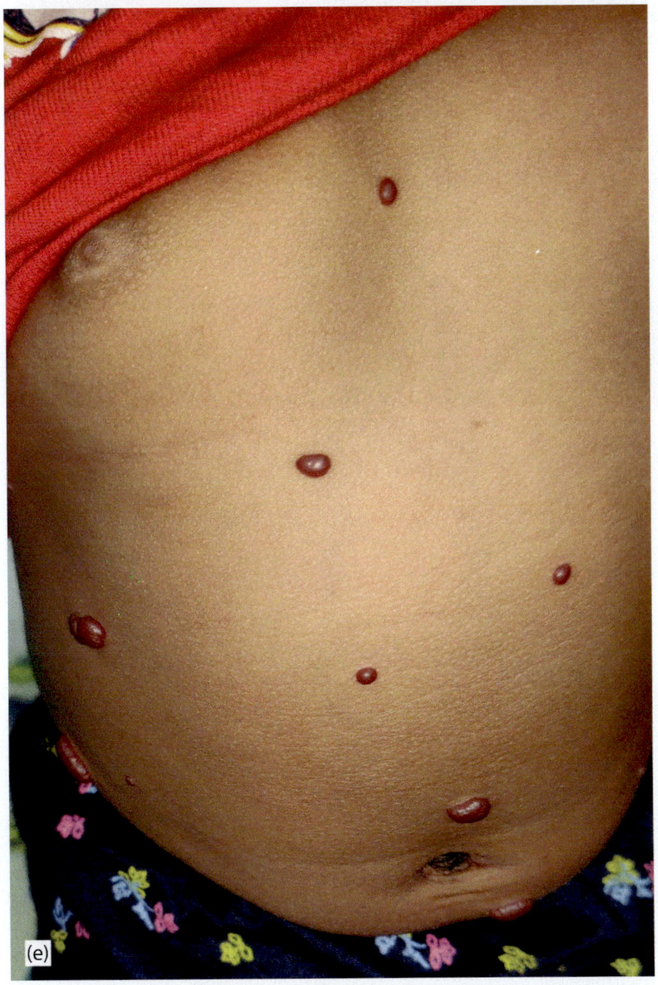


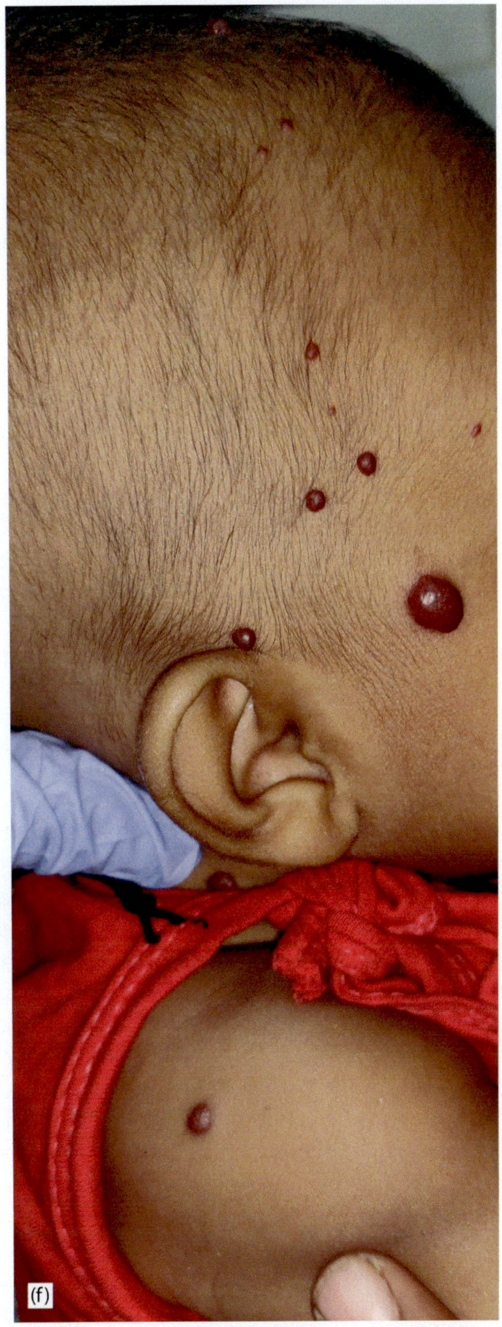


Figure 25.6 (*Continued*) **(d)** Rapidly proliferating lesion of infantile hemangioma may develop ulcerations. **(e)** Neonatal hemangiomatosis with multiple infantile hemangiomas on the abdomen. **(f)** Same child (Figure 25.6e) with facial lesions abdomen. (a–d – Courtesy: Dr. Piyush Kumar, Katihar, India; e,f – Courtesy: Dr. Soumyajit Roychoudhury, Berhampore, India.)

or mixed-type hemangiomas often show incomplete involution, with residual atrophic, wrinkled, telangiectatic, redundant skin (**Figure 25.6c**).

- Complications include ulcerations (**Figure 25.6d**), bleeding, heart failure, disfigurement, functional impairment (e.g., visual impairment), and airway obstruction.
- **Neonatal hemangiomatosis** is characterized by multiple (typically five or more) hemangiomas, affecting skin or mucosa (**Figure 25.6e,f**). Internal organs (liver, gastrointestinal tract, and brain) involvement may be seen (**Box 25.3**).
- Associated syndromes include PHACE/PHACES syndrome (posterior fossa brain malformations

## BOX 25.3: Neonatal hemangiomatosis

- Baby is born with multiple small hemangiomas that may number up to 100.
- Typically resembles infantile hemangioma, but size varies from 2 mm to 2 cm.
- Increases in size for the first few months, then starts involuting, and resolves by two to three years of age.
- More common in girls than boys.
- Multifocal/diffuse neonatal hemangiomatosis is a rare variant characterized by
  - Onset in the neonatal period
  - Lack of malignant transformation
  - Involvement of three or more organs
- The most common complications are congestive cardiac failure, hemorrhage, and multi-organ failure.
- The presence of heart failure and the involvement of five or more organs are associated with a higher mortality rate.
- The mortality of patients who received no treatment is quite high.

large segmental hemangiomas, arterial anomalies, cardiac anomalies and coarctation of the aorta, eye abnormalities and endocrine abnormalities, sternal cleft, supraumbilical raphe, or both), PELVIS syndrome (perineal hemangioma, external genitalia malformations, lipomyelomeningocele, vesicorenal abnormalities, imperforate anus, skin tag), SACRAL syndrome (spinal dysraphism, anogenital anomalies, cutaneous anomalies, renal and urologic anomalies, angioma of lumbosacral localization), and LUMBAR syndrome (lower body hemangioma, urogenital anomalies, ulceration, myelopathy, bony deformities, anorectal malformations, arterial anomalies, Renal anomalies).

- DD: Vascular malformations (**Table 25.4**), congenital hemangioma, pyogenic granuloma, tufted hemangioma.

Table 25.4 Vascular tumors and malformations

| Features | Infantile hemangioma | Vascular malformations |
|---|---|---|
| Sex predilection | Females more affected | No gender predilection |
| Onset | Congenital or acquired | Congenital |
| Growth | Grows in size | Increase in size in proportion to growth |
| Resolution | Spontaneous resolution may be seen | Do not involute |
| Consumption coagulopathy | Uncommon, seen in Kaposi hemangioendothelioma and tufted angioma | Common |
| Response to steroids | Yes | No |

### Congenital hemangioma

- Congenital hemangioma is different from IH, in being fully grown at birth, without having an accelerated/disproportionate postnatal growth and no gender preponderance.
- It is usually solitary, present on the head or limbs near a joint.
- It typically presents as a reddish, bluish, or purple plaque with telangiectasia and peripheral pallor, doughy in consistency and warm to touch.
- It has two forms – rapidly involuting congenital hemangiomas (RICH) and non-involuting congenital hemangiomas (NICH). RICH regresses rapidly, often by the first year of life with anetodermic skin atrophy. NICH has intrauterine growth, showing a plateau throughout life with no regression postnatally (**Figure 25.7**).
- Size may vary from a few to several centimeters.
- DD: Infantile hemangioma.

### Tufted angioma

- This is a rare tumor that occurs most commonly in prepubertal children.
- It is characterized by tender, red or purple indurated nodule or plaques with a size up to 20 cm. Lesions are

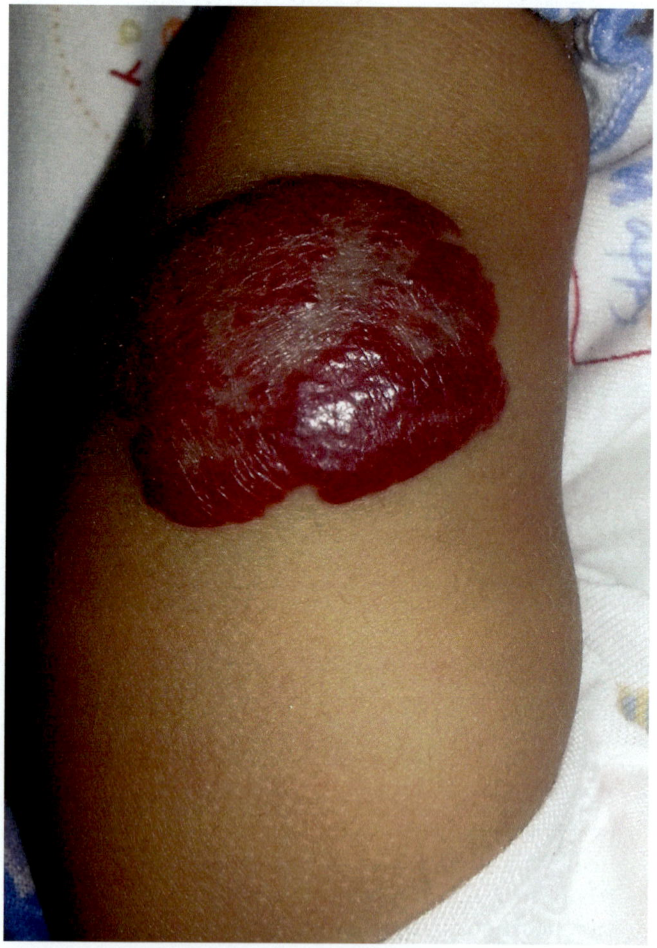

Figure 25.7 Non-involuting congenital hemangioma. (Courtesy: Dr. Hiral Shah, Baroda Medical College, Vadodara, India.)

most commonly seen on the upper thorax, neck, and shoulders (**Figure 25.8a**).
- They may have localized hypertrichosis or hyperhidrosis on their surface.
- Sometimes, lesions may assume annular configuration (**Figure 25.8b**) and may be multi-focal in origin.
- DD: Infantile hemangioma, Kaposiform hemangioendothelioma, venous malformation, glomuvenous malformation, subcutaneous fat necrosis of newborn.

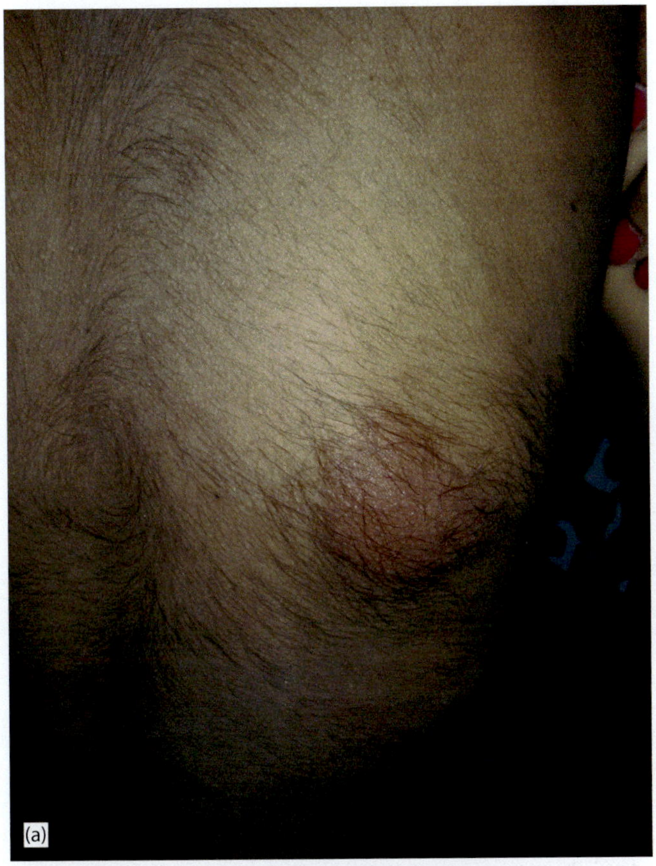


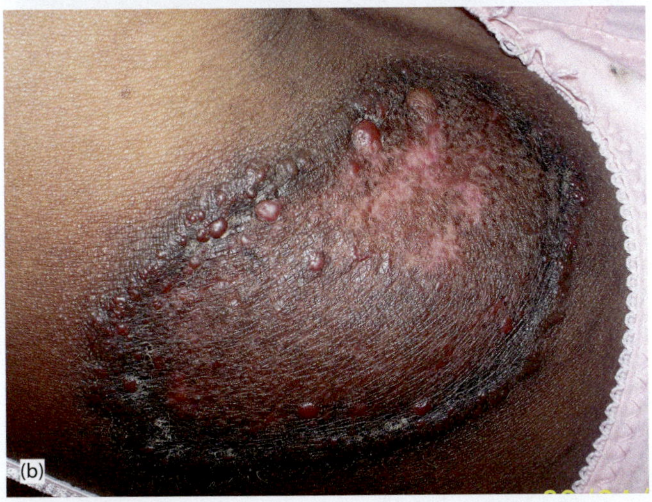


Figure 25.8 **(a)** Erythematous nodule of tufted angioma. **(b)** Annular tufted angioma on the trunk. The lesion expands at the periphery while the center heals with scarring. (b – Courtesy: Dr. Piyush Kumar, Katihar, India.)

## Hemangiopericytoma

- It rarely presents with cutaneous lesions.
- There are two types: infantile (congenital) and adult type.
- It typically presents as a lobulated mass deep in the subcutis, having red coloration, present anywhere on the body.
- It may resolve spontaneously, or excision may be needed.

## Reactive angioendotheliomatosis

- This is a rare and benign condition characterized by reactive intravascular proliferation of cells expressing endothelial cell markers.
- It presents with multiple erythematous and/or hemorrhagic macules, papules, and plaques on the trunk and limbs.
- Constitutional symptoms, such as fever with chills, malaise, weight loss, night sweats, arthralgia, and depression, are also present.
- It is associated with systemic diseases, including bacterial endocarditis, peripheral vascular atherosclerotic disease, cryoglobulinemia, liver and renal disease, antiphospholipid syndrome, amyloidosis, and sarcoidosis.
- DD: Acute cutaneous lupus erythematosus, sarcoidosis, Dabska tumor, bacillary angiomatosis, erythema nodosum, vasculitis.

## Kaposiform hemangioendothelioma

- This is a rare localized aggressive vascular proliferation of childhood that may either be retroperitoneal or cutaneous (superficial or deep).
- It usually manifests later than infantile hemangioma.
- It presents as a solitary vascular lesion that proliferates rapidly.
- Kasabach-Merritt phenomenon (KMP) is most commonly seen in this tumor (**Box 25.4**). Tufted angioma and hemangiopericytoma may also develop KMP.

### BOX 25.4: Kasabach-Merritt phenomenon (KMP)

- KMP is a potentially life-threatening consumption coagulopathy seen in certain rapidly proliferating vascular tumors.
- It is characterized by thrombocytopenia, microangiopathic hemolytic anemia, hypofibrinogenemia, and elevated fibrin split products.
- It is seen in Kaposiform hemangioendotheliomas, tufted angiomas, and sometimes other vascular tumors.
- With the onset of KMP, the lesion increases in size and becomes violaceous, ecchymotic, and indurated.
- Thrombocytopenia manifests as petechiae, painful bruising, and internal as well as external bleeding.

## Angiokeratoma

- This involves cutaneous hyperkeratotic vascular lesions that may be localized or diffuse.
- Localized forms are
  - Angiokeratoma circumscriptum
  - Angiokeratoma of Mibelli
  - Solitary papular angiokeratoma
  - Angiokeratoma of Fordyce
- The diffuse form is angiokeratoma corporis diffusum.
- Angiokeratoma circumscriptum
  - This is a rare condition, present from birth.
  - It appears as multiple aggregated bluish-black vascular papules forming a hyperkeratotic plaque, mostly on lower limbs, in a segmental pattern (**Figure 25.9a,b**).
  - Lesions do not remit with age.
  - With time, lesions become more warty but bleed after trauma.
  - It may be associated with soft tissue overgrowth – Klippel-Trenaunay Syndrome (KTS).
  - DD: Verrucous hemangioma (deeper vascular elements with capillary endothelial proliferation), microcystic lymphatic malformation (not hyperkeratotic), acral pseudolymphomatous angiokeratoma of children (more rare entity affecting the feet).
- Angiokeratoma of Mibelli
  - This appears late in childhood, between 10 and 15 years of age and is more common in girls than boys.

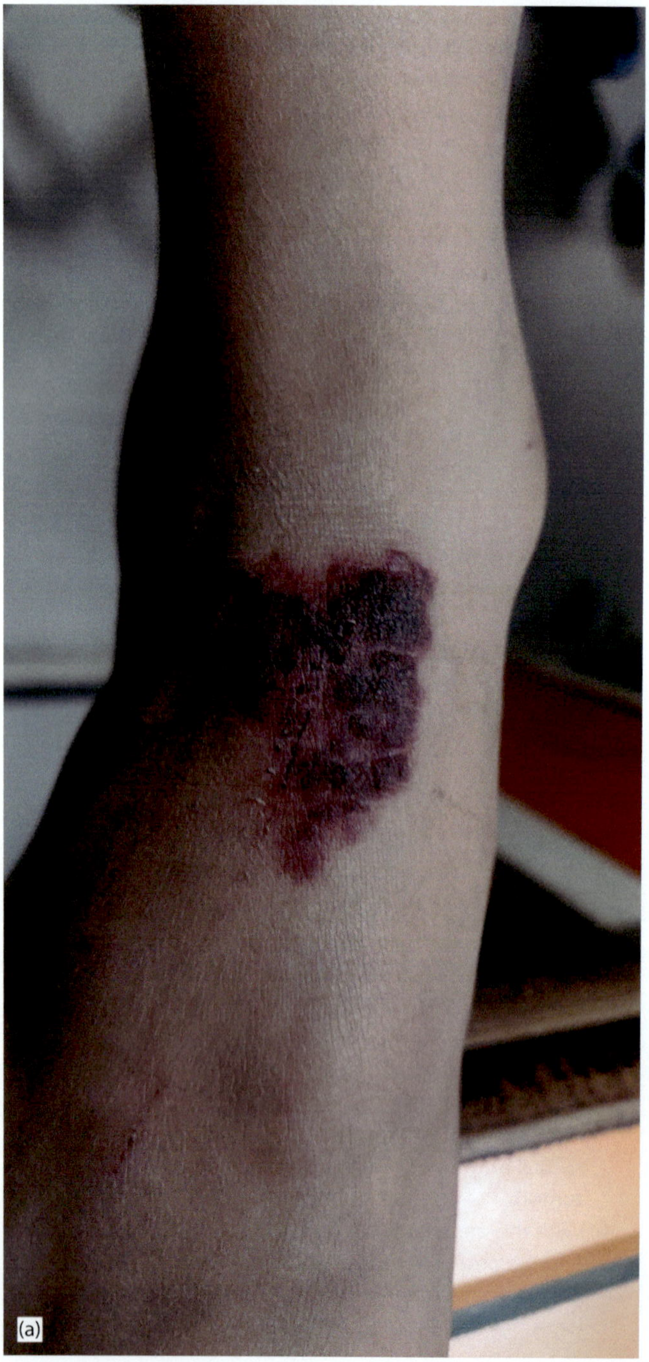


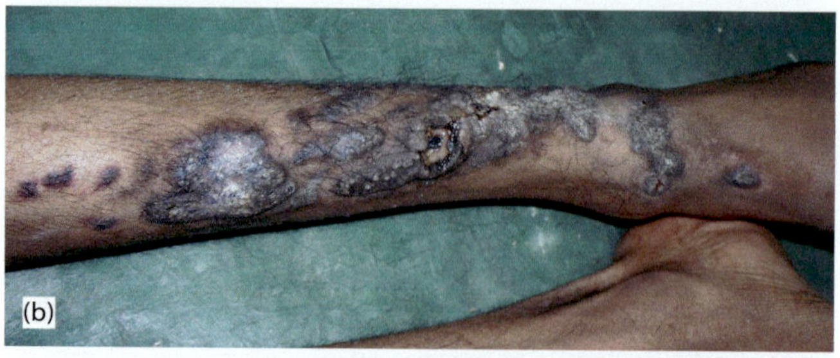


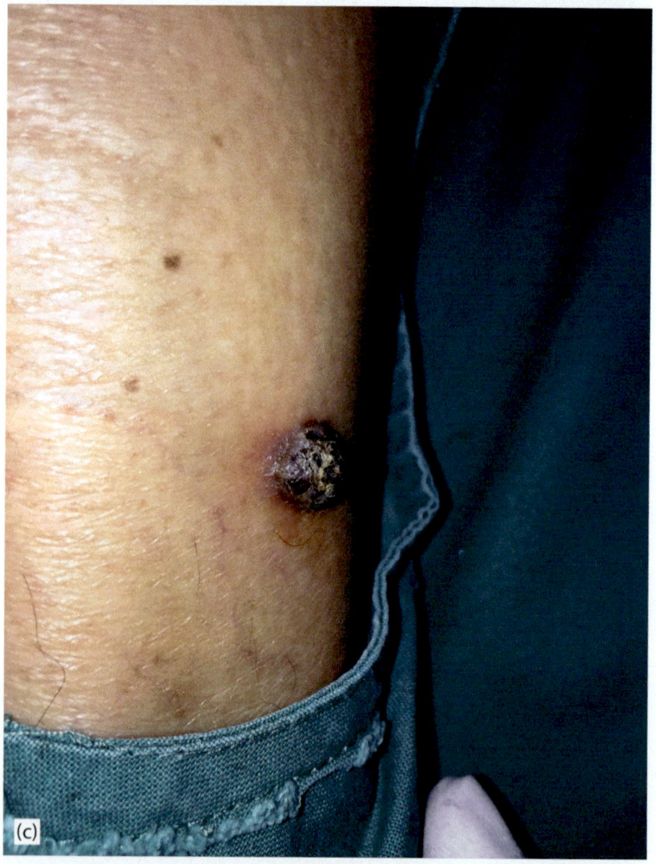


Figure 25.9 **(a)** Verrucous plaque on an erythematous background in angiokeratoma circumscriptum. **(b)** Red-blue plaques with hyperkeratotic surface and ulceration in angiokeratoma circumscriptum. **(c)** Solitary angiokeratoma presenting with erythematous lobulated nodule with verrucous surface. (*Continued*)

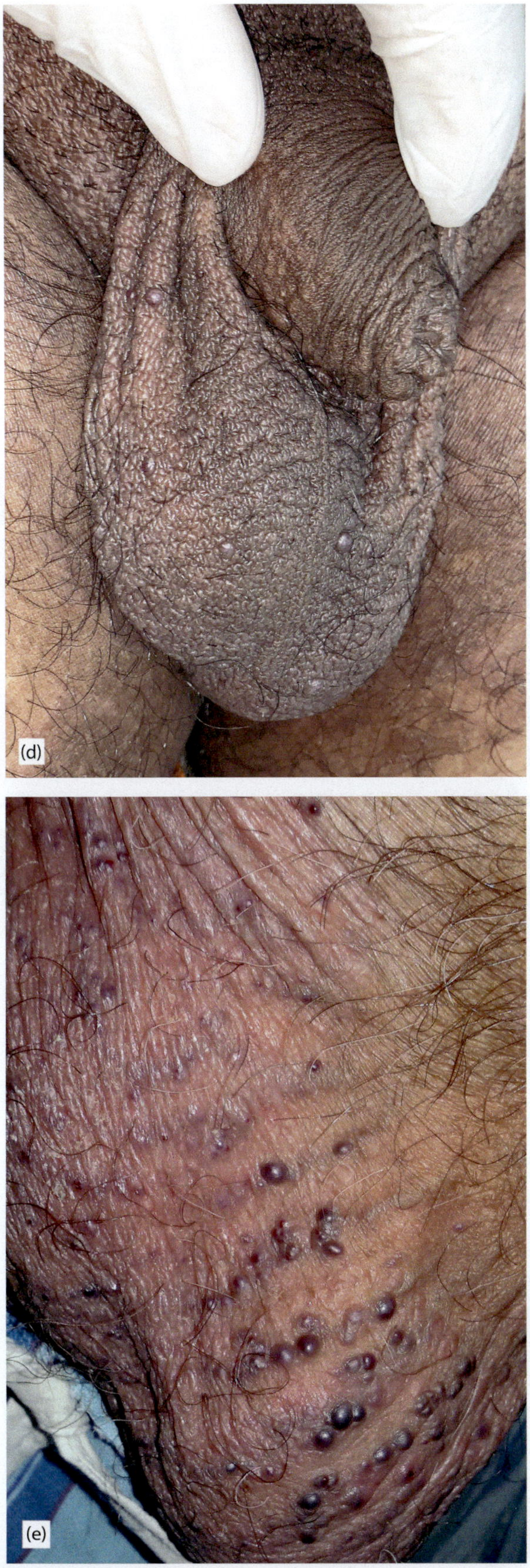

- Lesions are characterized by bright-red macules that slowly increase in size to become hyperkeratotic bluish papules and plaques.
- Usually there is a history of recurrent chilblains and acrocyanosis.
- Common sites are the dorsolateral aspects of fingers and toes.
- It is asymptomatic but may ulcerate.
- DD: Pyogenic granuloma, hemangioma, Kaposi sarcoma, melanocytic nevus verruca vulgaris.

- Solitary papular angiokeratoma
    - This is an acquired disorder arising after trauma. It is common in patients between 10 and 40 years of age.
    - A solitary lesion is indistinguishable from both angiokeratoma circumscriptum and angiokeratoma of Mibelli.
    - The lesion is characterized by a 2- to 10-mm dark-red to blue-black warty papule, usually solitary but sometimes multiple (**Figure 25.9c**).
    - It presents as a sudden enlargement and bleeding in a long-standing lesion on the legs.
    - DD: Viral wart, melanocytic nevi, and malignant melanoma.
- Angiokeratoma of the scrotum
    - Also called angiokeratoma of Fordyce, this is the most common angiokeratoma, generally seen in older age groups.
    - It is a degenerative disorder with local venous hypertension.
    - It clinically present as 1- to 4-mm bright-red vascular papules on the scrotum (**Figure 25.9d,e**). The lesions become bluish-black with aging. Discrete lesions are also present on the penis and groin area.
    - Itching, soreness, and bleeding are associated symptoms.
- Angiokeratoma corporis diffusum
    - It presents as clustered symmetrical erythematous papules on the "bathing trunk" area of the body (**Figure 25.9f**).
    - It is considered a cutaneous marker of lysosomal storage disorders, most notably Fabry disease. Other conditions associated with widespread

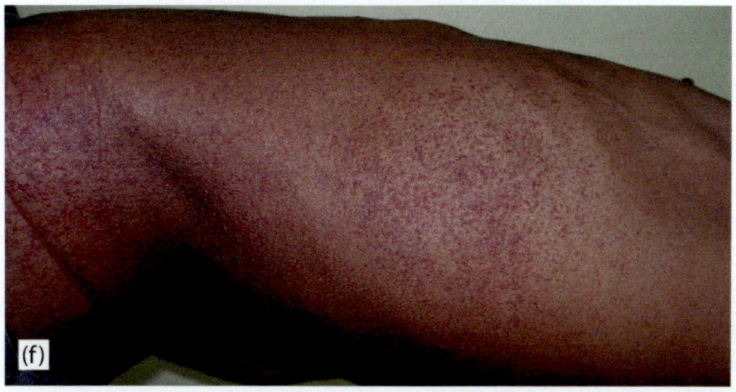

Figure 25.9 (*Continued*) **(d)** Angiokeratoma of Fordyce as erythematous papules. **(e)** Angiokeratoma of Fordyce. **(f)** Widespread erythematous papules in angiokeratoma corporis diffusum. (a – Courtesy: Dr. Anup Kumar Tiwary, Consultant Dermatologist, Yashoda Hospital and Research Center, Ghaziabad, India; b,d,f – Courtesy: Dr. Piyush Kumar, Katihar, India; c – Courtesy: Dr. Sushil S Savant, Mumbai, India.)

angiokeratomas are GM1 gangliosidosis, aspartylglucosaminuria, fucosidosis, β-mannosidosis, sialidosis, galactosialidosis, and Kanzaki disease.
- Rarely, it may be idiopathic without any associated systemic diseases.

## Verrucous hemangioma

- Congenital vascular lesions characterized by warty, deep-red papules and nodules (**Figure 25.10a,b**).

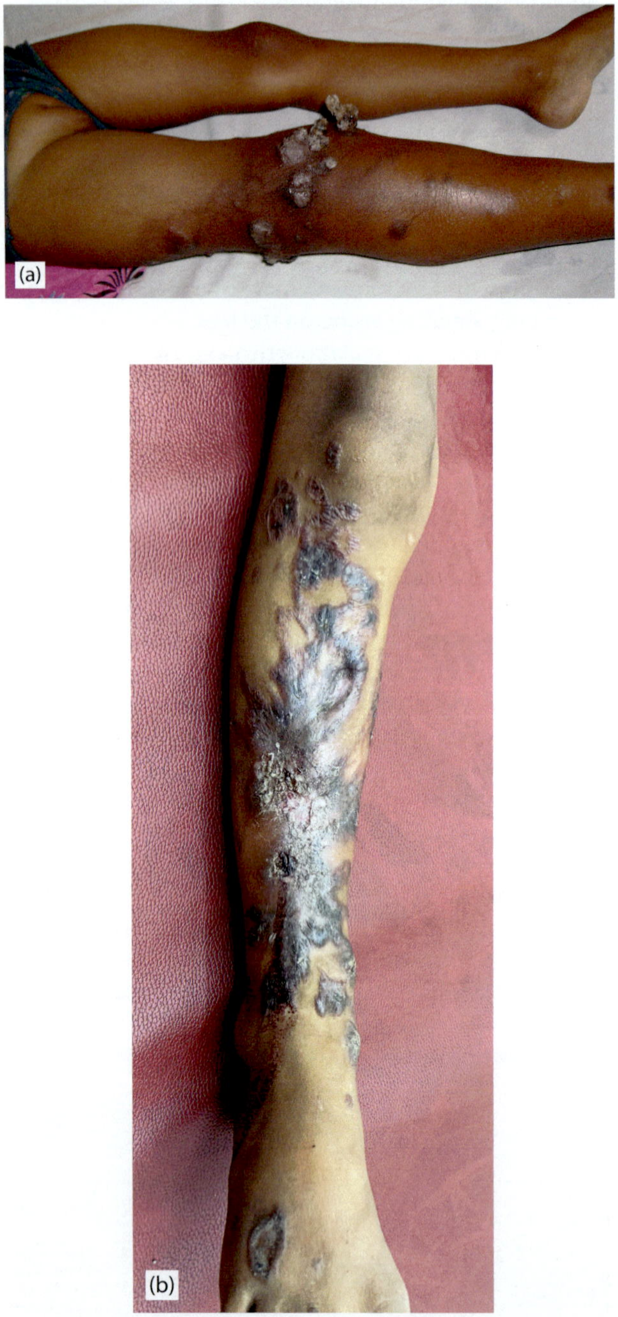

Figure 25.10 **(a)** Erythematous nodules with verrucous surface in verrucous hemangioma. Note soft-tissue overgrowth of the affected limb. **(b)** Verrucous hemangioma in a young child. (a – Courtesy: Dr. Hiral Shah, Baroda Medical College, Vadodara, India; b – Courtesy: Dr PC Das and Dr Piyush Kumar, Katihar, India.)

- Acral distribution is commonly present on lower limbs in a linear pattern. Oral mucosa is rarely involved.
- DD: Angiokeratoma.

## Microcystic lymphatic malformation (lymphangioma circumscriptum)

- Lymphatic malformation is the result of an embryologically disturbed lymphatic system.
- Lymphangioma circumscriptum is a microcystic lymphatic malformation.
- Characterized by clear or blood-stained vesicles in a plaque or area of diffuse swelling (**Figure 25.11a–d**).

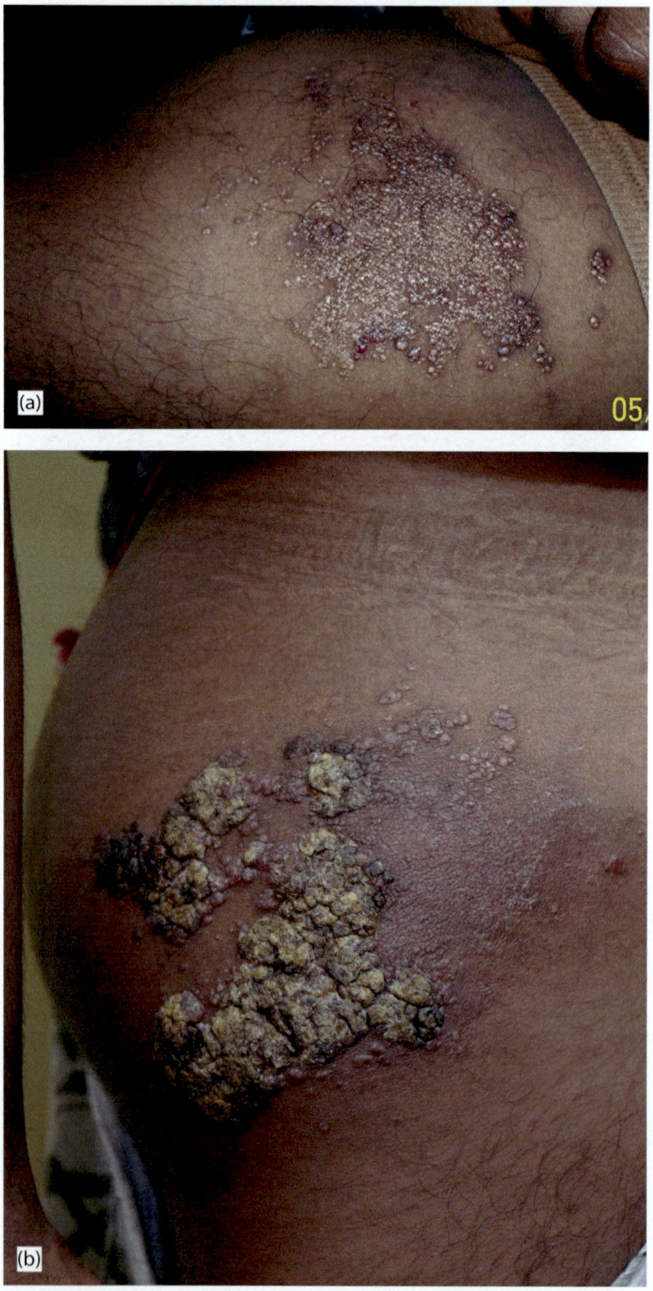

Figure 25.11 **(a)** Grouped clear-fluid–containing vesicles of lymphangioma circumscriptum. **(b)** Lymphangioma circumscriptum with crusted surface. (*Continued*)

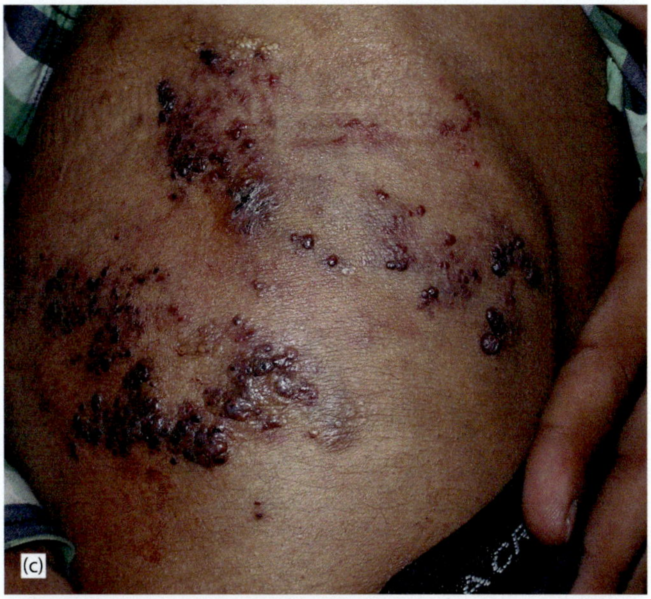


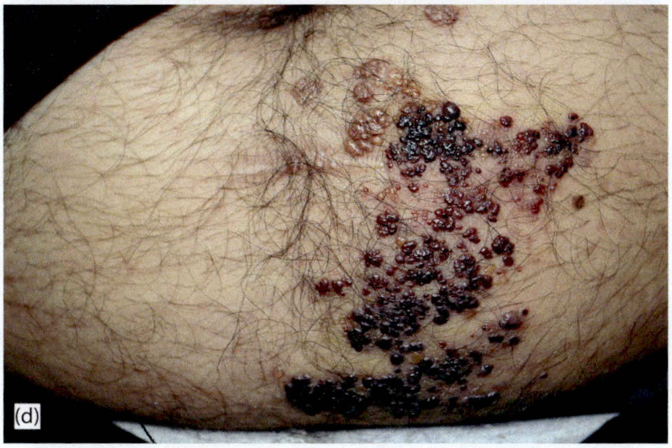


Figure 25.11 (*Continued*) **(c)** Bleeding into lymphangioma circumscriptum is common, and hemorrhagic vesicles are frequently noted. **(d)** Lymphangioma circumscriptum with lesions containing clear fluid and hemorrhagic fluid. (a–c – Courtesy: Dr. Piyush Kumar, Katihar, India; d – Courtesy: Dr. Shekhar Neema, Armed Forces Medical College, Pune, India.)

- Common sites are the mucosa and skin of the head and neck and sometimes the shoulders and waist area.
- Common complications are oozing with crusting and recurrent cellulitis.
- Extensive limb lymphatic malformation can lead to elephantiasis nostras verrucosa.
- DD: Venous malformation, deep hemangiomas, and infantile fibrosarcoma.

## Angiolymphoid hyperplasia with eosinophilia (epithelioid hemangioma/pseudopyogenic granuloma/histiocytoid hemangioma)

- This is a locally benign proliferation of blood vessels with distinctive large endothelial cells accompanied by a characteristic inflammatory infiltrate of eosinophils.
- It presents in young adults with a cluster of small, translucent, dome-shaped, smooth-surfaced nodules on the head and neck, particularly around the ear or the hairline. Rarely the hands, shoulders, breasts, penis, scrotum, and oral mucosa are involved (**Figure 25.12**).

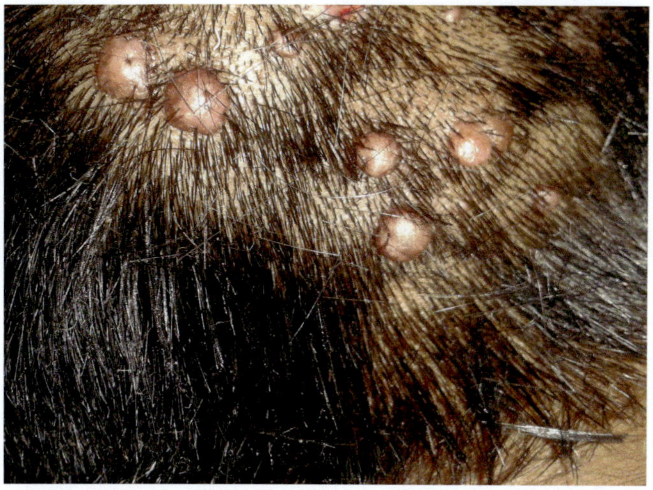

Figure 25.12 Smooth-surfaced, erythematous nodules of angiolymphoid hyperplasia with eosinophilia on the scalp.

- Extracutaneous sites include the orbit, peripheral arteries, the colon, the mandible, the lacrimal gland, the parotid gland, and throat.
- DD: Granuloma pyogenicum, sarcoidosis, lymphocytoma cutis, Kimura disease, Kaposi sarcoma, and granuloma faciale.

## Kimura disease

- It involves deeper tissues such as lymph nodes, salivary glands, and the subcutis.
- It has no initial overlying skin lesions and does not contain epithelioid endothelial cells.
- Peripheral blood eosinophilia is much more common in Kimura disease.
- It is strongly associated with nephrotic syndrome.

## Acroangiodermatitis of Mali (pseudo-Kaposi sarcoma)

- It is a hyperplasia of existing vasculature, as opposed to Kaposi sarcoma, in which the vascular proliferation is independent of the existing vessels.
- It is characterized by tiny purpuric macules that coalesce to form irregular plaques. The color of the lesions has varying shades of yellow (ochre) and brown from hemosiderin and other breakdown products (**Figure 25.13**). The epidermis may be normal or show mild eczematous changes, edema or ulceration.

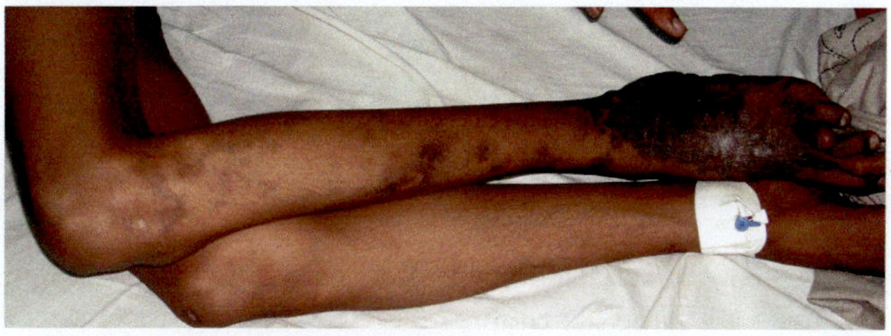

Figure 25.13 Brownish plaque of acroangiodermatitis of Mali in a patient with Klippel-Trenaunay syndrome.

- The lesions are commonly present on the lower legs and the dorsum of feet.
- It is associated with chronic venous insufficiency, vascular malformations (e.g., Klippel-Trenaunay syndrome, Stewart-Bluefarb syndrome, Prader-Labhart-Willi syndrome), protein-C deficiency, and symmetrical arteriovenous fistulae.
- It is also seen in amputees (especially in those with poorly fitting suction-type devices), in patients with paralyzed legs, in patients undergoing hemodialysis (from arteriovenous shunts distally), and in association with hepatitis C.

### Kaposi sarcoma (granuloma multiplex hemorrhagicum/idiopathic multiple pigmented sarcoma)

- This is a multifocal spindle cell tumor due to endothelial cell proliferation, predominantly involving the skin and other organs.
- There are four clinical types:
  1. Classic
  2. Endemic
  3. Iatrogenic
  4. HIV related
- Cutaneous lesions in Kaposi sarcoma are characterized by non-pruritic, brown, pink, red, or violaceous macules, papules, nodules, or plaque (**Figure 25.14a–c**).
- Common sites are the lower extremities, head and neck region, and mucous membrane (palate, gingiva, conjunctiva).
- It's size varies from several millimeters to several centimeters in diameter.
- Lesions may be discrete or confluent and typically appear in a linear, symmetrical distribution, following Langer lines.
- Tumor-associated lymphedema is typically manifested by lower extremity or facial involvement, due to obstruction of lymphatic channels.
- Visceral disease may occasionally precede cutaneous manifestations.
- DD: Bacillary angiomatosis, granuloma pyogenicum, hemangioma, capillaritis, dermatofibroma.

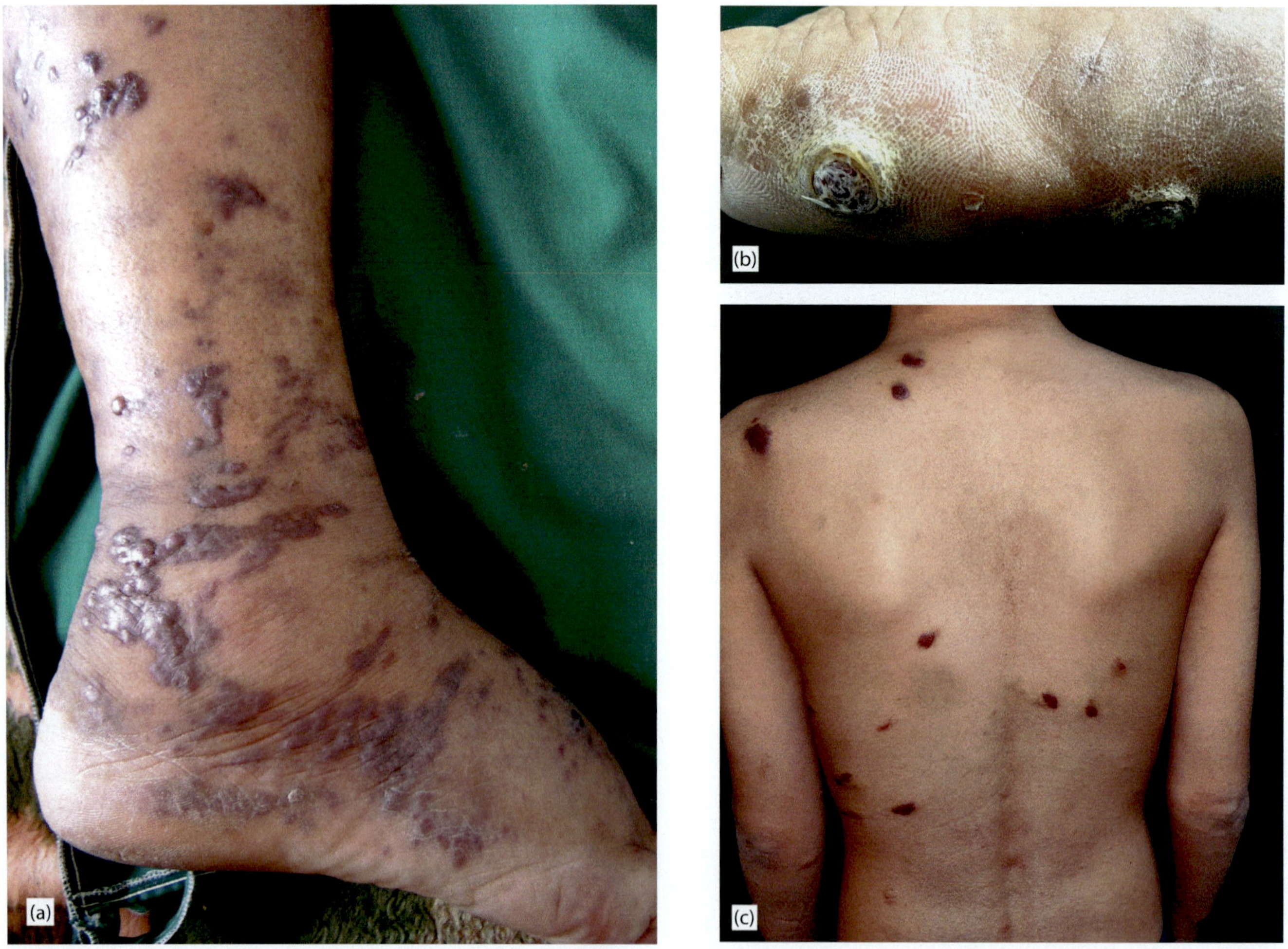


Figure 25.14 **(a)** Violaceous nodules and plaques on the leg in Kaposi sarcoma. **(b)** Violaceous nodules with scaly surface in Kaposi sarcoma. **(c)** Multiple violaceous plaques and nodules of Kaposi sarcoma on the back in an young adult with HIV infection. (a,b – Courtesy: Prof. Reza Yaghoobi, Dermatology, Ahvaz Jundishupor University of Medical Sciences, Iran; c – Courtesy: Dr. Shekhar Neema, Associate Professor, Dermatology, Armed Forces Medical College, Pune, India.)

### Targetoid hemosiderotic hemangioma (hobnail hemangioma)

- This is a benign and reactive vascular neoplasm characterized by dermal proliferation of small channels lined by endothelial cells with little cytoplasm and prominent dark nucleus (hobnail cells).
- Clinically it presents as a rapidly developing, asymptomatic, solitary, red, brown or violaceous papule and is surrounded by a pale brown halo (targetoid appearance) (**Figure 25.15a,b**).
- It is precipitated by trauma and seen on any body part.

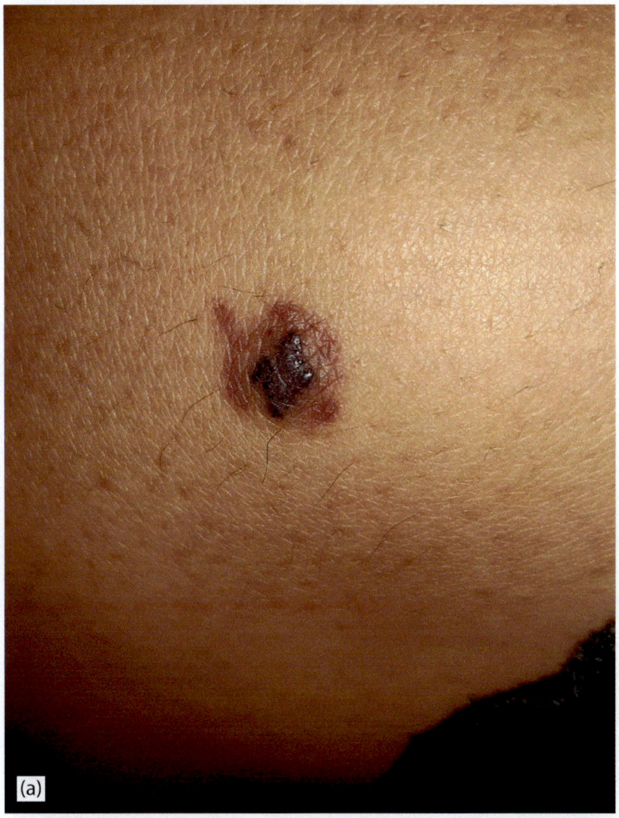

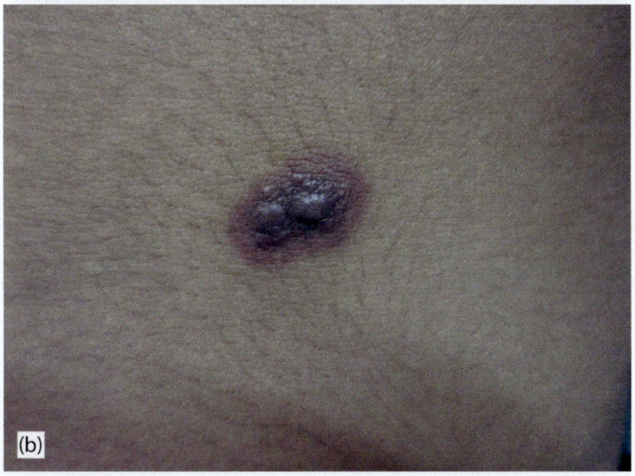

Figure 25.15 **(a)** Hobnail hemangioma with targetoid appearance. **(b)** Typical targetoid lesion of hobnail hemangioma. (a,b – Courtesy: Dr. Hiral Shah, Baroda Medical College, Vadodara, India.)

### Angiosarcoma (malignant hemangioendothelioma/hemangiosarcoma)

- This is a rare malignant neoplasm characterized by rapidly proliferating, extensively infiltrating anaplastic cells derived from blood vessels and lining irregular blood-filled spaces.
- Cutaneous angiosarcoma occurs in three settings:
  1. Idiopathic angiosarcoma of the face, scalp, and neck
  2. Angiosarcoma associated with chronic lymphoedema (Stewart-Treves syndrome)
  3. Post-irradiation angiosarcoma
- Clinically, it presents with an area of bruising initially (patient assumes it to be traumatic) followed by rapid development of dusky-blue or red nodules over it, and fresh, discrete nodules nearby.
- It is a multifocal malignant tumor in which dissemination occurs early.
- Angiosarcoma of face and scalp is more common in males and is invariably fatal.

### Dabska tumor (papillary intralymphatic angioendothelioma)

- It is a rare, low-grade angiosarcoma.
- It is commonly seen in infants and children.
- It presents as a slow-growing, asymptomatic, violaceous, pink or bluish-black plaque or nodule with a predilection for the limbs.

### Glomus tumor

- Glomus tumors are encapsulated proliferations of glomus cells (modified smooth-muscle cells that line endothelial walls of glomus bodies).
- The lesion is usually seen on distal extremities, with most cases involving subungual sites.
- Clinically, it presents as painful, blue-red papules or nodules. The pain is characteristically precipitated by cold temperature and pressure.

### Glomuvenous malformations (glomangioma)

- Glomuvenous malformations (GVMs) are venous malformations (VM) that are characterized by rows of glomus cells surrounding the distorted vascular channels of VM.
- GVMs present as blue-to-purple, partially compressible papules or nodules on extremities.
- The lesions may coalesce to form single or multiple plaques.
- Uncommonly, multiple lesions may be distributed randomly over the body.

### Venous lake

- This is a form of senile angioma.
- It presents as slow-growing, asymptomatic dark-blue compressible papules, caused by dilation of venules (**Figure 25.16**).

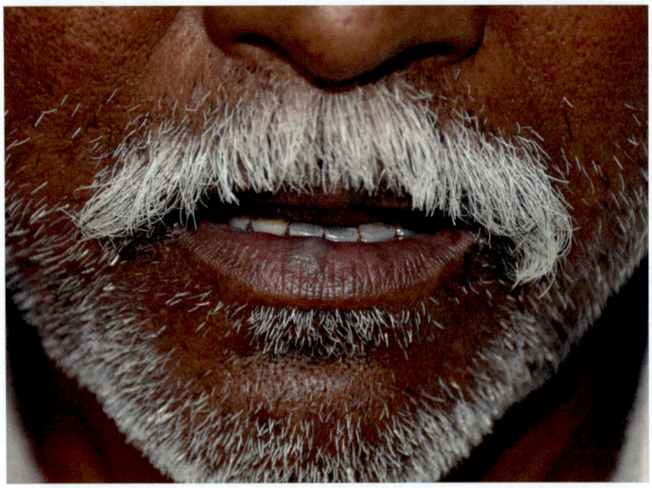

Figure 25.16 Bluish compressible swelling of venous lake on the lower lip. (Courtesy: Dr. Piyush Kumar, Katihar, India.)

- It is common on the face, lips, and ears of elderly patients.
- DD: Basal cell carcinoma, blue nevus, melanocytic nevus, lentigo, melanoma.

## Venous Malformation

- It is a slow-flow vascular malformation involving the veins.
- Clinically, it appears as bluish compressible nodules on the body due to the presence of ectatic veins between skin and bones (**Figure 25.17a,b**).

Table 25.5 Syndromes associated with venous malformations

| Syndrome | Cutaneous lesions | Other features |
|---|---|---|
| ***Maffucci's syndrome*** | • Multiple soft, bluish, tender nodules on hands and fingers since birth or in childhood.<br>• Involved hand/body part is grossly deformed. | Enchondroma (multiple ovoid, hard and radiolucent nodules) on the hands and fingers. |
| ***Blue rubber bleb nevus syndrome*** (Bean's syndrome) | • Blue/purple soft compressible "rubber blebs" nodules on the upper limbs and trunk.<br>• Mucosa may be affected. | Gastrointestinal tract involvement. |

- The most common symptoms are pain and burning sensations in involved muscles and bones due to thrombosis and hemarthrosis.
- Venous malformations tend to worsen later in childhood and adolescence.
- The most common site is the head and neck, leading to facial asymmetry.
- Life-threatening complications include intravascular coagulopathy, deep venous thrombosis, and pulmonary embolism.
- For associated syndromes see **Table 25.5**.

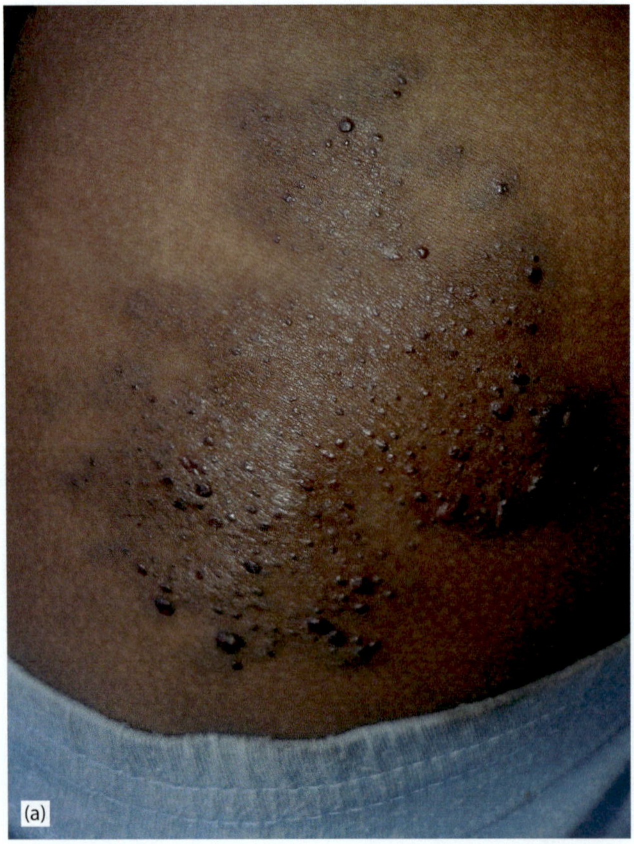


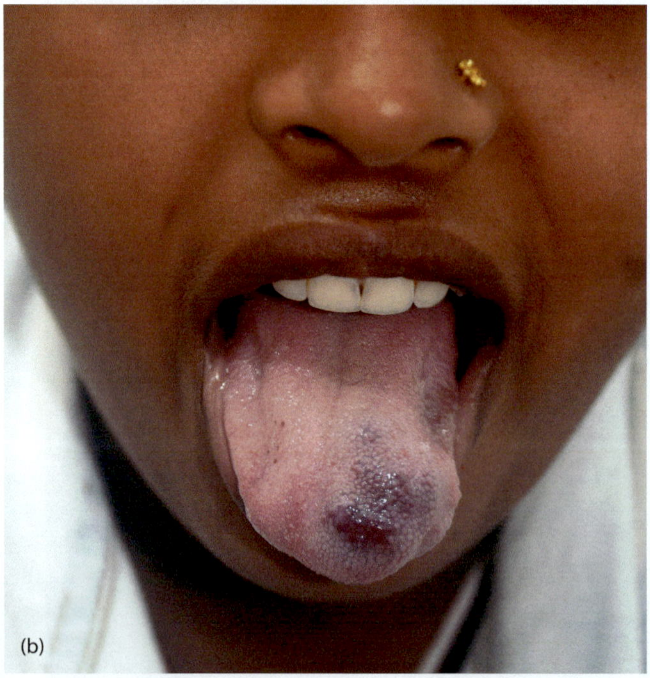


Figure 25.17 **(a)** Mixed capillary-venous malformation on the hip area. Venous malformation component is responsible for diffuse bluish discoloration and swelling of the skin. **(b)** Venous malformation affecting the tongue. (b – Courtesy: Dr Piyush Kumar, Katihar, India.)

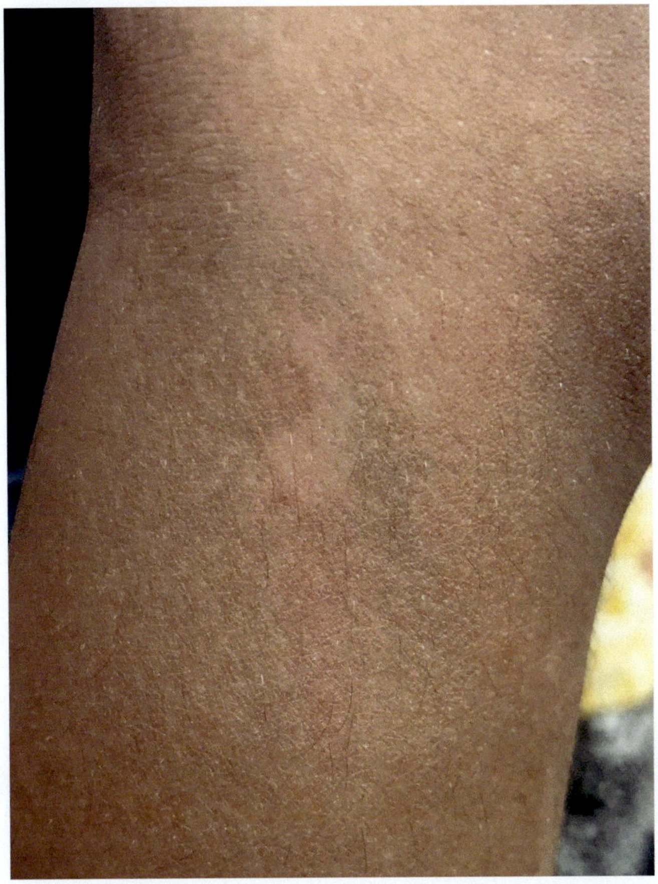

Figure 25.18 Nevus anemicus as hypopigmented patch with ill-defined margin.

### Arteriovenous malformation

- This is the most common high-flow vascular malformation.
- It is comprised of a communicating artery and vein, known as nidus.
- It develops during fetal life from primitive arteriovenous channels in the retiform plexus.
- Clinically, it presents as a red patch or nodule from birth, which are confused with capillary malformation or infantile hemangioma.
- Due to high vascularity, the affected body part becomes hyperplastic, showing asymmetry of the body.
- Parkes Weber syndrome is characterized by a congenital vascular stain with overgrowth of a limb. It is associated with a high-flow capillary arteriovenous malformation with multiple arteriovenous fistulae along the affected limb. The common differential diagnoses are Klippel-Trenaunay and Proteus syndrome, which lack true arteriovenous malformation.
- Wyburn–Mason syndrome is also known as Bonnet-Dechaume-Blanc syndrome. It is characterized by ipsilateral cerebral, retinal, and cutaneous arteriovenous malformation. The patient presents with headache, seizures, and visual disturbances.
- Cobb syndrome is a dermatomal pattern of arteriovenous malformation involving the skin and the segment of spinal cord in the same dermatome. It clinically presents as a segmental bright-red patch with spastic paralysis.

### Nevus anemicus

- This is a rare congenital localized vascular constriction.
- It presents at birth or in early childhood and persists unchanged throughout life.
- It is characterized by a pale or hypopigmented macule or patch with an ill-defined irregular border (**Figure 25.18**).
- It appears as a round or oval asymptomatic lesion, commonly on the trunk.
- If the lesion is examined by diascopy, the skin appears indistinguishable from the surrounding normal skin. Rubbing the skin causes reactive hyperemia in the adjacent skin but no change within the lesion itself. Both these features differentiate it from nevus depigmentosus.
- DD: Nevus depigmentosus, early vitiligo, pityriasis versicolor, ash-leaf macules, post inflammatory hypopigmentation.

## REFERENCES


1. Jahnke MN. Vascular lesions. Pediatr Ann 2016 Aug 1;45(8):e299–305.
2. Elluru RG. Cutaneous vascular lesions. Facial Plast Surg Clin North Am 2013;21(1):111–126.
3. Nosher JL, Murillo PG, Liszewski M, Gendel V, Gribbin CE. Vascular anomalies: A pictorial review of nomenclature, diagnosis and treatment. World J Radiol 2014;6(9):677–692.
4. Goss JA, Greene AK. Congenital vascular tumors. Otolaryngol Clin North Am 2018;51(1):89–97.
5. Levin LE, Lauren CT. Multifocal vascular lesions. Semin Cutan Med Surg 2016;35(3):153–160.
6. Nozaki T, Nosaka S, Miyazaki O, Makidono A, Yamamoto A, Niwa T, Tsutsumi Y, Aida N, Masaki H, Saida Y. Syndromes associated with vascular tumors and malformations: A pictorial review. Radiographics 2013;33(1):175–195.
7. Hagen SL, Hook KP. Overgrowth syndromes with vascular malformations. Semin Cutan Med Surg 2016;35(3):161–169.
8. Garzon MC, Huang JT, Enjolras O, Frieden IJ. Vascular malformations: Part I. J Am Acad Dermatol 2007 Mar;56(3):353–370.
9. Garzon MC, Huang JT, Enjolras O, Frieden IJ. Vascular malformations. Part II: Associated syndromes. J Am Acad Dermatol 2007;56(4):541–564.

# E48

# Vasculitis

SUNIL KUMAR GUPTA

## ABSTRACT

Vasculitis can be a challenging diagnosis for physicians, and recognition of cutaneous lesions helps physicians in assessing the caliber of vessels involved, which in turn provides some clue to the etiological diagnosis of vasculitis. This chapter discusses a clinical approach to the diagnosis of vasculitis.

The text of this chapter is available online at https://routledgetextbooks.com/textbooks/9781032399669/



DOI: 10.1201/9781351054225-78

# E49

# Neonatal dermatology

MANJUNATH M SHENOY, AMINA ASFIYA MI, GHALIYAH AZIZ KUTTY

## ABSTRACT

Neonates often exhibit a unique spectrum of dermatoses, and many dermatoses (e.g., birthmarks, developmental defects, cutaneous manifestations of various genetic diseases and transient physiological conditions) are particularly common in neonates. Additionally, various dermatoses may express themselves differently in neonates. Hence, neonatal dermatoses require a special attention as the dermatoses can range from benign birthmarks or physiological conditions to worrisome manifestations of a serious condition. Also, one should keep in mind that diagnosis of neonatal dermatoses rests on clinical examination and maternal (and obstetric) history. This chapter discusses the clinical approach to the diagnosis of various neonatal dermatoses.

The text of this chapter is available online at https://routledgetextbooks.com/textbooks/9781032399669/

DOI: 10.1201/9781351054225-79

# E50

# Geriatric dermatoses

RAJESH KUMAR MANDAL

## ABSTRACT

Skin diseases in old age are sometimes challenging regarding diagnosis as they may not present morphologically similar to their counterparts in young age. In this chapter the author has tried to classify the different common dermatological diseases according to their morphology, and emphasis is places on their morphological features, close differentials, and important differentiating points among them. This may help students and clinicians as a quick reference tool in their busy dermatology out-patient department.

The text of this chapter is available online at https://routledgetextbooks.com/textbooks/9781032399669/



DOI: 10.1201/9781351054225-80

E51

# Dermatoses of pregnancy

SWETALINA PRADHAN, GAURAV DASH

## ABSTRACT

The complex endocrinological, immunological, metabolic, and vascular changes associated with pregnancy result in characteristic skin, mucosal, hair, and nail changes. Some of these changes are common and of purely cosmetic concern and, hence, do not require any treatment. Such changes are called physiological changes. There are certain pregnancy specific disorders that are associated with maternal and/or fetal morbidity. Recognition of such pregnancy specific dermatoses can help physicians in identifying high-risk cases.

The text of this chapter is available online at https://routledgetextbooks.com/textbooks/9781032399669/

DOI: 10.1201/9781351054225-81

# 26

# Cutaneous adverse drug reactions

ABANTI SAHA, AMRITA SIL, NILAY KANTI DAS

## INTRODUCTION

Cutaneous adverse drug reactions (CADRs) may be defined as "unwanted reactions that are not characteristic of the desired pharmacodynamic effects and predict hazard for future administration of a particular drug." Some of the common causative drugs include non-steroidal anti-inflammatory drugs (NSAIDs), sulphonamides, fluoroquinolones, imidazoles, antiepileptics and allopurinol. Although the prognosis is good in most cases, 2% of CADRs are severe and can be lethal. Severe cutaneous adverse reactions (SCARs) comprise **D**rug **R**eaction with **E**osinophilia and **S**ystemic **S**ymptoms (DRESS), Stevens-Johnson syndrome/toxic epidermal necrolysis (TEN) and **A**cute **G**eneralized **E**xanthematous **P**ustulosis (AGEP). Pathologically, almost 80% are non-immunological (predictable and dose dependent) while the rest are immunological/hypersensitivity reactions. Clinically they can mimic any inflammatory disorder – "a great mimicker." Thus CADRs should be considered as a differential for any skin eruption of acute onset and causality association of a particular drug is assessed by the Naranjo Probability Scale and World Health Organization–Uppsala Monitoring Centre (WHO–UMC) Probability Scale (not discussed here) among others. This chapter discusses the clinical approach to various CADRs based on clinical presentation (**Table 26.1**).[1–8] The salient clinical features of these entities are discussed below, and detailed discussion of these CADRs is beyond the scope of this chapter. History of chemotherapy necessitates consideration of a separate set of CADRs unique to chemotherapy (**Table 26.2**), though common CADRs too can be observed in such patients.[9–11] Another subset of the population that requires specific consideration is persons on highly active antiretroviral therapy, but these are not covered in this chapter.

### Drug-induced phototoxic reaction

- Drug-induced photosensitivity may be of two types: phototoxic and photoallergic reactions.
- UV-A (320–400 nm) are more likely to cause drug-induced photosensitivity reactions, although occasionally UV-B (290–320 nm) can also be responsible for such effects.
- Phototoxic reaction clinically mimics sunburn and presents as painful erythematous, edematous, and sometimes scaly lesions on sun-exposed areas. In severe cases, vesicles and bullae may develop (**Figure 26.1a–d**).
- DD: Sunburn, photoallergic reaction (**Table 26.3**).
- Drugs causing phototoxic reactions are tetracyclines, fluoroquinolones, sulfonamides, ibuprofen, naproxen, furosemide, amiodarone, diltiazem, quinidine, etc.
- Drugs causing only photoallergic reactions are few in number, namely celecoxib, diaminodiphenyl sulfone (dapsone), and oral contraceptive pills. Among chemotherapeutic agents, flutamide (an antiandrogen) and tegafur may cause photoallergic reactions.
- Ketoprofen, hydrochlorothiazide, phenothiazines, itraconazole, and 5-FU cause both types of photosensitizing reactions.

### Fixed drug eruption

- Common causative drugs include fluoroquinolones and nitroimidazole fixed-dose combination or alone, non-steroidal anti-inflammatory drugs (NSAIDS), paracetamol, naproxen, sulphonamides, trimethoprim, antifungals, phenolphthalein, anticonvulsants, antibiotics, hydroxyzine, etc.
- Clinically, it presents as solitary or multiple, well-circumscribed, erythematous, bright-red or dusky-red itchy macules that evolve into an edematous plaque and finally resolve after few days to weeks, leaving residual grayish pigmentation. Bullous-type lesions may also appear (**Figure 26.2a–f**).
- Lesions may occur anywhere on the body. Oral mucosa and genitalia are commonly affected.



DOI: 10.1201/9781351054225-82

Table 26.1 Clinical approach to cutaneous adverse drug reactions.

| Morphology | Feature | Diseases |
|---|---|---|
| Erythema | Localized | • Sun-exposed area – phototoxic reaction<br>• Random distribution – fixed drug eruption (FDE) |
| | Generalized | • Flexures – symmetrical drug-related intertriginous and flexural exanthema (SDRIFE)<br>• With papules – morbilliform drug rash, drug rash with eosinophilia and systemic symptoms (DRESS)<br>• With scales – drug-induced erythroderma<br>• Without scales – early Stevens-Johnson syndrome/toxic epidermal necrolysis |
| Pigmentary changes | | Drug-induced hyperpigmentation<br>Drug-induced hypopigmentation |
| Papules | | Acneiform eruptions |
| Eczematous lesions | | Photoallergic drug reaction |
| Plaque | Non-scaly | Neutrophilic eccrine hidradenitis, pseudolympoma |
| | Scaly | Psoriasiform drug reaction<br>Lichenoid drug reaction<br>Pityriasis rosea<br>Drug-induced lupus |
| Vesicobullous lesions | With (variable) systemic features | • Target/targetoid lesions – erythema multiforme, Stevens-Johnson syndrome<br>• Sheets of epidermal necrosis – toxic epidermal necrolysis<br>• Palpable purpura – drug-induced vasculitis |
| | With minimal/absent systemic features | • With photosensitivity – phototoxic drug reaction, pseudoporphyria<br>• Without photosensitivity – bullous FDE, drug-induced pemphigus, drug-induced pemphigoid, linear IgA dermatosis |
| Pustules | | Acute generalized exanthematous pustulosis |
| Nodules | | Erythema nodosum |
| Scaling | | Drug-induced xerosis |
| Palpable purpura | | Drug-induced vasculitis |
| Urticaria lesions | | Drug-induced urticaria |
| Without skin lesions | | Drug-induced angioedema, drug-induced lupus |

Table 26.2 Cutaneous adverse reactions due to chemotherapeutic agents

| Morphology/ presentation | Feature | Diseases/chemotherapeutic agents |
|---|---|---|
| Pigmentation | Diffuse | • Fluorouracil, busulfan, methotrexate, procarbazine |
| | Flexural | • Bleomycin, cyclophosphamide, busulfan, and doxorubicin |
| | Sun-exposed area | • Fluorouracil, daunorubicin |
| | Trauma/pressure-prone areas | • Bleomycin, hydroxyurea, cisplatin |
| | Patterned | • Serpentine supravenous – fluorouracil, vincristine, docetaxel, CHOP regimen<br>• Linear (flagellate) – bleomycin<br>• Reticulate – paclitaxel, cytarabine, fluorouracil<br>• Annular/polycyclic – daunorubicin (scalp pigmentation) |
| | Local | • Site of application – topical fluorouracil, topical mechlorethamine<br>• Site of adhesives – docetaxel |
| | Mucosal | • Busulfan, cyclophosphamide (gingival, may be permanent), tegafur, doxorubicin, cisplatin, fluorouracil |

*(Continued)*

Table 26.2 Cutaneous adverse reactions due to chemotherapeutic agents (*Continued*)

| Morphology/ presentation | Feature | Diseases/chemotherapeutic agents |
|---|---|---|
| Erythematous patches | Localized | • Acral – hand-foot syndrome (acral erythema)<br>• Photoexposed area – phototoxic reaction |
| | Generalized | • Diffuse erythema – hydroxyurea, busulfan, and cladribine<br>• Erythroderma – cisplatin, methotrexate<br>• Stevens-Johnson syndrome/toxic epidermal necrolysis |
| Papules | Maculopapular eruptions | • Bortezomib, lenalidomide, cladribine, fludarabine, gemcitabine, pemetrexed, and cytarabine<br>• Drug reaction with eosinophilia and systemic symptoms |
| | Papulopustules | • Acneiform eruptions/chemotherapy-induced papulopustular eruptions – epidermal growth factor receptor (EGFR) inhibitors, tyrosine kinase inhibitors<br>• PRIDE complex |
| Plaques | Non-scaly | • Neutrophilic eccrine hidradenitis |
| | Scaly | • Drug-induced subacute cutaneous lupus erythematosus |
| | Inflamed plaques | • Inflammation of seborrheic keratosis |
| Vesicobullous lesions | Photo-exposed area | • Phototoxic reaction |
| | Acral area | • Hand-foot syndrome (acral erythema) |
| | Generalized | • Erythema multiforme<br>• Stevens-Johnson syndrome/toxic epidermal necrolysis |
| Eczematous lesions | Sun-exposed area | • Photoallergic reactions, photo recall |
| | Site of previous radiation | • Radiation recall dermatitis |
| Scaling/xerosis | | • Cetuximab |
| Scleroderma like changes | | • Bleomycin, gemcitabine, and docetaxel |

- On repeated exposure to a particular drug, lesions reappear on the same site and new lesions appear at different areas.
- Variants are generalized, non-pigmenting, with linear distribution.
- DD: Active lesions (erythema multiforme, irritant contact dermatitis), healed lesions (lichen planus pigmentosus).

## Symmetrical drug-related intertriginous and flexural exanthema (SDRIFE)

- This is characterized by erythema over the buttocks, thighs, groin, and flexural regions.
- It is most commonly associated with the use of beta-lactam antibiotics
- Diagnostic criteria are as follows:
  - Exposure to the systemic drug at first or repeated dose

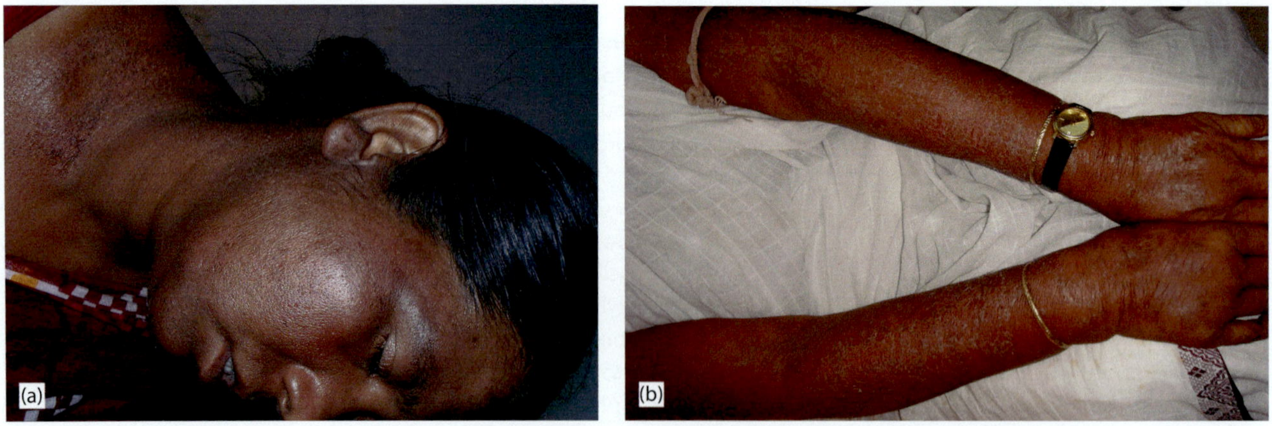

Figure 26.1 **(a)** Doxycycline-induced phototoxic reaction presenting as erythema and xerosis. **(b)** Phototoxic reaction causing erythema and dryness of extensor forearms. (*Continued*)

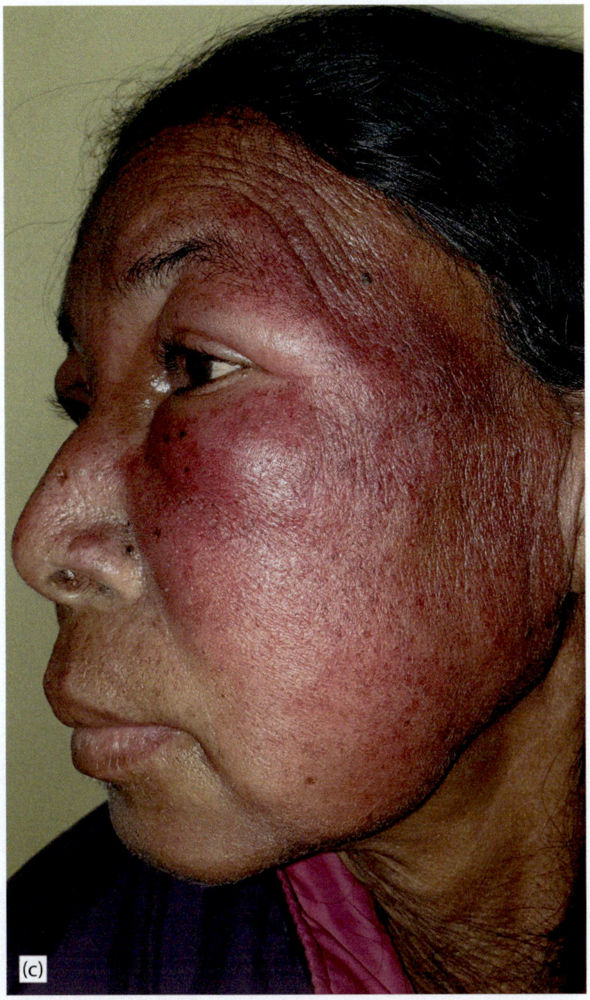


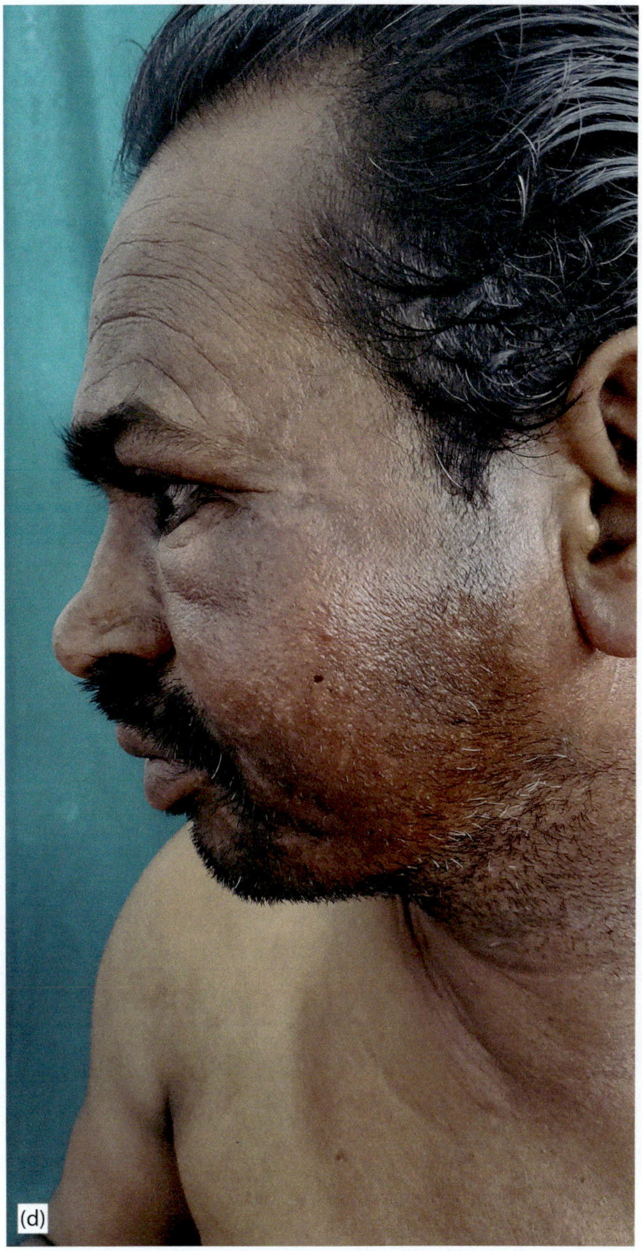


Figure 26.1 (Continued) **(c)** Imatinib-induced phototoxic reaction. **(d)** Griseofulvin-induced phototoxic reaction presenting as facial edema, erythema, and xerosis. (a,b – Courtesy: Dr. Piyush Kumar, Katihar, India; c – Courtesy: Dr. Rajesh Kumar Mandal, North Bengal Medical College and Hospital, India; d – Courtesy: Prof. Bhushan Madke, Jawaharlal Nehru Medical College, Datta Meghe Institute of Medical Sciences, India.)

Table 26.3 Phototoxic and photoallergic reaction.

| Phototoxic reaction | Photoallergic reaction |
|---|---|
| More common | Less common |
| Offending agent: large in amount | Offending agent: relatively small in amount |
| Immediate or early onset, even after single exposure | Occurs after 24 to 72 hours of exposure; more than one exposure is required for the lesion to develop |
| Sun-exposed parts | Sun-exposed as well as unexposed parts |
| Looks like exaggerated sunburn | Mimics dermatitis |

  - Erythema of the gluteal or perianal area and/or V-shaped erythema of the inguinal area involvement of at least one other intertriginous localization (**Figure 26.3**)
  - Symmetry of affected areas
  - Absence of systemic toxicity
- The most common drug association is beta-lactam antibiotics, particularly amoxicillin. Other well-documented medications include antihypertensives, radiocontrast media, and monoclonal antibodies intravenous immunoglobulin, barium sulphate, mitomycin C, oxycodone, rivastigmine.

## Morbilliform (exanthematous) drug reaction

- This is the most common cutaneous adverse reaction to drugs.
- Reaction rates are highest for antibiotics, ranging from 1%–8% of cases.

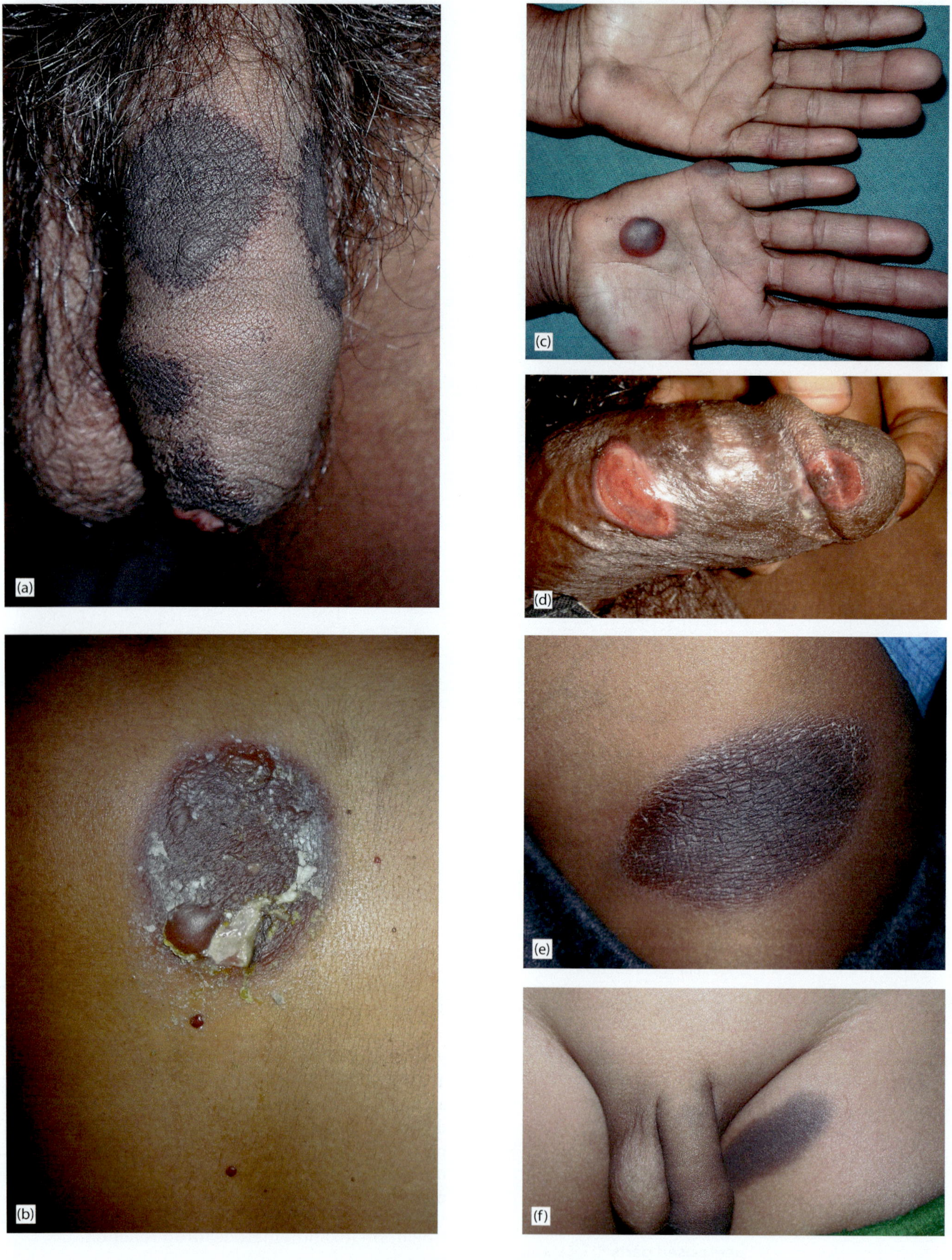

Figure 26.2 **(a)** Well-circumscribed, circular, dusky erythematous patches of fixed drug eruption. **(b)** Fixed drug eruption lesion developing bulla on its surface. **(c)** Bullous fixed drug eruption. **(d)** Bulla may rupture to leave erosions. **(e)** Older, dried-up lesion of fixed drug eruption. **(f)** Fixed drug reaction ultimately heals with post-inflammatory hyperpigmentation. (a–f – Courtesy: Dr. Piyush Kumar, Katihar, India.)

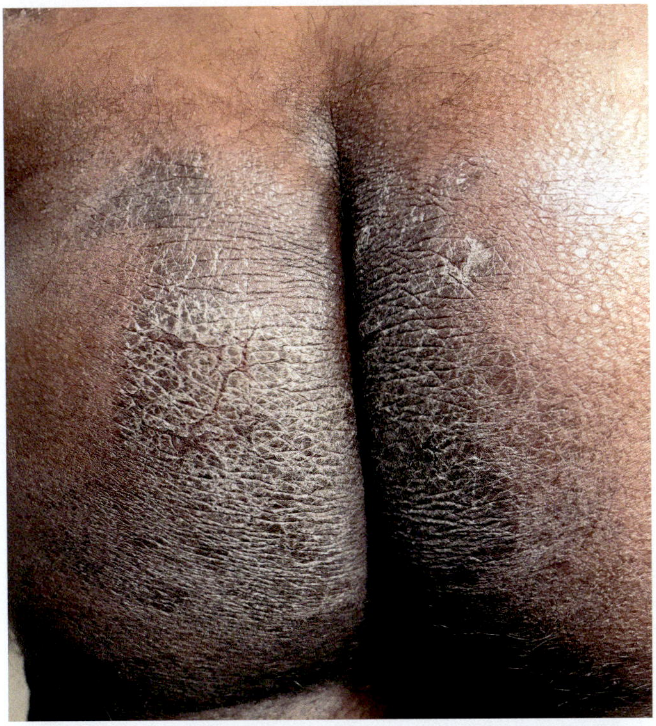

Figure 26.3 Symmetrical drug-related intertriginous and flexural exanthema presenting as symmetrical erythematous, scaly patches on the buttocks. (Courtesy: Dr. Chetan D Rajput, SBH Govt. Medical College, Dhule, Department of Skin and VD, Krishna Institute of Medical Sciences, Karad, India.)

- There is a profuse eruption of bright-red, symmetrically distributed, macules, papules, or both types of lesion (**Figure 26.4**).
- It heals within 10 to 14 days after withdrawal of the causative drug but can progress to exfoliative dermatitis if the drug is not withdrawn.
- Common causative drugs are penicillins, sulphonamides, antiepileptics, and non-nucleoside reverse transcriptase inhibitors.
- DD: Viral exanthem.

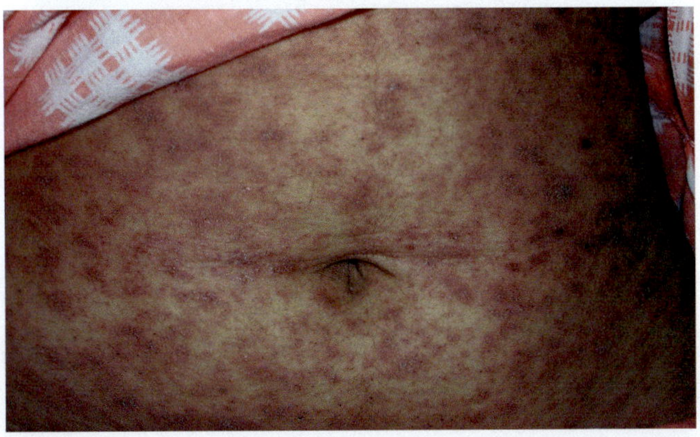

Figure 26.4 Amoxicillin-induced maculopapular eruption. (Courtesy: Dr. Piyush Kumar, Katihar, India.)

## Drug rash with eosinophilia and systemic symptoms (DRESS)/drug hypersensitivity syndrome (DHS)

- Synonyms for this condition are drug hypersensitivity syndrome, dapsone syndrome, febrile mucocutaneous syndrome, graft-vs-host disease-like illness, Kawasaki-like illness, drug-induced delayed multiorgan hypersensitivity syndrome (DIDMOHS).
- It is one of the severe forms of CADR (SCAR).
- It is characterized by a clinical triad of fever, skin rash, and internal organ involvement. Mucous membrane is rarely involved, and necrolysis of skin is never present.
- The cutaneous lesions start as maculopapular lesions on the face, trunk, and extremities and rapidly progress to diffuse and confluent erythema (**Figure 26.5**). The diagnosis of DRESS is considered when more than 50% body surface area is affected and there is facial edema, diffuse scaling, or purpura. In some cases, the disease may progress to erythroderma and vesicles and bulla, or pustules may be seen.
- Mucosal inflammation and pain are seen, but erosions are not observed.
- Characteristically it occurs with the first exposure to the drug but not with the first dose; an interval of 1 to 8 weeks with optimal dosage of the drug is required for the hypersensitivity to develop.
- Eosinophilia (90%) or mononucleosis-like atypical lymphocytosis (40%) is the hematological hallmark of this syndrome. Hence the acronym DRESS (**d**rug **r**ash with **e**osinophilia and **s**ystemic **s**ymptoms).
- It is A rare entity associated with considerable morbidity and mortality. Because of systemic involvement, it may mimic several other disorders.
- Common drugs involved are dapsone and other sulphonamides, carbamazepine, barbiturates,

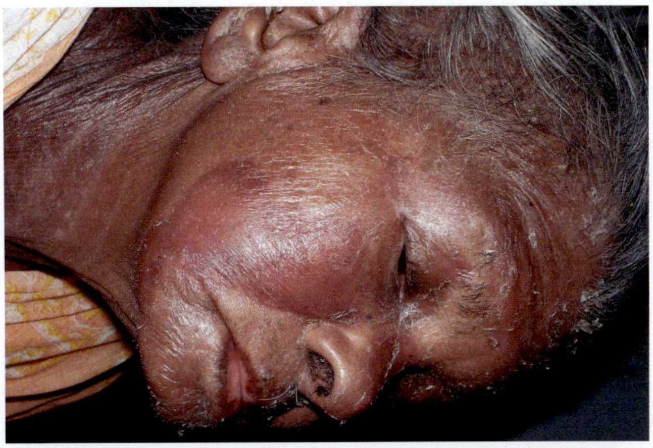

Figure 26.5 Diaminodiphenyl sulfone (dapsone)–induced drug hypersensitivity syndrome in a leprosy patient. Note erythematous plaque of leprosy on the face. (Courtesy: Dr. Piyush Kumar, Katihar, India.)

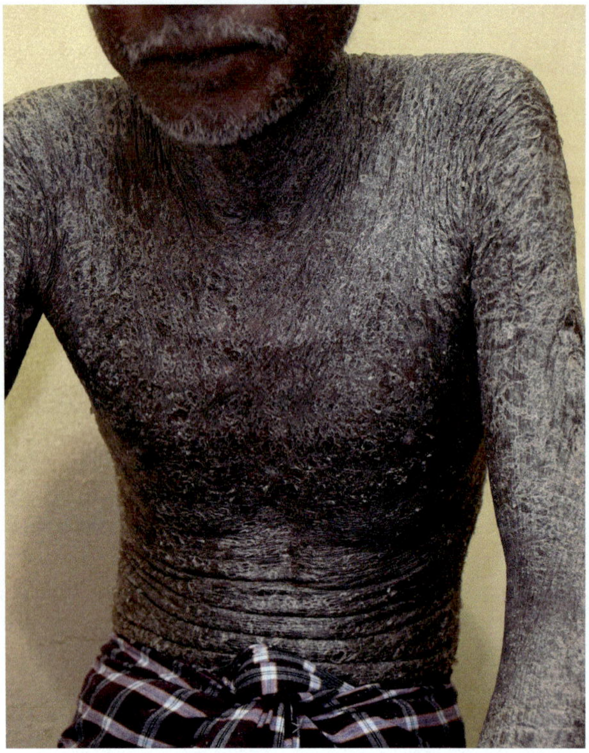

Figure 26.6 Drug-induced erythroderma. Patient was on highly active antiretroviral therapy for the previous six months and was started on antitubercular drugs one month back. (Courtesy: Dr. Piyush Kumar, Katihar, India.)

phenytoin, minocycline, azathioprine, allopurinol, and the antiretroviral drug abacavir.

- Offending chemotherapeutic drugs are chlorambucil and lenalidomide.

## Drug-induced erythroderma/exfoliative dermatitis

- This involves widespread inflammation of the skin with abrupt onset of erythema, edema, and scaling involving more than 90% of the body surface area. Lymphadenopathy hepatosplenomegaly, leukocytosis, eosinophilia, and anemia may be present (**Figure 26.6**).
- Common offending drugs include allopurinol, anticonvulsants, aspirin, barbiturates, captopril, carbamazepine, cefoxitin, chloroquine, chlorpromazine, cimetidine, diltiazem, griseofulvin, lithium, nitrofurantoin, omeprazole, phenytoin, sulfonamides, and thalidomide.
- Offending chemotherapeutic agents are cisplatin and methotrexate.

## Drug-induced pigmentation

- Drug-induced pigmentary abnormalities include (1) hyperpigmentation/melanosis, (2) hypopigmentation/leukoderma, and (3) dyspigmentation or occurrence of unusual skin color.
- The most commonly implicated medications are antimalarials, chemotherapeutic agents, heavy metals, amiodarone, zidovudine, minocycline, clofazimine (**Figure 26.7a–c**), psoralens, and psychotropic drugs.

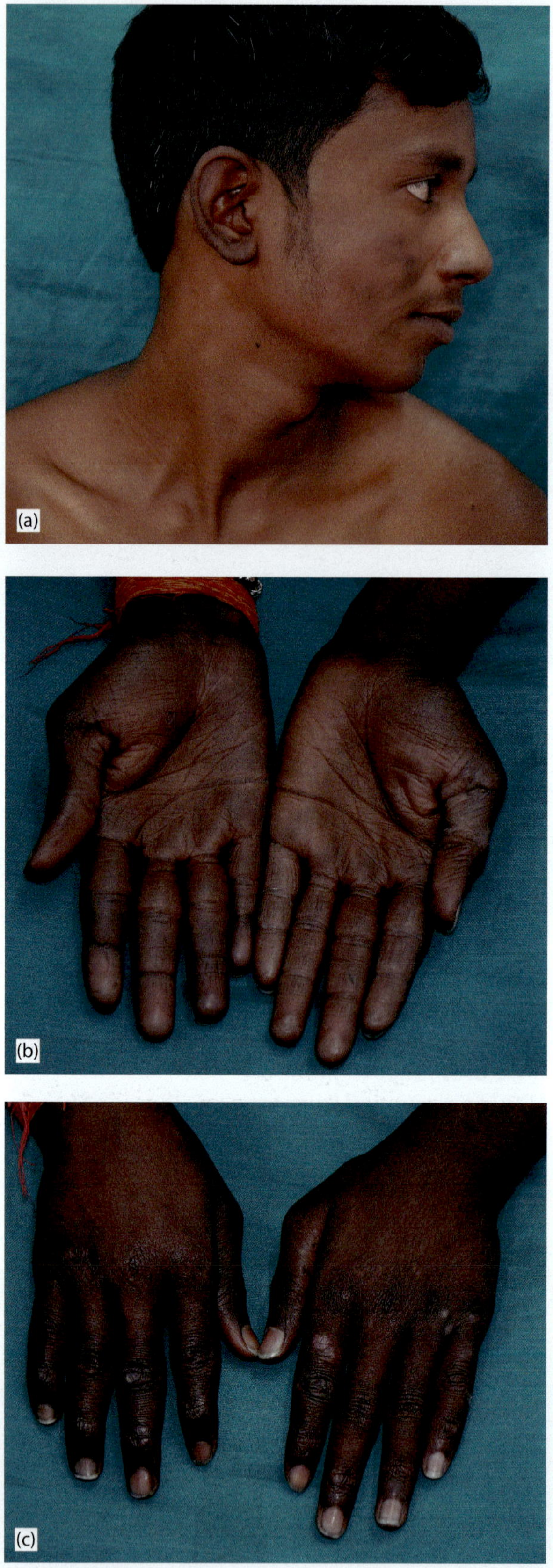



Figure 26.7 **(a)** Clofazimine-induced hyperpigmentation on the face. Note ear involvement. **(b)** Clofazimine-induced pigmentation of the palms. **(c)** Clofazimine-induced pigmentation of the dorsum of hands. (a–c – Courtesy: Dr. Piyush Kumar, Katihar, India.)

- Antimalarial-induced hyperpigmentation:
  - Affects almost one in four patients receiving antimalarials for at least four months.
  - Bluish-gray or purple pigmentation most frequently in the pretibial areas; can also involve the entire nail bed, nose, cheeks, forehead, ears, and oral mucosa (specifically the hard palate).
  - Reversible several months after stopping the inciting agent.
- Minocycline induced pigmentation:
  - **Type 1**: blue-black discoloration localized to scars and post-inflammatory sites.
  - **Type 2**: blue-gray pigmentation of normal skin on the extremities, especially the anterior shins mimicking antimalarial pigmentation.
  - **Type 3**: generalized "muddy" brown hyperpigmentation seen most prominently in sun-exposed skin

## Acneiform eruption

- This presents as monomorphic acne pattern lesions beyond the seborrheic areas (**Figure 26.8a**).
- It has an unusual age of onset.
- There is a resistance to conventional acne therapy and, of course, a history of recent drug introduction.
- Causative agents include corticosteroids (**Figure 26.8b,c**), neuro psychotherapeutic drugs like phenytoin, lithium, antituberculosis drugs like isoniazid, halogenated compounds, high-dose vitamin B-complex, epidermal growth factor receptor inhibitor (**Figure 26.8d**), and immunomodulating molecules.
- Disruption of the culprit drug is usually not required.

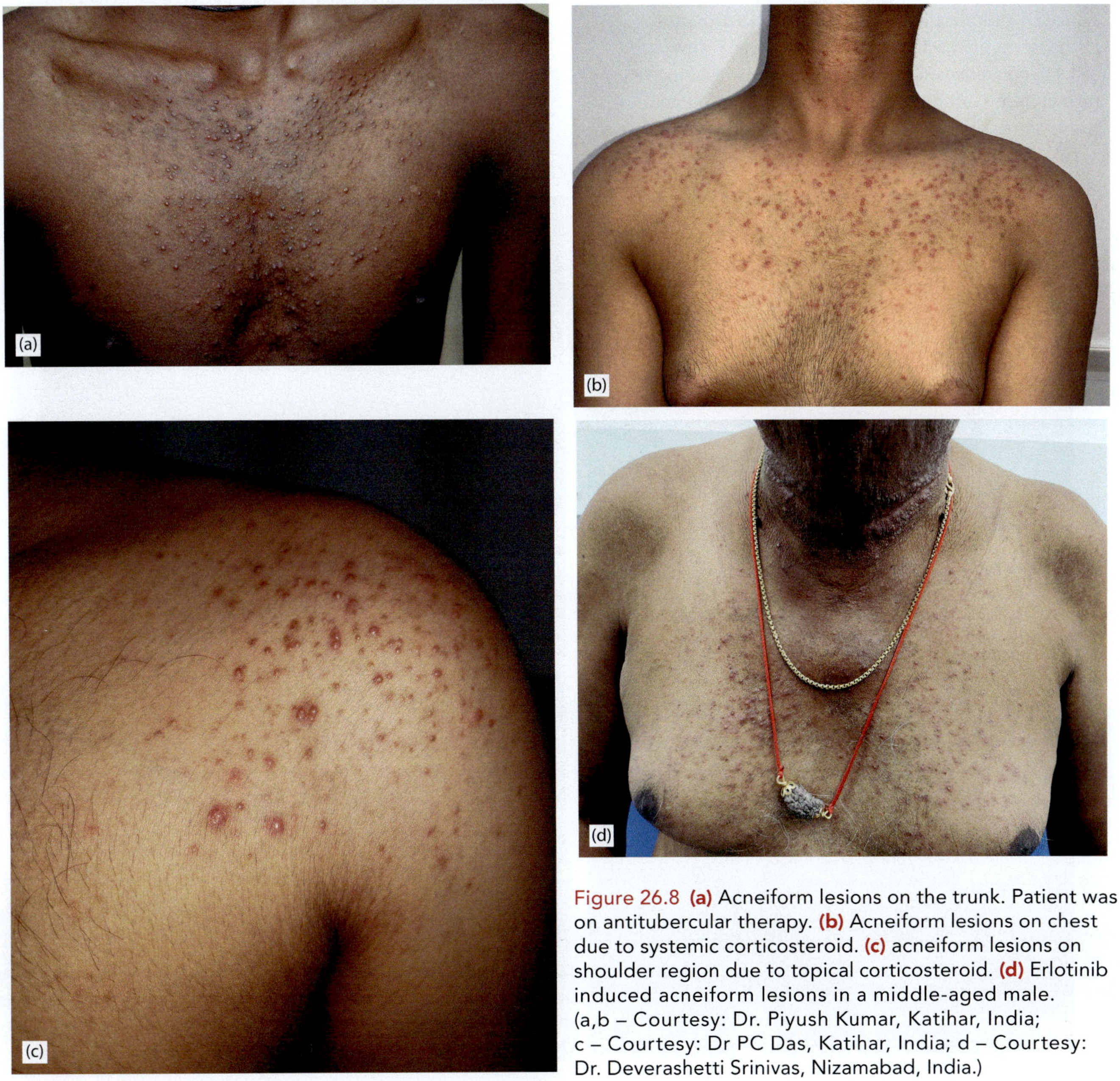


Figure 26.8 **(a)** Acneiform lesions on the trunk. Patient was on antitubercular therapy. **(b)** Acneiform lesions on chest due to systemic corticosteroid. **(c)** acneiform lesions on shoulder region due to topical corticosteroid. **(d)** Erlotinib induced acneiform lesions in a middle-aged male. (a,b – Courtesy: Dr. Piyush Kumar, Katihar, India; c – Courtesy: Dr PC Das, Katihar, India; d – Courtesy: Dr. Deverashetti Srinivas, Nizamabad, India.)

## Psoriasiform drug reaction

- This is an eruption of papulosquamous skin lesions, indistinguishable from lesions of idiopathic psoriasis vulgaris. The suspicion of the etiology arises only after seeing the temporal association.
- Drugs that can either precipitate or aggravate psoriasiform lesion include lithium, beta-blockers, antimalarials, ACE inhibitors, terbinafine, NSAIDS, aspirin, interleukins, and interferons.

## Lichenoid drug eruption

- Clinical features are similar to and indistinguishable from idiopathic lichen planus. However, lesions may not show flexural predilection and may be more scaly.
- Eruptions may be photodistributed without oral mucosal involvement and presence of eczematous or psoriasiform lesions (**Figure 26.9a,b**).
- It is caused by amlodipine, antimalarials, beta-blockers, captopril, diflunisal, diltiazem, enalapril, furosemide, glimepiride, gold, leflunomide, levamisole, L-thyroxine, orlistat, penicillamine, phenothiazine, pravastatin, proton pump inhibitors, rofecoxib, salsalate, sildenafil, tetracycline, thiazides, imatinib, and ursodeoxycholic acid.

## Drug-induced pityriasis rosea-like reaction

- Annular, circular to oval shaped scaly plaques are distributed mainly over the extremities and trunk with variable degrees of itching.
- Drugs involved include arsenicals, bismuth, gold, barbiturates, beta-blockers, clonidine, captopril, griseofulvin, isotretinoin, metronidazole, pyribenzamine, methoxypromazine and omeprazole.

## Drug-induced lupus erythematosus

- Drug-induced systemic lupus erythematosus (SLE) symptoms are identical to those of SLE, but skin findings are uncommon.
- Skin manifestations are common with drug-induced subacute cutaneous lupus erythematosus (SCLE), characterized by annular or psoriasiform, non-scarring lesions in a photodistributed pattern, identical with spontaneously occurring variant.
- In drug-induced SLE, hydralazine, procainamide and minocycline· beta-blockers, chlorpromazine, cimetidine, clonidine, estrogens, isoniazid, lithium, lovastatin, methyldopa, oral contraceptives, quinidine,

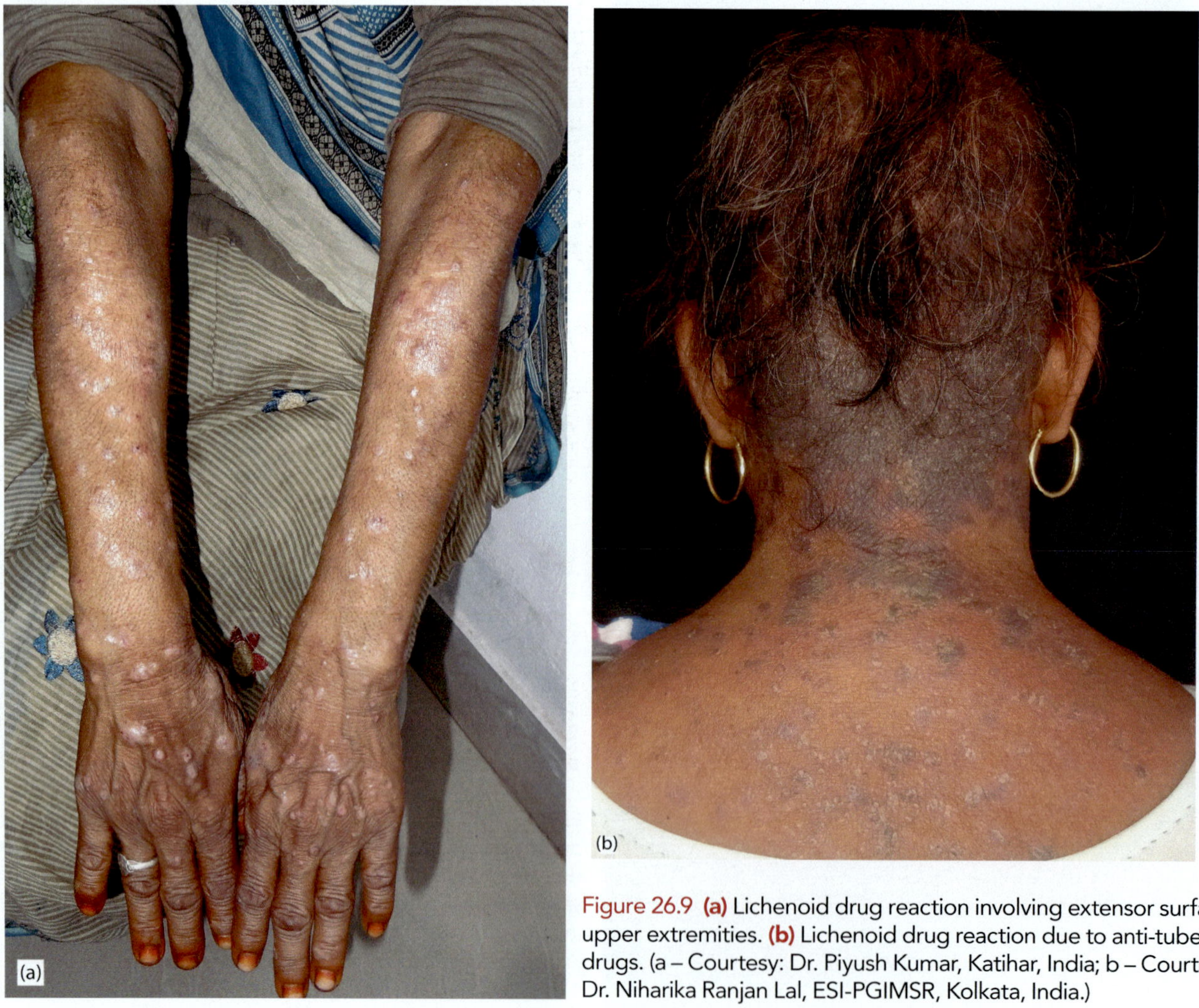


Figure 26.9 **(a)** Lichenoid drug reaction involving extensor surface of upper extremities. **(b)** Lichenoid drug reaction due to anti-tubercular drugs. (a – Courtesy: Dr. Piyush Kumar, Katihar, India; b – Courtesy: Dr. Niharika Ranjan Lal, ESI-PGIMSR, Kolkata, India.)

sulfonamides, tetracyclines, and tumor necrosis factor (TNF)–alpha inhibitors have been reported.
- Drug-induced SCLE involves hydrochlorothiazide (most common), calcium channel blockers, cimetidine, griseofulvin, leflunomide, terbinafine, and TNF-alpha inhibitors.
    - Offending chemotherapeutic agents include taxanes, fluorouracil and capecitabine, doxorubicin plus cyclophosphamide, and gemcitabine.

## Erythema multiforme

- Acrally distributed lesions present as papules or plaques of erythema surrounding an area of central clearing with a central hemorrhagic crust or vesicles; the lesions may enlarge and eventually form the typical target lesions. They might then evolve further, resulting in more confluent patches or annular lesions (**Figure 26.10a,b**). Mucosal involvement is in the form of oral or genital erosions.
- Bullous lesions are also seen.
- Offending chemotherapeutic drugs include busulfan, chlorambucil, cyclophosphamide, docetaxel, hydroxyurea, and tamoxifen.
- DD: Other factors causing erythema multiforme, including viral infections, bacterial infections, histoplasmosis, systemic lupus erythematosus, Wegener's granulomatosis, X-ray therapy.

## Stevens-Johnson syndrome (SJS), toxic epidermal necrolysis (TEN) and SJS-TEN overlap (Lyell's syndrome)

- This is a life-threatening cutaneous adverse reactions to drugs (SCAR).
- SJS is clinically characterized by widespread, flat, targetoid lesions with blisters arising on erythematous or purpuric macules and/or ulceration of the conjunctiva and the oral and genital mucosae, with systemic upset, a prodromal

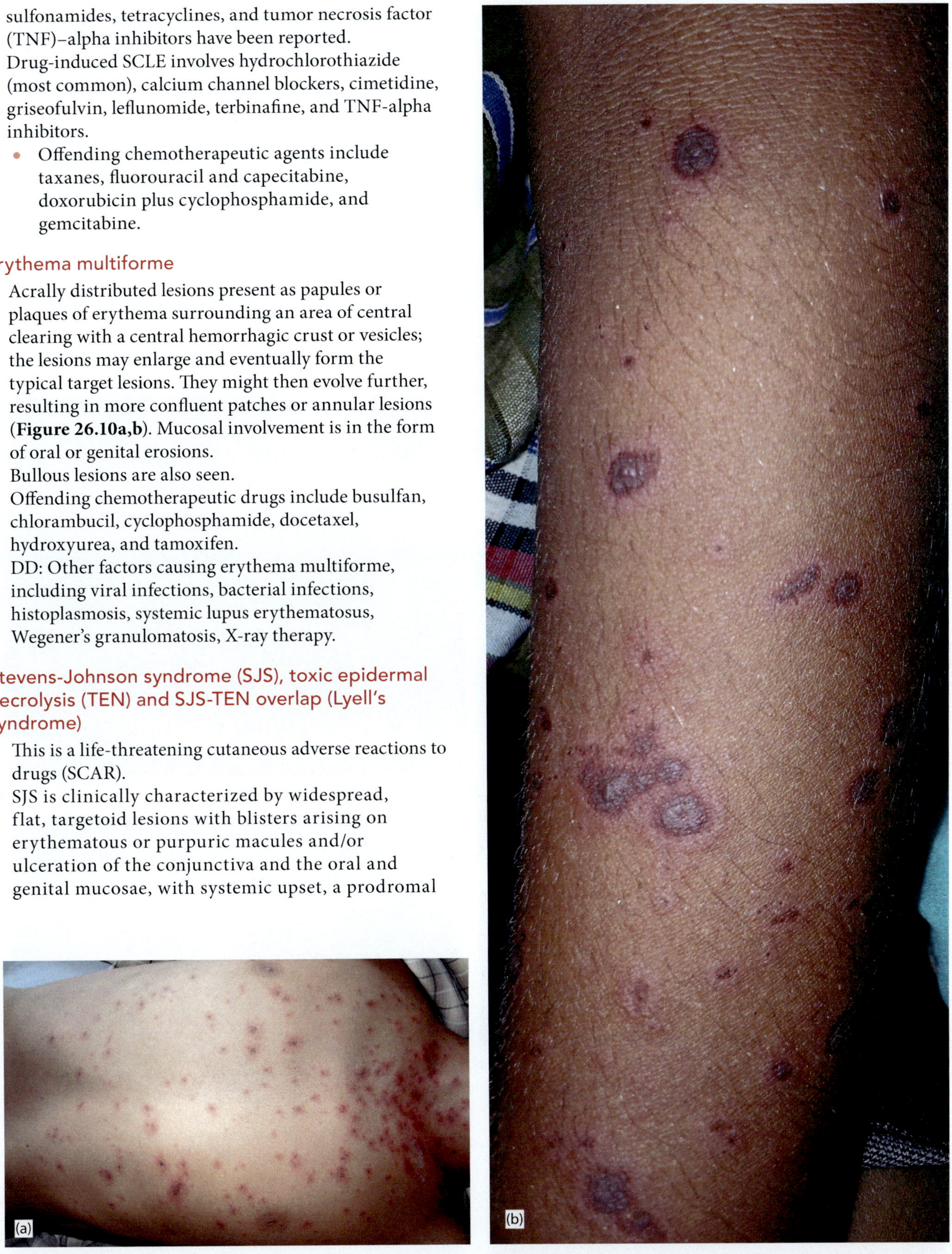

(a) (b)

Figure 26.10 **(a)** Extensive lesions of drug-induced erythema multiforme. **(b)** Erythema multiforme with central dusky erythematous skin (indicating damaged epidermis). (a,b – Courtesy: Dr. Piyush Kumar, Katihar, India.)

phase of fever, sore throat, and stinging eyes for one to three days (**Figure 26.11a,b**). Nikolsky's sign may be positive.

- TEN starts as dusky-red macules and patches that progress rapidly to full-thickness epidermal necrosis and dermal–epidermal detachment. The lesions become confluent and widespread erosions develop (**Figure 26.11c,d**). Prominent erosive mucositis is often present.
- SJS and TEN are considered a spectrum of drug-induced skin diseases having the same pathogenesis and are characterized by epidermal detachment ranging from mild (up to 10% of total body surface area in SJS), moderate (10–30% in SJS/TEN overlap), and severe (>30% in TEN). They are hence distinct from erythema multiforme.
- Mucous membrane erosions also affect the trachea, bronchi, and gastrointestinal tract.
- Offending drugs include sulfonamides, phenobarbital, phenytoin, carbamazepine, valproic acid, oxicam, non-steroidal anti-inflammatory drugs, chlormezanone, allopurinol, acetaminophen, imidazole, antifungal agents, corticosteroids for systemic use, aminopenicillins, cephalosporins, quinolones, and tetracyclines, and COX-2 inhibitors.
- Offending chemotherapeutic drugs include bleomycin, capecitabine, doxorubicin, etoposide, lenalidomide, methotrexate, and procarbazine.

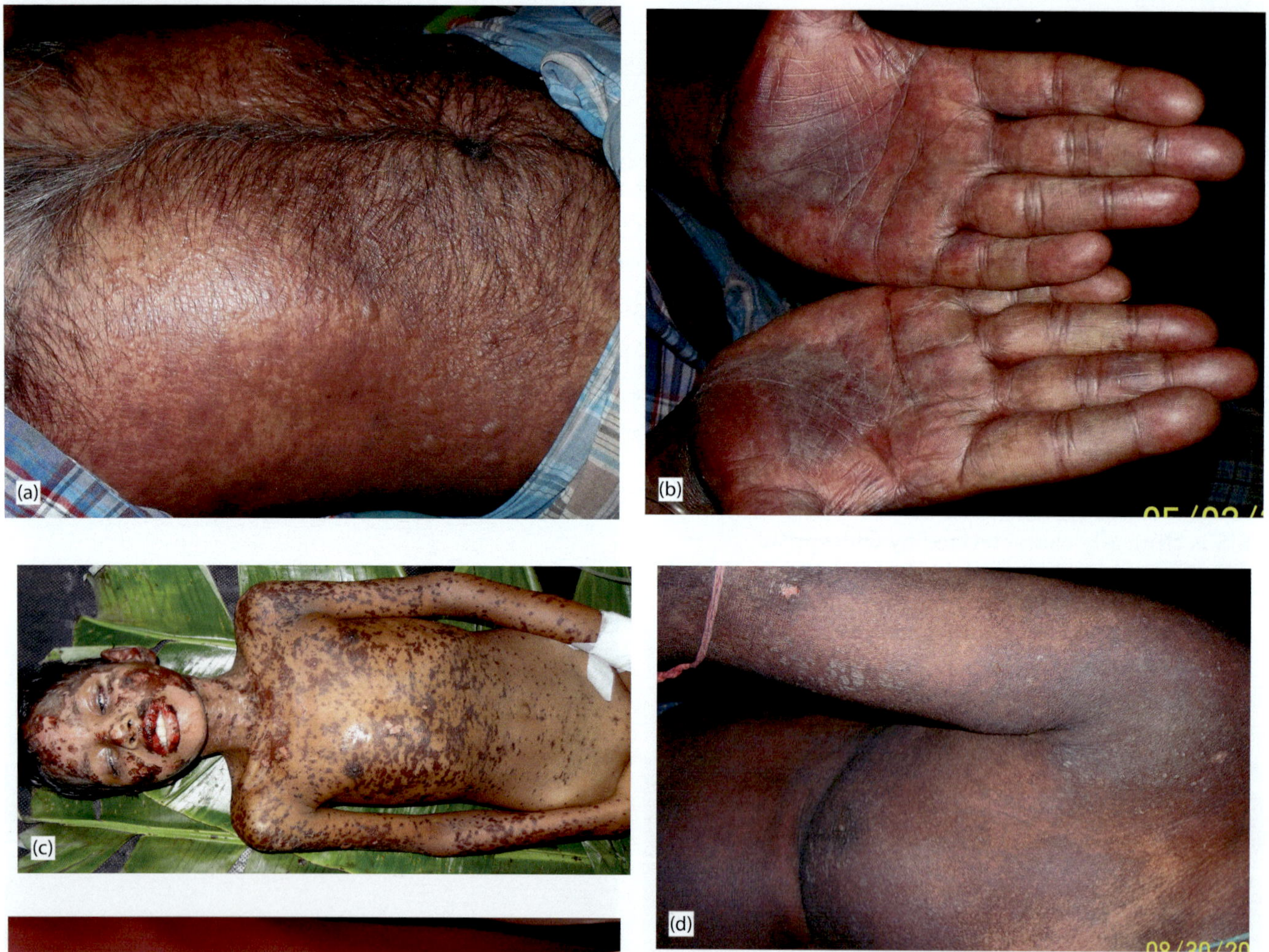


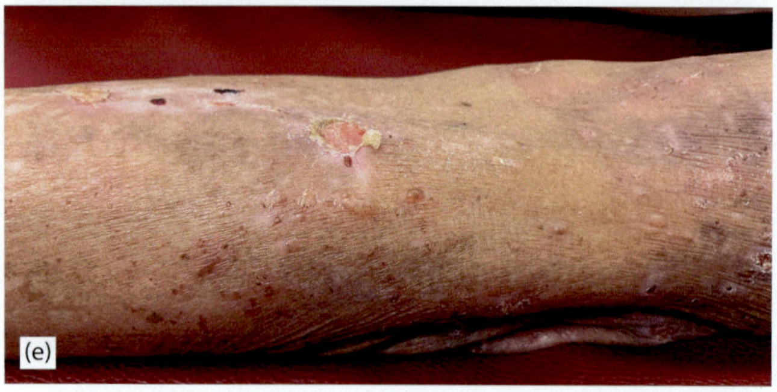


Figure 26.11 **(a)** Stevens-Johnson syndrome with vesicobullous lesions over an erythematous base. **(b)** Erythematous and purpuric lesion on the palm in Stevens-Johnson syndrome. **(c)** Toxic epidermal necrolysis with widespread dusky erythematous lesions on the body and erosive mucositis. **(d)** Toxic epidermal necrolysis with confluent dusky erythematous lesions with vesiculation due to epidermal detachment. **(e)** Vildagliptin induced bullous pemphigoid in a 76-year-old male. (a-e – Courtesy: Dr. Piyush Kumar, Katihar, India.)

- DD: Erythema multiforme (typical target lesions with elevated atypical target lesions).

## Drug-induced pseudoporphyria

- This is characterized by formation of vesiculobullous drugs with skin fragility without any blood or urine abnormalities. History of offending drug is an additional clue.
- Clinical features to differentiate it from porphyria cutanea tarda (PCT), its commonest differential, are as follows:
  - Present both in PCT and pseudoporphyria: photosensitivity, skin fragility, and blistering of the hands and forearms and sometimes milia.
  - Not seen in pseudoporphyria: hypertrichosis, dyspigmentation, and skin sclerosis.
- True PCT may be precipitated by barbiturates, estrogens, griseofulvin, rifampicin, and sulfonamides.
- Pseudoporphyria can be induced by furosemide, nabumetone, nalidixic acid, naproxen, oxaprozin, tetracycline, and voriconazole.

## Drug-induced pemphigus

- Drug-induced pemphigus needs to be differentiated from drug-triggered pemphigus. (**Table 26.4**).

Table 26.4 Drug-induced and drug triggered pemphigus

| Drug-induced pemphigus | Drug-triggered pemphigus |
|---|---|
| Exposure to drugs only, no genetic predisposition. | Genetic predisposition. |
| No such association. | Autoimmune disorders such as lupus, bullous pemphigoid, and myasthenia gravis may already be present. |
| Thiol drugs (–SH or sulfhydryl group), which are present in drugs like penicillamine, captopril, pyritinol, piroxicam, and thiopronine, are the most common agent implicated in drug-induced pemphigus. | Drugs known to trigger pemphigus include amoxicillin, ampicillin, cephalosporins, penicillin, rifampicin, propranolol, phenytoin, and phenobarbitone. |
| Thiol-drug–induced pemphigus foliaceus an average of 11 months after commencing treatment and regress spontaneously after discontinuation of the drug. | Pemphigus vulgaris commonly occurs following therapy with non-thiol drugs for a an average of four months. Spontaneous recovery is lower in non-thiol–induced pemphigus (only 15%) after stopping the drug. |

## Drug-induced bullous pemphigoid

- Patients are commonly younger than patients with idiopathic pemphigoid.
- Itching is common.
- Involvement of the epiglottis may lead to acute airway obstruction.
- Tense bullae occur on normal skin or on an erythematous base.
- Denuded areas heal spontaneously.
- There are erythematous patches, urticarial plaques, and targetoid lesions on face, trunk, limbs, palms, soles, and mucous membranes (**Figure 26.11e**).
- Nikolsky's sign may be positive, unlike in idiopathic pemphigoid.
- Causative drugs include furosemide, gliptins, amoxicillin, ampicillin, phenacetin, penicillin, penicillamine, psoralen-ultraviolet-A light, and beta-blockers.
- Cicatricial pemphigoid occurred after the use of practolol, topical echothiophate, D-penicillamine, clonidine, topical pilocarpine, topical demecarium, indomethacin, topical glaucoma, and sulfadoxine. Oral terbinafine has been associated with the development of bullous pemphigoid.

## Linear IgA bullous dermatoses (LAD)

- The clinical presentation of drug-induced LAD differs from other causes of LAD in that mucosal involvement may be less likely in drug-induced cases.
- Usually develops within one to two weeks of exposure to offending agent.
- Patients may complain of severe burning and pruritus.
- The most common presentations include urticated plaques, papulovesicles resembling dermatitis herpetiformis, targetoid lesions as in EM, and bullae that may be hemorrhagic resembling bullous pemphigoid.
- Common sites are the trunk and limbs.
- Drugs known to cause LAD include vancomycin (most common) diclofenac, somatostatin, lithium, phenytoin, captopril, amiodarone, cefamandole, amoxicillin, and ampicillin-sulbactam.

## Acute generalized exanthematous pustulosis (AGEP)

- This is a rare disease; more than 90% of cases are caused by drugs.
- Myriad disseminated, non-follicular, sterile pustules occur on a background of diffuse erythematous skin; the patient may have a fever (**Figure 26.12a–d**).
- Common offending drugs include beta-lactam antibiotics, aminopenicillins, sulfonamides, diltiazem, anticonvulsants, and antifungals.
- There is a localized variant.
- DD: Pustular psoriasis (differentiating points are acute onset, temporal relationship with drug and rapid resolution following drug withdrawal within 10 to 15 days).

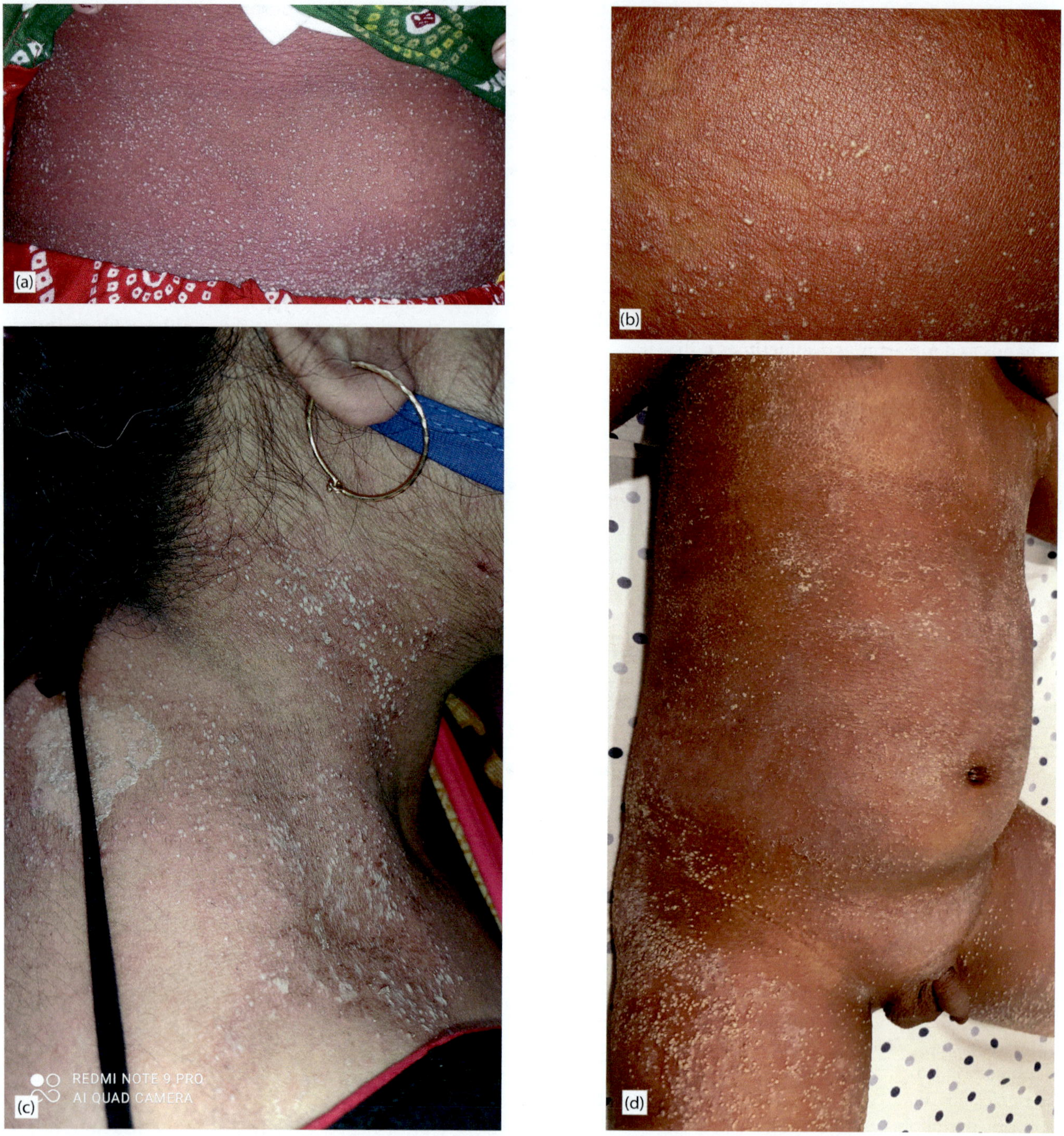


Figure 26.12 **(a)** Acute generalized exanthematous pustulosis with numerous tiny pustules over an erythematous background. **(b)** Close-up of acute generalized exanthematous pustulosis lesions. **(c)** Discrete and confluent pustules in acute generalized exanthematous pustulosis. **(d)** Extensive pustules and scaling on an erythematous skin in acute generalized exanthematous pustulosis. (a,b – Courtesy: Dr. Piyush Kumar, Katihar, India; c – Courtesy: Dr. Supratim Karmakar and Dr. Shiladitya Chowdhury, Medical College and Hospital, Kolkata, India; d – Courtesy: Dr. Guruvani Ravu, Sunshine hospital, Hyderabad, India.)

## Drug-induced erythema nodosum

- This is characterized by tender, red, subcutaneous nodules that typically appear on the anterior aspect of the legs.
- Lesions do not suppurate or ulcerate.
- Drugs involved include oral contraceptives (most common), halogens, penicillin, sulfonamides, analgesics, potassium iodide, and tetracycline.

## Drug-induced xerosis

- This is commonly seen with statins, isoniazid, retinoids, butyrophenones, cimetidine, allopurinol, and clofazimine (**Figure 26.13**).

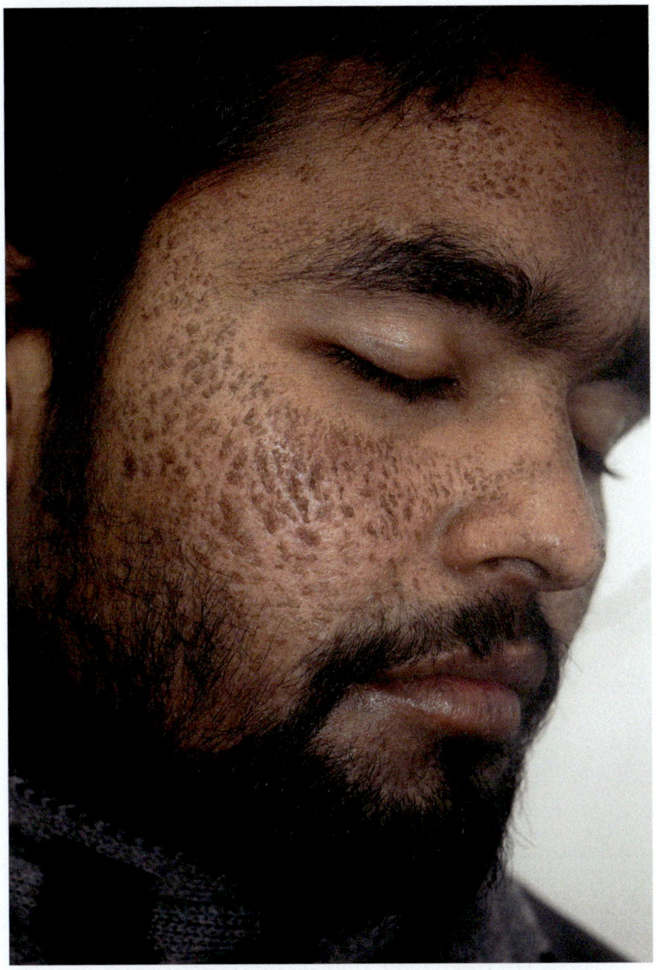

Figure 26.13 Isotretinoin-induced xerosis of the face. (Courtesy: Dr. Piyush Kumar, Katihar, India.)

## Drug-induced vasculitis (DIV)

- It is a relatively common drug eruption in clinical practice.
- Clinical features include blanching erythematous macules, quickly followed by palpable purpura. Fever, myalgias, arthritis, and abdominal pain may accompany (**Figure 26.14**).
- It typically develops 7 to 21 days after the onset of drug therapy.
- Hemorrhagic blisters, urticaria, ulcers, nodules, Raynaud's phenomenon, and digital necrosis are less frequent.
- Propylthiouracil induces a distinct type of vasculitis in which the face and earlobes are involved. Antineutrophil cytoplasmic antibodies (ANCA) and antinuclear antibodies may be produced in this particular type of DIV.
- Common drugs causing vasculitis include adalimumab, allopurinol, aspirin/NSAIDs, aminopenicillins, cimetidine, gold, hydralazine, leflunomide, levofloxacin, minocycline, montelukast, phenytoin, proton pump inhibitors, quinolones, ramipril, sulfonamide, tetracycline, thiazides, and thioridazine.

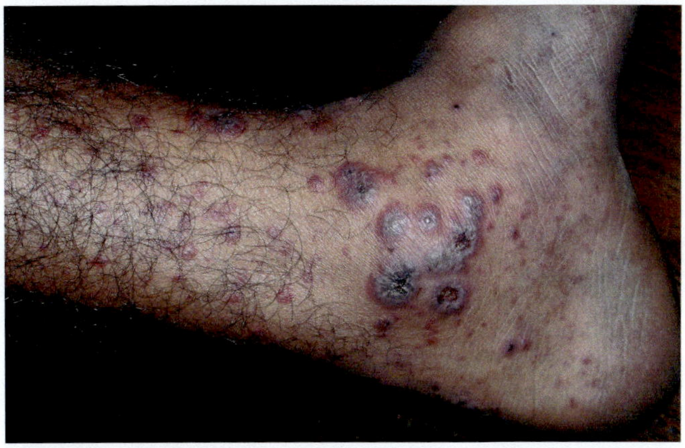

Figure 26.14 Drug-induced vasculitis with palpable purpura and necrotic lesions. (Courtesy: Dr. Piyush Kumar, Katihar, India.)

## Drug-induced urticaria/angioedema

- This is another common type of CADR.
- It appears within 36 hours of drug administration but on rechallenge may develop within minutes.
- Two-thirds of patients have associated extensive morbilliform rash.
- Common drugs include ACE inhibitors, NSAIDs, ketoconazole, fluconazole, penicillin, cephalosporins, aspirin, codeine, hydantoin, hydralazine, and cetirizine.
- DD: Urticaria and angioedema due to other causes, urticarial vasculitis.

## Flagellate dermatoses

- This is an uncommon figurate dermatoses characterized by a parallel linear or curvilinear arrangement simulating the marks of whiplashes.
- It is originally seen with bleomycin, but can be seen with peplomycin and docetaxel too.
- Other causes are shiitake mushroom ingestion, poison ivy, dermatogtraphism, religious punishment, torture, child abuse, dermatitis artefacta, etc.

## Acral erythema/palmar-plantar erythrodysesthesia/hand-foot syndrome (HFS)

- It is a dose-limiting adverse effect and is related to both the peak blood level and the cumulative dose of chemotherapy drug. The lesions may recur with increasing severity with successive cycles of chemotherapy.
- The lesions start as painful, well-defined erythema on palms and soles, and are associated with tingling, numbness, and stiffness of digits. In severe cases, blisters and ulceration may develop. Onycholysis may accompany HFS. The lesions usually resolve over two to four weeks (**Figure 26.15**).
- In darker skin, the skin becomes dry, darker, and thicker. It interferes with daily activities.

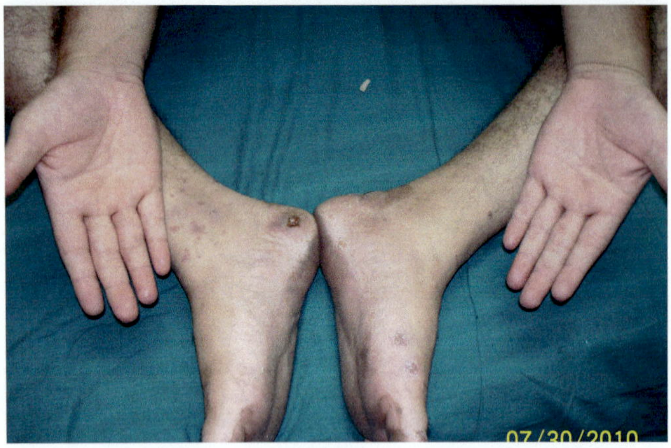

Figure 26.15 Imatinib-induced hand-foot syndrome with erythema and isolated pustular lesions. (Courtesy: Dr. Piyush Kumar, Katihar, India.)

- Causative drugs include cytarabine, doxorubicin hydrochloride, fluorouracil, and docetaxel. Nowadays targeted therapy drugs such as sorafenib, sunitinib, and other multikinase inhibitors are implicated more frequently.
- DD: Graft-vs-host disease.

## Neutrophilic eccrine hidradenitis (drug-induced eccrine hidradenitis)

- Clinical features include dusky-red or violaceous papules, plaques, and nodules, commonly occurring on the face, back, trunk, and extremities. The lesions may be asymptomatic or may be associated with pain and tenderness (**Figure 26.16**).
- It generally follows the administration of chemotherapy by 2 to 21 days, particularly during treatment of acute and chronic myeloid leukemias. It may appear in chemotherapy-naïve patients too.
- It is most commonly associated with the use of cytarabine (Ara-C) and/or anthracyclines. This cutaneous reaction is not a contraindication to further administration of the suspected agent.
- It may be seen with non-chemotherapy drugs (including minocycline, granulocyte colony-stimulating factors, cyclophosphamide, carbamazepine, antiretroviral medications) too.
- DD: Sweet syndrome, graft-vs-host disease, erythema nodosum, erythema multiforme.

## Inflammation of actinic keratoses

- Inflammation of actinic keratoses occurs due to systemic chemotherapy.
- Originally it was observed with fluorouracil.
- Doxorubicin, dactinomycin, dacarbazine, vincristine, deoxycoformycin, fludarabine, and cisplatin, may also be responsible.
- This particular reaction may even be considered to be beneficial. Once the acute reaction has subsided, chemotherapy may be reinstituted.

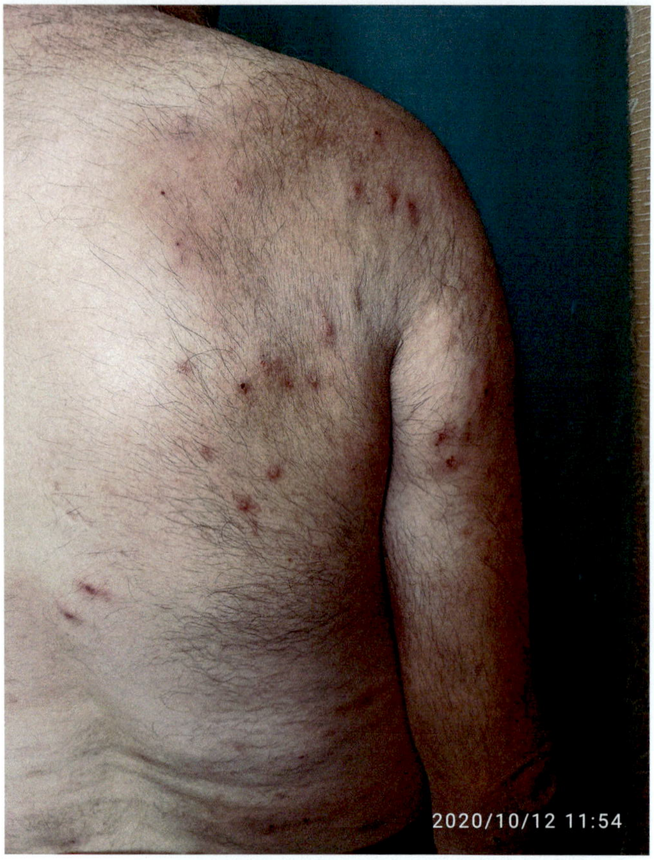


Figure 26.16 Erythematous papules and nodules of Neutrophilic eccrine hidradenitis in an elderly male. (Courtesy: Dr. Hiral Shah, Baroda Medical College, Vadodara, India.)

## PRIDE complex

- This is a spectrum of cutaneous adverse reactions known as the PRIDE complex (**p**apulopustules and/or paronychia, **r**egulatory abnormalities of hair growth, **i**tching, **d**ryness due to **E**GFR inhibitors). It is considered to correlate positively with the effectiveness of the EGFR treatment.
- Lesions appear around 8 days to 15 weeks after the onset of treatment.
- Itchy, follicular papulopustular eruptions over the seborrheic area (sparing palms and soles) appear earliest, but xerosis is most common adverse effect (**Figure 26.17**).
- Other manifestations include maculopapular rash, mucositis, trichomegaly, telangiectasia, and hyperpigmentation.
- Epidermal growth factor receptor (EGFR) inhibitor therapy comprises erlotinib and gefitinib and monoclonal antibody (cetuximab).
- Impaired growth and migration of keratinocytes, and inflammatory chemokine expression lead to inflammatory cell recruitment and subsequent cutaneous injury, which accounts for the majority of symptoms.

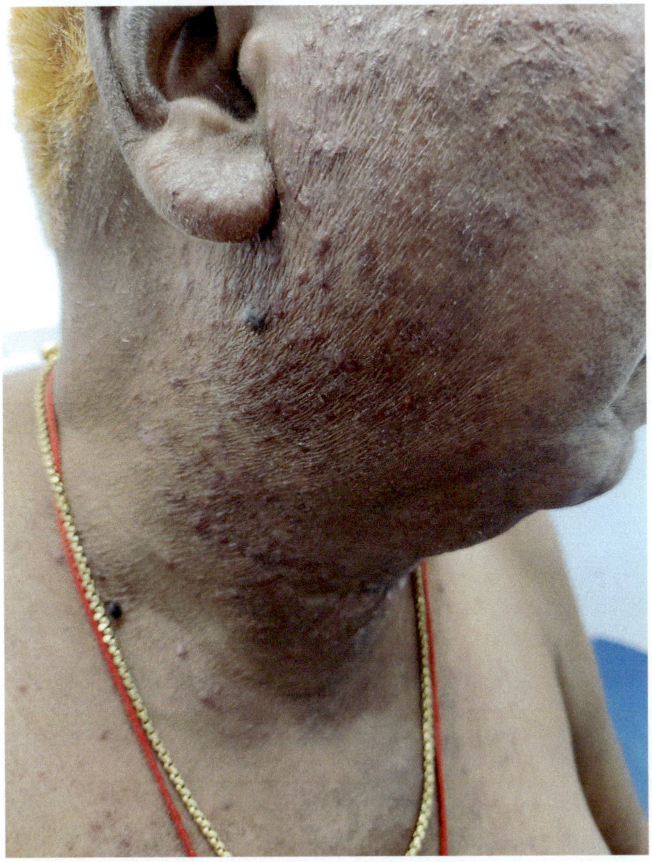

Figure 26.17 Erlotinib induced itchy scaly papular lesions on the face. (Courtesy: Dr. Deverashetti Srinivas, Nizamabad, India.)

- There are abnormalities in keratinocyte differentiation (i.e., premature expression of keratin 1 and signal transducer and activator of transcription 3 [STAT3]) causing defective stratum corneum responsible for xerosis and pruritus.
- Management of these dermatological adverse effects rarely requires discontinuation of targeted therapy and can be managed symptomatically.

### Photo recall phenomenon

- It is an acute inflammatory reaction in a previously sunburned area after the administration of systemic chemotherapeutic agents without further sun exposure.
- It is commonly seen after the intake of methotrexate and paclitaxel (taxanes).
- Antibiotics like cefazolin, gentamicin sulphate and tobramycin, piperacillin and ciprofloxacin too may cause a photo recall phenomenon.
- The latent period may vary from a couple of days to weeks.

### Radiation recall dermatitis

- Radiation recall dermatitis refers to an acute inflammatory reaction of the skin at the site of previous irradiation.
- Patients clinically present with itchy and/or painful, maculopapular eruptions with erythema, edema, vesicle formation, and exfoliation. Severe cases may develop necrosis of the skin.
- It usually starts within days to weeks after exposure to the precipitating drug.
- Common culprit drugs are actinomycin-D, 5-fluorouracil, hydroxyurea, vinblastine, methotrexate, adriamycin, etoposide, tamoxifen, bleomycin, melphalan, paclitaxel, docetaxel, gemcitabine, and pegylated liposomal doxorubicin.
- Among non-chemotherapeutic drugs, antituberculous drugs and simvastatin can cause radiation recall dermatitis.

## REFERENCES


1. Valeyrie-Allanore L, Obeid G, Revuz J. Drug Reactions. In: Bolognia JL, Schaffer JV, Cerroni L, editors. Dermatology. 4th edition. North York: Elsevier Limited; 2018. P. 348–375.
2. Hötzenecker W, Prins C, French LE. Erythema Multiforme, Stevens–Johnson Syndrome, and Toxic Epidermal Necrolysis. In: Bolognia JL, Schaffer JV, Cerroni L, editors. Dermatology. 4th edition. North York: Elsevier Limited; 2018. P. 332–347.
3. Ardern-Jones MR, Lee HY. Benign Cutaneous Adverse Reactions to Drugs. In: Griffiths CEM, Barker J, Bleiker T, Chalmers R, Creamer D, editors. Rook's Textbook of Dermatology. 9th edition. West Sussex: John Wiley & Sons; 2016. P. 118.1–118.17.
4. Walsh S, Lee HY, Creamer D. Severe Cutaneous Adverse Reactions to Drugs. In: Griffiths CEM, Barker J, Bleiker T, Chalmers R, Creamer D, editors. Rook's Textbook of Dermatology. 9th edition. West Sussex: John Wiley & Sons; 2016. P. 119.1–119.23.
5. Heelan K, Sibbald C, Shear NH. Cutaneous reactions to drugs. In: Kang S, Amagai M, Bruckner AL, Enk AH, Margolis DJ, McMichael AJ, Orringer JS, editors. Fitzpatrick's Dermatology. 9th edition. New York, NY: McGraw-Hill Education; 2019. P. 749–764.
6. Mockenhaupt M, Roujeau JC. Epidermal Necrolysis (Stevens-Johnson Syndrome and Toxic Epidermal Necrolysis). In: Kang S, Amagai M, Bruckner AL, Enk AH, Margolis DJ, McMichael AJ, Orringer JS, editors. Fitzpatrick's Dermatology. 9th edition. New York, NY: McGraw-Hill Education; 2019. P. 733–748.
7. Sengupta SR, Das NK. Cutaneous adverse drug reaction to systemic drugs: Recent updates. In: Ghosh S, editor. Recent advances in Dermatology: Volume 3. 1st edition. New Delhi: Jaypee Brothers Medical Publishers Ltd; 2004: P. 88–114.
8. Masatkar V, Nagure A, Gupta LK. Unusual and interesting adverse cutaneous drug reactions. Indian J Dermatol 2018;63:107–116.
9. Wyatt AJ, Leonard GD, Sachs DL. Cutaneous reactions to chemotherapy and their management. Am J Clin Dermatol 2006;7(1):45–63.
10. Kaul S, Kaffenberger BH, Choi JN, Kwatra SG. Cutaneous adverse reactions of anticancer agents. Dermatol Clin 2019;37(4):555–568.
11. Payne AS, Savarese DMF. Cutaneous side effects of conventional chemotherapy agents. In: Drews RE, Corona R, editors. [UpToDate]. https://www.uptodate.com/contents/cutaneous-side-effects-of-conventional-chemotherapy-agents/print

# E52

# Dermatitis artefacta, dermatitis neglecta, and terra firma-forme dermatosis

SAUMYA PANDA, RASHID SHAHID

## ABSTRACT

Dermatitis artefacta refers to cutaneous lesions produced by a patient's or caretaker's act and mimics many common dermatoses. Dermatitis neglecta results from inadequate cleansing and usually presents with localized flakes and/or crust. Terra firma-forme dermatosis mimics dermatitis neglecta closely.

The text of this chapter is available online at https://routledgetextbooks.com/textbooks/9781032399669/



DOI: 10.1201/9781351054225-83

E53

# Pruritus Sine Materia

ANURADHA PRIYADARSHINI

## ABSTRACT

Pruritus sine materia refers to chronic pruritus without any associated primary skin lesions, and patients may exhibit secondary lesions (e.g., excoriations only on clinical examination). Pruritus in such patients is of systemic, neurological, or psychiatric origin and requires thorough evaluation to arrive at a diagnosis. This chapter discusses the clinical approach to pruritus sine materia.

The text of this chapter is available online at https://routledgetextbooks.com/textbooks/9781032399669/

DOI: 10.1201/9781351054225-84

# E54

# Hyperhidrosis

ANKAN GUPTA, NAVYA HANDA

## ABSTRACT

Hyperhidrosis is a clinical condition characterized by excessive sweating, compared to the general population. It can be localized to a particular anatomical site or generalized. It can be physiological or associated with metabolic disorders, endocrine disorders, and more sinister neurologic disorders and malignancy, apart from drugs and addiction. Some cases, called primary hyperhidrosis, have no discernible cause. A thorough investigation is required about this condition, as it constitutes an important reason for dermatologic consultation, for psychological and even occupational problems.

The text of this chapter is available online at https://routledgetextbooks.com/textbooks/9781032399669/


DOI: 10.1201/9781351054225-85

# E55

# Anhidrosis

SABHA MUSHTAQ

## ABSTRACT

Hypohidrosis and anhidrosis refer to diminished and absence of sweating respectively, in response to appropriate stimuli. Depending on the presentation, it can either be localized or generalized. There are several causes, viz. exogenous (localized damage to skin and sweat glands or systemic medications) and endogenous (dermatological and neurologic disorders). This chapter focuses on the clinical entities of diminished sweating, their important causes, and a brief framework to approach such a patient.

The text of this chapter is available online at https://routledgetextbooks.com/textbooks/9781032399669/

DOI: 10.1201/9781351054225-86

# 27

# Photosensitivity in children

RESHAM VASANI

## INTRODUCTION

Photosensitivity is an abnormal or adverse reaction of the skin on exposure to ordinary light that includes ultraviolet (UV) light or visible radiation. It usually follows sunlight but can also be caused by artificial light sources. Photosensitivity in children (**Box 27.1**) may be seen in a diverse group of hereditary and genodermatoses, idiopathic photodermatoses, and metabolic dermatoses, or may be induced by exogenous agents. The clinical approach to photosensitivity disorders in children has been summarized in **Table 27.1**.[1-3]

Salient features of commonly occurring photodermatoses in children are given below.[1-4]

### Neonatal Lupus erythematosus (NLE)

- NLE is characterized by development of cutaneous, cardiac, and systemic abnormalities in newborn infants born of mothers having autoantibodies against Ro/SSA and La/SSB.
- It may present at birth or within weeks of birth.
- The lesions can be exacerbated by UV exposure, but sun exposure is not required for the development of the lesions and they can be seen at birth prior to any sun exposure.
- Classically, NLE occurs in the periorbital area and the scalp as erythematous annular or polycyclic scaly plaques (**Figure 27.1**). The lesions are typically non-scarring and resemble subacute lupus erythematosus. Periorbital erythema ("raccoon eye" or "owl eye") is a characteristic feature. Bullous lesions may develop, especially on the soles.
- The lesions are self-limiting within one year of life after the clearance of the anti Ro antibody acquired transplacentally.
- Telangiectasia may be noted and is the sole cutaneous manifestation reported in some patients. The atrophic telangiectatic changes are most evident near the temples and scalp.
- These infants should be monitored for congenital heart block as well as hepatic and hematologic manifestations.
- DD: Seborrheic dermatitis, atopic dermatitis, Langerhans cell histiocytosis, Bloom syndrome, Rothmund-Thomson syndrome.

**BOX 27.1: When to suspect photosensitivity in a child**

1. Subjective symptoms: sunburn reaction/swelling/intense itching after exposure to sunlight
2. Objective symptoms: skin eruption/skin fragility/scarring, predominantly over the sun-exposed areas – face/V of the neck/dorsa of hands and arms

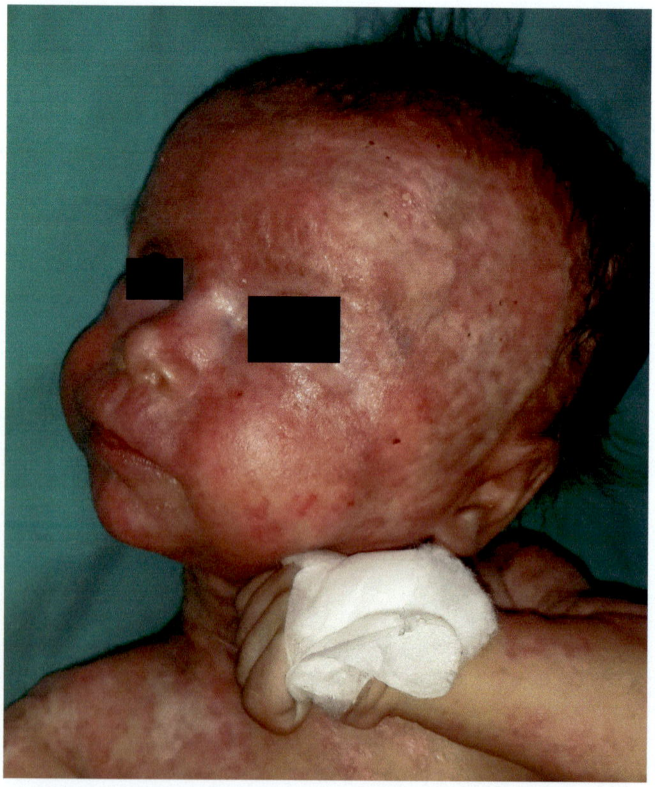

Figure 27.1 Case of neonatal lupus erythematosus presenting with erythematous telangiectatic atrophic plaques on the face.



DOI: 10.1201/9781351054225-87

Table 27.1 Approach to pediatric patients with photosensitivity

| Step 1: What is the age of onset of the disease? | | | |
|---|---|---|---|
| **At birth** | **< 1 year** | **1–5 years** | **School age** |
| Neonatal, LE<br>CEP & HEP | RTS, BS<br>XP, CS (type II), TTD<br>phenylketonuria<br>neonatal LE | AT Hartnup disease<br>EPP<br>Kindler syndrome<br>CS (Type I) | PLE, JSE, HV, SU, AP childhood LE<br>juvenile DM<br>BS (cutaneous features)<br>TTD<br>Phytophotodermatitis, pellagra |
| **Step 2: What is the predominant clinical manifestation?** | | | |
| **Pigment dilution**<br>Albinism, PKU | **Butterfly erythema**<br>BS, RTS, CS, SLE, pellagra, Hartnup disease | **Dermatitis**<br>Pellagra, Hartnup disease, PLE, phytophotodermatitis | **Papulonodular lesions**<br>Actinic prurigo |
| **Vesicobullous lesions**<br>SLE, RTS, BS, porphyrias, hydroa vacciniforme | **Wheals**<br>Solar urticaria<br><br>**Hypertrichosis**<br>porphyrias<br>juvenile DM | **Telangiectasia**<br>RTS, BS, XP, AT, SLE, juvenile DM | **Poikiloderma**<br>RTS, juvenile DM |
| **Step 3: What are the associated clinical features?** | | | |
| **Neurological features**<br>• Cerebellar ataxia with psychiatric disturbances – Hartnup disease<br>• Cerebellar ataxia with nystagmus – AT<br>• Mental retardation – Hartnup disease, PKU, AT, CS, XP<br>• Seizures, psychosis – SLE | | **Growth retardation**<br>BS, PKU, porphyria, AT, CS, XP | **Immunodeficiency**<br>BS, RTS, AT, PKU |
| **Dark Urine**<br>Hepatoerythropoetic porphyria<br>staining of Diapers – CEP | | **Malignancies**<br>BS, XP, RTS | **Ophthalmic involvement**<br>XP, BS, RTS |

*Abbreviations:* LE, lupus erythematosus; CEP, congenital erythropoietic porphyria; HEP, hepatoerythropoietic porphyria; XP, xeroderma pigmentosum; CS, Cockayne syndrome; TTD, trichothiodystrophy; RTS, Rothmund-Thomson syndrome; EPP, erythropoietic protoporphyria; PMLE, polymorphous light eruption; AP, actinic prurigo; JSE, juvenile spring eruption; HV, hydroa vacciniforme; DM, dermatomyositis; SU, solar urticaria.

## Porphyria

- Porphyrias are a group of disorders resulting from deficiency of various enzymes involved in heme (part of haemoglobin) biosynthesis, resulting in accumulation and excretion of precursors of heme called porphyrins.
- Porphyrias with cutaneous involvement include the following (**Table 27.2**).
    - Congenital erythropoietic porphyria (CEP)
    - Erythropoietic protoporphyria (EPP)
    - Porphyria cutanea tarda (PCT)

Table 27.2 Childhood porphyria of dermatological importance

| Type of Porphyria | Age of onset | Clinical features |
|---|---|---|
| Porphyria cutanea tarda | Type 1 (sporadic) – Third to fourth decade of life, usually not before puberty<br>Type II – Adulthood<br>Type III – Childhood | Cutaneous manifestations in sun-exposed areas, including skin fragility, erosions, crusts, vesicles and bullae, milia, scarring, hyperpigmentation and hypertrichosis |
| Erythropoietic protoporphyria | Early childhood (1 to 4 years) | Erythema, edema, crusts, purpura, skin thickening and waxy scars, primarily on dorsal hands and face |
| Congenital erythropoietic porphyria | Infancy/first decade of life | Vesicles, bullae, erosions, ulcerations, crusts, milia, scarring, hyperpigmentation, hypertrichosis, mutilation, hemolytic anemia, hepatosplenomegaly, porphyrin deposition in the teeth (erythrodontia), pink, red, or violet staining of diapers |

- Hereditary coproporphyria
- Variegate porphyria
- Varied clinical presentations occur because of the differences in water solubility of the intermediate porphyrins. Childhood onset of hereditary coproporphyria and variegate porphyria are only rarely reported and are outside the scope of this chapter.
- **Congenital erythropoietic porphyria** (Gunther disease)
  - This is an autosomal recessive condition caused by deficiency of uroporphyrinogen III synthase. It is associated with a significant decrease in life expectancy.
  - The most disfiguring form of porphyrias is mutilation of facial skin and cartilage.
  - It presents in infancy as discomfort on sun exposure or generalized blistering on phototherapy. Dark-colored urine (**Figure 27.2a**) and staining of diapers with red fluorescence on Wood's lamp is noted.
  - In childhood, patients exhibit severe photosensitivity with blistering (tense) on the photo-exposed areas, healing with scarring, and mutilation. Red- or brown-colored teeth (**Figure 27.2b**) that fluoresce red orange on Wood's lamp examination, hypertrichosis (**Figure 27.2c**), and hyperpigmentation are additional findings.
  - Ocular involvement results in photophobia, corneal scarring, ulcerative keratoconjunctivitis, and cataracts.
  - Bone involvement manifests as osteolysis with osteoporosis, bone fragility, and fractures.
  - Other common findings are hemolytic anemia, hypercellular bone marrow, and splenomegaly.
  - DD: Porphyria cutanea tarda, variegate porphyria, epidermolysis bullosa.

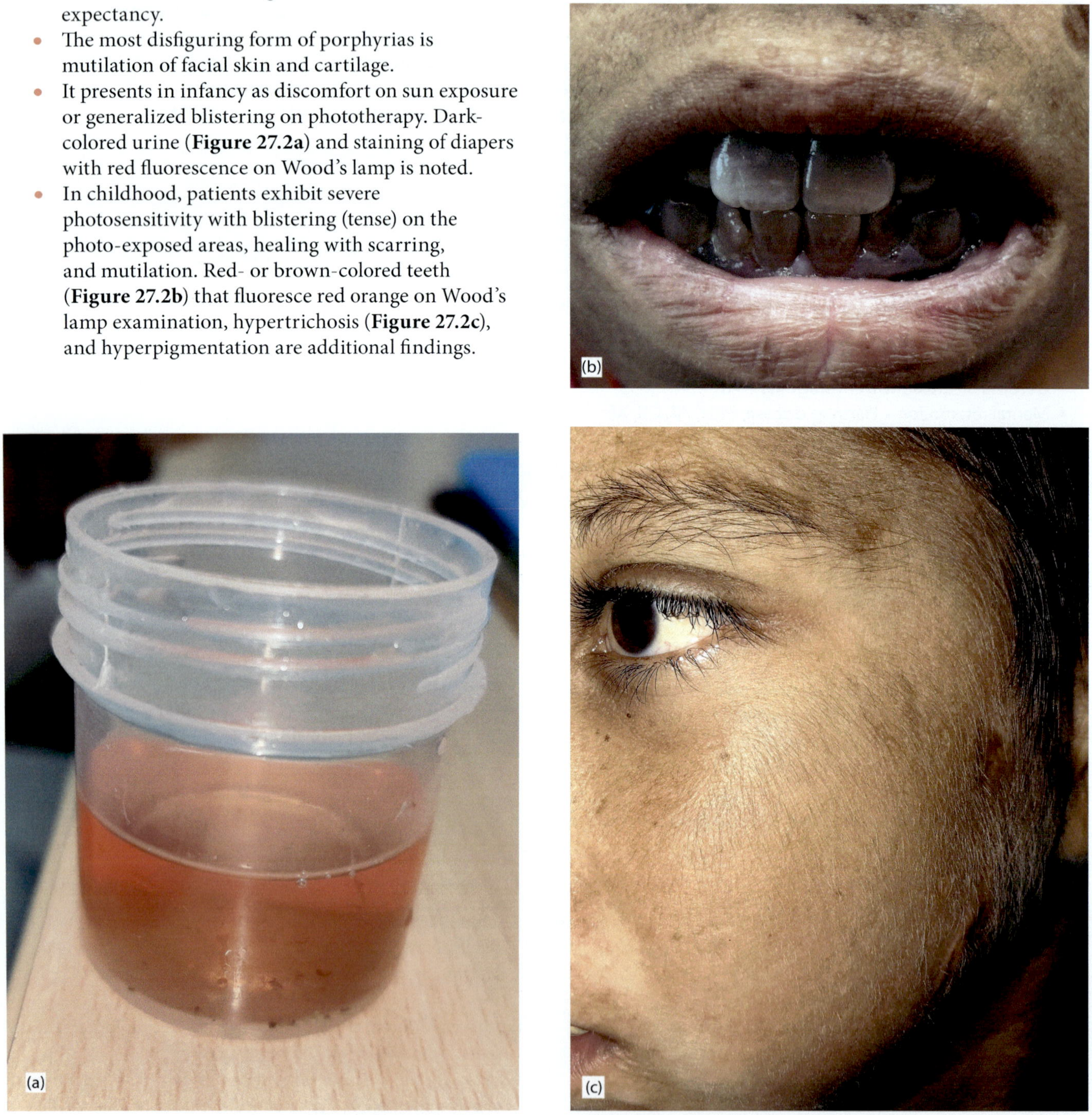

Figure 27.2 **(a)** Dark-colored urine of a child with congenital erythropoietic porphyria. **(b)** Erythrodontia in congenital erythropoietic porphyria. **(c)** Hypertrichosis in a case of porphyria. *(Continued)*

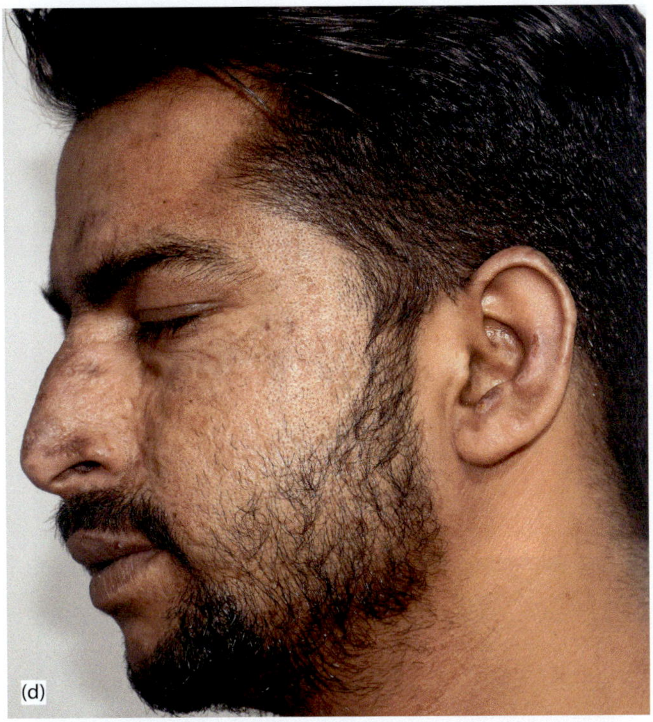


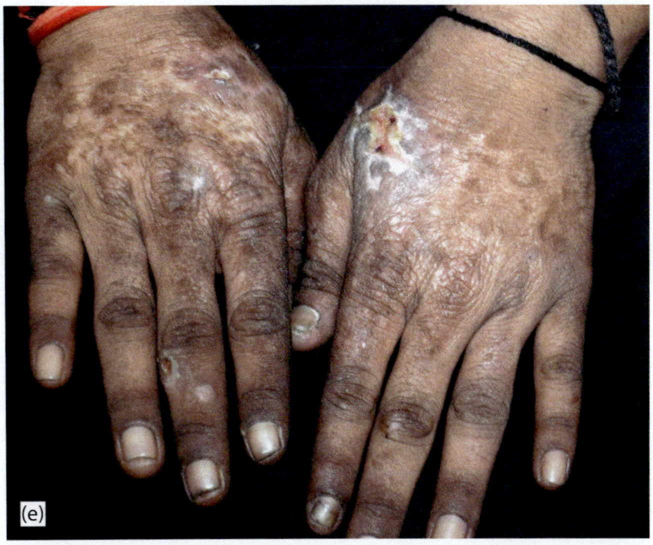


Figure 27.2 (*Continued*) **(d)** Atrophic scarring on the face and erosions on the ear in a case of erythropoietic protoporphyria. **(e)** Atrophic scarring and ulcer on the dorsum of hand in erythropoietic protoporphyria. (a,b – Courtesy: Dr. Sunil Kumar Gupta, AIIMS Gorakhpur, India; c,e – Courtesy: Dr. Piyush Kumar, Katihar, India.)

- **Erythropoietic protoporphyria**
  - This is the most common porphyria in childhood.
  - It is an autosomal recessive condition caused by partial deficiency of enzyme ferrochelatase.
  - EPP is characterized by an immediate painful reaction within minutes of sun exposure. Erythema and edema with severe burning pain over the exposed areas, especially on the dorsal surfaces of the hands, feet, and face, are noted (**Figure 27.2d**). The burning pain responds only to cold air and cold water. Photo-onycholysis may be observed.
  - Vesicobullous lesions typical of other cutaneous porphyrias are uncommon.
  - In chronic cases, thickening of skin on knuckles with subtle scarring on the bridge of the nose is observed (**Figure 27.2e**).
  - Liver dysfunction and hypochromic microcytic anemia are major systemic features.
  - DD: Phototoxic drug reactions, contact dermatitis, other cutaneous porphyrias.
- **Porphyria cutanea tarda (PCT)**
  - PCT usually presents in adulthood; patients with homozygous mutations (type III, Hepatoerythropoietic porphyria) in enzyme (uroporphyrinogen decarboxylase) may present in childhood. In fact, it is the second most common porphyria in childhood.
  - PCT presents with cutaneous symptoms only. Erosions, vesicles or bullae on sun exposed cutaneous surfaces, especially dorsa of hands and forearms are noted (**Figure 27.3a**). Lesions heal with hyperpigmentation, atrophic scarring and milia formation (**Figure 27.3b**). Periorbital hypertrichosis can occur.
  - Sclerodermoid changes can occur in photo exposed and non-photo–exposed areas (**Figure 27.3c**).
  - Ocular involvement may be seen and includes ocular pain and photophobia.
  - Liver dysfunction may be noted.

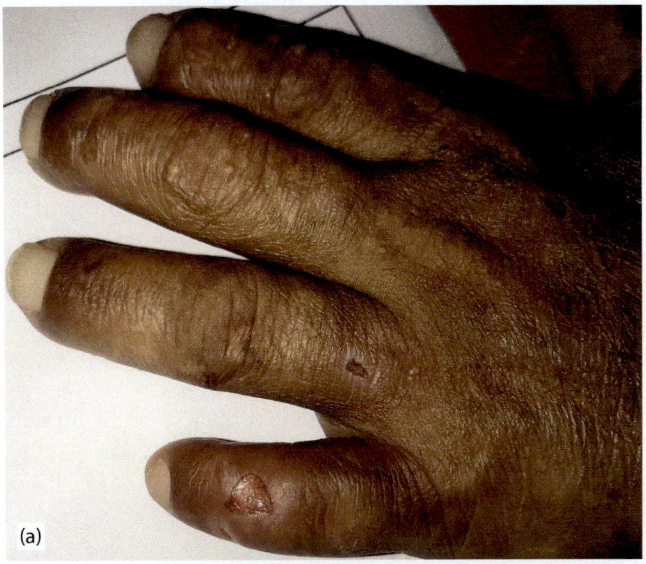


Figure 27.3 **(a)** Erosion on the dorsum of the finger in a case of porphyria cutanea tarda. (*Continued*)

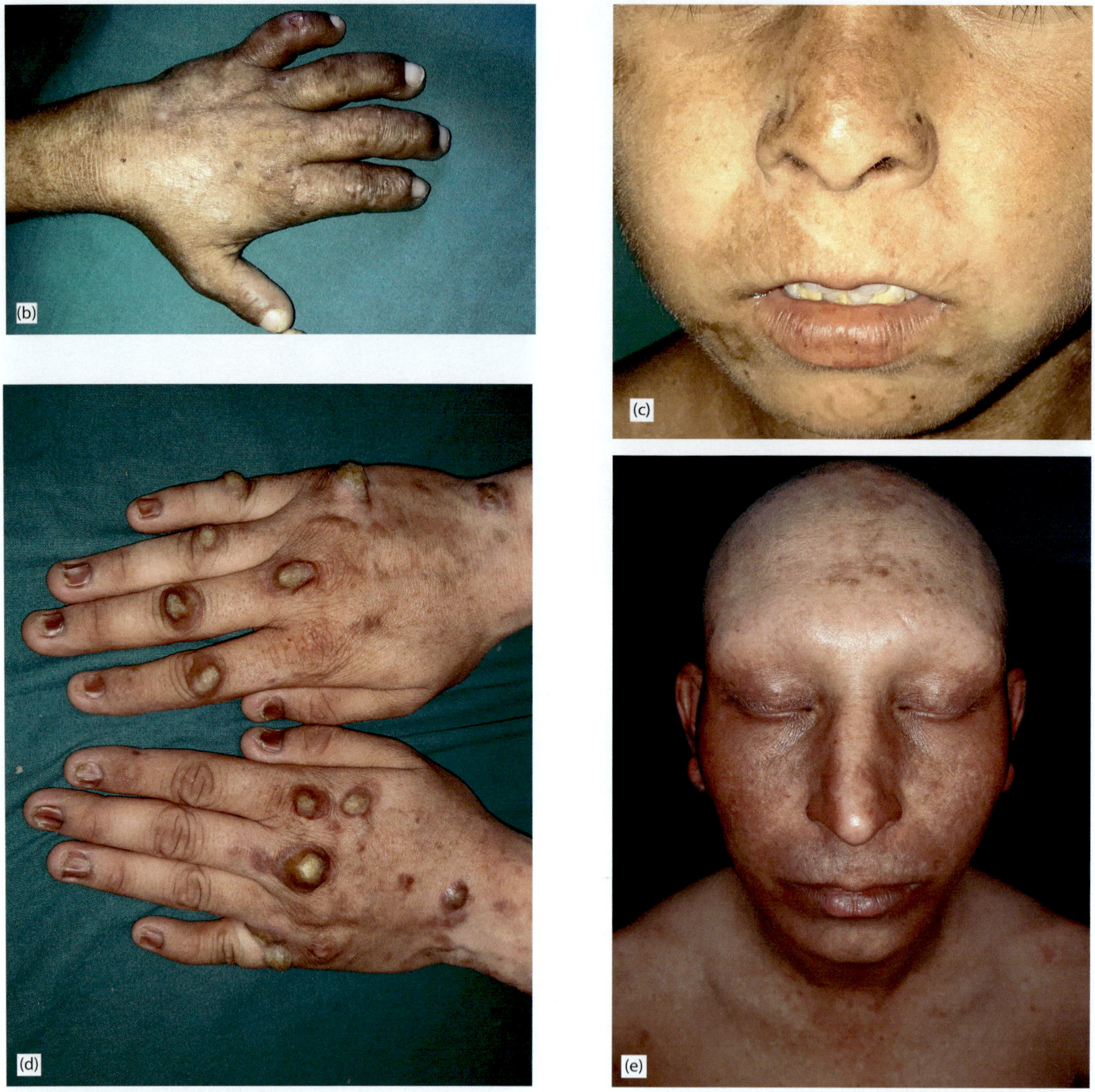

Figure 27.3 (*Continued*) **(b)** Multiple milia on the dorsa of the hand in a case of porphyria cutanea tarda. **(c)** Pinched nose and pseudo rhagades in a case of porphyria cutanea tarda. **(d)** Keratotic lesions on the dorsum of hands in Rothmund-Thomson syndrome. **(e)** Bird like facies of Rothmund-Thomson syndrome with sparse hairs and poikiloderma. (d,e – Courtesy: Dr Hiral Shah, Baroda Medical College, Vadodara, India.)

- DD: Epidermolysis bullosa, bullous systemic lupus erythematosus, other cutaneous porphyrias.

### Rothmund-Thomson syndrome (poikiloderma congenitale)

- This is an autosomal recessive condition caused by mutations in the RECQL4 gene, which encodes an enzyme RecQ DNA helicase, involved in DNA replication and repair.
- Skin changes develop in first year of life, usually in first three to six months.
- In infancy, children develop erythema, swelling, and blistering of face. Gradually, reticulated hyperpigmented and hypopigmented patches, and telangiectasia within areas of punctate atrophy (poikiloderma) appear over face, extensor extremities, and buttocks. The trunk and abdomen are usually spared.

- Keratotic lesions most commonly occur on elbows, knees, hands, and feet (**Figure 27.3d**). Palmoplantar keratoderma can occur.
- Additional findings include sparse hair, sparse eyelashes, and bird-like facies (**Figure 27.3e**).
- Systemic features include skeletal abnormalities (short stature, disproportionately small hands and feet, bilateral thumb aplasia, etc.), juvenile cataracts, sexual abnormalities, and increased risk of cancers (osteosarcomas, non-melanoma skin cancers, etc.).
- DD: Bloom's syndrome, Cockayne syndrome, dyskeratosis congenita, Kindler syndrome.

### Bloom syndrome (congenital telangiectatic erythema)

- This is an autosomal recessive condition caused by mutations in gene BLM, which encodes an enzyme (RecQ family of helicases) involved in DNA recombination and repair.
- The affected child presents with failure to thrive and stunted growth in infancy and early life. Cutaneous features develop late in childhood.
- Characteristic facies is a long and narrow face, an underdeveloped malar area, retrognathia or micrognathia, and prominent nose and/or ears.
- Patients develop erythematous patches and telangiectasia on sun-exposed areas of face in a butterfly distribution. The rash spreads to other photo-distributed areas – ears, extensor of forearms, and dorsa of the hands. In severe cases, blisters, hemorrhage and crusts may develop. In dark-skinned individuals, skin findings may be subtle or absent.
- Other mucocutaneous findings include cheilitis (lower lip), poikiloderma, and eyebrow or eyelash hair loss.
- Severe pre- and post-natal growth retardation, stunted growth with long limbs and disproportionately large hands and feet, and sparseness of subcutaneous tissue (wasted appearance) are among the most prominent features.
- Other important findings include type 2 diabetes, ocular disease (scleral telangiectasias, bulbar conjunctival telangiectasia), infertility (in males) and subfertility (in females), deficiency of immunoglobulin A (leading to recurrent respiratory and gastrointestinal infections), and increased predisposition to cancers (lymphomas, leukemia, oral/esophageal squamous cell carcinoma, etc.).
- DD: Cockayne syndrome, childhood lupus erythematosus.

### Xeroderma pigmentosum (XP)

- This is an autosomal recessive condition caused by a genetic defect in nucleotide excision repair, leading to impaired repair of DNA damaged by UV radiation.
- Presents at one to two years of age.
- The disease starts as an acute sunburn-like reaction with blistering or persistent erythema after minimal UV exposure, and scaling, usually at six months of life. Freckling is marked by the age of two years (**Figure 27.4a,b**).
- As age advances, chronic actinic damage results in dry and parchment-like skin with mottled pigmentation, poikiloderma (**Figure 27.4c**), and premalignant lesions such as actinic keratosis and Bowen's disease.
- The most dreaded cutaneous complications are accelerated photoaging and a 1000-fold increased risk of development of cutaneous malignancies. Squamous cell carcinoma, basal cell carcinoma, and

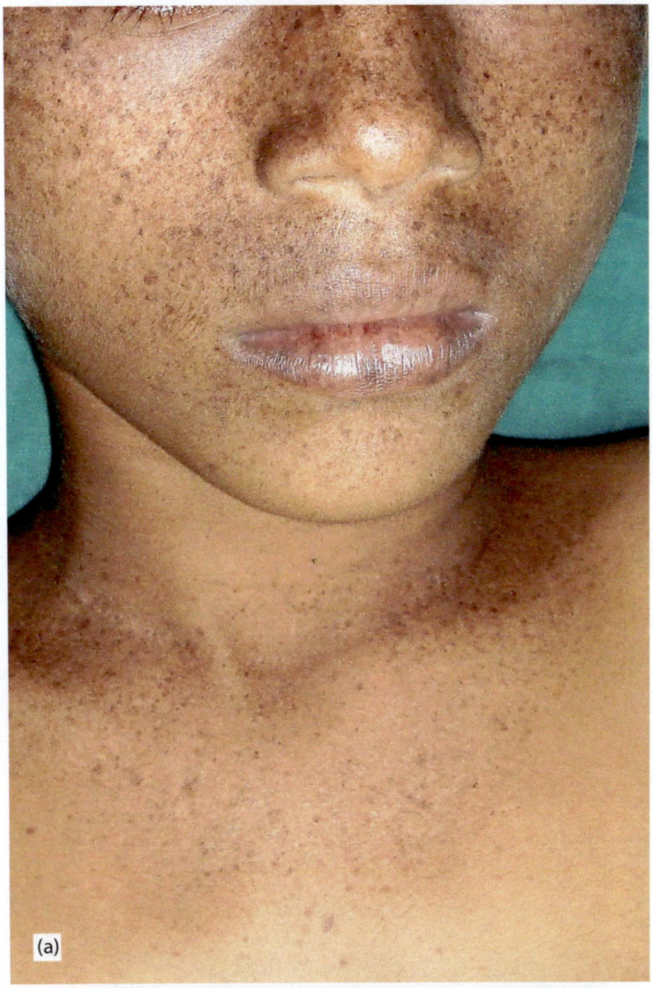


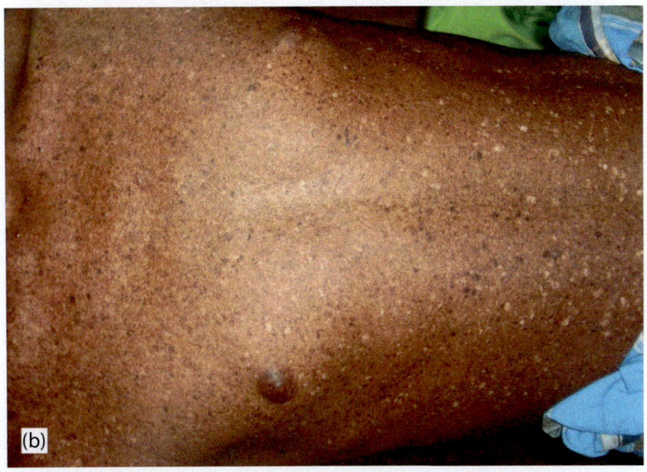


Figure 27.4 **(a)** Freckling on the photo-exposed areas of the face, including the lips and the V of the neck, in a case of Xeroderma pigmentosum. **(b)** Extensive freckling in xeroderma pigmentosum. Note depigmented macules causing a mottled appearance. (*Continued*)

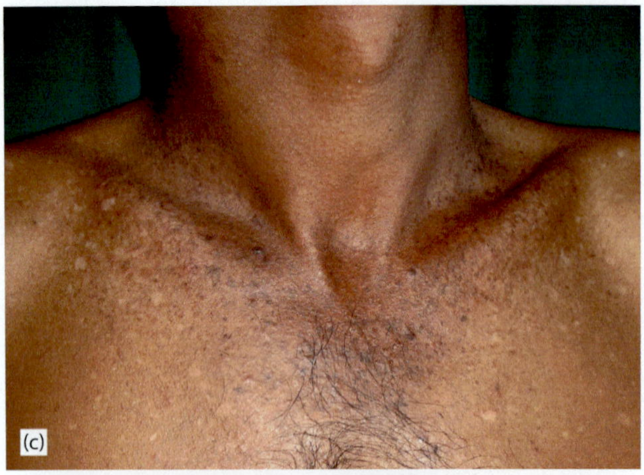


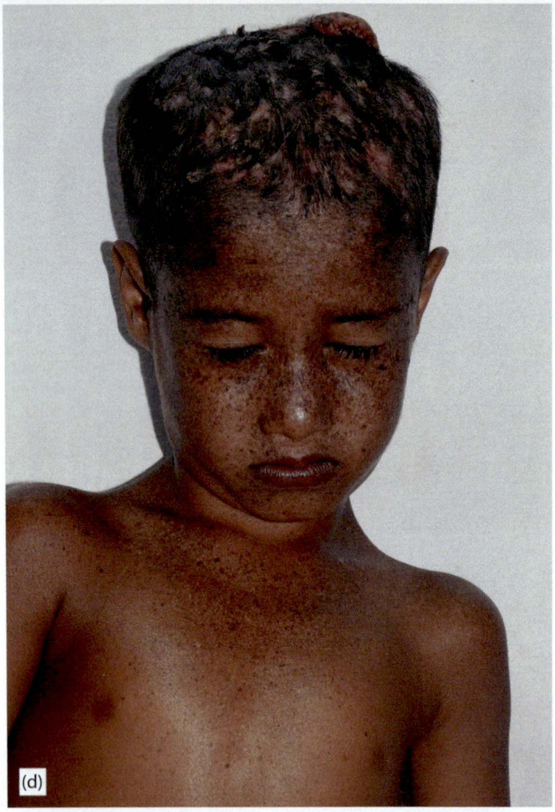


Figure 27.4 (*Continued*) **(c)** Dyspigmentation with hyper and hypopigmented macules on the V area of the chest in a case of xeroderma pigmentosum (XP). **(d)** Squamous cell carcinoma on the scalp in a child with xeroderma pigmentosum. Note extensive freckling on the sun-exposed areas. **(e)** Multiple cutaneous malignancies and premalignant lesions in an older child with xeroderma pigmentosum. **(f)** Corneal scarring in a case of xeroderma pigmentosum. **(g)** Keratoacanthoma in a case of xeroderma pigmentosum. (b,d,e – Courtesy: Dr. Piyush Kumar, Katihar, India.)

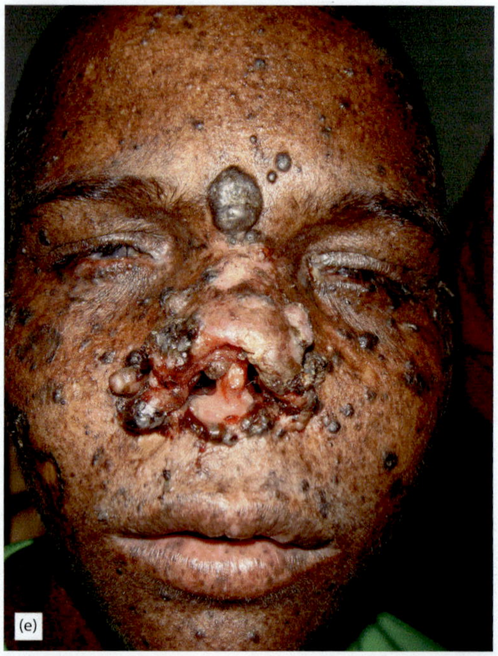


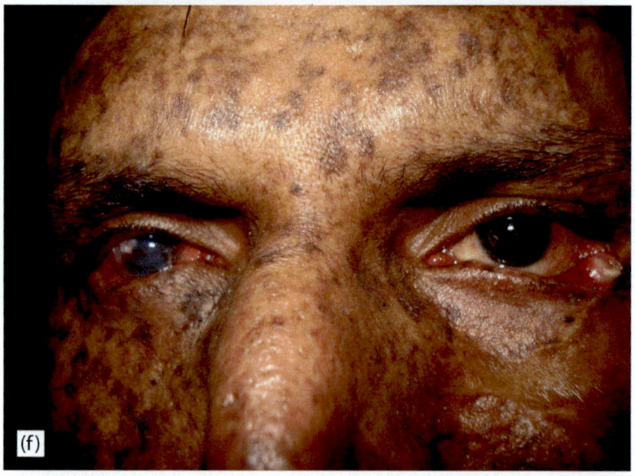


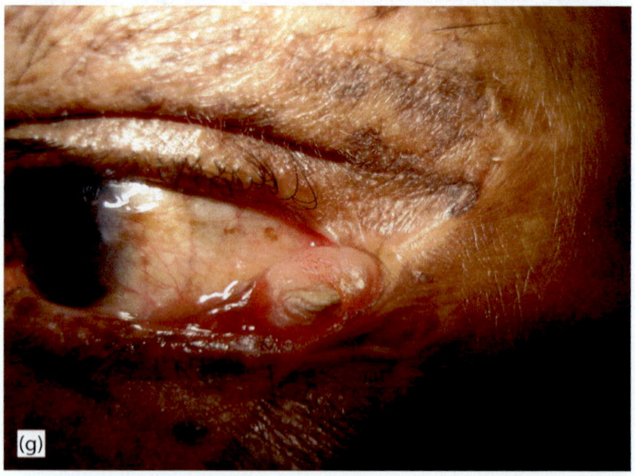


melanoma may develop as early as three to five years of life and are predominantly seen on sun-exposed areas (**Figure 27.4d,e**).

- Ophthalmologic involvement is very prominent and manifests as
  - Chronic UV-induced conjunctivitis and keratitis – corneal opacification and vascularization (**Figure 27.4f**)
  - Pinguecula and pterygium
  - Atrophy of the skin of the eyelids, resulting in ectropion, entropion, and in severe cases complete loss of eyelids
  - Epithelioma, squamous cell carcinoma, and melanoma of the UV-exposed portions of the eye (**Figure 27.4g**)

- Neurological involvement is seen in 30% of cases. Spasticity, hyporeflexia, areflexia, ataxia, chorea, motor neuron signs, segmental demyelination and mental retardation may be seen.
- DD: Rothmund-Thomson syndrome, Werner syndrome, LEOPARD syndrome.

## Cockayne syndrome (CS)

- This is an autosomal recessive condition caused by genetic cellular sensitivity to ultraviolet (UV) mediated DNA damage.
- Two types are recognized: Type I (classical, presents in childhood, death by second or third decade of life) and Type II (severe, presents at birth/in infancy, death by six to seven years of age).
- Characteristic facies includes microcephaly, deep-set eyes, prominent ears, and a shrivelled facial appearance – Mickey Mouse facies (**Figure 27.5a**).
- Loss of subcutaneous fat gives a wasted appearance.
- Photosensitivity is manifested as erythema and scales in acute cases and as hyperpigmentation, telangiectasia, and atrophy in chronic cases.
- Other prominent features include postnatal growth failure and cachexic dwarfism, long limbs with large hands and feet, absent or hypoplastic teeth and delayed teeth eruption, neurological degeneration, pigmentary retinopathy, cataracts, sensorineural hearing loss, etc.
- Metronidazole administration in CS patients may cause potentially fatal liver failure.
- Rare cases with combined clinical features of XP and CS (XP-CS complex) are known (**Figure 27.5b**).
- DD: Bloom syndrome, Rothmund-Thomson syndrome, Werner Syndrome, xeroderma pigmentosum.

## Trichothiodystrophy (TTD)[5]

- This is an autosomal recessive condition caused by genetic abnormalities in the general transcription factor IIH (TFIIH) complex, participating in the repair of UV-induced DNA damage.
- TTD is a heterogenous group of disorders characterized by sulphur-deficient (cysteine and methionine) brittle hairs and neuroectodermal manifestations. A detailed discussion of different types of TTD is beyond the scope of this book.
- The cutaneous manifestations include ichthyosis (including lamellar ichthyosis), dry skin, and photosensitivity.
- Hairs are characteristically sparse, short, dry, and brittle, or there may be complete loss of hairs. Light microscopy of hairs shows a wavy, irregular outline and a flattened shaft that twists like a folded ribbon. Polarizing microscopy shows characteristic alternating dark and light bands "tiger tail appearance."
- Nail findings include onychodystrophy, splitting, and ridging or thickening.
- Systemic findings include growth retardation, skeletal manifestations (peripheral osteopenia and central osteosclerosis), neurological manifestations (developmental defects, microcephaly, intellectual impairment and ataxia), and decreased fertility.
- XP-TTD overlap is called PIBIDS syndrome – **p**hotosensitivity, **i**chthyosis, **b**rittle hairs, **i**mpaired

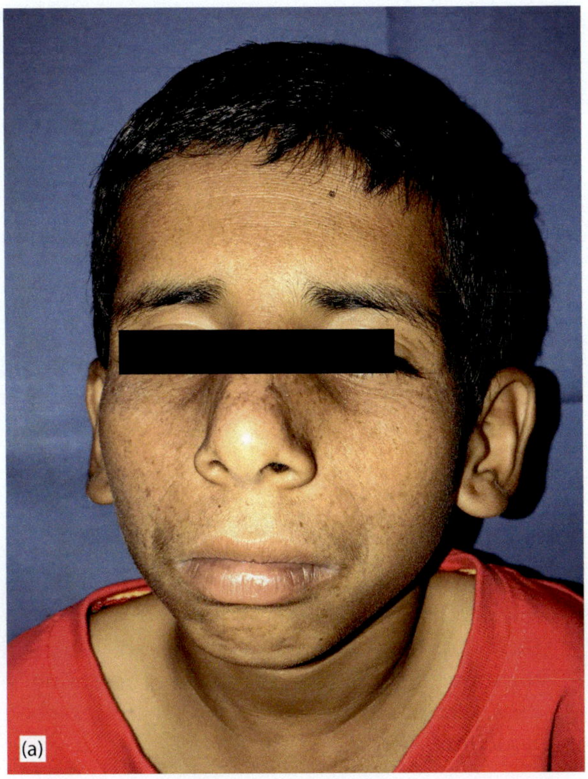


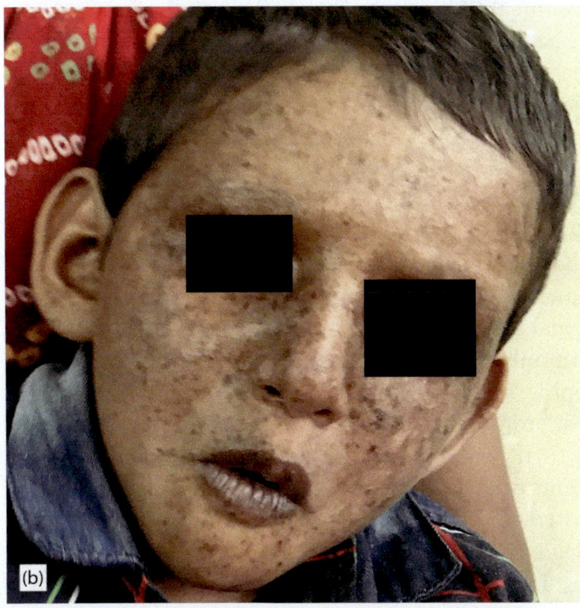


Figure 27.5 **(a)** Pinched narrow face and a beaked thin nose and large ears suggestive of Mickey Mouse facies in a case of Cockayne syndrome. **(b)** Cockayne XP overlap syndrome presenting with freckling of the photo-exposed areas with facial features of Cockayne syndrome.

physical and mental development, **d**ecreased fertility and **s**hort stature. Unlike XP, patients with TDD do not show freckle-like pigmentation and the high frequency of light-induced skin cancer.
- DD: Congenital alopecias.

### Phenylketonuria (PKU)

- This is an autosomal recessive disorder of amino acid metabolism caused by deficiency of phenylalanine hydroxylase enzyme, causing accumulation of phenylalanine.
- The clinical manifestations of the disease may be minimal if diagnosed and treated early (low phenylalanine diet).
- There is widespread pigmentary dilution of skin, hairs, and eyes. Patients often exhibit photosensitivity and may develop sclerodermoid plaques, if left untreated.
- Developmental delay and mental retardation are other prominent features. Other findings include mousy odor, eczematous lesions, seizures, self-mutilation, and severe behavioral disorders.
- DD: Tetrahydrobiopterin deficiency, tyrosinemia.

### Ataxia telangiectasia

- This is an autosomal recessive condition caused by mutations in ATM gene, which encodes protein kinase ATM. Protein kinase ATM plays a key role in repair of double-strand breaks in DNA.
- Ataxia, the hallmark of disease, has its onset in the first year of life and becomes appreciable as the child grows. Oculocutaneous telangiectasia starts appearing at the three to six years (sometimes delayed till adolescence).
- The clinical findings are heterogenous – four groups have been identified. Also, the rate of progression of the disease varies.
- Facies is relaxed, dull, sad, and seemingly inattentive, contrasting with cheerful, alert appearance during the slow-spreading smile.
- Ocular telangiectasia is a prominent finding and starts at the angles of both eyes, spreading toward the cornea. Eyelids too may be affected.
- Cutaneous telangiectasia may appear on the face, internal ears, cubital and popliteal fossae, and, less commonly, elsewhere. Gradually patients develop atrophic, sclerodermoid skin changes and poikiloderma (most prominent on facial skin) in adolescence. Hairs may turn gray, and ears may become inelastic.
- Patients often have a prematurely aged appearance –wasted face, scattered gray hairs, oculocutaneous telangiectasia, and stooped posture.
- Neurological changes (ataxia, abnormal eye movements, choreoathetosis, etc.) appear before cutaneous telangiectasia and progress relentlessly, making the child wheelchair-bound by the age of ten to eleven years. Deep tendon reflexes may be preserved till seven to eight years and are lost thereafter.
- Children assume a characteristic posture – stooping, with the shoulders drooped and the head sunk forward and usually tilted to one side.
- Increased risk of lymphoid malignancies (Hodgkin and non-Hodgkin lymphoma, leukemia) and solid tumors (stomach cancer, breast cancer, medulloblastoma, basal-cell carcinoma, hepatoma, etc.) is noted.
- DD: Hartnup disease, Refsum disease, Gaucher disease.

### Hartnup disease

- This is an autosomal recessive metabolic disorder caused by impaired gastrointestinal and renal transport of neutral amino acids, including tryptophan, leading to a consequent decrease in nicotinic acid synthesis eventuating in a pellagra-like presentation.
- Onset of the disease is usually at three to nine years of age.
- The affected children may be asymptomatic or may develop episodic worsening of the cutaneous and neurological symptoms. The symptoms progress over several days and last one to four weeks before spontaneous resolution. The frequency of episodes decreases with age.
- With milder sun exposures, erythema and scaling develop over the sun-exposed areas. In severe cases, dry scaly well-marginated patches (resembling pellagra) develop over the forehead, cheeks, periorbital regions, dorsal surfaces of the hands, and other light-exposed areas. Lesions on the face may resemble the malar rash of childhood LE. The skin lesions resolve with dyspigmentation.
- Other pellagra-like features include photophobia; gingivitis, stomatitis, and glossitis; and diarrhea.
- Neurological symptoms may be observed and include ataxia, spasticity, anxiety, mood changes and mental retardation.
- DD: Pellagra, phototoxic reaction, childhood LE, ataxia-telangiectasia.

### Kindler syndrome

- This is an autosomal recessive subtype of epidermolysis bullosa
- It is characterized by poikiloderma (**Figure 27.6a**), trauma-induced acral blistering, and subsequent cigarette paper thinning of the skin (**Figure 27.6b**), mucosal fragility, photosensitivity, and an increased predisposition to cancer.

### Polymorphous light eruption (PLE)

- This presents from childhood to late adulthood.
- The prevalence is inversely related to latitude – high prevalence in Scandinavia, the U.K., and northern U.S., and low in Australia and equatorial regions.
- There is seasonal variation – maximally seen at the beginning of the summer season and becoming less severe as the summer season progresses (photo hardening).

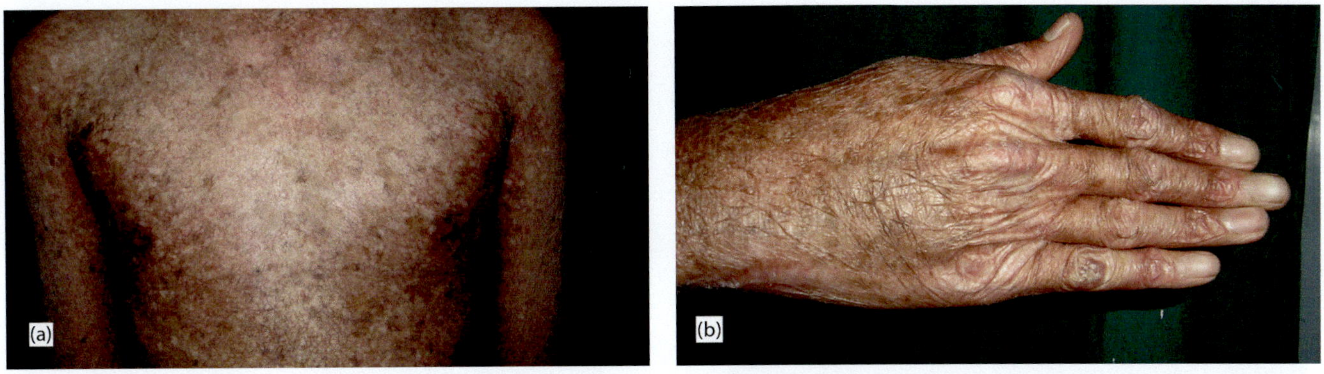

Figure 27.6 **(a)** Atrophy, dyspigmentation and telangiectasia suggestive of poikiloderma in a case of Kindler syndrome. **(b)** Cigarette paper thinning of the skin on the dorsum of the hand in a case of Kindler syndrome.

- Appears within 20–30 minutes or one to two days after sun exposure.
- The lesions appear in a patchy manner over sun-exposed areas of the extensors of forearms and nape of the neck and upper back. The face, which is always exposed to sunlight, is usually, but not always, spared.
- The most common presentation in dark skin is pinhead-sized, grouped, pruritic papules (**Figure 27.7a,b**). These may coalesce to form a plaque (**Figure 27.7c**). These lesions typically heal without scarring, leaving hypopigmentation and mild scaling (**Figure 27.7d**).
- Other presentations include eczematous lesions, variably sized papules, large plaques, papulovesicles, vesicles, urticarial lesions, hemorrhagic, insect-bite–like and erythema multiforme-like lesions.
- DD: Atopic dermatitis (AD), photoallergic reactions.

## Juvenile spring eruption (JSE)

- This is a variant of PLE seen mostly in young boys (5 to 12 years).
- Lesions are classically seen on the top of the ears as pruritic erythematous papules that are usually confined to

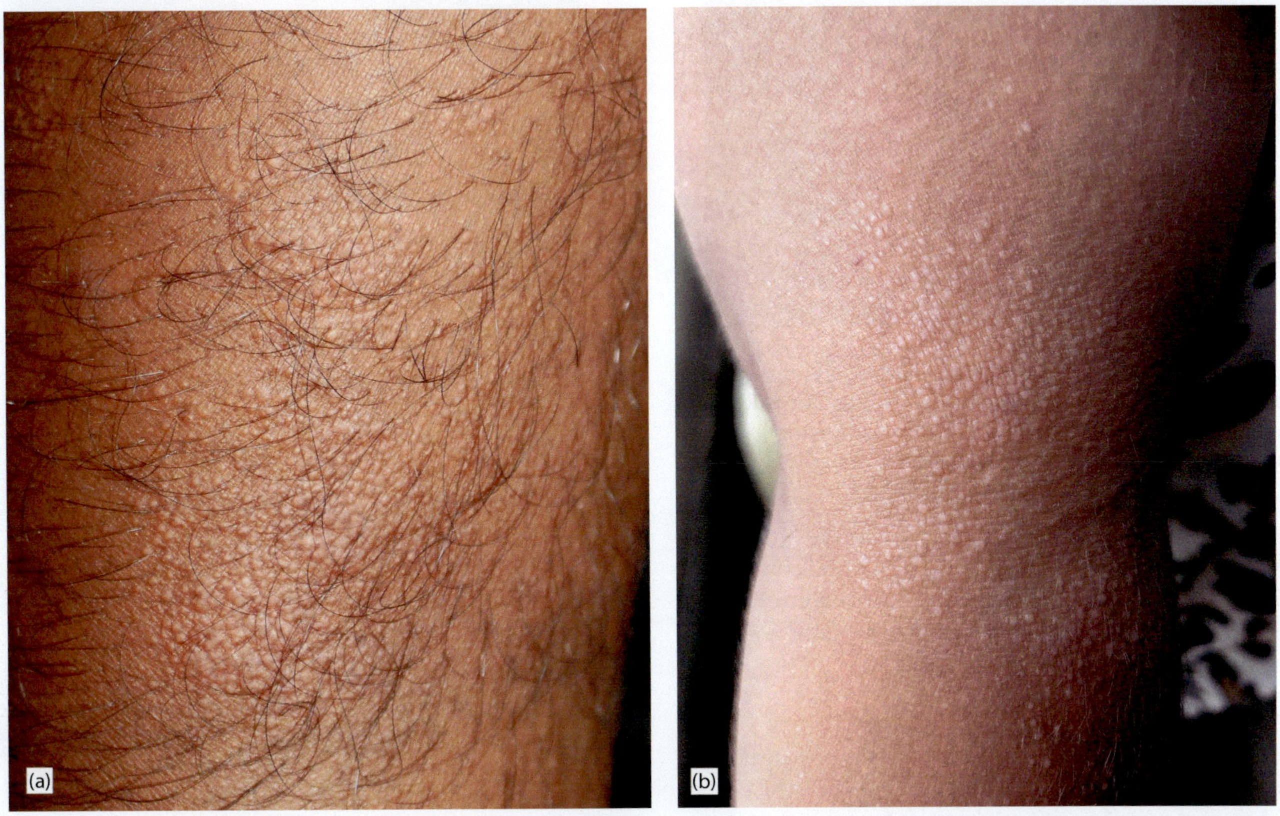

Figure 27.7 **(a)** Multiple pinhead-sized skin colored papules tending to coalesce on the forearm in a case of polymorphous light eruption. **(b)** Lichen-nitidus–like hypopigmented micropapules over the forearm and arm in a case of polymorphous light eruption.*(Continued)*

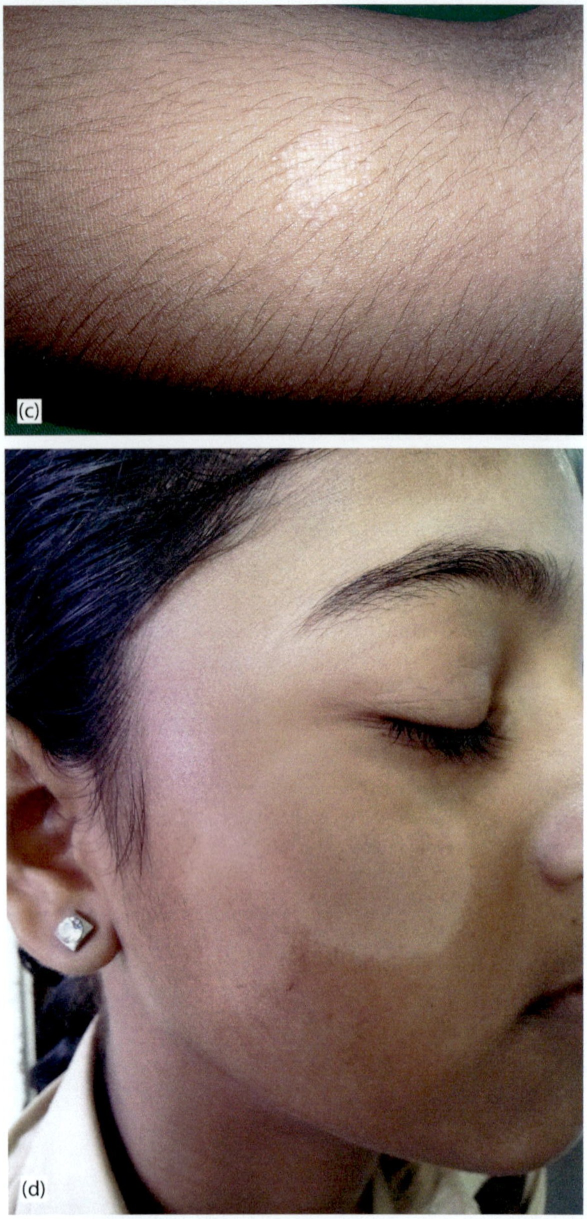


Figure 27.7 (*Continued*) **(c)** Pinhead-sized papules coalesced to form a hypopigmented plaque-like polymorphous light eruption. **(d)** Case of polymorphous light eruption healed with post-inflammatory hypopigmentation on the face of a schoolgirl.

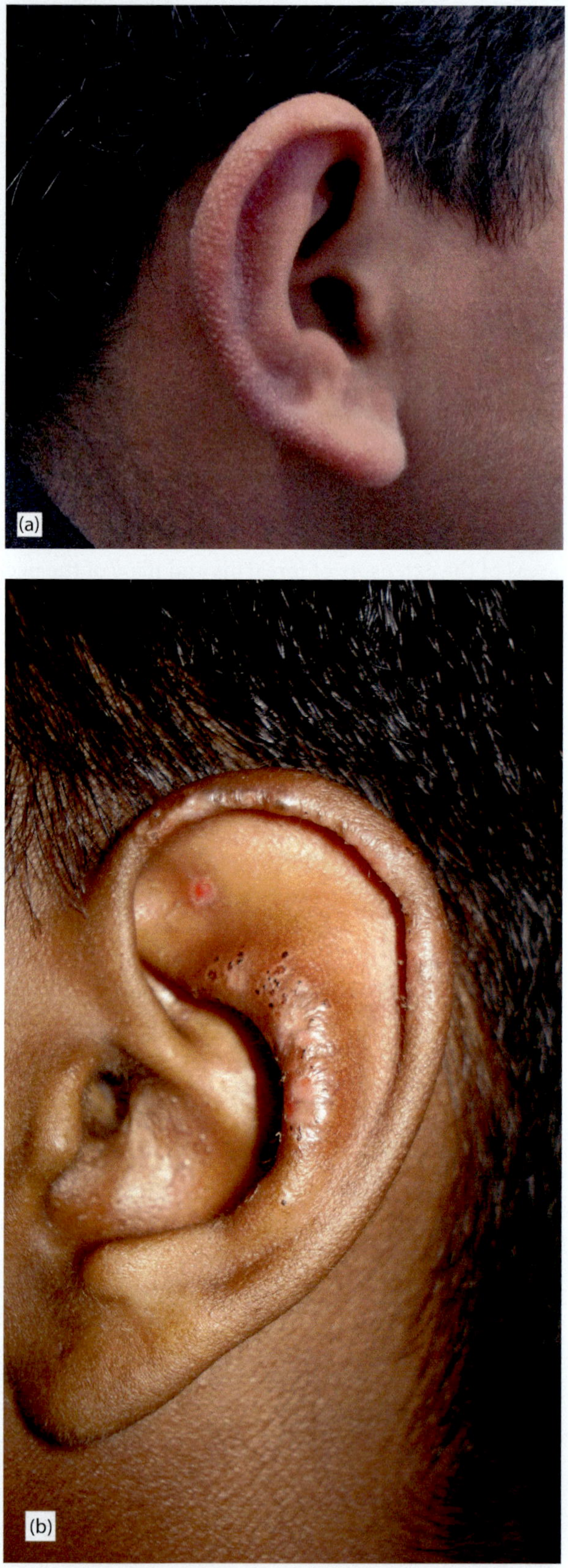


Figure 27.8 **(a)** Multiple skin-colored micropapules located on the external pinna in a case of juvenile spring eruption. **(b)** Multiple papulovesicular lesions on the pinna with a few lesions topped with hemorrhagic crusts and healing with scarring in a case of juvenile spring eruption.

the helices of ears and evolve into vesicles and crusts. The lesions heal with minimal or no scarring (**Figure 27.8a,b**).
- Rarely, systemic symptoms such as fever, general malaise, and headache may be seen.

## Hydroa vacciniforme (HV)

- HV is a rare, idiopathic photodermatosis principally affecting children. Rarely, adults may be affected. The mean age of onset is eight years (range is three to fifteen years). The disease resolves spontaneously in adolescence or young adulthood.
- A history of summer aggravation is seen.

- Lesions appear within hours to a day after exposure to sun.
- There may be an itching and burning sensation with mild constitutional symptoms preceding the eruption.
- HV is characterized by recurrent crops of discrete 2- to 3-mm sized erythematous macules and papules on the face and dorsa of hands. The lesions progress to blisters and umbilicated, necrotic papules and eventually heal with pitted varioliform scarring.
- Keratoconjunctivitis, uveitis, blistering of lips and photo-onycholysis can accompany it.
- DD: EPP, vesicular PLE, bullous SLE, porphyria cutanea tarda (PCT).

### Solar urticaria

- The age of is variable; it can present as early as one week to as late as the eighth decade.
- There is seasonal variation: it is aggravated in summer.
- It appears within five to ten minutes after exposure to sun.
- It is clinically characterized by the appearance of wheals and flares associated with pruritus and a burning sensation appearing soon after sun exposure; it resolves within 24 hours without any residual changes.
- Headache, nausea, wheezing, syncope, and anaphylactic shock can accompany the eruption.
- DD: Acute urticaria, acute cutaneous lupus erythematosus, cholinergic urticaria, urticarial vasculitis, polymorphous light eruption.

### Actinic prurigo (Hutchinson's summer prurigo)

- The disease appears to be common in dark-skinned populations and people living at higher altitudes.
- Childhood cases have onset before puberty, but it can appear anytime between 2 to 43 years of age. Spontaneous remission may occur in adolescence, but persistence is common. Childhood cases have equal gender distribution, but adult onset cases show female preponderance.
- There is seasonal variation – summer exacerbation, with persistence of pruritus throughout the year.
- Clinically, it presents as intensely itchy papules, plaques, and nodules with excoriation and scars on the sun-exposed areas. Sometimes, in long-standing cases the covered areas too may be affected. Secondary eczematization and lichenification is common.
- Very shallow linear, flat, or punctate scars may occur on the face. There can be associated cheilitis, conjunctivitis, and pseudopterygium.
- DD: Atopic dermatitis, prurigo nodularis, lichen planus.

### Childhood systemic lupus erythematosus (CSLE)

- CSLE appears to be less common in whites than in non-whites.
- It presents during childhood, between 11 and 15 years of age. CSLE is rare under five years of age.
- The cutaneous and systemic manifestations are similar to adulthood onset SLE (discussed in Chapter E35). Some key differences have been highlighted here.[6]
    - In general, CSLE has a more severe and more aggressive course than adulthood SLE.
    - Raynaud's phenomenon is less common in CSLE. On the other hand, avascular necrosis is more common in affected children.
    - Renal diseases and central nervous system involvement is more frequent in CSLE.
    - Compared to adults, children with discoid LE are more likely to progress to SLE.
- Malar rash (**Figure 27.9a**) is the most common cutaneous manifestation of SLE in children. Rarely photo-exacerbated annular and psoriasiform lesions of subacute cutaneous lupus erythematosus and lesions of discoid lupus erythematosus, though uncommon, may be seen in the pediatric age group (**Figure 27.9b**).

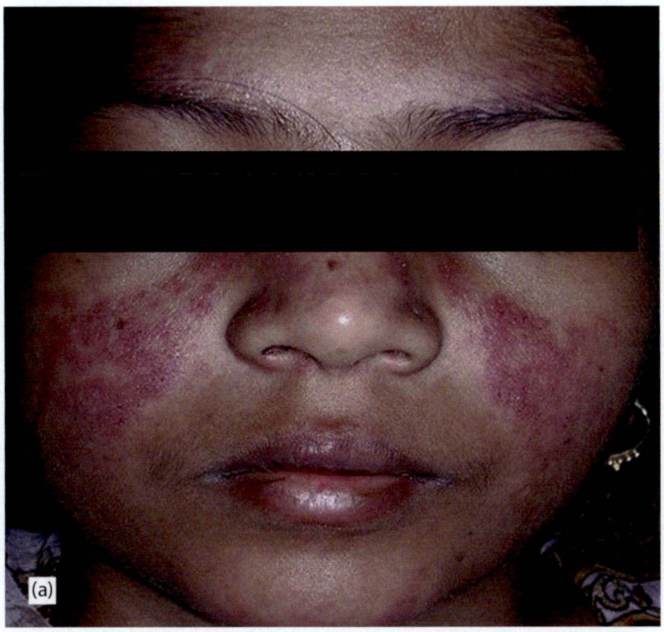


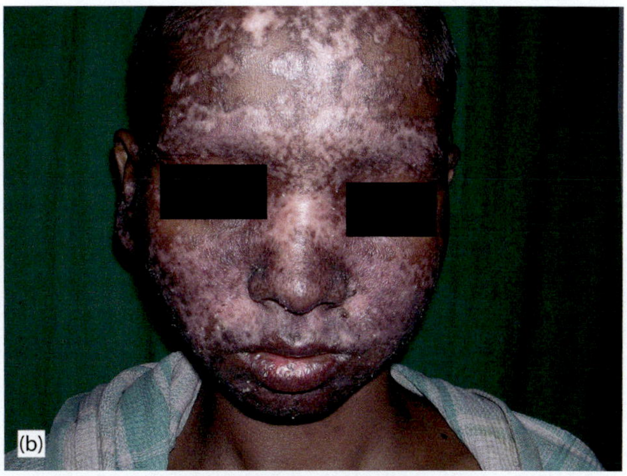


Figure 27.9 **(a)** Erythematous well-demarcated eruption that occurs on bridge of the nose and cheeks, classically sparing the naso labial fold in a case of systemic lupus erythematosus. **(b)** Discoid lupus erythematosus lesions on the face in a case of systemic lupus erythematosus.

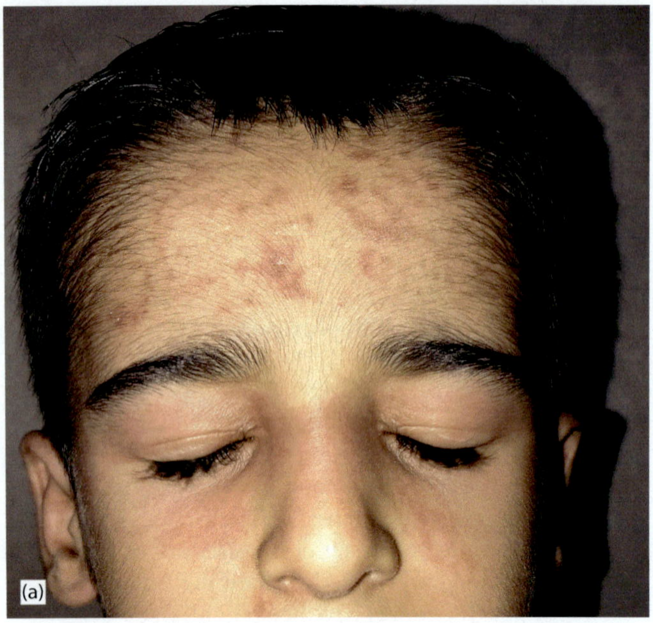


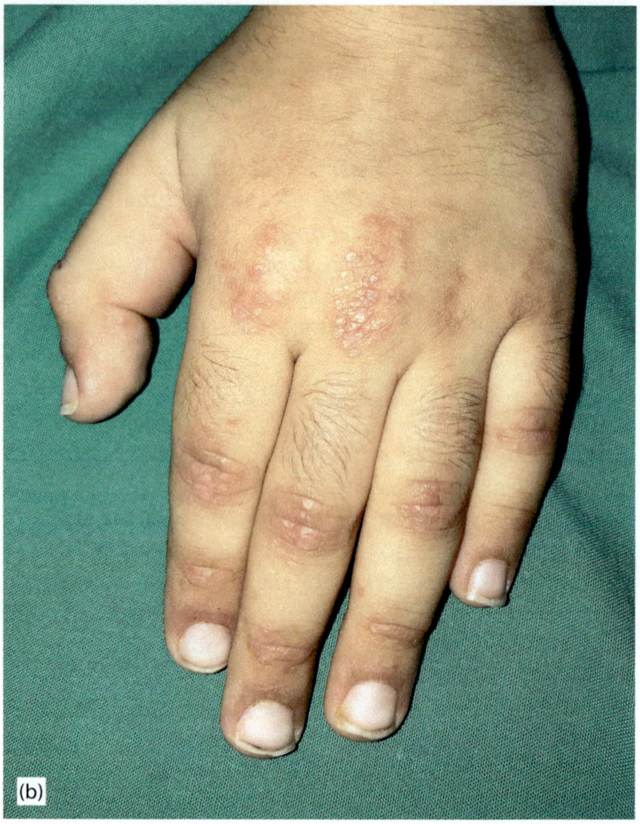


Figure 27.10 **(a)** Violaceous erythema with edema over the periorbital area, suggestive of the heliotrope rash in a case of juvenile dermatomyositis. **(b)** Violaceous flat-topped papules over the knuckles and the metacarpophalangeal joints, suggestive of Gottron papules in a case of juvenile dermatomyositis.

- DD: Juvenile dermatomyositis, acute rheumatic fever, leukemia.

## Juvenile dermatomyositis (JDM)

- The common age of presentation is seven years.
- The clinical features of JDM are similar to those of adult DM. Some salient differences include the following:[7]
    - The cutaneous rash of JDM can occur anywhere on the body and is more frequently associated with ulcerative change.
    - Interstitial lung disease and malignancy are less common in JDM. Conversely, calcinosis cutis is more common in children.
    - JDM appears to have a better prognosis compared to adult DM.
- Cutaneous findings include photo-distributed rash on the face with periorbital violaceous erythema and edema (Heliotrope rash) (**Figure 27.10a**), with involvement of V of the neck, Gottron papules (**Figure 27.10b**), and calcinosis cutis.
- DD: Childhood SLE.

## Photosensitivity to exogenous chemicals

- Photosensitivity caused by exogenous agents is relatively rare in children. It can manifest as a phototoxic or a photoallergic reaction.
- Phototoxic reactions
    - Plant-induced photosensitivity (phytophotodermatitis) caused by furocoumarins is the most common cause of phototoxic reactions in the pediatric age group. It usually begins a day after exposure to furocoumarin and sunlight. Mild erythema to severe blistering eventuate in a characteristic hyperpigmentation. Linear streaks of hyperpigmentation on the face, chest, hands, and lower legs are characteristic. Hyperpigmentation can occur over one to two weeks and can persist over 6 to 12 months. Phototoxic reactions are also commonly seen due to topical applications of psoralens prescribed in vitiligo (**Figure 27.11a–c**).

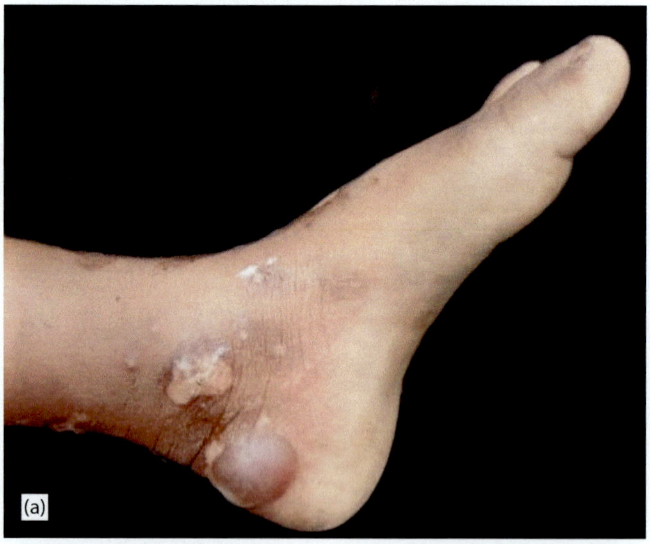


Figure 27.11 **(a)** Phototoxic reaction due to use of topical psoralen followed by sun exposure in a case of vitiligo. (*Continued*)

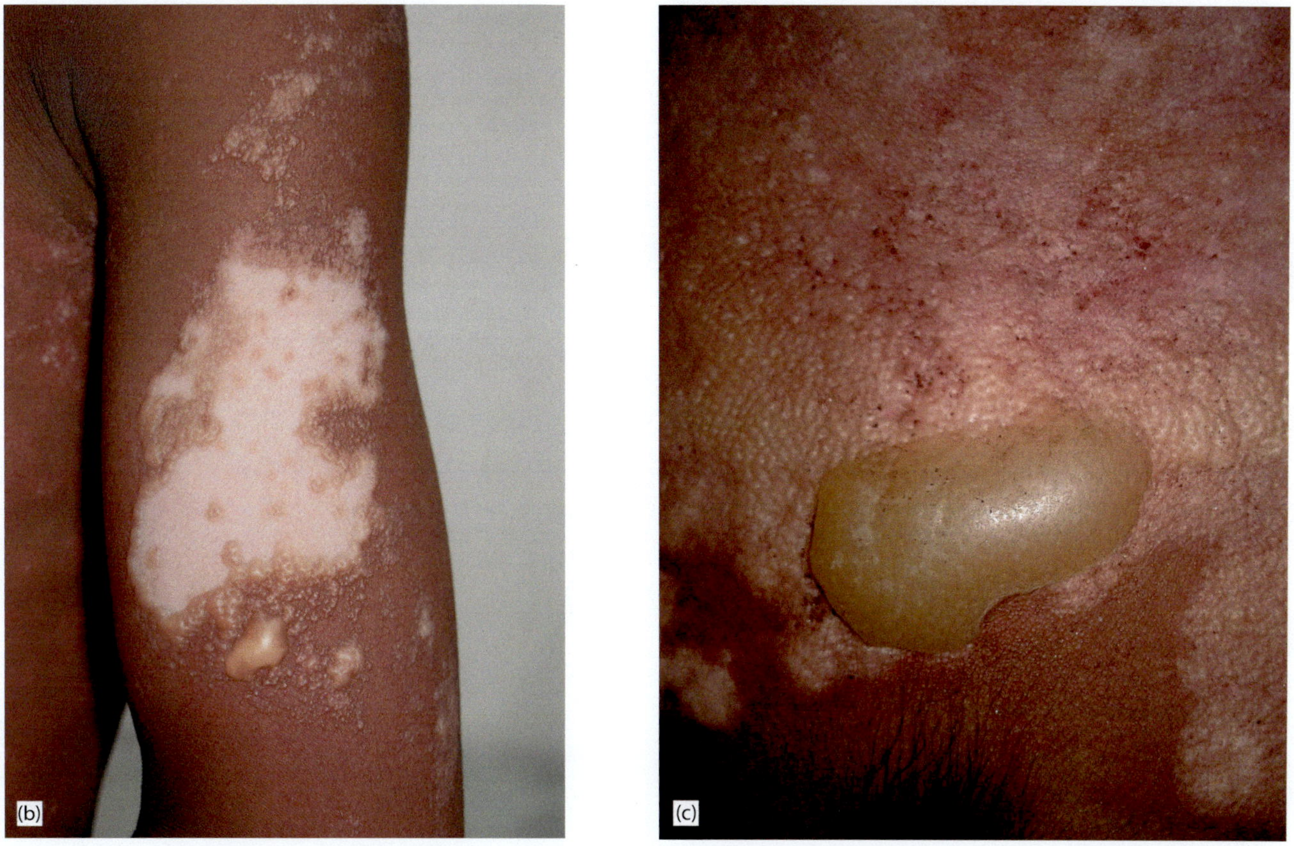


Figure 27.11 (*Continued*) **(b)** Severe phototoxic reaction due to excessive sun exposure after topical psoralen application in a case with vitiligo. **(c)** Bulla in phototoxic reaction following topical PUVA therapy. (b – Courtesy: Dr. Piyush Kumar, Consultant Dermatologist, Katihar, India; c – Courtesy: Dr. PC Das, Consultant Dermatologist, Katihar, India.)

    - Systemic phototoxicity, though rare, can be caused by systemic antibacterial agents (doxycycline, tetracycline, sulphonamides, nalidixic acid and fluoroquinolones), antifungal agents (griseofulvin), sulfonylurea antidiabetics, furosemide, non-steroidal anti-inflammatory drugs, amiodarone, quinine, isoniazid, and the thiazide group of drugs.
- Photoallergic reactions
    - Photoallergic reactions are rare in the pediatric age group, and organic components of sunscreens, such as octocrylene, benzophenone -3, and butyl methoxydibenzoylmethane, are known photosensitizers in the western population.

## Pellagra

- Pellagra is caused by an acquired deficiency of niacin or its precursor, tryptophan. It is primarily a disorder of adults but may be seen in children too.
- The clinical findings in pediatric pellagra are similar to those in adult disease.
- Cutaneous lesions are characterized by sharply demarcated and symmetric, tender erythematous edematous plaques over sun-exposed areas especially the dorsa hands, forearms, face, and neck, accompanied by pruritus and burning (**Figure 27.12**).

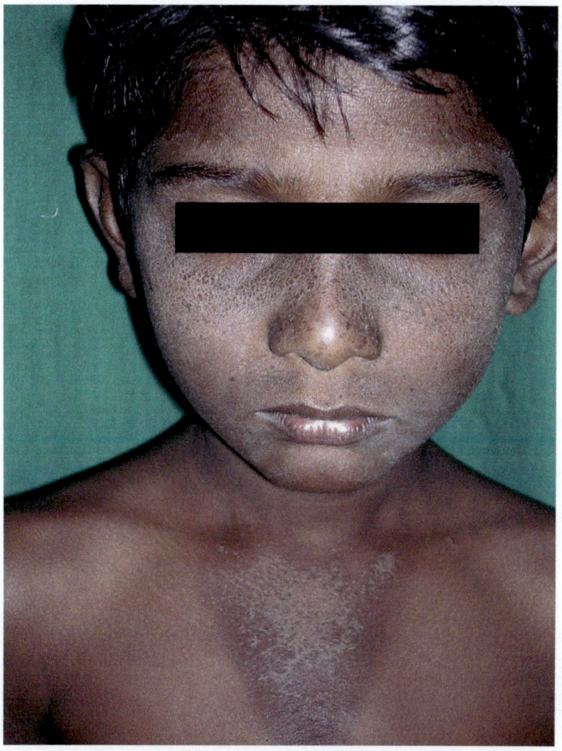

Figure 27.12 Burned skin-like appearance on the photo-exposed areas in a case of pellagra.

Lesions may develop vesicles and erosions, and eventually the affected skin thickens and becomes hyperpigmented.

- DD: Pediatric SLE, phototoxic reaction.

## REFERENCES


1. Inamadar AC, Palit A. Photosensitivity in children: An approach to diagnosis and management. Indian J Dermatol Venereol Leprol 2005;71:73–79.
2. Chantorn R, Lim HW, Shwayder TA. Photosensitivity disorders in children: Part I. J Am Acad Dermatol 2012;67(6):1093.e1–18.
3. Chantorn R, Lim HW, Shwayder TA. Photosensitivity disorders in children: Part II. J Am Acad Dermatol 2012;67(6):1113.e1–15.
4. Grossberg AL. Update on pediatric photosensitivity disorders. Curr Opin Pediatr 2013;25(4):474–479.
5. Faghri S, Tamura D, Kraemer KH, DiGiovanna JJ. Trichothiodystrophy: A systematic review of 112 published cases characterises a wide spectrum of clinical manifestations. J Med Genet 2008;45:609–621.
6. Papadimitraki ED, Isenberg DA. Childhood-and adult-onset lupus: An update of similarities and differences. Expert Rev Clin Immunol 2009;5(4):391–403.
7. Tansley SL, McHugh NJ, Wedderburn LR. Adult and juvenile dermatomyositis: are the distinct clinical features explained by our current understanding of serological subgroups and pathogenic mechanisms? Arthritis Res Ther 2013;15(2):211.

# E56

# Photosensitivity in adults

SANTOSHDEV P RATHOD, KALGI BAXI

## ABSTRACT

Photosensitivity refers to precipitation or aggravation of skin disorders by ultraviolet rays and sometimes by visible light too. Photosensitive skin disorders may be congenital or acquired later in life. This chapter focuses on clinical aspects of acquired photosensitive disorders.

The text of this chapter is available online at https://routledgetextbooks.com/textbooks/9781032399669/

DOI: 10.1201/9781351054225-88

# E57

# Maculopapular rash

PREETI SHARMA

## ABSTRACT

The differential diagnosis for maculopapular rash is extensive. Evaluating the patients with such a rash can be challenging because the differential diagnosis is extensive and includes benign self-limiting (roseola) as well as life-threatening illnesses (Kawasaki disease). The key features that help in clinical diagnosis are mode of onset (acute/chronic/relapsing), distribution (localized or generalized, central or peripheral), evolution (some conditions begin with morbilliform rash but evolve into different morphology, e.g., vesicles in varicella), and presence or absence of systemic features, along with family history and drug history.

The text of this chapter is available online at https://routledgetextbooks.com/textbooks/9781032399669/


DOI: 10.1201/9781351054225-89

E58

# Fever with rash in children

BHUMESH KUMAR KATAKAM

## ABSTRACT

Fever with rash in children is seen by dermatologists as well as pediatricians. Usually the most common cause is viral exanthem, which is self-resolving, but it is important to know the signs and symptoms of other serious illnesses for timely diagnosis and treatment.

The text of this chapter is available online at https://routledgetextbooks.com/textbooks/9781032399669/

DOI: 10.1201/9781351054225-90

# Index

Note: Locators in *italics* represent figures and **bold** indicate tables in the text

## A

## B

## C

## D

## E

## F

## G

## H

## I

## M

## O

## Q



## R

## S

## T

## U

## V

## W

## X



## Y



## Z